Topley & Wilson's

MICROBIOLOGY
AND MICROBIAL
INFECTIONS

First published in Great Britain 1929
Second edition1936
Third edition 1946
Fourth edition 1955
Fifth edition 1964
Sixth edition 1975
Seventh edition 1983 and 1984
Eighth edition 1990
Ninth edition published in Great Britain 1998
by Arnold, a member of the Hodder Headline Group,
338 Euston Road, London NW1 3BH

Co-published in the United States of America by
Oxford University Press, Inc.,
198 Madison Avenue, New York, NY 10016
Oxford is a registered trademark of Oxford University Press

Whilst the advice and information in this book is believed to be true and
accurate at the date of going to press, neither the authors nor the publisher
can accept any legal responsibility or liability for any errors or omissions
that may be made. In particular (but without limiting the generality of the
preceding disclaimer) every effort has been made to check drug dosages;
however it is still possible that errors have been missed. Furthermore,
dosage schedules are constantly being revised and new side-effects
recognized. For these reasons the reader is strongly urged to consult the
drug companies' printed instructions before administering any of the drugs
recommended in this book.

British Library Cataloguing in Publication Data
A catalogue record for this book is available from the British Library

Library of Congress Cataloging-in-Publication Data
A catalog record for this book is available from the Library of Congress

ISBN 0 340 663200 (Volume 5)
ISBN 0 340 614706 (Set)

Publisher:	Georgina Bentliff
Project Editor:	Sophie Oliver
Project Coordinator:	Melissa Morton
Production Controller:	Helen Whitehorn

Copy Editors:	Kathleen Lyle; Jennifer Glasspool
Proofreader:	Elizabeth Weaver
Indexer:	Jan Ross

Typeset in 9.5/11pt New Baskerville by Photo·graphics
Printed and bound in Great Britain at The Bath Press, Avon

Topley & Wilson's

MICROBIOLOGY AND MICROBIAL INFECTIONS

NINTH EDITION

Leslie Collier
Albert Balows • **Max Sussman**

VOLUME 5

PARASITOLOGY

VOLUME EDITORS
Francis EG Cox • **Julius P Kreier** • **Derek Wakelin**

A member of the Hodder Headline Group
LONDON • SYDNEY • AUCKLAND
Co-published in the USA by Oxford University Press, Inc., New York

Editor-in-Chief

Leslie Collier MD, DSc, FRCP, FRCPath

Professor Emeritus of Virology, The London Hospital Medical College, London;
formerly Director, Vaccines and Sera Laboratories, The Lister Institute of Preventive
Medicine, Elstree, Hertfordshire, UK

General Editors

Albert Balows AB, MS, PhD, ABMM

Professor Emeritus, Emory University School of Medicine and Georgia State
University; Former Director at The Center for Infectious Diseases, Centers for Disease
Control and Prevention, Atlanta, Georgia, USA

Max Sussman BSc, PhD, CBiol, FIBiol, FRCPath

Professor Emeritus of Bacteriology, Department of Microbiology, The Medical School,
Newcastle upon Tyne, UK

Volume Editors

Francis EG Cox PhD, DSc

Professor of Parasite Immunology, School of Life, Basic Medical and Health Sciences,
King's College London, London, UK

Julius P Kreier VMD, MSc, PhD

Emeritus Professor of Microbiology, The Ohio State University, Columbus, Ohio, USA

Derek Wakelin BSc, PhD, DSc, FRCPath

Professor of Zoology, Department of Life Science, University of Nottingham,
Nottingham, UK

CONTENTS OF VOLUME 5
PARASITOLOGY

Contents of Volumes 1, 2, 3 and 4

VOLUME 3: BACTERIAL INFECTIONS

CONTRIBUTORS

Masamichi Aikawa MD, PhD
Professor, The Research Institute of Medical Sciences, Tokai University, Boseidai, Isehara, Kanagawa, Japan

Libero Ajello PhD
Adjunct Professor, Department of Ophthalmology, Emory University Eye Center, Atlanta, Georgia, USA

RP Allaker BSc, PhD
Lecturer in Oral Microbiology, Department of Oral Microbiology, St Bartholomew's and the Royal London School of Medicine and Dentistry, London, UK

Stephen D Allen MA, MD
Director, Division of Clinical Microbiology, Director of Laboratories, Department of Pathology and Laboratory Medicine, Indiana University School of Medicine, and Director, Disease Control Laboratories, Indiana State Department of Health, Indianapolis, Indiana, USA

Martin Altwegg PhD
Professor of Medical Microbiology, Head of Molecular Diagnostics Unit, Department of Medical Microbiology, University of Zurich, Zurich, Switzerland

Daniel Amsterdam PhD
Professor of Microbiology and Pathology, Associate Professor of Medicine, Director of Clinical Microbiology and Immunology, Director, Department of Laboratory Medicine, Erie County Medical Center, University of Buffalo Medical School, Buffalo, New York, USA

Larry J Anderson MD
Chief, Respiratory and Enteric Viruses Branch, Centers for Disease Control and Prevention, Atlanta, Georgia, USA

Roy M Anderson BSc, PhD, FRS
Director, Wellcome Trust Centre for the Epidemiology of Infectious Disease; Linacre Professor and Head, Department of Zoology, University of Oxford, Oxford, UK

Jørn Andreassen PhD
Assistant Professor, Department of Population Biology, Zoological Institute, University of Copenhagen, Copenhagen, Denmark

Masanori Aoki MS
Professor of Physics, School of Health Sciences, Faculty of Medicine, Kanazawa University, Kanazawa, Ishikawa, Japan

Sarath N Arseculeratne MBBS, DipBact, DPhil
Professor of Microbiology, Faculty of Medicine, University of Peradeniya, Sri Lanka

RW Ashford PhD, DSc
Professor of Medical Zoology, The Liverpool School of Tropical Medicine, Liverpool, UK

Hazel M Aucken MA, PhD
Clinical Microbiologist, Laboratory of Hospital Infection, Central Public Health Laboratory, Colindale, London, UK

L Andrew Ball D Phil
Professor of Microbiology, Department of Microbiology, University of Alabama at Birmingham, Birmingham, Alabama, USA

Albert Balows AB, MS, PhD, ABMM
Professor Emeritus, Emory University School of Medicine and Georgia State University; Former Director at The Center for Infectious Diseases, Centers for Disease Control and Prevention, Atlanta, Georgia, USA

Jangu E Banatvala MA, MD, FRCP, FRCPath, DCH, DPH
Professor of Clinical Virology, Department of Virology, United Medical and Dental Schools of Guy's and St Thomas's, St Thomas's Hospital, London, UK

PA Bates BA, PhD
Lecturer in Medical Parasitology, The Liverpool School of Tropical Medicine, Liverpool, UK

Derrick Baxby BSc, PhD, FRCPath, FRSA
Senior Lecturer in Medical Microbiology, Department
of Medical Microbiology and Genitourinary Medicine,
Liverpool University, Liverpool, UK

Norman T Begg MBCLB, DTM&H, FFPHH
Consultant Epidemiologist, Public Health Laboratory
Service Communicable Diseases Surveillance Centre,
London, UK

William J Bellini PhD
Chief, Measles Virus Section, Respiratory and
Enterovirus Branch, Centers for Disease Control and
Prevention, Atlanta, Georgia, USA

PM Bennett BSc, PhD
Reader in Bacteriology, Department of Pathology and
Microbiology, School of Medical Sciences, University of
Bristol, Bristol, UK

Ruth L Berkelman MD
Deputy Director, National Center for Infectious
Diseases, Centers for Disease Control and Prevention,
Atlanta, Georgia, USA

Jennifer M Best PhD, FRCPath
Reader in Virology, Department of Virology, United
Medical and Dental Schools of Guy's and St Thomas's,
St Thomas's Hospital, London, UK

Jochen Bockemühl MD, PhD
Head, Division of Bacteriology, Institute of Hygiene,
Hamburg, Germany

SP Borriello BSc, PhD, FRCPath
Director, Central Public Health Laboratory, Colindale,
London, UK

Edward J Bottone PhD
Director, Consultative Microbiology, Division of
Infectious Diseases, Department of Medicine, Mount
Sinai Hospital, Mount Sinai School of Medicine, New
York, New York, USA

George HW Bowden PhD
Professor, Department of Oral Biology, Faculty of
Dentistry, University of Manitoba, Winnipeg, Manitoba,
Canada

Janet M Bradbury BSc, MSc, PhD
Reader, Department of Veterinary Pathology, University
of Liverpool, Leahurst, Neston, South Wirral, UK

William J Britt MD
Professor, Department of Pediatrics, University of
Alabama at Birmingham, Birmingham, Alabama, USA

B Kay Buchanan PhD
Microbiology and Immunology Director, Microbiology
Laboratory, Sarasota Memorial Hospital, Sarasota,
Florida, USA

Donald E Burgess PhD
Associate Professor, Veterinary Molecular Biology
Laboratory, College of Agriculture, Agricultural
Experiment Station, Montana State University,
Bozeman, Montana, USA

James P Burnie MD, PhD, MSc, MA, MRCP,
FRCPath
Head of Department, Department of Medical
Microbiology, Manchester Royal Infirmary, Manchester,
UK

Colin K Campbell BSc, MSc, PhD
Clinical Scientist, Mycology Reference Laboratory,
Bristol, UK

Richard Campbell BSc, MSc, PhD
Senior Lecturer, School of Biological Sciences, Bristol,
UK

Michael Cappello MD
Assistant Professor, Pediatric Infectious Diseases,
Laboratory of Epidemiology and Public Health, Yale
University School of Medicine, New Haven,
Connecticut, USA

Keith AV Cartwright MA, BM, FRCPath
Group Director, Public Health Laboratory Service,
South West, Gloucester Royal Hospital, Gloucester, UK

Pascal Cassinotti PhD
Deputy Head, Molecular Biology Division, Institute for
Clinical Microbiology and Immunology, St Gallen,
Switzerland

E Owen Caul FIBMS, PhD, FRCPath
Deputy Director, Head of Virology, Regional Virus
Laboratory, Public Health Laboratory, Bristol, UK

Glenn H Chambliss BSc, MSc, PhD
Professor and Chair, Department of Bacteriology,
Madison, Wisconsin, USA

Francis W Chandler DVM, PhD
Professor of Pathology, Department of Pathology,
Medical College of Georgia, Augusta, Georgia, USA

Ken Charlton DVM, PhD
Formerly Research Scientist, Animal Diseases Research
Institute, Nepean, Ontario, Canada

T Cheasty BSc
Head, *E. coli* and *Shigella* Reference Unit, Laboratory of
Enteric Pathogens, Central Public Health Laboratory,
Colindale, London, UK

Ian L Chrystie TD, PhD
Lecturer, Department of Virology, United Medical and
Dental Hospitals of Guy's and St Thomas's, St
Thomas's Hospital, London, UK

Ian N Clarke BSc, PhD
Senior Lecturer in Microbiology, Molecular
Microbiology, University Medical School, Southampton
General Hospital, Southampton, UK

Jill E Clarridge PhD, ABMM
Chief, Microbiology Section, Veterans Administration
Medical Center; Associate Professor, Baylor College of
Medicine, Houston, Texas, USA

Timothy J Cleary PhD
Director of Clinical Microbiology, Department of
Pathology, University of Miami, Jackson Memorial
Hospital, Miami, Florida, USA

J Barklie Clements BSc, PhD, FRSE
Professor of Virology, Department of Virology, Institute
of Virology, University of Glasgow, Glasgow, UK

Leslie Collier MD, DSc, FRCP, FRCPath
Professor Emeritus of Virology, The London Hospital
Medical College, London; formerly Director, Vaccines
and Sera Laboratories, The Lister Institute of
Preventive Medicine, Elstree, Hertfordshire, UK

Michael J Corbel PhD, DSc, MRCPath, CBiol,
FIBiol
Head, Division of Bacteriology, National Institute for
Biological Standards and Control, Potters Bar,
Hertfordshire, UK

CS Cox BSc, PhD
Research Leader, DERA, Chemical and Biological
Defence, Porton Down, Salisbury, Wiltshire, UK

Francis EG Cox PhD, DSc
Professor of Parasite Immunology, School of Life, Basic
Medical and Health Sciences, King's College London,
London, UK

Gary M Cox MD
Assistant Professor of Medicine, Duke University
Medical Center, Durham, North Carolina, USA

Nancy J Cox PhD
Chief, Influenza Branch, Division of Viral and
Rickettsial Disease, Centers for Disease Control and
Prevention, Atlanta, Georgia, USA

Marie B Coyle PhD
Professor of Laboratory Medicine and Microbiology,
Department of Laboratory Medicine, Harbor View
Medical Center, University of Washington, Seattle,
Washington, USA

Dorothy H Crawford PhD, MD, MRCPath, DSc
Professor of Microbiology, Department of Medical
Microbiology, University of Edinburgh, Medical School,
Edinburgh, UK

DWT Crompton MA, PhD, ScD, FRSE
John Graham Kerr Professor of Zoology, Division of
Environmental and Evolutionary Biology, Institute of
Biomedical and Life Sciences, University of Glasgow,
Glasgow, UK

William L Current BS, MS, PhD
Senior Research Scientist, Infectious Diseases Research,
Lilly Research Laboratories, Eli Lilly and Company,
Indianapolis, Indiana, USA

A Curry BSc, PhD
Top Grade Clinical Scientist, Public Health Laboratory,
Withington Hospital, Manchester, UK

Melanie T Cushion PhD
Associate Professor of Medicine, Division of Infectious
Diseases, Department of Internal Medicine, University
of Cincinnati College of Medicine, Cincinnati, Ohio,
USA

William Cushley BSc, PhD
Senior Lecturer, Division of Biochemistry and
Molecular Biology, Institute of Biomedical and Life
Sciences, University of Glasgow, Glasgow, UK

David AB Dance MB, ChB, MSc, FRCPath,
DTM&H
Director/Consultant Microbiologist, Public Health
Laboratory Service, Derriford Hospital, Plymouth, UK

Gregory A Dasch BA, PhD
Senior Microbiologist, Viral and Rickettsial Diseases
Program, Infectious Diseases Department, Naval ·
Medical Research Institute, Bethesda, Maryland, USA

AJ Davison MA, PhD
Senior Scientist, MRC Virology Unit, Institute of
Virology, Glasgow, UK

Martin Day BSc, PhD
Reader in Microbial Genetics, School of Pure and
Applied Biology, University College Wales, Cardiff, UK

DD Despommier BS, MS, PhD
Professor of Public Health and Microbiology, Division
of Environmental Health Sciences, Faculty of Medicine,
School of Public Health, Columbia University, New
York, New York, USA

Ulrich Desselberger MD, FRCPath, FRCP
Director, Clinical Microbiology and Public Health
Laboratory, Addenbrooke's Hospital, Cambridge, UK

Arthur F DiSalvo MD
Director, Nevada State Health Laboratory, Reno,
Nevada, USA

Edouard Drouhet MD
Professor of Mycology, Pasteur Institute, Mycology Unit,
Pasteur Institute, Paris, France

JP Dubey MVSC, PhD
Senior Scientist/Microbiologist, Parasite Biology and
Epidemiology Laboratory, US Department of
Agriculture, Beltsville, Maryland, USA

Brian I Duerden BSc, MD, FRCPath
Professor and Head, Department of Medical
Microbiology, University of Wales College of Medicine,
Cardiff; Deputy Director, Public Health Laboratory
Service, London, UK

Lee M Dunster PhD
Co-ordinator, Viral Haemorrhagic Fever/Arbovirus
Surveillance, Kenya Medical Research Institute, Virus
Research Centre, Nairobi, Kenya

Daniel Elad DVM, PhD
Head, General Bacteriologic and Mycologic Diagnostics
Division, Kimron Veterinary Institute, Beit Dagan, Israel

David B Elkins MSPH, PhD
Senior Research Fellow, Australian Centre for
International and Tropical Medicine and Nutrition,
Queensland Institute of Medical Research, Brisbane,
Queensland, Australia

David H Ellis BSc, MSc, PhD
Associate Professor, Department of Microbiology and
Immunology, University of Adelaide and Head,
Mycology Unit, Women's and Children's Hospital,
North Adelaide, Australia

Gisela Enders MD
Professor Dr, Institut für Virologie und Epidemiologie,
Stuttgart, Germany

Sir MA Epstein CBE, MA, MD, PhD, DSc, FRCPath,
FRS
Professor, Nuffield Department of Clinical Medicine,
University of Oxford, John Radcliffe Hospital, Oxford,
UK

Martha Espinosa Cantellano MD, DSc
Associate Professor, Department of Experimental
Pathology, Center for Research and Advanced Studies,
Mexico City, Mexico

SJ Eykyn FRCP, FRCS, FRCPath
Reader (Hon Consultant) in Clinical Microbiology,
Division of Infection, United Medical and Dental
School of Guy's and St Thomas's, St Thomas's Hospital,
London, UK

Richard R Facklam PhD
Chief, Streptococcus Laboratory, Centers for Disease
Control and Prevention, Atlanta, Georgia, USA

S Faine MD, DPhil, FRCPA, FASM
Emeritus Professor, Department of Microbiology,
Monash University, Melbourne, Australia Armadale,
Victoria, Australia

Heinz Feldmann MD
Assistant Professor, Institut für Virologie, Philipps
University Marburg, Marburg, Germany

Hugh J Field ScD, FRCPath
Lecturer in Virology, Centre for Veterinary Science,
University of Cambridge, Cambridge, UK

Roger G Finch FRCP, FRCPath, FFPM
Professor of Infectious Diseases, Department of
Microbiology and Infectious Diseases, Nottingham City
Hospital, University of Nottingham, Nottingham, UK

Sydney M Finegold MD
Professor of Medicine; Professor of Microbiology and
Immunology, UCLA School of Medicine; Staff
Physician, Infectious Diseases Section, Veteran Affairs
Medical Center, Los Angeles, California, USA

Michelle Nett Fiordalisi PhD
Fellow, William W McLendon Clinical Immunology
Laboratory, University of North Carolina Hospitals,
Chapel Hill, North Carolina, USA

Ana Flisser BS, PhD
Director, National Institute for Epidemiological
Diagnosis and Reference, Ministry of Health, Carpio,
Mexico City, Mexico

James D Folds PhD
Professor, Pathology and Laboratory Medicine;
Director, McLendon Clinical Laboratories, University of
North Carolina Hospitals, Chapel Hill, North Carolina,
USA

Thomas M Folks BA, MS, PhD
Chief, HIV/Retrovirus Diseases Branch, DASTLR,
Centers for Disease Control and Prevention, Atlanta,
Georgia, USA

Edward AC Follett BSc, PhD, FRCPath
Adviser in Microbiology, Scottish National Blood
Transfusion Service, Regional Virus Laboratory, Ruchill
Hospital, Glasgow, UK

Jocelyn RL Forsyth MB ChB, Dip Bact, MD,
FRCPA
Senior Associate, Department of Microbiology, The
University of Melbourne, Parkville, Victoria, Australia

Hisashi Fujioka PhD
Assistant Professor of Pathology, Institute of Pathology,
Case Western Reserve University, Cleveland, Ohio, USA

Guido Funke MD, FAMH
Consultant in Medical Microbiology, Department of
Medical Microbiology, University of Zurich, Zurich,
Switzerland

Kenneth L Gage PhD
Plague Section Chief, Bacterial Zoonoses Branch,
Division of Vector-Borne Infectious Diseases, Centers
for Disease Control and Prevention, Fort Collins,
Colorado, USA

N Spence Galbraith CBE, MB, FRCP, FFPHM,
DPH
Formerly Director, Public Health Laboratory Service,
Communicable Disease Surveillance Centre, Colindale,
London, UK

Lynne S Garcia MS, F(AAM)
Manager, UCLA Brentwood Facility Laboratory,
Pathology and Laboratory Medicine, University of
California at Los Angeles Medical Center, Los Angeles,
California, USA

Nigel J Gay MA, MSc
Mathematical Modeller, Immunisation Division, Public
Health Laboratory Service, Communicable Disease
Surveillance Centre, London, UK

Edwin E Geldreich AB, MS
Microbiology Consultant in Drinking Water, Cincinnati,
Ohio, USA

Caroline Attardo Genco PhD
Associate Professor, Department of Microbiology and
Immunology, Morehouse School of Medicine, Atlanta,
Georgia, USA

Wolfram H Gerlich PhD
Professor, Institute of Medical Virology, Giessen,
Germany

Saheer E Gharbia BSc, PhD
Research Fellow (Hon), National Collection of Type
Cultures, Public Health Laboratory Service, Colindale,
London, UK

David I Gibson PhD, DSc
Head, Parasitic Worms Division, Department of
Zoology, The Natural History Museum, London, UK

RJ Gilbert MPharm, PhD, DipBact, FRCPath
Director, Food Hygiene Laboratory, Central Public
Health Laboratory, London, UK

Herbert M Gilles MSc, MD, DSc, DMedSc, FRCP,
FFPHM
Emeritus Professor, Liverpool School of Tropical
Medicine, Liverpool, UK

Youri Glupczynski MD, PhD
Head, Department of Clinical Microbiology, Centre
Hospitalier Universitaire André Vésale, Montigny-le-
Tilleul, Belgium

Robert C Good BA, MS, PhD
Guest Researcher, TB/Mycobacteriology Branch,
Division of AIDS, STD and TB Laboratory Research,
Centers for Disease Control and Prevention, Atlanta,
Georgia, USA

Michael Goodfellow PhD, DSc, CBiol, FIBiol
Professor of Microbial Systematics, Department of
Microbiology, The Medical School, Newcastle upon
Tyne, UK

Norman L Goodman PhD
Professor and Director of Clinical Microbiology
Laboratory, Department of Pathology, College of
Medicine, University of Kentucky, Lexington, Kentucky,
USA

Michael C Goodnough PhD
Assistant Scientist, Department of Food Microbiology
and Toxicology, University of Wisconsin, Madison,
Wisconsin, USA

Alexander WC von Graevenitz MD
Professor of Medical Microbiology; Director,
Department of Medical Microbiology, Department of
Medical Microbiology, Zurich University, Zurich,
Switzerland

JM Grange MD, MSc
Reader in Clinical Microbiology, Imperial College
School of Medicine, National Heart and Lung Institute,
London, UK

John R Graybill MD
Chief, Infectious Diseases Division, Audie Murphy
Veterans, Administration Hospital; and University of
Texas Health Science Center, San Antonio, Texas, USA

David Greenwood PhD, DSc, FRCPath
Professor of Antimicrobial Science, Division of
Microbiology and Infectious Diseases, Department of
Clinical Laboratory Sciences, University Hospital,
Queen's Medical Centre, Nottingham, UK

Duane J Gubler ScD, MS
Director, Division of Vector-Borne Infectious Diseases,
Centers for Disease Control and Prevention, Fort
Collins, Colorado, USA

Eveline Guého PhD
Researcher at INSERM, Unité de Mycologie, Institut
Pasteur, Paris, France

Jacques Guillot DVM, PhD
Assistant Professor of Parasitology-Mycology, Unité de
Parasitologie-Mycologie, URA-INRA Immunopathologie
Cellulaire et Moleculaire, Ecole National Vétérinaire
d'Alfort, Maisons-Alfort, France

Stephen C Hadler MD
Director, Epidemiology and Surveillance Division,
National Immunization Program, Centers for Disease
Control and Prevention, Atlanta, Georgia, USA

Thomas L Hale PhD
Department Chief, Department of Enteric Infections,
Walter Reed Army Institute of Research, Washington
DC, USA

Pekka E Halonen MD
Emeritus Professor of Virology, Medicity and
Department of Virology, University of Turku, Turku,
Finland

JM Hardie BDS, PhD, DipBact, FRCPath
Professor of Oral Microbiology, Department of Oral
Microbiology, St Bartholomew's and the Royal London
School of Medicine and Dentistry, London, UK

Melissa R Haswell-Elkins BA, MSc, PhD
Senior Research Fellow, Indigenous Health
Programme, Australian Centre for International and
Tropical Health and Nutrition, University of
Queensland, Royal Brisbane Hospital, Brisbane,
Queensland, Australia

Charles L Hatheway PhD
Chief, Botulism Laboratory, Centers for Disease Control
and Prevention, Atlanta, Georgia, USA

Harald zur Hausen MD, DSc
Managing Director, Deutsches Krebsforschungszentrum,
Heidelberg, Germany

Sir David L Hawksworth CBE, DSc, FDhc, CBiol,
FIBiol, FLS
President, International Union of Biological Sciences;
Visiting Professor, Universities of Kent, London and
Reading; Director, International Mycological Institute,
Egham, Surrey, UK

Roderick J Hay DM, FRCP, FRCPath
Mary Dunhill Professor of Cutaneous Medicine, St
John's Institute of Dermatology, United Medical and
Dental Schools of Guy's and St Thomas's, Guy's
Hospital, London, UK

John C Hierholzer PhD
Former Supervisory Research Microbiologist, Centers for Disease Control and Prevention, Atlanta, Georgia, USA

Tor Hofstad MD, PhD
Professor of Medical Microbiology, Department of Microbiology and Immunology, The Gade Institute, University of Bergen, Bergen, Norway

John J Holland PhD
Professor Emeritus, Biology Department, University of California at San Diego, La Jolla, California, USA

Barry Holmes PhD, DSc, FIBiol
Clinical Scientist, National Collection of Type Cultures, Central Public Health Laboratory, Colindale, London, UK

Stanley C Holt PhD
Professor of Microbiology, Department of Microbiology, University of Texas Health Science Center at San Antonio, San Antonio, Texas, USA

Marcel Hommel MD, PhD
Alfred Jones and Warrington Yorke Professor of Tropical Medicine, Liverpool School of Tropical Medicine, Liverpool, UK

GS de Hoog PhD
Professor of Mycology, Centraalbureau voor Schimmelcultures, Baarn, The Netherlands

Douglas B Hornick MD
Associate Professor of Pulmonary and Critical Care Medicine, Department of Medicine, University of Iowa School of Medicine, Iowa City, Iowa, USA

Peter J Hotez MD, PhD
Associate Professor, Department of Pediatrics and Epidemiology, Yale University School of Medicine, New Haven, Connecticut, USA

TGB Howe MD, PhD
Senior Lecturer in Bacteriology, Department of Pathology and Microbiology, School of Medical Sciences, University of Bristol, Bristol, UK

TJ Humphrey BSc, PhD, MRCPath
Professor; Head of Public Health Laboratory Service Food Microbiology Research Unit, Heavitree, Exeter, Devon, UK

Hilary Humphreys MD, FRCPI, FRCPath
Consultant Microbiologist, Federated Dublin Voluntary Hospitals, Dublin, Ireland

Charles J Hunter MD
Fellow, Department of Pathology, Division of Infectious Diseases, University of Virginia Health Science Center, Charlottesville, Virginia, USA

Thomas J Inzana PhD
Professor of Microbiology, Department of Biomedical Sciences and Pathobiology, Virginia-Maryland Regional College of Veterinary Medicine, Blacksburg, Virginia, USA

Michael J Janda BSc, MS, PhD
Chief, Enterics and Special Pathogens Section, Microbial Diseases Laboratory, California Department of Health Services, Berkeley, California, USA

AE Jephcott MA, MD, FRCPath, DipBact
Director, Public Health Laboratory, Bristol, UK

Robert C Jerris PhD
Assistant Professor, Department of Pathology and Laboratory Medicine, Emory University School of Medicine, Atlanta, Georgia, USA

David T John MSPH, PhD
Professor of Microbiology/Parasitology; Associate Dean for Basic Sciences, Department of Biochemistry and Microbiology, Oklahoma State University, College of Osteopathic Medicine, Tulsa, Oklahoma, USA

Elizabeth M Johnson BSc, PhD
Clinical Scientist, Mycology Reference Laboratory, Bristol, UK

Eric A Johnson ScD
Professor of Food Microbiology and Toxicology, Food Research Institute, College of Agricultrual and Life Sciences, University of Wisconsin, Madison, Wisconsin, USA

Russell C Johnson PhD
Professor of Microbiology, Department of Microbiology, University of Minnesota, Minneapolis, Minnesota, USA

Dorothy Jones BSc, MSc, PhD, DipBact
Honorary Fellow, Department of Microbiology and Immunology, University of Leicester, Leicester, UK

J Zoe Jordens BSc, PhD
Clinical Scientist/Honorary Senior Lecturer, Haemophilus Reference Laboratory, Oxford Public Health Laboratory and Nuffield Department of Pathology & Bacteriology, John Radcliffe Hospital, Headington, Oxford, UK

Stephen L Josephson PhD
Director, Microbiology/Virology, APC 1136, Rhode Island Hospital, Providence, Rhode Island, USA

Kimberly L Kane BSc, PhD
Postdoctoral Fellow, Clinical Microbiology–Immunology Laboratories, University of North Carolina Hospitals, Chapel Hill, North Carolina, USA

Michael Kann MD
Research Fellow, Institute of Medical Virology, Justus-Liebig-Universität Giessen, Giessen, Germany

SHE Kaufmann PhD
Professor and Head of Immunology, Department of Immunology, University of Ulm, Ulm, Germany

Yoshihiro Kawaoka PhD
Professor, Department of Pathobiological Science, School of Veterinary Medicine, University of Wisconsin-Madison, Madison, Wisconsin, USA

Masako Kawasaki PhD
Instructor, Department of Dermatology, Kanazawa
Medical University, Uchinada, Ishikawa, Japan

Rima F Khabbaz MD
Associate Director for Medical Science, Division of Viral
and Rickettsial Diseases, National Center for Infectious
Diseases, Centers for Disease Control and Prevention,
Atlanta, Georgia, USA

Michael P Kiley BS, MS, PhD
Senior Scientific Adviser, Federal Laboratories for
Health Canada and Agriculture and Agri-Food Canada,
Winnipeg, Manitoba, Canada

Mogens Kilian DMD, DSc
Professor of Microbiology, Head, Department of
Medical Microbiology and Immunology, University of
Aarhus, Aarhus, Denmark

Hans-Dieter Klenk MD
Professor of Virology, Head, Department of Hygiene
and Medical Microbiology, Institute for Virology,
Philipps-University Marburg, Marburg, Germany

Wesley E Kloos PhD
Professor of Genetics and Microbiology, Department of
Genetics, North Carolina State University, Raleigh,
North Carolina, USA

Somei Kojima MD, PhD
Professor of Parasitology, Department of Parasitology,
University of Tokyo, Minato-ku, Tokyo, Japan

Paul E Kolenbrander PhD
Research Microbiologist, National Institute of Dental
Research, National Institutes of Health, Bethesda,
Maryland, USA

Myriam S Künzi PhD
Postdoctoral Fellow, John Hopkins Oncology Center,
Baltimore, Maryland, USA

Ralph Lainson OBE, FRS, AFTWAS, DSc
Professor (Honoris Causa), Federal University of Pará,
ex Director, The Wellcome Belém Leishmaniasis Unit,
Departamento de Parasitologia, Instituto Evandro
Chagas, Belém, Pará, Brazil

Paul R Lambden BSc, PhD
Senior Research Fellow, Molecular Microbiology,
University Medical School, Southampton General
Hospital, Southampton, UK

Sandra A Larsen MS, PhD
Guest Researcher, Bacterial STD Branch, Division of
AIDS, Sexually Transmitted Diseases and Tuberculosis
Laboratory Research, National Center for Infectious
Diseases, Centers for Disease Control and Prevention,
Atlanta, Georgia, USA

Edward R Leadbetter PhD
Professor of Microbiology, Department of Molecular
and Cell Biology, University of Connecticut, Storrs,
Connecticut, USA

James W LeDuc PhD
Associate Director, Global Health, National Center for
Infectious Diseases, Centers for Disease Control and
Prevention, Atlanta, Georgia, USA

Paul F Lehmann PhD
Professor of Microbiology and Immunology,
Microbiology Department, Medical College of Ohio,
Toledo, Ohio, USA

Stanley M Lemon MD
Professor of Microbiology and Immunology and
Internal Medicine, Chairman, Department of
Microbiology and Immunology, University of Texas
Medical Branch at Galveston, Galveston, Texas, USA

Lony Chong-Leong Lim PhD
Fellow, William W McLendon Clinical Immunology
Laboratory, University of North Carolina Hospitals,
Chapel Hill, North Carolina, USA

Graham Lloyd BSc, MSc, PhD
Head of Diagnosis, Centre for Applied Microbiology
and Research, Porton Down, Salisbury, Wiltshire, UK

Alberto T Londero MD
Emeritus Professor, Department of Microbiology,
Session Medical Mycology, School of Medicine, Federal
University of Santa Maria, Santa Maria, RS, Brazil

Francisco J López-Antuñano MD, MPH
Consultant, Instituto Nacional de Salud, Morelos,
Mexico

Mario Lozano Chiu PhD
Postdoctoral Fellow, University of Texas Medical
School, Houston, Texas, USA

David M MacLaren MA, MD, FRCP, FRCPath
Emeritus Professor of Medical Bacteriology, Moidart
House, Bodicote, Banbury, Oxford, UK

Alastair P MacMillan BVSc, MSc, MRCVS
Head, FAO/WHO Collaborating Centre for Reference
and Research on Brucellosis, Central Veterinary
Laboratory, Addlestone, Surrey, UK

CR Madeley MD, FRCPath
Consultant Virologist, Public Health Laboratory Service,
Institute of Pathology, Newcastle General Hospital,
Newcastle upon Tyne, UK

John T Magee PhD, MSc, FIMLS
Top Grade Scientific Officer, Department of Medical
Microbiology and Public Health Laboratory, University
of Wales College of Medicine, Cardiff, UK

Brian WJ Mahy PhD, ScD
Director, Division of Viral and Rickettsial Diseases,
National Center for Infectious Diseases, Centers for
Disease Control and Prevention, Atlanta, Georgia, USA

Scott A Martin BS, MS, PhD
Professor, Department of Animal and Dairy Science,
College of Agriculture, Livestock and Poultry,
University of Georgia, Athens, Georgia, USA

William J Martin PhD
Director, Scientific Resources Program, National Center for Infectious Diseases, Centers for Disease Control and Prevention, Atlanta, Georgia, USA

Adolfo Martínez-Palomo MD, DSc
Director General, Centro de Investigación y de Estudios Avanzados, Mexico City, Mexico

Tadahiko Matsumoto MD, DMSc
Director, Department of Dermatology, Toshiba Hospital, Higashi-oi, Shinagawa-ku, Tokyo, Japan

Ruth Matthews MD, PhD, MSc, FRCPath
Reader in Medical Microbiology, Department of Medical Microbiology, Manchester Royal Infirmary, Manchester, UK

Joseph E McDade PhD
Associate Director for Laboratory Science, National Center for Infectious Diseases, Centers for Disease Control and Prevention, Atlanta, Georgia, USA

Michael R McGinnis PhD
Director, Medical Mycology Research Center, Associate Director, University of Texas at Galveston-WHO Collaborating Center for Tropical Diseases, and Professor, Department of Pathology, University of Texas Medical Branch at Galveston, Galveston, Texas, USA

Jim McLauchlin PhD
Clinical Scientist, Central Public Health Laboratory, Colindale, London, UK

Heinz Mehlhorn PhD
Professor of Parasitologie, Institut für Zoomorphologie, Zellbiologie und Parasitologie, Heinrich-Heine-Universität, Düsseldorf, Germany

A Leonel Mendoza MS, PhD
Assistant Professor, Department of Microbiology, Medical Technology Program, Michigan State University, East Lansing, Michigan, USA

Volker ter Meulen MD
Chairman, Institute for Virology and Immunobiology, University of Würzberg, Würzberg, Germany

Gillian Midgley BSc, PhD
Lecturer in Medical Mycology, Department of Medical Mycology, St John's Institute of Dermatology, United Medical and Dental School of Guy's and St Thomas's, St Thomas's Hospital, London, UK

Michael A Miles MSc, PhD, DSc
Professor of Medical Parasitology and Head, Applied Molecular Biology Unit, Department of Medical Parasitology, London School of Hygiene and Tropical Medicine, London, UK

J Michael Miller PhD, ABMM
Chief, Diagnostic Microbiology Section, Hospital Infections Program, National Center for Infectious Diseases, Centers for Disease Control and Prevention, Atlanta, Georgia, USA

P Minor BA, PhD
Head, Division of Virology, National Institute for Biological Standard and Control, Potters Bar, Hertfordshire, UK

AC Minson BSc, PhD
Professor of Virology, Virology Division, Department of Pathology, University of Cambridge, Cambridge, UK

DH Molyneux MA, PhD, DSc
Director, Professor of Tropical Health Sciences, Liverpool School of Tropical Medicine, Liverpool, UK

Arnold S Monto MD
Professor of Epidemiology, School of Public Health, University of Michigan, Ann Arbor, Michigan, USA

Stephen A Morse MSPH, PhD
Associate Director for Science, Division of AIDS, STD and Tuberculosis Laboratory Research, Centers for Disease Control and Prevention, Atlanta, Georgia, USA

RP Mortlock BS, PhD
Professor of Microbiology, Section of Microbiology, Cornell University, Ithaca, New York, USA

Ralph Muller DSc, PhD, BSc, FIBiol
Formerly Director, International Institute of Parasitology, St Albans, Hertfordshire, UK

David A Murdoch MA, MBBS, MSc, MD, MRCPath
Honorary Clinical Research Fellow, Department of Microbiology, Southmead Health Services NHS Trust, Westbury-on-Trym, Bristol, UK

Frederick A Murphy DVM, PhD
Professor, School of Veterinary Medicine, University of California, Davis, California, USA

RP Murray PhD
Professor, Division of Laboratory Medicine, Departments of Pathology and Medicine, Washington University School of Medicine, St Louis, Missouri, USA

David Mutimer MBBS
Senior Lecturer, Birmingham University Department of Medicine; Honorary Consultant Physician, Liver and Hepatobiliary Unit, Queen Elizabeth Hospital, Edgbaston, Birmingham, UK

Irving I Nachamkin PhD
Professor of Pathology and Laboratory Medicine, Department of Pathology and Laboratory Medicine, University of Pennsylvania School of Medicine, Philadelphia, Pennsylvania, USA

Francis E Nano PhD
Associate Professor, Department of Biochemistry and Microbiology, University of Victoria, Victoria, British Columbia, Canada

AA Nash BSc, MSc, PhD
Professor, Department of Veterinary Pathology, University of Edinburgh, Edinburgh, UK

Neal Nathanson MD
Professor and Chair Emeritus, Department of
Microbiology, University of Pennsylvania Medical
Center, Philadelphia, Pennsylvania, USA

James C Neil BSc, PhD
Professor of Virology and Molecular Oncology,
Department of Veterinary Pathology, University of
Glasgow, Glasgow, UK

WC Noble DSc, FRCPath
Professor of Microbiology, Department of Microbial
Diseases, St John's Institute of Dermatology, United
Medical and Dental Schools of Guy's and St Thomas's,
St Thomas's Hospital, London, UK

Steven J Norris PhD
Professor of Pathology and Laboratory Medicine,
Microbiology and Molecular Genetics, Department of
Pathology, University of Texas Health Science Center,
Houston, Texas, USA

David C Old PhD, DSc, FIBiol, FRCPath
Reader in Medical Microbiology, Department of
Medical Microbiology, Ninewells Hospital and Medical
School, Dundee, UK

Arvind A Padhye PhD
Chief, Fungus Reference Laboratory, Emerging
Bacterial and Mycotic Diseases Branch, Division of
Bacterial and Mycotic Diseases, Centers for Disease
Control and Prevention, Atlanta, Georgia, USA

Norberto J Palleroni PhD
Professor of Microbiology, Center for Agricultural
Molecular Biology, Cooke College, Rutgers University,
New Brunswick, New Jersey, USA

Stephen R Palmer MA, MB, BChir, FFPHM
Professor & Director, Welsh Combined Centres for
Public Health, University of Wales College of Medicine;
Head, Communicable Disease Surveillance Centre
Welsh Unit, Cardiff, UK

Demosthenes Pappagianis PhD, MD
Professor of Medical Biology and Immunology,
Department of Medical Microbiology and Immunology,
University of California, Davis, California, USA

M Thomas Parker MD, FRCPath, DipBact
Formerly Director, Cross-Infection Reference
Laboratory, Central Public Health Laboratory,
Colindale, London, UK

D Parratt MD, FRCPath
Senior Lecturer, Department of Medical Microbiology,
Ninewells Hospital, Dundee, UK

Roger Parton BSc, PhD
Senior Lecturer, Division of Infection and Immunity,
Institute of Biomedical and Life Sciences, University of
Glasgow, Glasgow, UK

Thomas F Patterson MD
Associate Professor of Medicine, Division of Infectious
Diseases, Department of Medicine, University of Texas
Health Science Center, San Antonio, Texas, USA

Charles W Penn BSc, PhD
Reader in Microbiology, School of Biological Sciences,
University of Birmingham, Edgbaston, Birmingham, UK

T Hugh Pennington MB, BS, PhD, FRCPath, FRSE
Professor of Bacteriology, Department of Medical
Microbiology, University of Aberdeen, Aberdeen, UK

John R Perfect MD
Professor of Medicine, Duke University Medical Center,
Durham, North Carolina, USA

William A Petri Jnr MD, PhD
Professor, Department of Infectious Diseases, University
of Virginia Health Sciences Center, Charlottesville,
Virginia, USA

Paula M Pitha BS, MS, PhD
Professor of Oncology, Oncology Center and
Department of Molecular Biology and Genetics,
Baltimore, Maryland, USA

Tyrone L Pitt MPhil, PhD
Deputy Director, Laboratory of Hospital Infection,
Central Public Health Laboratory, Colindale, London,
UK

Tanja Popovic MD, PhD
Principal Investigator, Diphtheria Research Project,
Childhood and Respiratory Diseases Branch, Division of
Bacterial and Mycotic Diseases, National Center for
Infectious Diseases, Centers for Disease Control and
Prevention, Atlanta, Georgia, USA

R Scott Pore PhD
Professor of Microbiology and Immunology,
Department of Microbiology and Immunology, West
Virginia University School of Medicine, Morgantown,
West Virginia, USA

Roger Pradinaud MD
Directeur, Service de Dermato-Vénéreo-Leprologie,
Centre Hospitalier de Cayenne, Guyane Française

Craig R Pringle BSc, PhD
Professor of Biological Sciences, Biological Sciences
Department, University of Warwick, Coventry,
Warwickshire, UK

Stanley B Prusiner AB, MD
Professor of Neurology, Biochemistry and Biophysics,
Department of Neurology, University of California, San
Francisco, California, USA

Thomas J Quan PhD, MPH
Microbiologist, Imu-Tek Animal Health Inc, Fort
Collins, Colorado, USA

CP Quinn BSc, PhD
Head, Biotherapy Unit, Centre for Applied
Microbiology and Research, Porton Down, Salisbury,
Wiltshire, UK

Sharath K Rai PhD
Postdoctoral Fellow, Department of Molecular
Immunology, Bristol Myers Squibb PRI, Seattle,
Washington, USA

Anita Rampling MA, PhD, MB ChB, FRCPath
Director, Public Health Laboratory, Department of
Pathology, West Dorset Hospital, Dorchester, UK

Robert C Read MD, MRCP
Senior Clinical Lecturer in Infectious Diseases,
Department of Medical Microbiology, University of
Sheffield Medical School, Sheffield, UK

Stephen C Redd MD
Chief, Measles Elimination Activity, Epidemiology and
Surveillance Division, Centers for Disease Control and
Prevention, Atlanta, Georgia, USA

Sanjay G Revankar MD
Infectious Diseases Fellow, Department of Medicine,
Division of Infectious Diseases, University of Texas
Health Science Center, San Antonio, Texas, USA

John H Rex MD
Associate Professor, University of Texas Medical School,
Houston, Texas, USA

Malcolm D Richardson BSc, PhD, CBiol, MIBiol,
FRCPath
Director, Regional Mycology Reference Laboratory,
Department of Dermatology, Glasgow, UK

Geoffrey L Ridgway MD, BSc, MRCP, FRCPath
Consultant Microbiologist, Department of Clinical
Microbiology, University College London Hospitals;
Honorary Senior Lecturer, University College Hospital,
London, UK

Glenn D Roberts PhD
Director, Clinical Mycology and Mycobacteriology
Laboratories; Professor of Microbiology and Laboratory
Medicine, Mayo Medical School, Division of Clinical
Microbiology, Mayo Clinic, Rochester, Minnesota, USA

Betty H Robertson PhD
Chief, Virology Section, Hepatitis Branch, Division of
Viral and Rickettsial Diseases, Centers for Disease
Control and Prevention, Hepatitis Branch, Atlanta,
Georgia, USA

Frank G Rodgers PhD
Professor of Microbiology; Editor, Journal of Clinical
Microbiology, Department of Microbiology, Rudman
Hall, University of New Hampshire, Durham, New
Hampshire, USA

John T Roehrig PhD
Chief, Arbovirus Diseases Branch, Division of Vector-
Borne Infectious Diseases, National Center for
Infectious Diseases, Centers for Disease Control and
Prevention, Fort Collins, Colorado, USA

MJ Rosovitz BSc
Research Assistant, Department of Bacteriology,
University of Wisconsin-Madison, Madison, Wisconsin,
USA

Paul A Rota PhD
Research Microbiologist, Measles Virus Section, Centers
for Disease Control and Prevention, Atlanta, Georgia,
USA

Andrew H Rudolph MD
Clinical Professor of Dermatology, Dermatology
Department, Baylor College of Medicine, Houston
Texas, USA

Kathryn L Ruoff PhD
Assistant Professor of Pathology, Harvard Medical
School; Assistant Director, Microbiology Laboratories,
Massachusetts General Hospital, Boston, Massachusetts,
USA

A Denver Russell BPharm, PhD, DSc, FRCPath,
FRPharmS
Professor, Welsh School of Pharmacy, University of
Wales at Cardiff, Cardiff, UK

WC Russell BSc, PhD, FRSE
Emeritus Research Professor, School of Biological and
Medical Sciences, University of St Andrews, St Andrews,
Fife, UK

Maria S Salvato PhD
Assistant Professor, Department of Pathology and
Laboratory Medicine, Services Memorial Institute,
University of Wisconsin Medical School, Madison,
Wisconsin, USA

Anthony Sanchez PhD
Special Pathogens Branch, Division of Viral and
Rickettsial Diseases, National Center for Infectious
Diseases, Centers for Disease Control and Prevention,
Atlanta, Georgia, USA

Klaus P Schaal MD
Director, Professor of Medical Microbiology, Institute
for Medical Microbiology and Immunology, University
of Bonn, Bonn, Germany

Julius Schachter PhD
Professor of Laboratory Medicine, World Health
Organization Collaborating Centre for References and
Research on Chlamydia, Chlamydia Research
Laboratory, Department of Laboratory Medicine, San
Francisco General Hospital, San Francisco, California,
USA

Wiley A Schell MSc
Research Associate, Department of Medicine, Duke
University Medical Center, Durham, North Carolina,
USA

Walter F Schlech III MD
Professor of Medicine, Faculty of Medicine, Dalhousie
University, QE II HSC, Halifax, Nova Scotia, Canada

L Schlesinger MD
Associate Professor of Medicine, Department of
Medicine, Division of Infectious Diseases, University of
Iowa, Iowa City, Iowa, USA

Connie S Schmaljohn PhD
Chief, Department of Molecular Virology, US Army
Medical Research Institute of Infectious Diseases, Fort
Detrick, Maryland, USA

Gabriel A Schmunis MD, PhD
Coordinator, Communicable Diseases Program, Pan American Health Organization, Washington, DC, USA

Sibylle Schneider-Schaulies PhD
Lecturer, Institut für Virologie und Immunbiologie, Universität Würzberg, Würzberg, Germany

John Richard Seed PhD
Professor, Department of Epidemiology, School of Public Health, University of North Carolina, Chapel Hill, North Carolina, USA

Esther Segal PhD
Professor of Microbiology/Mycology, Department of Human Microbiology, Sackler School of Medicine, Tel Aviv University, Ramat Aviv, Tel Aviv, Israel

Bernard W Senior BSc, PhD, FRCPath
Lecturer in Medical Microbiology, Department of Medical Microbiology, Dundee University Medical School, Ninewells Hospital and Medical School, Dundee, UK

Haroun N Shah BSc, PhD, FRCPath
Head, Identification Services Unit, National Collection of Type Cultures, Central Public Health Laboratory, Colindale, London, UK

Jeffrey J Shaw PhD, DSc
Professor, Departamento de Parasitologia, Instituto de Ciências Biomédicas, Universidade de São Paulo, São Paulo, Brazil

Thomas M Shinnick PhD
Chief, Tuberculosis/Mycobacteriology Branch, Centers for Disease Control and Prevention, Atlanta, Georgia, USA

Stuart G Siddell BSc, PhD
Professor of Virology, Institute of Virology, University of Würzburg, Würzburg, Germany

Gunter O Siegl PhD
Professor and Head, Institute for Clinical Microbiology and Immunology, St Gallen, Switzerland

Lynne Sigler MSc
Curator and Associate Professor, University of Alberta Microfungus Collection and Herbarium, Devonian Botanic Garden, Edmonton, Alberta, Canada

RB Sim BSc, DPhil
MRC Scientific Staff, MRC Immunochemistry Unit, Department of Biochemistry, University of Oxford, Oxford, UK

Peter Simmonds BM, PhD, MRCPath
Senior Lecturer, Department of Medical Microbiology, University of Edinburgh Medical School, Edinburgh, UK

Anthony Simmons MA, MB, BChir, PhD, FRCPath
Senior Medical Specialist, Infectious Diseases Laboratories, Institute of Medical and Veterinary Science, Adelaide, Australia

Martin B Skirrow MB, ChB, PhD, FRCPath, DTM&H
Consultant Medical Microbiologist, Public Health Laboratory, Gloucestershire Royal Hospital, Gloucester, UK

Mary PE Slack MA, MB, FRCPath
Lecturer (Honorary Consultant) in Bacteriology, Haemophilus Reference Laboratory, Oxford Public Health Laboratory and Nuffield Department of Pathology and Bacteriology, John Radcliffe Hospital, Oxford, UK

Henry R Smith MA, PhD
Deputy Director, Laboratory of Enteric Pathogens, Central Public Health Laboratory, Colindale, London, UK

Eric J Snijder PhD
Assistant Professor, Department of Virology, Institute of Medical Microbiology, Leiden University, Leiden, The Netherlands

Phyllis H Sparling DVM, MS
Liaison, Centers for Disease Control and Prevention, Atlanta, Georgia, USA

David CE Speller MA, BM, BCh, FRCP, FRCPath
Emeritus Professor of Clinical Microbiology, University of Bristol, Bristol, UK

Carol A Spiegel PhD
Associate Professor, Department of Pathology and Laboratory Medicine, University of Wisconsin, Madison, Wisconsin, USA

Andrew Spielman ScD
Professor of Tropical Public Health, Department of Tropical Public Health, Harvard School of Public Health, Boston, Massachusetts, USA

Bret M Steiner PhD
Chief, Treponemal Pathogenesis, Division of Sexually Transmitted Diseases, Centers for Disease Control and Prevention, Atlanta, Georgia, USA

Scott J Stewart BS
Formerly of National Institute of Allergies and Infectious Diseases; 344 Roaring Lion Road, Hamilton, Montana, USA

Max Sussman BSc, PhD, CBiol, FIBiol, FRCPath
Emeritus Professor of Bacteriology, Department of Microbiology, The Medical School, Newcastle upon Tyne, UK

Roland W Sutter MD, MPH, TM
Deputy Chief for Technical Affairs, Polio Eradication Activity, National Immunization Program, Centers for Disease Control and Prevention, Atlanta, Georgia, USA

Bala Swaminathan PhD
Chief, Foodborne and Diarrhoeal Diseases Laboratory 333 Section, Foodborne and Diarrhoeal Diseases Branch, Centers for Disease Control and Prevention, Atlanta, Georgia, USA

Robert V Tauxe MD, MPH
Chief, Foodborne and Diarrhoeal Diseases Branch,
Division of Bacterial and Mycotic Diseases, Centers for
Disease Control and Prevention, Atlanta, Georgia, USA

David J Taylor MA, VetMB, PhD, MRCVS
Reader in Veterinary Microbiology, Department of
Veterinary Pathology, University of Glasgow, School of
Veterinary Medicine, Bearsden, Glasgow, UK

John M Taylor PhD
Senior Member, Fox Chase Cancer Center,
Philadelphia, Pennsylvania, USA

David Taylor-Robinson MD, MRCP, FRCPath
Emeritus Professor of Microbiology and Genitourinary
Medicine, Department of Genitourinary Medicine, St
Mary's Hospital, London, UK

Lucia Martins Teixeira PhD
Associate Professor, Universidade Federal do Rio de
Janeiro, Instituto de Microbiologia, Rio de Janeiro,
Brazil

Sam Rountree Telford III DSc
Lecturer in Tropical Health, Department of Tropical
Public Health, Harvard University, Boston,
Massachusetts, USA

Ram P Tewari PhD
Professor of Microbiology, Department of Medical
Microbiology and Immunology, Southern Illinois
University, Springfield, Illinois School of Medicine,
Springfield, Illinois, USA

E John Threlfall BSc, PhD
Grade C Clinical Scientist, Laboratory of Enteric
Pathogens, Central Public Health Laboratory,
Colindale, London, UK

Richard C Tilton BS, MS, PhD
Senior Vice President, Chief Scientific Director, BBI
Clinical Laboratories, New Britain, Connecticut, USA

Noel Tordo PhD
Head, Laboratoire de Lyssavirus, Institut Pasteur, Paris,
France

Anna Maria Tortorano PhD
Associate Professor of Hygiene, Laboratory of Medical
Microbiology, Institute of Hygiene and Preventive
Medicine, School of Medicine, Università degli Studi di
Milano, Milano, Italy

Kevin J Towner BSc, PhD
Consultant Clinical Scientist, Public Health Laboratory,
University Hospital, Queen's Medical Centre,
Nottingham, UK

JG Tully BS, MS, PhD
Chief, Mycoplasma Section, Laboratory of Molecular
Microbiology, National Institute of Allergy and
Infectious Diseases, National Institutes of Health,
Frederick, Maryland, USA

Peter C B Turnbull BSc, MS, PhD
Head, Anthrax Section, Centre for Applied
Microbiology and Research, Porton Down, Salisbury,
Wiltshire, UK

Kenneth L Tyler MD
Professor of Neurology, Medicine, Microbiology and
Immunology, Department of Neurology, University of
Colorado Health Sciences Center, and Chief,
Neurology Service Denver Veteran Affairs Medical
Center, Denver, Colorado, USA

Edward J Usherwood MA, PhD
Research Fellow, Department of Veterinary Pathology,
Edinburgh, UK

Maria Anna Viviani MD
Associate Professor of Hygiene, Laboratory of Medical
Microbiology, Institute of Hygiene and Preventive
Medicine, School of Medicine, Università degli Studi di
Milano, Milano, Italy

Martin I Voskuil BA
Research Scientist, Department of Bacteriology,
University of Wisconsin-Madison, Madison, Wisconsin,
USA

William G Wade BSc, PhD
Richard Dickinson Professor of Oral Microbiology,
Head of Oral Biology Unit, Department of Oral
Medicine and Pathology, United Medical and Dental
Schools of Guy's and St Thomas's, Guy's Hospital,
London, UK

Derek Wakelin BSc, PhD, DSc, FRCPath
Professor of Zoology, Department of Life Science,
University of Nottingham, Nottingham, UK

Alexander Wandeler MSc, PhD
Head of Rabies Unit, Animal Diseases Research
Institute, Nepean, Ontario, Canada

Audrey R Wanger PhD
Assistant Professor, Department of Pathology and
Laboratory Medicine, University of Texas Medical
School at Houston, Houston, Texas, USA

Bodo Wanke PhD, MD
Head of Laboratório de Micologia Médica, Laboratório
de Micologia, Hospital Evandro Chagas, Rio de Janeiro,
Brazil

ME Ward BSc, PhD
Professor of Medical Microbiology, Molecular
Microbiology, Southampton University School of
Medicine, Southampton General Hospital,
Southampton, UK

MFR Waters OBE, MB, FRCP, FRCPath
Formerly Consultant Leprologist and Physician,
Hospital for Tropical Diseases, London, UK

Emilio Weiss BS, MS, PhD
Emeritus Chair of Science, Naval Medical Research
Institute, Bethesda, Maryland, USA

Irene Weitzman PhD
Assistant Director, Clinical Microbiology Service, and
Associate Professor of Clinical Pathology in Medicine,
Columbia Presbyterian Medical Center, New York, New
York, USA

Lawrence J Wheat MD
Professor of Medicine, Infectious Disease Division,
Wishard Memorial Hospital, Indianapolis, Indiana, USA

Richard J Whitley MD
Professor of Pediatrics, Microbiology and Medicine,
Department of Pediatrics, University of Alabama at
Birmingham, Birmingham, Alabama, USA

James Whitworth MD, FRCP, DTM&H
Team Leader, MRC Programme on AIDS, Entebbe,
Uganda

Louis A Wilson BS, MSc, MD, FACS
Professor of Ophthalmology, Emory University School
of Medicine and Adjunct Professor of Microbiology,
Georgia State University, Atlanta, Georgia, USA

John A Wyke MA, VetMB, PhD, MRCVS, FRSE
Director of Research, Beatson Institute, Honorary
Professor at University of Glasgow, Beatson Institute for
Cancer Research, Glasgow, UK

Kentaro Yoshimura BVM, DVM, PhD
Professor of Parasitology, Chairman, Department of
Parasitology, Akita University School of Medicine, Akita,
Japan

Viqar Zaman MBBS, DSc, DTM&H, FRCPath
Professor, Department of Microbiology, The Aga Khan
University, Karachi, Pakistan

Stephen H Zinder BA, MS, PhD
Professor of Microbiology, Section of Microbiology,
Cornell University, Ithaca, New York, USA

EDITOR-IN-CHIEF'S PREFACE

The period since publication of the first edition in 1929 has seen various modifications in the form and content of *Topley and Wilson*, perhaps the most important of which was the change with the 7th edition to a multi-author work in four volumes. This, the 9th edition, marks three spectacular departures from past policy.

First, and most obviously, the work now covers every class of pathogen: viruses, bacteria, fungi and parasites, including the helminths. The arrangement is in order of complexity, ranging from *Virology* in Volume 1 through *Systematic Bacteriology* and *Bacterial Infections* in Volumes 2 and 3, *Medical Mycology* in Volume 4 and *Parasitology* in Volume 5. Each has its own index, and a general index to the entire work is provided in Volume 6.

This major expansion called for a change in authorship, which previously was almost entirely British. Clearly, the range of expertise now needed to cover every aspect of medical microbiology, including mycology and parasitology, can no longer be provided from any one country and we have been fortunate in recruiting leading experts from many parts of the world for this expanded edition. In all, there are 234 chapters, of which the USA has provided 45% and the UK 35%; the remainder come from 20 other countries.

The third important new feature is the appearance of an electronic version alongside the printed work, which will facilitate information retrieval, cross-referencing and, most important, a continual programme of revision and updating.

During the planning phase, surveys of known and potential readers indicated a majority demand for more detailed referencing than hitherto, and the provision of factual material rather than the more speculative and discursive treatment characteristic of the early editions. This trend has become increasingly apparent with successive editions, and there is now no justification for retaining the word 'Principles' in the title. Despite this change in emphasis, the readership

for whom the work is intended remains the same; it comprises primarily microbiologists working in research, diagnostic and public health laboratories and those teaching both undergraduates and postgraduates. Although it is first and foremost a treatise on microbiology, the comprehensive coverage of the clinical and pathological features of infection makes it also an invaluable source of reference for physicians dealing with infective disease.

The 8th edition comprised four volumes of text, of which the first covered *General Bacteriology and Immunity*, and was intended to service those dealing with the more specialized topics. This arrangement did not, however, prove satisfactory; the 9th edition is therefore designed to make the volumes more self-contained, and descriptions of the immune response as it relates respectively to viruses, bacteria and the eukaryotic parasites are provided in the appropriate volumes.

The arrangement of the *Virology* volume is similar to that in the 8th edition, except that it is divided into five rather than two parts. Accounts of the general characteristics of bacteria and of bacteria in the environment will now be found in Volume 2 (*Systematic Bacteriology*). Both this and Volume 3 (*Bacterial Infections*) can be read individually, but, as in past editions, they obviously complement each other. The quantity of information now available has meant a further increase in size of Volumes 1, 2 and 3, which now contain about 30% more material than did the whole of the 8th edition. The two new volumes, dealing respectively with *Medical Mycology* and *Parasitology*, greatly enhance the value of the work as a whole. Whether to include the helminths under the title *Microbiology and Microbial Infections* was a debatable point, which succeeded on the grounds that to omit them would impair coverage of the entire gamut of infection, and that a separate mention in the title would have made it unwieldy.

Some points of editorial policy deserve mention. As in previous editions, the emphasis throughout is on infections of humans; animal diseases are given much less prominence, usually receiving mention only when they cause zoonoses, serve as models of pathogenesis or are of economic importance. Sections likely to be of interest only to the more specialized reader are indicated by the use of a small typeface, and the location and cross-referencing of specific sections are now made easier by numbering them.

The standard of the illustrations, many of which are now in colour, is considerably higher than in previous editions; in particular, there is a wealth of excellent drawings and photographs in Volumes 4 and 5. The quality of the references has been greatly improved by providing the titles of papers and both first and last pages; and the international provenance of the contributors has resulted in broader surveys of the world literature than is usual in predominantly British or American texts.

In conclusion, I take this opportunity of saying how much I appreciate the efforts of all those concerned with bringing this large and complex work to fruition. Almost by definition, the more distinguished the author, the more he or she will have other pressing commitments, a consideration that applies to most of our contributors. Sincere thanks are due to them for their participation and for providing the huge fund of learning and expertise that is apparent throughout the edition. I gladly take this opportunity of expressing my gratitude to all my colleagues on the editorial team for the intensive and sustained effort they have devoted to bringing this large and complex publication to fruition. It would be invidious to single out individuals among the copy-editors and the staff at Arnold who have laboured so devotedly behind the scenes, but to each of them my gratitude is also due for their competent help and unfailing support during the preparation of this edition.

LC

VOLUME EDITORS' PREFACE

The inclusion of a volume devoted to parasitic infections is a new initiative for *Topley and Wilson*. Strictly speaking, the term parasite can be applied to any infectious agent but, by convention, is generally restricted to infections caused by protozoa and helminths and excludes the viruses and prokaryotic organisms traditionally covered in these volumes. The grouping together of protozoa and helminths is not entirely satisfactory because, from the point of view of systematics, they have little in common except their eukaryotic nature, the former being unicellular and the latter multicellular. In fact, infections caused by protozoa have more in common with viral and bacterial infections than with those caused by helminths; modern epidemiological concepts therefore tend to group protozoa with viruses and bacteria as microparasites – characteristically, small organisms that multiply within their vertebrate hosts – and regard helminths as macroparasites that are characteristically large and usually do not do so. Nevertheless, parasitology is a well established and inclusive discipline: parasitology textbooks, courses, societies and international meetings all continue to embrace both protozoa and helminths, a tradition followed in this volume.

Until relatively recently, parasitic infections in humans were regarded mainly as exotic problems of concern only to those living in the tropics and subtropics, but in 1976 WHO drew attention to the magnitude of the problem that these diseases cause and listed five parasitic infections – malaria, trypanosomiasis, leishmaniasis, schistosomiasis and filariasis – among six diseases presenting the greatest challenges in the developing world (the sixth being leprosy).

The impact of parasitic diseases in developing countries is enormous, but they are no longer confined to such areas. The rapid spread of quick and affordable international travel has meant that parasitic infections are frequently imported into more temperate regions by immigrants and returning travellers; a number of parasites are now world wide in their distribution and many infections once thought to be harmless are now known to be life-threatening in immunocompromised individuals.

The chapters that follow summarize what is known about the most important parasitic diseases of humans, some caused by one species and some, like leishmaniasis, by several. Many of these parasites use a vector or one or more intermediate hosts in their complex life cycles and these are also described. Of particular interest is the fact that parasites have developed many ways to survive in hostile environments. This adaptability includes the capacity to evade the immune response: thus, most parasitic infections are of long duration and cause chronic diseases; many helminth infections last for 2–10 years; and some protozoan infections persist for the lifetimes of their hosts. Partly because of the ability of parasites to evade the immune response, there is currently no vaccine against any parasitic infection in humans. Parasites also have the capacity to develop resistance to the few effective drugs available, resistance to antimalarials being the most spectacular, presenting problems also common in bacterial infections. Furthermore, attempts to control parasites by attacking their vectors have been hampered by the development of insecticide resistance. Parasitic infections, therefore, present enormous challenges, many of which are outlined in the chapters that follow, but there have been successes: guinea worm has all but been eliminated by the provision of clean water and onchocerciasis in Africa is one of the few infections that have almost totally succumbed to chemotherapeutic intervention. On the other hand, the news is not all good and several parasites are included in the growing list of those causing emerging infections, particularly in people infected with HIV or undergoing immunosuppressive therapy. Prominent among these are the microsporidians, several species of which have been recovered only from immunocompromised patients. Toxoplasmosis and cryptosporidiosis are other examples of parasitic diseases encountered mainly in immunosuppressed individuals as is pneumocystosis, the causative agent of which, *Pneumocystis carinii*, is included in this volume for completeness because, although now clearly established as a fungus (see Volume 4, Chapter 34) it has in the past been classified with the Protozoa and is often included in the protozoological literature.

The overall objective of this volume is to enhance, update and strengthen the literature familiar to those working with tropical diseases and to introduce parasitic infections to those in all parts of the world who are less well versed in their importance.

FC
JK
DW

ABBREVIATIONS

ABR	annual biting rate	**DALYs**	disability adjusted life years
ADCC	antibody dependent cell-mediated cytotoxicity	**DAT**	direct agglutination test
		DCL	diffuse cutaneous leishmaniasis
ADCL	anergic diffuse cutaneous leishmaniasis	**DDT**	dichlorodiphenyltrichloroethane
ADH	alcohol dehydrogenase	**DEC**	diethylcarbamazine
ADP	adenosine diphosphate	**DEET**	diethyltoluamide
AEC	alveolar epithelial cells	**DFMO**	difluoromethylornithine (eflornithine)
AIDS	acquired immunodeficiency syndrome	**DHFR**	dihydrofolate reductase
ALDH	aldehyde dehydrogenase	**DHPS**	dihydropteroate synthetase
ALS	antilymphocyte serum	**DTH**	delayed-type hypersensitivity
AP	aerosolized pentamidine	**EBA**	erythrocyte binding antigen
APC	antigen-presenting cell	**ECG**	electrocardiogram
ARC	AIDS-related complex	**ECM**	extracellular matrix components
ARDS	adult respiratory distress syndrome	**ECP**	eosinophil cationic protein
ATP	adenosine triphosphate; annual transmission potential	**EDN**	eosinophil-derived neurotoxin
		EDTA	ethylenediamine tetraacetic acid
AV	atrioventricular	**EEG**	electroencephalogram
AVL	American visceral leishmaniasis	**ELISA**	enzyme-linked immunosorbent assay
BCG	Bacille Calmette–Guérin	**EMP**	Embden–Meyerhof–Parnas
BGG	bovine G globulin	**ENT**	ear, nose and throat
BHC	benzene hexachloride	**EPA**	Environmental Protection Agency
CAA	circulating anodic antigen	**EPI**	expanded programme of immunization
CAEP	ceramide aminoethyl phosphonate	**EPO**	eosinophil peroxidase
CAT	computerized axial tomography	**EPX**	eosinophil protein X
CATT	card agglutination test for trypanosomiasis	**ER**	endoplasmic reticulum
CCA	circulating cathodic antigen	**E-S**	excretory-secretory
CDC	Centers for Disease Control	**FAD**	flavin adenine dinucleotide
cDNA	complimentary DNA	**FECT**	formalin-ethyl acetate concentration
CDT	cytidine diphosphate	**FILCO**	Filariasis Control Movement
CFA	circulating filarial antigen	**G6PD**	glucose-6-phosphate-dehydrogenase
CFT	complement fixation test	**GABA**	γ-aminobutyric acid
CIE	counter-immunoelectrophoresis	**GAE**	granulomatous amoebic encephalitis
CL	cutaneous leishmaniasis	**GAPDH**	glyceraldehyde-3-phosphate dehydrogenase
CLM	cutaneous larva migrans		
CMFL	community microfilarial load	**GIPLs**	glycosylphosphatidylinositols
CMP	cytidine monophosphate	**GMP**	guanosine 5′-monophosphate
CNS	central nervous system	**Gp**	glycoprotein
COP	circumoval precipitin	**gpA**	glycoprotein A
CRP	cysteine-rich surface protein	**GPI**	glycosyl-phosphatidylinositol
CS	circumsporozoite	**GR**	glutathione reductase
CSF	cerebrospinal fluid	**gRNA**	guide RNA
CSP	circumsporozoite protein	**GSH**	glutathione
CT	computed tomography	**GSSG**	GR (glutathione reductase) substrate glutathione disulphide
CTC	capillary tube centrifugation		
CTP	cytidine triphosphate	**GST**	glutathione S-transferase

IFA	immunofluorescence assay	**MMR**	measles/mumps/rubella
IFN	interferon	**MMTV**	mouse mammary tumour virus
Ig	immunoglobulin	**MMV**	mice minute virus
IHA	indirect haemagglutination	**moi**	multiplicity of infection
IL	interleukin	**MPGN**	membranoproliferative glomerulonephritis
IM	infectious mononucleosis	**mRNA**	messenger RNA
iNOS	inducible nitric oxide synthetase	**MuLV**	murine leukaemia virus
INV	intracellular naked virus	**MuV**	mumps virus
IP	immunoperoxidase	**MV**	measles virus
IPA	immunoperoxidase assay	**MVC**	minute virus of canine
IPV	inactivated polio vaccine	**MVE**	Murray Valley encephalitis
IR	inverted repeat	**NA**	neuraminidase
IRES	internal ribosome entry site	**NAAT**	nucleic acid amplification technique
ISCOM	immuno-stimulating complex	**NANB**	non-A, non-B [hepatitis]
ISG	immune serum globulin; interferon-stimulated gene	**NASBA**	nucleic acid sequence-based amplification
ISRE	interferon-specific response element	**NDV**	Newcastle disease virus
ISVP	intermediate subviral particle	**NFT**	neurofibrillary tangles
ITR	inverted terminal repeat/repetition	**NGF**	nerve growth factor
IVDU	intravenous drug user	**NK**	natural killer
IVIG	intravenous immunoglobulin	**NLS**	nuclear localization site
JAK	Janus kinase	**NNSV**	non-segmented negative-strand [RNA] virus
JcDNV	*Junonia coenia* densovirus	**NP**	nucleoprotein
JCV	JC virus	**NPC**	nasopharyngeal carcinoma
JE	Japanese encephalitis	**NPS**	nasopharyngeal secretion
JHMV	murine coronavirus JHM	**NSI**	non-syncytia inducer
JLP	juvenile laryngeal papillomatosis	**NSP**	non-structural protein
kDa	kilodalton	**nt**	nucleotide
KRV	Kilham rat virus	**NTR**	non-translated region; non-translated RNA
KSHV	Kaposi's sarcoma herpesvirus	**OAAV**	ovine adenoassociated virus
LA	latex agglutination	**2′,5′-OAS**	2′,5′-oligoadenylate synthetase
LAT	latency-associated transcript	**OPV**	oral poliovirus
LAV	lymphadenopathy-associated virus	**ORF**	open reading frame
LCL	lymphoid cell line	**ORS**	oral rehydration salt
LCMV	lymphocytic choriomeningitis virus	**P & I**	pneumonia and influenza
LCR	ligase chain reaction	**PAGE**	polyacrylamide gel electrophoresis
LDL	low density lipoprotein	**PBMC**	peripheral blood mononuclear cell
LDV	lactate dehydrogenase-elevating virus	**PBS**	phosphate-buffered saline; primer binding site
LIP	lymphoid interstitial pneumonitis	**PCP**	papain-like cysteine proteinase; *Pneumocystis carinii* pneumonia
LMP	last menstrual period; latent membrane protein		
LNYV	lettuce necrotic yellows virus	**PCR**	polymerase chain reaction
LOD	logarithm of odds	**PCV**	penciclovir
LPD	lymphoproliferative disease	**PEDV**	porcine epidemic diarrhoea virus
LPV	lapine parvovirus	**PFA**	phosphonoformate
LSD	lumpy skin disease	**pfu**	plaque-forming unit
LTR	long terminal repeat	**PHA**	phytohaemagglutinin
LUIIV	LUIII virus	**PHC**	primary hepatocellular carcinoma
M	matrix/membrane [protein]	**pHSA**	polymerized human serum albumin
M-MuLV	Moloney murine leukaemia virus	**PK**	[cytoplasmic] protein kinase
MAb	monoclonal antibody	**PKC**	cellular protein kinase
MACRIA	M-antibody capture radioimmunoassay	**PKR**	protein kinase dsRNA
MADT	morphological alteration and disintegration test	**PMKC**	primary [cynomolgus/rhesus] monkey kidney cell
MAI	*Mycobacterium avium* intracellular [infection]	**PML**	progressive multifocal leucoencephalopathy
MAR	monoclonal antibody-resistant	**PPD**	purified protein derivative
MBP	mannose-binding protein; myelin basic protein	**PPV**	porcine parvovirus
		PRCV	porcine respiratory coronavirus
MDCK	Madin–Darby canine kidney [cell]	**PRRSV**	porcine reproductive and respiratory syndrome virus
ME	myalgic encephalomyelitis		
MEV	mink enteritis virus	**PTA**	phosphotungstic acid
MGF	myxoma growth factor	**PTB**	polypyrimidine tract binding [protein]
MHC	major histocompatibility complex	**pTP**	precursor of terminal protein
MHV	murine hepatitis virus; murine herpesvirus	**PVR**	poliovirus receptor
MIBE	measles inclusion body encephalitis	**RbCV**	rabbit coronavirus
MK	monkey kidney	**RCV**	rat coronavirus
MM	maintenance medium	**RdRp**	RNA-dependent RNA polymerase

REA	restriction enzyme analysis		**TAC**	transient aplastic crisis
RER	rough endoplasmic reticulum		**TAP**	transporter associated with antigen processing
RF	replicative form			
RHDV	rabbit haemorrhagic disease virus		**TBEV**	tick-borne encephalitis virus
RI	replicative intermediate		**Tc**	cytotoxic T cell
RIA	radioimmunoassay		**3TC**	2′-deoxy-3′-thiacytidine
RIPA	radioimmunoprecipitation assay		**TCID50**	median tissue culture infectious dose
RK	receptor kinase		**TCR**	T cell receptor
RNP	ribonucleoprotein		**TCV**	turkey coronavirus
RPV	raccoon parvovirus		**TF**	transcription factor
RR	ribonucleotide reductase; Ross River		**TFT**	trifluorothymidine
RRE	rev-responsive element		**Tg**	transgenic
RREID	rapid rabies enzyme immunodiagnosis		**TGEV**	transmissible gastroenteritis virus
RRV	rhesus rotavirus		**TGF**	transforming growth factor
RSSV	Russian spring–summer encephalitis		**Th**	T helper [cell]
RSV	respiratory syncytial virus; Rous sarcoma virus		**TIBO**	tetrahydro-imidazo[4,5,1-jk][1,4]-benzodiazepin-2H(1H)-thione
RT	reverse transcriptase		**α-TIF**	α-*trans*-inducing factor
RT-PCR	reverse transcriptase polymerase chain reaction		**TK**	thymidine kinase
			TMEV	Theiler's murine encephalomyelitis virus
RTPV	RT parvovirus		**TMV**	tobacco mosaic virus
RV	rabies virus; rubella virus		**TNF**	tumour necrosis factor
SAR	secondary attack rate; structure–activity relationship		**TP**	terminal protein
			TR-FIA	time-resolved fluoroimmunoassay
SCID	severe combined immunodeficiency		**TRIS**	tris(hydroxymethyl)amino-methane
SCR	short consensus repeat		**TRTV**	turkey rhinotracheitis virus
SDAV	sialodacryoadenitis virus		*ts*	temperature sensitive
SDS-PAGE	sodium dodecyl sulphate–polyacrylamide gel electrophoresis		**TS**	thymidylate synthase
			TSP/HAM	tropical spastic paraparesis/HTLV-I-associated myelopathy
sec	secretion factor			
serpin	serine protease inhibitor		**TTP**	thymidine triphosphate
SF	Semliki Forest		**TUT**	terminal uridylate transferase
SFGF	Shope fibroma growth factor		**TVX**	tumour virus X
SFV	Semliki Forest virus		**UTR**	untranslated region
SHFV	simian haemorrhagic fever virus		**V-RG**	vaccinia-rabies glycoprotein
SI	syncytia inducer		**VA**	virus associated
SIRSV	swine infertility and respiratory syndrome virus		**VACV**	valaciclovir
			VAP	virus attachment protein
SIV	simian immunodeficiency virus		**VCA**	viral capsid antigen
SKIF	specific PKR inhibitory factor		**VCAM**	vascular cell adhesion molecule
SLE	St Louis encephalitis		**VEE**	Venezuelan equine encephalitis
SN	serum neutralization		**VETF**	viral early transcription factor
SNV	Sin Nombre virus		**VEV**	vesicular exanthem virus
SP-A	surfactant protein A		**vIL**	viral interleukin
SP-D	surfactant protein D		**VLA**	very late antigen
SPIEM	solid phase immunoelectron microscopy		**VLP**	virus-like particle
SRH	single radial haemolysis		**VN**	virus neutralization
SRP	signal recognition particle		**VNA**	virus-neutralizing antibody
SRSV	small round structured virus		**vRNA**	virion RNA
SRV	small round virus		**VSV**	vesicular stomatitis virus
ss	single-stranded		**VV**	vaccinia virus
SSPE	subacute sclerosing panencephalitis		**VZIG**	varicella-zoster immune globulin
Stat	signal transducers and activators of transcription		**VZV**	varicella-zoster virus
			WB	Western blot
STD	sexually transmitted disease		**WEE**	western equine encephalitis
STLV	simian T cell leukaemia virus		**WG**	week of gestation
SV	subvirion		**WHV**	woodchuck hepatitis virus
SV40	simian virus 40		**WKA**	Wistar–King–Aptekman
SVD	swine vesicular disease		**WV**	whole virus
SVDV	swine vesicular disease virus		**XLA**	X-linked agammaglobulinaemia
SVP	subviral particle		**XLPS**	X-linked lymphoproliferative syndrome (Duncan syndrome)
SYNV	sonchus yellow net virus			
T1L	type 1 Lang [virus]		**YFV**	yellow fever virus
T3D	type 3 Dearing [virus]		**ZIG**	zoster immunoglobulin

Part I

General Considerations

HISTORY OF HUMAN PARASITOLOGY

F E G Cox

1 Introduction	3 Protozoa and protozoal infections
2 Helminths and helminth infections	4 Summary and conclusions

1 INTRODUCTION

The history of parasitology is a long and distinguished one that embraces 3 interconnected fields: zoology, with its interest in parasites for their own sakes; medicine, in particular tropical medicine; and veterinary medicine. The history of human parasitology parallels the history of other diseases about which there are many excellent books, the most comprehensive and useful being the 'Encyclopaedia of the History of Medicine' (Bynum and Porter 1993) and Cambridge World History of Human Diseases' (Kiple 1993). The lavishly illustrated 'Medicine: An Illustrated History' (Lyons and Petrucelli 1978) is an excellent overall introduction to the subject.

It was recognized nearly a century ago that most tropical diseases are caused by infectious agents (Manson 1898). As infectious diseases existed before humans evolved, their history is not only long but shrouded in mystery. Nevertheless, it is possible to see some evidence of the presence of tropical diseases before written history began; characteristic lesions have been depicted in early sculptures and the eggs of parasitic worms have been found in Egyptian mummies and among other human remains. The first written records date from a period of Egyptian medicine between 3000 and 400 BC, particularly the papyri of 1500 BC discovered by Georg Ebers at Thebes (Bryan 1930). Many diseases, specifically fevers, are described in detail in the writings of Greek physicians produced between 800 and 300 BC, including descriptions written by Hippocrates in 'Airs, Waters and Places' in the 5th century BC (Jones and Whithington 1948–1953). Significant contributions to our understanding of parasitic diseases have also been made by physicians from other civilizations, such as China 3000–300 BC, India 2500–200 BC, Rome 700 BC–AD 400 and the Arab Empire in the latter part of the first millennium. In particular, the Arab authors Rhazes (850–923) and Avicenna 980–1037) wrote important medical works that contain a great deal of information about diseases caused by parasites.

In Europe, the Dark and Middle Ages were characterized by religious and superstitious beliefs that held back medical progress until the Renaissance; this era released a flurry of activity, culminating in the great discoveries that characterized the end of the nineteenth century. The turning point was the evolution of the 'germ theory', which involved the following key figures: Louis Pasteur, whose experiments demolished the theory of spontaneous generation and showed that diseases could be caused by bacteria; Robert Koch, who introduced methods of preventing diseases caused by micro-organisms; and Patrick Manson who incriminated vectors in the transmission of parasites.

Most commentators date the origin of tropical diseases as a distinct branch of medicine to 1898, when the first edition of 'Tropical Diseases' was published by Sir Patrick Manson, now universally regarded as the 'father of tropical medicine'. The important tropical diseases described by Manson included a number caused by parasites: malaria, sleeping sickness, amoebic dysentery, kala azar and bilharzia. He discussed these parasitic diseases in the same way as non-parasitic diseases such as leprosy, plague, cholera, brucellosis, yaws, yellow fever, dengue fever and beri beri. At the turn of the century, the causes of most of these diseases were unknown but the explosion of discoveries that occurred during the first decade of this century necessitated the publication of 5 more editions of Manson's book by the time he died in 1922.

Warboys has pointed out that 'the dominant tradition of the history of tropical diseases has been to celebrate the discoveries of the aetiologies of the classic group of vector-borne parasitic diseases in the period 1870–1920' (Warboys 1993). It is now clear that the work of those who investigated parasitic diseases in the centuries before Manson should not be dismissed as irrelevant to our understanding of these diseases. Nor should the discoveries of the 20th century workers be regarded as mere finishing touches to previous knowledge. Scientific progress during any period of history depends on the availability of techniques and of individuals capable of using and interpreting the information that becomes available. The remarkable thing about the turn of the century was the coming together of so many ideas and personalities and this chapter is concerned with some of these.

Parasitic diseases have always held a fascination for travellers, clinicians and scientists. Some, such as sleeping sickness, are unique to the tropics whereas others, such as malaria, are of particular importance in the tropics but also extend into more temperate regions. Finally, some parasites, such as hookworm, have world-wide distribution (either now or in the past). The present distribution of parasitic diseases reflects the success of hygiene and control measures in the more developed parts of the world rather than any clear geographical or climatic restriction. Thus many parasites that were once widespread are now found in only the warmer and poorer parts of the world and are considered as 'exotic' diseases when imported into the cooler northern and southern latitudes where they were once prevalent.

The history of parasitology has been well served in the scientific literature particularly in works devoted to tropical medicine. As well as the works already mentioned there is a considerable amount of information about the history of parasitology in Scott (1939), Ackernecht (1965), Brothwell and Sandison (1967), Ransford (1983), Campbell, Hall and Klausner (1992), Chernin (1977), Mack (1991), Norman (1991), Ranger and Slack (1992) and Cox (1996). More specifically, there are a number of publications dedicated to the history of parasitology including those of Foster (1965), Garnham (1970), Hoeppli (1956, 1959), Warboys (1983) and Kean, Mott and Russell (1978). The most comprehensive work on the history of any aspect of parasitology, one that will be impossible to emulate, is 'A History of Human Helminthology' (Grove 1990), which contains over 800 pages of detailed accounts of all the discoveries in human helminthology and allied fields. 'The Wellcome Trust Illustrated History of Tropical Diseases' (Cox 1996) contains chapters on most of the important human parasitic infections but excludes some that are not specifically tropical, e.g. toxoplasmosis and cestodiasis. Foster's 'A History of Parasitology' (Foster 1965) covers some, but not all, important parasitic infections. In addition, there are a number of important monographs mainly relating to the associations between parasitic infections and human endeavour and welfare and these will be mentioned in the appropriate places.

In the history of parasitology, discoveries about the helminths and protozoa have tended to run in parallel paths which briefly converged at the turn of the century when one man, Patrick Manson, introduced the medical and veterinary world to the concept of vector-borne parasitic diseases. Helminth worms are large and easily recognizable and are common parasites of domesticated and wild animals. Thus they attracted the attention of zoologists who, schooled in the concepts of comparative zoology, treated parasites in the same way as any other group of animals and tended to ignore the fact that they also caused disease. However, veterinarians and clinicians were quick to note the implications of these infections and to draw parallels between parasitic infections in domesticated animals and humans and discoveries in the field of zoology. To this day, helminthology is usually regarded as a branch of zoology. Protozoa, being microscopic, had to await the development of the microscope before they were first recognized; the history of these parasites parallels that of other micro-organisms and has largely been the province of medicine rather than zoology. There is thus a dichotomy that is not always apparent in that the interest of most helminthologists has centred on the worms themselves and, to a lesser extent, the diseases they cause. In contrast, protozoologists have tended to focus predominantly on diseases. There are other obvious reasons for this dichotomy; for example the fact that helminths are multicellular organisms and can be examined outside their hosts has facilitated physiological and biochemical studies whereas isolating protozoa from their host cells has proved to be very difficult. These differences in approach have had a marked effect on our understanding and interpretation of the history of parasitology.

The history of parasitology embraces some of the most exciting discoveries ever made in medicine and these findings have had an impact well outside their immediate field. For example, the discovery of the vector-borne nature of the filarial worms influenced ideas about the transmission of malaria which, in turn, led to discovery of the mosquito-borne transmission of yellow fever; the whole field of arboviruses; and the implication of other vectors in trypanosomiasis, relapsing fever and plague. Similarly, the discovery that trypanosomes caused diseases in both animals and humans opened up a new field of zoonoses (infections common to animals and humans) and the study of reservoir hosts for a number of infections.

Remarkably, many of the great discoveries in parasitology were made over a relatively short period, in the 30 years between 1885 and 1915, a time when major advances were also being made concerning other infectious diseases. The great personalities of this period made discoveries in a number of fields and their findings and ideas fed off one another. The names of Pasteur, Koch, Bruce, Manson and Ross occur time and time again in the history of parasitology and microbiology.

The history of parasitic diseases can be considered as a number of phases; the recognition of the disease; the discovery of the organism involved; the connection between the organism and the disease; the consolidation of all these strands; and the application of this knowledge to control schemes.

So vast is the field of human parasitology, with its many and far-reaching discoveries, that it is not possible to do justice to the whole subject and in the rest of this chapter only the most significant aspects will be discussed. No attempt is made to discuss the parasites or the diseases they cause other than briefly and the reader is referred to other chapters in this volume to provide the necessary background information and details.

2 HELMINTHS AND HELMINTH INFECTIONS

2.1 Discovery of the organisms

Given the ubiquitous nature and large size of the helminth worms, it would be surprising if our earliest ancestors had not been aware of the more common types; evidence for this assumption comes from the fact that in primitive tribes in Sarawak and North Borneo most people are aware of their intestinal roundworms and tapeworms (Hoeppli 1959). Much has been made of quotations from the bible on this subject but these are often open to several interpretations; the only conclusion that can be safely drawn is that those who contributed to the bible were aware of the existence of parasitic worms (i.e. we cannot conclude that they possessed any detailed knowledge of the subject). With the first written records we are on firmer ground and the Egyptian medical papyrus, usually referred to as the 'Papyrus Ebers', dating from c. 1500 BC, refers to intestinal worms and these records are backed by the discovery of calcified helminth eggs in mummies dating from 1200 BC. The Greeks, Aristotle (384–322 BC) in particular, were familiar with a range of parasites from fishes, domesticated animals and humans. The writings of the Greek and Roman physicians, including Hippocrates (460–375 BC), Celsus (25 BC–AD 50) and Galen (AD 129–200), indicate that they were also familiar with the human roundworms, *Ascaris lumbricoides* and *Enterobius vermicularis,* and tapeworms belonging to the genus *Taenia.* In fact, the terms 'roundworm' (helmins strongyle) and 'ribbon worm' (helmins taenia) can be traced back to the earliest Greek records (Grove 1990). Paulus Aegineta (625–690) clearly described *Ascaris, Enterobius* and tapeworms and gave good clinical descriptions of the infections they caused. With the decline and fall of the Roman empire, the study of medicine switched to Arabic physicians. Avicenna (981–1037) recognized not only *Ascaris, Enterobius* and tapeworms but also the guinea worm, *Dracunculus medinensis;* by that time this worm been recorded in parts of the Arab world, particularly around the Red Sea, for over 1000 years.

The medical literature of the Middle Ages is very limited but the existence of parasitic worms was widely recorded and, in many cases, these were regarded as the causes of a number of diseases. Unfortunately, many of these 'worms' were fictitious as were the symptoms ascribed to their presence, for example toothache and heart attacks (Hoeppli 1959). On the other hand, the Chinese believed that humans should harbour at least 3 worms to be in good health and this

belief that worms were beneficial also extended into Europe (Foster 1965).

The history of helminthology really took off in the 17th and 18th centuries following the re-emergence of science and scholarship during the Renaissance. In his 'Systema Naturae', Linnaeus described 6 helminth worms: *A. lumbricoides, A. vermicularis* (= *Enterobius vermicularis*), *Gordius medinensis* (= *Dracunculus medinensis*), *Fasciola hepatica, Taenia solium* and *Taenia lata* (= *Diphyllobothrium latum*) (Linnaeus 1758). Thereafter there was a gradual accretion of new species; there were 9 species identified by 1782, with the addition of *Trichuris trichiura, Taenia saginata* and *Echinococcus granulosus.* This number remained virtually unchanged in various texts published between 1800 and 1819 but was subsequently extended by the inclusion of: *Trichinella spiralis* and *Loa loa* by 1845; *Ancylostoma duodenale, Schistosoma mansoni* and *Hymenolepis nana* by 1855; *Strongylus stercoralis, Wuchereria bancrofti, Clonorchis sinensis, Fasciolopsis buski, Paragonimus westermani, Heterophyes heterophyes, Schistosoma haematobium* and *Dipylidium caninum* between 1885 and 1890 (see Grove 1990).

By the beginning of the 20th century, 28 species had been recorded in humans, a number that has grown to over 80 today, of which c. 20 are common. Including accidental and very rare records, >340 species have been recorded in humans (Coombs and Crompton 1991). Now, at the end of the 20th century, the description of a new species of helminth worm in humans is a rare event. Nevertheless, advances in biochemistry and molecular biology are permitting the identification of minute but significant differences between parasites that are likely to lead to the creation of many more species and subspecies from within the current list.

Our understanding of parasitology could not progress until the theory of spontaneous generation had been disproved. Doubts had been raised about the validity of this concept in the 17th century but it still persisted until the definitive experiments of Pasteur at the end of the 19th century (see Vallery-Radot 1906). A number of helminthologists were among those who began to doubt the concept and they included Francisco Redi and Edward Tyson who, in the 17th century, went so far as to describe sexual reproduction in worms. It was Pasteur who indirectly enabled the study of helminthology to progress and also acted as a midwife for the birth of the new subject of protozoology.

2.2 *Ascaris* and ascariasis

Human infection with the large roundworm *Ascaris lumbricoides* is world wide with >250 million people infected. The presence of this worm, which is often voided in the faeces, is very obvious and its existence has been recorded from the following: Egyptian medical papyri of 1500 BC; the works of Hippocrates in the 5th century BC; Chinese writings of the 2nd and 3rd centuries BC; and the texts of Roman and Arabic physicians (see Grove 1990 and Goodwin 1996b). Eggs of

Ascaris have been detected in human remains from 800 BC. *Ascaris lumbricoides* is one of the 6 worms listed by Linnaeus (1758) and its name has remained unchanged ever since. The detailed anatomy of the worm was described by Tyson (1683) and Redi (1684) but the mode of infection by the ingestion of eggs was not established until nearly 200 years later (Grassi 1881) and the whole life-cycle, including the migration of the larval stages around the body, was elaborated only in 1922 (Koino 1922).

2.3 *Trichinella* and trichinosis

Trichinosis, also known as trichinellosis and trichina infection, is caused by the nematode worm *Trichinella spiralis* and is usually acquired by eating infected pork. Foster (1965) considers this to be one of the most interesting parasitic infections and more likely to be responsible for the Mosaic and Mohammedan traditions of avoiding pork than the possibility of tapeworm infection (see section 2.11). Although the association with pigs had been recognized since the earliest times, the encysted larvae in the muscle were not seen until 1822 and even then their presence was not associated with disease. The story of the association between the worm and human infection, described in full by Foster (1965) and Grove (1990) can only be summarized here. It revolves around the discovery of the worm in humans in 1835 by James Paget, a medical student at St Bartholomew's Hospital in London; this discovery led to intensive investigations by some of the world's most important parasitologists including Rudolf Leuckart, Rudolph Virchow, Thomas Cobbold, Richard Owen and Gottlob Küchenmeister. Although the discovery was made by Paget, much of the credit has been attributed to Owen who not only wrote the definitive report (Owen 1835) but also played down Paget's role. Owen and subsequent writers did not recognize the worm in human muscle as a larval stage although this had been suspected by French and German workers in the 1840s. The adult worm was discovered by Rudolph Virchow and Friedrich Zenker and it was the latter who finally recognized the clinical significance of the infection (see Grove 1990 and Bundy and Michael 1996).

2.4 Hookworms and hookworm infection

Human hookworm infections caused by *Ancylostoma duodenale* and *Necator americanus*, the former originating in Asia and the latter in Africa, have been associated with humans for over 5000 years (Hoeppli 1959). Hookworms reached America before the 5th century BC and larvae have been found in coprolites dating from this period (Ferreira, Araujo and Confalonieri 1980). Hookworm disease has been recognized since the earliest records began and the Egyptian papyrus of 1500 BC, the works of Hippocrates in the 5th century BC and Avicenna in the 10th century all give accurate descriptions of the disease; its history has been reviewed by Foster (1965) Grove (1990) and Ball (1996). Adult *A. duodenale* worms were first recognized by Angelo Dubini in 1843 (Dubini 1843) and credit for the discovery that humans become infected through the skin goes to Arthur Looss who accidentally infected himself (Looss 1898).

The major contributions made in the 20th century have been the determination of blood loss that causes the anaemia associated with the disease and the valiant efforts of the Rockefeller Foundation to control the disease. This activity led to the establishment of a number of Schools of Public Health and the creation of the World Health Organization (Ettling 1990).

2.5 Lymphatic filariasis

Lymphatic filariasis is caused by infection with the nematode worms *Wuchereria bancrofti*, *Brugia malayi* and *B. timori*, which are transmitted by mosquitoes. The discovery of the life-cycle by Patrick Manson in 1877 is widely regarded as the most significant discovery in tropical medicine with implications that reached far beyond helminthology into such diverse areas as malaria and the arboviruses. The massive swellings of the limbs associated with lymphatic filariasis cannot have gone unnoticed by our early ancestors and descriptions of what was almost certainly this disease date back to 2000 BC in Egypt and to Nok sculptures of the Sudan and West Africa from AD 500 (see Grove 1990, Nelson 1996). The larval stages of the filarial worms, microfilariae, were first seen in the blood of dogs in 1843 (Gruby and Delafond 1843) and in humans by Demarquay (1863). This latter discovery attracted the attention of a number of eminent parasitologists, including Wilhelm Greisinger, Theodor Bilharz and Otto Wucher, but it was a relatively unknown Scottish clinician, Timothy Lewis, who realized that the worms were associated with filariasis (Lewis 1872). The mode of transmission remained a mystery until Patrick Manson discovered that the mosquito was involved (Manson 1878).

The story of Manson's discoveries has been told many times (see Manson-Bahr 1962, Foster 1965, Service and Wilmott 1978, Chernin 1983, Grove 1990, Eldridge 1992, Nelson 1996). Manson, then working in Amoy in China, found microfilariae in the blood of dogs and humans; he hypothesized that these parasites in the blood might be transmitted by bloodsucking insects. Accordingly, he fed mosquitoes on the blood of his gardener, who was harbouring the parasites, and subsequently was able to detect larval stages in the mosquitoes (Manson 1878). Manson mistakenly believed that the parasite escaped from the mosquito into water and that human infections were acquired through contaminated material; the actual mode of transmission was not established until suggestions by the Australian parasitologist, Thomas Bancroft, were followed up by Manson's assistant George Carmichael Low (Low 1900). In a footnote to the history of parasitology, Manson founded the Royal Society of Tropical Medicine and Hygiene in London and the lecture theatre at the Society's premises, Manson House, is now named after Low.

2.6 *Onchocerca* and onchocerciasis

The history of onchocerciasis, or river blindness, caused by the nematode worm *Onchocerca volvulus* is a relatively short one and there are few reliable early records. This is partly because there are so many causes of blindness in the tropics with which this condition can be confused. Accounts of the history of onchocerciasis are given by Grove (1990) and Muller (1996b). The skin lesions associated with this infection were well known in West Africa and called 'craw craw' by the time John O'Neill first identified nematode parasites in the lesions of those suffering from this condition in 1875 (O'Neill 1875). Adult worms were not seen until some years later when Rudolf Leuckart received specimens from a German doctor in Ghana and sent them to Patrick Manson who, with due acknowledgements, described them in Davidson's 'Hygiene and Diseases of Warm Climates' (Manson 1893).

For a number of years, this parasite was considered to be a rare curiosity until the connection between the worm and the skin lesions was made by Rodolfo Robles in Central America in 1916 (Robles 1917). Robles was also the first person to incriminate black-flies in the transmission of the infection but the conclusive experiments were not carried out until 1923–1926 by Donald Breadalbane Blacklock (Blacklock 1926). The role of *Onchocerca* as a cause of blindness was recognized 2 years later (Ochoterena 1928). The 20th century has been one of triumph over this disease, first with the use of insecticides to control the blackfly larvae and later with the development and free distribution of a very effective drug, ivermectin.

2.7 Loiasis

Loa loa, the nematode that causes loiasis, is a large worm that occasionally passes through the eye and that must have been recognized from the earliest times. There are few early records but there is no doubt that Huighen van Linschoten became aware of this worm during the course of his researches into guinea worm at the end of the 16th century (van Linschoten 1610). The adult worm was first seen by a French surgeon, Mongin, in 1770 (Mongin 1770) and the microfilariae were seen in 1890 by Stephen Mackenzie who sought Patrick Manson's views on the subject (see Manson 1891). The mode of transmission remained a mystery until the work of Argyll-Robertson who, in 1895, predicted that the vector would be a blood-sucking insect. This idea was based on Manson's earlier work on lymphatic filariasis, but Argyll-Robertson failed to find any parasites in his suspected insect hosts. It was not until 1912 that Robert Leiper showed that the vectors were actually tabanid flies belonging to the genus *Chrysops* (Leiper 1913).

2.8 *Dracunculus* and dracunculiasis (Guinea worm disease)

Dracunculiasis, caused by the nematode *Dracunculus medinensis*, is the only parasitic infection of which a good description is given in the bible; most observers agree that the 'fiery serpents' that afflicted the children of Israel in the region of the Red Sea between 1300 and 1234 BC were dracunculus worms (The Bible Numbers 21 Verse 6, Foster 1965). There are also numerous records of this worm in second millennium papyri from Egypt; writings from Mesopotamia in the 7th century BC; and later records by Greek, Roman and Arabic physicians (see Grove 1990, Tayeh 1996). One of the best descriptions is that by Avicenna in his book 'Al Canon fe al Tib'. Avicenna recognized that this was a worm and not a rotten vein as had previously been maintained (hence the old name 'Medina vein'). The Dutch navigator Huighen van Linschoten recorded that the mode of transmission was through drinking water (van Linschoten 1610). The presence of the worm in the leg was recognized by Thomas Herbert as long ago as 1643 (Herbert 1643). Throughout the 18th and early 19th centuries the conviction strengthened that dracunculiasis was caused by the worm *Dracunculus medinensis* (listed as *Gordius medinensis* by Linnaeus in 1758) and that infection was acquired through drinking water. George Busk (Busk 1846) and H. J. Carter (Carter 1855) argued that the infection could be acquired through the skin. The actual life-cycle was unravelled by a Russian scientist, Aleksej Fedchenko, who suspected that water fleas, *Cyclops*, were involved and that infection was acquired by accidentally consuming these invertebrates. He was, however, unable to induce infections in experimental animals by feeding them infected water fleas (Fedchenko 1870). It was not until 1905 that Robert Leiper demonstrated that *Dracunculus* larvae could survive in digestive juices (Leiper 1906) and the whole life-cycle was finally elaborated by Dyneshvar Turkhud in 1913 (Turkhud 1914). The 20th century has been one of considerable success in controlling this infection which is on course to be eradicated by the end of the century.

2.9 Schistosomes and schistosomiasis

Human schistosomiasis, or bilharzia, affects between 200 and 300 million people and is caused by several species of *Schistosoma* each giving rise to a characteristic form of the disease. The most obvious sign of urinary schistosomiasis, caused by *S. haematobium*, is blood in the urine; this attracted the attention of the ancient Egyptians who described the disease as 'a-a-a' disease and recorded it in over 50 early papyri, including the Papyrus Ebers. Calcified eggs have been found in Egyptian mummies dating from 1250 to 1000 BC (Contis and David 1996). The *S. haematobium* worm was first described by Theodor Bilharz in 1851 and the popular name for all forms of schistosomiasis is now 'bilharzia' in honour of his discovery (Bilharz and von Siebold 1852–53).

The search for the intermediate stages in the life-cycle of this parasite took a long time. Although it was known that other flukes employed a snail vector, a number of experienced parasitologists working at the end of the 19th century, including Arthur Looss, Prospero Sonsino and Thomas Cobbold, all failed to infect snails with this parasite. It was not until 1915 that Robert Leiper demonstrated the complete life-cycle in the snail host (Leiper 1916).

In contrast to urinary schistosomiasis, our knowledge of the history of intestinal schistosomiasis, caused by *S. mansoni*, is of relatively recent origin; it dates back to conclusions reached by Patrick Manson in 1902 (Manson 1902) that there were 2 species of *Schistosoma* in humans although there had been suggestions that this was the case earlier in the previous century. Manson's ideas were not universally accepted and it was Leiper who firmly established the existence of *S. mansoni* as a separate species in 1915 (Leiper 1916). The third important form of schistosomiasis, Katayama disease, caused by *S. japonicum*, was first recognized by a Japanese parasitologist, Akira Fujinami, in 1847 in a report that did not become available until 1909 (Fujinami and Nakamura 1909 cited by Warren 1973). Although schistosome eggs have been found in bodies buried in Japan over 200 years ago, the worm itself was discovered by Fujiro Katsurada only in 1904 (Katsurada 1904). Development in the snail host was described by Miyairi and Suzuki in 1913, 2 years before Leiper independently described the life-cycle of *S. haematobium*.

The history of such an important disease as schistosomiasis involves a great number of observations, events and individuals and a detailed account of the history is given by Grove (1990). There are shorter accounts by Hoeppli (1959), Foster (1965) and Goodwin (1996a). A full bibliography is given by Warren (1973) and an account of schistosomiasis in the context of British and American imperialism is given by Farley (1991).

The 20th century has been largely concerned with the discovery of further species of schistosomes, *S. intercalatum* and *S. mekongi*, and the development of control measures including effective drugs, particularly praziquantel. Detailed studies of the immunology and immunopathology of schistosomiasis are now providing hope of a vaccine against this important complex of diseases.

2.10 Liver and lung flukes

Several flatworms or flukes infect humans, the most important of which are *Paragonimus westermani*, causing paragonimiasis, *Clonorchis sinensis*, causing clonorchiasis, and *Opisthorchis* spp. causing opisthorchiasis. Virtually all the important discoveries about the parasites themselves were made over a period of less than 45 years, between 1874 and 1918, and all were based on observations that had been made on other parasitic flukes such as *Fasciola hepatica* in sheep and others of zoological rather than medical interest. The various discoveries were made by a large number of people

and often reported in obscure publications and no attempt will be made here to list the individual achievements; for this the reader is referred to Grove (1990) and Muller (1996a).

The histories of these infections as diseases begin with the discovery of the worms and continue with the elaboration of the various life-cycles. *Paragonimus westermani* was discovered in the lungs of a human by Ringer in 1879 and the presence of eggs in the sputum was recognized independently by Manson and Erwin von Baelz in 1880 (see Manson 1881). Manson, in 1881, also postulated that a snail might act as an intermediate host and a number of Japanese workers, including Koan Nakagawa, Sadamu Yokogawa, Harujiro Kobayashi and Keinosuke Miyairi, reported on the whole life-cycle in the snail *Semisulcospira* between 1916 and 1922 (see Grove 1990).

The human liver fluke, *Clonorchis sinensis*, was first recognized by James McConnell in 1875 and the snail host by Masatomo Muto in 1918. It was the discovery in 1915 by Kobayashi of a second intermediate host, an important food fish from which human infections are acquired, that had the greatest impact on the control of this infection.

The first records of *Opisthorchis* in humans were made by Konstantin Wingradoff in 1892 and the snail and fish hosts were described by Hans Vogel in 1934.

2.11 Cestodes and cestodiasis

Humans harbour a number of tapeworm infections, of which the most important are the adults of *Diphyllobothrium latum* (the broad tapeworm), *Taenia solium* (the pork tapeworm) and *T. saginata* (the beef tapeworm) and the larval stages of the dog tapeworm, *Echinococcus granulosus*. The large size of these adult worms and their common occurrence attracted the attention of all the major medical writers including the authors of the Papyrus Ebers, Hippocrates, Celsus and Avicenna. By the beginning of the 17th century it was realized that there were 2 different kinds of tapeworm (broad and taeniid) in humans (see Grove 1990).

It is generally held that the broad tapeworm *D. latum* was first recognized by Felix Platter at the beginning of 17th the century (see Foster 1965, Grove 1990). By the middle of the 18th century it was apparent that those harbouring *D. latum* were those whose diet was mainly fish, but it was not until the life-cycles of other tapeworms of zoological interest had been elaborated that further progress became possible. The existence of 3 hosts in the life-cycle of *D. latum* (human, fish and copepod) confused the issue and it was not until 1917 that Janicki and Rosen independently worked out the whole of the life-cycle (Janicki and Rosen 1917). Platter had already provided an excellent description of the disease and the only significant subsequent discovery was made in 1948 when it was realized that this worm has an affinity for vitamin B_{12} thus accounting for the pernicious anaemia associated with this infection (see von Bonsdorff

1977). The history of diphyllobothriasis is reviewed in detail by Grove (1990).

The scientific study of the taeniid tapeworms can be traced to the work of Edward Tyson who, in the late 17th century, studied not only the tapeworms of humans but also those of dogs and other animals. This gave him the opportunity to recognize the 'head' (scolex) of a tapeworm for the first time; to describe the anatomy and physiology of the adult worms (Tyson 1683); and to lay the foundations for our knowledge of the biology of the taeniid tapeworms of humans. The existence of 2 species of *Taenia* in humans presented problems because, even to the trained eye, the distinctions between *T. solium* and *T. saginata* are not obvious. This led to confusion between the 2 worms until a century after the work of Tyson when, in 1782, Johann Goeze noted the similarities between the heads of tapeworms in humans and pigs (Goeze 1782). The presence of cysts in pork had been noted throughout recorded history and is mentioned by Aristotle in the 4th century BC, Hippocrates and Galen (see Foster 1965 and Groves 1990). It was not until 1855 that Gottlob Küchenmeister demonstrated experimentally that eating infected pork gave rise to tapeworms in humans (see Grove 1990).

The history of *T. saginata* parallels that of *T. solium,* scientists such as Goeze and Küchenmeister being credited with recognising the differences between the 2 species of *Taenia* in humans. In 1868–9, Oliver noted tapeworm infections in individuals who had eaten 'measly' beef (Oliver 1871) and this was confirmed in a more controlled experiment by Perroncito in 1877. Together with observations on the pork tapeworm, these discoveries had a massive impact on the control of tapeworm infections in humans, as they led to restriction of the amount of infected meat consumed by humans.

Humans are also host to 2 important kinds of larval tapeworm, cysticerci of the pork tapeworm *T. solium* and hydatid cysts of the dog tapeworm *E. granulosus.* The demonstration of the life-cycle of *T. solium* threw new light on the nature of cysticercosis and it was soon apparent that humans could become infected with the larval stages of *T. solium* when they ingested eggs. This made humans, in effect, dead-end intermediate hosts for this parasite that also used humans as its definitive hosts. Although, for ethical reasons, the conclusive experiments could not be carried out, by the middle of the 19th century various experiments with animals and observations on humans had established without doubt that cysticercosis was caused by the ingestion of the eggs of *T. solium* (Küchenmeister 1860).

Infections with the larval stages of the dog tapeworm *E. granulosus* cause hydatid disease in humans and these cysts have been recognized from the earliest times and there are accurate descriptions by Hippocrates and Galen, among others (see Grove 1990). It was not until the 17th century that Francesco Redi recognized the parasitic nature of these cysts (in 1684) and in 1853 Carl von Siebold demonstrated that echinococcus cysts from sheep gave rise to adult tapeworms when fed to dogs (von Siebold 1853).

The whole story was completed in 1863 when Bernhard Naunyn found adult tapeworms in dogs fed with hydatid cysts from a human (Naunyn 1863).

In the 20th century a number of other accidental infections of humans with a variety of tapeworm larvae have been recorded (see Coombs and Crompton 1991) and the main advances have been concerned with preventive measures and the development of effective drugs.

3 PROTOZOA AND PROTOZOAL INFECTIONS

3.1 Discovery of the organisms

Because of their small size, it was not possible to see protozoa until the invention of the microscope; it was not until Antony van Leeuwenhoek's observations towards the end of the 17th century (Dobell 1960) that they were recognized at all and they were only recognized as a phylum of the Animal kingdom a century later (Müller 1786). Protozoology as a discipline in its own right emerged from the discovery of bacteria and the birth of the germ theory, promulgated by Pasteur and his colleagues at the end of the last century. Protozoa have seldom been classified with the other micro-organisms where they naturally belong; they have long been the province of zoologists who have tended to regard them as a particularly interesting subdivision of the Animal kingdom. This attitude is rapidly changing. Advances in elucidating the morphological characteristics of these organisms began with the elaboration of the cell theory in 1839, a process that is still going on today. Current research in traditional protozoology includes attempts to derive natural phylogenetic trees from a very heterogeneous group of organisms and the use of biochemical and molecular markers to classify particular organisms.

All commentators agree that the first person to see a parasitic protozoan was Leeuwenhoek, who observed *Giardia* in his own stools. His written descriptions and his clinical observations leave little doubt that this flagellate is indeed the organism that he saw (Dobell 1960). Any doubt must be dispelled by the fact that Leeuwenhoek was an accurate observer, as testified by his unambiguous descriptions of protozoan parasites of frogs. Curiously, it was not until over 140 years later that other parasitic protozoa were described and these were the large and conspicuous gregarines of insects (Dufour 1828), the beloved introduction to parasitic protozoology of generations of parasitologists. Among the conspicuous parasites in the blood are the trypanosomes and the first to be recognized was from the blood of a fish (Valentin 1841); it is interesting to note that it was more than 50 years before similar parasites were seen in humans. The first associations between blood parasites and disease were those recorded by Griffiths Evans, who found trypanosomes in the blood of horses suffering from surra (Evans

1881). David Bruce found similar organisms in cattle suffering from nagana in 1895 (see Bruce 1915). Amoebae are also conspicuous protozoa and those in humans were first seen in 1849 by Gros who recognized the non-pathogenic *Entamoeba gingivalis* from the mouth (see Dobell 1919); the pathogenic *E. histolytica* was recognized for the first time by Alexandrovitch Lösch in 1875 (Lösch 1875).

The detection of protozoa living in red blood cells was not possible until the development of adequate staining techniques; the first to be seen were malaria parasites by Charles Laveran in 1880; *Babesia* in cattle by Smith and Kilbourne in 1893 (Smith and Kilbourne 1893); and *Theileria* in cattle by Koch in 1989 (see Koch 1903).

Leishmania parasites were discovered independently by P.F. Borovsky in 1898, William Leishman in 1903, Charles Donovan in 1903 and James Homer Wright in 1903. The first leishmania parasites associated with New World leishmaniasis were discovered by Gaspar Vianna in 1911.

The remaining important protozoan parasites of humans were not detected until the beginning of this century when, in a flurry of activity, *Trypanosoma cruzi* was identified as the cause of the condition that is now called Chagas disease (Chagas 1909). In a remarkable discovery that was to have much wider implications, *Toxoplasma gondii*, a parasite with the widest known host range including humans, was found in an obscure mammal, the gundi, by Charles Nicolle and Louis Manceaux in 1909.

3.2 Amoebae and amoebiasis

Humans harbour 5 or 6 species of amoebae of which only one, *E. histolytica*, is a pathogen. *E. histolytica* causes 2 forms of the same disease: amoebic dysentery, resulting from the invasion of the gut wall; and hepatic amoebiasis caused by extra-intestinal amoebae in the liver. There is circumstantial evidence that both forms of the disease were recognized from the earliest times but there are so many causes of both dysentery and liver disease that these records are open to other interpretations (see Bray 1996). The history of amoebiasis has been described by Dobell (1919), Foster (1965) and Bray (1996). James Annersley (1828) is credited with the first accurate descriptions of both forms of the disease and was the first to suggest the connection between them. From the middle of the 19th century, several workers observed amoebae in the stools of patients with amoebic dysentery but credit for the discovery of *E. histolytica* is now given to Alexandrovitch Lösch (Lösch 1875). The association between the amoeba and liver abscesses was finally determined shortly afterwards when Kartulis demonstrated amoebae in both the intestine and liver (Kartulis 1886). Many workers did not believe that *E. histolytica* could cause disease, as this species was generally thought to be harmless. It was therefore suggested that humans might harbour 2 morphologically similar amoebae, one pathogenic and one not (see Dobell 1919). This situation was only resolved much later using biochemi-

cal techniques that clearly show that there are indeed 2 species; *E. histolytica*, that can cause disease, and *E. dispar* that cannot (see Chapter 8).

3.3 *Giardia* and giardiasis

Giardia holds a special place in the affection of all protozoologists because the parasite that causes giardiasis, *Giardia lamblia* (also known as *G. intestinalis* or *G. duodenalis*) was the first parasitic protozoan ever to be seen (see p. 9). An account of the history of giardiasis is given by Farthing (1996).

The first good illustrations of *Giardia* were those of Vilém Lambl in 1859 but the parasite received very little attention until the second world war; returning troops with diarrhoea were found to have *Giardia* parasites in their faeces, the cysts of which caused similar disease in laboratory animals (Fantham and Porter 1916). In 1921 the distinguished British protozoologist, Clifford Dobell, suggested that *Giardia* could be a serious pathogen (Dobell 1921). It was another 30 years before this fact became widely recognized, when the detailed studies of Robert Rendtorff produced unambiguous evidence linking the parasite with the disease (Rendtorff 1954).

In the 300 years since *Giardia* was first discovered it has become recognized as a common and serious pathogen world wide. It is still not known how many species infect humans and what role, if any, is played by reservoir hosts in the epidemiology of the infection.

3.4 African trypanosomes and sleeping sickness

The story of African sleeping sickness is told briefly by Hoare (1972) and in more detail by Foster (1965), Nash (1969), Lyons (1992) and Williams (1996). The early records of African trypanosomiasis or sleeping sickness are vague and the first definitive accounts are those given by an English naval surgeon, John Atkins, in 1721 (see Atkins 1734) and Thomas Winterbottom, who coined the term 'negro lethargy', in 1803 (Winterbottom 1803). Many explanations were put forward as causes of sleeping sickness but the real basis of the disease was not forthcoming until Pasteur had established the germ theory towards the end of the 19th century. The first clues came from observations on the horse disease, surra, and the cattle disease, nagana. Although trypanosomes had been seen in the blood of fishes, frogs and mammals several years before, it was not until 1881 that Griffith Evans found trypanosomes in the blood of horses and camels suffering from surra and suggested that the parasites might be the cause of the condition (Evans 1881).

In 1894, David Bruce, a British army surgeon, was sent to Zululand to investigate an outbreak of nagana in cattle (a century ago the demarcation between the appropriate subject matter for medical, veterinary or scientific investigation was not as rigid as it is today). Given the scientific climate of the period, Bruce suspected a bacterial cause but instead found trypanosomes in the blood of diseased cattle; he later demonstrated that these caused nagana in cattle, horses and dogs. Bruce also noticed that infected cattle had spent some time in the fly-infested 'tsetse belt' and that the disease was similar to that in humans suffering from 'negro lethargy' and the 'fly disease' of hunters (see Bruce 1915). Using this information, Bruce soon showed that the infection was acquired from tsetse flies, but he mistakenly thought that transmission was purely mechanical.

It was later discovered that the trypanosomes that cause nagana and surra are not the same as those that cause human sleeping sickness. Although organisms that were certainly trypanosomes had been seen in human blood by Gustave Nepveu in 1891 (see Nepveu 1898), it was not until 1902 that Everett Dutton found the trypanosome that causes Gambian or chronic sleeping sickness (*Trypanosoma brucei gambiense*) in humans (Dutton 1902). In 1910 *T. b. rhodesiense*, the cause of Rhodesian or acute sleeping sickness, was described by J.W.W Stephens and Harold Fantham (Stephens and Fantham 1910). The role of the tsetse fly in the transmission of sleeping sickness remained controversial until Friedrich Kleine, a colleague of Robert Koch, demonstrated cyclical transmission, but he mistakenly thought that there was a sexual stage in the life-cycle (Kleine 1909).

The persistence of trypanosomes in the blood and the existence of successive waves of parasitaemia have attracted the attention of all those who have worked with trypanosomiasis. This phenomenon was described in detail by Ronald Ross and D. Thompson in 1911 (Ross and Thompson 1911). The underlying mechanism and the way in which the parasite evades the immune response, now called 'antigenic variation', were not elaborated until the work of Keith Vickerman in 1969 (Vickerman and Luckins 1969); this discovery precipitated a vast amount of interest in trypanosomes as cells and not only as causes of disease. Other 20th century investigations have been concerned with refining the early discoveries and establishing the epidemiology of African sleeping sickness, leading to the development of methods for the control of both the human and animal forms of trypanosomiasis and the development of new and effective drugs. Trypanosomes have also become firm favourites for molecular biologists working on a number of biochemical and genetic problems unrelated to parasitic diseases.

3.5 South American trypanosomiasis: Chagas disease

The earliest records of Chagas disease in South America are from 2000-year-old mummies that show clear signs of the destructive nature of the disease. There are also a number of early written records but the signs and symptoms of Chagas disease are so vague that it is difficult to know whether or not many of the conditions attributed to this infection are really valid. The early history of Chagas disease is described by Guerra (1970) and Miles (1996) and is passed over here because, from a scientific and medical viewpoint,

the history really begins with a remarkable series of discoveries that were made between 1907 and 1912 by Carlos Chagas. Chagas not only discovered the trypanosome that causes the disease but also demonstrated its life-cycle in the bugs that transmit it and described the disease which, although it affected millions of people, had until then remained enigmatic. Chagas's discoveries have been extensively described elsewhere (Scott 1939, Guerra 1970, Lewinsohn 1979, Kean, Mott and Russell 1978, Leonard 1990, Miles 1996). Briefly, Chagas, who was then in charge of an anti-malaria campaign in Brazil, noticed that the bugs that infested the poorly constructed houses harboured flagellated protozoa; these could experimentally infect monkeys and guinea pigs, in the blood of which a new trypanosome, *Trypanosoma cruzi*, was subsequently detected (Chagas 1909). Chagas suspected that these bugs might also transmit the parasite to humans and found the trypanosomes in the blood of children suffering from an acute febrile condition (Chagas 1911). In addition, in 1912, Chagas demonstrated that *T. cruzi* was maintained in a number of reservoir hosts (Chagas 1912) thus completing in less than 5 years a cycle of discovery that had taken many years for earlier workers in other fields. The disease that affects some 18 million people now commemorates his name.

The one thing that Chagas did not get right was the actual mode of transmission by the bug as he thought that the trypanosomes were transmitted via the bite of the insect; it was left to Emile Brumpt to demonstrate that transmission was via the faecal route (Brumpt 1912). The links between infection with *T. cruzi* and the various signs of Chagas disease, such as megacolon, megaoesophagus and cardiac failure, were not determined until the work of Fritz Koberle in the 1960s (Koberle 1968). Exactly how the damage to heart and nerves is caused and whether or not there is an autoimmune component are still controversial issues.

3.6 *Leishmania* and leishmaniasis

Leishmaniasis, caused by several species of *Leishmania*, is transmitted by sandflies and occurs in various forms in both the Old World and New World. Human leishmaniasis was, and still is in some cases, acquired accidentally from naturally infected wild animals; the conspicuous lesions have been the subject of numerous records dating back to 2500–1000 BC (see Manson-Bahr 1996). Detailed descriptions of the Old World forms are given by the Arab physicians including Avicenna in the 10th century and missionaries were well aware of this disease in the New World in the 16th century (see Lainson 1996).

The history of Old World leishmaniasis is described by Hoare (1938), Garnham (1987) and Manson-Bahr (1996). The discovery of the parasite responsible for the Old World cutaneous disease has been a matter of some controversy and credit for its discovery is usually given to an American, James Homer Wright (Wright 1903). There is no doubt that the organism was actually seen nearly 20 years previously in 1885 by

David Cunningham and in 1898 by a Russian military surgeon, P.F. Borovsky (Borovsky 1898). Credit for the discovery of *Leishmania donovani*, the parasite that causes visceral leishmaniasis (kala azar) goes to William Leishman and Charles Donovan who independently discovered the parasite in the tissues of patients suffering from this condition (Leishman 1903, Donovan 1903). Borovsky's discoveries were unknown to Wright and to Leishman and Donovan but the names of the 2 latter workers are commemorated in the popular designation of the intracellular parasites as Leishman-Donovan bodies.

The search for a vector was a long one partly because of the small size of the sandfly vectors. Although enough epidemiological evidence to incriminate sandflies belonging to the genus *Phlebotomus* had accumulated by the mid 1910s, it was not until 1921 that the experimental proof of transmission to humans from a sandfly was demonstrated by the Sergent brothers, Edouard and Etienne (Sergent *et al.* 1921). Infection through the bite of a sandfly was not finally demonstrated until 1941 (Adler and Ber 1941).

Leishmaniasis also occurs in the New World and the disfiguring conditions caused have been recognized in sculptures since the 5th century and in the writings of the Spanish missionaries in the 16th century (see Lainson 1996). Until 1911, it was thought that the New World forms of leishmaniasis were the same as in the Old World but in that year Gaspar Vianna found that the parasites in South America differed from those in Africa and India and created a new species, *Leishmania braziliensis* (Vianna 1911). Since then a number of other species unique to the New World have been found (see Chapter 13). There is some controversy about the status of New World visceral leishmaniasis which was once thought to be caused by *L. donovani*, a species imported from the Old World possibly with the Spanish military and missionaries. Since 1937 it has been regarded as a separate species, *L. chagasi*, named in honour of the great Brazilian parasitologist, Carlos Chagas, and the validity of this species has since been confirmed by biochemical and molecular studies (see Chapter 13).

Following the discovery of the sandfly transmission of Old World leishmaniasis, the vectors in the Old World were also thought to belong to the same genus, *Phlebotomus*, but in 1922 it was discovered that the genus involved was actually *Lutzomyia*. Over the last 2 decades the complex pattern of species of parasite, vector, reservoir host and disease has been painstakingly elaborated by Ralph Lainson and his colleagues (Lainson 1996).

Fig. 1.1 (a) Sir Patrick Manson (1844–1922) the Scottish physician who is universally regarded as the 'father of tropical Medicine' and who spent his early years working in China. In 1877 he discovered that filarial worms were transmitted by mosquitoes and thus opened up the whole field of vector-borne diseases. In 1894 he initiated the successful search for the mosquito vector of malaria and was the inspiration behind Ross's discoveries of the life-cycle of the malaria parasite. He also made a number of other discoveries, including the identification the eggs of *Paragonimus westermani* in sputum, and was influential in the discoveries of the larval and adult stages of *Loa loa* and the larval stages of *Onchocerca volvulus*. Manson helped to found, and was the first Dean of, the Medical School of what is now the University of Hong Kong. He also founded the Royal Society of Tropical Medicine and Hygiene in London. He received the Nobel Prize for Medicine in 1902. (Reproduced by kind permission of the Royal Society of Tropical Medicine and Hygiene). (b) Francesco Redi (1626–1697) the Italian physician who began to destroy the theory of spontaneous generation by demonstrating that flies did not arise *de novo* from rotting meat. His main parasitological contributions were detailed studies of *Ascaris lumbricoides* and recognition of the parasitic nature of *Echinococcus* cysts. (From *Parasitology* **13**, 1921 and reproduced by kind permission of Cambridge University Press). (c) Arthur Looss (1861–1923) the influential German parasitologist, who worked for much of his life in Egypt. He discovered that hookworm infections occurred through the skin when he accidentally infected himself and made a number of other important contributions to helminthology (From *Parasitology*, **16**, 1924 and reproduced by kind permission of Cambridge University Press). (d) Carl Georg Friedrich Rudolf Leuckart (1822–1898) the German physician and zoologist who made a number of important contributions to both invertebrate biology and helminthology, including the discovery that *Paragonimus* in humans and animals was the same and elucidation of the life-cycle of *Trichinella spiralis*. He was also instrumental in passing on the first specimens of *Onchocerca* to Manson. (From *Parasitology*, **14**, 1922 and reproduced by kind permission of Cambridge University Press). (e) Robert Thomas Leiper (1881–1969) the Scottish physician and helminthologist who made numerous contributions to parasitology including the discovery that *Dracunculus* larvae could survive in gastric juices, that tabanid flies were the vectors of loiasis and that *Schistosoma mansoni* was a separate species in 1905. He also determined the life-cycle of *Schistosoma haematobium* in its snail host in 1916. (Reproduced by kind permission of the London School of Hygiene and Tropical Medicine). (f) Theodor Bilharz (1825–1862) the German physician who first described the worm *Schistosoma haematobium* in 1851 and whose memory is commemorated in the common name for schistosomiasis, bilharzia. (From *Parasitology*, **16**, 1924 and reproduced by kind permission of Cambridge University Press). (g) Carl Theodor von Siebold (1804–1885) the German physician who was involved, with Theodor Bilharz, in the discovery of the schistosome worm and whose major discovery (in 1853) was that echinococcus cysts in sheep developed into adult tapeworms in their definitive hosts. (From *Parasitology*, **14**, 1922 and reproduced by kind permission of Cambridge University Press). (h) Vilém Lambl (1824–1895) the Czech pathologist who made a number of contributions to anatomy, pathology and gynaecology but only published 2 papers on parasitology, one of which contained the first detailed description of *Giardia*. (From *Parasitology*, **32**, 1940 and reproduced by kind permission of Cambridge University Press). (i) Sir David Bruce (1855–1931) the Scottish army surgeon who found trypanosomes in cattle suffering from nagana; realised that trypanosomes caused human sleeping sickness; and incriminated the tsetse fly in the transmission of these diseases. (Reproduced by kind permission of the Royal Society of Tropical Medicine and Hygiene).

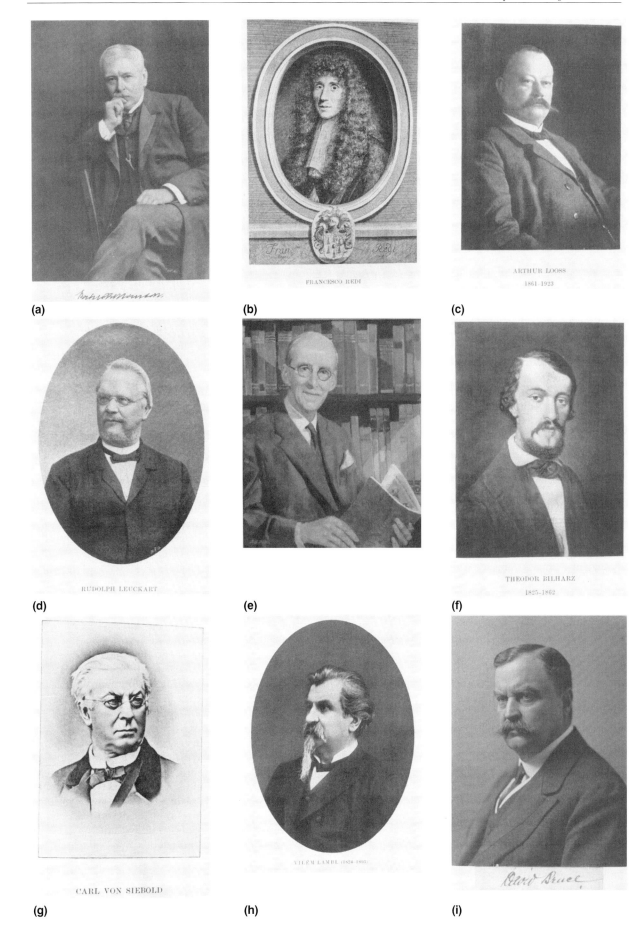

(a)

(b)

FRANCESCO REDI

(c)

ARTHUR LOOSS
1861–1923

(d)

RUDOLPH LEUCKART

(e)

(f)

THEODOR BILHARZ
1825–1862

(g)

CARL VON SIEBOLD

(h)

VILÉM LAMBL (1824–1895)

(i)

3.7 Malaria

Malaria ranks among the most important infectious diseases in the world. Its history extends into antiquity and has been reviewed many times by, for example, Garnham (1966), Harrison (1978), Bruce-Chwatt (1985, 1988) and McGregor (1996). Malaria almost certainly evolved with humans during our development from our primate ancestors; similar parasites are common in monkeys and apes. The disease probably originated in Africa and spread with human migrations, first throughout the tropics, subtropics and temperate regions of the Old World and then to the New World with explorers, missionaries and slaves. The periodic fevers of malaria are characteristic and are mentioned in the records of every civilized society from China in 2700 BC, through the writings of Greek, Roman, Assyrian, Indian, Arabic and European physicians up to the 19th century. The earliest detailed accounts are those of Hippocrates in the 5th century BC and for the next 700 years much of what we know about malaria relates to the disease in Greece, Italy and throughout the Roman Empire. Thereafter, references to malaria become commonplace in Europe and elsewhere.

The science of malariology could not take off until the end of the 19th century, with the establishment of the germ theory and the birth of microbiology; a start was then made in earnest to discover the cause of the disease that was threatening many parts of the European empires. The story of the discovery of the malaria parasite and its mode of transmission is one of the most exciting in the history of infectious diseases and, like all good stories, is full of triumphs, disappointments and rivalries (see McGregor 1996).

In 1880, a French army surgeon, Charles Laveran, looking for a bacterial cause of malaria, found and described malarial parasites in human blood and the parasite was immediately causally linked with the disease (Laveran 1880). The mode of transmission was not at all clear and numerous suggestions were put forward, none of which stood up to any detailed analysis. The actual incrimination of the mosquito as a vector was largely due to the intuition of one man, Patrick Manson. In 1877, Manson had demonstrated the mosquito transmission of lymphatic filariasis and Bruce, in 1894, had implicated tsetse flies in the transmission of African trypanosomiasis. Thus, it was evident to Manson that a vector might be involved in the transmission of malaria and he postulated that it could be a mosquito (Manson 1894). Manson, however, was unable to undertake this investigation himself and secured the services of Ronald Ross, an army surgeon working in India. After several false starts using the wrong kinds of mosquito, *Culex* and *Aedes* instead of *Anopheles*, Ross found developing parasites in a mosquito fed on the blood of a patient suffering from malaria (Ross 1897). The rest of the life-cycle in the mosquito was worked out by the Italian scientists Amico Bignami, Battista Grassi and Giovanni Bastianelli a few years later (Bastianelli and Bignami 1900). The life-cycle in humans, however, remained incom-

pletely understood and nobody knew where the parasites developed during the first 10 days after infection, as they could not be found in the blood. In part this was due to too much reliance on a mistake by the influential German scientist Fritz Schaudinn who in 1903 described the direct penetration of red blood cells by the infective sporozoites injected by the mosquito. The question was not resolved until 1947 when Henry Shortt and Cecil Garnham, working in London, showed that a phase of division in the liver preceded the development of parasites in the blood (Shortt and Garnham 1948); thus the whole life-cycle had taken over 50 years to elucidate.

The last 50 years have been dominated by the control of the malaria parasite and its vectors by drugs and insecticides and the search for a vaccine. For a fascinating and amusing insight into the problems, solutions, intrigues and personalities involved the reader is referred to the popular book 'The Malaria Capers' by Robert Desowitz (Desowitz 1991).

3.8 *Toxoplasma*, toxoplasmosis and infections caused by related organisms

The history of toxoplasmosis is a relatively recent one despite the fact that the organism that causes the disease, *Toxoplasma gondii*, is the most common human parasite world wide and one that infects the widest range of hosts (see Chapter 16). The history of toxoplasmosis has largely escaped the attention of the major reference books but the basic events are well covered by Dubey and Beattie (1988) and Moulin (1993). *T. gondii* was discovered, largely by accident, by Charles Nicolle while searching for a reservoir host of *Leishmania* in a North African rodent, *Ctenodactylus gondi* (Nicolle and Manceaux 1909). At about the same time, Alfonso Splendore, working in Sao Paulo, discovered the same parasite in rabbits (Splendore 1909) and subsequently there have been numerous records from mammals and birds both in the wild and in captivity. The association with human disease was not made until 1937 when Wolf and Cowen reported on a congenital infection (Wolf and Cowen 1937). This report stimulated a vast amount of research, quickly leading to the knowledge that *T. gondii* is actually a very common parasite of humans but rarely causes disease and that the parasite can cross the placenta and damage the foetus. The life-cycle of *T. gondii* remained elusive until 1970 when William Hutchison and his colleagues demonstrated that this parasite is a stage in the life-cycle of a common intestinal coccidian of cats (Hutchison et al. 1970) an observation quickly confirmed by other workers. The parasitological significance of this discovery was that until then it had been assumed that the intestinal coccidians of vertebrates had only one host. The discovery of the *T. gondii* life-cycle initiated a massive search for similar phases in the life-cycles of other coccidian parasites. As a result, a number of protozoa that had not been properly identified could be classified as stages in the life-cycle of other poorly understood coccidians; in many cases transmission depended on a predator-prey relationship (see Chapter 17). Toxoplasmosis subsequently took on a new significance as a serious concomitant of HIV infections.

3.9 Other important protozoa

A number of other important protozoan parasites of humans have come to light over the past few years including *Cryptosporidium parvum*, *Cyclospora cayetanensis* and several species of microsporidians, mainly as concomitant infections with HIV; it is likely that other new species will follow. It is too early to discuss the history of these parasites and the infections they cause and the salient points are covered in the appropriate chapters elsewhere in this volume.

4 SUMMARY AND CONCLUSIONS

The history of parasitology is a fascinating one and parasites have been the subject of some of the most exciting discoveries in the field of medicine. In this chapter, it has not been possible to do more than merely touch on the major events, each one of which has represented the culmination of years of observation, conjecture and experimentation. The personalities involved were among the most eminent of their generations but the cooperation and competition that existed between them would require a book on its own. The history of parasitology to a large extent reflects the availability of new concepts and techniques; thus each discovery has been the product of its own time and has been possible only because particular individuals have been willing and able to exploit new knowledge as it became accessible. There is more to the history of parasitology than this because most of the great discoveries were made by individuals who were not looking in the same direction as everybody else. The conviction that diseases arose from decay and the air we breathe held back the discovery of the microbial causes of diseases despite the fact that, with hindsight, all the clues were there. Had the helminthologists been able to persuade others not only

that worms do not arise *de novo,* but also that they cause disease, then the germ theory would have emerged 2 centuries earlier. The germ theory, with its emphasis on the search for bacterial causes of disease, held back the discovery of the protozoal causes of disease; in another context, it also inhibited a logical approach to nutritional disorders. Those who broke through the barriers of preconceived ideas, no matter how fashionable, were the ones who made the greatest discoveries. The history of 20th century medicine will pinpoint the mistakes made in the study of AIDS and BSE and will, almost certainly, tell us that our approaches to such subjects as vaccines and drugs were misplaced. For the present, it is widely assumed that all the important discoveries have been made; moreover, the climate of research at the end of the 20th century favours large teams working on relatively small projects. It is difficult to imagine that any future discoveries in the field of parasitology will engender the excitement of many of those outlined in this chapter but there will certainly be new inventions and developments. There will, for example, be new drugs and new vaccines, new species will be described and molecular techniques will be used to unravel details about both the parasites and the diseases they cause. These developments will bring fame and fortune, membership of learned societies and possibly Nobel Prizes, but the most important achievements will probably go unsung. The eradication of Guinea worm is on course for the end of this century, the end is in sight for river blindness and malaria is being controlled by the use of insecticide-impregnated bed nets. These events, which will probably not be mentioned in any publications other than specialized reports, will be much more important to those suffering from these diseases than any other more spectacular discoveries or advances. The future history of parasitology will be, and should be, written in terms of the development of the underprivileged parts of the world that have borne the burden of these diseases for far too long.

Figure 1 shows a number of the important figures in the history of human parasitology.

REFERENCES

Ackernecht EH, 1965, *History and Geography of the Most Important Diseases*, Hufner, New York.

Adler S, Ber M, 1941, The transmission of *Leishmania tropica* by the bite of *Phlebotomus papatasi, Indian J Med Res,* **122:** 803–9.

Annersley J, 1828, *Researches into the Causes, Nature and Treatment of the More Prevalent Diseases of Warm Climates Generally*, Longman, Rees, Orme, Brown and Green, London.

Argyll-Robertson DM, 1895, Case of *Filaria loa* in which the parasite was removed from under the conjunctiva, *Trans Ophthalmol Soc,* **15:** 137–67.

Atkins J, 1734, *The Navy Surgeon or a Practical System of Surgery*, Caesar Ward and Richard Chandler, London.

Avicenna, c1000, *Al Canon fi al Tib.*

Ball PAJ, 1996, Hookworm disease, *The Wellcome Trust Illustrated History of Tropical Diseases*, ed Cox FEG, The Wellcome Trust, London, 318–25.

Bastianelli G, Bignami A, 1900, Malaria and mosquitoes, *Lancet,* **1:** 79–83.

The Bible, Numbers, verse 6.

Bilharz T, von Siebold CT, 1852–1853, Ein Beitrag zur Helminhographia humana, aus brieflichen Mitteilungen des Dr. Bilharz in Cairo, nebst Bermerkungen von Prof. C. Th. von Siebold in Breslau, *Z Wiss Zool,* **4:** 53–76.

Blacklock B, 1926, The development of *Onchocerca volvulus* in *Simulium damnosum, Ann Trop Med Parasitol,* **20:** 1–48.

von Bonsdorff G, 1977, *Diphyllobothriasis in Man*, Academic Press, London.

Borovsky PF, 1898, Cited in Hoare (1938).

Bray RS, 1996, Amoebiasis, *The Wellcome Trust Illustrated History of Tropical Diseases*, ed Cox FEG, The Wellcome Trust, London, 170–7.

Brothwell D, Sandison AT, eds, 1967, *Diseases in Antiquity*, CT Thomas, Springfield Illinois.

Bruce D, 1915, Croonian lectures, *Br Med J,* **1:** 1073–8.

Bruce-Chwatt LJ, 1985, *Essential Malariology*, 2nd edn, Heinemann, London.

Bruce-Chwatt LJ, 1988, History of malaria from prehistory to eradication, *Malaria: Principles and Practice of Malariology*, vol 1, eds Wernsdorfer WH, McGregor I, Churchill Livingstone, Edinburgh, 1–59.

Brumpt E, 1912, Le *Trypanosoma cruzi* évolué chez *Conorhinus megistus, Cimex lectularis, Cimex boueti, Ornithodorus moubata.* Cycle évolutif de ce parasite, *Bull Soc Pathol Exot Filiales,* **5:** 360–7.

Bryan CP, 1930, *The Papyrus Ebers (translated from the German),* Geoffrey Bles, London.

Bundy DAP, Michael E, 1996, Trichinosis, *The Wellcome Trust Illustrated History of Tropical Diseases,* ed Cox FEG, The Wellcome Trust, London, 310–17.

Busk G, 1846, Observations on the structure and nature of the *Filaria medinensis* or Guinea Worm, *Trans Micr Soc,* **2:** 65–80.

Bynum W F, Porter R, eds, 1993, *Encyclopedia of the History of Medicine,* vols 1 and 2, Routledge, London and New York.

Campbell S, Hall B, Klausner D, eds, 1992, *Health, Disease and Healing in Medieval Culture,* Macmillan, London.

Carter HJ, 1855, Notes on dracunculus in the island of Bombay, *Trans Med Phys Soc Bombay,* **2:** 45–6.

Chagas C, 1909, Nova tripanosomiase humana. Estudos sobre e morfologia e o ciclo evolutivo do *Schizotrypanum cruzi* n.gen. n.sp. agente etiologico de nova entidade morbida do homem, *Mem Inst Oswaldo Cruz,* **1:** 159–218.

Chagas C, 1911, Nova entidade morbida do homem. Rezumo geral de estudios etiologicos e clinicos, *Mem Inst Oswaldo Cruz,* **3:** 276–94.

Chagas C, 1912, Sobre un trypanosomo do tatu, *Tatusia novemcincta,* transmitido pela *Triatoma geniculata* Latr. (1811), Possibilidade do ser o tatu um depositario do *Trypanosoma cruzi* no mundo exterior, *Brasil Médico,* **26:** 305–6.

Chernin E, 1977, Milestones in the history of tropical medicine and hygiene, *Am J Trop Med Hyg,* **26:** 1053–104.

Chernin J, 1983, Sir Patrick Manson's studies on the transmission and biology of filariasis, *Rev Infect Dis,* **5:** 148–66.

Contis G, David AR, 1996, The epidemiology of bilharzia in ancient Egypt: 5000 years of schistosomiasis, *Parasitol Today,* **12:** 253–5.

Coombs I, Crompton DWT, 1991, *A Guide to Human Helminthology,* Taylor and Francis, London.

Cox FEG, ed, 1996, *The Wellcome Trust Illustrated History of Tropical Diseases,* The Wellcome Trust, London.

Demarquay JN, 1863, Sur une tumeur des bourses contenant un liquide laiteux (galactocèle de Vidal) et renferment des petits entres vermiformes que l'on peut considerée comme des helminthes hematoides a l'état d'embryon, *Gaz Med Paris,* **18:** 665–7.

Desowitz RS, 1991, *The Malaria Capers,* Norton, New York.

Dobell C, 1919, *The Amoebae Living in Man,* John Bale Sons and Danielsson, London.

Dobell C, 1921, *A Report on the Occurrence of Intestinal Parasites in the Inhabitants of Britain with Special Reference to* Entamoeba histolytica. *Medical Research Council Special Report Series No 59,* His Majesty's Stationery Office, London.

Dobell C, 1960, *Antony van Leeuwenhoek and His 'Little Animals',* Dover Publications, New York.

Donovan C, 1903, The etiology of the heterogeneous fevers in India, *Br Med J,* **2:** 1401.

Dubey JP, Beattie CP, 1988, *Toxoplasmosis of Animals and Man,* CRC Press, Boca Raton.

Dubini A, 1843, Nuovo verme intestinal umano (*Agchylostoma duodenale*) constituente un sesto genere dei nematoidea propri dell'uomo, *Ann Universali Med,* **106:** 5–13.

Dufour L, 1828, Note sur la Grégarine, nouveau genre de ver qui vit en troupeau dans les intestines de divers insectes, *Ann Soc Nat,* **13:** 366–9.

Dutton JE, 1902, Preliminary note upon a trypanosome occurring in the blood of man, *Thompson Yates Lab Rep,* **4:** 455–68.

Eldridge BF, 1992, Patrick Manson and the discovery age of vector biology, *J Am Mosq Control Assoc,* **8:** 215–20.

Ettling J, 1990, The role of the Rockefeller Foundation in hookworm research and control, *Hookworm Disease: Current Studies and New Directions,* eds Schad G, Warren KS, Taylor and Francis, London, 3–14.

Evans G, 1881, On a horse disease in India known as 'Surra' probably due to a haematozoon, *Vet J Ann Comp Path,* **13:** 1–10, 82–8, 180–200, 326–33.

Fantham HB, Porter A, 1916, The pathogenicity of *Giardia (Lamblia) intestinalis* to men and experimental animals, *Br Med J,* **2:** 139–41.

Farley J, 1991, *Bilharzia. A History of Imperial Tropical Medicine,* Cambridge University Press, Cambridge.

Farthing MJG, 1996, Giardiasis, *The Wellcome Trust Illustrated History of Tropical Diseases,* ed Cox FEG, The Wellcome Trust, London, 248–55.

Fedchenko AP, 1870, Concerning the structure and reproduction of the Guinea Worm *Filaria medinensis* (translated from the Russian), *Am J Trop Med Hyg,* **20 (1971):** 511–23.

Ferreira LF, Araujo AGE, Confalonieri UEC, 1980, The finding of eggs and larvae of parasitic helminths in archaeological material from Unai, Minas Gerais, Brazil, *Trans R Soc Trop Med Hyg,* **174:** 798–800.

Foster WD, 1965, *A History of Parasitology,* Livingstone, Edinburgh.

Fujinami A, Nakamura A, 1909, [The mode of transmission of Katayama disease of Hiroshima Prefecture. Japanese schistosomiasis, the development of the causative worm and the disease in animals caused by it] (in Japanese), *Hiroshima Iji Geppo,* **132:** 324–41.

Garnham PCC, 1966, *Malaria Parasites and other Haemosporidia,* Blackwell Scientific Publications, Oxford.

Garnham PCC, 1970, *Progress in Parasitology,* Athlone Press, London.

Garnham PCC, 1987, Introduction, *The Leishmaniases in Biology and Medicine,* vol 1, eds Peters W, Killick-Kendrick R, Academic Press, London, 8–15.

Goeze JAE, 1782, *Versuch einer Naturgeschichte der Eingeweidewürmer thierischer Körper,* P Pape, Blankenberg.

Goodwin L, 1996a, Schistosomiasis, *The Wellcome Trust Illustrated History of Tropical Diseases,* ed Cox FEG, The Wellcome Trust, London, 264–73.

Goodwin L, 1996b, Ascariasis, *The Wellcome Trust Illustrated History of Tropical Diseases,* ed Cox FEG, The Wellcome Trust, London, 326–31.

Grassi B, 1881, Noto interno ad alcuni parassiti dell'uomo III. Interno all'Ascaris lumbricoides, *Gaz Ospital Milano,* **2:** 432.

Grove DI, 1990, *A History of Human Helminthology,* CAB International, Wallingford.

Gruby D, Delafond HM, 1843, Note sur une altération vermineuse de sang d'un chien determiné par un grand nombre d'hematozoaires du genre filaire, *C R Acad Sci,* **16:** 325–35.

Guerra F, 1970, American trypanosomiasis. An historical and human lesson, *J Trop Med Hyg,* **72:** 83–118.

Harrison G, 1978, *Mosquitoes, Malaria and Man,* John Murray, London.

Herbert T, 1634, *A Relation of Some Yeares Travaile into Afrique, Asia, Indies,* Da Capo, Amsterdam.

Hoare CA, 1938, Early discoveries regarding the parasites of oriental sore, *Trans R Soc Trop Med Hyg,* **32:** 67–92.

Hoare CA, 1972, *The Trypanosomes of Mammals,* Blackwell Scientific Publications, Oxford, 3–5.

Hoeppli R, 1956, The knowledge of parasites and parasitic infections from ancient times to the 17th century, *Exp Parasitol,* **5:** 398–419.

Hoeppli R, 1959, *Parasites and Parasitic Infections in Early Science and Medicine,* University of Malaya Press, Singapore.

Hutchison WM, Dunachie JF et al, 1970, Coccidian-like nature of *Toxoplasma gondii, Br Med J,* **1:** 142–4.

Janicki C, Rosen F, 1917, Le cycle évolutif du *Bothriocephalus latus* L., *Bull Soc Neuchateloise Sci Nat,* **42:** 19–21.

Jones WH, Withington ET, 1948–1953, *Works of Hippocrates*, vols 1–4, Loeb Classical Library, Heinemann, London.

Kartulis S, 1886, Zur aetiologie der dysenterie in Aegyptien, *Arch Pathol Anat*, **105**: 521–31.

Katsurada F, 1904, [The etiology of a parasitic disease] (in Japanese translated in Kean, Mott and Russell 1978), *Iji Shinbun*, **669**: 1325–32.

Kean BH Mott KE, Russell AJ, eds, 1978, *Tropical Medicine and Parasitology: Classic Investigations*, vols 1, 2, Ithaca, Cornell University Press.

Kiple K, ed, 1993, *The Cambridge World History of Human Disease*, Cambridge University Press, Cambridge.

Kleine FK, 1909, Positiv Infektionversuche mit *Trypanosoma brucei* durch *Glossina palpalis*, *Dtsch Med Wochenschr*, **35**: 469–70.

Kobayashi H, 1915, On the life history and morphology of *Clonorchis sinensis*, *Cent Bakt Parasit Infekt*, **75**: 299–317.

Koberle F, 1968, Chagas' disease and Chagas' disease syndrome: the pathology of American trypanosomiasis, *Adv Parasitol*, **6**: 63–116.

Koch R, 1903, *Interim Report on Rhodesian Redwater or 'African Coast Fever'*, Argus Printing and Publishing, Salisbury Rhodesia.

Koino S, 1922, Experimental infection of the human body with ascarides, *Japan Med World*, **15**: 317–20.

Küchenmeister F, 1855, Offenes Sendschreiben an die k.k. Gesellschaft der Aertze zu Wien. Experimenteller Nachweis dass *Cysticercus cellulosae* innerhalb des menschlichen Damarkanales sich in *Taenia solium* umwandelt, *Wien Med Wochenschr*, **5**: 1–4.

Küchenmeister F, 1860, Erneuter Versuch der Umwandlung des *Cysticercus cellulosae* in *Taenia solium hominis*, *Dtsch Klinik*, **12**: 187–9.

Lainson R, 1996, New World leishmaniasis, *The Wellcome Trust Illustrated History of Tropical Diseases*, ed Cox FEG, The Wellcome Trust, London, 218–29.

Lambl V, 1859, Microscopische untersuchungen der darmexcrete. Beitrag zur pathologisches des darmes und zur diagnostik am krankenbette, *Viert Prakt Heilkunde (Prague)*, **61**: 1–57.

Laveran A, 1880, Note sur un nouveau parasite trouvé dans le sang de plusieurs malades atteints de fièvre palustre, *Bull Acad Méd*, **9**: 1235–6.

Leiper RT, 1906, The influence of acid on Guinea worm larvae encysted in *Cyclops*, *Br Med J*, **1**: 19–20.

Leiper RT, 1913, Report to the advisory committee of the Tropical Diseases Research Fund, Colonial Office London, *Trop Dis Bull*, **2**: 195–6.

Leiper RT, 1916, On the relation between the terminal-spined and lateral-spined eggs of bilharzia, *Br Med J*, **1**: 411.

Leishman WB, 1903, On the possibility of the occurrence of trypanosomiasis in India, *Br Med J*, **1**: 1252–4.

Leonard J, 1990, Carlos Chagas, health pioneer of the Brazilian backlands, *Bull Pan Am Health Organ*, **24**: 226–39.

Lewinsohn R, 1979, The discovery of *Trypanosoma cruzi* and of American trypanosomiasis (foot-note to the history of Chagas' disease), *Trans R Soc Trop Med Hyg*, **73**: 513–23.

Lewis TR, 1872, On a haematozoon inhabiting human blood, its relation to chyluria and other diseases, *8th Annual Report Sanitary Commission Government of India*, **8**: 241–66.

Linnaeus C, 1758, *Systema Naturae, sive regina tria naturae systematice proposita por classes, ordines, genera, species cum characteribus differentiis synonymis, locis*, 10, L Salvi, Holmiae.

van Linschoten JH, 1610, *Histoire de la Navigaation de JHL*, Amsterdam.

Looss A, 1898, Zur Lebensgeschichte des *Ankylostoma duodenale*, *Cent Bakt Parasit Infekt*, **24**: 483–8.

Lösch FA, 1875, Massive development of amebas in the large intestine (translated from the Russian), *Am J Trop Med Hyg*, **24 (1975)**: 383–92.

Low GC, 1900, A recent observation on *Filaria nocturna* in *Culex*, probable mode of infection in man, *Br Med J*, **1**: 1456–7.

Lyons AS, Petrucelli RJ, 1978, *Medicine: An Illustrated History*, Abrams, New York.

Lyons M, 1992, *A Colonial Disease: A Social History of Sleeping Sickness in Northern Zaire 1900–1940*, Cambridge University Press, Cambridge.

McConnell JF, 1875, Remarks on the anatomy and pathological relations of a new species of liver-fluke, *Lancet*, **2**: 271–4.

McGregor I, 1996, Malaria, *The Wellcome Trust Illustrated History of Tropical Diseases*, ed Cox FEG, The Wellcome Trust, London, 230–47.

Mack A, 1991, *In time of Plague: the History and Social Consequences of Lethal Epidemic Disease*, New York University Press, New York.

Manson P, 1878, On the development of *Filaria sanguis hominis* and on the mosquito considered as a nurse, *J Linn Soc (Zool)*, **14**: 304–11.

Manson P, 1881, *Distoma ringeri*, *Med Times Gaz*, **2**: 8–9.

Manson P, 1891, The *Filaria sanguinis hominis major* and *minor*, two new species of haematozoa, *Lancet*, **1**: 4–8.

Manson P, 1893, Diseases of the skin in tropical climates, *Hygiene and Diseases of Warm Climates*, ed Davidson AH, Young J Pentland, London.

Manson P, 1894, On the nature and significance of crescentic and flagellated bodies in malarial blood, *Br Med J*, **2**: 1306–8.

Manson P, 1898, *Tropical Diseases*, 1st edn, Cassell, London.

Manson P, 1902, Report of a case of bilharzia from the West Indies, *Br Med J*, **2**: 1894–5.

Manson-Bahr P, 1962, *Patrick Manson: the Father of Tropical Medicine*, Thomas Nelson, London.

Manson-Bahr PEC, 1996, Old World leishmaniasis, *The Wellcome Trust Illustrated History of Tropical Diseases*, ed Cox FEG, The Wellcome Trust, London, 206–17.

Miles MA, 1996, New World trypanosomiasis, *The Wellcome Trust Illustrated History of Tropical Diseases*, ed Cox FEG, The Wellcome Trust, London, 192–205.

Miyairi K, Suzuki M, 1913, [On the development of *Schistosoma japonicum*] (in Japanese translated in Kean, Mott and Russell 1978), *Tokyo Iji Shinshi*, **1836**: 1–5.

Mongin, 1770, Sur un ver trouvé sous la conjunctive à Maribarou, isle Saint-Dominique, *J Méd Chir Pharm*, **32**: 338–9.

Moulin AM, 1993, Historical introduction: the Institut Pasteur's contribution, *Res Immunol*, **144**: 8–13.

Müller OF, 1786, *Animalcula Infusoria Fluviatilia et Marina*, Hauniae.

Muller R, 1996a, Liver and lung flukes, *The Wellcome Trust Illustrated History of Tropical Diseases*, ed Cox FEG, The Wellcome Trust, London, 274–85.

Muller R, 1996b, Onchocerciasis, *The Wellcome Trust Illustrated History of Tropical Diseases*, ed Cox FEG, The Wellcome Trust, London, 304–9.

Muto M, 1918, [On the primary intermediate host of *Clonorchis sinensis*] (in Japanese translated in Kean, Mott and Russell 1978), *Chuo Igakkai Zasshi*, **25**: 49–52.

Nash TAM, 1969, *Africa's Bane. The Tsetse Fly*, Collins, London.

Naunyn B, 1863, Ueber die zu *Echinococcus hominis* gehörige täen, *Arch Anat Physiol Wiss Med*, 412–16.

Nelson G, 1996, Lymphatic filariasis, *The Wellcome Trust Illustrated History of Tropical Diseases*, ed Cox FEG, The Wellcome Trust, London, 294–303.

Nepveu G, 1898, Sur un trypanosome dans le sang de l'homme, *C R Soc Biol (Marseilles)*, **5**: 1172–4.

Nicolle C, Manceaux L, 1909, Sur un protozoaire nouveau du gondi, *Arch Inst Pasteur*, **2**: 97–103.

Norman JM, 1991, *Morton's Medical Bibliography. An Annotated Check List of Texts Illustrating the History of Medicine (Garrison and Morton)*, 5, Scolar Press, Aldershot.

Ochoterna B, 1928, Contribucíon para el conocimento de la onchocercosis en Mexico, *Arb Tropenkrank*, Festschrift Bernhard Nocht, 386–9.

Oliver JH, 1871, *Seventh Annual Report of the Sanitary Commissioner*

(1870) of the Government of India, Government Printing House, Calcutta, 82–83.

O'Neill J, 1875, On the presence of a filaria in 'craw craw', *Lancet*, **1**: 265–6.

Owen R, 1835, Description of a microsopic entozoon infesting the muscles of the human body, *London Med Gaz*, **16**: 125–7.

Perroncito E, 1877, On the tenacity of life of the cysticercus in the flesh of oxen and on the rapid development of the corresponding *Taenia mediocanellata* in the human body, *The Veterinarian*, **50**: 817–18.

Ranger T, Slack P, eds, 1992, *Epidemics and Ideas*, Cambridge University Press, Cambridge.

Ransford O, 1983, *Bid the Sickness Cease: Disease in the History of Black Africa*, John Murray, London.

Redi F, 1684, *Osservazione intorno agli animali viventi che si trouvano negli animali viventi*, Pietro Martini, Florence.

Rendtorff RC, 1954, The experimental transmission of human protozoan parasites. II *Giardia lamblia* cysts given in capsules, *J Hyg*, **59**: 209–20.

Rhazes (abu Bakr Muhammad ibn-Zakariya-al-Razi), c900, *Al-Hawi (A Summary of Medical Knowledge)*.

Robles R, 1917, Enfermedad neuva en Guatemala, *Juventid Medica*, **17**: 97–115.

Ross R, 1897, On some peculiar pigmented cells found in two mosquitoes fed on malarial blood, *Br Med J*, **2**: 1736–88.

Ross R, Thompson D, 1911, A case of sleeping sickness studied by precise enumerative methods: further observations, *Ann Trop Med Parasitol*, **4**: 395–415.

Schaudinn F, 1903, Studien über krankheitserregende Protozoen II. *Plasmodium vivax* (Grassi et Feletti) der Erreger des Tertianfiebers beim Menschen, *Arb Kaiserlichen Gesund*, **19**: 169–250.

Scott HH, 1939, *A History of Tropical Medicine*, vols 1, 2, Edward Arnold, London.

Sergent ED, Sergent ET et al, 1921, Transmission du clou de Biskra par le phlebotome *Phlebotomus papatasi* Scop., *C R Seanc Soc Biol*, **73**: 1030–2.

Service MW, Wilmott S, eds, 1978, *Medical Entomology Centenary Symposium Proceedings*, Royal Society of Tropical Medicine and Hygiene, London.

Shortt HE, Garnham PCC, 1948, Pre-erythrocytic stages in mammalian malaria parasites, *Nature (London)*, **161**: 126.

von Siebold CT, 1853, Ueber die Verwandlung der *Echinococcus*-brut in Taenien, *Z Wissen Zool*, **4**: 409–25.

Smith T, Kilbourne FC, 1893, Investigations into the nature, causation and prevention of Texas or Southern fever, *Bull Bureau Animal Indust US Dept Agric*, **1**: 177–304.

Splendore A, 1909, Sur un nouveau protozoaire parasite du lapin, deuxième note préliminaire, *Bull Soc Pathol Exot Filiales*, **2**: 462–5.

Stephens JWW, Fantham HB, 1910, On the peculiar morphology of a trypanosome from a case of sleeping sickness and the possibility of its being a new species (*T. rhodesiense*), *Proc R Soc Lond (Biol)*, **83**: 28–33.

Tayeh A, 1996, Dracunculiasis, *The Wellcome Trust Illustrated History of Tropical Diseases*, ed Cox FEG, The Wellcome Trust, London, 286–303.

Turkhud DA, 1914, *Report of the Bombay Bacteriological Laboratory for the Year 1913*, Government Central Press, Bombay, 14–16.

Tyson E, 1683, *Lumbricus teres*, or some anatomical observations on the round worm bred in human bodies, *Philos Trans R Soc Lond (Biol)*, **13**: 153–61.

Valentin GG, 1841, Ueber ein Entozoon im Blut von *Salmo fario*, *Muller's Archives fur 1841*, 435–6.

Vallery-Radot R, 1906, *The Life of Pasteur (translated from the French)*, McClure Phillips, New York.

Vianna G, 1911, Sobre uma nova espécie de *Leishmania*, *Brasil Médico*, **25**: 411.

Vickerman K, Luckins AG, 1969, Localization of variable antigens in the surface coat of *Trypanosoma brucei* using ferritin conjugated antibody, *Nature (London)*, **224**: 1125–6.

Vogel H, 1934, Der Entwicklungszyklus von *Opisthorchis felineus* (Riv.) nebst Bemerkungen über Systematik und Epidemiologie, *Zoologica*, **33**: 1–103.

Warboys M, 1983, The emergence and early development of parasitology, *In Parasitology: a Global Perspective*, eds Warren KS, Bowers JZ, Springer-Verlag, New York, 1–18.

Warboys M, 1993, Tropical diseases, *Encyclopedia of the History of Medicine*, vol 1, eds Bynum WF, Porter R, Routledge, London and New York, 512–536.

Warren KS, 1973, *Schistosomiasis. The Evolution of a Medical Literature*, MIT Press, Cambridge Mass.

Williams BI, 1996, African trypanosomiasis, *The Wellcome Trust Illustrated History of Tropical Diseases*, ed Cox FEG, The Wellcome Trust, London, 178–91.

Winogradoff K, 1892, [On a new species of distomum [*Distomum sibiricum*] in the human liver] (abstracted from the Russian), *Cent Allgem Path Anat*, **3**: 910–11.

Winterbottom TM, 1803, *An Account of the Native Africans in the Neighbourhood of Sierra Leone to Which is Added an Account of the Present State of Medicine Among Them*, vol 2, C Whittingham, London, 29–31.

Wolf A, Cowen D, 1937, Granulomatous encephalomyelitis due to an encephalitozoon (encephalitozoic encephomyelitis). A new protozoan disease of man, *Bull Neurol Inst N Y*, **6**: 306–71.

Wright JH, 1903, Protozoa in a case of tropical ulcer, *J Med Res*, **10**: 472–82.

Chapter 2

WORLD-WIDE IMPORTANCE OF PARASITES

G A Schmunis and F J López Antuñano

1 Parasitic diseases and global health	**3** Some significant parasitic diseases: new and
2 Some significant parasitic diseases: the old	expanding threats
threats	**4** Conclusion

1 PARASITIC DISEASES AND GLOBAL HEALTH

1.1 Introduction

This chapter describes the prevalence and overall distribution of parasitic infections in the world, the burden they constitute to the human population and the costs they represent to individuals and society.

In 1993, life expectancy in the least developed countries of the world was 43 years, compared with 73 years in developed countries. Although life expectancy is projected to increase to 79 years by the year 2000 in developed countries it is expected to remain <60 years in 45 developing countries (WHO 1995a).

About 51 million people died in the world in 1993, 39 million of them in the developing countries. World wide, communicable diseases were responsible for c. 40% of the total number of deaths (20 million). In contrast, 80% (16 million) of deaths in developing countries were due to infectious and parasitic diseases (WHO 1995a).

Parasitic diseases occur world wide. Poverty and its accompanying features (lack of sanitation, malnutrition, illiteracy and overcrowding) are all causes and consequences of most of the parasitic diseases of public health importance. Although infectious and parasitic diseases are more significant causes of morbidity and mortality among the poor, no one is exempt from infection. Internal and external parasites are among the most common pathogens world wide and anyone can be exposed to them at home or when they travel.

1.2 The burden of parasitic diseases

A comprehensive study by the World Bank (1993a) attempted to measure the burden that diseases, as a group or individually, represent in different regions of the world. The measurement took into account both losses from premature death (defined as the difference between the actual age of death and the age at which death would have occurred in a population with a low mortality) and the effects of losses caused by weakened health. The effects of the loss of healthy life were quantified for the diseases listed in the 109 categories included in the International Classification of Diseases (WHO 1977) and for approximately 95% of possible causes of disability (World Bank 1993a). To evaluate losses from illness, the incidence of cases by age, sex and demographic region was estimated and the number of years of healthy life lost was obtained by multiplying the expected duration of the disease by a severity weight that estimated the severity of the disability in comparison with loss of life caused by the illness (World Bank 1993a). The global burden of disease estimated in this manner was quantified into units called the disability adjusted life years (DALYs). The relative global burden of a specific disease was estimated by comparing the DALYs lost from different diseases or groups of diseases.

In many areas of the world communicable diseases continue to impose a significant burden that is greater in developing countries than in countries with established market economies. Injuries also cause greater losses in developing countries than in developed countries (Fig. 2.1).

Parasitic diseases contribute heavily to the burden produced by communicable diseases, their contribution being comparable with such common diseases as tuberculosis, sexually transmitted diseases, diseases preventable by vaccination and acute respiratory infections. Malaria is the parasitic disease responsible for the greatest burden world wide; in Africa its burden is almost as great as that produced by acute respiratory infections. Worm infections are also a significant burden in Africa and some other regions (Fig. 2.2) (World Bank 1993b).

The burden of infectious diseases, including para-

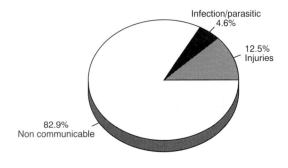

Established market economies

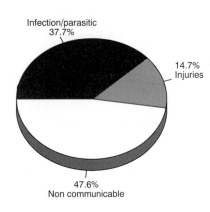

Developing countries

Fig. 2.1 Percentage distribution of DALYs lost by overall cause in countries with established market economies and developing countries. (Data from World Bank, 1993b.)

sitic infections, is borne mainly by the poorest people in the poorest countries of the world. Parasitic diseases are thus contributing to inequalities that exist both within and between societies (Evans and Jamison 1994).

In Fig. 2.3 the DALYs lost as a result of infectious diseases of microbial and viral origin are compared with the losses caused by parasitic diseases in developing countries and in countries with established market economies. Although the burdens produced by diseases of viral or microbial origin are the highest, the burden produced by parasitic diseases is also great (World Bank 1993b).

The effects and burdens produced by parasitic diseases vary greatly from region to region. Different parasitic diseases are responsible for the bulk of the burden in different geographical areas, for example, malaria and schistosomiasis are the diseases that cause the highest burden globally, but Chagas disease produces the highest burden in Latin America and the Caribbean (Fig. 2.4).

The burden of different parasitic diseases also varies with age. Malaria produces the highest burden in children <5 years of age but intestinal worms produce the

highest burden in children aged 5–14 years (Table 2.1).

Disease burdens vary not only with age and geographical region but also among demographic groups. Not surprisingly, a significant proportion of the deaths caused by parasites occurs in developing countries (Table 2.2) and the individuals at greatest risk are those living in rural areas and in urban squatter settlements. Such people are usually poor and lack adequate housing, safe water supplies and good waste disposal systems. Workers involved in mining and timber exploitation are also often exposed to parasitic diseases as an occupational hazard (Rosenfield, Golladay and Davidson 1984).

1.3 Population movement and parasitic diseases

Population movements have helped to raise awareness of parasites as a world wide public health problem. In the early 1990s, 500 million people crossed international borders by air, 18–20 million refugees were generated from conflicts and 20–30 million people were displaced for other reasons (Wilson 1995, WHO 1995b). Of the 5.2 billion people in the world one out of every 134 was forced to leave their home in 1992 (WHO 1995b) and an estimated 70 million people, mostly from developing countries, work in countries to which they have migrated (Wilson 1995). Many of these people have carried parasites to their new homes, sometimes requiring treatment themselves and sometimes serving as sources of infection to others. As a result of these population shifts, medical personnel in many advanced countries have gained personal experience of parasitic diseases for the first time.

In addition to international migration, many people also migrate beween regions of a country; in the last 6 decades economic hardship in the rural areas of developing countries has stimulated migration to urban areas within the same country. As a result, c. 45% of the world's population now live in cities and diseases that were traditionally considered to be 'rural' have spread into the cities, usually affecting the most deprived populations. This phenomenon has brought many people within the orbit of public health services for the first time and diseases previously not noticed have now made themselves apparent. It has also increased demands on already overburdened public health services. From their bridgeheads in the slums the parasites may spread to other urban areas, reaching new hosts through vectors, through fecal contamination of soil, food and water and through transfused blood.

Transfusion-acquired malaria (particularly *Plasmodium vivax* malaria) and Chagas disease pose particular problems as they are both easily transmitted by blood transfusion. Other parasites, such as the African trypanosomes (particularly *Trypanosoma gambiense*), *Babesia microti* and the filarial worms such as *Brugia malayi*, *Loa loa*, *Wuchereria bancrofti*, *Mansonella ozzardi* and *M. perstans*, may also be transmitted by blood

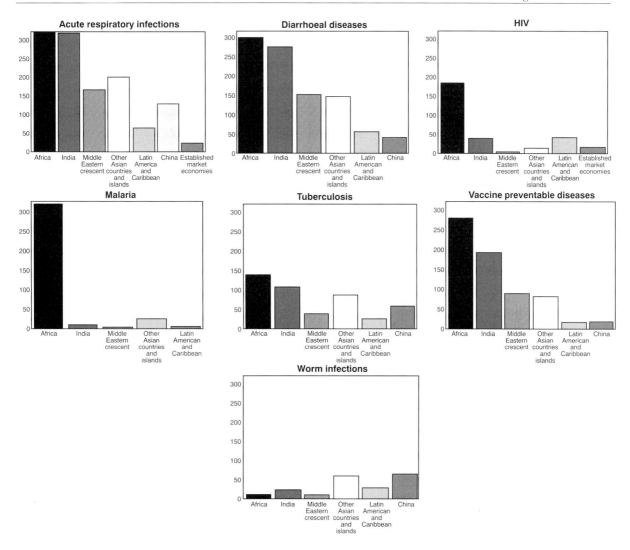

Fig. 2.2 Distribution of DALYs lost by selected communicable diseases by region, 1990 (in hundred of thousands of DALYs lost). (Data from World Bank, 1993b.)

transfusion but fortunately this mode of transmission is rare even in the endemic countries.

It is not surprising that malaria has resulted from blood transfusion as plasmodia can remain viable in refrigerated blood for up to 10 days. In developing countries, transfusion malaria is most common in people who have received blood sold by low income donors, whereas in developed countries transfusion malaria results from the migration of carriers from endemic areas. To avoid such infections, blood donation is not permitted in some countries from those who have had malaria or who have visited or lived in malarious areas.

Individuals with positive serology for *T. cruzi*, the causative agent of Chagas diseases, have been found among the 7 million or more legal immigrants from South and Central America to the USA. Their presence poses a risk of transmission of Chagas disease by blood transfusion. A similar risk exists in Europe where >250 000 immigrants from Central and South America now live (Schmunis 1994). Transfusion-transmitted *T. cruzi* infection has been reported in

Canada, the USA and Spain (Villalba et al. 1992, Schmunis 1991). Infection may occur in non-endemic areas by means other than transfusion, for example, infection in a migrant was the cause of a case of congenital *T. cruzi* infection in Sweden.

As air travel has become more common, imported malaria has been seen with increasing frequency in Canada, the Caribbean, Europe, Oceania and the USA and it has been stated that patients with malaria are now more often seen in temperate London (England) than in tropical Jamaica (West Indies) (Alleyne 1983). For travellers in most areas of Asia, the species of *Plasmodium* responsible for malaria is usually *P. vivax*, whereas for travellers in Africa and some parts of Asia it is *P. falciparum* and either or both species may occur in travellers in the Americas. There is a constant risk that travellers infected with plasmodia who return to areas where there are *Anopheles* mosquitoes susceptible to infection may start local transmission (Maldonado et al. 1986, Phillips-Howard 1991, Lopez Antuñano and Schmunis 1993). Malaria has also been reported in individuals living in non-malarious areas who have

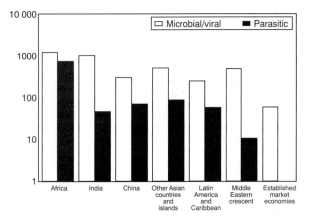

Fig. 2.3 Burden of disease caused by parasites (including malaria, African and American trypanosomiasis, schistosomiasis, leishmaniasis, filariasis, onchocerciasis, ascariasis, trichuris, and hookworm) and by microbial and viral infections (including tuberculosis, sexually transmitted diseases, HIV, diarrhoeal diseases, pertussis, poliomyelitis, diphtheria, measles, tetanus, meningitis, hepatitis, and acute respiratory infections) by region, 1990 (in hundreds of thousands of DALYs lost). (Data from World Bank, 1993b.)

never left that area and have never had a blood transfusion. Most cases have been acquired by people living near or passing through airports and have been attributed to bites from infected mosquitoes transported on aeroplanes.

Food-borne trematodes, such as *Opisthorchis* spp., are responsible for diseases in migrants from South

East Asia and the eastern Pacific and a high prevalence has been reported in refugees in camps in Cambodia and Laos and in Thai immigrant workers in Kuwait and China. Pulmonary paragonimiasis has been diagnosed in refugees from South East Asia residing in France and in the USA. Liver flukes have been found in immigrants from Asia to Europe and the USA (WHO 1995b). Ethiopian refugees in Israel also harbour liver flukes. The round worm *Strongyloides stercoralis* and the protozoa *Giardia duodenalis* and *Entamoeba histolytica* are among the parasites often acquired by migrants and by travellers to developing countries.

2   SOME SIGNIFICANT PARASITIC DISEASES: THE OLD THREATS

2.1   Blood protozoa

AFRICAN TRYPANOSOMIASIS (SLEEPING SICKNESS)

Trypanosomiasis, caused by *T. gambiense* and *T. rhodesiense*, is endemic in rural areas of 36 countries of sub-Saharan Africa, particularly in west, central and east Africa in areas where the tsetse fly is present. Sleeping sickness caused by the trypanosomes has eliminated entire communities in Africa. Outbreaks of sleeping sickness produced by *T. gambiense* continue to occur in Angola, Congo, Sudan, Uganda and Zaire and *T. rhodensiense* is a serious threat in Tanzania and Mozambique. Sporadic cases of sleeping sickness have also

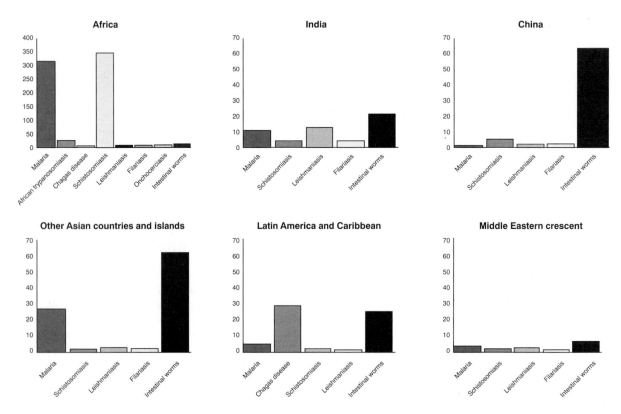

Fig. 3.4 Burden of disease caused by various parasitic diseases by regions, 1990 (in hundreds of thousands of DALYs lost). (Data from World Bank, 1993b.)

Table 2.1 Main causes of disease burden in children from developing countries. 1990[a]

Diseases	≤4 years old[b]	%	Diseases	5–14 years old[b]	%
Acute respiratory infections	93.2	18	Intestinal helminths[d]	16.8	11.8
Diarrhoeal diseases	82.5	16	Vaccine preventable diseases	11.8	8.3
Vaccine preventable diseases[c]	55.1	10.6	Acute respiratory infections	10.4	7.36
Malaria	24.3	4.7	Diarrhoeal diseases	9.3	6.5
Tuberculosis	2.6	0.5	Tuberculosis	6.8	4.85
Sexually transmitted diseases and HIV	5.0	1.0	Malaria	6.5	4.57
Total DALYs lost in millions[e]	518.0			142.0	

[a]Adapted from World Bank, 1993b.
[b]Millions of DALY's lost.
[c]Pertussis, polio, measles and tetanus.
[d]Ascaris and trichuris.
[e]Communicable, non communicable, and injuries DALYs lost.

Table 2.2 Deaths by cause and demographic group[a] according to types of country and age group. 1990

Diseases	Developing countries		Formerly socialist economies of Europe and established market economies		World
	≤4 y	≥5 y	≤4 y	≥5 y	
Acute respiratory infections	2710	1274	21	309	4314
Diarrhoeal diseases	2474	392	4	3	2873
Tuberculosis	71	1907	0	38	2016
Malaria	633	294	0	0	926
African trypanosomiasis	5	51	0	0	55
Chagas disease	0	23	0	0	23
Schistosomiasis	1	37	0	0	38
Leishmaniasis	7	46	0	0	54
Onchocerciasis	0	29	0	0	30
Ascaris	0	13	0	0	0
Trichuris	0	10	0	0	9
Hookworm	0	6	0	0	0
Lymphatic filariasis	0	0	0	0	0

[a]In thousands—data obtained from World Bank, 1993b.

been reported from some southern African countries (WHO 1986 and 1994a). It is estimated that over 55 million people are at risk of acquiring sleeping sickness and that 250 000–300 000 people are infected. The yearly incidence is difficult to ascertain because surveillance is poor in the c. 200 confirmed foci of endemic sleeping sickness. The number of cases reported annually varies from 20 000 to 25 000 (WHO 1986 and 1994a).

Projects for economic development, if planned without proper consideration for their effects on the environment and on health, can cause unexpected health problems. Development projects for producing electricity and improving agriculture may change the local ecology and facilitate the spread of trypanosomiasis and other parasitic infections. For instance, they may encourage people to migrate to areas where their contact with parasites and their vectors is increased. Dams may displace villages, forcing people into tsetse-infested grasslands. Extensive lake margins may encourage growth of vegetation in which tsetse flies

can breed, increasing the risk of bites among people who come to collect water. Such exposures may cause recrudescences of infection and even bring about full blown epidemics (WHO 1986). Political upheavals and droughts may also stimulate life-style changes, many of which facilitate the spread of diseases. One of the most common consequences of civil disorder and of drought is the mass movement of people. While in transit, they are vulnerable to disease and many may become infected if they migrate into or across trypanosomiasis endemic areas.

If untreated, both forms of African trypanosomiasis are lethal, but there are important differences between the 2 forms of the disease. *T. gambiense* infections may run a protracted course of several years duration and infected individuals may serve as sources of infection if they migrate to areas where susceptible hosts and vectors are present. The disease caused by *T. rhodesiense* in east Africa causes death in weeks or at most in a few months and therefore carriers pose less of a threat to individuals in uninfected areas.

Programmes for control of sleeping sickness are based on a combination of active and passive medical surveillance and on vector control. Costs include those incurred as a result of death and loss of productivity due to illness and those incurred as a result of the cost of treatment and disease control. The estimated cost from loss of income due to premature death from sleeping sickness is US$615–761 per person, varying in different areas and among different segments of society; cost per individual is higher for those with a higher income. In 1984–85, the cost of surveillance was estimated at US$0.79–1.39 per person depending on the strategy used. The cost of treatment, including hospitalization, was US$35, US$88 and US$133 per person for treatment with pentamidine, suramin and melarsoprol, respectively. Costs for prevention using screens and traps varied from US$2.30 to US$11.50 per person. Ground spraying costs were estimated at US$200–1000 km^{-2}. The cost per person protected by screens and traps depended on the number of people served per screen or trap and on the density of the population in the area under surveillance (WHO 1986).

AMERICAN TRYPANOSOMIASIS (CHAGAS DISEASE)

Chagas disease occurs frequently in South and Central America, from Mexico in the north to Argentina and Chile in the south. Most of the 16–18 million people infected with *T. cruzi* in this region live in poor rural or semi-urban areas. Infected individuals have been detected in all Central and South American countries, including a few in French Guiana, Guyana and Surinam. The only Spanish-speaking countries in the western Hemisphere where human *T. cruzi* infections have not been found are Cuba and the Dominican Republic. American trypanosomiasis also occurs as a zoonotic disease in the USA, where its range extends to Northern California in the west and to Maryland in the east.

The majority of cases of human infection occur in rural areas, particularly where houses are colonized by the triatome bugs that transmit the infection. The extent of vector transmission in the human population is related to socioeconomic status, poor people living in inadequate housing being most commonly infected. The infection persists wherever living conditions permit intimate contact between the triatome bugs and the human host. Congenital transmission also occurs in at least 3% of babies born to infected mothers (Schmunis 1994). Many infected individuals show few or no clinical symptoms of disease and thus may not seek treatment. Infected individuals who are untreated remain infected throughout their lives.

Transfusion is the second most common mode of acquiring the infection. Infection rates in blood donors vary from 6 to 12% in some areas of Argentina, Brazil and Chile and from 2% in Honduras to 48% in Bolivia. Prevalence in the general population is 0.34% in Ecuador, 1.25% in Uruguay, 11.5% in Paraguay and 22.2% in Bolivia. Incidence estimates range from 4030 for Costa Rica to 179703 for Venezuela (Table 2.3) (Hayes and Schofield 1990, Schmunis 1994).

Chagas disease is a debilitating and incapacitating chronic condition that develops in 20% of those infected with *T. cruzi*, killing 45000 people every year. Chagasic cardiopathy ranked third as a cause of disability in a rural area of Brazil where *T. cruzi* infection is endemic (Dias et al. 1985a) and was also the main cause of early retirement in the region (Lopes and Chapadeiro 1986). In another endemic area of Brazil, 4–9% of all incapacity benefits received by individuals 30–50 years old were attributed to the effects of Chagas disease (Zicker and Zicker 1985). The number of productive years lost because of the disease among individuals 15–64 years of age in endemic areas of Brazil was estimated to be 2.275 and 1.369 per 100000 population for males and females respectively (Pereira 1984).

Using data from the World Bank study and from other sources it is possible to compare the burden and general costs of Chagas disease with those of other diseases (World Bank 1993b). The disease burdens produced by malaria (35700000 DALYs) and schistosomiasis (4500000 DALYs) world wide are higher than that produced by Chagas disease (2740000 DALYs), but the Chagas disease burden is higher than those produced by leishmaniasis, African trypanosomiasis, leprosy, filariasis and onchocerciasis (Fig. 2.4). In Latin America, the burden of Chagas disease exceeds that of the so-called tropical diseases (i.e. malaria, schistosomiasis and leishmaniasis) and intestinal worms. In Latin America tropical diseases together produced a disease burden that was only about one-quarter of that caused by Chagas disease. The disease burden caused by Chagas disease is moreover the fourth highest among all infectious diseases which occur in the region. Only acute respiratory infections, diarrhoea and AIDS produced higher disease burdens.

As the affected population is mostly of a low socioeconomic level, the cost of treatment is usually provided by the State. In Brazil in 1987, the estimated cost for pacemakers and surgery to correct enlarged viscera was US$250 million and the cost of lost labour by the 75000 chagasic workers represented a loss of another US$625 million (Dias 1987). These costs did not include consultation, care and supportive treatment, costs for which amounted to another US$1000 per patient per year (Schofield and Dias 1991), or disability payments which in one Brazilian State in 1987 were US$400000 (Dias 1987). In Argentina, the cost for 30 months of treatment of 128 patients who had cardiac lesions was US$350000 (Evequoz 1993). Bolivia spends US$215000 each year for treatment of patients with acute Chagas disease; US$21 million for treatment of chronic disease and US$186000 for treatment of congenital disease. In 1994, direct costs to Bolivia as a result of deaths from the disease were US$343000 per year and annual indirect costs of morbidity and mortality were estimated at US$43.8 and 57.5 million, respectively (Human Development Ministry 1994). In Chile, the yearly cost of the disease was estimated at US$37 million in addition to the cost of

Table 2.3   Infection by *Trypanosoma cruzi* in the Americas[a]

Country	Endemic[b] area in km^2	Percentage of total country area	Estimated population at risk		Estimated infected population		Estimated yearly incidence
			Number[b,c]	As a percentage of the total population	Number[b]	As a percentage of the total population	
Argentina	1946	70	6 900	23	2333	7.2	[d]
Bolivia	1300	100	2 834	55	1134	22.2	86 676
Brazil	3615	42	41 054	32	5000	4.3	[d]
Chile	350		1 800	15	1239	10.6	[d]
Colombia	200	18	3 000	10	900	3.3	39 162
Costa Rica	ND	...	1 112	45	130	5.3	4 030
Ecuador	100	35	3 823	41	30	0.34	7 488
El Salvador	ND	...	21	43	322	6.9	10 048
Guatemala	ND	...	4 022	52	730	9.8	30 076
Honduras	ND	...	1 824	42	300	7.4	9 891
Mexico	ND	...	...	...	...	...	142 880
Nicaragua	ND	...	...	...	...	...	5 016
Panama	ND	...	898	42	220	10.6	7 130
Paraguay	ND	...	1 475	45	397	11.59	14 680
Peru	120	9	6 766	34	643	3.47	24 320
Uruguay	125	71	975	33	37	1.25	[d]
Venezuela	697	76	11 392	68	1200	7.42	179 703

[a]Data for 1980–1985; ND: No data. [b]In thousands. [c]Total population the year the study was made or average population for the years the study was made. (Schmunis 1994). [d]Incidence from these countries are not included because the beneficial effect of control programmes is not considered in the calculation. (Hayes and Schofield 1990).

pacemakers and surgery for implantation of pacemakers (Apt 1991).

In addition to the costs of treatment, there are also costs associated with the control of vectors responsible for Chagas disease. The annual cost for vector control through insecticide spraying, housing improvement and health education in countries infested with the vector *T. infestans* is large: US$100 000 for Uruguay; US$300 000 for Chile; US$18 million for Argentina and US$25 million for Brazil.

LEISHMANIASIS

Leishmaniasis is considered to be endemic in Africa, in most countries of the Americas and Asia and in many countries of Europe. Most cases of cutaneous leishmaniasis (>90%) occur in Afghanistan, Brazil, Iran, Peru, Saudi Arabia and Syria. More than 90% of visceral leishmaniasis cases occur in Bangladesh, India, Nepal and Sudan (WHO 1994b). In all its forms there are 12–13 million cases of leishmaniasis world wide; the annual incidence is 600 000 new clinical cases and 350 million people are at risk of infection. Leishmaniasis is transmitted by sandflies and the clinical manifestations of infection vary depending on the species of *Leishmania* involved (WHO 1990a).

Cutaneous leishmaniasis is characterized by skin ulcers that heal slowly and leave scars. The species causing cutaneous leishmaniasis in the Old World are *L. tropica*, *L. major* and *L. aethiopica*; the latter is also the aetiological agent of diffuse leishmaniasis. In the New World, cutaneous leishmaniasis is mainly caused

by *L. braziliensis, L. mexicana, L. amazonensis, L. venezuelensis, L. panamensis* and *L. guyanensis. L. braziliensis* and *L. panamensis* are mainly responsible for mucocutaneous leishmaniasis, a condition in which cutaneous lesions spread to the mucosa of the mouth and nose and *L. mexicana* and related forms are responsible for diffuse cutaneous leishmaniasis in the New World (WHO 1990a, Rey 1991).

The development of new territories, explosive migration, rapid urbanization and the associated environmental changes are expanding the areas where human cutaneous leishmaniasis commonly occurs.

Cutaneous leishmaniasis is not usually life threatening, but clinical visceral leishmaniasis (kala azar) is often fatal if untreated. Visceral leishmaniasis is caused by *L. donovani* and *L. infantum* in the Old World and *L. chagasi* in the New World. Although most infections are asymptomatic or subclinical, those associated with malnourishment often result in severe disease. In the Indian subcontinent 400 000 new cases are estimated to have occurred each year with a case fatality rate of 5–7%. Large epidemics of kala azar occurred in India in 1978, 1982 and 1987 (WHO 1990a). An epidemic in Southern Sudan was first recognized in mid 1988 and by 1993, 300 000–400 000 people were at risk of infection and 40 000 were thought to have died. In some villages, the population decreased by 30–40% as a consequence of the epidemic (WHO 1993a).

Prevention of cutaneous leishmaniasis is based on

(1) case detection and treatment; (2) the destruction of sandflies and their breeding places; and (3) the prevention of contact between humans and sandflies. In addition to these measures, the canine reservoir must also be eliminated to prevent visceral leishmaniasis in the Mediterranean and American regions. Treatment costs (drug only) for cutaneous and mucocutaneous leishmaniasis vary from US$60 to US$70 per person, in different regions. Control costs for visceral leishmaniasis are US$100 per person. When other related costs are included, the cost of each case of visceral leishmaniasis amounts to US$250. When treatment with amphotericin is needed (because of failure of other drugs to bring about cure) the cost of each case increases by US$45 (WHO 1990a, WHO 1993a).

MALARIA

Malaria is the most important protozoan disease affecting humans. People suffering from malaria mostly live in poverty in rural areas where *Anopheles* mosquitoes are present. Over 40% of the world's population remains exposed to varying degrees of risk from malaria and one or more types of malaria occur in 90 regions of the world (WHO 1994c, 1994d, 1994e). The global incidence of malaria is c. 120 million clinical cases each year, the parasite being carried by 300–400 million people. Countries in tropical Africa account for >80% of all clinical cases and >90% of all carriers (WHO 1992a and 1995a). The reporting of incidence figures for large regions tends to mask trends within countries and among countries in a region. The malaria situation has improved in some countries but has deteriorated in others. In India, the reduction in reported malaria cases from 9 million to 5 million between 1976 and 1984 was largely due to a return to levels that had occurred before a peak just prior to 1976.

Some areas are particularly susceptible to epidemics of malaria. These include the 'frontier areas' in South East Asia and South America which have experienced substantial population increases and are now being rapidly developed. In the highly endemic areas of Africa, there has been little change in levels of infection, but epidemics associated with weather and population movement have occurred in areas of low endemicity (WHO 1992a). Malaria distribution in the world and major problem areas are shown in Fig. 2.5 (WHO 1993b).

Of the 5.3 million cases reported to the World Health Organization in 1992 (excluding the African Region), 75% were concentrated in 6 countries: Afghanistan, Brazil, Colombia, India, Sri Lanka and Vietnam (Table 2.4) (WHO 1994c). Within these countries, malaria is concentrated in certain areas (WHO 1992a).

Severe and fatal malaria infections are usually caused by *P. falciparum*, the predominant species of malaria in tropical Africa. In the rest of the world, *P. falciparum* is less common. For certain areas, including 'frontier areas' and areas with civil war or other conflicts, illegal trade and mass movements of refugees, malaria mortality is probably greatly underestimated

(WHO 1994c). For example, a total of 1 428 deaths from malaria was reported from the Americas in 1986 but the annual malaria mortality for the Brazilian Amazon region alone (a 'frontier area') was between 6000 and 10 000. The vast majority of deaths from malaria occur in Africa, where the death toll caused by malaria is now estimated to be 1 million per year in children (WHO 1993b). Between 1970 and 1975 malaria was responsible for 20–30% of infant mortality in Kenya and Nigeria, and in the Gambia mortality from malaria was 6.3 per 1000 per year in infants and 10.7 per 1000 per year in children <4 years of age (WHO 1992a).

Resistance of *P. falciparum* to the antimalarial drug chloroquine was detected almost simultaneously in Brazil, Colombia, Venezuela and Thailand in the late 1950s and the 1960s. Several countries have now reported the widespread presence of *P. falciparum* strains resistant not only to chloroquine but also to amodiaquine, pyrimethamine in combination with long-acting sulphonamides and to other drugs. The degree of resistance varies from country to country (Lopez Antuñano and Schmunis 1993).

P. falciparum has a high prevalence in areas that border jungles where the population is very mobile owing to expansion of agricultural and mining activities. In South America, these areas also have a high frequency of infection with *P. falciparum* strains resistant to antimalarial drugs. In such areas, migration favours contact between carriers and others who are susceptible to the infection. Exposure of large numbers of susceptible people to infected vectors gives rise to epidemics with high rates of morbidity and mortality. In these areas, the breakdown of the social structure, the absence of health service facilities and the resultant failure of diagnosis and treatment of infected people adds to the risk of infection and death from malaria.

In many of the nations that are promoting national development and experiencing expanding populations, new roads are opened into jungle areas that are undergoing agricultural development and from which natural resources are being extracted. One of the detrimental consequences of such development is an increase in the incidence of malaria, mainly because of internal migrations. The destinations of the migrants are often determined by roads planned by development officers in remote cities without any thought for public health considerations. The migrants use the new roads to penetrate into jungle areas where disease vectors abound; here they often construct temporary dwellings that lack even minimum sanitary facilities. These areas often lack basic health and education programmes as well as political and administrative organization, leaving the impoverished migrants vulnerable to disease. Some types of development programme are particularly likely to increase the risk of malaria, for example, flood-based irrigation systems used for growing rice and banana crops. Poorly built roads, dams and irrigation canals can also produce anopheline breeding sites, particularly during long periods of rain.

In areas where the population is relatively stable,

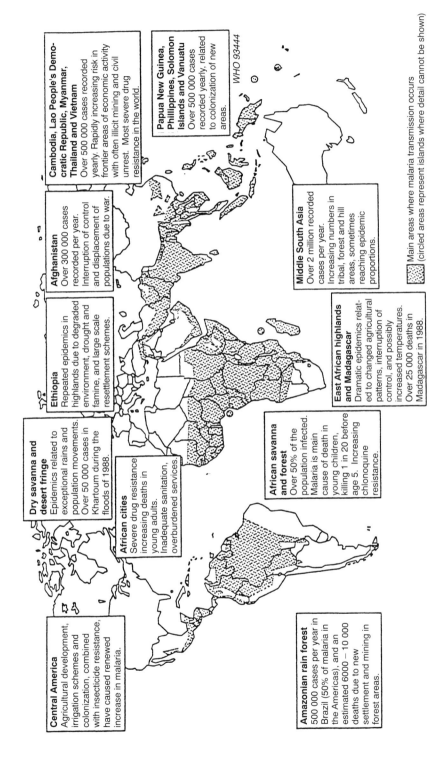

Central America
Agricultural development, irrigation schemes and colonization, combined with insecticide resistance, have caused renewed increase in malaria.

Dry savanna and desert fringe
Epidemics related to exceptional rains and population movements. Over 50 000 cases in Khartoum during the floods of 1988.

African cities
Severe drug resistance increasing deaths in young adults. Inadequate sanitation, overburdened services.

Ethiopia
Repeated epidemics in highlands due to degraded environment, drought and famine, and large scale resettlement schemes.

Afghanistan
Over 300 000 cases recorded per year. Interruption of control and displacement of populations due to war.

Cambodia, Lao People's Democratic Republic, Myanmar, Thailand and Vietnam
Over 500 000 cases recorded yearly. Rapidly increasing risk in frontier areas of economic activity with often illicit mining and civil unrest. Most severe drug resistance in the world.

Papua New Guinea, Phillippines, Solomon Islands and Vanuatu
Over 500 000 cases recorded yearly, related to colonization of new areas.

WHO 93444

Middle South Asia
Over 2 million recorded cases per year. Increasing numbers in tribal, forest and hill areas, sometimes reaching epidemic proportions.

East African highlands and Madagascar
Dramatic epidemics related to changed agricultural patterns, interruption of control, and possibly increased temperatures. Over 25 000 deaths in Madagascar in 1988.

African savanna and forest
Over 50% of the population infected. Malaria is main cause of death in young children, killing 1 in 20 before age 5. Increasing chloroquine resistance.

Amazonian rain forest
500 000 cases per year in Brazil (50% of malaria in the Americas), and an estimated 6000 – 10 000 deaths due to new settlement and mining in forest areas.

Main areas where malaria transmission occurs (circled areas represent islands where detail cannot be shown)

Fig. 2.5 Malaria distribution and problem areas. (Reproduced by permission of World Health Organization from World Health Organization 1993b.)

Table 2.4 Countries with the highest numbers of malaria cases. 1992[a,b]

Country	Number of cases
Afghanistan	297 000
Brazil	609 860
Colombia	184 023
India	2 125 800
Sri Lanka	399 349
Vietnam	212 000

[a]Data from WHO 1994c.
[b]Excluding Africa.

malaria can often be controlled by vector source reduction and by protection of households from vectors by various methods including spraying with residual insecticides. For migrant populations, the best approach for prevention and control is promotion of the use of self-protection devices such as screened tents, mosquito nets impregnated with insecticide and insect repellents. In all situations, early case detection and treatment will decrease morbidity and prevent mortality. Selection of the appropriate control measures requires assessment of the risk factors present in the area. In most cases it is necessary to use several control measures in an integrated fashion (López Antuñano and Schmunis 1993).

For most countries the cost of malaria has been enormous. In the USA, it was estimated to be US$500 million in 1938 (Williams 1938). In Greece prior to the 1940s, the annual costs of malaria were huge: US$12 million for the loss of working days and earnings (using the minimum wage for the calculations), US$3.5 million for treatment and US$7.5 million for deaths (Livadas and Athanassatos 1963). In India, annual costs were US$50, US$60 and US$340 million, respectively (Sinton 1938). In the 1950s lost wages amounted to US$60 million per year in Indonesia and US$14 million per year in the Philippines, where treatment costs were US$25 million per year and costs due to deaths were US$15 million per year (Wernsdorfer and Wernsdorfer 1988). In Paraguay, the economic potential of a family with malaria was 74–86% of the potential of families without the disease (Conly 1975).

High malaria prevalence with its concomitant high social and economic costs interferes with the productivity and stability of agricultural settlements (Sawyer 1993). In Thailand in 1952, at the beginning of the intensification of the antimalarial programme, the loss in agricultural production caused by malaria was US$1.52–1.90 million. Fourteen years later, this figure had decreased to US$0.30–0.37 million per year (Kuhner 1971). The cost of deaths associated with malaria was estimated at US$157 million in Mexico for the period 1949–1963 (Wernsdorfer and Wernsdorfer 1988). In 1985 in Africa a malaria episode in a person cost US$1.80 directly and US$9.80 indirectly. Another study showed that the cost of providing treatment was US$0.21 per child and US$0.63 per adult. The direct expenditures incurred as a result of malaria by low and high income households during a year in Malawi

were US$19.13 and US$19.84, respectively and the indirect costs were US$2.13 and US$20.61, respectively (Ettling et al. 1994). Thus, it is not surprising that direct and indirect costs of malaria in Africa as a whole were US$800 million in 1987 (WHO 1993b) and were predicted to reach US$1.8 billion by 1995 (WHO 1995a). High costs caused by malaria are not limited to Africa. In Thailand, for example, the cost of the malaria control programme was US$17 million in 1980 (Kaewsonthi and Harding 1984). Resistance to (1) DDT and other insecticides and (2) to chloroquine and other drugs has significantly increased the costs associated with malaria prevention and control. In the Americas, good records of the cost of malaria control programmes have been kept for several years and these indicate a continuous increase in the funds spent on antimalarial activities. Unfortunately, funding from international organizations and bilateral agencies has steadily decreased (Fig. 2.6) (López Antuñano and Schmunis 1993, PAHO 1994 and 1995). From 1979 to 1982, expenditures by the 21 American countries with active control programmes exceeded US$500 million (Lopez Antuñano and Schmunis 1993).

Table 2.5 shows the overall budget for the health sector, the budget devoted to public health and the budget for malaria control programmes in countries of the Americas (PAHO 1994). Despite high expenditures for malaria control, the problem of malaria in the Americas remains unsolved.

INTESTINAL PROTOZOA

Intestinal protozoa are the aetiological agents of several widespread parasitic diseases, the most common of which are caused by *E. histolytica* and *G. duodenalis* (also known as *G. lamblia*).

Amoebiasis, caused by *E. histolytica*, is a cosmopolitan infection transmitted by the faecal-oral route. Its greatest impact is in Africa and Asia. In Africa, Egypt, Morocco and countries located between 10°N and 10°S are severely affected. Prevalence is high in Asia,

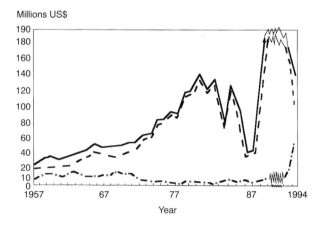

Fig. 2.6 Funds for malaria programs in the Americas, 1957-1993. Total funds ——; funds provided by local governments - - -; funds provided by international or bilateral aid agencies -.-. (Data from Lopez Antuñano and Schmunis 1993, PAHO 1994 and 1995.)

Table 2.5 Funds assigned to the health sector, public health and malaria prevention and control programmes from the countries of the Americas 1993[a]

Countries (by geographical sub-regions)	Budget for health sector	Budget for public health	Percentage assigned for public health	Budget for malaria programmes	% of health sector	Loans or grants for malaria programmes
Mexico	13 376 794 032	1 494 709 452	11.17	28 441 613	0.21	—
Belize	9 717 172	1 655 934	17.04	477 919	4.92	100 000
Costa Rica	1 166 108 757	50 479 687	4.33	1 714 017	0.15	344 310
El Salvador	887 956 536	84 883 721	9.56	1 220 930	0.14	1 023 255
Guatemala	134 204 319	93 324 434	69.54	2 434 719	1.81	166 985
Honduras	805 829 807	83 904 586	10.41	2 016 013	0.25	283 072
Nicaragua d)	…	…	…	…	…	301 647
Panama	344 163 190	172 081 595	50.00	3 719 976	1.08	71 000
Haiti	973 600	…	…	20 000	2.05	250 000
Dominican Republic	…	…	…	599 334	…	517 815
French Guiana	…	…	…	538 535	…	—
Guyana	…	…	…	91 973	…	—
Brazil	…	1 130 947 000	…	97 124 000	…	5 500 000
Bolivia	96 404 722	35 846 246	37.18	187 066	0.19	—
Colombia	…	738 829 332	…	13 524 381	…	—
Ecuador	204 632 124	100 307 839	4.90	4 963 244	0.24	—
Peru	5 380 095 982	…	…	…	…	—
Venezuela	10 735 841 686	851 385 818	7.93	6 976 914	0.06	4 600 000
Argentina	…	…	…	1 826 000	…	—
Paraguay	225 233 859 410	83 547 789 813	37.09	6 405 522	0.003	—
Total	260 218 581 338	88 386 145 456	33.97	172 282 156	0.066	13 158 084

[a]US dollar conversion based on United National exchange rates as of 31 Dec. 1993 (Pan American Health Organization 1994).

particularly in Bangladesh, Myanmar (formerly Burma), China, India, Iraq, the Republic of Korea and Vietnam. The amoebae in these countries are highly pathogenic. Amoebiasis is also a problem in Mexico and other Latin American countries. On the other hand, in Europe and the USA amoebic infection is often asymptomatic or benign in spite of prevalence rates as high as 2–5% (WHO 1981). In 1984 it was estimated that 500 million people world wide were infected with *E. histolytica* and that 40–50 million individuals had clinical symptoms of amoebiasis, including diarrhoea, dysentery and liver disease. World-wide amoebiasis causes 40–100 thousand deaths per year (WHO 1981, 1987, 1993c).

The highest prevalence of *G. duodenalis* occurs in the tropics and subtropics where sanitation is poor. Transmission may be direct by ingestion of faeces or indirect through ingestion of contaminated water or food. Travellers to tropical Africa, Mexico, Russia, South East Asia, southern Asia and western South America are at a high risk of acquiring giardiasis (Wolfe 1992). Giardiasis may infect 200 million people world wide and may produce symptoms in 500 000 individuals every year (Walsh and Warren 1979, WHO 1987, 1993c).

In developing countries, *G. duodenalis* is one of the first pathogens to infect infants and peak prevalence rates of 15–20% occur in children <10 years old (Hill 1993). In developed countries, outbreaks frequently occur in child care settings (Thompson 1994) and in adults who drink contaminated water. From 1977 to 1988, giardiasis was the leading cause of outbreaks of water-borne disease in the USA, causing an estimated 4 600 hospital admissions annually (Lengerich, Adiss and Juranek 1994). Homosexual males constitute a special risk group.

G. duodenalis may cause acute or chronic diarrhoea, steatorrhoea, loose stools, malabsorption of fat (Benenson 1990) and growth retardation and malnutrition in children (Farthing et al. 1986). Its major impact is on children <3 years old, the undernourished and the immunocompromised. It is also a cause of morbidity in adults (Farthing 1993).

Prevention of amoebiasis and giardiasis is based on the implementation of good personal hygiene, appropriate disposal of human waste and adequate handling and treatment of water supplies. The combination of filtration and chlorination usually eliminates these organism from water, but higher concentrations of chlorine and longer exposure times are needed than those required for the elimination of bacteria. Boiling is an effective method of purifying drinking water for personal use.

There are few estimates of the cost of amoebiasis, but one calculation suggested that in Mexico in 1984 expenditure for the treatment of invasive amoebiasis was 1.6% of the budget of the Health Ministry (WHO 1987). In the developing countries, the costs associated with giardiasis are difficult to estimate because there are no hard data on the number of cases of diarrhoea induced by giardiasis. An estimate made on the basis of the number of admissions to hospitals for giardiasis in the USA suggests direct costs of US$3–5 million annually.

2.2 The helminth worms

Dracunculiasis (Guinea worm disease)

Dracunculiasis occurs in 16 sub-Saharan countries in Africa, as well as in India and Pakistan. It afflicts the 10 African countries considered to be among the least developed countries of the world, where the gross domestic product ranges from US$450 to US$550 per inhabitant per year. The number of cases reported in the 1980s world wide was 5–10 million and this decreased to 3 million in 1992, to 229 773 in 1993 and to 164 973 in 1994. Niger, Nigeria and Sudan accounted for two-thirds of all cases from Africa (WHO 1993c and 1995c).

Dracunculiasis causes disability as a result of the migration of the parasite through the host. This migration results in localized pain, mainly in the areas around the joints. When the worm emerges through the skin, the pain at the site is severe and is accompanied by general symptoms of fever, nausea and vomiting. There is a painful oedema followed by a blister and then an ulcer at the site of penetration. Extraction of the worm may cause disability for 2–4 weeks.

The success of the eradication campaign now underway in many countries is based on the provision of potable drinking water through the construction of safe wells. In infected areas, prevention is implemented through health education programmes that convey the message that drinking contaminated water is the origin of the disease, that individuals with open blisters and ulcers should not be permitted to come into contact with any source of drinking water and that water must be treated (by boiling, chlorinating or filtering) to eliminate the larvae of the crustaceans that act as the intermediate hosts. In Nigeria, control of the intermediate host costs US$3.00 per household for water filters and US$1 per capita for cement ring wells. This amounts to c. 30% of the estimated potential losses suffered in a season due to incapacity caused by the disease (Guyatt and Evans 1992).

Filariasis

About 750 million people in 76 countries live in areas of endemic filariasis, an estimated 90 million of them are infected with filariae. Of these, 72.8 million are infected with *W. bancrofti* and 5.8 million are infected with a variety of species of *Brugia* (WHO 1993c). There are 300 000 individuals infected with filariae in 7 countries of the Americas; 48.6 million in 8 countries of South East Asia (4.8 million infected with *Brugia*); 3.9 million in 14 countries or territories of the western Pacific (1 million infected with *Brugia*); and 25.6 million in 40 countries in Africa (WHO 1992b). Almost 40 million people world wide suffer from lymphoedema, elephantiasis or hydrocoele caused by bancroftian filariasis, 14 million of them in Africa and 21 million in South East Asia. World wide, *Brugia* is believed to cause lymphoedema and elephan-

tiasis in 2.8 million people of which 1 900 000 are in South East Asia and 900 000 are in the western Pacific (WHO 1994f).

Clinical manifestations of bancroftian and brugian filariasis vary widely in different geographical areas from asymptomatic microfilaraemia and malaise to acute symptoms characterized by adenolymphagitis with fever, hydrocele, lymphoedema, elephantiasis and chyluria, the last 4 being characteristic of chronic bancroftian filariasis (WHO 1992b). In India, it is estimated that an infected person suffers 4.47 acute attacks per year if they have bancroftian filariasis and 2.20 acute attacks per year if they have brugian filariasis. Each attack has an average duration of 4 days and the numbers of working days lost per year per person are 17.43 and 8.91, for bancroftian and brugian filariasis respectively (WHO 1992b).

The vectors of filariasis are *Culex, Anopheles, Aedes* and *Mansonia* mosquitoes. Slum dwellers with poor housing and sanitation are at the highest risk of bancroftian filariasis transmitted by *C. quinquefasciatus* whereas the rural poor suffer more from filariasis transmitted by other mosquitoes. Control measures are directed towards reduction of vector density and interruption of contact between human and vector by the application of a combination of chemical or biological control measures, environmental management and personal protection measures (WHO 1992b). Treatment is another factor in control and involves annual administration of a single dose of diethylcarbamazine (DEC) or a combination of DEC and ivermectin (WHO 1994g). Control costs vary with the scope of coverage and the strategy, or combination of strategies, used. Control costs are US$1.8 million in China; US$1 million in India and Thailand; US$500 000 in Egypt and Malaysia; and from US$27 000 to US$300 000 in French Polynesia, Papua New Guinea and Sri Lanka (WHO 1994g).

Between 75 million and 122.9 million people are at risk of onchocerciasis (river blindness), which is endemic in 28 countries in Africa and 6 countries in the Americas. In Africa 17.7 million people are infected with *O. volvulus*, of whom 500 000 have damaged vision and 267 000 are blind. In the Americas, 140 000 people are infected with *Onchocerca* of whom 750 are blind (WHO 1995d).

Many individuals infected with *O. volvulus* are asymptomatic. Symptoms of acute dermal or ocular infection are rare clinical manifestations of chronic established infection, the most severe consequences of which are reduction of the visual field and blindness. The impact of the disease is seen mainly in sub-Saharan countries where in some areas up to 40% of adults may have severe visual impairment. This results in an inability of the family to support itself and a decrease in agricultural output that leads to unstable communities (WHO 1995d).

Control activities were originally based on control of the black fly *Simulium*, the vector of onchocerciasis, but are now based on yearly administration of single doses of ivermectin to people at risk. Vector control has been successful in many areas and has resulted in the virtual interruption of transmission in 11 countries of west Africa. Levels of infection in children have been significantly reduced and the numbers of infected people decreased from 1 million in 1975 to 10 000 in 1992. Since the inception of the prevention programme, 100 000 people have avoided blindness. Costs of ivermectin distribution vary from US$0.10 to US$5 per person per year (WHO 1995d).

FOOD-BORNE TREMATODE INFECTIONS

Food-borne trematode infections have their highest prevalence in South East Asia and in the western Pacific; they are also present in areas of Africa, the Americas and Europe. The geographical areas involved are expanding as are the populations at risk as a result of improvements in transportation that favour population movements and trade. It is estimated that food-borne trematode infections affect 40 million people throughout the world (WHO 1995b). The food-borne parasites of greatest public health importance are *Fasciola, Clonorchis, Paragonimus* and *Opisthorchis.*

Human fascioliasis, caused by *F. hepatica* and *F. gigantica*, has been reported from Bolivia, China, Ecuador, Egypt, Iran, Peru, Portugal and Spain, 2.4 million people being infected altogether. Clonorchiasis has been observed in China, Hong Kong, Macao, Republic of Korea, Russia and Vietnam and estimates suggest that 7 million people are infected. Opisthorchiasis, caused by *O. viverrini* and *O. felinus*, occurs in Kazakhstan, Laos, Russia, Thailand and Ukraine; 10 million people are infected. Of less importance from the public health viewpoint are the intestinal flukes that cause echinostomiasis, fasciolopsiasis, heterophyiasis, metagonimiasis and nanophyetiasis. These infections are found in China, Egypt, Japan, Republic of Korea, Russia and Thailand and c. 1.2 million people are infected (WHO 1995b).

The epidemiology of these diseases is determined by ecological and environmental factors. Aquatic or semiterrestrial snails are the intermediate hosts and the reservoir hosts are fish, crustaceans or mammals. Human infection occurs from ingestion of raw or uncooked fish, shellfish or aquatic plants that harbour the infective metacercariae (Fig. 2.7). In some areas, industrial production of cultured fish and shellfish may be related to the spread of food-borne trematodes (Benenson 1990, WHO 1995b).

To prevent human *Fasciola* infection, infection of livestock must also be controlled, as humans are only accidental hosts. The consumption of watercress or other aquatic plants from areas where sheep or cattle graze should be avoided, as should be the use of animal faeces for fertilizing water plants. Mollusc hosts should be eliminated when possible. The best method for prevention of infection with *Clonorchis* and *Opisthorchis* is to avoid eating raw fish and to use sanitary methods for disposal of faeces. Infection with these parasites is serious as they not only produce liver disease but also increase the risk of cholangiocarcinoma. *P. westermani* and several other related species cause lung fluke disease. These parasites have freshwater crabs as their intermediate hosts and prevention is effected by thoroughly cooking crustacea, by disposal of sputum and faeces in a sanitary manner and by snail control when feasible (Benenson 1990). In migrants to developed nations lung fluke infection is often misdiagnosed as tuberculosis. Programmes for control of food-borne trematodes should be multisectoral, integrating the activities related to human health, food safety, aquaculture, agriculture and education (WHO 1995b).

The economic burden of these diseases stems from a number of direct and indirect costs associated with the infections, including morbidity, loss of productivity, absenteeism and cost of health care in infected people as well as losses in agricultural and aquacultural enterprises. The wages lost annually in Thailand as a result of opisthorchiasis in 15–60 year olds are estimated at US$60 million and the cost of medical care is US$19.4 million. In addition, the cost of control for a 6 year period (1988–1993) (with a coverage of 3 million people) was US$8.3 million, including costs for faecal examinations, drugs and the promotion and training of personnel for community participation in control programmes. In the Republic of Korea, control programmes provide medical examinations and treatment for 15 million people and cost an estimated US$2.5 million per year (WHO 1995b).

INTESTINAL WORMS: *ASCARIS* AND *TRICHURIS*

Ascaris lumbricoides infections have been reported during the last few years from >150 of the 208 states and countries of the world. Hookworms and the whipworm, *Trichuris trichura*, are as widely distributed as *Ascaris* (Bundy and Cooper 1989, WHO 1987). These parasites are soil-transmitted helminths of global importance. Strongyloidosis has a patchy global distribution and is less prevalent than ascariasis. *Ascaris* has high prevalence in the subtropical and tropical areas of Africa, Asia and the Latin American countries. Although common in humid parts of the world, *Trichuris* is also found in temperate climates. Hookworm infection has almost been eradicated from Europe and the USA. The hookworm *Necator americanus* occurs in the Americas, equatorial Africa, southern Asia, South East Asia, Polynesia and Australia. *Ancylostoma duodenale*, another hookworm, is more common in Africa and in northern and south-western Asia. The ranges of both species of hookworm (and of other parasites of global importance) often overlap.

During 1977–1978, 800 million–1000 million people were infected with *Ascaris* and of these 1 million had symptoms; hookworm infected 700–900 million people, of whom 1.5 million had symptoms; and *Trichuris* affected 500 million people of whom 100 000 had symptoms. The number of deaths due annually to *Ascaris* and hookworms in this period were approximately 20 000 and 50 000 respectively (WHO 1993c). Subsequently, it was reported that *Ascaris* and *Trichuris* cause clinical symptoms in 214 and 133 million people, respectively and that hookworm causes clinical symptoms in 96 million (WHO 1995a).

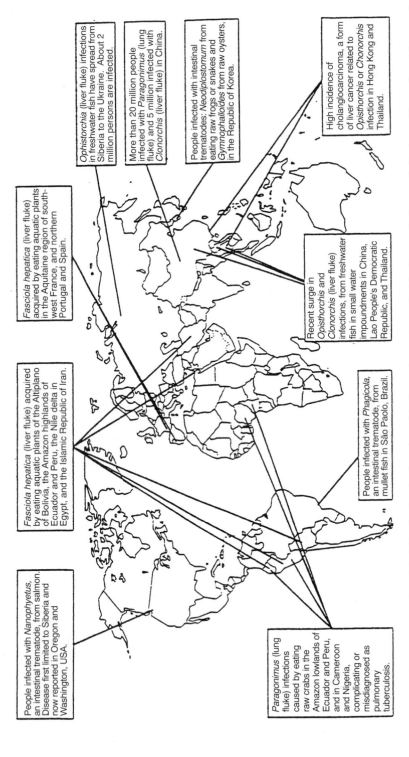

People infected with *Nanophyetus*, an intestinal trematode, from salmon. Disease first limited to Siberia and now reported in Oregon and Washington, USA.

Fasciola hepatica (liver fluke) acquired by eating aquatic plants in the Aquitaine region of south-west France, and northern Portugal and Spain.

Ophistorchia (liver fluke) infections in freshwater fish have spread from Siberia to the Ukraine. About 2 million persons are infected.

More than 20 million people infected with *Paragonimus* (lung fluke) and 5 million infected with *Clonorchis* (liver fluke) in China.

People infected with intestinal trematodes: *Neodiplostomum* from eating raw frogs or snakes and *Gymnophalloides* from raw oysters, in the Republic of Korea.

High incidence of cholanglocarcinoma, a form of liver cancer related to *Opisthorchis* or *Chonorchis* infection in Hong Kong and Thailand.

Fasciola hepatica (liver fluke), acquired by eating aquatic plants of the Altiplano of Bolivia, the Amazon highlands of Ecuador and Peru, the Nile delta in Egypt, and the Islamic Republic of Iran.

Recent surge in *Opisthorchis* and *Clonorchis* (liver fluke) infections, from freshwater fish in small water impoundments in China, Lao People's Democratic Republic, and Thailand.

People infected with *Phagicola*, an intestinal trematode, from mullet fish in São Paolo, Brazil.

Paragonimus (lung fluke) infections caused by eating raw crabs in the Amazon lowlands of Ecuador and Peru, and in Cameroon and Nigeria, complicating or misdiagnosed as pulmonary tuberculosis.

Fig. 2.7 Food-borne trematode infections: the global distribution is changing with the environment and with changes in human behaviour. (Reproduced by permission of the World Health Organization from World Health Organization 1995b.)

The impact of these parasites on public health is related to the severity of the infection; heavy infections cause malabsorption and large blood and protein losses which are compounded in the context of poor nutritional status. Heavily infected people are also at risk of developing complications such as intestinal obstruction or anaemia. The impact of these parasitic diseases is difficult to evaluate, as they may cause effects such as retarded physical growth, retarded development of cognitive skills, low participation in education and poor performance (Evans and Jamison 1994). None of these effects is easy to isolate and measure routinely. Although there is a relationship between parasitic infections and human malnutrition, it is sometimes difficult to determine which is the primary factor because there are similarities in the socioeconomic conditions in which these conditions both occur (Crompton and Nesheim 1982).

Ascaris is mainly prevalent in young people, i.e. children aged 6–12 years. *Trichuris* infections peak in early life and then generally remain steady, whereas hookworm prevalence peaks in adolescence. Heavy worm burdens of *Ascaris* and *Trichuris* are found in children of primary school age (WHO 1981 and 1987).

In many communities 15% of the infected population harbour >60% of the worms. As morbidity is usually related to intensity of infection, heavily infected individuals have a greater risk of developing disease symptoms, and they also cause the most contamination of the environment (Anderson 1986). In addition, individuals with a heavy worm burden are more likely to re-acquire heavy infection after treatment and to suffer from polyparasitism (Anderson and Medley 1985, Bundy and Cooper 1989).

The growth and nutrition of children are adversely affected by *Ascaris* and *Trichuris* infection and there are remarkable improvements in appetite, food intake, digestion, absorption and growth in infected children who receive treatment (Cooper et al. 1990, Stephenson et al. 1989). Hookworm infection often causes iron deficiency anaemia which may reduce productivity in affected individuals. The infection and the resulting anaemia may impair mental development in children, negatively influencing their cognitive performance. Infection may also complicate pregnancy (Stephenson 1984, Prescott and Jancloes 1984, WHO 1987).

The cost of infection by intestinal worms is huge. In the late 1970s US$4.4 million was lost in Kenya annually by worm infested people in the form of nutrients wasted as unabsorbed food. In the same country in 1976 the cost incurred by the government for treatment of parasitic intestinal infections was US$339 000 (costs for examining patients and for drugs) and the cost incurred by affected families US$394 000 (cost for drugs, lost wages and for transportation). These figures seem to be low as 88 804 patients were admitted to hospitals that year as a result of ascariasis in Kenya (Stephenson 1984, WHO 1987).

Programmes for prevention of infection with intestinal worms must be based on the use of several strategies, focusing on improvements in basic sanitation, waste disposal, health education and health services. In the short term, immediate action can be taken by administering the drug albendazole, which decreases morbidity and mortality. One strategy is to select the target population and then treat only those who are infected. This approach requires screening the entire population. It has been estimated that in Rwanda, application of this strategy would cost US$600 000 in salaries excluding costs for the collection and handling of samples. Treatment of infected individuals (about two-thirds of the population for round worms and one-third for flat worms) would cost US$64 000 per year. An alternative programme using chemotherapy (piperazine and niclosamide) on all individuals has been estimated to cost US$440 000 per year (de Schaepdryver 1984). Improving basic environmental sanitation and treatment facilities would be considerably more expensive than either of these policies. Control of these parasites requires a massive effort to raise the standard of living of the affected population if the benefits of any treatment programmes are to have a lasting effect.

SCHISTOSOMIASIS

Schistosomiasis is the most important and prevalent of the water-borne parasitic diseases. It is a major health risk in the rural areas of 74 developing countries. Five species of *Schistosoma* affect humans: (1) *S. mansoni* occurs in 36 countries in Africa, 9 in the Americas and 7 in the east Mediterranean; (2) *S. japonicum* is found in China, Indonesia, the Philippines and Thailand (3) *S. mekongi* occurs in Cambodia and Laos; (4) *S. intercalatum* is present in 5 Central African countries; and (5) *S. haematobium* is prevalent in 51 eastern Mediterranean and African countries and in India and Turkey.

The first 4 species listed cause intestinal schistosomiasis and *S. haematobium* causes urinary schistosomiasis.

It is estimated that >200 million people residing in rural and agricultural areas are infected with schistosomes and that 500–600 million people are exposed to infection. The estimated mortality rate is about 200 000 per year (WHO 1985, 1993d and 1994h).

The prevalence of schistosomiasis within a country varies widely; in some countries the entire population is exposed, in others, there are only scattered foci of disease. Morbidity also varies widely, the foci of clinical disease usually being highly localized. The incidence of clinical schistosomiasis may be significantly higher in countries where the prevalence of the infection is >40% (WHO 1985). In the past 10 years, the incidence and prevalence of schistosome infection have decreased in some areas but the infection become more widespread in other areas. Large hydroelectric and agricultural irrigation projects (some involving the creation of artificial water reservoirs) and associated population movements are considered to be responsible for many of the increases.

Rates of infection with schistosomes are higher for men than for women because cultural and social biases in behaviour and occupation cause men to be more exposed to contaminated water.

Of the individuals infected with *S. haemotobium*, 60–70% are aged 5–14 years and this group is also the most heavily infected group in areas where *S. haemotobium* is endemic. Haematuria is present in 80% of infected children. The prevalence and intensity of urinary disease is lower in older age groups. In contrast, *Schistosoma japonicum* infection has no typical age prevalence and intensity distribution (WHO 1985 and 1993d).

In areas endemic for *S. mansoni*, the highest prevalence of infection is in those aged 10–24 years, but the prevalence in older groups may also be high. Usually, the most heavily infected individuals are those aged 10–14 years. A significant proportion of these individuals (those with an egg count of <800 eggs/g of faeces) have hepatomegaly and splenomegaly (WHO 1985 and 1993d). Poverty, ignorance, substandard housing and poor sanitation are the main factors that maintain these endemic foci.

Several studies have been made on the public health impact of the schistosomiasis. In these studies, the following parameters have been assessed: school performance, physical fitness, growth, productivity and earnings. Although results have not been conclusive (Tanner 1989) there is consensus that in north-eastern Brazil, Egypt and Sudan there is a severe reduction of the work capacity of the rural population as a consequence of schistosomiasis (WHO 1994h).

The economic impact of schistosomiasis is partly a result of the large number of working days lost per infected person per year. This loss is 4.4 and 40 days per year per person for those infected with *S. haematobium* and *S. japonicum*, respectively. About 10% of people infected with *S. mansoni* develop severe symptoms. The number of days of life lost because of schistosomiasis is c. 600–1000 per case (Walsh and Warren 1979). The global burden caused by schistosomiasis amounts to 4 500 000 DALYs (World Bank 1993b).

The annual per capita cost for control of schistosomiasis depends on the nature of the programme used; for example, in the case of Saint Lucia these costs were US$1.10 per person per year for chemotherapy, US$3.70 for snail control and US$4.50 for a clean water supply (US Congress 1985). Costs per protected person were estimated at US$0.70–3.10 per year in 3 African countries. This amount may seem small, but it should be taken into account that total health expenditures per person in these countries varied from US$1 to US$3 per person per year (Gryseels 1989). Case detection of infected individuals in Sudan cost US$0.03 per capita per year, just for operating the health services. In Brazil the costs, including laboratory diagnosis, consultation and drugs, were US$3.73 (Guyatt and Evans 1992). The introduction of specialized programmes, instead of using the general health services for control of schistosomiasis, increased the annual cost per person from US$1.50 to US$6.53 (WHO 1993d). A schistosomiasis control programme for control of *S. haematobium* or *S. mansoni*

in a rural area with a population of 100 000 will have a 5 year cost from US$3.70 to US$25.91 per capita. The variation is determined by the prevalence, intensity and rate of infection in the population (Rohde 1989).

MISCELLANEOUS WORMS OF REGIONAL IMPORTANCE

In addition to the parasites of global importance, there are others of regional or national relevance. These are the roundworms *Capillaria philippinensis*, *Enterobius vermicularis* and *S. stercoralis*, the cestodes *Hymenolepis nana*, *Taenia saginata*, *T. solium* and *Diphyllobothrium latum* and the trematode *Fasciolopsis buski* (WHO 1987). The most widespread of these is *S. stercoralis* which is prevalent in tropical and subtropical areas and is a severe problem in South America and the Caribbean. *Enterobius* is cosmopolitan, but human infections are most common in temperate regions and it is often found in developed countries in the northern hemisphere (WHO 1981 and 1987). Morbidity is usually low. Taeniasis, caused by *T. saginata*, is also cosmopolitan but is most prevalent in African countries south of the Sahara, eastern Mediterranean countries and in parts of the former Soviet Union. Lower prevalences are found in Europe, India and southern Asia, Japan, the Philippines and much of Latin America. The lowest prevalences are found in Australia, Canada and the USA (WHO 1979). *T. solium* is mainly restricted to low socioeconomic areas of central and southern Africa, Mexico, Central and South America and southern Asia. Sporadic cases are found in southern Europe (WHO 1979). Human cysticercosis, caused by the larval stages of *T. solium* in tissues, is far more important as a public health problem than is human taeniasis, i.e. the adult form in the intestine. The highest prevalences of human cysticercosis are found in some areas of Africa, Asia and South America (WHO 1981 and 1987). It has been estimated that there are 80–100 million cases of *Strongyloides*, 400 million of *Enterobius* and 78 million of *Taenia* world wide (WHO 1990b, Warren et al. 1993).

3 SOME SIGNIFICANT PARASITIC DISEASES: NEW AND EXPANDING THREATS

New diseases may emerge as a result of changes in ecology, human demographics and human behaviour. Factors such as international travel and commerce; introduction of new technology and industry; microbial adaptation and change; breakdown of public health measures; and social disorder all affect human health (Institute of Medicine 1992, Morse 1995). As a result, several parasites, such as *Anisakis*, *Babesia*, *Cryptosporidium*, cyclospora, *Giardia*, microsporidians, *Plasmodium*, *Pneumocystis carinii*, *S. stercolaris* and *Toxoplasma gondii* may be poised for an increase in importance (Institute of Medicine 1992, Wurtz 1994). This list could also be extended to include a number of other parasites. Some of these parasites (i.e. *Giardia*,

Plasmodium, Strongyloides and *Schistosoma*) and the factors that favour their emergence or reemergence, have been mentioned before. For example, schistosomiasis has increased in incidence in many areas after the construction of dams. A brief review of the others follows.

Anisakis is a common parasite of marine mammals and fish and the aetiological agent of herring worm disease (anisakiasis) in humans, who are incidental hosts. Humans are infected by larvae present in undercooked fish, squid or octopus. The larvae localize in the gastrointestinal tract and then migrate upwards, attaching to the oropharynx. Many cases have been observed in Japan, where it is customary to consume raw fish. Infected fish can be transported around the world and the incidence of infection is increasing because of the growing trend in the consumption of raw fish. Cases have been reported in the Americas, Asia, Europe and the South Pacific (WHO 1987, Benenson 1990, Institute of Medicine 1992). Prevention is effected by not eating raw fish.

Babesia microti is a protozoan transmitted by nymphs of the *Ixodes* tick. It infects red blood cells and is carried mainly by deer mice. Human babesiosis is usually a result of infection by *B. microti* but other species of *Babesia* have also been implicated. Babesiosis in humans has been observed in Mexico, Europe and the USA. The emergence of cases in the USA is linked to reforestation and a resultant increase in the deer population and the number of deer mice. Preventive measures include the elimination of deer mice in the vicinity of human habitations and the use of tick repellents (Benenson 1990).

The coccidian *Cryptosporidium parvum* was recognized as a human pathogen <20 years ago. Cryptosporidia live intracellularly in the gut cells of humans and domestic animals such as cattle. Transmission is by the faecal to oral route with direct person to person and animal to person and indirect waterborne transmission occurring. The parasite is found world wide and its importance as a human pathogen was recognized as a result of several small outbreaks that were either water-borne or food-borne and a massive outbreak associated with drinking water which affected more than 400 000 people in Wisconsin, USA. In immunocompetent individuals the infection may be asymptomatic or it may produce an acute or persistent diarrhoea. Individuals immunosuppressed because of HIV infection or from other causes have been the most severely affected, experiencing crytosporidiosis as an aggressively opportunistic infection. Prevention should be achieved by improving surveillance of water purification plants to detect malfunction and by applying high standards of personal hygiene. Appropriate measures include the sanitary disposal of human faeces and animal excreta. Chemical disinfection of water is ineffective against cryptosporidia because the oocysts (the infective stage) are very resistant to chlorine (Benenson 1990, Fraser 1994, Colley 1995).

Although described in 1979, *Cyclospora cayetanensis*, another coccidia, is now recognized as producing long lasting diarrhoea in humans in North, Central and South America and the Caribbean, as well as in southeast Asia and Eastern Europe. It is transmitted through contaminated water or food, but is highly unlikely to be transmitted from person to person because oocysts require days or weeks to sporulate becoming infectious (Ortega 1993, Wurtz 1994). A recent outbreak of *c.* 850 cases occurred recently in Canada and USA (Centers for Disease Control 1996). *C. cayetanensis* may be the origin of persistent diarrhoea in immunocompromised patients with AIDS. Prevention is similar to that of the other food or water borne diseases.

Microsporidia are normally parasites of animals other than humans. Four genera of microsporidia, *Encephalitozoon, Enterocytozoon, Nosema* and *Trachipleistophora*, have been recognized as human pathogens world wide, usually affecting the immunosuppressed, including those with HIV. *Encephalitozoon* has been reported to cause systemic infection with central nervous system and kidney involvement; *Nosema* is considered to be the cause of keratitis; and *Trachipleistophora* has been recognized as an agent of myositis. *Enterocytozoon*, which causes the majority of microsporidial infections in humans, produces chronic diarrhoea in AIDS patients. Parasites of a fifth genus *Septata* have also been found to infect the epithelial cells of humans and to produce systemic infections in AIDS patients. The mode of transmission of microsporidia to humans is unknown (Desportes et al. 1985, Canning and Hollister 1987, Shadduck and Greeley 1989, Centers for Disease Control 1990, Orenstein et al. 1990, Cali et al. 1991, Madi et al. 1991, Molina et al. 1993, Pol, Romana and Richard 1993).

Immunocompromised individuals throughout the world are at high risk of acquiring *Pneumocystis carinii* pneumonia. This parasite is carried by >50% of HIV patients. Also at risk are individuals who are debilitated, malnourished or chronically ill and premature infants. *Pneumocystis* transmission is probably by the airborne route (Satler 1994). In immunosuppressed carriers, prophylactic treatment is used to suppress infection.

Toxoplasma gondii is a coccidian parasite of cats that produces disease opportunistically in immunosuppressed humans on all continents. Infection is also common in immunocompetent individuals, but most of them are asymptomatic. Infection occurs as a result of eating infected raw or undercooked meat from the intermediate hosts (sheep, swine, chicken, goats, cattle or birds) or by ingestion of food or water contaminated with oocysts from cat faeces. Transplacental infection occurs when pregnant women acquire the infection during pregnancy. Prevention is based on personal hygiene, avoiding eating raw or undercooked meat and avoiding contact with cat faeces. Patients with AIDS must receive prophylactic treatment to prevent disease caused by *Toxoplasma* (Benenson 1990, Wong and Remington 1994).

Table 2.6 Global estimates of parasitic infections[a,b]

	Infected population	No. of cases	Population at risk	Annual deaths
African trypanosomes[c]	250–300[b]	250–300[b]	50–55[a]	55[b]
American trypanosomes[d,e]	16–18[a]	3.2–3.6[a]	60[a]	45[b]
Amoebiasis[f]	500[a]	40–50[a]		40–100[b]
Ascariasis[g]	785–1150[a]	1[a]–214[a]		20–60[b]
Clonorchiasis[h]	7[a]		289.3[a]	
Dracunculiasis[i]	164[b]		100[a]	
Enterobiasis[j]	400[a]			
Fascioliasis[h]	2.4[a]		180[a]	
Filariasis[k]	78.6–90[a]	5[a,l]	751[a]	
Giardiasis[m]	200[a]	500[b]		
Hookworms[n]	750–1000[a]	1.5[a]–96[a]		50–90[b]
Intestinal flukes[h]	1.3[a]			
Leishmaniasis[o]	12–13[a]	600[b]	350[a]	80[b]
Malaria[p]	500[a]	250–450[a]	2400[a]	2[a]
Onchocerciasis[q]	17.5[a]	270[b,r]	75–80[a]	
Opisthorchiasis[h]	10.3[a]		63.5[a]	
Paragonimiasis[h]	20.5[a]		194.8[a]	
Schistosomiasis[s]	200[a]		400–500[a]	200[b]
Strongyloidosis[j]	80–100[a]			
Taeniasis[t]	70[a]			
Trichuriasis[v]	750–100[a]	1[b]–133[a]		

[a]Millions; [b]Thousands; [c]WHO 1994d and 1995a; [d]Schmunis 1994; [e]400 000 cases of heart and hollow viscera disease annually, WHO 1995a; [f]WHO 1987 and 1993c; [g]WHO 1990b, 1993c and 1995a; [h]WHO 1995b; [i]WHO 1995c; [j]WHO 1990b; [k]WHO 1992b, 1993c and 1994f; [l]disabled; [m]WHO 1987 and 1993c; [n]WHO 1993c and 1995a; [o]WHO 1990a, 1993c and 1995a; [p]WHO 1993b and 1995a; [q]WHO 1995c; [r]Blind; [s]WHO 1985, 1993d and 1994h; [t]Warren et al. 1993; [v]WHO 1990b, 1993c and 1995a.

4 CONCLUSION

Infectious disease must be viewed as a global problem, a problem exacerbated by dynamic ecological changes brought about by technological, socioeconomic, environmental and demographic changes as well as by microbial change and adaptation (Institute of Medicine 1992). The mobility of modern humans and the evolution of parasites (including drug resistant strains) mean that parasitic diseases are a threat in both developing and developed regions.

Parasitic infections cause human suffering and economic losses world wide but the burden is greatest in the underdeveloped countries. Millions of people are at risk of infection, disease and death from protozoan and metazoan parasites. These parasites cause social problems and their effects are increased by the conditions in disordered societies. Their presence hampers educational, political and economic development, imposing a tremendous burden on the already precarious health services in the poor areas of the world. This situation constitutes a serious public health concern and inhibits the healthy development of individuals and social groups (Table 2.6).

In developed countries, worms and protozoa present increased threats because of population movement, trade and changing life-styles. To make a comparison with a viral disease, the AIDS epidemic is a classic example of the result of human mobility and the effect of life-style choices. Implementation of prevention and control strategies requires a systematic multidisciplinary and multisectoral approach.

For many diseases there is sufficient knowledge to develop successful control programmes. The following factors are vital: (1) knowledge of the means of spread of the parasite and of any reservoirs; (2) a means of detecting both clinically apparent and asymptomatic infection; and (3) a system of treatment or a method of interrupting spread. In addition, it is also neccesary to have the political will to implement control programmes, and this is often lacking in societies that lack cohesion and where social and economic chaos prevail. Meanwhile, failure to use classic public health measures while waiting for a 'miraculous' system of cure will retard progress. Because of the complexity and cost of controlling infectious diseases, the worldwide burden caused by parasitic infections is only likely to decrease in the context of both social and economic development.

REFERENCES

Alleyne GAO, 1983, What is the role of institutions in the developing world, *New Developments in Tropical Medicine*, vol 2, eds Simpson TW, Strickland GT, Mercer MA, Ntl Council Intl Hlth, Washington DC, 9–14.

Anderson RM, 1986, The population dynamics and epidemiology of intestinal nematode infections, *Trans R Soc Trop Med Hyg*, **80:** 706–18.

Anderson RM, Medley GF, 1985, Community control of helminth infections of man by mass and selective therapy, *Parasitology*, **90:** 629–60.

Apt WB, 1991, Aspectos clínicos de la enfermedad de chagas en Chile y sus repercusiones económicas, *Programa de actividades. Taller sobre erradicación o control de la enfermedad de Chagas en Chile, Santiago*, 8.

Benenson AS, 1990, *Control of Communicable Diseases in Man*, 15th edn, Pub Hlth Ass, Washington DC, 96, 97, 112, 163, 183 and 440.

Bundy DAP, Cooper ES, 1989, Human trichuris and trichuriasis, *Adv Parasitol*, vol 29, Academic Press, London and New York, 107–73.

Cali A, Meisler DM, Rutherford I et al., 1991, Corneal microsporidiosis in a patient with AIDS, *Am J Trop Med Hyg*, **44:** 463–8.

Canning EU, Hollinster WS, 1987, Microsporidia of mammals – widespread pathogens or opportunistic curiosities? *Parasitol Today*, **3:** 262–73.

Centers for Disease Control, 1990, Microsporidian keratoconjunctivitis in patients with AIDS, *Morbid Mortal Weekly Rep*, **39:** 188–9.

Centers for Disease Control, 1996, Update: outbreaks of Cyclospora cayetanensis infection – United States and Canada, 1996, *Morbid Mortal Weekly Rep*, **45:** 611–2.

Colley DG, 1995, Waterborne cryptosporidiosis threat addressed, *Emerg Infect Dis*, **1:** 67–8.

Conly GN, 1975, *The Impact of Malaria on Economic Development: A Case Study*, Sci Pub 297, Pan Am Hlth Org, Washington, DC.

Cooper ES, Bundy DA, Mac Donald TT et al., 1990, Growth suppression in the trichuris dysentery syndrome, *Eur J Clin Nutr*, **44:** 285–91.

Crompton DWT, Nesheim MC, 1982, Nutritional science and parasitology: a case for collaboration, *BioScience*, **32:** 677–80.

De Schaepdryver A, 1984, Costs of training and maintenance of expert man-power vs costs of drugs. Priorities in the field of helminthic diseases in developing countries, *Soc Sci Med*, **19:** 1113–16.

Desportes I, Le Charpentier Y, Galian A et al., 1985, Occurrence of a new microsporidian: *Enterocytozoon bieneusi* n.g. n.sp., in the enterocytes of human patient with AIDS, *J Protozool*, **32:** 250–4.

Dias JCP, 1987, Control of chagas' disease in Brazil, *Parasitol Today*, **3:** 336–41.

Dias JCP, Loyola CCP, Brener S, 1985, Doença de Chagas em Minas Gerais: Situação actual e perspectivas, *Rev Bras Malariol Doencas Trop*, **37:** 7–28.

Ettling M, McFarland DA, Schultz LJ et al., 1994, Economic impact of malaria in Malawian households, *Trop Med Parasitol*, **45:** 74–9.

Evans DB, Jamison DT, 1994, Economics and the argument for parasitic disease control, *Science*, **264:** 1866–7.

Evequoz MC, 1993, *Evaluación de la Miocardiopatia Chagásica. Grados II y III. Estimación de costos*, Tesis. Universidad Nacional de Córdoba. Facultad de Medicina. Escuela de Salud Pública Córdoba, Argentina.

Farthing MJG, 1993, Diarrhoeal disease: Current concepts and future challenges. Pathogenesis of giardiasis, *Trans R Soc Trop Med Hyg*, **3:** 17–21.

Farthing MJG, Mata L, Urrutia JJ et al., 1986, Natural history of giardia infection in infants and children in rural Guatemala and its impact on physical growth, *Am J Clin Nutr*, **43:** 395–405.

Fraser D, 1994, Epidemiology of *Giardia lamblia* and cryptosporidium infections in childhood, *Isr J Med Sci*, **30:** 356–61.

Gryseels B, 1989, The relevance of schistosomiasis for public health, *Trop Med Parasitol*, **40:** 134–42.

Guyatt HL, Evans D, 1992, Economic considerations for helminth control, *Parasitol Today*, **18:** 397–402.

Hayes, RJ Schofield C, 1990, Estimación de las tasas de incidencia de infecciones y parasitosis crónicas a partir de la prevalencia: la enfermedad de chagas en América Latina, *Bol Of Sanit Panam*, **108:** 308–16.

Hill DR, 1993, Giardiasis. Issues in diagnosis and management, *Infect Dis Clin North Am*, **7:** 503–25.

Human Development Ministry, 1994, *Chagas in Bolivia*, US Agency International Development, La Paz, Bolivia, 81–90.

Institute of Medicine, 1992, *Emerging Infections*, Institute of Medicine, Natural Academy Press, Washington DC.

Kaewsonthi S, Harding A, 1984, Cost and performance of malaria surveillance in Thailand, *Soc Sci Med*, **19:** 1081–97.

Kühner A, 1971, The impact of public health programs on economic development, *Int J Health Serv*, **1:** 285–92.

Lengerich EJ, Adiss DG, Juranek DD, 1994, Severe giardiasis in the United States, *Clin Infect Dis*, **18:** 760–3.

Livadas GA, Athanassatos D,, 1963, The economic benefits of malaria eradication in Greece, *Riv Malariol*, **42:** 177–87.

Lopes ER, Chapadeiro E, 1986, Doenca de Chagas no Triangulo Mineiro, *Rev Goiana Med*, **32:** 109–13.

López-Antuñano FJ, Schmunis GA, 1993, Plasmodia of humans, *Parasitic Protozoa*, 2nd edn, ed Kreier JP, Academic Press, San Diego, 135–266.

Madi K, Trajman A, Silva CF et al., 1991, Jejunal biopsy in HIV-infected patients, *J Acquired Immune Defic Syndr*, **4:** 930–7.

Maldonado YA, Nahlen BL, Roberto RR et al., 1986, Transmission of *Plasmodium vivax* malaria in San Diego County California, *Am J Trop Med Hyg*, **42:** 3–9.

Molina JM, Sarfati C, Beauvais B et al., 1993, Intestinal microsporidiosis in human immunodeficiency virus-infected patients with chronic unexplained diarrhoea: prevalence and clinical and biological features, *J Infect Dis*, **167:** 217–21.

Morse SM, 1995, Factors in the emergence of infectious diseases, *Emerg Infect Dis*, **1:** 7–15.

Orenstein J, Chiang J, Steinberg W et al., 1990, Intestinal microsporidiosis as a cause of diarrhoea in human immunodeficiency virus-infected patients: a report of 20 cases, *Hum Pathol*, **21:** 475–81.

Ortega YR, Sterling C et al, 1993, Cyclospora species – a new protozoan pathogen of humans, *N Engl J Med*, **328:** 1308–12.

Pan American Health Organization, 1994, *Status of Malaria Programs in the Americas*, XLII Report, Pan Am Hlth Org CSP24/INF/2, Washington DC.

Pan American Health Organization, 1995, *Status of Malaria Programs in the Americas*, XLIII Report, Pan Am Hlth Org CD38/INF/2, Washington DC.

Pereira MG, 1984, Caracteristicas da mortalidade urbana por Doença de Chagas Distrito Federal, Brasil, *Bol Of Sanit Panam*, **104:** 213–20.

Phillips-Howard P, 1991, Travellers beware, *World Health*, **Sep–Oct:** 24–5.

Pol S, Romana CA, Richard S, 1993, Microsporidia infection in patients with the human immunodeficiency virus and unexplained cholangitis, *N Engl J Med*, **328:** 95–9.

Prescott N, Jancloes MF, 1984, Selected economic issues in helminth control, *Soc Sci Med*, **19:** 1060–84.

Rey L, 1991, *Parasitologia*, 2nd edn, Guanabara Koogan, Rio de Janeiro, 182–215.

Rohde R, 1989, Schistosomiasis control: an estimation of costs, *Trop Med Parasitol*, **40:** 240–4.

Rosenfield PL, Golladay F, Davidson RK, 1984, The economics of parasitic diseases: research priorities, *Soc Sci Med*, **19:** 1117–26.

Sattler FR, 1994, Pneumocystis carinii pneumonia, *Textbook of*

AIDS Medicine, eds Broder S, Merigan TC, Bolognesi D, Williams and Wilkins, Baltimore, 193–221.

Sawyer D, 1993, Economic and social consequences of malaria in new colonization projects in Brazil, *Soc Sci Med*, **37**: 1131–6.

Schmunis GA, 1991, *Trypanosoma cruzi*, the etiologic agent of chagas' disease: status in the blood supply in endemic and non endemic countries, *Transfusion*, **31**: 547–57.

Schmunis GA, 1994, American trypanosomiasis as a public health problem, *Chagas Disease and the Nervous System*, 547, Pan Am Hlth Org Sci Pub, Washington, DC, 3–29.

Schofield CJ, Dias JCP, 1991, A cost benefit analysis of Chagas' disease control, *Mem Inst Oswaldo Cruz*, **86**: 285–95.

Shadduck JA, Greeley E, 1989, Microsporidia and human infections, *Clin Microbiol Rev*, **2**: 158–69.

Sinton, 1938, What malaria cost India, *Govt India Hlth Bull*, **26**.

Stephenson LS, 1984, Methods to evaluate nutritional and economic implications of ascaris infections, *Soc Sci Med*, **19**: 1061–5.

Stephenson LS, Latham MC, Kurz KM et al., 1989, Treatment with a single dose of albendazole improves growth of Kenyan school children with hookworm, *Trichuris trichura*, and *Ascaris lumbricoides* infections, *Am J Trop Med Hyg*, **41**: 78–87.

Tanner M, 1989, Evaluation of public health impact of schistosomiasis, *Trop Med Parasitol*, **40**: 143–8.

Thompson SC, 1994, *Giardia lamblia* in children and the child care setting: A review of the literature, *J Pediatr Child Health*, **30**: 202–9.

US Congress, 1985, *Status of Biomedical Research and Related Technology for Tropical Diseases*, US Congress office of technological assessment OTA H-258, US Govt Print Off, Washington DC, 101–2.

Villalba R, Fornes G, Alvarez MA et al., 1992, Acute Chagas disease in a recipient of a bone marrow transplant in Spain: case report, *Clin Infect Dis*, **14**: 594–5.

Walsh JA, Warren KS, 1979, Selective primary health care. An interim strategy for disease control in developing countries, *N Engl J Med*, **301**: 967–74.

Warren KS, Bundy DAP, Anderson RM et al., 1993, Helminth infections, *Disease Control Priorities in Developing Countries*, eds Jamison DT, Mosley WH, Measham AR, Bobadilla JL, Oxford Medical Publications, Oxford, 131–60.

Wernsdorfer G, Wernsdorfer WH, 1988, Social and economic implications of malaria and its control, *Principles and Practices of Malariology*, vol 2, Churchill Livingstone, New York, 1421–71.

Williams LL, 1938, Economic importance of malaria control, *New Jersey Mosq Extermin Ass*, **25**: 148–51.

Wilson ME, 1995, Travel and the emergence of infectious diseases, *Emerg Infect Dis*, **1**: 39–46.

Wolfe MS, 1992, Giardiasis, *Clin Microbiol Rev*, **5**: 93–100.

Wong SV, Remington JS, 1994, Toxoplasmosis and the setting of AIDS, *Textbook of AIDS Medicine*, eds Broder S, Merigan TC, Bolognesi D, Williams and Wilkins, Baltimore, 233–57.

World Bank, 1993a, *World Development Report 1993a, Investing in Health. World Development Indicators*, Oxford University Press, Oxford, 25–36.

World Bank, 1993b, *World Development Report 1993b, Investing in Health. World Development Indicators*, Oxford University Press, Oxford, 213–25.

World Health Organization, 1977, *Manual of the International Statistical Classification of Diseases Injuries and Causes of Death*, WHO, Geneva.

World Health Organization, 1979, Parasitic zoonosis, *W H O Tech Rep Ser*, **637**.

World Health Organization, 1981, Intestinal protozoan and helminthic infections, *W H O Tech Rep Ser*, **666**.

World Health Organization, 1985, The control of schistosomiasis, *W H O Tech Rep Ser*, **728**.

World Health Organization, 1986, Epidemiology and control of African trypanosomiasis, *W H O Tech Rep Ser*, **739**.

World Health Organization, 1987, Prevention and control of intestinal parasitic infection, *W H O Tech Rep Ser*, **749**.

World Health Organization, 1990a, Control of the leishmaniases, *W H O Tech Rep Ser*, **793**.

World Health Organization, 1990b, *Informal Consultation on Intestinal Helminth Infections*, W H O /CDS/IPI/90.1, WHO, Geneva.

World Health Organization, 1992a, World malaria situation in 1990, Part I, *W H O Wkly Epidemiol*, **67**: 161–8.

World Health Organization, 1992b, Lymphatic filariasis: the disease and its control, *W H O Tech Rep Ser*, **821**.

World Health Organization, 1993a, Leishmaniasis epidemic in Southern Sudan, *W H O Weekly Epid Rec*, **68**: 41–2.

World Health Organization, 1993b, A global strategy for malaria control, World Health Organization, Geneva.

World Health Organization, 1993c, Global health situation IV. Selected infectious and parasitic diseases due to identified organisms, *W H O Wkly Epidemiol Rec*, **68**: 43–4.

World Health Organization, 1993d, The control of schistosomiasis, *W H O Tech Rep Ser*, **830**.

World Health Organization, 1994a, *Control of Tropical Diseases, 1. Progress Report*, W H O, CTD/MIP/94.4, W H O, Geneva, 41–4.

World Health Organization, 1994b, *Control of Tropical Diseases 1. Progress Report*, W H O STD/MIP/94.4, W H O, Geneva, 33–5.

World Health Organization, 1994c, World malaria situation in 1992, *W H O Wkly Epidem Rec*, **42**: 309–14.

World Health Organization, 1994d, World malaria situation in 1992, *W H O Wkly Epidemic Rec*, **43**: 317–21.

World Health Organization, 1994e, World malaria situation in 1992, *W H O Wkly Epidem Rec*, **44**: 325–30.

World Health Organization, 1994f, *Control of Tropical Diseases, 1. Progress Report*, W H O , CTD/MIP/94.4, W H O , Geneva, 27–31.

World Health Organization, 1994g, *Lymphatic Filariasis Infection and Disease: Control Strategies*, W H O TDR/CTD/FIL/Penang/94.1, W H O , Penang, Malaysia.

World Health Organization, 1994h, *Control of Tropical Diseases, 1. Progress Report*, W H O CTD/MIP/94.4, W H O, Geneva, 23–6.

World Health Organization, 1995a, *The World Health Report. Bridging the Gap. Executive Summary*, W H O, Geneva, 1–5.

World Health Organization, 1995b, Control of food borne trematode infections, *W H O Tech Rep Ser*, **849**.

World Health Organization, 1995c, Dracunculiasis, *W H O Wkly Epidemiol Rec*, **70**: 125–32.

World Health Organization, 1995d, Onchocerciasis and its control, *W H O Tech Rep Ser*, **852**.

Wurtz R, 1994, Cyclospora: a newly identified intestinal pathogen of humans, *Clin Infect Dis*, **18**: 620–3.

Zicker F, Zicker EM, 1985, Beneficios providenciarios por incapacidade como indicador de morbidade. Estudo da doenca de Chagas em Goias, *Rev Goiana Med*, **31**: 125–36.

EPIDEMIOLOGY OF PARASITIC INFECTIONS

R M Anderson

1 INTRODUCTION

Epidemiology is the study of patterns of infection and associated disease within populations or defined communities. It is interdisciplinary in character, drawing on concepts and methods from a wide variety of biomedical fields including molecular biology, immunology, genetics, population biology, statistics and mathematics, plus the specific fields associated with a particular infection such as virology, bacteriology, parasitology and vector biology. It is a quantitative field of medicine relying on accurate surveillance and measurement of infection plus disease, and dependent on statistical methods for hypothesis testing, parameter measurement and description plus mathematical techniques for the provision of a theoretical template to facilitate the interpretation of observed pattern or experimental outcome. A sound and detailed knowledge of the biology of the host and infectious agent, however, is an essential prerequisite for the successful application of such quantitative tools.

The past decade has witnessed significant changes in the manner in which epidemiological research is conducted, largely arising from the availability of new methods of measurement or detection of infection or disease linked to rapid advances in the disciplines of molecular biology and immunology. One example is the use of polymerase chain reaction (PCR) methods to detect the presence of very low concentrations of a particular pathogen within the human host. Such techniques enable quantitative measures to be made of parasite load or burdens within infected patients, in addition to the more precise determination of the prevalence (proportion of hosts infected) of infection. New immunological tools greatly facilitate the detection of current or past infection with non-invasive sample collection procedures (such as saliva-based assays for antibodies specific to viral, bacterial and

parasite infections) being of particular value in field based studies.

Advances in other areas have also made very important contributions to epidemiology, particularly in the field of genetics. Molecular methods and the increased availability of genome sequence data for both pathogen and host open new avenues for the study of the determinants of pathogenesis and the coevolution of the parasite and its human or vector host. Increasingly, linkage or segregation analyses are beginning to find associations between the occurrence of disease, or persistent infection, and particular genotypes within human populations. Molecular or genetic epidemiology will undoubtedly be a major growth area in the coming decade. Associated population genetic studies can define the frequency of predisposition to infection or disease within defined populations.

There has also been a growing realization amongst researchers in this area that conventional statistical approaches to epidemiology, which have been so successful in improving understanding of non-infectious disease problems, are less appropriate for the study of the population level consequences of infection and immunity. Increasingly, concepts and methods that have evolved in evolutionary biology, ecology and population genetics are being used to study the population biology, transmission dynamics and evolution of infectious diseases within human communities. Such approaches recognize that the interaction between parasite and host is a very dynamic one, in terms of transmission and persistence, and of the evolution of both organisms (with that of the pathogen having the potential to take place much more rapidly than that of the human host).

Observed patterns of infection and disease in human communities are determined by the interplay between the variables that control susceptibility to infection, its typical course and the likelihood of serious disease within an individual, and the variables that control the rate of transmission between people. The former include innate susceptibility, the distribution of latent and infectious periods plus the duration of acquired immunity, while the latter include behavioural, social, environmental and demographic factors. Researchers are typically concerned with the recondite biological and clinical details that make each infection unique. This chapter focuses on the principles that determine observed epidemiological patterns, independent of the type of infectious agent under study. Historically work on infectious disease is often compartmentalized into distinct areas based on the taxonomy of the infectious agent, namely, virology, bacteriology and parasitology. However, the principles governing the spread, persistence and evolution of all infectious agents are the same. A simple example is provided by the notion of reproductive or transmission success. If we consider the host as the basic unit of study, then the reproductive number of an infection (R_0) is the average number of secondary cases of infection generated by one primary case in a susceptible host population (Anderson and May 1991). The magnitude of this parameter reflects the potential for transmission and evolution, and the degree to which control measures must inhibit transmission if an infection is to be eradicated in a given population.

The real world is of course replete with complications – economic and social as well as biological – and it is easy to lose sight of generalities when grappling with the details that ultimately make each infectious agent unique. However, it is often the case in epidemiology that the influence of a few factors dominates the generation of observed pattern. Understanding the key principles that underpin spread and persistence helps in the identification of these factors.

This chapter highlights the key processes that influence the transmission, persistence and control of protozoan and helminth parasites with a focus on malaria, intestinal nematodes, schistosome flukes and the filarial worms. Bear in mind, however, that the principles are equally relevant to the study of viral and bacterial infections (Anderson and May 1979).

2 BASIC CONCEPTS

2.1 Microparasites and macroparasites

A distinction is made between **microparasites** and **macroparasites** to cut across conventional taxonomic lines in order to focus on the population biology of the infectious agent.

MICROPARASITES

Microparasites may be thought of as those agents which have direct reproduction – usually at very high rates – within the host (Anderson and May 1979). They tend to be characterized by small size and a short generation time. Recovery from infection is usually associated with acquired immunity against reinfection with the same strain of parasite for some time, and

often for life. For many viruses, bacteria and protozoa, however, immunity may be highly strain specific although a degree of cross-protection may arise via shared antigens. Although there are important exceptions, the duration of infection is typically short relative to the expected life span of the human host. This feature, combined with acquired immunity, means that microparasite infections are typically of a transient nature in individual hosts. Most viral, bacterial and (in a less certain manner) many protozoan parasites fall broadly into the microparasitic category.

For such infectious agents, it makes sense to stratify the host population into a few classes namely: susceptibles, infecteds but latent (i.e. non-infectious), infecteds and infectious, and immune individuals. A reasonable operational definition of a microparasite is an organism whose population biology can, to a sensible first approximation, be described by such a compartmental model. An essential feature of the framework is that no account is taken of the degree or severity of the infection (i.e. the abundance of the infectious agent within the host). The reality of heterogeneity between individuals with respect to genetic background, behaviour and environment is replaced by the abstraction of some average 'infected' or 'immune' individual.

It is often necessary to distinguish between infection and disease. The period between the point of infection and the appearance of symptoms of disease is termed the **incubation period.** The duration of symptoms of disease is not necessarily synchronous with the period during which an infected host is infectious to susceptible individuals. Furthermore, the host may be infected but not infectious. The period from the point of infection to the beginning of the state of infectiousness is termed the **latent period**. For some infections such as malaria, intermittent bouts of infectiousness may occur. For others, such as HIV, the degree of infectiousness may vary widely throughout the incubation period. The sum of the latent and infectious periods is referred to as the average **generation time** of the infection. The term average refers to the fact that latent, infectious and incubation periods are often very variable between individuals due to a variety of factors such as host and parasite genetic background and the size of the infecting inoculum of the infectious agent.

Most epidemiological and demographic parameters – human birth and death rates, disease-induced death rate, recovery rates, rate of loss of immunity – can be measured directly by appropriate observational studies. The transmission rate, however, combines many biological, social and environmental factors, and is thus rarely amenable to direct measurement. The best way is to infer this rate indirectly via longitudinal or cross-sectional cohort based studies to directly measure the incidence of infection.

MACROPARASITES

Macroparasites may be thought of as those having no direct reproduction within the definitive host. This category embraces helminths and arthropods, where transmission stages produced within or on the host pass to the exterior to complete development to the next stage of often complex life cycles which may involve more than one host (e.g. the schistosome flukes and the filarial worms). Macroparasites are typically larger than microparasites and have much longer generation times, often being an appreciable fraction of the human host's life span. When an immune response is elicited, it usually depends on the past and present number of parasites harboured, and tends to be of a relatively short duration once parasites are removed (e.g. by chemotherapy) from the host. Thus macroparasitic infections are typically persistent in character, with hosts continually being reinfected. The evocation of an immune response and the pathology induced by infection both depend on the burden of parasites harboured by the host. This means that to quantify levels of infection and morbidity in the population it is necessary to measure the distribution between individuals of parasite numbers per host. As shown in Fig. 3.1 parasite numbers are rarely uniformly or randomly distributed. Typically, the distributions are highly heterogeneous with most people harbouring few parasites and a few harbouring many. Compartmental models based on divisions into susceptible and infected persons are therefore inappropriate descriptions of the epidemiology of macroparasitic infections. The appropriate framework for study is one that records the prevalence (fraction infected) of infection, the average intensity of infection and the distribution of parasite numbers within the human population.

The division into microparasites and macroparasites is rather crude. Many infectious agents are not easily forced into this dichotomous scheme. Many protozoan parasites such as the *Plasmodium* species that induce the disease malaria may, to a good approximation, have their epidemiology described by a microparasitic compartmental framework (i.e. prevalence of infecteds, susceptibles and immunes), although their patterns of persistence within the human population, with individuals being repeatedly

infected, are characteristic of macroparasites. However, the dichotomy serves as a useful starting point for highlighting the population biology and epidemiology, as opposed to emphasizing conventional taxonomic categorizations.

2.2 Basic reproductive number of infection, R_0

For a microparasite the basic or case reproductive rate, R_0, is defined as the average number of secondary cases of infection produced by one primary case in a susceptible population. When a microparasitic infection first invades a human community, the fraction susceptible decreases over time. Eventually some sort of equilibrium state is reached (**endemic infection**) which may involve oscillatory fluctuations in prevalence or incidence of a seasonal or longer term nature. At this equilibrium (or oscillating equilibrium) the rate at which susceptible infants or children are infected is exactly balanced by the rate at which new susceptibles are born into the community and each infection will on average produce exactly one secondary case. That is, at equilibrium, the effective reproductive rate $R = 1$. If we assume that the human community mixes homogeneously (independent of age, sex, residence location, etc), the effective reproductive rate R is equal to the basic reproductive rate, R_0, discounted by x, the fraction of the human community that is susceptible, R, is equal to $R_0 x$. Given that at equilibrium $R = 1$, then

$$R_0 = 1/x \qquad (2.1)$$

where x is the fraction susceptible at equilibrium. This simple relationship provides a method of estimating the value of R_0 from serological or other data on age-specific susceptibility.

For a macroparasite, R_0 is the average number of female offspring (in the case of a dioecious parasite) produced throughout the lifetime of a mature female parasite, which themselves achieve reproducive maturity in the absence of density-dependent constraints. In the absence of these constraints, which include competition for space or other resources within the human host and acquired immunity dependent on parasite load, parasite numbers within the population would grow exponentially provided $R_0 > 1$. In practice macroparasite populations tend to be rather stable through time and a variety of density-dependent factors act to generate such stability.

For most common viral and bacterial infections and some protozoa (e.g. *Toxoplasma*), serological tools are available to establish whether or not a person has acquired and recovered from infection at some time in their past. Age-stratified cross-sectional serological surveys or longitudinal cohort studies provide the best information for estimating the magnitude of R_0 in a given community. A diagrammatic serological profile is shown in Fig. 3.2. The magnitude of R_0 can either be estimated from this profile by calculating the fraction of the total population susceptible to infection or equally simply from the following expression:

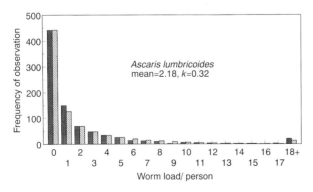

Fig. 3.1 The frequency distribution of *Ascaris lumbricoides* in a fishing community in Pulicat, Tamil Nadu, India (after Elkins et al. 1986). The negative binomial probability distribution provides a good empirical description of the observed pattern with mean = 2.8 worms per person and $k = 0.32$. Dark bars, observed value; hatched bars, expected value.

$$R_0 = (L - M)/(A - M) \qquad (2.2)$$

where L is life expectancy, M is the average duration of maternal antibody derived protection (typically 6 months for many common viral infections such as measles) and A is the average age at infection. The key quantity is A, which can be estimated directly from the serological profile (Grenfell and Anderson 1985). If the value of A is small, R_0 is large, and the infection has high transmission efficiency, while, conversely, if A is large, R_0 is small, and the infection has low reproductive success. Transmission success of a given parasite can vary widely in value between different locations and at different times of the year.

Serological surveys provide a wealth of information about the transmission dynamics of infectious agents. They not only provide information on the values of M (duration of maternally derived protection) and A (average age at infection) but they can also guide decisions on the optimum age at which to vaccinate and on the fraction who should be immunized to block transmission. Carrying out large-scale surveys to include infants, children and adults can be difficult if blood samples are required to extract serum for the evaluation of the presence or absence of antibodies specific to particular antigens. Techniques based on the testing of saliva for secreted antibodies (Perry et al. 1993) have been developed for a variety of infectious agents and these provide epidemiologists with a powerful tool for the study of transmission. Serum or saliva samples must be collected at random within the community, taking due note of important stratifications within the population such as age, sex, ethnic background, residence location, etc. However, problems can arise if the duration of measurable antibody production following infection is not life long. This is thought to be the case for many bacterial and protozoan infections which makes serological surveys of less value in determining past and current patterns of transmission. We require more sophisticated techniques to detect immunological markers of past infection with antigenically variable parasitic organisms. In general, however, the collection of serological data, finely stratified according to age, is of vital importance in any quantitative assessment of transmission and the potential impact of control measures. Ideally, age-stratified cross-sectional surveys should be conducted each year such that a profile of herd immunity can be constructed prior to and post the introduction of any intervention programme.

The measurement and interpretation of the magnitude of R_0 can be made complicated by genetic variability within the parasite population when such variability is reflected by different phenotypic properties such as transmissibility or antigenic characteristics (Gupta and Day 1994). Consider a protozoan that induces lifelong immunity in those who recover from infection. In such cases R_0 is inversely related to the average age at infection, A, by a simple relationship

$$R_0 = L/A \qquad (2.3)$$

where L is human life expectancy. However, lifelong immunity is rarely observed in parasitic protozoa due largely to the existence of many distinct antigenic strains of a particular parasite species. In such cases recovery from infection by one strain may or may not confer a degree of resistance to another strain depending on their degree of 'antigenic' relatedness. Immunity may then only develop as a consequence of exposure to many different antigenic types or strains circulating in a given locality. This appears to be the case for the malaria parasite *Plasmodium falciparum.* Young children in hyperendemic malaria zones may experience many clinical attacks of malaria per year (Greenwood, Marsh and Snow 1991). Although older children develop a functional but non-sterilizing immunity manifest as a reduction in clinical episodes, a substantial reduction in parasite load is only observed in adults after a long period of exposure to the genetical diverse population of parasites. If the delay in the development of immunity is a direct consequence of the antigenic diversity within the parasite population (as opposed to parasite evasion or modulation of the host's immunological attack) then we would expect to see a slower rise by age of immunological (seroepidemiology) evidence of exposure to a particular strain, but a much faster rise in the exposure to 'malaria', where the latter is defined as the experience of any one of several strains. When n strains are independently circulating in a defined population, the average age on first exposure to malaria, A_n, is

$$A_n = 1 / \sum_{i=1}^{n} R_{0i} \qquad (2.4)$$

Here it assumed that strain-specific immunity is life-long and R_{0i} defines the case reproductive number of strain i. This equation makes clear that a low average age at first infection (often the case for *P. falciparum*) can arise when the transmissibilities of each of many strains circulating is low. These conclusions are well supported by field observation on the rise with age in

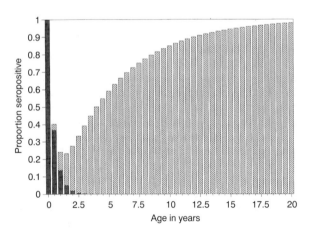

Fig. 3.2 Diagrammatic representation of a cross-sectional seroepidemiological survey, stratified by age, for the presence of antibodies specific to parasite antigens. Dark bars, maternal antibodies; hatched bars, antibodies from infection.

the fraction of a population in Madang, Papua New Guinea who had experienced infection with 5 antigenically distinct strains of *P. falciparum* (Gupta et al. 1994) (Fig. 3.3).

2.3 The relationship between prevalence and intensity of infection

We have briefly noted that many sources of heterogeneity influence the distribution of parasites within a human community (Fig. 3.1). The precise degree of heterogeneity, measured either by a statistic such as the variance/mean ratio (V/M) of parasite load per host, or the aggregation parameter, k (which varies inversely with the degree of aggregation) of the negative binomial probability distribution (which provides a good empirical model of many observed distributions), determines the relationship between the prevalence and mean intensity of infection (Fig. 3.4a). As the degree of contagion or aggregation increases the prevalence reaches to a plateau, well below 100%, as the mean parasite load rises. For a given species of parasite, observed patterns of heterogeneity are often remarkably constant independent of the study community or geographical region (Anderson and May 1985, see Fig. 3.4b). For helminth parasites in particular, worm load is directly correlated with the likelihood of symptoms of disease. As such parasite aggregation determines the prevailing burden of disease in a given population for a fixed mean worm load, the greater the degree of parasite aggregation the smaller the number of individuals in the population showing symptoms of disease. However, for extreme aggregation the severity of disease will be greater in those showing symptoms due to their very high worm loads.

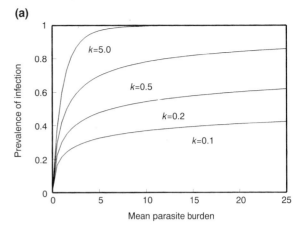

(a)

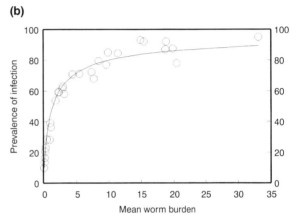

(b)

Fig. 3.4 (a) The relationship between the prevalence and mean intensity of infection predicted by the negative binomial distribution for different values of the aggregation parameter k (where $k \rightarrow 0$ reflects extreme aggregation and $k \rightarrow 5$ reflects a random distribution of parasite numbers per host). (b) A comparison of the observed and expected (on the basis of the negative binomial model with $k = 0.586$) relationship between the prevalence and intensity of infection with *Ascaris lumbricoides* in different human communities. The circles represent observed values; the continuous line is the expected value (after Guyatt et al. 1990).

2.4 Heterogeneity and predisposition to infection

The epidemiological measures of prevalence and average intensity of infection are summary statistics of the frequency distribution of parasite numbers per host (Fig. 3.1). The form of these distributions is of great significance to the burden of disease in a population and the regulating constraints acting on the net rate of parasite transmission. For helminths and protozoa the distributions are highly aggregated or contagious in form such that most individuals harbour few parasites and a few individuals harbour many. In other words, the variance in parasite load is much greater in value than the mean.

Parasite aggregation may arise as a consequence of a wide variety of factors, either acting alone or concomitantly (Anderson and Gordon 1982). These include heterogeneity in exposure to infection (due

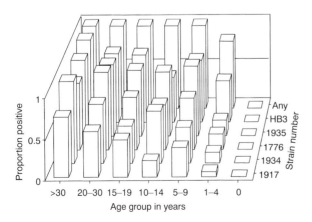

Fig. 3.3 Age-stratified serological survey for presence of past infection by a series of distinct isolates or strains (serotypes) of *Plasmodium falciparum* from a community in Papua New Guinea (data from Gupta, Trenholme et al. 1994). The isolates differ in parasite induced erythrocyte surface antigens (PIESAs). The proportion exposed to any type is recorded at the back of the graph (= Any).

to social, environmental or behavioural factors, or to aggregation in the spatial distribution of infective stages or infected intermediate hosts), differences in susceptibility to infection (due to genetic or nutritional factors, or to varying past experience of infection) or to variability in parasite survival within different individuals (due to genetic, immunological, or nutritional factors). Which factors are of major importance as determinants of observed patterns is often difficult to ascertain in particular settings. Heterogeneity in the human behavioural patterns associated with exposure to infection is often very important as well illustrated by water contact patterns in relation to *Schistosoma mansoni* transmission (Fulford et al. 1996) (see Fig. 3.6). However, host genetic background is undoubtedly of greater importance as well illustrated by the practice of using inbred strains of rodent hosts in the experimental study of many parasitic infections in order to reduce variability in the typical course of infection.

A growing number of studies are pointing to genetic factors in human communities as key determinants of susceptibility to infection and disease. For example, severe clinical disease in schistosomiasis is typically the consequence of heavy infection, the occurrence of which is determined largely by the susceptibility or resistence of individuals (Wilkins et al. 1987). The intensity of infection in a particular study site in Brazil has been shown to be influenced by a major gene leading to the hypothesis that worm burden is largely controlled by the genetic background of the human host concomitant with the degree of exposure to infection (Abel et al. 1991). The gene, referred to as *sm1*, is located on chromosome 5 and the region in which segregation analysis indicates it lies contains several candidate genes that encode immunological molecules that are known to play important roles in the acquisition of resistance to *S. mansoni* (Marquet et al. 1996).

The discovery of a clear genetic marker for predisposition to heavy infection in the study of Marquet et al. (1996) in the case of schistosomes may point the way to a better understanding in general of predisposition to helminth infection and associated disease. Epidemiological studies based on the quantification of worm load, chemotherapeutic treatment and the monitoring of patterns of reinfection post treatment, have provided firm evidence of predisposition to heavy infection for a variety of parasites including *Ascaris lumbroides* (Elkins et al. 1986), *Necator americanus* (Schad and Anderson 1985), *Trichuris trichiura* (Bundy et al. 1987) and *Schistosoma mansoni* (Bensted Smith et al. 1987). Undoubtedly, however, genetic factors act concomitantly with the host behaviours to determine parasite load.

Aggregated distributions of parasite numbers per host are also of importance for protozoans such as the malarial parasites. Observed heterogeneities include the distribution of oocysts in mosquito populations, the number of distinct antigenic types or strains per human host or per mosquito, and the frequency distribution of mosquito bites per person (Paul et al. 1995,

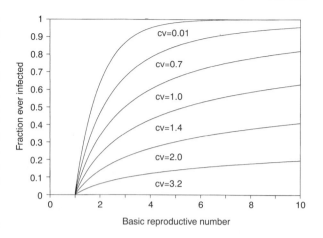

Fig. 3.5 The predicted relationship between the fraction of a population infected by a microparasite over the course of an epidemic in a virgin population and the degree of heterogeneity in the human behaviours that dictate exposure to infection as measured by the coefficient of variation (cv) where cv = 0 reflects a random distribution (see Anderson and May 1991).

Dye and Hasibeder 1986, Anderson 1994). If there is significant heterogeneity in exposure/susceptibility to infection then in epidemic situations, the fraction of the population infected will depend critically on the degree of heterogeneity in exposure. This point is illustrated in Fig. 3.5 which records the relationship between the fraction infected in an epidemic and the magnitude of transmission success of the parasite (R_0), as a function of the degree of heterogeneity in the rate of exposure to infection defined by the coefficient of variation (where cv = 0 reflects a random distribution of exposure) of the frequency distribution. An example of variation in exposure to infection is shown in Fig. 3.6.

Irrespective of the generative mechanisms of such patterns, aggregation of parasites within human communities has important implications for the epidemi-

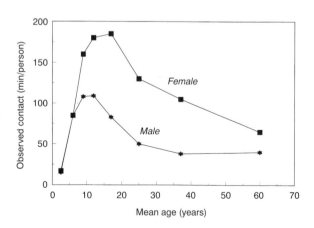

Fig. 3.6 Recorded water contact rates, stratified by age and sex in a Kenyan community where *Schistosoma mansoni* is endemic. The vertical axis records the arithmetic mean duration of water contact per individual (Kintengei community (1990–1992), after Fulford et al. 1996).

ology and control of these infections. First, it enhances the likelihood of an individual parasite finding a mate of the opposite sex (Fig. 3.7). It therefore enhances the net reproductive rate of the total parasite population. Second, it increases the net regulatory impact of density-dependent constraints on parasite establishment, survival and reproduction (often immunologically mediated). Third, it results in severe symptoms of disease typically occurring in a relatively small fraction of the total population. Finally, it has important implications for the design of control programmes (i.e. chemotherapy can be focused on those predisposed to heavy infection). If host genetic background has a major influence on immunocompetence, however, as suggested by work on *S. mansoni* (Marquet et al. 1996), then work towards vaccine development must take account of the fact that the aim of immunization must be to protect those least able to acquire immunity.

3 TRANSMISSION DYNAMICS

Observed epidemiological pattern is generated by the population or transmission dynamics of the parasite within a defined community. Before turning to the key processes influencing transmission, brief comment is made on observed patterns of prevalence and intensity of infection.

3.1 Cross-sectional surveys of prevalence and intensity of infection

A variety of methods may be employed to assess the manner in which the prevalence or intensity of infection changes over time or between different strata (such as age groups) of the population, depending on the type of infectious agent under study. These range from molecular and immunological methods to the direct counting of either parasite eggs in faecal material (intestinal nematodes) or infected red blood cells in blood samples (i.e. for *Plasmodium*). The majority of published studies are cross-sectional and stratified by age owing to the long period of study required to monitor longitudinal changes in a cohort of people over their average life span.

As illustrated in Figs 3.8, 3.9 and 3.10, changes in both prevalence and intensity with age (= time) are typically convex in form with the latter showing a greater degree of convexity than the former. Changes in prevalence as individuals age are a poor reflection of average parasite load due to the high degree of heterogeneity in the frequency distribution of parasite numbers per person. Convex patterns of change with age may arise either as a result of age-related changes in exposure to infection (due to behavioural factors) (see Fig. 3.6) and/or increased resistance to infection (where acquired immunity may influence establishment or parasite survival once in the host) in older individuals with considerable past experience of infection. With respect to convexity in prevalence an additional factor may be of importance. A decay in prevalence in older age groups could arise, independent of any change in the average worm load, if the degree of parasite aggregation increases with age. Much evidence supports this notion and it may arise due to heterogeneity in genetic make-up within the host population where some individuals develop a good degree of immunity after limited exposure while others remain predisposed to heavy infection. In general convexity is a common feature for all of the major parasitic infections and may arise from ecological (= behavioural) or immunological processes, or a combination of both.

Studies in which age-related changes in exposure have been quantified (i.e. water contact patterns in the case of schistosomes, vector biting rates for malaria and the filarial worms) suggest that a combination of both factors acts to determine the observed convex profiles. A good indication of the significance of the slow build up of immunity with repeated exposure as individuals age is provided by comparative studies of the degree of convexity as a function of the overall net intensity of transmission in a defined community. For intestinal nematodes (Anderson and May 1991), schistosomes (Anderson 1987) and malaria (Boyd 1949), the degree of convexity is greater in areas of high transmission intensity and less in areas of low average exposure (Fig. 3.11). The issue of why immunity to parasite infection builds up slowly as individuals age is discussed later in this chapter.

In summary, observed patterns of infection with parasitic organisms tend to reveal 3 key points, namely, heterogeneity in parasite burdens per person, predisposition to heavy or light infection and convexity in the manner prevalence or intensity change as individuals age.

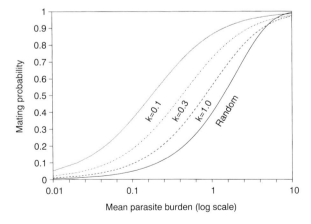

Fig. 3.7 The dependence of the probability that a female worm is mated, on the mean worm burden per person, for various assumptions concerning the distribution of parasite numbers per host for a monogamous parasite. The distributions are the negative binomial (= aggregated) with various *k* values and the Poisson (= random) distribution (after May 1977).

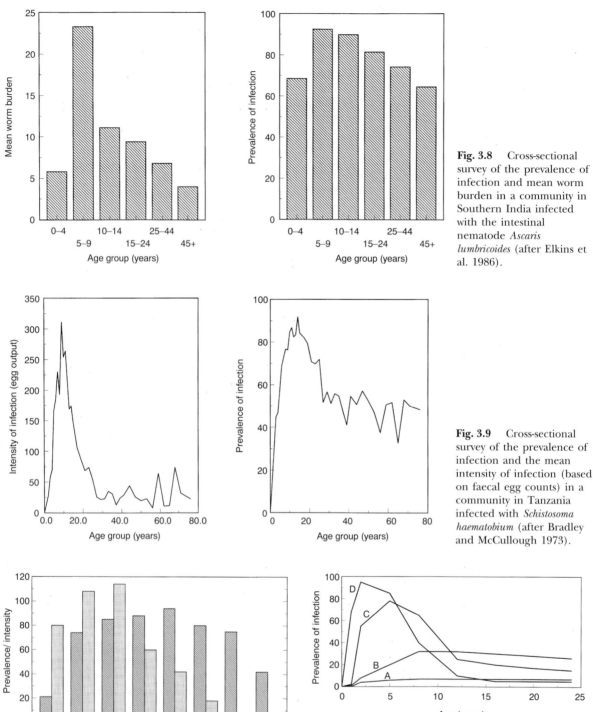

Fig. 3.8 Cross-sectional survey of the prevalence of infection and mean worm burden in a community in Southern India infected with the intestinal nematode *Ascaris lumbricoides* (after Elkins et al. 1986).

Fig. 3.9 Cross-sectional survey of the prevalence of infection and the mean intensity of infection (based on faecal egg counts) in a community in Tanzania infected with *Schistosoma haematobium* (after Bradley and McCullough 1973).

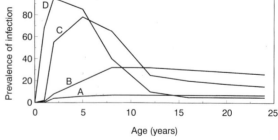

Fig. 3.11 Prevalence of acute malaria infection versus age in years in populations with differing levels of endemicity. A, low endemicity; B, moderate endemicity; C, high endemicity; D, hyperendemicity (after Boyd 1949).

Fig. 3.10 Cross-sectional survey of the prevalence (dark bars) and intensity (lighter bars) of *Plasmodium falciparum* (after Davidson and Draper 1953).

3.2 Life cycles and reproductive success

Microparasite and macroparasite life or developmental cycles may be direct or indirect. In the latter case one or more intermediate hosts may be involved, such as the molluscan intermediate host of the schistosomes and the mosquito vector of the malaria parasites. The transmission potential of a parasite with a complex life cycle is determined by many distinct population-determining rate processes that influence the many distinct developmental stages. Examples of

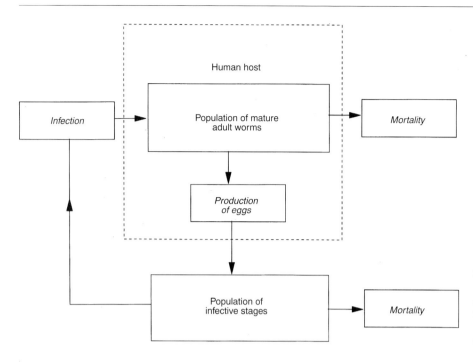

Fig. 3.12 Flow chart of the principal population and rate processes involved in the life cycle of a directly transmitted intestinal nematode (macroparasite).

the population and rate processes involved in some direct (intestinal nematodes) and indirect cycles are portrayed in Figs 3.12–3.14. The overall transmission or reproductive success is best defined by the basic reproductive number, R_0, of the parasite. For a direct life cycle intestinal nematode with a free-living larval or egg stage as the transmission stage (Fig. 3.12), the magnitude of R_0 in a human community of size N is defined as follows (see Anderson and May 1991):

$$R_0 = [s\lambda\beta N d_1 d_2]/[(\mu + \mu_1)(\mu_2 + \beta N)] \quad (3.1)$$

The individual parameters are defined in Table 3.1. Provided $R_0 > 1$ the parasite population will persist in the host population. However, unlike many directly transmitted viral or bacterial infections, the critical host density for persistence of most protozoa and helminths is typically very low. Infections such as intestinal nematodes or malaria parasites were therefore able to persist endemically in small hunter-gatherer societies in areas such as the Amazon basin or Papua New Guinea (Tyrell 1980) prior to the encroachment of civilization into remote rain forest habitats.

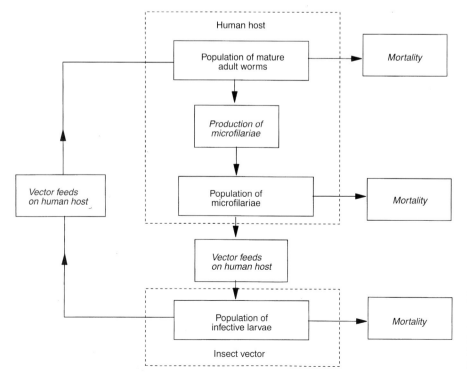

Fig. 3.13 Flow chart of the principal populations and rate processes involved in the life cycle of an indirectly transmitted filarial nematode (macroparasite).

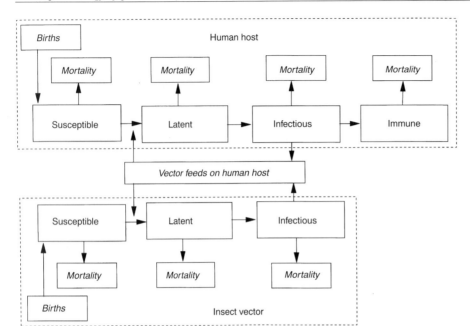

Fig. 3.14 Flow chart of the principal population and rate processes involved in the life cycle of a malarial parasite (vector transmitted microparasite).

Table 3.1 The rate processes that determine the magnitude of the basic reproductive number, R_0, of a direct life cycle intestinal nematode (see Anderson and May, 1991)

Parameter	Definition
s	Sex rate of adult worms
λ	Per capita fecundity of female worms
β	Per capita transmission rate of infective stages to the human host
d_1	Proportion of adult worms that attain sexual maturity
d_2	Proportion of transmission stages that survive to the infective stage
μ^{-1}	Life expectancy of the human host
μ_1^{-1}	Life expectancy of adult worms
μ_2^{-1}	Life expectancy of infective larvae
N	Human population size

Table 3.2 Helminth parasite life expectancy in the human host (see Anderson and May 1985 for source references)

Parasite	Life expectancy (years)[a]
Enterobius vermicularis	<1
Trichuris trichiura	1–2
Ascaris lumbricoides	1–2
Necatur americanus	2–3
Ancylostoma duodenale	2–3
Schistosoma mansoni	3–6
Schistosoma haematobium	3–6
Wuchereria bancrofti	3–5
Onchocerca volvulus	8–10

[a]Rough approximations, owing to the practical difficulties inherent in estimation.

In the absence of regulating constraints on population growth the parasite population growth rate Λ is given approximately by:

$$\Lambda = (R_0 - 1)/(\mu^{-1} + \mu_1^{-1}) \quad (3.2)$$

This expression makes clear the role of net reproductive success (R_0) and adult parasite life expectancy μ_1^{-1} as important determinants of reinfection rates, or parasite population recovery, post the cessation of control measures. Populations of short lived parasites (i.e. malaria) will bounce back rapidly to pre-controlled levels once control measures cease, while long-lived species may take many years to recover (Table 3.2).

For microparasites with indirect life cycles (Fig. 3.14) such as the *Plasmodium* species, the magnitude of R_0 is determined by rate processes acting on the human and vector populations. For malaria R_0 is defined as follows (see Aron and May 1982):

$$R_0 = [ma^2bc/\mu_2\gamma] \exp(-\mu_1 T_1 - \mu T_2) \quad (3.3)$$

where m is the ratio of female mosquitos per human host, a is the rate of biting on humans by a single mosquito (the 'human biting rate' defined as the number of bites per unit of time), b is the proportion of infectious bites that produce a patent infection, γ^{-1} is the average duration of infectiousness over the course of infection in the human host, c is the proportion of bites by a susceptible mosquito on infected people that produce a patent infection in the vector, μ_1^{-1} is mosquito life expectancy, μ_2^{-1} is human life expectancy, T_2 is the latent period in the mosquito (before it becomes infectious to humans) and T_1 is the latent period in humans (before gametocytes appear) (Table 3.3). In practice the effective time the insect vector has to transmit is much shorter than its life expectancy due to the fact that the latent period of infection in the vector is often long by comparison with life expectancy (Table 3.3). This is the reason why the prevalence of infection in vectors is often very low (a few per cent or less), since few survive long enough for the infection to mature. If $R_0 > 1$ the infection is endemic in the human population.

Vector densities often fluctuate widely over the different seasons of a year due to the influence of environmental factors such as rainfall on breeding success and life expectancy. The magnitude of m in equation (3.3) may therefore fluctuate widely such that at certain times of the year $R_0 > 1$ whilst at others (the dry season) it falls below unity in value. In such circumstances the endemic persistence of malaria depends on the survival of the infection in the human host. Areas of low transmission are much more sensitive to seasonal changes in mosquito or vector density.

More generally, the longest lived stage in the parasite's life cycle plays a key role in ensuring the long persistence of the organism. Control measures aimed at different stages in the cycle (e.g. insecticides acting on the vector or chemotherapeutic agents acting on the infection in the human host) may have similar effects on transmission success but very different effects on the ability of the parasite population to recover rapidly post the cessation or interruption of control measures.

3.3 Regulating constraints on parasite population growth

A characteristic of many parasitic infections is their stability or robustness to perturbation, whether induced by environmental changes or control interventions. Helminth infections are particularly remarkable in this sense, where post the cessation of mass chemotherapy, parasite abundance typically returns, over a time span of a year or so, to pre-control levels. In part this is a consequence of their transmission potential (e.g. very high fecundity) and in part due to the long life expectancy of the mature worms in the human host (Table 3.2). In the absence of density-dependent constraints on population growth, however, provided $R_0 > 1$, their abundance would grow exponentially. As originally noted by Malthus in the context of human population, resource limitation must eventually regulate the rate of growth until some sort of equilibrium is attained. This may be oscillating in character but for most parasites, if we ignore short term seasonal fluctuations, endemic states appear to

be stable and non-oscillatory. For parasites occupying an environment created by another living organism, the constraints on growth are many and varied and act on establishment, fecundity and survival. An example is presented in Fig. 3.15 where the fecundity of *S. mansoni* is plotted as a function of the intensity of infection. They may arise via competition for limiting resources such as food or space or, more commonly, as a result of the non-linear action of the host's immunological responses. The non-linear nature of such responses is reflected by modest or little response at very low parasite densities, and strong responses at high densities. At very high parasite (or antigen) densities in some cases the effectiveness of the immune response decays as depicted in Fig. 3.16 where T cell proliferation in response to different concentrations of *P. falciparum* antigens is plotted. This may be due to modulation by the parasite, the accumulation of parasite secreted toxins or some sort of malfunctioning of the host induced regulatory constraints on the immune response.

3.4 Immunity to parasitic infections

One of the major features of the epidemiology of parasite infections is evidence for repeated infection as individuals age in areas of endemic exposure despite abundant evidence of immune recognition

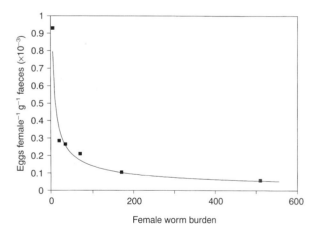

Fig. 3.15   Density-dependent fecundity in *Schistosoma mansoni* based on autopsy data collected by Cheever (1968) (see Medley and Anderson 1985).

Table 3.3   Latent periods and vector life expectancies (see Anderson and May 1991 for source references)

Parasite	Latent period (days)	Vector	Life expectancy (days)
Plasmodium falciparum	11 days (24°C)	*Anopheles gambiae*	8–15
Trypanosoma brucei	15–35	*Glossina morsitans*	28–32
Yellow fever virus	10–12	*Aedes aegypti*	8–14
Onchocerca volvulus	14	*Simulium damnosum*	10–20
Wuchereria bancrofti	13–15	*Anopheles funestus*	10–15
Schistosoma mansoni	20–42 (22°C)	*Biomphalaria glabrata*	7–42

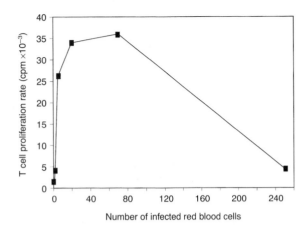

Fig. 3.16 Dose response curve of the influence of antigen concentration (number of *P. falciparum* infected red blood cells) on T-cell proliferation rates (after Jones et al. 1990).

and attack. This is a puzzle of both practical and fundamental significance. Protozoa and helminths have complex genomes and elaborate developmental cycles, and have evolved a wide array of mechanisms to evade or modulate immunological attack (Maizels et al. 1993 and Chapter 4).

As mentioned earlier, the observed aggregated distributions of parasite number per host may reflect differences in innate susceptibility to infection or in the ability to mount effective immunological responses. Work on the population dynamics of the interaction between subsets of T helper cells (Th1 and Th2 subsets) suggests that early exposure to infection in infancy (or even in the womb via maternal experience) may in part determine predisposition to heavy or light infection where high exposure generates tolerance with elevated Th2 responses concomitant with high helminth loads (Schweitzer and Anderson 1992). The quantitative details of the host's ability to recognize and respond to particular parasite antigens (influenced by the genetic make-up of the host) is of importance in determining whether the host is persistently susceptible or develops protective immunity.

To tease out the factors that control observed patterns of infection and immunity in communities, epidemiological study must turn more and more to detailed longitudinal studies of changes in parasite numbers and immunological responses specific to parasite antigens. For the blood-dwelling schistosome flukes in humans (*S. mansoni* and *S. haematobium*) circulating specific and non-specific serum IgE correlates both positively with accumulated past experience of infection and negatively with reinfection rates after drug treatment (Hagan et al. 1987). For the gut dwelling nematode *Trichuris trichiura* comparison of age-dependent isotope responses and the age-profile of worm burden in 2 endemic communities with very different levels of transmission suggests that parasite-specific secretory IgA responses best reflect accumulated past experience of infection, whereas serum IgG

isotopes simply correlate positively with current worm burden (Needham et al. 1994) (Fig. 3.17).

How specific immunological responses to protozoa and helminths operate to generate resistance (effector mechanisms) is poorly understood. Some information can be drawn from epidemiological studies via association of parasite load with different types of response, or by following immune responses post drug treatment and during reinfection. A general pattern seems to be that individual responses mounted to protozoan and helminths rarely operate in isolation and resistance is typically a multi-component response (see chapter 4).

The many and exciting opportunities presented by advances in molecular biology for the study of immunity to parasites are parallelled by the challenge of an ever-expanding descriptive literature. At present our understanding of how immunity (as reflected by resistance to infection and increased rates of parasite clearance from the host) works for any single protozoan or helminth parasite of humans is limited despite abundant descriptive study (see chapter 4). The population ecology of the immune system is a very non-linear world and future research will need to emphasize the measurement and quantification of the many rate parameters that control the humoral and cellular responses to parasite antigens, and the functional dependencies between parasite and immune system variables that determine the dynamics of infection both within the host and in the community of hosts. To achieve this for the major infections of human communities will require more detailed longitudinal studies that combine conventional measures of parasite burden with immunological and molecular studies of parasite genetic diversity and the dynamics of immune responses under repeated exposure to infection.

3.5 Antigen diversity and strain structure in parasite populations

The maintenance of antigenic diversity is a key strat-

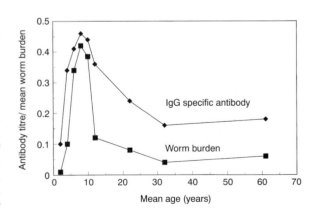

Fig. 3.17 Age-related changes in the burden of *Trichuris trichiura* and IgG antibodies specific to parasite antigens in a community in St Lucia, West Indies (after Needham et al. 1994).

egy adopted by many infectious agents to evade immunological attack in the host and to facilitate the invasion of hosts who have prior experience of infection. Advances in molecular biology have provided many new tools for the study of genetic diversity within parasite populations and these have stimulated a shift in emphasis in epidemiological research towards a more evolutionary approach to the study of infection and immunity. Evolution is at the core of the relationship between host and pathogen. In seeking explanations of observed epidemiological pattern, in the search for new drugs and vaccines, or indeed in the study of immunological responses to infection, the enormous potential of viruses, bacteria, protozoa and helminths to evolve rapidly (either via mutation or recombination events) on timescales much shorter than the generation time of the human host, is often inadequately appreciated. In many cases, particularly for microparasites, such evolution may take place on a timescale faster than that required to mount an effective immunological response. Genetic variation in microparasites, via antigenic change, is often a central pillar of the pathogen's strategy to persist in the host in the face of immunological attack. Persistence enhances the likelihood of transmission to new hosts in the population. This strategy is particularly common amongst persistent viral or protozoan infections such as HIV or *Plasmodium* or *Trypanosoma* species, where the immune system acts as the main selective force driving the emergence and reproductive success of 'escape' antigenic variants. One spin-off of the rapidly expanding databases on the antigenic diversity of important human pathogens (sequence data bases), has been the development of statistical techniques to examine relatedness between different parasite isolates via the construction of phylogenetic trees (Harvey 1996). These techniques often enable inferences to be drawn (about who acquired infection from whom) via sequence data from parasite isolates from different patients. In the coming decade sequence information on genetic variation within pathogen populations will increasingly be linked to phenotype, as mirrored by reproductive success of the parasite or the pathogenesis induced by different genetic variants.

At the between-host level, antigenic variation for both the microparasites and macroparasites may permit repeated infection of individual hosts as is evident in *P. falciparum* infection in humans. The slow build up of cross-reactive (across parasite strains) immunological responses after repeated exposure to different antigenic strains will influence the duration of infection, the infectiousness of a person and in some cases the likelihood of the occurrence of disease. In many cases the delay in the development of immunity to parasitic infection may be a consequence of the antigenic diversity of the parasite in which protective immunity only develops after exposure to many different antigenic types or strains circulating in a given locality. The antigenic genetic constitution of a parasite population may vary from one locality to another (Gupta and Day 1994).

Where many strains persist in a given community the question arises of how this diversity is maintained A simple view might be that the strain with the greatest reproductive success would, over time, competitively displace other strains. However, recent work shows that this is not necessarily the case, provided a degree of cross-immunity builds up to antigens shared by all strains. In the case of complete cross-immunity competitive exclusion occurs, while in the case of no cross-immunity (unlikely in reality) all strains can persist since they circulate independently in the host population (Gupta et al. 1994). For intermediate cases (probably the norm) coexistence is possible provided the reproductive successes (the R_0's) of the various strains do not differ too widely in magnitude (Fig. 3.18). Long term studies of temporal and spatial trends in the prevalence of different parasite strains (e.g. *P. falciparum*, African trypanosomes and some helminth species) are in progress but as yet little is understood about longitudinal trends in parasite diversity within defined human communities (Anderson 1994, Snow et al. 1993). What has become clear, however, is that superinfection of an infected host by a new strain appears common for many of the microparasitic organisms, including HIV and malaria (Paul et al. 1995, Robertson et al. 1995).

The observation that many distinct strains persist in human communities over long periods of time raises a further question concerning the role of genetic exchange in the maintenance of parasite strain structure. Many parasites have the opportunity for the exchange of genetic material because of, for example, sexual processes in the case of *P. falciparum*, coinfection of the same host cell for HIV, or transformation in bacteria. The persistence of strain structure plus the frequent opportunity for genetic exchange appears paradoxical because it would seem that the former would be lost rapidly as a result of genetic recombination. This issue has recently been resolved by theoretical and observational studies which reveal that

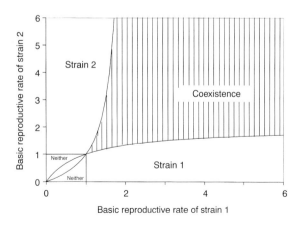

Fig. 3.18 The influence of the degree of cross-immunity ($c = 0$, total cross-immunity, $c = 1$, no cross-immunity, with c set at 0.5) on the pattern of coexistence of two strains of a microparasite as a function of their respective transmission success as measured by the basic reproductive number, R_0 (after Gupta, Swinton and Anderson 1994).

dominant polymorphic antigenic determinants (that is, those that elicit the most effective immune responses) will be organized into non-overlapping combinations of antigenic determinants as a result of selection by the host's immune system, thereby defining a set of distinctive independently transmitted strains (Gupta et al. 1996). Dominant polymorphic antigen determinants will be in linkage disequilibrium, despite frequent genetic exchange, even though they may be encoded by several unlinked genes. By contrast, weaker polymorphic determinants within the same parasite population will be in linkage equilibrium. This suggests that the detection of non-random association between epitope regions of parasite antigens can be employed as a strategy for identifying the dominant polymorphic antigens. To date analyses of linkage disequilibrium patterns within infectious agent populations have, for the most part, only addressed the question of clonality (Walliker 1989, Tibayrenc et al. 1990).

The population dynamics and genetics of a parasite population that is structured into strains by a dominant immune response may be influenced at other levels by weaker responses to both conserved and other polymorphic determinants. For example, the typical age-distribution of *P. falciparum* prevalence (see Fig. 3.10) suggest that although the variant surface antigens (VSAs) (which undergo antigenic variation within the host) categorize the population into strains (each with a given repertoire of expressed antigens), some degree of infection blocking immunity to all strains is eventually established after repeated exposure to a conserved antigen (Gupta and Day 1994).

More generally, these and other studies reveal the importance of a better understanding of the population genetics of parasite and host populations for the interpretation of epidemiological patterns. Molecular epidemiological studies that address the question of the linkage between genetic diversity in the parasite and the incidence of infection and associated disease are likely to be a major focus in the epidemiology of infectious diseases in the coming decade. The occurrence of disease in infected patients may often be linked to the subtle interplay between the genetic background of the host and that of the invading pathogen.

4   CONTROL OF INFECTION AND DISEASE

At present the options for the community-based control of the major tropical parasitic infections are either chemotherapy (e.g. for malaria and the helminth infections) or interventions to prevent exposure to infection (e.g. impregnated bed nets to prevent contact with biting vectors, safe water supplies and good sanitation to reduce contact with the transmission stages of intestinal nematodes). Vaccines are not available for any of the key parasitic infections and early trial results with candidate products have been disap-

pointing. To date no effective vaccine has been developed for an antigenically variable infectious agent that provides long protection duration, irrespective of whether the target agent is a virus, bacterium or protozoan. In research on candidate vaccines most attention is directed at achieving high efficacy. However, duration of protection is of equal significance in terms of potential effectiveness within a community-based immunization programme.

For both chemotherapy and interventions to reduce the likelihood of transmission, the difficulty of the task of achieving long term control is related to the magnitude of the transmission intensity in a defined community as measured by R_0. To block or prevent transmission the magnitude of R_0 must be reduced to less than unity in value. As control measures are introduced, and the value of R_0 progressively declines over time, significant changes in the prevalence of infection are only likely to occur as the critical point of $R_0 = 1$ is approached (Fig. 3.19).

For microparasite infections, community-based chemotherapy or chemoprophylaxis (in the case of malaria) is expensive and beyond the reach of most communities in poor tropical regions. In addition treatment tends to select for resistant strains of the parasite as well illustrated by malaria. In many regions of the world, but particularly in South-East Asia, multi-drug resistant strains of *P. falciparum* are a major cause of morbidity and mortality. Some take a pessimistic view that with the decline in the rate of development of new antimalarials (because of drug development costs and the endemism of the infection in poor developing as opposed to wealthy developed countries) the battle to control malaria by community-based drug use is likely to be futile in the longer term. As such, many see the future in terms of vaccines although current progress does not promote optimism for rapid advances in this area. The main hope at present lies in an integrated approach involving vector control by insecticides, the promotion of community-wide impregnated bed net use and drug treatment to prevent mortality (see chapter 5).

Epidemiological study of the emergence and persist-

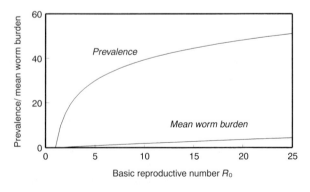

Fig. 3.19   The relationship between the prevalence and intensity of a macroparasitic infection as a function of the magnitude of transmission success as measured by R_0. Below the point $R_0 = 1$, the parasite is unable to persist in the host population.

ence of drug resistant parasites has been limited in scope and scale to date. Detailed long term longitudinal studies (ideally cohort based) are required in defined areas to measure the frequency of the genes that determine resistance to defined drugs. In parallel with such molecular epidemiological studies, quantitative information must be acquired on patterns of drug use to define the intensity of selection that induces the observed change in resistance frequency. Much more thought must be given to defining optimum methods for the use of a number of different drugs, both for the individual patient and for the community, to maximize the effective life expectancy of a drug and minimize the rate of evolution of resistance.

A more encouraging picture emerges for the helminth infections where community-wide use of anthelmintics (often targeted at the child age groups in which the intensity of infection and associated morbidity is greatest) has been very effective in parasite control. To reduce R_0 to less than unity in value, the proportion of the population that must be treated per unit of time (i.e. monthly or yearly) must exceed a critical value, g, where

$$g = 1 - \exp\left[(1 - R_0)/A\right]/h \qquad (4.1)$$

Here A is the life expectancy of the parasite in the human host, and h is the efficacy of the drug (Anderson and May 1991). To take a specific example, namely *Ascaris lumbricoides* for R_0 values around 3 and with $A = 1$ year, a drug of 95% efficacy would have to be administered to more than 91% of the population each year to eradicate the infection (Fig. 3.20). However, if morbidity control is the aim, a much more targeted programme of treatment of heavy infection in schoolchildren would suffice. Recent studies show that additional benefits accrue from the treatment of heavy infection, such as improved rates of growth in children, improved cognitive function and a net reduction in transmission in the community as a whole (Nokes and Bundy 1994). A major practical advantage of targeting treatment to children is their accessibility during school attendance. The frequency of treatment post the introduction of control will depend on rates of reinfection as defined by the magnitude of R_0. For long lived species with limited transmission success, such as the schistosome and filarial worms, intervals of a few to many years may suffice (Butterworth et al. 1991). Conversely, for the short-lived worms such as the intestinal parasites, yearly or more frequent treatment is required (Thien-Hliang et al. 1984).

Long term control of all parasites in areas of endemic infection will require continual intervention or chemotherapeutic treatment unless the intensity of control is sufficient to eradicate the parasite. For the important infections in tropical regions, eradication is difficult to envisage given limited resources for public health measures. Vaccines are ideally required and their development must remain a research priority in the coming years (see chapter 5).

The scientific assessment of the effectiveness of a given intervention programme in both epidemiolog-

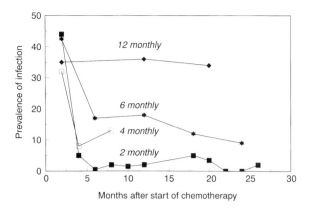

Fig. 3.20 The influence of different monthly intervals between rounds of mass chemotherapy on the prevalence of *Ascaris lumbricoides* in a study population in Korea (after Seo et al. 1980).

ical and economic terms, is often poor despite large expenditure in the implementation of a specific programme. More rigorous approaches to intervention study design and evaluation are required that meld quantitative epidemiology study pre- and post intervention, with assessments of cost and benefit. Cost-benefit analyses of different control options must be based on a framework that captures the interaction between the transmission dynamics of the parasite and the intensity of the control measure. This relationship is invariably non-linear and hence intuition alone will not suffice to accurately deduce the potential impact of a given policy. The key problem, however, is often in the design of the intervention programme. Detailed statistical analyses are required to determine the correct sample size (whether in units of people or communities) required to detect a defined level of change in the incidence of infection or disease post intervention.

The practical aspects of the control of parasitic diseases are discussed in more detail in chapter 5.

5 Conclusions

The interdisciplinary character of epidemiological research implies that advances in a wide variety of disciplines will influence our understanding of the processes that control the spread and persistence of infectious agents in human communities in the coming years. These include those in molecular biology, immunology, mathematics, genetics and information handling, storage and retrieval. Modern desktop computers plus associated software provide a striking illustration of how advances in one field of science can influence progress in epidemiological study. Database construction and handling for a large cohort intervention study is now a simple task, as are comparative studies of sequence data from different patients or pathogen isolates, or detailed statistical analyses seeking associations between host and parasite variables.

However, in parallel with such technical advances,

whether in data management or the measurement plus detection of infection or immunity, there is an associated need to broaden the conceptual template on which epidemiological study is based. Until recently, much epidemiological research on infectious agents ignored the very dynamic nature of the interaction between host and parasite populations, both with respect to the dynamics of transmission and evolution. A failure to take account of population biology and evolution may even influence the more practical end of epidemiology, namely, cost–benefit analyses of different control interventions. Such analyses must be based on measures of the impact of control on both transmission success and parasite evolution.

Direct and indirect benefits arise from vaccinating or drug treating individual patients. The direct benefits to the patient are obvious but the indirect benefits relate to the removal of a host that can potentially pass infection to others. As such, net benefit to the community includes an element related to the reduction in transmission success of the parasite. Drug use may promote the rate of spread of drug resistant parasite strains and hence reduce the period over which a given drug is an effective treatment.

A key problem in all epidemiological studies is the interpretation of heterogeneity in patterns of infection and disease within human communities. It is in this area that recent advances in biological research, particularly at the molecular genetic level, are likely to promote the greatest change in epidemiological research. Genetic diversity in host and pathogen populations is now measurable on the scale required for population-based comparisons and linkage analyses. There seems little doubt that such work will begin to provide answers to such fundamental questions as to why some are predisposed to specific infections and associated disease, while others are not.

REFERENCES

Abel L, Demenai F et al., 1991, Evidence for the segregation of a major gene in human susceptibility/resistance to infection by *Schistosoma mansoni*, *Am J Hum Genet*, **48**: 959–70.

Anderson RM, 1987, Determinants of infection in human schistosomiasis, *Baillière's Clinics in Tropical Medicine and Communicable Diseases. Schistosomiasis.*, vol. 2, ed. Mahmoud AF, Baillère Tindall London, 278–300.

Anderson RM, 1994, The Croonian Lecture. Populations, infectious disease and immunity: a very nonlinear world, *Phil Trans R Soc Lond B*, **346**: 457–505.

Anderson RM, Gordon DM, 1982, Processes influencing the distribution of parasite numbers within host populations with special emphasis on parasite-induced host mortalities, *Parasitology*, **85**: 373–98.

Anderson RM, May RM, 1985, Helminth infections of humans: mathematical models, population dynamics and control, *Adv Parasitol*, **24**: 1–101.

Anderson RM, May RM, 1991, *Infectious Diseases of Humans; Dynamics and Control*, Oxford University Press, Oxford.

Aron JL, May RM, 1982, The population dynamics of malaria, *The Population Dynamics of Infectious Diseases: Theory and Applications*, ed. Anderson RM, chapter 5, Chapman & Hall, London, 139–79.

Bensted-Smith R, Anderson RM et al., 1987, Evidence for predisposition of individual patients to reinfection with *Schistosoma mansoni* after treatment, *Trans R Soc Trop Med Hyg*, **81**: 651–6.

Boyd MF (ed.), 1949, Malariology, Saunders, Philadelphia.

Bradley DJ, McCullough FS, 1973, Egg output stability and the epidemiology of *Schistosoma haematobium*. Part II. An analysis of the epidemiology of endemic *S. haemotobium*, *Trans R Soc Trop Med Hyg*, **67**: 491–500.

Bundy DAP, Cooper ES et al., 1987, Predisposition to *Trichuris trichiura* infection in humans, *Epidemiol Infect*, **98**: 65–72.

Butterworth AE, Sturrock RF et al., 1991, Comparison of different chemotherapy strategies against *Schistosoma mansoni* in Machakos District, Kenya: effects on human infection and morbidity, *Parasitology*, **103**: 339–55.

Cheever AW, 1968, A quantitative post-mortem study of *Schistosoma mansoni* in man, *Am J Trop Med Hyg*, **17**: 38–64.

Davidson G, Draper CC, 1953, Field study of some of the basic factors concerned in the transmission of malaria, *Trans R Soc Trop Med Hyg*, **47**: 522–35.

Dye CM, Hasibeder HG, 1986, Population dynamics of mosquito-borne disease: effects of flies which bite some people more than others, *Trans R Soc Trop Med Hyg*, **83**: 69–77.

Elkins D, Haswell-Elkins M et al, 1986, The epidemiology and control of intestinal helminths in the Publicat Lake region of Southern India. I. Study design and pre- and post- treatment on *Ascaris lumbricoides* infection, *Trans R Soc Trop Med Hyg*, **80**: 774–92.

Fulford AJC, Ouma JH et al., 1996, Water contact observations in Kenyan communities endemic for schistosomiasis: methodology and patterns of behaviour, *Parasitology*, **113**: 223–24.

Gupta SD, Day KP, 1994, A strain theory of malarial transmission, *Parasitol Today*, **10**: 476–81.

Gupta S, Maiden MCJ et al., 1996, The maintenance of strain structure in populations of recombining infectious agents, *Nature Medicine*, **2**: 437–42.

Gupta S, Swinton J, Anderson RM, 1994, Theoretical studies of the effects of heterogeneity in the parasite population on the transmission dynamics of malaria, *Proc R Soc London B*, **256**: 231–8.

Gupta S, Trenholme K et al., 1994, Antigenic diversity and the transmission dynamics of *P. falciparum*, *Science*, **263**: 961–963.

Grenfell BT, Anderson RM, 1985, The estimation of age-related rates of infection from case notifications and serological data, *J Hyg (Cambridge)*, **95**: 419–36.

Guyatt HL, Bundy DAP et al., 1990, The relationship between the frequency distribution of *Ascaris lumbricoides* and the prevalence and intensity of infection in human communities, *Parasitology*, **101**: 139–43.

Hagan P, Blumenthal UJ et al., 1987, Resistance to infection with *Schistosma haematobium* in Gambian children: analysis of their immune response, *Trans R Soc Trop Med Hyg*, **81**: 938–46.

Harvey PH, 1996, Phylogenies for ecologists, *J Anim Ecol*, **65**: 255–63.

Jones KR, Hickling JK et al., 1990, Polyclonal in vitro proliferative responses from non-immune donors to *Plasmodium falciparum* malaria antigens require UCHL+(memory) T cells, *Eur J Immunol*, **20**: 307–15.

Maizels RM, Bundy DAP et al, 1993, Immunological modulation and evasion by helminth parasites in human populations, *Nature (London)*, **365**: 686–805.

Marquet S, Abel I et al., 1996, Genetic control of a locus controlling the intensity of infection by *Schistosoma mansoni* on chromosome 5q31-q33, *Nature Genetics*, **14**: 181–4.

May RM, 1977, Togetherness among schistosomes: its effects on the dynamics of the infection, *Math Biosci*, **35**: 301–43.

Medley G, Anderson RM, 1985, Density-dependent fecundity in *Schistosoma mansoni* infections in man, *Trans R Soc Trop Med Hyg*, **79**: 532–4.

Needham CS, Lillywhite JE et al., 1994, Temporal changes in

Trichuris trichiura infection intensity and serum isotype responses in children, *Parasitology*, **109**: 197–200.

Nokes CB, Bundy DAP, 1994, Does helminth infection affect mental processing and educational achievment?, *Parasitol Today*, **10**: 14–18.

Paul REL, Packer MJ et al., 1995, Mating patterns in malaria parasite populations of Papua New Guinea, *Science*, **269**: 1709–11.

Perry KR, Brown DWG et al., 1993, Detection of measles, mumps and rubella antibodies in saliva using capture radioimmuno-assay, *J Med Virol*, **40**: 235–40.

Robertson DL, Sharp PM et al., 1995, Recombination in HIV-1, *Nature (London)*, **374**: 124–6.

Schad GA, Anderson RM, 1985, Predisposition to hookworm infection in man, *Science*, **228**: 1537–40.

Schweitzer N, Anderson RM, 1992, The regulation of immuno-logical responses to parasitic infections and the development of tolerance, *Proc R Soc London B*, **247**: 107–12.

Seo B, Chai J, 1980, Comparative efficacy of various internal mass treatment of *Ascaris lumbricoides* infection in Korea, *Korean J Parasitol*, **18**: 145–51.

Snow RW, Schellenberg JRMA et al, 1993, Periodicity and space-time clustering of severe childhood malaria on the coast of Kenya, *Trans R Soc Trop Med Hyg*, **87**: 386–90.

Thein-Hliang, Saur J et al., 1984, Epidemiology and transmission dynamics of *Ascaris lumbricoides* in Okpo, rural Burma, *Trans R Soc Trop Med Hyg*, **78**: 497–504.

Tibayrenc M, Kjellberg F, Ayala FJA, 1990, A clonal theory of parasitic protozoa:the population structure of *Entamoeba, Giardia, Leishmania, Naegleria, Plasmodium, Trichomonas* and *Trypanosoma* and their medical significance, *Proc Natl Acad Sci USA*, **87**: 2414–18.

Tyrrell DAJ, 1977, Aspects of infection in isolated communities, *Infectious Diseases in Isolated Communities*, CIBA Foundation, London, 137–53.

Walliker D, 1989, Genetic recombination in malaria parasites, *Exp Parasitol*, **69**: 303–9.

Wilkins HA, Blumenthal UJ et al., 1987, Resistance to infection after treatment of urinary schistomisasis, *Trans R Soc Trop Med Hyg*, **81**: 29–35.

Chapter 4

IMMUNOLOGY AND IMMUNOPATHOLOGY OF HUMAN PARASITIC INFECTIONS

F E G Cox and D Wakelin

1 Introduction	**3 Immunity to protozoa**
2 Immune responses to parasitic infections	**4 Immunity to helminths**

1 INTRODUCTION

Parasites affect over half the world's population and are a major cause of mortality in the developing world; in the developed world, they represent a threat to those undergoing immunosuppressive therapy or suffering from HIV infections. All parasitic infections induce some kind of immune response which in some cases is protective and in others causes pathological changes. In order to understand the nature of immunity to parasites it is first necessary to consider the immune response as a whole. The human immune system is concerned with defence against invading organisms and the removal of malignant cells. Over the last 25 years the immune response has been subjected to detailed studies, using the most advanced techniques of biochemistry and molecular biology, as a result of which most of the processes involved are now clearly understood. It is now possible to view most aspects of the immune response in terms of dogma rather than hypothesis and to understand it in terms of a small number of well defined processes operating sequentially or concurrently. Initially, our understanding of the immune response was limited to experimental situations in which a simple antigen elicited a single response in a particular strain of inbred mouse, but within a remarkably short period of time our knowledge has extended to complex antigens in humans and we now know that immunity to infectious agents follows the same rules that apply to immune responses to simple antigens. All infectious agents, particularly protozoan and helminth parasites, act as very complex antigens and elicit a range of immune responses, a proportion of which are relevant to protection. Our interest now is not so much in determining whether or not an immune response occurs but instead is largely concerned with unravelling the complex interplay between invader and invaded, which results in either protection or pathology or a combination of both. The practical aim on one hand is to determine what is actually responsible for protection and how this can be induced artificially and, on the other, to determine what causes pathology and how this can be ameliorated.

The role of the immune system is to deliver an appropriate immune response at the right time and place and it is not surprising that different infectious agents should elicit different immune responses. In order to understand the nature of infectious agents, particularly parasites, it is necessary to distinguish between microparasites and macroparasites (see Chapter 3). Microparasites are small and multiply within their vertebrate host, often inside cells, thus posing an immediate threat unless contained by an appropriate immune response. Viruses, bacteria and protozoa are microparasites, typically inducing an infection in which the host becomes infected, then experiences the following: a latent period during which the parasites multiply; a period of disease and discomfort during which the immune response brings the infection under control; and finally a gradual recovery and long term resistance to reinfection. Macroparasites (i.e. helminths) are large and do not multiply within their vertebrate host. Thus they do not present an immediate threat after initial infection, but the host must protect itself from large infections and reinvasion by infective stages and can only do so by eliciting an appropriate immune response. Immune responses to protozoa, which are microparasites, and helminths, which are macroparasites, are therefore very different from one another.

Although protozoa and helminths are very different in terms of the immune responses they elicit, the infections they cause have a great deal in common, usually being very long-lasting and, over a period of years, inducing immunopathological changes which may be more dangerous than the infection itself. In short, the parasite invades the host, is recognized as foreign and elicits an apparently appropriate immune response. But parasites are very complex and highly evolved, with life cycles involving different stages and occupying different sites. In addition, all have evolved mechanisms for evading the immune response. The net result is a situation in which the infection is partially controlled but the parasite may not be eliminated so the host continues to mount increasingly complex immune responses until the parasite wins, the host wins or there is an uneasy compromise. During the course of all infections, parasites die or are killed and parasite molecules are deposited on host tissues. These may elicit autoimmune responses which, in turn, contribute to the pathology of the infection. In addition, some parasites evade the immune response by mimicking host molecules which, if effective, can be very successful but, if unsuccessful, can initiate an autoimmune reaction. The majority of parasitic infections also elicit powerful inflammatory responses that may alter, render non-functional or even destroy host tissues.

Virtually all parasitic infections are long-term and chronic and are accompanied by immunopathological changes and periods of immunodepression. Because of this it was believed for many years that there were no effective immune responses against the majority of parasites, but it is now clear that immunity is the rule. The evidence for this comes from a number of sources: (1) in endemic areas the majority of people experience clinical immunity to parasitic infections and the prevalence of infection falls with age whereas immunological parameters increase; (2) the uneasy compromise that exists after recovery can be broken, for example by immunosuppressive drugs or concomitant infections; and (3) in every experimental model investigated immunity can be demonstrated and there is no reason why humans should be different.

The study of the immunology of parasitic infections has generated a vast literature which can only be touched on in this chapter but there are a number of authoritative multi-author works available in English including Behnke (1990), Warren (1993), Kierszenbaum (1994) and Boothroyd and Komuniecki (1995) and there is a very useful review in Spanish by Barriga (1994).

2 IMMUNE RESPONSES TO PARASITIC INFECTIONS

2.1 The overall immune response

The immune response to any parasite, as with any other infectious agent, begins when the host becomes infected and the parasite is recognized by the cells of the immune system. In order to initiate an immune response, molecules of the parasite must come into contact with the cells of the immune system and if this

does not happen, then no immune response will be initiated. It is easy to see how this occurs with parasites that invade the internal tissues and organs of the body. Many intestinal parasites invade internal tissues before reaching their final location and thus come into direct contact with the immune system. Even in the intestinal parasites that do not breach the integrity of gut wall, such as the nematode worm *Enterobius vermicularis* and the non-pathogenic strains of the amoeba, *Entamoeba histolytica*, there is the potential for direct antigen uptake across the mucosa and they therefore can also initiate an immune response. Once a parasite is recognized as foreign the next series of events is initiated. The events involved in recognition are complex and much of what we know about them is concerned with peptide antigens; this chapter will contain no detailed discussion of carbohydrate antigens, although these play an important role in many anti-parasite responses. In the simplest situation, the first event is when a parasite, or a fragment of it, is taken up by an antigen-presenting cell (APC), such as a macrophage, as part of the normal process of phagocytosis, and is then broken down into short peptides by proteolytic enzymes in the phagolysosome. Certain of these peptides are then transported to the surface of the macrophage in combination with specific class II major histocompatibility complex (MHC) molecules. The whole complex, consisting of the MHC molecule and the peptide, which can now be considered as the antigen, is recognized by antigen receptors on helper T lymphocytes and the immune response proper is initiated. These early steps are known as antigen 'processing' and 'presentation' and these events determine the eventual outcome of the immune response. A number of cells can act as antigen presenting cells but in most, if not all, parasitic infections, macrophages or related cells are the only cells normally considered. As the antigen on the surface of the antigen presenting cell binds to the receptor on the helper T lymphocyte, the macrophage releases a T cell activating cytokine, interleukin 1 (IL-1), and in response the helper T cell produces other cytokines that, in their turn, activate the effector cells of the immune system, cytotoxic T cells, natural killer (NK) cells, activated macrophages, B lymphocytes and a variety of inflammatory cells (Fig. 4.1).

Each of these cells has its own specific role in the immune response and can act concurrently or sequentially, with or without other cells, to bring about the immobilization or destruction of the invading organism. The specific target of the immune attack is the antigen that initiated the immune response in the first place but parasites, particularly helminths, represent very large targets and the immune response can normally recognize a large number of surface antigens. Not all of these are involved in protection and some are even able to deflect the immune response away from more vulnerable targets. Much research has been devoted to the identification and characterization of protective antigens in order to try to understand how the immune response to parasites works and to target vaccines to relevant molecules. Many

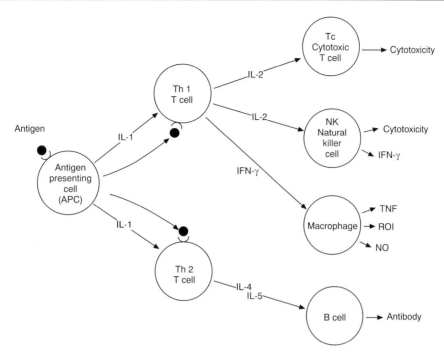

Fig. 4.1 Diagrammatic representation of the main features of the overall immune response. Antigen is recognized and processed by antigen presenting cells (APC), in this case macrophages, and presented to Th1 or Th2 cells that carry receptors for the antigen. At the same time the APCs release the cytokine IL-1 which activates resting Th1 and Th2 cells. Activated Th1 cells produce a number of cytokines including IL-2 which in turn activates cytotoxic T (Tc) or natural killer (NK) cells. Cytotoxic T cells kill target cells carrying the original antigen in an MHC restricted manner whereas NK cells kill target cells non-specifically. Another important Th1 cell product is INF-γ, which activates resting macrophages making them more phagocytic and causing them to release a variety of molecules, including tumour necrosis factor (TNF), reactive oxygen intermediates (ROI) and nitric oxide (NO). ROI and NO are involved in intracellular killing of ingested parasites or the destruction of parasites in close proximity to the activated macrophage. Th2 cells release a different set of cytokines, including IL-4 and IL-5, that are involved in B cell differentiation and activation and the release of antibodies specific to the antigen. IL-5 also activates eosinophils. Antibodies may act in cooperation with cells such as macrophages and eosinophils by acting as a bridge bringing the activated cell and the parasite together and facilitating the release of toxic molecules directly onto the surface of the parasite.

efforts have also been made to identify the antigens that are irrelevant to protection or even counter-protective and are involved in the evasion of the immune response and possibly contribute to the pathology of the disease.

It is known that the immune responses to parasites are complex but that individual components are relatively simple and that there is nothing unique or special about these responses to parasites except for their complexity. In this context, it is convenient to consider the protective immune response as having 4 arms: cytotoxic T cells, NK cells, activated macrophages and antibody, the first 3 constituting what is conventionally called 'cell mediated immunity' and the last constituting 'humoral immunity' (Fig. 4.1). Cytotoxic T cells (Tc cells) engage target cells expressing antigens in combination with class I MHC molecules and effect their cytotoxic activity by creating pores in the membrane of the target cell, which then ruptures. Cytotoxic T cells are frequently involved in viral infections but are seldom implicated in parasitic infections. Natural killer (NK) cells constitute a heterogeneous collection of lymphocytes that are neither B nor T cells, are not specific to a particular antigen and do not involve MHC class I molecules. NK cells

seem to be able to kill target cells directly and pores are formed in the target cell, which ruptures as in cytotoxic T cell killing. It is still not clearly understood what actually constitutes NK cell killing, but NK cells are being increasingly implicated in protection against parasitic infections.

Activated macrophages, i.e. macrophages that have been sensitized and triggered by signals such as lipopolysaccharide and interferon-γ–(IFN-γ), are among the most important cells involved in protection against parasites and can kill target cells either intracellularly or extracellularly. If it is small, the target cell can be phagocytosed and destroyed in the phagolysosome via a number of pathways, including proteolytic enzymes as described for antigen processing. Macrophages also produce toxic molecules, including the reactive oxygen intermediates, superoxide, hydrogen peroxide and hydroxyl radicals, that destroy the target cell though a process of lipid peroxidation, and nitric oxide (NO) which reacts with the superoxide anion to produce highly toxic peroxynitrite and hydroxyl radicals, which, among other things, interfere with mitochondrial function. Macrophages also produce tumour necrosis factor (TNF) which synergises with NO and, either on its own or together with other molecules, is effective in damaging target cells. One of the key features of the activation of macrophages is that the various toxic molecules produced are released not only into the phagolysosome but also extracellularly and are thus able to destroy cells in the close vicinity of the activated macrophage. Macrophages are therefore able to kill large cells or multicellular organisms, especially if the macrophage is closely bound to the target via, for example, an antibody bridge as described below. These toxic molecules can also damage host cells and their release in an inappropriate place or in excess is a major cause of immunopathology.

The humoral immune response is concerned with B cells products, i.e. antibodies. The 4 major classes, IgA, IgG, IgM and IgE, occur in different situations and are effective against parasites in different ways although there is some sharing of functions. Antibodies are effective against invading organisms in 4 main ways: neutralization, agglutination, complement activation and facilitated opsonization. IgA occurs as 2 subclasses, IgA1 and IgA2, each of which can occur in a monomeric, dimeric or, occasionally,· polymeric form. IgA is essentially an antibody found in secretions where it protects the mucous surfaces of the gut, respiratory tract and urinogenital tract; it also occurs in breast milk. Its main functions are the neutralization of bacterial toxins and the inhibition of the invasion of the mucosa, either by agglutinating the infectious agents or blocking attachment to host cells. IgG and IgM are found in the serum and extravascular spaces. IgM, a pentameric immunoglobulin which occurs as a single subclass, is the first antibody to be produced in response to antigenic stimulation and is very good at agglutinating micro-organisms with repeated epitopes and activating complement via the classic pathway. IgG, which occurs as 4 subclasses, IgG1, IgG2, IgG3 and IgG4, and usually replaces IgM, is the most common antibody in secondary immune responses. All subclasses can agglutinate micro-organisms. IgG1, IgG2 and IgG3 can activate complement, IgG3 being the most effective. IgG1 and IgG4 can pass across the placenta and IgG1 and IgG3 can bind to macrophages and neutrophils via their Fc portions. IgE has an affinity for mast cells, basophils and eosinophils, to which it binds via the Fc portion; when bound to an antigen it causes cross-linking, resulting in the release of pharmacologically active substances from the cells to which it is bound.

Antibodies seldom work in isolation from other components of the immune system. IgG and IgM fix complement and initiate the complement mediated lysis of the target cell. Both IgG and IgE bind to effector cells, usually activated macrophages or eosinophils respectively, via the Fc portion, and to the target cell by the Fab portion and thus facilitate the destruction of the target cell, a process known as 'antibody dependent cell mediated cytotoxicity' (ADCC).

With respect to immunity to parasites, the important fact is that the immune responses evoked are not unusual and are essentially the same as those involved in immunity to other infectious organisms.

What is different is the complexity of the immune response in reaction to diverse antigens expressed by different stages of complicated life cycles often in different situations in the host. This leads to a plethora of antibody independent and antibody dependent responses which, over a period of time, can give rise to misdirected immune responses leading to pathological changes instead of protection. For example, in malaria the production of TNF is beneficial but an excess is detrimental and in schistosomiasis potentially protective responses lead to the formation of harmful granulomas around non-threatening eggs deposited in tissues. For these reasons, current interest in immunity to parasites is being concentrated on an understanding of the overall control of the immune response which is brought about by the interactions of the various cytokines involved in a cytokine network.

2.2   The cytokine network in parasitic infections

The cytokine network consists of a number of peptide hormones that act as signals between the cells of the immune system, the cells that produce them and the cells on which they act. Many are growth or activation factors and without them the immune system could not function. An understanding of the cytokine network has permitted immunologists to unravel the interactions that come into play during an immune response and to consider individual components separately before considering them in the context of the response as a whole. Many cell types produce cytokines, but T lymphocytes of the T helper (Th) subset are a major source. Central to our understanding of the cytokine network was the discovery that there are 2 distinct types of T helper lymphocytes. Both carry the same surface CD4+ marker, but cytokines from one, Th1, drive the immune response towards antibody independent immune responses whereas those from the other, Th2, drive it towards antibody production. The overall features of the cytokine network are shown in Fig. 4.2.

T helper cell subsets and the cytokine network were originally identified and defined in mice (Mossman and Coffman 1989) but virtually every component has since been shown to apply to humans as well (Romagnani 1991), parasitic infections providing the first evidence for a similar T helper cell dichotomy. Currently, extrapolations are made from mouse to humans and are tested before any assumptions are made. It is important to understand the cytokine system in parasitic infections because of the complexity of the immune responses involved. Through an understanding of the system, it is possible to interpret events leading to protection on one hand and pathology on the other.

Infections with *Leishmania* species in inbred strains of mice have become the paradigms for studies on T cell subsets and the cytokine network as a whole, and the approaches used with these models have been extended to the study of many other infections, including those in humans. Such studies have also

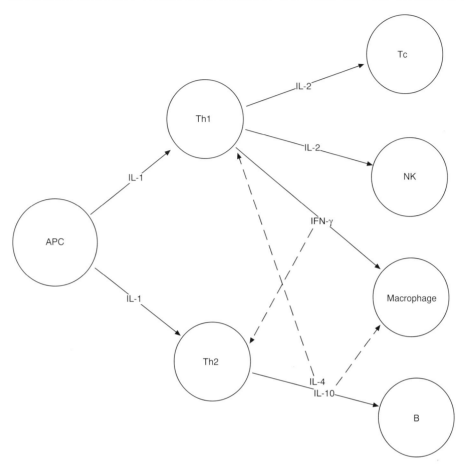

Fig. 4.2 Diagrammatic representation of the cytokine control of the immune response. IFN-γ, as well as having a positive role in the activation of macrophages (Th1 response), also has a negative effect on Th2 responses. Similarly, the Th2 cell products IL-4 and IL-10 inhibit Th1 responses. Positive pathways are indicated by solid lines and negative pathways by broken lines.

shown that there is a considerable degree of antagonism between the products of Th1 and Th2 cells and that in many immune responses to infections either the Th1 or the Th2 cell response is protective whereas the other is counter-protective leading to pathological changes or the switching off of part of the immune response. An overview of the cytokine network in parasitic infections is given by Cox and Liew (1992) and reviews of the roles of cytokines in malaria, leishmaniasis, trypanosomiasis and helminth infections can be found in Mustafa et al. (1996).

In a number of cases the outcomes of parasitic infections are known to be under the control of the 2 T cell subsets. By the beginning of the 1990s a general pattern emerged in which it appeared that, in the majority of protozoal infections in experimental models, Th1 cells were protective and Th2 cells were counter-protective, whereas in helminth infections the reverse was the case, Th2 cells were protective and Th1 cells counter-protective (Cox and Liew 1992). There have been several important developments in knowledge since 1992, for example: (1) human T cell responses are basically similar to murine ones, (2) there are 2 subsets of CD8+ cells based on the cytokines they produce, (3) Natural Killer (NK) cells are involved in the immune response, (4) IL-12 plays an important role in the immune response, (5) the nature of the immune response is determined by cytokines present and (6) in many infections the mol-

ecule NO plays a major role in protection and pathology.

HUMAN T CELLS

The human cytokine response shows the same functional dichotomy as in mice, but for IL-2, IL-6, IL-10 and IL-13 the dichotomy is not so absolute. Nevertheless, we can now be confident that the situation in humans is similar to that in mice (Mosmann and Sad 1996).

CD8+ T CELLS

The main feature of CD8+ T cells is that the cytokines produced by Tc1 and Tc2 cells are essentially the same as for Th1 and Th2 cells. We do not yet know what the situation is in humans but it is probably safe to assume that it is the same or very similar. The important point here is that we had previously assumed that CD8+ cells were primarily effector cells involved in target cell killing but now we know that they are also involved in the control of the immune response.

NK CELLS

Like cytotoxic T cells, NK cells were assumed to be effector cells that kill target cells including micro-organisms in a non-MHC restricted manner. Subsequent studies showed that NK cells are able to activate cytotoxic T cells and are also important producers of IFN-γ and thus they also strongly influence the outcome of the immune response. NK cells are activated by IL-12.

IL-12

The nature and role of IL-12, which has only been elaborated over the past 5 years, now occupies a central role in our understanding of immunity to parasitic infections. IL-12 is produced by macrophages and was originally called 'NK stimulatory factor' (NKSF), being thought to be mainly responsible for the activation of NK cells. This does seem to be one of its major roles but the most important roles of IL-12 are now thought to be the regulation of IFN-γ and the growth and differentiation of Th1 T cells. IL-12 and NK cells therefore have a major role in Th1-type responses against parasitic infections (Scott and Trinchieri 1995, Lamont and Adorini 1996).

We now have a much more detailed picture of the cross-regulation between Th1 and Th2 cells, which determines the outcome of the immune response. The Th1 product, IFN-γ, downregulates Th2 responses whereas the Th2 products, IL-10, and to a lesser extent IL-4, downregulate Th1 responses. IL-4 produced by Tc2 cells downregulates Tc1 responses although there is no evidence that Tc1 cells are able to downregulate Tc2 cells. In addition to these negative influences, IL-12 and IFN-γ upregulate the activity of Th1 cells and IL-4 upregulates the activity of Th2 cells. In this context it is interesting that NK cells produce IFN-γ which both upregulates the Th1 response and downregulates the Th2 response. Presumably, the activities of the various cytokines produced by Th1, Th2, Tc1 and Tc2 cells are the same, thus the immune response is controlled by a network of cytokines some driving the immune response one way and some driving it the other (Fig. 4.3).

NO has assumed a central role in our understanding of the immunology and immunopathology of parasitic infections. It is a reactive gas with many functions. Its role in cell signalling has been known for a long time but it is only in the past few years that its role in immunity to infection has been understood (Clark and Rockett 1996). There are 2 important iso-

forms of NO, constitutive and inducible. Constitutive NO is found in a variety of cells. Inducible NO is produced by macrophages under the control of the enzyme inducible NO synthase (iNOS). NO is a powerful anti-microbial compound and is capable of killing a range of organisms including bacteria, protozoa and helminth worms. NO acts on iron-sulphur clusters in macromolecules and represses DNA synthesis and iron-containing enzymes, including those involved in respiration. Nitric oxide synthase is upregulated by IFN-γ and TNF and is downregulated by IL-4, IL-5 and IL-10. NO is, therefore, a key molecule in the immune response to parasitic infections and its production and activity are favoured by Th1 responses and inhibited by Th2 responses (James 1995).

Our interpretations of the immune response to parasites of only a few years ago now seem very simplistic and the new discoveries have called for a reinterpretation of many of the facts observed. On the other hand, these new discoveries have enabled us to understand many of the phenomena observed much more clearly. In the remainder of this chapter an attempt will be made to illustrate these points by reference to a selected number of parasitic infections and to interpret these in terms of the human diseases.

CYTOKINES IN PROTOZOAL INFECTIONS

Until relatively recently, protozoal infections created problems for immunologists because they appeared not to obey any of the rules of immunology. Unlike most viral and bacterial infections, protozoal infections tend to be long and chronic and to be associated with inappropriate immune responses, immunodepression to superimposed infections and immunopathological damage. This pattern was regarded as unusual and the only parallels were the mycobacterial infections, leprosy and tuberculosis, in which most individuals usually develop some immunity to the clinical disease whilst never actually eliminating the

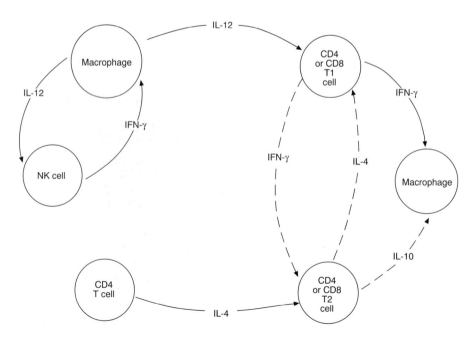

Fig. 4.3 Diagrammatic representation of part of the overall control of the immune response showing the involvement of both CD4+ and CD8+ T cells, NK cells and IL-12. Positive pathways are indicated by solid lines and negative pathways by broken lines.

infection altogether. It was not until the AIDS virus was recognized that it became clear that there were similarities between infections caused by parasitic protozoa and HIV. The present situation is that leprosy, tuberculosis, AIDS and many protozoal infections present similar problems and the study of protozoa is now providing important clues as to what is happening in other infections. Our increasing knowledge of immune responses to protozoa is also beginning to explain the immunopathology associated with such infections, because the long chronic infections continually stimulate the immune system which then gets out of control and eventually begins to attack the body itself.

Studies with the protozoan *Leishmania major* in strains of inbred mice have provided a paradigm by which parasitologists have been able to understand the nature of immune responses to a number of parasitic infections. *Leishmania* parasites live and divide in macrophages. The protective immune response seen in certain strains of mice involves IFN-γ activated macrophages that kill the intracellular parasites, but in other strains this immune response is inhibited by IL-4 and IL-10, which inhibit the production of IFN-γ. The net result is the accumulation of macrophages at the site of infection, uncontrolled growth of the lesions and a massive amount of antibody that has no protective effect.

The fundamental observations that protection is afforded by Th1 cells and that Th2 responses are counter-protective still stand, but we now know that the effector molecule responsible for parasite killing is NO and that the production of this molecule can be enhanced by the presence of IFN-γ and other Th1 cell promoting cytokines (Liew and O'Donnell 1993). In humans, there is now abundant evidence for a similar pattern of cytokine activation (see Chapters 12 and 13). Patients with localized cutaneous lesions tend to have high levels of IFN-γ whereas those with disseminated infections or mucocutaneous leishmaniasis tend to have high levels of IL-4 (Kemp, Theander and Kharazmi 1996). These cytokines are also predictive of the outcome of the cutaneous forms of leishmaniasis; those with high levels of IFN-γ tend to have a better prognosis than those with high levels of IL-4. The situation is not so simple in the case of visceral leishmaniasis, in which levels of IFN-γ and IL-10, normally antagonistic, are both elevated. Overall, it seems as if the outcome of leishmaniasis infections in humans depends on a balance between those factors promoting a Th1 response and those promoting a Th2 response.

Toxoplasma gondii is also a parasite of macrophages and, like *Leishmania*, is killed by IFN-γ activated macrophages, TNF synergising with IFN-γ in this killing. Interestingly, both CD4+ and CD8+ cells contribute to the production of IFN-γ but in mice without CD8+ cells, NK cells take over this role. *T. gondii* itself is able to stimulate the production of IL-12 which in turn stimulates NK cells to produce IFN-γ and the actual parasite killing involves NO (Sher 1995).

Malaria is a complex infection and immunity seems to involve both Th1 and Th2 responses (see Chapter 20). Parasite killing involves NO but it is not at all clear how this gets into the infected red cell. One of the most interesting aspects of the role of NO in malaria is as a possible cause of the coma associated with cerebral malaria. This suggests that cerebral malaria might be prevented by inhibiting NO synthesis and there is evidence that this can be done by treating comatose children with antibody against TNF, one of the co-stimulators of NO production (Grau 1996). Malaria also demonstrates one of the fundamental problems in trying to control parasitic infections, getting the balance between protection and counterprotection right (Clark and Rockett 1996).

CYTOKINES IN HELMINTH INFECTIONS

Knowledge of cytokine responses in helminth infections was derived initially from a number of detailed studies of experimental systems in rodents, but is increasingly being extended to infections in humans. Both experimental and human studies can provide direct data on cytokine production in terms of increased cytokine-specific mRNA in cells from infected hosts or of cytokine protein released from cells stimulated with antigen in vitro. Experimental systems have the additional advantage of allowing direct manipulation of in vivo responsiveness by injection of recombinant cytokines or monoclonal anti-cytokine antibodies, as well as through the use of genetically modified hosts. Reliable indications of cytokine-mediated influences on the immune response to helminths can also be gained indirectly by measuring levels of isotype-specific anti-parasite antibodies and of particular inflammatory responses.

Both in rodents (Sher and Coffman 1992, Locksley 1994) and in humans (Del Prete et al. 1991, Mahanty et al. 1993), helminth antigens elicit responses that are predominantly mediated through cytokines released from cells of the Th2 subset. Th2-dependent antibody responses to helminths characteristically include the isotype IgE, which is regulated by IL-4 and IL-13. The IgG isotypes IgG4 in humans and IgG1 in mice are also Th2-dependent, whereas IgG2a in mice is a marker of Th1-dominated responsiveness, being regulated by IFN-γ. The cellular inflammatory responses most often associated with helminths are eosinophilia and mucosal mastocyosis, both of which are dependent on Th2 cytokines such as IL-4, IL-5 and IL-9, although a number of other cytokines (e.g. IL-3) also contribute. The emphasis of experimental studies has largely been on associations between particular cytokine profiles and resistance or susceptibility to infection. Human studies have placed an equal emphasis on cytokine correlates of immunopathological responses. The most valuable rodent model systems have been those involving schistosomes, filarial and intestinal nematodes.

Schistosomes can be maintained in the laboratory in several species of rodent, but detailed immunological studies primarily concern infections in rats and mice (Capron et al. 1992). In rats, immunity to schistosomes involves a strong Th2 component, being mediated through ADCC mechanisms involving IgE and eosinophils. In mice, the Th response is dramatically switched to the Th2 subset once egg production begins, Th1 responses being down-regulated by IL-10. The IgE-eosinophil axis does not provide effective immunity in infected mice, which sustain long-term infections. Vaccinated mice express a resistance that is Th1-mediated and can be enhanced by administration of IL-12, which has the effect of down regulating Th2 responses.

Infections with filarial nematodes such as *Brugia pahangi* in mice, although unnatural host-parasite associations, have shown striking differences between Th subset responses to infections involving the microfilaria and adult stages (Lawrence 1996). Microfilaria elicit Th1 responses whereas adult females elicit Th2 responses. Immunity elicited by irradiated L3 larvae seems to involve Th2 activity, but genetically modified (knock-out) mice that are incapable of producing IL-4 can still respond protectively.

Intestinal nematodes elicit Th2 subset responses in local lymphoid populations, levels of IL-4, IL-5 and IL-9, as well as IL-3, being elevated (Urban et al. 1992). This helps to explain the almost inevitable association of such infections with IgE, eosinophilia and mastocytosis. In some cases, the initial response is Th1 biased, later switching to Th2. It is possible that non-T cell sources of type 1 cytokines, such as NK cells, release IFN-γ in response to IL-12 production and so promote the initial Th1 response. It is equally possible that non-T cell sources of type 2 cytokines, such as mast cells, basophils, and possibly B cells, then release IL-10, thus switching off the Th1 response and inducing a Th2 response. Although Th2-mediated responses correlate with the development and expression of protective immunity, it is still unclear, in many cases, what the causal connection is between these responses and the events that provide the host with protection. Model systems vary considerably, but it is generally true that neither removal of the capacity to produce IgE nor depletion of eosinophil responses by giving anti-IL-5 antibody have significant effects on immunity. In contrast, reduced resistance has been shown when mast cell responses are depleted or when anti-IL-4 antibody or the cytokine IL-12 (both enhancing Th1 responses) are administered (Finkelman et al. 1994, Donaldson et al. 1995).

One of the most interesting experimental models of intestinal nematode infection is that using the nematode *Trichuris muris* in mice where, as with *Leishmania*, there is a reciprocal relationship between Th subset response and immunity, Th2 activity leading to resistance and Th1 activity to continuing susceptibility. The dependence of the host response on specific cytokines is elegantly demonstrated by the fact that the phenotypes of genetically susceptible and resistant mice can be reversed by injection of the appropriate cytokines or anti-cytokine reagents (Else et al. 1994). This relationship between Th subsets and resistance to *T muris* is, of course, the reverse of that seen in the mouse-*Leishmania* model.

The most detailed human studies on the roles of Th subsets in helminth infections have been those involving schistosomes and filarial nematodes. In both, immunoepidemiological studies on populations in endemic areas have thrown light on correlations between particular immune responses and patient status, which have then been explored in detail using a variety of in vivo and in vitro techniques. These long-term infections are associated with reduced T cell responsiveness that seems preferentially to affect the Th1 subset, whilst Th2 activity remains unaffected or is substantially increased. These imbalances are parasite-induced and are usually reversed after successful chemotherapy. They often result from an IL-10-mediated down regulation of Th1 cells.

In human schistosomiasis, in which it has long been recognized that immunity is slow to develop, it has been shown that resistance is correlated with production of IgE antibodies, which can contribute to the operation of effector mechanisms, such as ADCC involving eosinophils (see Chapter 25). In younger children, IgE-mediated ADCC is thought to be blocked by competitive interactions between target epitopes and other isotypes, of which IgG4 is one of the most important (Hagan et al. 1991). Both IgG4 and IgE are Th2-regulated isotypes, but clearly there are additional factors that influence the production of each. As children age, the relative proportions of parasite-specific IgG4 and IgE alter, in favour of the latter, and resistance becomes effective in reducing further infection. During chronic infections, Th1 responses are down-regulated, presumably as a result of the activity of Th2 cytokines such as IL-10.

Much attention has been focused on the role of T cells in immunopathological responses to schistosome infection (Stadecker 1994). Granuloma formation around trapped eggs is a major cause of pathology and is triggered by cytokines derived from T cells and other sources. With time, the size of newly formed granulomata is reduced. Although there is some debate, studies in mice have implicated Th2 cells in granuloma formation and Th1 cells, through the release of IFN-γ, in modulation of the response. Up-regulation of Th1 responses by injection of IL-12 has been suggested as the basis of an anti-pathology vaccine. Interestingly, in SCID mice, which lack all T cells, granuloma formation can be initiated by injection of TNF-alpha (Amiri and Locksley 1992).

Filariasis, like schistosomiasis, is a chronic infection and is associated with high prevalence in endemic areas. Patients fall into a number of categories based on parasitological and pathological criteria, from those who show heavy infections (as assessed by the degree of microfilaraemia, which is the number of microfilaria larvae in the bloodstream) but are asymptomatic, to those who are parasitologically negative but show severe pathology such as elephantiasis (Maizels et al. 1995) (see Chapter 32). IgE and IgG4 antibodies are found in both, implying Th2 activity, but in the former the ratio between the isotypes is biased to IgG4 and in the latter to IgE. Asymptomatic microfilaraemia is associated with a T cell anergy, which appears to be due to downregulation of Th1 responsiveness by Th2 cells. Both Th1 and Th2 responses appear (or at least have the potential) to be involved in anti-parasite activity. There is, therefore, a complex, parasite-induced interplay between Th cell subsets that results in modulation of both antibody and cellular responsiveness and determines both the parasitological and pathological outcomes of infection.

3 IMMUNITY TO PROTOZOA

As pointed out in Section 1 of this chapter, protozoa are microparasites that multiply within their vertebrate hosts. They do this by dividing at a genetically determined rate; thus no matter how small the initial infective dose, unless it is controlled, the infection will eventually overwhelm the host. The only ways in which the rate of multiplication can be curtailed are by exhausting the number of cells available for infection or by the intervention of an immune response. In protozoal infections, some kind of acquired immunity is the rule and the main reason why this does not eliminate the infection is because all protozoan parasites have evolved ways of evading the consequences of the immune responses that they themselves have evoked. Protozoal infections, therefore, tend to be long and chronic and the general pattern is typically a latent period during which few or no parasites can be detected, a phase of logarithmic increase, a crisis and a rapid or gradual decline leading to a chronic infection with the possibility of subsequent recrudescences.

Protozoal infections are accompanied by a number of immunological changes including the production of specific antibodies, usually IgM followed by IgG, and cell mediated responses measured in various ways. It is often not appreciated that many of these immunological responses have little or nothing to do with protection. All protozoa are antigenically complex and are therefore recognized as foreign and a variety of immune responses are inevitably initiated. These responses are often either due to irrelevant antigens or to relevant antigens that the parasite is able to use as part of its repertoire of immune evasion techniques. For example, antibodies to the dominant antigen of the malaria sporozoite merely deflect the immune response away from more vulnerable targets and, in leishmaniasis, antibodies merely represent the stimulation of a counter-protective Th2 response. In reality, these non-protective immune responses are no different from those produced against any experimental antigen such as bovine γ globulin (BGG), keyhole limpet haemocyanin (KLH) or the purified protein derivative (PPD) of mycobacteria.

In summary, protozoal infections are accompanied by changes in immunological parameters that, in some cases, mirror recovery but do not necessarily represent any protective mechanism. Unfortunately, a vast amount of the literature on the immunology of protozoal infections is devoted to these 'Will-o-the-wisps' and this has tended to obscure valid and relevant observations.

The importance of protective immune responses to protozoa has been highlighted by the consequences of co-infections with HIV and protozoal infections such as cryptosporidiosis and microsporidiosis. These were once thought to be rare and harmless, but are now recognized as concomitants of AIDS with major pathologic potential (see Chapters 18 and 21). Similarly, the occurrence of such infections in immunosuppressed and immunocompromised patients has become an important aspect in the management of these patients. HIV is known to depress the immune response to a number of protozoal infections including leishmaniasis, microsporidiosis, toxoplasmosis, pneumocystosis (Ambroise-Thomas and Grillot 1995) and also amoebiasis, cryptosporidiosis and Chagas disease, but does not seem to affect the outcome of malaria or African trypanosomiasis. Thus, in many parts of the world, an understanding of the immune response to parasitic protozoa has taken on a new significance.

3.1 Immunity to intestinal protozoa

The gastrointestinal tract serves as a habitat for a number of organisms including viruses, bacteria, protozoa and helminth worms. In normal, healthy individuals the mucus layer of the gastrointestinal tract passively protects the underlying cells from invasion. In addition there is a specialized mucosal immune system consisting of mucosa-associated lymphoid tissue (MALT), intra-epithelial lymphocytes, macrophages, T and B lymphocytes in the lamina propria and a secreted non-complement fixing immunoglobulin, IgA. Singly or together these elements provide the first line of defence against invading organisms that gain entry to the body via the alimentary tract, thus the immunology of the gut can be considered as a discrete component of the overall immune system. Once an organism has broached the intestinal defences it effectively no longer occupies the gastrointestinal compartment of the body and becomes subject to attack by other components of the immune system. It is necessary to consider immunity to intestinal protozoa against this background. In this context, it is important to note that many experimental studies have involved the administration of parasite antigens by routes other than the intestinal one; thus the immune responses generated have not necessarily been appropriate. The literature on immune responses to intestinal protozoa has been confused by results of such experiments and many of the conclusions drawn probably have little validity. This section, therefore, stresses what is known about immunity to intestinal protozoa in humans and underemphasises the contributions made by animal and in vitro studies. The comprehensive reviews available will be cited.

INTESTINAL AMOEBAE

Entamoeba histolytica is the only amoeba of importance and about which anything concerning the immunology is known (see Chapter 8). Most strains of *E.*

histolytica are non-pathogenic and live as harmless commensals in the large intestine where they do not appear to elicit any immune response. There are some pathogenic forms that can invade the mucosa and submucosa forming ulcers; they may be carried to the liver where they form large abscesses. Immune responses, indicated by the production of specific antibodies, are elicited at various stages after invasion but there is no evidence that recovery from infection induces any protection against subsequent infections nor, at the population level, is there any age-dependent diminution in prevalence that can be ascribed to the acquisition of immunity (reviewed by Kretschmer 1993, Martínez-Palomo, Kretschmer and Meza Gomez Palacio 1993). In patients with invasive amoebiasis there is a transient secretory immune response followed by the production of serum antibodies (Peréz Montfort and Kretschmer 1990). The secretory immunoglobulin is IgA, which occurs in colostrum, breast milk and saliva, but its role in amoebiasis is not known. There is no correlation between serum antibodies, predominantly IgG, and the severity of the infection or recovery. It is not clear whether the apparent absence of acquired immunity is due to some defect in the immune system or to the fact that the amoebae have evolved ways of evading the humoral immune response. These include the capacity to degrade secretory IgA, to resist complement lysis and to redistribute or shed surface antigens. Nor is it clear what, if any, is the role of cellular immune responses. In some, but not all, individuals with invasive amoebiasis, there is transient cell mediated immune response as detected by skin tests, but it is not known what this actually means. It is possible that potentially protective cell mediated responses can be aborted and in vitro studies show that amoebae can lyse target cells, including those of the immune system, by inserting ion channels called amoebapores into their membranes. In conclusion, there is little evidence that humans mount an effective immune response against *E. histolytica* but the fact that recurrences of amoebic ulcers are rare warrants some attention. (See also Chapter 8).

INTESTINAL FLAGELLATES

Giardia intestinalis has been long considered to be a harmless commensal of the small intestine but increasing evidence that it can cause malabsorption and severe diarrhoea has stimulated interest in immune responses to this parasite (see Chapter 10). Experimental studies with *G. muris* in mice clearly demonstrate that there is acquired immunity and protection against subsequent challenge (Roberts-Thomson et al. 1976). In humans, the evidence for acquired immunity is more circumstantial but comes from a number of sources. There is usually spontaneous clearance and resistance to reinfection and those living in endemic areas are less affected than visitors. Young children are more affected than older ones or adults and immunodepressed individuals tend to experience long chronic infections (reviewed by Janoff and Smith 1990, Nash 1994, Kulda and Nohynkova 1995 and Faubert 1996 and see also Chapter 10). All the available evidence

suggests that the effector mechanism or mechanisms involve secretory IgA but the case is by no means proven. IgA is the most characteristic *Giardia*-specific antibody in patients with acute giardiasis and individuals with hypogammaglobulaemia tend to experience chronic infections, but there is little direct evidence of any IgA anti-parasitic effects. On the other hand, specific antibodies are found in human milk and saliva; breast-fed infants in endemic areas seem to acquire some degree of protection (Walterspiel et al. 1994). Other antibodies may also be involved, for example, current infections are accompanied by high levels of specific IgM but this is quickly replaced by IgA in acute infections and after re-exposure. Overall, it seems that immunity to giardiasis is similar to immunity to a number of bacterial infections in which secretory IgA in breast milk protects the new born infant until it can produce its own IgA. This antibody, which cannot fix complement, presumably adversely affects the parasites indirectly by preventing attachment to the villi. *G. intestinalis* can undergo antigenic variation although the actual mechanism is not understood, nor is it known how this might affect the acquisition of immunity to this parasite (Nash 1995). There have been reports of giardiasis in AIDS patients, but *Giardia* is not considered to be a major concomitant of HIV infections (Janoff, Smith and Blaser 1988).

Although the human intestine is parasitized by a number of other flagellates, *Chilomasitx mesnili*, *Dientamoeba fragilis*, *Trichomonas gingivalis* and *T. hominis*, these are not normally regarded as important pathogens and virtually nothing is known about any immunological responses to them.

INTESTINAL COCCIDIANS

Little is known about the immune responses of humans to any of the 3 intestinal coccidians, *Cryptosporidium parvum*, *Isospora belli* or *Cyclospora cayetanensis*. Cryptosporidiosis is the only important disease caused by any of these parasites and has only been recognized as such during the last 20 years (reviewed by Martins and Guerrant 1995 and see Chapter 18). In healthy individuals, the infection is an unpleasant but self-limiting one, lasting less than a month, characterized by mild to severe watery diarrhoea, but in AIDS patients the infections are more persistent and the symptoms much more severe and death may result (Adal Sterling and Guerrant 1995). This suggests that normally there is immune involvement and specific antibodies have been detected in the serum of infected individuals; characteristically IgM is produced first and this is replaced by IgG, levels of which begin to decline after about a year. Nothing is known about the possible mechanisms or relevance of these immunological responses.

INTESTINAL CILIATES

The only intestinal ciliate of humans is *Balantidium coli*, which is comparatively rare. Nothing is known about the immune responses to this ciliate and, by analogy with *Entamoeba histolytica*, it is unlikely that there is any reaction unless the mucosa and submucosa are invaded.

3.2 Immunity to protozoa inhabiting the urinogenital tract

The only protozoan that inhabits the human urinogenital tract is *Trichomonas vaginalis*, which parasitizes both men and women. The nature of the infection and the disease caused in men is poorly documented, but vaginitis caused by this parasite is an important sexually transmitted disease in women, in whom it persists for long periods unless treated (reviewed by Honigberg and Burgess 1994 and see Chapter 11). There are no really appropriate animal models of human trichomoniasis and, although experimental infections in guinea pigs and mice have provided some information (e.g. complement-dependent and complement-independent killing in animals given intraperitoneal, intradermal or subcutaneous injections), little that is really relevant can be derived from these observations (Ackers 1989). Similarly, observations on *T. foetus* in cattle have been largely irrelevant to human trichomoniasis. In humans, secretory IgA antibodies to *T. vaginalis* have been detected in vaginal secretions. Antibodies produced in response to infection diminish with time and do not appear to confer any protection against reinfection. Epidemiological evidence derived from many studies in sexually transmitted disease clinics, suggest that infections with *T. vaginalis* tend to be persistent, that reinfection frequently occurs after cure and that the prevalence of the infection does not plateau or fall off in the older age groups, suggesting that there is little or no acquired immunity and that specific immune responses play an insignificant role in limiting this infection. The reasons why there appears to be no immunity to *T. vaginalis* are not clear although it has been suggested that this parasite has considerable antigenic diversity; whether or not it can also undergo antigenic variation is an open question (Alderete 1983).

3.3 Immunity to macrophage-inhabiting protozoa

INTRODUCTION

Three groups of parasitic protozoa inhabit macrophages at some stage during their life cycles, *Leishmania spp.*, *Trypanosoma cruzi* and *Toxoplasma gondii*. Each has evolved its own way of evading the destructive mechanisms of the macrophage: leishmanias survive in the fused phagolysosome; *T. cruzi* escapes from the phagosome into the macrophage cytoplasm; and *T. gondii* prevents phagosome-lysosome fusion. In addition, all these parasites also possess enzymes that counteract the various toxic molecules present in the phagolysosome. Because of their ability to avoid destruction by macrophages, these parasites escape from attack by one of the main arms of the immune system and this enables them to give rise to long,

chronic infections. On the other hand, none of these parasites is able to survive in IFN-γ activated macrophages, thus they live on a knife edge by inhabiting cells that can sustain them but which also have the capacity to destroy them. *Leishmania* spp. are totally dependent on macrophages whereas *T. cruzi* and *T. gondii* are also able to parasitize other cell types. This section deals with immunity to *Leishmania* spp. and the other 2 parasites will be discussed under the heading of tissue-inhabiting protozoa.

LEISHMANIA spp.

Twenty species of *Leishmania* infect humans, 14 in the New World and 6 in the Old World, and the number is gradually increasing. Leishmaniasis can be conveniently classified into 3 forms, cutaneous, mucocutaneous and visceral, but these categories are not absolute (see Chapters 12 and 13). As these parasites are very common and as the majority of those infected (particularly with the cutaneous forms) do recover, albeit slowly, the immunology of these parasites has been intensively studied, mainly with the ultimate aim of producing a vaccine. *Leishmania major*, the causative agent of Old World cutaneous leishmaniasis, and *L. donovani*, the causative agent of visceral leishmaniasis, have been the most intensively studied species, mainly because of the ease with which they can be maintained in genetically characterized laboratory mice (reviewed by Liew 1990, Alexander and Russell 1992, Liew and O'Donnell 1993 and Sacks et al. 1993). The *Leishmania major*-mouse model has become a paradigm for all leishmanial infections and extrapolations to the human situation have tended to confirm the universal nature of the immune response involved. Leishmania parasites survive and multiply within normal macrophages but are killed by IFN-γ activated macrophages through a mechanism involving NO. Tumour necrosis factor and TNF-inducers play a secondary role in this process by upregulating the IFN-γ-induced NO killing. In contrast, NO activity is downregulated by IL-4 and IL-10. Thus, resistant strains of mice have high levels of IFN-γ and low levels of IL-4 and IL-10, whereas the reverse is the case in susceptible strains. The overall control of the immune response depends on the activation of one of 2 subsets of T lymphocytes, Th1 cells produce IFN-γ and protection whereas Th2 cells produce IL-4 and IL-10 and are counter-protective (see Reiner and Locksley 1995, Scott 1996).

Although the distinctions between Th1 and Th2 subsets are not so clear cut as in mice this pattern is also true for human leishmaniasis (Kemp, Theander and Kharazmi 1996). In those with fulminating *L. donovani* infections, IL-4 and IL-10 levels tend to be high and IFN-γ levels low, in cutaneous infections (in which recovery is normally the rule) IFN-γ levels are high and in chronic mucocutaneous infections IL-4 levels are high. All these facts are in accordance with well established clinical observations, for example: the development of strong delayed type hypersensitivity (DTH), indicating macrophage activation, correlates with recovery from cutaneous leishmaniasis; diffuse cutaneous leishmaniasis is characterized by the absence of DTH; and high levels of non-protective IgM and IgG antibodies (resulting from Th2 cell activity) are seen in visceral leishmaniasis (see Blackwell 1993). In localized mucocutaneous leishmaniasis, Th1 cytokines predominate whereas in the more destructive forms there is a mixture of Th1 and Th2 responses although the Th2 cytokine, IL-4, tends to predominate in accordance with the well established paradigm (Pirmez et al. 1993).

There have been a number of experimental vaccines developed against leishmaniasis and there have been some encouraging results in humans (see Mayrinck et al. 1986, Greenblatt 1988, Convit et al. 1989), but there are no commercial vaccines in the pipeline, although the WHO is optimistic that some will eventually be available for clinical trials (Modabber 1995).

3.4 Immunity to blood-inhabiting protozoa

INTRODUCTION

Four important groups of protozoan parasites inhabit the human bloodstream: the African trypanosomes, *Trypanosoma brucei gambiense* and *T. b. rhodesiense*; the South American trypanosome, *Trypanosoma cruzi*; the malaria parasites, *Plasmodium falciparum*, *P. malariae*, *P. ovale* and *P. vivax*; and rare and accidental infections with *Babesia* spp. *Trypanosoma cruzi* makes only a transient appearance in the blood and is best regarded as a tissue parasite. The bloodstream is a dangerous place for a parasite to live, as there is continual and intimate contact with the cells and molecules of the immune system, particularly IgM and IgG antibodies and phagocytic cells. This ability to survive in what should be a very hostile environment has attracted the attention of numerous scientists. African trypanosomes and malaria parasites have been particularly intensively studied in laboratory animals and this activity has generated a vast literature much of it, unfortunately, largely irrelevant to the human disease. In this section, only those aspects of the immune response directly concerned with human infections will be discussed.

AFRICAN TRYPANOSOMES

The African trypanosomes that infect humans are *Trypanosoma brucei gambiense* and *T. b. rhodesiense*, both related to *T. b. brucei*, a trypanosome of wildlife and domesticated animals that does not infect humans (see Chapter 14). Little is known about the acquisition of immunity to trypanosomes in humans but there is epidemiological evidence that immunity to Gambian sleeping sickness does develop, albeit slowly, in human populations (Khonde et al. 1995). Because of the similarities between these parasites *T. b. brucei* has been widely used as a model for both the human and animal disease, largely because it is the only one that is easy to maintain in laboratory mice. Infections with all 3 subspecies are similar; the parasites live and multiply in the blood and infections are characterized by successive peaks of parasitaemia representing different antigenic variants. Each trypanosome is covered with a thick glycoprotein coat, the variant surface glycoprotein (VSG). There is an almost limitless repertoire of VSGs, each known as a variable antigen type (VAT), and the normal pattern of events is that the parasites multiply in the blood, are destroyed by an antibody-mediated immune response specific to the major VAT, and are replaced by another population of parasites carrying a new VAT. The main antibody involved in human infections is IgM and the actual killing mechanism involves agglutinating antibodies, complement mediated lysis and phagocytosis (see Pearson 1993, Vickerman, Myler and Stuart 1993, Kirchoff 1994). The killing and lysis of trypanosomes brings about the release of numerous internal and external antigens and toxic factors that circulate in the body giving rise to immune complex-mediated damage accompanied by the production of pharmacologically active substances that affect smooth muscle contraction and vascular permeability. These phenomena have been well characterized in rabbits and, although it is impossible to study the situation in humans in the same way, the clinical picture suggests that similar processes do occur in humans.

The whole field of the immunology of trypanosome infections is a very controversial one and the traditional view that anti-VSG antibody is responsible for the remission of the infection, albeit temporarily, has been challenged by several workers including Mansfield (1994) and de Baetselier (1996) based on in vitro observations and studies in mice. Mansfield suggests that macrophage-derived NO affects the survival of the trypanosomes and also inhibits T cell function, leading to immunodepression. Baetselier maintains that the trypanosomes induce CD8+ T lymphocytes to produce IFN-γ and macrophages to produce TNF and that these synergise to produce toxic molecules that both adversely affect the trypanosomes and cause immunodepression. It is, however, not at all clear what the situation is in humans, whether or not there is any immunodepression or, if so, whether it has any affect with respect to intercurrent infections such as HIV.

MALARIA PARASITES

Malaria is generally recognized as the most important parasitic disease, both in terms of mortality and morbidity (see Chapter 20). It affects some 350–500 million people in the tropics and subtropics, killing 2–3 million annually, mainly children in sub-Saharan Africa. Humans harbour 4 species, *Plasmodium falciparum*, *P. vivax*, *P. malariae* and *P. ovale*, in order of clinical importance. *P. falciparum* is the most intensively studied parasite and, unless otherwise specified, is the only one to be considered here. The control of malaria has largely depended on the combined use of insecticides and drugs but resistance has made these ineffective and attention has turned to the possibility of developing a vaccine. An important spin-off of this work has been the realization that much of the pathology of malaria is closely associated with immunity, in particular the involvement of cytokines. Research into immunity and immunopathology has resulted in a massive literature reaching tens of thousands of papers, mostly based on rodent models and in vitro systems and much of it, particularly many of the extrapolations made, irrelevant or peripheral to the human situation (Cox 1988). Studies using simian malaria parasites have been more rewarding (Collins 1988) but our knowledge of immunity to human malaria is very limited (Houba 1988, McGregor and Wilson 1988). The immunology of malaria has been extensively reviewed (López-Antuñano and Schumis 1993, Melancon-Kaplan et al. 1993, Perlmann, Berzins and Wahlgren 1993, Good and Langhorne 1994, Riley, Hviid and Theander 1994 and see also Chapter 20). The following facts are known:

1   malaria infections are long-lived, 1–2 y in the case *P. falciparum* and 3–50 y for *P. malariae*
2   individuals can be reinfected after natural recovery or cure
3   there is a gradual build up of immunity over a period of many years
4   any immunity fades quickly
5   immunity is largely strain-specific.

In summary, immunity to malaria can be considered to be the rule, although it is often incomplete and may take many years and numerous exposures to the bite of infected mosquitoes to develop. Thus there is evidence of some immunity and the real challenge is to try to improve on this.

It has been generally assumed that the malaria parasite is relatively free from attack while it is intracellular so the only points at which it should be fully susceptible are: (1) when the sporozoite is circulating in the blood; (2) when merozoites are liberated from the liver into the bloodstream and before they invade the red blood cell; and (3) when merozoites have been released from red blood cells. The sporozoite is the obvious target for immune attack. It is the first stage in the infection and the parasites are free in the blood for up to 30 min. The sporozoite possesses an immunodominant 40–60 kDa protein surface coat, covering the whole of the parasite, called the 'circumsporozoite protein' (CSP). The most interesting thing about the CSP molecule is that it possesses a dominant epitope consisting of 4 amino acids repeated 37 times and 3 or 4 copies of a smaller repeat dispersed throughout the molecule. In *P. falciparum*, the amino acids of the dominant repeat are Asparagine-Alanine-Asparagine-Proline, usually written as $(NANP)_{37}$, and the minor repeat is Asparagine-Valine-Aspartate-Proline (NVDP). Other malaria parasites have similar repeat regions but with different amino acid sequences. The CSP is very antigenic and elicits a strong antibody response and has, therefore, been a favourite for vaccination studies. When exposed to antibody, however, the surface molecules are crosslinked and the sporozoite sheds the coat and escapes; thus it is now thought that the repeat sequence is a mechanism whereby the parasite evades the immune response by putting up a powerful 'smoke screen' that deflects the response away from more important targets. The sporozoite has not been abandoned as a

possible target for immune attack and current research is now concentrated on antigens from the non-repeat regions of the CSP and those involved in the penetration of the liver hepatocytes. It was previously thought that, once in the liver, the parasite was safe from immune attack as there is no sign of inflammation or lymphocyte infiltration even after c. 10 days. In murine malaria models, there is now evidence that there is a cytotoxic T cell response to the early stage in the liver and that what is recognized is parasite antigen in the presence of a liver cell MHC class I molecule. We do not know what happens in humans but there is evidence that in West Africa the outcome of infection is controlled by the MHC class I molecules; there is no evidence that this is the case elsewhere.

The erythrocytic stages, particularly the merozoites, have received the most attention. They are the easiest to study, they are responsible for the disease and they are obvious targets for attack. A vast amount of information about these stages has accumulated and many of the antigens involved have been characterized and cloned. Interestingly, most of them are also characterized by the presence of repeats of amino acids, suggesting that these also are involved in immune evasion. The best studied antigen is the Major Surface Protein (MSP) associated with the merozoite. MSP-1 is found in all the malaria parasites studied to date, and is a glycoprotein with a molecular mass of c. 190–195 kDa. Experimentally, antibodies against MSP-1 block red blood cell invasion, thus this could be a major target for immune attack and for exploitation as a vaccine. Unfortunately, there is considerable diversity in MSP-1 between isolates and immunity to one isolate does not confer immunity to another. The same applies to other antigens including the 155 kDa Ring Infected Erythrocyte Surface Antigen (RESA), found on the surface of newly invaded red cells, which has been used in experimental vaccination studies. Other *P. falciparum* antigens of importance are Apical Membrane Antigen (AMA-1), Erythrocyte Binding Antigen (EBA-175) and Serine Rich Antigen (SERA), all of which are involved in binding to or invading red blood cells. The Mature Infected Erythrocyte Surface Antigen (MESA or PfEMP-2), found on the surface of late-infected red cells, seems to be involved in cytoadherence but does not seem to be susceptible to antibody attack. The actual mechanisms involved in immunity are not at all clear.

The antigens associated with the sexual stages would seem to be unlikely targets for immune attack but, in fact, they are very important. There are a number of antigens associated with the gametocytes, the male and female gametes and the zygote and, unlike most of the other antigens of malaria parasites, they are very susceptible to antibody attack. This only happens when the gametocytes are taken up by a mosquito together with antibodies in the serum. When the gametocytes escape from the infected red cell they are recognized by the antibody and, by an unexplained mechanism, they are either killed or inactivated. In either case, the infection in the mosquito cannot continue. The antigens of interest are: a 250 kDa antigen on the gametocytes, gametes and zygote; a 25 kDa antigen on the gametes and zygote; and a 48 kDa antigen on the zygote and oocyst.

A major problem in malaria is that all the stages in the life cycle are antigenically distinct so the acquisition of immunity must involve a number of components working together or in sequence. Potential exists for something to go wrong with the control of such complex reactions and one of the problems is that much of the pathology is associated with the protective immune response (Fig. 4.4).

The complexity of the immune response means that inevitably some of the reactions will be adverse ones and some of the symptoms of cerebral malaria are caused by NO elicited as part of the immune response. Such knowledge can be used to devise ways of halting or reversing these adverse reactions; for example TNF contributes to the production of NO and anti-TNF antibodies have been successfully used to treat children with cerebral malaria. Other approaches involve anti-disease vaccines targeted against the toxins released when the infected red cells in the blood rupture.

A vaccine against malaria is one of the greatest goals of immunologists but it has proved very difficult to design one (Berzins 1994). A vaccine should be possible for a number of reasons. First, most people do recover and out of the 350 million or so infected, <1% die and those that do recover are subsequently resistant to the most serious forms of the disease, if not infection. Secondly, in a very large number of animal

experiments, it has proved possible to induce some degree of protection artificially and this has provided hope that this might also happen in humans. The problems are that: (1) immunity in humans is slow to develop and often incomplete in that reinfections do occur although they are less life-threatening; (2) immunity in humans is usually specific to local strains of the parasite; and (3) experimental immunization is rarely completely successful and often involves the use of methods of vaccination that would be unacceptable for human use.

The development of a vaccine must take into consideration what stage of the life cycle of the parasite to attack and what kind of antigens to use. The malaria life cycle is very complex and includes a number of stages that are biochemically and immunologically distinct. Immune responses against all these stages have been detected but immunity against one does not protect against the next. In effect, malaria infections consist of a sequence of different infections, not just one.

The antigens are also complex as each stage possesses a large number of different antigens some of which are protective and some of which are not. In addition, malaria parasites have evolved several ways to evade the immune response, so some of the antigens identified could be counter-protective. The current approach is to identify and characterise potentially protective surface antigens and to use these as: (1) subunit antigens on their own; (2) as recombinant molecules expressed in a suitable vector; or (3) as a basis for synthetic vaccines. All 3 methods have been

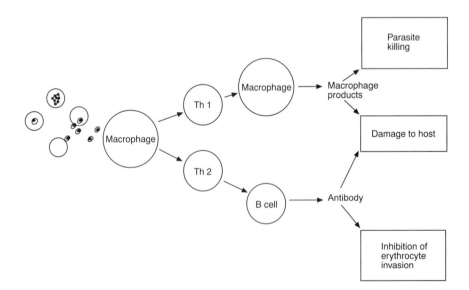

Fig. 4.4 Diagrammatic representation of the balance between protection and pathology in malaria infections. Parasite killing is brought about by a combination of antibody and cell mediated responses but both have adverse side effects resulting in pathological changes. In this diagram, the erythrocytic stage of the infection initiates the immune response when parasites or parasite products are processed and presented by macrophages. Both Th1 and Th2 cells are involved. The Th1 pathway results in the activation of macrophages and the release of TNF, ROI and NO which act in sequence or together and constitute a non-specific arm of the immune response. These molecules also have adverse effects as they can damage host cells and thus contribute to the pathology associated with malaria. Similarly, the Th2 arm results in the activation of B cells and the release of antibodies, some of which inhibit erythrocyte invasion and are protective. Other antibodies form antigen-antibody complexes that can cause local damage and also stimulate macrophage activity, with the release of more toxic molecules and consequent damage. Similar patterns exist in other infections.

tried with varying success and this subject has been extensively reviewed (Cox 1991, Berzins 1994, Corradin, Engers and Trigg 1994, Jones and Hoffman 1994, Targett 1995a, 1995b).

Sporozoites are obvious targets, being the first stages to enter the body and circulating in the blood for a short time before entering the liver. A vaccine against the sporozoite would prevent infection. Early experiments showed that irradiated sporozoites would protect mice quite well and were partly protective in humans. The major surface peptide of the sporozoite (CSP) has been used as a basis for recombinant vaccine expressed in *E. coli* and for synthetic vaccines. A number of trials were initially promising, about 20–30% of volunteers being protected, but they revealed no correlation between antibody levels and protection. It is now widely accepted that the sporozoite repeat antigen is not a good vaccine candidate because if even one sporozoite escaped into the liver an infection would be initiated and the epidemiological evidence does not support the concept that a sporozoite vaccine would work. The sporozoite surface antigen is easily shed from the sporozoite and the repeated epitope probably represents a non-protective target that acts as a 'smoke-screen', diverting the immune response away from more protective targets. A number of other more promising sporozoite antigens are now receiving attention.

Liver stages are also possible targets. It was once thought that there was no immune response against the liver stages, but it is now apparent that there are immune responses in the liver, probably blocking the invasion of the hepatocytes. These responses involve sporozoite antigens outside the repeat region and antigens unique to the liver stage. Although several liver stage antigens that are possible targets for immune attack have been recognized, there is currently no serious attempt to develop a vaccine against them.

Blood stages are obvious targets because there are so many of them and because they cause the disease. A number of potential antigens have been recognized either associated with the infected red cell, intra-erythrocytic parasites or merozoites or secreted soluble antigens. MSP-1 (MSA-1) is currently being considered for Phase I and Phase II (safety and efficacy) trials. Trials are also under way using AMA-1, an antigen associated with the rhoptry of the parasite, and EBA-175, a merozoite antigen, both involved in binding to red blood cells and blocking red cell invasion and SERA released when the schizont bursts; this is protective in monkeys by an unknown mechanism.

Currently, the only vaccine that is undergoing extensive field trials is SPf66, a synthetic vaccine consisting of a polymer of 3 merozoite antigens (Pf83 (an 83 kDa peptide representing part of MSP-1), Pf55 and Pf35, neither of which has been identified with any of the known major malaria antigens) linked by the sporozoite antigen NANP (Tanner, Teuscher and Alonso 1995). The first trials involved safety and immunogenicity in over 15 000 individuals in the Tumaco region of Colombia, where malaria is endemic; the next involved 751 soldiers in the same area. Although the numbers of infected individuals were very small, episodes of malaria were reduced by c. 60–80%. The vaccine was safe and immunogenic and, although it did not prevent malaria, it reduced the number of malaria episodes.

SPf66 is the only malaria vaccine approved by the WHO and is currently undergoing more extensive trials in natural populations of adults and children in South America, Africa and Thailand. It is too early to say whether or not this vaccine is effective. The minimum efficacy of 33% suggested by the WHO is far from being achieved at present. On the other hand, this vaccine can be regarded as a first generation one. It also represents a change of approach towards reducing the burden of malaria and the number of episodes, rather than trying to prevent infection altogether. It also depends on repeated re-infection in order to boost the immunity, thus the more people are exposed to infection, the stronger their immunity becomes.

The only other vaccine currently being considered is one that targets the sexual stages in the mosquito (Targett 1995a). At first this might seem to be a very strange approach but it is both logical and feasible. The principle is to immunize individuals with sexual stage antigens, which will inactivate the sexual stages when taken up by a mosquito. This has been called the 'transmission blocking' or 'altruistic' vaccine because it does not protect the person immunized, but does prevent transmission. Pfs25, an antigen on the surface of the malaria zygote, is the most favoured candidate for such a vaccine. Until now, the idea of such a vaccine would have been unthinkable, but if current opinion favours a vaccine that reduces the burden of malaria without actually preventing it, there is no reason why such a transmission-blocking antigen should not be added to SPf66 as a 'cocktail'. Numerous other possibilities are currently being pursued and it will probably be necessary to have a multi-pronged approach. Once the concept of a cocktail vaccine that does not necessarily produce sterile immunity but does reduce the severity of the infection has been accepted it should be possible to consider novel approaches such as vaccinating against the disease rather than the infection; there is evidence that it is possible to immunize laboratory animals against the toxins produced by malaria parasites (Playfair et al. 1990). Other approaches still at the experimental stage involve multiple antigen peptides incorporating T and B cell epitopes, antigens expressed in viruses and *Salmonella* and naked DNA.

BABESIAL INFECTIONS

Babesiosis, although common in wild and domesticated animals, is a rare accidental infection in humans (see Chapter 19). Little is known about immune responses in humans except that immunologically intact individuals are susceptible to infection with the rodent babesia, *Babesia microti*. Such infections are accompanied by raised specific antibody levels, even in the presence of persisting parasitaemias, a phenomenon common in many protozoal infections. Babesiosis caused by *B. microti* is more serious in immunologically compromised patients and the European form, caused by *B. bovis*, has been reported from only splenectomized individuals, suggesting that an intact immune system is required to keep this infection under control (see Telford et al. 1993).

3.5 Immunity to tissue-inhabiting protozoa

Several parasitic protozoa occur in human tissues, including the following: (1) the ubiquitous coccidian, *Toxoplasma gondii*, in a variety of nucleated cells, including macrophages, and the brain; (2) *Trypanosoma cruzi* in muscle and nerve cells; (3) *Sarcocystis* spp. in muscle; (4) microsporidians; and (5) opportunistic amoebae in the brain. Of these, *T. gondii* and *T. cruzi* are the most important and, partly because of the ease with which they can be maintained in laboratory animals, have been the most intensively studied. Apart from *T. cruzi*, most of these tissue-inhabiting protozoa cause long, chronic and usually harmless infections but these may become fulminating in immunologically compromised individuals such as those co-infected with HIV.

TOXOPLASMA GONDII

Toxoplasma gondii is a common parasite of cats, which can be transmitted to virtually all warm-blooded animals (Dubey and Beattie 1988; see also Chapter 16). The parasite infects macrophages, in which it survives by preventing phagosome-lysosome fusion, and undergoes rapid division as a merozoite known as a 'tachyzoite'. After a short time, division slows down and the parasites transform into slowly dividing bradyzoites which remain dormant in cysts, mainly in the brain, where they may die and become calcified. If the infected individual is subsequently immunocompromised in some way, the parasites in the dormant cysts may become activated and give rise to a fulminating infection. In humans, most infections are benign or inapparent but if the parasite passes across the placenta it can seriously damage the fetus. *Toxoplasma gondii* infections are also now becoming serious concomitants of AIDS (Ambroise-Thomas and Pelloux 1993). Most individuals acquire the infection relatively early in life and recover from the infection after which they are immune to reinfection. Acute infections are characterized by specific IgM and chronic or recovered infections are characterized by IgG. Much of what is known about immunity to toxoplasmosis has been derived from studies in mice (Gazzinelli, Denkers and Sher 1993) although there have also been numerous studies using sheep, as toxoplasmosis is a serious veterinary problem associated with abortions. The key cells in the immune response are macrophages and there are 2 patterns of immune response. In the first, tachyzoites are coated with antibody and are either prevented from invading host macrophages or are unable to prevent phagosome-lysosome fusion if they are successful. In the second, intracellular parasites are killed by IFN-γ-activated macrophages. The actual mechanisms involved are far from clear but, from murine models, they seem to be Th1-type responses involving CD8+ lymphocytes, CD4+ lymphocytes and NK cells operating in synergy to produce IFN-γ which, in combination with TNF, initiates macrophage-mediated killing via reactive oxygen molecules and NO (Sibley et al. 1991, Hunter, Subauste and Remington 1994, Darcy and Santoro 1994). There is also increasing evidence that IL-12 is involved in immunity during the acute phases of experimental toxoplasmosis (Gazzinelli, Denkers and Sher 1993). IFN-γ plays a central role in toxoplasmosis as it induces microbicidal activity, promotes cyst formation and prevents cyst rupture. In common with other infections controlled by Th1-type responses, IL-4 causes exacerbated infections. On the other hand, IL-10 ameliorates the inflammatory response and is therefore beneficial to the host (Burke et al. 1994). It is not easy to make direct extrapolations to humans but the available evidence suggests that the mechanisms of immunity are similar to those in mice, for example IFN-γ inhibits replication of the tachyzoites in macrophages from infected AIDS patients (Delemarre et al. 1994). Whatever the mechanism, immunity is clearly very important in humans, given that the majority of the world's population will be infected at some time and that those that are immunoincompetent (e.g. the fetus) or immunodepressed are at particular risk from a fulminating infection. Toxoplasmosis is now regarded as the most common cause of focal central nervous system infection in AIDS patients (Mariuz, Bosler and Luft 1994).

There is no vaccine against toxoplasmosis in humans and, although one based on an attenuated strain of *T. gondii* for use in sheep is commercially available (Buxton 1993), this would be unacceptable for human use. There is some optimism that a more acceptable vaccine could be developed in the future (Araujo 1994).

CHAGAS DISEASE (NEW WORLD TRYPANOSOMIASIS)

Chagas disease, caused by the trypanosome *Trypanosoma cruzi*, is confined to South and Central America where 65–90 million people are at risk and 12–24 million are infected (see Dusanic 1991 and Chapter 15). *T. cruzi* infects >150 species of mammals and most of the research done with this parasite has been carried out in rodents, particularly mice, in which the pattern of immunity that emerges is complex and is influenced by the genetic make up of both the parasite and host. Chagas disease is one of the most insidious of all the parasitic diseases. The infection is transmitted by biting bugs and is typically acquired in childhood; the victim experiences little more than a localized swelling and a transient fever. In some individuals the infection may be acute and it is life-threatening in 2–8% of those infected. The trypanosomes divide at the site of the bite and circulate briefly in the blood before entering macrophages, in which they survive by escaping from the phagolysosome and multiplying in the cytoplasm of the cell. From here they escape and invade a variety of other nucleated cell types, including muscle cells (particularly cardiac muscle) and nerve cells. The infection is life-long and usually chronic but is accompanied by the gradual destruction of the infected cells, giving rise to cardiac failure and loss of control of the digestive system later in life, possibly 20–30 y later. It is difficult and dangerous to work with *T. cruzi* and the mechanisms of pathogenesis have not been fully elucidated, but there is general agreement that the destruction of host cells is an autoimmune phenomenon. Whether it is initiated by the antigens of host or parasite origin is still a matter of speculation. Some parasite antigens may be absorbed by host cells, which are damaged by the immune response releasing further antigens and accelerating the autoimmune reactions. Some antigens may be shared by the parasite and host neural cells and cardiac cells, for example laminin is found in both the heart and the trypanosome surface.

A number of immunological defence mechanisms have been identified mainly from rodent and in vitro studies (reviewed by Takle and Snary 1993, Kierszenbaum and Sztein 1994 and Kirchoff 1994). Macrophages activated by IFN-γ or IL-12 represent a major defence mechanism and NO is a powerful killing agent, but macrophage activity can be inhibited by IL-4, IL-10 and TGF-β (Monoz-Fernandez, Fernandez and Fresno 1992, Gazzinelli et al. 1992, Reed 1995).

T. cruzi employs a variety of immune evasion mechanisms and these contribute to the longevity of the infection and to the associated pathological changes. In this context it might be to the advantage of the parasite to mimic host cells, but the inevitable outcome of the possession of shared antigens is autoimmunity which is characteristic of this infection. As well as escaping from the phagolysosome, the parasites themselves produce a number of products that inhibit the immune response. These include inhibitors of CD3, CD4, CD8 and IL-2 receptors and factors that induce the production of IL-10 and TGF-β (Sztein, Cuna and Kierszenbaum 1990).

In summary, immunity to *T. cruzi* involves some of the most complex immunological responses encountered in any infection and the interplay between immunity, immune evasion and autoimmunity is likely to take many years to elucidate. In the meantime, although some experimental vaccines have been developed, the possibility of a protective vaccine that does not cause any autoimmunity against this important human pathogen seems remote.

Microsporidians

Microsporidiosis, caused by at least 8 species belonging to 5 genera (see Chapter 21) is a rare but increasingly recognized condition in immunologically compromised patients, particularly those suffering from AIDS (Bryan 1995, Deraedt and Molina 1995). As the condition is virtually unknown in immunologically competent individuals, there must be some immune response that keeps these infections under control, but definite evidence for this, and its mech-

anisms, are lacking. Apart from the epidemiological evidence, most of our knowledge comes from animal and in vitro studies, which might not be relevant to what happens in humans. It is clear that perturbation of T cell function is a major cause of immunological failure leading to microsporidiosis, but as T cells are central to so many immunological responses it is difficult to draw firm conclusions about the nature of natural or acquired immunity to microsporidiosis in humans.

Sarcocystis and related organisms

Little is known of these rare infections in humans (described in Chapter 17) in terms of the immune responses that they evoke in their natural hosts, laboratory animals or humans. All form thick-walled cysts with few signs of any immunological reaction or immunopathology.

Opportunistic amoebae

Although these free-living amoebae (belonging to the genera *Acanthamoeba*, *Balamuthia* and *Naegleria*) are sometimes grouped with the intestinal amoebae, it is convenient to consider them briefly here. As there have been relatively few human infections, there is very little information available and it is not known whether or not individuals mount a protective immune response. If they do, it is not clear whether this protects against subsequent infection (which, in any case, would be very unlikely). Virtually all that is known is that specific antibodies have been detected in the sera of infected individuals (See Chapter 9). Information that has accrued from observations in animal models has been reviewed by John (1993).

4 Immunity to helminths

4.1 Characteristics of helminths in relation to the immune response

Helminths (worm parasites) confront the immune system with problems that are quite different from those posed by protozoans. These problems are largely the consequences of greater size and structural complexity, but are compounded by 3 additional factors:

1 worms have the ability to move actively through the body of the host
2 as part of their life cycles, many undergo sequential developmental changes in the host, during which their structure and antigenic make-up may change dramatically
3 their bodies are covered by layers that are more complex and less vulnerable to immune attack than conventional plasma membranes.

Thus, although helminths occupy many of the sites in the body that are exploited by protozoans (other than the truly intracellular), the immune mechanisms required to destroy them in, or remove them from, these sites must often be qualitatively different. Unlike protozoans, the majority of helminths do not replicate within the host. In these circumstances, an increase in the worm burden carried (and the associated danger of pathology) occurs only when the host is repeatedly infected. Under conditions of natural infection, immune responses are therefore most important in preventing or reducing reinfection. There are, however, some helminths in which the numbers of parasite stages present in the body do increase after infection. These include: tapeworms such as *Taenia solium* and *Echinococcus*, in which an initial infection may produce large numbers of larval stages; the blood flukes (*Schistosoma*) in which eggs become trapped in tissues; and the nematodes *Strongyloides* and *Trichinella*, in which larvae accumulate in the body. In such cases the development of the immune response can be considered analogous to that which occurs in protozoan infections.

Adult stages of helminths range in length from a few millimetres to several metres. Larval stages may be <1mm in length, but even the smallest larva is too large to be phagocytosed or lysed by a single cell; cytotoxic activity therefore requires multiple interactions between the parasite surface and inflammatory cells. Such interactions can be mediated by both complement and antibody, antibody-dependent cellular cytotoxicity (ADCC) being a common response to invasion by worms.

In addition to being large, helminths are complex multicellular organisms with well developed organs and tissues. When alive they present the immune system with a diverse range of antigens, both on their surfaces and in excretory and secretory products. When they die, many more antigens may be released. Although immune responses are made to the majority of these antigens, they may have little or no effect upon the parasite for some or all of the following reasons:

1 the molecules concerned may not be essential for worm survival
2 in the living worm these molecules may be inaccessible to effector mechanisms
3 the response to released antigens may take place at a considerable distance from the parasite
4 the parasite may actively move away from the immune response generated at a particular site
5 the antigens may elicit inappropriate immune responses
6 the parasite may evade, inactivate or down-regulate immune effectors.

In general then, although there are important exceptions involving larval stages, worms are likely to be much less easily controlled by immediate interactions with immune effector mechanisms than are protozoans. Binding of antibodies, or surface activation of complement, rarely kills worms directly; effective immunity is more often the indirect result of immunologically specific recognition events. Among the more important of these are ADCC, immune-mediated inflammation and antibody-mediated inhibition of enzyme activity.

The result of ADCC reactions is the adherence of large numbers of cells and the release onto the surface of a variety of enzymes and short-range mediators. These may harm the parasite directly, either by destroying the integrity of the surface layer or by causing damage to deeper tissues. The effectiveness of such attack is influenced by the nature of the surface available. For example, whereas flukes such as schistosomes have relatively delicate cytoplasmic surfaces, nematodes have tougher collagenous cuticles that provide them with considerable protection against external damage. Larval nematodes may be killed by ADCC, but adults are often unaffected. Even the theoretically more vulnerable schistosomes have multiple evasion strategies that result in their surfaces being difficult to damage. In addition, effective ADCC requires not only that cells bind to the target, but also that they maintain contact, which is sometimes difficult when the target is an active worm.

By mechanisms that are not fully understood, the range of immune responses elicited by infections with helminths typically show a number of important differences from those generated by protozoan infections. The majority of worm infections are associated with responses that reflect release of cytokines from Th2 cells (see 2.2). Prominent among these responses are the increased production of reaginic antibody (IgE), mast cells and eosinophils. Immediate hypersensitivity reactions, in which these components are involved, are therefore characteristic accompaniments of worm infections, but rare in protozoans. The inflammatory consequences of such reactions can be very effective forms of host defence and provide substantial resistance to infection. They result in structural, functional and biochemical changes in the tissues surrounding the worms and lead to the release of powerful biologically active mediators. If antigenic stimulation and inflammation persist, worms may become the focus of cellular accumulations that trap them and that may ultimately kill them. Unfortunately, such chronic reactions can also cause severe pathology.

With the important exceptions of tapeworms and acanthocephalans, most helminths feed actively and digest their food source enzymatically, either within their own intestines or externally before uptake. The enzymes used in these processes can be important targets for the host immune response, as are those used by worms to penetrate the host and to move through its tissues. The interaction of antibodies with target parasite enzymes can inhibit their activity, which can prevent successful invasion, migration, growth and development and may result in worm death. Indeed, the complex nutritional, environmental and behavioural requirements of worms makes any host-mediated interference with normal function a potential means of increasing resistance.

It should therefore be clear that, although protozoa and helminths are grouped together as 'parasites' and both are powerfully immunogenic to the hosts, if they are to be successfully controlled by immune responses rather different strategies are required and quite distinct mechanisms may be involved.

4.2 Immunity to intestinal helminths

The characteristics of the intestine as an environment for parasites have already been described (section 3.1). Despite the many defences that can act there, the intestine is one of the commonest environments for parasitic worms and it is colonized by representatives of all the major groups: digeneans (flukes), cestodes (tapeworms) and nematodes (roundworms). Relatively little is known of immune responses to flukes and tapeworms in humans. More is known about nematodes, but most of this information concerns responses that can be measured peripherally, i.e. antibodies, proliferative and cytokine responses of circulating lymphocytes, delayed hypersensitivity and inflammatory responses. For an insight into responses operative at the intestinal level we are heavily dependent on data obtained from work with experimental models.

INTESTINAL NEMATODES

A very large number of nematode species live in or infect via the intestine (see Chapters 29, 30, 31). Collectively, they are among the commonest of all parasites, infecting an estimated one-quarter of the world's population (Maizels et al. 1993). The major intestinal nematodes of humans (*Ascaris*, hookworms, *Strongyloides* and *Trichuris*) all mature in the intestine, but reach that site in a variety of ways. *Trichuris* infections are established by ingestion of eggs and the worms develop directly in the large intestine. *Ascaris* also infects orally, but after hatching, the larval stages penetrate the intestinal mucosa and migrate via the liver and lungs before returning to the small intestine to mature. The larvae of hookworms and *Strongyloides* characteristically infect through the skin and then migrate to the small intestine. In addition to the intestine itself, immunity to worms with migratory stages may therefore operate at several sites in the body. The mechanisms likely to be effective will be determined by the characteristics of each organ system involved. Immune and inflammatory responses in parenteral sites such as the skin, liver and lungs share a number of common features. Worms moving through these sites are likely to be in intimate contact with potential effectors, such as antibodies (IgM, IgG), complement, biologically active mediators and cytotoxic cells, and can therefore be damaged directly. In contrast, worms living in the intestine itself may have a quite different relationship with the immune system. Not only does the intestine have distinctive immune mechanisms, but unless worms penetrate into the mucosa they are unlikely to be accessible to some of the effector mechanisms that operate in the tissues. Those effectors that may affect intestinal worms include the antibody isotypes that are secreted into the lumen (IgA and IgM) or leak from the mucosa (IgG), and mediators such as amines, prostaglandins, leukotrienes and reactive oxygen and nitrogen metabolites that are produced by inflammatory cells. Intestinal worms, like all parasites, are wholly dependent upon the physical and physicochemical characteristics of their environment,

and these conditions may change dramatically when the intestine is inflamed as a result of infection. Such changes can themselves contribute to immunity by making the local habitats of the parasites unsuitable for their continued survival. As already mentioned (2.2 and 4.1) worm infections selectively elicit Th2 subset responses and the cytokines produced by these cells generate powerful inflammatory responses, 3 components of which (IgE, mast cells and eosinophils) are known to be potent mediators of intestinal inflammation.

Experimental systems in laboratory animals show that intestinal worms can be very effectively controlled by host immune responses (Wakelin, Harnett and Parkhouse 1993). It is much less clear whether intestinal worms in humans are similarly controlled. Infections are not only very common, but they are often persistent. Individuals may acquire worms early in life, retain worms for long periods and be easily reinfected. Epidemiological studies indicate that although the prevalence of infections often remains high as people age, the intensity of infection (numbers of worms) can decline significantly (Bundy 1995). This may indicate the operation of protective immune responses, although it is obvious that behavioural changes will also be involved, as transmission of all the major intestinal worms is dependent upon some degree of contact with faecal, or faecally contaminated, material. Cross-sectional analysis of infected populations shows that the parasite burden is aggregated into relatively few individuals, most having small numbers of worms. Again this may indicate an effective immunity or may reflect behavioural influences. It is well established that individuals are predisposed to a particular level of infection, i.e. they reacquire worm burdens after chemotherapy that are similar to those existing before treatment. In some, this predisposition results in heavy infections (i.e. the individuals are susceptible); in others only light infections are acquired (i.e. they appear resistant). Predisposition suggests the operation of genetically determined levels of immunity to infection, although alternative explanations still cannot be ruled out.

Knowledge of immune responses to intestinal nematodes of humans is much less detailed than that of responses to the other major helminth groups (see 4.3 and 4.4) and is mainly derived from correlative immunoepidemiological studies. In general, serological responses correlate positively with intensity and duration of infection, but certain isotypes do show correlations that suggest an involvement in protective immunity. These include IgA responses in *Trichuris* infections (Bundy and Medley 1992) and IgE responses in hookworm (*Necator*) infections (Pritchard, Quinnell and Walsh 1995). The functional roles of anti-worm antibodies are uncertain. ADCC responses may be generated against stages migrating through tissues, but the adults in the intestine are large and well protected organisms. Antibodies may interfere with feeding activities, particularly where, as in hookworms and possibly *Trichuris*, these depend upon the worm releasing enzymes into the host's tissues. Antibodies may also reduce the effectiveness of worm secretions that interfere with the operation of host defence mechanisms, such as anti-enzymes, anti-oxidants and immunomodulators (Pritchard 1995). Little direct information is available about cellular responses, but data showing correlations between HLA haplotypes and putative resistance to infection confirm the relevance of T cell activity (Bundy and Medley 1992, Holland et al. 1992).

Considerable attention has been paid to allergic responses to intestinal nematodes, in particular to those associated with *Ascaris,* for which a major allergen has been defined. Significantly increased levels of IgE are common in all infections, except *Trichuris,* but the protective attributes of this isotype are poorly defined in humans.

Experimental studies in rodents have given much more detailed pictures of the nature and operation of immune responses against intestinal nematodes. These may operate during the course of primary infections to expel worms from the intestine. On reinfection, protective responses operate more quickly and may prevent the establishment of infection almost completely. In all cases, immunity is T helper cell-dependent, and Th2 cells play the major role (Urban et al. 1992). In manipulative experiments it has been shown that IFN-γ can prevent, and IL-4 can promote, the normal expression of immunity (Urban et al. 1993, 1995). Responses to infection are accompanied by acute inflammatory changes that result in structural and functional modifications of the intestinal mucosa. With some species (e.g. *Nippostrongylus, Strongyloides, Trichinella*) inflammation is the single most important effector mechanism, mediators from mast cells or mucus from goblet cells acting indirectly or directly to eliminate worms (Nawa et al. 1994). Although IgE antibodies and eosinophilia accompany the intestinal inflammation, they do not seem to have a significant role, and deletion of these responses by using antibodies against the relevant cytokines does not affect the expression of immunity. In other parasites (e.g. *Trichuris*) anti-worm IgA and IgG1 antibodies seem to be important, probably by interfering with important metabolic or behavioural activities. In worms that migrate through the tissues to reach the intestine (*Nippostrongylus, Strongyloides*), immunity acts against the intestinal stages during a primary infection, but against tissue stages in subsequent infections, larvae being trapped in eosinophil-rich inflammatory foci in the lungs or the skin. Similar mechanisms act against migrating larval hookworms in immune mice (Wilkinson, Wells and Behnke 1990).

Experimental models have not only allowed the study of protective responses, they have also shed light on situations in which immunity does not operate or operates at best ineffectively. Some nematodes in mice (like nematodes in humans) establish chronic, long-term infections (Behnke, Barnard and Wakelin 1992). With one species (*Heligmosomoides polygyrus*) this is due to immunomodulatory influences exerted by adult worms, which effectively suppress the potentially protective responses elicited by the larval stages. Immuno-modulation is associated with the release of particular molecules in the secretions of adult worms. Full expression of this immune suppression is under strong host genetic influences, which determine the speed and nature of anti-parasite responses. *Trichuris muris* can also establish chronic infections in certain strains of inbred mice. In most strains, infection elicits Th2 responses that result in effective immunity and worms are lost before they can become mature. In certain strains, the initial Th2 response is switched, possibly by worm-derived molecules, to a Th1 response and the host is then not only unable to eliminate the existing infection but remains susceptible to subsequent infections as well, a situation that has many parallels with human *Trichuris* infections (Grencis 1996). Chronic worm infections are often associated with immuno-pathological changes to the intestine, which almost certainly reflect the effects of persisting, inappropriate immune responses.

4.3 Immunity to filarial nematodes

Filarial nematodes (members of the Filarioidea) are important human parasites in many subtropical and tropical countries (see Chapters 32, 33). All are transmitted by insect vectors, which act as intermediate hosts allowing development of larvae to the infective stage. These larvae are transmitted when the insect bites, the initial stages of infection therefore involving the skin and dermal tissues. In some species the adults remain in the superficial layers of the body, but in others the adult worms live within much deeper tissues; both are therefore, theoretically, susceptible to direct interaction with immune effectors such as antibody, complement and cytotoxic cells. There are several species of filariae that infect humans, many of which are of low pathogenicity or of only local significance. The most important species are those in which the adult worm lives in the lymphatic tissues (the genera *Wuchereria* and *Brugia*) and those in which the adults live in the skin (*Onchocerca*). In the former, adult females liberate embryos (microfilaria larvae) that circulate in the blood; female *Onchocerca* release microfilaria into the skin. Biting insects pick up these larvae while feeding, the larvae undergo moults to reach the infective third stage, and these then re-enter the human at the next blood meal. In the lymphatic species, pathology is caused by the adult stages, whereas in *Onchocerca* microfilaria are the primary cause of pathology.

It is characteristic of all filarial infections that they are long-lived, worms surviving for many years and releasing millions of microfilaria. Many individuals in areas where these infections are endemic continue to accumulate worms over long periods. These 2 features suggest that there is little or no immunity, but more detailed epidemiological studies, particularly those concerned with lymphatic filariases, suggest otherwise (Ottesen 1992, Maizels et al. 1995); similar data are available for onchocerciasis (Elson et al. 1994). Even in areas where the overall prevalence is high, some individuals are parasitologically negative, show no pathology but do have anti-parasite immune responses, indicating exposure to infection. The majority show signs of infection, of pathology or both. Some are heavily infected, with many circulating microfilaria, but may have relatively little overt pathology; some have severe pathology but may have few or no microfilaria in the blood; others may have low microfilaraemia but show abnormal pathology indicative of hypersensitivity reactions. Collectively, these data show that filarial infections do stimulate immune responses; in some individuals these responses appear to be fully protective, but in others, immune responses contribute to the development of pathologic changes. This spectrum of responsiveness probably reflects a variety of patterns of T helper cell and cytokine activity, most clearly reflected in levels of T cell reactivity to parasite antigen and in levels of particular antibody isotypes (Maizels et al. 1995).

Analysis of protective responses to filarial nematodes has been carried out (1) in vitro, using human cells and sera, and (2) in vivo, using a variety of animal models. It has been shown in several cases that immunity can effectively operate through ADCC reactions directed against antigens present on the cuticular surface. The filarial cuticle is relatively delicate, compared with that of the intestinal nematodes, for example, and may play a significant role in the uptake of nutrients. Antigens on the cuticle are known to be targets for antibodies, particularly IgG and IgE isotypes, and these facilitate adherence of cells such as eosinophils, macrophages and neutrophils. Under experimental conditions, ADCC reactions can kill all stages, from microfilaria to adult; under conditions of natural infection it is most likely that a primary target is the incoming infective larva.

Although the cuticle appears to be a major target for immune responses, other antigens have also been identified. For example, antigens derived from internal tissues can elicit protective responses when used to immunize experimental animals. Two of the most interesting of these are the muscle proteins, paramyosin (used to immunize jirds, *Meriones unguiculatus*, against *B. malayi*) (Li, Chandrashekar and Weil 1993) and tropomyosin (used to immunize mice against *O. volvulus*) (Taylor, Jenkins and Bianco 1996).

Immunity to filaria is T cell dependent and involves the activity of T helper cells, according to evidence from a variety of sources. In humans, putative immunity correlates with production of T-dependent antibody isotypes (IgE and IgG3), and these isotypes are also required for effective ADCC. Production of eosinophils, a major contributor to cytotoxicity, is also T dependent. Studies in experimental animals have not only confirmed the need for T helper cell activity, but have also indicated that in some cases the Th2 subset is functionally important (Lawrence 1996). There are some interesting exceptions to these conclusions (e.g. Rajan et al. 1994) and these raise the perennial problem as to how representative of human responses are those measured in experimental animals.

Some of the most interesting data concerning immune responses to filarial infections in humans are those which attempt to correlate patient status with particular components of the immune system. It is now widely accepted that, both for lymphatic filariasis and onchocerciasis, there are individuals in populations in endemic areas who neither develop patent infections nor show any signs of diseases, yet they are immunologically positive in the sense of having anti-parasite antibodies and antigen-specific T cell activity. Such individuals are often referred to as 'endemic normals', although the use of this term is debatable (Day 1991). The fact that these individuals remain parasitologically negative despite exposure to infected vectors implies effective control of incoming infections and it is thought that this control operates against the infective larval stages. Experimental data from *Brugia* infections in cats, as well as data from rodent models, supports this interpretation; indeed there is good evidence that irradiated infective larvae can induce an effective immunity when used as a vaccine and that this immunity is Th2-dependent (Bancroft et al. 1994).

The suggestion that some individuals do develop immunity to filarial infections raises the question of why the majority apparently do not, despite evidence for immune responses to the parasites. Those who show parasitological or pathological evidence of infection can be divided into a number of categories (King and Nutman 1991). In lymphatic filariasis the extremes are patients who are microfilaraemic and asymptomatic, and those who are microfilaria negative but show obstructive pathology. Another category shows atypical allergic hyper-responsiveness (tropical pulmonary eosinophilia). The lymphocytes of those with high microfilaraemia often appear to be unresponsive to parasite antigens when tested in vitro (as is also the case with cells from patients with heavy skin burdens of the microfilaria of *Onchocerca*). There is some evidence that released parasite products themselves can be directly immunosuppressive, but much attention has focused on altered T cell-subset activity and cytokine production as contributory factors (Maizels et al. 1995). The unresponsiveness observed in vitro has been linked to an altered balance between Th1 and Th2 activity, leading to depression of Th1 responsiveness and enhancement of Th2. One consequence of the latter is the high levels of circulating anti-worm IgG4 and IgE. These isotypes are found in both microfilaraemic and elephantiasis patients, but in the former the ratio between the isotypes is biased to IgG4 and in the latter the bias is towards IgE. The high levels of IgG4 may inhibit allergic responsiveness in the microfilaremic patients, whereas high IgE may promote pathological responses leading to obstructive pathology. IgE may therefore be important in protection against larval stages, through mediation of ADCC, but it may also contribute to immunopathology via hypersensitivity reactions to adult worms. Other IgG isotypes are low in microfilaraemic individuals but more prominent in the elephantiasis group, in whom they may again contribute to pathology.

The T cell anergy seen in patients heavily infected

with lymphatic filarias or with *Onchocerca* appears to be due to downregulation of Th1 responsiveness by the cytokine IL-10 (King and Nutman 1991, Mahanty and Nutman 1995). This is released from both Th2 cells, monocytes and macrophages, but predominantly the latter. T cells from microfilaraemic individuals release little IFN-γ, but much IL-4, whereas cells from individuals with elephantiasis (who are parasite-negative) produce both IFN-γ and IL-4, as do cells from those who show neither pathology nor infection. Microfilaraemic patients show high IL-10 production and low antigen-specific T cell proliferation; symptomatic patients produce little IL-10 and their T cells proliferate well when exposed to parasite antigen. These results suggest that Th1 responses are somehow involved in anti-parasite activity, which may be both beneficial, giving immunity against larvae, and harmful, via inflammatory responses to adult worms. IL-4 secretion appears to be linked with that of IL-5, lymphatic filariasis being characterized by high peripheral eosinophilia. In filarial infections there is, therefore, a complex, parasite-induced interplay between Th subsets that results in modulation of antibody and cellular responsiveness and determines both the parasitological and pathological outcomes of infection (Fig 4.5).

4.4 Immunity to flukes

Several species of digenenan Platyhelminthes are parasitic in humans. They can be divided into 4 categories, based on their locations within the body: the lung flukes (*Paragonimus*); liver flukes (e.g. *Clonorchis/Opisthorchis*); intestinal flukes (many genera); and the blood flukes (*Schistosoma*). Both lung and liver flukes can be highly pathogenic, infections resulting in severe tissue damage (see Chapter 26). Serological and cellular responses to these parasites are well described, but are not easily correlated with protective immunity. Little is known of immune responses to the human intestinal flukes, although infections of mice with *Echinostoma* have shown that an effective immunity can operate. The most intensively studied flukes are the schistosomes.

Schistosomes

Adult schistosomes live in the blood vessels of the host. Infections are initiated by penetration through the skin of larval stages that have developed in aquatic snails. To reach their final location, the larvae (schistosomula) migrate from the skin via the lungs to the liver, where they develop into mature male and female worms. These form permanent pairs, and then move to the mesenteric veins around the intestine or the vesical veins around the bladder. Once there, the worms can survive for prolonged periods (possibly years) during which time the female releases large numbers of eggs. These must leave the body and hatch in water so that larvae can find and penetrate a suitable snail. Eggs develop in the host's body and the contained larvae release enzymes that facilitate their passage out of blood vessels, through tissues into the lumen of the gut or bladder. Release from the body therefore occurs with faeces or urine. There are 3 major species infecting humans: *Schistosoma japonicum*, *S. mansoni* (both in mesenteric veins), and *S. haematobium* (vesical veins).

Schistosomiasis is a multifaceted, immunopathological disease, but the most important components are the hypersensitivity responses initiated by eggs that are trapped in tissues (see Chapter 25). Granulomata form around the eggs, particularly those in the liver, and cause considerable local tissue damage. By blocking blood flow, granulomata can cause portal hypertension and serious vascular abnormalities, some of which (e.g. oesophageal varices) may be life threatening.

Schistosome infections are common wherever climatic and environmental conditions favour snail development and where socio-economic conditions allow faecal and urinary contamination of water that is used for drinking, bathing, washing or working. Infections are acquired early in life and are long-lasting; the disease is most serious in older children and young adults. The intensity of infection declines with age; it is now accepted that this decline has an immunological as well as a behavioural component. Experimental work in animals initially suggested that powerful protective immune responses could effectively control infection (Newport and Colley 1993).

Experimental models have primarily used *S. mansoni*, which will infect a variety of rodents and primates. Early primate work defined the phenomenon of 'concomitant immunity' (the host is immune to reinfection whilst continuing to harbour the adult worms from an initial infection). Concomitant immunity was interpreted as showing that resistance mechanisms operated against the early schistosomula stage, but that adult worms were unaffected. In essence this view still holds, although there is evidence that adults may also be affected by immunity (Hagan and Wilkins 1993). Early studies also focused on effector mechanisms that resulted in damage to the tegumental surface, which, in the larval stages at least, appeared vulnerable to direct damage by complement-mediated mechanisms and to damage brought about by antibody-dependent cellular cytotoxicity (ADCC). The ability of adult worms (and indeed later larval stages) to survive in the face of responses capable of destroying early schistosomula depends upon the following: intrinsic changes in the tegument itself, rendering it less easily damaged; the acquisition of host molecules (including immunglobulin and glycolipids) that provide an immunological 'disguise'; and a number of active evasion strategies that interfere with host immune mechanisms.

Experimental models indicate that there are multiple mechanisms through which resistance can be expressed. The experiments that have defined these mechanisms have been carried out (1) in vitro, using cells, sera and larval stages; and (2) in vivo, in animals that have been immunized by infection or by vaccination with irradiated larvae. This variety of approaches in a different host species has inevitably

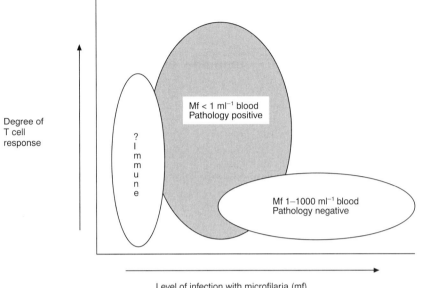

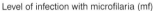

Level of infection with microfilaria (mf)

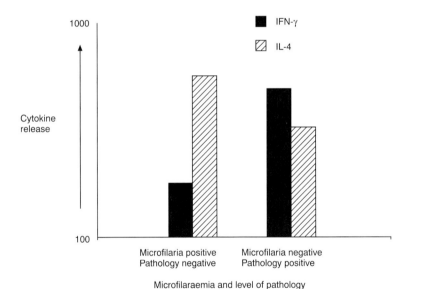

Microfilaraemia and level of pathology

Fig. 4.5 Diagrammatic representation of the variations in T cell responsiveness and T helper cell subset activity in patients infected with the lymphatic filaria *Brugia malayi*. T cell responses, reflected in level of proliferation when stimulated in vitro with antigen, are much higher in individuals without obvious infection (putatively immune) and in patients showing obstructive pathology than in those showing heavy microfilaraemia but little pathology. Cytokine profiles (as measured by in vitro cytokine production) indicate that heavy microfilaraemia is associated with a predominant T helper 2 response (i.e. IL-4 production) whereas pathology in the absence of microfilaraemia is associated with a predominant T helper 1 response (i.e. IFN-γ is the major cytokine). Data from Maizels et al. 1995.

meant that there is still no clear consensus about the mechanisms underlying protective immunity, although it seems clear that ADCC can be an important component of protective immunity. Several antibody isotypes and cell populations can participate in this response; eosinophils are major killer cells and IgG, IgE and IgA are important isotypes. Interactions between parasites and macrophages may also be important, both in terms of ADCC and through the release of mediators capable of damaging the worms. A major difficulty, which has still to be resolved, is the relevance of data from animal experiments and from in vitro studies to the immune responses likely to occur in humans living in endemic areas (Butterworth 1994).

The antigens that can initiate immunity include molecules present at the surface of the tegument, the targets for ADCC (Abath and Werkhauser 1996). Internal antigens are also important. The latter include structural proteins, e.g. paramyosin, as well as a number with enzyme activity, e.g. glutathione S-transferase (GST) and triosephosphate isomerase (Bergquist 1995). Several antigens have been defined and produced as recombinant or synthetic molecules and some, particularly GST, are now being exploited as vaccine candidates. Trials have been carried out in rodents, bovines and primates, with some degree of success achieved, largely in terms of reducing worm egg production and thus reducing egg-induced pathology (Dunne, Hagan and Abath 1995).

The demonstration that immunity does play a part in determining the age-related decline in infection seen in endemic areas has come from detailed population surveys; these have monitored levels of reinfection after chemotherapy, as well as degrees of water contact. They have shown that individuals may effectively resist reinfection despite frequent contact with infected waters. Immunological studies on these populations have identified significant correlations between protective immunity and levels of anti-worm IgE, but have also shown that other isotypes (particularly IgM, IgG2 and IgG4) can act as blocking antibodies and interfere with the expression of immunity (Newport and Colley 1993). In young children (<10 years) blocking antibodies predominate, in older children protective IgE predominates. It is assumed that IgE may act in ADCC and that blocking antibodies interfere with the optimal operation of this protective mechanism.

These associations between immunity, susceptibility and particular isotypes highlight the complex roles of Th1 and Th2 responses against schistosome infection (Sher and Coffman 1992). Experimental models show that there is a switch between Th1 and Th2 responses when the adult worms begin to release eggs, schistosome egg antigens being potent stimulators of IL-4 release from non-lymphoid cells, which is thought to drive Th2 subset development (Sabin and Pearce 1995). Data from infected humans suggest a similar phenomenon. Production of both IgE and eosinophils require help from Th2 cells, as does production of the blocking isotype IgG4; thus it is not possible to explain immunity as a simple Th2-dependent phenomenon. In humans, Th1 responses correlate strongly with pathology and morbidity, although Th2 cytokines can also contribute to granuloma formation, but in mice it seems that vaccine-induced protection is Th1 dependent.

Invasion and development of schistosomes are associated with distinct immunopathological phases. Penetration of the skin by cercariae causes a dermatitis, which may be severe in individuals sensitized by prior infection. The developmental stages may also be associated with allergic symptoms. This is particularly true in the case of *S. japonicum* infection, in which fever, eosinophilia, lymphadenopathy, splenomegaly and intestinal disturbances form the syndrome known as 'Katayama fever'. The hypersensitivity responses that lead to granuloma formation around trapped eggs have been studied in great detail, particularly in *S. mansoni* infections (Wynn and Cheever 1995). The development of granulomata is T cell dependent and involves a complex set of interactions between cytokines, chemokines and a variety of inflammatory cells, of which eosinophils are particularly important. Both Th1 and Th2 cells contribute to granuloma formation, but down-regulation of Th2 activity occurs as infection progresses and this results in modulation of granuloma formation.

S. mansoni and *S. japonicum* eggs leave the host's body via the intestine, which may become extensively damaged as tissues become sensitized to the eggs. In *S. haematobium*, the eggs of which leave via the bladder, inflammatory responses may produce severe pathological changes. There is a definite, but unexplained, association between such changes and the development of bladder cancers.

4.5   Immunity to tapeworms

Humans may act as hosts for adult stages of a number of tapeworm species. Some of these (e.g. *Taenia saginata* and *T. solium*) occur only in humans, others (e.g. *Diphyllobothrium latum*) occur in other hosts as well. Infections with adult tapeworms are acquired, in almost all cases, by ingestion of larval stages present in the bodies of intermediate hosts; e.g. in the case of *T. saginata* by ingesting cysticerci present in infected beef and in the case of *D. latum* by ingesting plerocercoids present in infected fish. One species, *Hymenolepis nana*, has a unique life cycle in which development from the egg to the adult can take place within a single host. This species can therefore be locally quite common, particularly in children. Very little is known of immune responses to adult tapeworms in humans; experimental studies with *H. nana* and other hymenolepids in rodents have shown that protective responses can act in the intestine against the adult stage.

LARVAL TAPEWORMS

In general, adult cestodes cause relatively little pathology, whereas larval tapeworms (metacestodes) can be highly pathogenic. In most cases, larvae are acquired by the accidental ingestion of eggs released from adult tapeworms in the intestines of other host species or from larval stages carried in transport hosts used for food. Larvae of the pork tapeworm *T. solium*, however, can develop from eggs released by adults in the intestine of the same or other humans.

The larval infections of greatest clinical importance are those caused by *T. solium* (cysticercosis, *Echinococcus granulosus*), hydatid disease and *E. multilocularis* (alveolar echinococcosis) (see Chapter 28). In all of these the metacestodes form cyst-like structures in host tissues. Cysticercosis occurs wherever *T. solium* infections are common in the natural intermediate host, the pig. If infected pig meat is eaten raw or undercooked the larval stages (cysticerci) become activated in the intestine, attach to the mucosa and transform into the adult worm. When mature, the adult begins to shed segments (proglottids) that pass out with faeces. As these decay, they release infective eggs that may contaminate water or vegetables, which then become a source of human infection. It is also thought that eggs can hatch directly in the intestine of a host harbouring an adult worm (autoinfection). By whatever route infection is achieved, eggs hatch, then larvae penetrate the intestinal wall and migrate via the bloodstream. Cysticerci can form in the muscles, where they are relatively harmless, and in the CNS, where they can cause severe symptoms.

Larvae of *Echinococcus* spp. are acquired by accidental ingestion of eggs deposited in the faeces of dogs or wild carnivores such as foxes. The eggs hatch in the small intestine, the larvae penetrate the mucosa and migrate via the blood, and develop in internal organs such as the lungs, liver, peritoneal cavity and CNS. Larvae of *E. granulosus* grow into large fluid-filled cysts (hydatid cysts), whereas larvae of *E. multilocularis* form a pseudo-malignant mass of proliferating vesicular structures.

The immunological relationships between larval tapeworms and their hosts are complex and not well understood. Metacestodes often elicit little inflammation, they can persist for long periods and some can metastasize. All of these characteristics imply minimal or ineffective immune responses, yet it quite clear that infections are immunogenic. There are many descriptions of cellular and serological responses to metacestodes in humans, from which some correlations with protective immunity can be drawn. There has been considerable work on infections in animal models, from which have come more precise insights into determinants of resistance and susceptibility (Dixon and Jenkins 1995a). Immune responses can be considered as operative early or late in infection. The term 'early' describes responses against the hexacanth larva or onchosphere that is released from the egg and which undertakes the initial migration into the tissues; 'late' describes responses against the subsequent developing cystic metacestode stages (Lightowlers et al. 1993)

In the early stages of larval development, the tapeworms have an unprotected external layer called the 'tegument'. They are therefore susceptible to damage by complement-fixing antibodies (e.g. IgG1 and IgG2 isotypes in mice; IgG2a in rats) and by complement- and antibody-mediated cellular cytotoxicity. Experimental studies show that host immunity can destroy larvae as they cross the mucosa or after they penetrate into other organs, but killing does not occur during an initial infection and the larvae become successfully established; early immunity is therefore most effective against reinfection. As the larvae develop, they acquire an external protective layer formed of both host and parasite components. They also produce sulphated polysaccharides and proteoglycans that interfere with host complement activation. In consequence the larvae become insusceptible to the responses that can damage earlier life cycle stages. Late immunity appears to operate exclusively through cytotoxic mechanisms, though these have little significant effect on larvae when they are fully developed. Larval tapeworm infections, like schistosome infections, therefore show concomitant immunity, the host harbouring fully developed primary infection larvae whilst being resistant to reinfection.

There is considerable evidence that larval tapeworms exert a variety of immunosuppressive effects on the host (Dixon and Jenkins 1995b). For example, larval secretions inhibit T cell proliferative responses and IL-2 production, prevent the accumulation of inflammatory cells, and interfere with normal macrophage functions. Infections, particularly with *E. granulosus*, generate powerful hypersensitivity responses, which can be life threatening if there is release of cyst fluid during surgical removal procedures.

Studies with *E. multilocularis* in experimental rodents and in humans are beginning to identify some of the key immunological events that may determine the outcome of infection (Gottstein and Felleisen 1995). As with many infections, there are striking genetically determined differences in the susceptibility and resistance of different strains of mice to this parasite. Mice that have greater resistance show responses that seem to indicate a dominant influence of Th1 cells, and the granulomata that develop around the mass of larval tissue contain a high proportion of CD8+ T cells. In contrast, more susceptible mice, in which parasite growth is unchecked, have Th2-dominated responses and a high proportion of CD4+ T cells in the granulomata. It is suggestive that similar data have come from studies of humans in endemic areas, some of whom, though susceptible to infection, seem to be resistant to disease. In these individuals, CD8+ T cell numbers in the granulomata are high and peripheral lymphocytes secrete large amounts of the Th2 cytokine IL-5.

There is no immediate prospect of immunoprophylaxis against larval tapeworm infections in humans, but a recombinant vaccine has been introduced to immunize sheep against the larval stages of *Taenia ovis* (Rickard 1995) and recombinant antigens of *E. granulosus* are being tested in sheep (Lightowlers et al. 1996). The most important practical application of immunological studies at present is the development of improved immunodiagnosis; larval tapeworm infections being difficult to diagnose definitively, even with modern scanning techniques.

REFERENCES

Abath FGC, Werkhauser RC, 1996, The tegument of *Schistosoma mansoni*: functional and immunological features, *Parasite Immunol*, **18**: 15–20.

Ackers JP, 1989, Immunologic aspects of human trichomoniasis, *Trichomonads Parasitic in Humans*, ed Honigberg BM, Springer Verlag, New York, 36–52.

Adal KA, Sterling CR, Guerrant RL, 1995, *Cryptosporidium* and related species, *Infections of the Gastrointestinal Tract*, ed Blaser MJ, Smith PD et al., Raven Press, New York, 1107–28.

Alderete JF, 1983, Antigen analysis of several pathogenic strains of *Trichomonas vaginalis*, *Infect Immun*, **39**: 1041–7.

Alexander J, Russell DG, 1992, The interaction of *Leishmania* with macrophages, *Adv Parasitol*, **31**: 175–254.

Ambroise-Thomas P, Grillot R, 1995, Une étape très actuelle de destin des malades infectieuses: les infections opportunistes parasitaires et fongiques, *Bull Acad Natl Med*, **179**: 798–803.

Ambroise-Thomas P, Pelloux H, 1993, Toxoplasmosis – congenital and in immunocompromised patients: a parallel, *Parasitol Today*, **9**: 61–3.

Amiri P, Locksley RM, 1992, Tumour necrosis factor restores granulomas and induces parasite egg-laying in schistosoma infected SCID mice, *Nature (London)*, **356**: 604–7.

Araujo FG, 1994, Immunization against *Toxoplasma gondii*, *Parasitol Today*, **10**: 358–60.

De Baetselier P, 1996, Mechanisms underlying trypanosome-induced T-cell immunosuppression, *T-cell Subsets and Cytokine Interplay in Infectious Diseases*, eds Mustafa AS, Al-Attiyah RJ et al., Karger, Basel, 124–39.

Bancroft AJ, Grencis RK et al., 1994, The role of CD4 cells in protective immunity to *Brugia pahangi*, *Parasite Immunol*, **16:** 385–7.

Barriga OO, 1994, Inmunoparasitología, *Rev Invest Pecuaris*, **7:** 1–24.

Behnke JM, ed, 1990, *Parasites: Immunity and Pathology*, Taylor and Francis, London.

Behnke JM, Barnard CJ, Wakelin D, 1992, Understanding chronic nematode infections: evolutionary considerations, current hypotheses and the way forward, *Int J Parasitol*, **22:** 861–907.

Bergquist NR, 1995, Controlling schistosomiasis by vaccination: a realistic option?, *Parasitol Today*, **11:** 191–4.

Berzins K, 1994, Development of vaccines against malaria, *Int J Immunopharmacol*, **16:** 385–94.

Blackwell JM, 1993, Immunology of leishmaniasis, *Clinical Aspects of Allergy*, 5th edn, eds Lachmann PJ, Peters K et al., Blackwell Scientific Publications, Oxford, 1575–97.

Boothroyd JC, Komuniecki R, 1995, *Molecular Approaches to Parasitology*, Wiley Liss, New York.

Bryan RT, 1995, Microsporidiosis as an AIDS-related opportunistic infection, *Clin Infect Dis*, **21 (Suppl. 1):** s62–5.

Bundy DAP, 1995, Epidemiology and transmission of intestinal helminths, *Enteric Infection 2: Intestinal Helminths*, eds Farthing MJG, Keusch GT, Wakelin D, Chapman and Hall Medical, London, 5–24.

Bundy DAP, Medley GF, 1992, Immunoepidemiology of human geohelminthiasis: ecological and immunoogical determinants of worm burden, *Parasitology*, **104:** S105–19.

Burke JM, Roberts CW et al., 1994, Temporal differences in the expression of mRNA for IL-10 and IFN-gamma in the brains and spleens of C57BL/10 mice infected with *Toxoplasma gondii*, *Parasite Immunol*, **16:** 305–14.

Buxton D, 1993, Toxoplasmosis: the first commercial vaccine, *Parasitol Today*, **9:** 335–7.

Capron A, Dessaint JP et al., 1992, Schistosomiasis: from effector and regulation mechanisms in rodents to vaccine strategies in humans, *Immunol Invest*, **1992:** 409–22.

Clark IA, Rockett KA, 1996, Nitric oxide and parasitic disease, *Adv Parasitol*, **37:** 1–56.

Collins WE, 1988, Major animal models in malaria research: simian, *Malaria: Principles and Practice of Malariology*, vol 2, eds Wernsdorfer WH, McGregor I, Heinemann, London, 1473–501.

Convit J, Castellanos P et al., 1989, Immunotherapy of localized, intermediate, and diffuse forms of American cutaneous leishmaniasis, *J Infect Dis*, **160:** 104–15.

Corradin G, Engers H, Trigg PI, 1994, Malaria vaccines: current status, *Clin Immunother*, **1:** 191–8.

Cox FEG, 1988, Major animal models in malaria research: rodent, *Malaria: Principles and Practice of Malariology*, vol 2, eds Wernsdorfer WH, McGregor I, Heinemann, London, 1503–43.

Cox FEG, 1991, Malaria vaccines – progress and problems, *Trends Biotech*, **9:** 389–94.

Cox FEG, Liew FY, 1992, T-cell subsets and cytokines in parasitic infections, *Immunol Today*, **13:** 445–8.

Darcy F, Santoro F, 1994, Toxoplasmosis, *Parasitic Infections and the Immune System*, ed Kierszenbaum F, Academic Press, San Diego, 163–201.

Day KP, 1991, The endemic normal in lymphatic filariasis: a static concept, *Parasitol Today*, **7:** 341–3.

Delemarre FGA, Stevenhagen A et al., 1994, Effect of IFN-gamma on the proliferation of *Toxoplasma gondii* in monocytes and monocyte-derived macrophages from AIDS patients, *Immunology*, **83:** 646–50.

Del Prete GF, De Carli M et al., 1991, Purified protein derivative of *Mycobacterium tuberculosis* and excretory-secretory antigen(s) of *Toxocara canis* expand in vitro human T cells with stable and opposite (type 1 T helper or type 2 T helper) profiles of cytokine production, *J Clin Invest*, **32:** 284–8.

Deraedt S, Molina JM, 1995, Les microsporidioses en pathologie humaine, *Méd Mal Infect*, **25:** 570–6.

Dixon JB, Jenkins P, 1995a, Immunology of mammalian metacestode infections. I. Antigens, protective immunity and immunopathology, *Helminthol Abstr*, **64:** 533–42.

Dixon JB, Jenkins P, 1995b, Immunology of mammalian metacestode infections. II. Immune recognition and effector function, *Helminthol Abstr*, **64:** 599–613.

Donaldson LE, Schmitt E et al., 1995, A critical role for stem cell factor (SCF) and *c-kit* in host-protective immunity to an intestinal helminth, *Int Immunol*, **8:** 559–67.

Dubey JP, Beattie CP, 1988, *Toxoplasmosis of Animals and Man*, CRC Press, Boca Raton.

Dunne DW, Hagan P, Abath FGC, 1995, Prospects for the immunological control of schistosomiasis, *Lancet*, **345:** 1488–92.

Dusanic DG, 1991, *Trypanosoma (Schizotrypanum) cruzi*, *Parasitic Protozoa*, 2nd edn, vol 1, eds Kreier JP, Baker JR, Academic Press, San Diego, 137–94.

Else KJ, Finkelman FD et al., 1994, Cytokine-mediated regulation of chronic intesinal helminth infection, *J Exp Med*, **179:** 347–51.

Elson LH, Guderian R et al., 1994, Immunity to Onchocerciasis: identification of a putative immune population in a hyperendmic area of Ecuador, *J Infect Dis*, **169:** 588–94.

Faubert GM, 1996, The immune response to *Giardia*, *Parasitol Today*, **12:** 140–5.

Finkelman FD, Madden KB et al., 1994, Effects of interleukin 12 on immune response and host protection in mice infected with intestinal nematode parasites, *J Exp Med*, **179:** 1563–72.

Gazzinelli RT, Denkers EY, Sher A, 1993, Host resistance to *Toxoplasma gondii*: A model for studying the selective induction of cell-mediated immunity by intracellular parasites, *Infect Agents Dis*, **2:** 139–50.

Gazzinelli RT, Oswald IP et al., 1992, The microbicidal activity of interferon-gamma treated macrophages against *Trypanosoma cruzi* involves a L-arginine dependent mechanism inhibitable by interleukin-10 and transforming growth factor-β, *Eur J Immunol*, **22:** 2501–6.

Good MF, Langhorne J, eds, 1994, *59th Forum in Immunology: T-Cell Immunity to Malaria*, Malaria Program Naval Medical Research Institute, Bethesda MD.

Gottstein B, Felleisen R, 1995, Protective immune mechanisms against the metacestode of *Echinococcus multilocularis*, *Parasitol Today*, **11:** 320–6.

Grau GE, 1996, T-cell subsets and effector mechanisms of pathology in cerebral malaria, *T-Cell Subsets and Cytokine Interplay in Infectious Diseases*, eds Mustafa AS, Al-Attiyah RJ et al., Karger, Basel, 63–71.

Greenblatt CL, 1988, Cutaneous leishmaniasis: the prospects for a killed vaccine, *Parasitol Today*, **4:** 53–5.

Grencis RK, 1996, T cell and cytokine basis of host variability in response to intestinal nematode infections, *Parasitology*, **112:** S31–7.

Hagan P, Wilkins HA, 1993, Concomitatnt immunity in schistosomiasis, *Parasitol Today*, **9:** 3–6.

Hagan P, Blumenthal UJ et al., 1991, Human IgE, IgG4 and resistance to reinfection with *Schistosoma haematobium*, *Nature (London)*, **349:** 243–5.

Holland CV, Crompton DWT et al., 1992, A possible genetic factor influencing protection from infection with *Ascaris lumbricoides* in Nigerian children, *J Parasitol*, **78:** 915–16.

Honigberg BM, Burgess DE, 1994, Trichomonads of importance in human medicine including *Dientamoeba fragilis*, *Parasitic Protozoa*, 2nd edn, vol 9, ed Kreier JP, Academic Press, San Diego, 1–109.

Houba V, 1988, Specific immunity: immunopathology and immunosuppression, *Malaria: Principles and Practice of Malariology*, vol 1, eds Wernsdorfer WH, McGregor I, Heinemann, London, 621–37.

Hunter CA, Subauste CS, Remington JS, 1994, The role of cytokines in toxoplasmosis, *Biotherapy*, **7**: 237–47.

James SL, 1995, Role of nitric oxide in parasitic infections, *Microbiol Rev*, **59**: 533–47.

Janoff EN, Smith PD, 1990, The role of immunity in *Giardia* infections, *Giardiasis*, ed Meyer EA, Elsevier, Amsterdam, 215–37.

Janoff EN, Smith PD, Blaser MJ, 1988, Acute antibody responses to *Giardia lamblia* are depressed in patients with AIDS, *J Infect Dis*, **157**: 798–804.

John DT, 1993, Opportunistically pathogenic free-living amebae, *Parasitic Protozoa*, 2nd edn, vol 3, ed Kreier JP, Academic Press, San Diego, 143–246.

Jones TR, Hoffman SL, 1994, Malaria vaccine development, *Clin Microbiol Rev*, **7**: 301–10.

Kemp M, Theander TG, Kharazmi A, 1996, The contrasting roles of CD4+ T cells in intracellular infections in humans: leishmaniasis as an example, *Immunol Today*, **17**: 13–16.

Khonde N, Pepin J et al., 1995, Epidemiological evidence for immunity following *Trypanosoma brucei gambiense* sleeping sickness, *Trans R Soc Trop Med Hyg*, **89**: 607–11.

Kierszenbaum F, ed, 1994, *Parasitic Infections and the Immune System*, Academic Press, San Diego.

Kierszenbaum F, Sztein MB, 1994, Chagas' disease (American trypanosomiasis), *Parasitic Infections and the Immune System*, ed Kierszenbaum F, Academic Press, San Diego, 53–85.

King CL, Nutman TB, 1991, Regulation of the immune responses in lymphatic filariasis and onchocerciasis, *Immunoparasitol Today*, eds Ash C, Gallagher RB, Elsevier Trends Journals, Cambridge, A54–8.

Kirchoff LV, 1994, American trypanosomiasis (Chagas' disease) and American trypanosomiasis (Sleeping sickness), *Curr Opin Immunol*, **7**: 542–6.

Kretschmer RR, 1993, Immunology of amoebiasis and giardiasis, *Clinical Aspects of Allergy*, eds Lachmann PJ, Peters K et al., Blackwell Scientific Publications, Oxford, 1613–26.

Kulda J, Nohynkova E, 1995, Giardia in humans and animals, *Parasitic Protozoa*, 2nd edn, vol 10, ed Kreier JP, Academic Press, San Diego, 225–422.

Lamont AC, Adorini L, 1966, IL-12: a key cytokine in immune regulation, *Immunol Today*, **17**: 214–17.

Lawrence RA, 1996, Lymphatic filariasis: what mice can tell us, *Parasitol Today*, **12**: 267–71.

Li B-W, Chandrashekar R, Weil GJ, 1993, Vaccination with recombinant filarial paramyosin induces partial immunity to *Brugia malayi* in jirds, *J Immunol*, **150**: 1881–5.

Liew FY, 1990, Regulation of cell-mediated immunity in leishmaniasis, *Curr Top Microbiol Immunol*, **155**: 54–64.

Liew FY, O'Donnell CA, 1993, Immunology of leishmaniasis, *Adv Parasitol*, **32**: 161–81.

Lightowlers MW, Mitchell GF, Rickard MD, 1993, Cestodes, *Immunology and Molecular Biology of Parasitic Infections*, ed Warren KS, Blackwell Scientific Publications, Oxford, 438–72.

Lightowlers MW, Lawrence SB et al., 1996, Vaccination against hydatidosis using a defined recombinant antigen, *Parasite Immunol*, **18**: 457–62.

Locksley RM, 1994, Th2 cells: help for helminths, *J Exp Med*, 1405–7.

López-Antuñano FJ, Schumis GA, 1993, Plasmodia of humans, *Parasitic Protozoa*, 2nd edn, vol 5, ed Kreier JP, Academic Press, San Diego, 135–266.

McGregor IA, Wilson RJM, 1988, Specific acquired immunity in man, *Malaria: Principles and Practice of Malariology*, vol 1, eds Wernsdorfer WH, McGregor I, Heinemann, London, 1559–619.

Mahanty S, King CL et al., 1993, IL-4 and IL-5-secreting lymphocyte populations are preferentially stimulated by parasite-derived antigens in human tissue invasive nematode infections, *J Immunol*, **151**: 3704–11.

Mahanty S, Nutman TB, 1995, Immunoregulation in human lym-

phatic filariasis: the role of interleukin 10, *Parasite Immunol*, **17**: 385–92.

Maizels RM, Bundy DAP et al., 1993, Immunological modulation and evasion by helminth parasites in human populations, *Nature (London)*, **365**: 797–805.

Maizels RM, Sartono E et al., 1995, T-cell activation and the balance of antibody isotypes in human lymphatic filariasis, *Parasitol Today*, **11**: 50–6.

Mansfield JM, 1994, T-cell responses to the trypanosome variant surface glycoprotein: A new paradigm?, *Parasitol Today*, **10**: 267–70.

Mariuz P, Bosler EM, Luft BJ, 1994, Toxoplasmosis in individuals with AIDS, *Infect Dis Clin North Am*, **8**: 365–81.

Martínez-Palomo A, Kretschmer RR, Meza Gomez Palacio I, 1993, *Entamoeba histolytica* and amebiasis, *Immunology and Molecular Biology of Parasitic Infections*, ed Warren KS, Blackwell Scientific Publications, Oxford, 143–56.

Martins CAP, Guerrant RL, 1995, *Cryptosporidium* and cryptosporidiosis, *Parasitol Today*, **11**: 434–5.

Mayrinck W, Atunes CMF et al., 1986, Further trials of a vaccine against American cutaneous leishmaniasis, *Trans R Soc Trop Med Hyg*, **73**: 385–7.

Melancon-Kaplan J, Burns JM et al., 1993, Malaria, *Immunology and Molecular Biology of Parasitic Infections*, ed Warren KS, Blackwell Scientific Publications, Oxford, 302–51.

Modabber F, 1995, Vaccines against leishmaniasis, *Ann Trop Med Parasitol*, **89**: 83–8.

Mossman TR, Coffman RI, 1989, Heterogeneity of cytokine secretion patterns and functions of helper T-cells, *Adv Immunol*, **46**: 111–47.

Mossman TR, Sad S, 1996, The expanding universe of T-cell subsets, *Immunol Today*, **17**: 138–46.

Munoz-Fernandez MA, Fernandez MA, Fresno M, 1992, Activation of human macrophages for the killing of intracellular *Trypanosoma cruzi* by TNF-alpha and IFN-gamma through a nitric oxide dependent mechanism, *Immunol Lett*, **33**: 35–40.

Mustafa AS, Al-Attiyah et al. eds, 1996, *T-Cell Subsets and Cytokines in Infectious Diseases*, Karger, Basel.

Nash TE, 1994, Immunology: the role of the parasite, *Giardia: From Molecules to Disease*, eds Thompson RCA, Reynoldson JA, Lymbery AJ, CAB International, Wallingford, 139–54.

Nash TE, 1995, Antigenic variation in *Giardia lamblia*, eds Boothroyd JC, Komuniecki R, Wiley-Liss, New York, 31–42.

Nawa Y, Ishikawa N et al., 1994, Selective effector mechanims for the expulsion of intestinal helminths, *Parasite Immunol*, **16**: 333–8.

Newport GR, Colley DG, 1993, Schistosomiasis, *Immunology and Molecular Biology of Parasitic Infections*, Warren KS, Blackwell Scientific Publications, Oxford, 387–437.

Ottesen EA, 1992, Infection and disease in lymphatic filariasis: an immunological perspective, *Parasitology*, **104**: S71–9.

Pearson TW, 1993, The immunology of African trypanosomiasis, *Clinical Aspects of Allergy*, 5th edn, eds Lachmann PJ, Peters K et al., Blackwell Scientific Publications, Oxford, 1599–612.

Pérez-Montford R, Kretschmer RR, 1990, Humoral immune responses, *Amebiasis: Infection and Disease by Entamoeba histolytica*, ed Kretschmer RR, CRC Press, Boca Raton, 91–103.

Perlmann P, Berzins K, Wahlgren M, 1993, Malaria, *Clinical Aspects of Allergy*, eds Lachmann PJ, Peters K et al., Blackwell Scientific Publications, Oxford, 1535–73.

Pirmez C et al., 1993, Cytokine patterns in the pathogenesis of human leishmaniasis, *J Clin Invest*, **91**: 1390–5.

Playfair JHL, Taverne J et al., 1990, The malaria vaccine: anti-parasite or anti-disease?, *Immunol Today*, **11**: 25–7.

Pritchard DI, 1995, The survival strategies of hookworms, *Parasitol Today*, **11**: 255–9.

Pritchard DI, Quinnell RJ, Walsh EA, 1995, Immunity in humans to *Necator americanus*: IgE, parasite weight and fecundity, *Parasite Immunol*, **17**: 71–5.

Rajan TV, Nelson FK et al., 1994, CD4⁺ T-lymphocytes are not required for murine resistance to the human filarial parasite, *Brugia malayi*, *Exp Parasitol*, **78:** 352–360.

Reed SG, 1995, Cytokine control of *Leishmania* and *T. cruzi*, *Molecular Approaches to Parasitology*, eds Boothroyd JC, Komuniecki R, Wiley-Liss, New York, 443–53.

Reiner SL, Locksley RM, 1995, The regulation of immunity to *Leishmania major*, *Annu Rev Immunol*, **13:** 151–77.

Rickard MD, 1995, *Taenia ovis* recombinant vaccine-'quo vadis'?, *Parasitology*, **110:** S5–9.

Riley EM, Hviid L, Theander TG, 1994, Malaria, *Parasitic Infections and the Immune System*, ed Kierszenbaum F, Academic Press, San Diego, 119–43.

Roberts-Thomson IC, Stevens DP et al., 1976, Giardiasis in the mouse: an animal model, *Gastroenterology*, **71:** 57–61.

Romagnani S, 1991, Human Th1 and Th2 subsets: doubts no more, *Immunol Today*, **12:** 256–7.

Sabin EA, Pearce EJ, 1995, Early IL-4 production by non-CD4[+] cells at the site of antigen deposition predicts the development of a Thelper 2 cell response to *Schistosoma mansoni* eggs, *J Immunol*, **155:** 4844–53.

Sacks DL, Louis JA et al., 1993, Leishmaniasis, *Immunology and Molecular Biology of Parasitic Infections*, ed Warren KS, Blackwell Scientific Publications, London, 237–68.

Scott P, 1996, Th cell development and regulation in experimental cutaneous leishmaniasis, *Th1 and Th2 Cells in Health and Disease*, ed Romagnani S, Karger, Basel, 98–114.

Scott P, Trinchieri G, 1995, The role of natural killer cells in host-parasite interactions, *Curr Opin Immunol*, **7:** 34–40.

Sher A, 1995, Regulation of cell-mediated immunity by parasites: the ups and downs of an important host adaptation, *Molecular Approaches to Parasitology*, eds Boothroyd JC, Komuniecki R, Wiley-Liss, New York, 431–42.

Sher A, Coffman RL, 1992, Regulation of immunity to parasites by T cells and T cell-derived cytokines, *Ann Rev Immunol*, **10:** 385–409.

Sibley LD, Adams LB et al., 1991, Tumor necrosis factor-alpha triggers antitoxoplasmal activity of IFN-γ primed macrophages, *J Immunol*, **147:** 2340–5.

Stadecker MK, 1994, The shrinking schistosomal egg granuloma: how accessory cells control T cell-mediated pathology, *Exp Parasitol*, **79:** 198–201.

Sztein MB, Cuna WR, Kierszenbaum F, 1990, *Trypanosoma cruzi* inhibits the expression of CD3, CD4, CD8 and IL2R by mitogen activated and cytotoxic human Lymphocytes, *J Immunol*, **144:** 3558–62.

Takle GB, Snary D, 1993, South American trypanosomiasis (Chagas' disease), *Immunology and Molecular Biology of Parasitic Infections*, ed Warren KS, Blackwell Scientific Publications, 213–36.

Tanner M, Teuscher T, Alonso PL, 1995, SPf66 - the first malaria vaccine, *Parasitol Today*, **11:** 10–13.

Targett GAT, 1995a, Malaria - advances in vaccines, *Curr Opin Infect Dis*, **8:** 322–7.

Targett GAT, 1995b, Malaria vaccines – now and the future, *Trans R Soc Trop Med Hyg*, **89:** 585–7.

Taylor MJ, Jenkins RE, Bianco AE, 1996, Protective immunity induced by vaccination with *Onchocerca volvulus* tropomyosin in rodents, *Parasite Immunol*, **18:** 219–25.

Telford SR, Gorenflot A et al., 1993, Babesial infections in humans and wildlife, *Parasitic Protozoa*, 2nd edn, vol 5, ed Kreier JP, Academic Press, San Diego, 1–47.

Urban JF, Madden KB et al., 1992, The importance of Th2 cytokines in protective immunity to nematodes, *Immunol Rev*, **127:** 205–20.

Urban JF, Madden KB et al., 1993, IFN inhibits inflammatory responses and protective immunity in mice infected with the nematode parasite, *Nippostrongylus brasiliensis*, *J Immunol*, **151:** 7086–94.

Urban JF, Maliszewski CR et al., 1995, IL-4 treatment can cure established gastrointestinal nematode infection in immunocompetent and immunodeficient mice, *J Immunol*, **154:** 4675–80.

Vickerman K, Myler PJ, Stuart KD, 1993, African trypanosomiasis, *Immunology and Molecular Biology of Parasitic Infections*, ed Warren KS, Blackwell Scientific Publications, 170–212.

Wakelin D, Harnett W, Parkhouse RME, 1993, Nematodes, *Immunology and Molecular Biology of Parasitic Infections*, Warren KS, Blackwell Scientific Publications, Oxford, 496–526.

Walterspiel JN, Morrow AL et al., 1994, Secretory anti-*Giardia lamblia* antibodies in human milk: protective effects against diarrhoea, *Pediatrics*, **93:** 28–31.

Warren KS, ed, 1993, *Immunology and Molecular Biology of Parasitic Infections*, Blackwell Scientific Publications, Oxford.

Wilkinson M, Wells, C, Behnke JM, 1990, *Necator americanus* in the mouse: histopathological changes associated with the passage of larvae through the lungs of mice exposed to primary and secondary infection, *Parasitol Res*, **76:** 386–92.

Wynn TA Cheever AW, 1995, Cytokine regulation of granuloma formation in schistosomiasis, *Curr Opin Immunol*, **7:** 505–11.

CONTROL OF PARASITES, PARASITIC INFECTIONS AND PARASITIC DISEASES

D H Molyneux

1 **Introduction**	4 **Stratification of parasitic diseases in relation**
2 **Concepts of control and eradication**	**to epidemiology and control**
3 **Components of control**	5 **Approaches to control**

1 INTRODUCTION

The World Development Report (WDR) 'Investing in Health' (World Bank 1993) provides a background to health issues and addresses the comparative importance of all causes of ill health, i.e. communicable and non-communicable diseases and accidents: parasitic infections fall into the category of communicable diseases. The importance of each disease is expressed in terms of 'disability adjusted life years' (DALYs) lost, a combined measure of morbidity and mortality (Murray and Lopez 1994). Although the emphasis of the report is considered by some authorities to provide an unfair reflection of the problems of communicable diseases, its approach is valuable for determining broad health sector policies and for guiding investment in health. Data for each of the major parasitic diseases, referred to in the report as the 'tropical cluster', have been disputed by parties interested in particular diseases, who suggest that the published figures are flawed or underestimated. It has also been pointed out that certain diseases have a deleterious impact in terms of suffering, disfigurement and socioeconomic consequences that cannot be measured in DALYs. The relevant figures produced by the World Bank are shown in Table 5.1, with appropriate updates from other sources if available (World Bank 1993, Murray and Lopez 1994).

The WDR recommends major changes in approaches to health policy that will inevitably have an impact on traditional methods of controlling parasitic infections. Whilst implementation of the report may take several decades, its influence on health policy will be felt rapidly, as World Bank funded restructuring of the health sector is introduced. This will be particularly true in sub-Saharan Africa where the burden of communicable disease remains the most severe and is likely to remain so for the next 40–50 years (Murray and Lopez 1994). Parasite disease control programmes will be integrated into overall strategies for health gain, as the trend away from vertical programmes gathers momentum. This will be driven by the policies and priorities of major donors, as reflected in the 1994 publication 'Better Health in Africa' (World Bank 1994); this publication is likely to act as a blueprint for health sector investment, despite the reservations of some major healthcare contributors. Some non-governmental organizations (NGOs) see the document as too prescriptive and insufficiently focused on those in the poverty trap with no access to healthcare. In addition, the total breakdown of health services in countries suffering conflict or undergoing rehabilitation (e.g. Afghanistan, Liberia, Angola, Sudan, Somalia and Mozambique) or where government structures are in abeyance (e.g. Zaire) has provoked a reconsideration of how healthcare can best be delivered outside of governmental control. Africa is identified in the WDR as the continent where improved health is most needed, where the communicable disease burden is proportionately greatest and where the 'epidemiological transition' (an increased proportion of morbidity and mortality resulting from non-communicable disease or accidents) has not yet been seen. Despite these facts, absolute disease burden may be greater in India because of the larger population.

Neither the WDR nor 'Better Health in Africa' (World Bank 1993, 1994) takes into account the increasing problem of epidemic disease and the effects of epidemics on governments and other health providers. Epidemics may be provoked by ecological, climatic and environmental change, urbanization,

Table 5.1 Overview of public health importance of parasitic infection

	Population at risk	No. of endemic countries	No. of infected/ prevalence	Estimated deaths mortality/y humans × 1000 (or million)	DALYs Female	DALYs Male	Total DALYs
Malaria	2000m	90	300–500m	1.5–2.7 million	182.3	17.5	357.3
Leishmaniasis	350m	82	12m	53.7	12	8.6	20.6
Lymphatic filariasis	750m	65	119m		5.6	2.9	7.5
Guinea worm	140m	18	c. 120 000				
Onchocerciasis	122m	34	17.6m	29.8	3.7	2.7	6.4
African trypanosomes	50m	36	20 000– >300 000	55.1	9	8.8	17.8
Chagas disease	90m	19	16m	23.1	14.8	12.6	27.4
Schistosomiasis	500–600m	74	200m	37.6	29.9	15.4	45.3
Ascaris			1000m		53.8	51.4	105.2
Trichuris			900m		32.2	30.9	63.1
Hookworm			500m		5.8	5.6	11.4
Entamoeba			500m	40–100 000			
Giardia			200m				
Taeniasis	40m		15m				
Neurocystocercosis			50m	50 000			
Food-borne trematodes			500m				
Fascioliasis	180.25m	8	2.39m				
Clonorchiasis	289.26m	6	7.0m				
Opisthorchiasis	63.6m	5	10.3m				
Paragonimiasis	194.8m	5	20.6m				
Other intestinal flukes		6	1.28m				

human population movement resulting from civil unrest and conflict, reduced surveillance and drug or insecticide resistance. It is recommended by these reports that health systems are restructured to include: a generalized 'horizontal' pattern of healthcare; insurance systems and user charges; and decentralization of management to district level (or equivalent). Such restructuring reduces the ability of the system to respond to factors that lead to epidemics. It must be borne in mind that vertical parasitic disease control activities, such as onchocerciasis control and Guinea worm eradication programmes, have been remarkably successful, the former being judged particularly cost effective (Benton and Skinner 1990). Because of the complexity of the biological systems inherent in parasitic infections, particularly those that are vector-borne, such diseases are not easily amenable to control by a horizontal approach.

This chapter seeks to draw together information on the control of parasites, parasitic infections and the diseases caused by parasites, providing an overview of the chapters in this volume. The title represents a deliberate attempt to distinguish between the control of an organism (parasite, vector or ectoparasite) at the level of the individual and at the level of the community, the latter being a more desirable goal. An example of this paradox is the conflict between the treatment of individual malaria patients compared with the need to control or even eradicate the disease. It is important to emphasize these distinctions as they

are frequently ignored by policy makers, health workers and scientists seeking to develop new approaches and tools for control.

The changing health environment has already been emphasized, but it is important to recognize that approaches to control are dependent on an accurate knowledge of the problem. This requires biological, medical and epidemiological inputs to define the aetiology (causative organisms), the vectors (if vector-borne), the parameters and mode of transmission (vector-borne, water-borne, aerosol, orofaecal, venereal). Systems of surveillance and evaluation are required to define prevalence and trends of infection and disease (Molyneux 1993). Without such fundamental information a control strategy cannot be appropriately designed and implemented. Biological information needs to be supplemented by consideration of issues such as logistics; cost effectiveness; potential for integration within existing programmes; past successes or failures; input from governmental sectors other than health (agriculture, forestry, education, water, other natural resources, wildlife); acceptability of an intervention to the target communities; potential for ecological damage; priority rating afforded by the Ministry of Health (MOH); availability of human resources for implementation; and potential of research to provide improved products within a particular timescale. The overall framework of approaches towards parasitic disease control is summarized in Fig. 5.1.

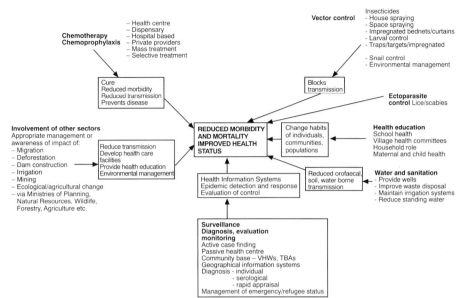

Fig. 5.1 A framework for control of parasitic disease.

2 CONCEPTS OF CONTROL AND ERADICATION

A distinction must be maintained between the terms 'control' and 'eradication'; the latter term is often used inappropriately and it should be employed with caution. In 1988 the International Task Force for Disease Eradication (ITFDE) was formed to evaluate systematically the potential for eradication of candidate diseases and to identify specific barriers to eradication. The ITFDE defined eradication as 'reduction of the world-wide incidence of a disease to zero as a result of deliberate efforts obviating the necessity for further control measures'. The group reviewed more than 90 diseases, 30 of them in depth, and concluded that dracunculiasis, rubella, poliomyelitis, mumps, lymphatic filariasis and cysticercosis could probably be eradicated using existing technology. The more appropriate term 'elimination' is increasingly being used to replace the term 'eradication'. The Task Force also considered that the public health manifestations of 7 other diseases could be eliminated and pointed out that additional diseases could be eradicated in time, depending on appropriate progress in research.

The classic eradication programme was that of smallpox which achieved its target in the mid 1970s. To date, no parasitic disease has been totally eradicated, although attempts to eradicate Guinea worm are underway, through the programme Global 2000. Nevertheless, successful local eradication has been achieved in some restricted geographical or epidemiological situations. For example, onchocerciasis has been eliminated from several parts of Kenya and from the Nile at Jinja in Uganda, by using DDT to remove the local vectors (*Simulium neavei* and *S. damnosum*, respectively). The Onchocerciasis Control Programme (OCP) in West Africa has achieved the same goal by targeting particular cytoforms of the *S. damnosum* complex using aerial application of insecticides. The following local eradications have also been achieved; the

malaria vector *Anopheles gambiae* from Brazil in the late 1930s; animal trypanosomiasis from parts of North East Nigeria; *Aedes aegypti*, the vector of the non-parasitic disease yellow fever, in Central and South America. Local anti-mosquito spraying has eradicated lymphatic filariasis in the Solomon Islands whereas chemotherapeutic approaches have eliminated this disease from Japan, South Korea and Taiwan (WHO 1994). A long eradication programme has finally been successful against hydatid disease in Iceland, and malaria has been eradicated from Sardinia by DDT spraying.

One noticeable feature of eradication successes is that most examples refer to islands. Clearly the advantages of isolation and a greater ability to control population movements are important. Eradication of any disease on a wider scale (regional or continental) is more difficult to achieve.

The high cost of eradication programmes may be justified as they are time limited whereas disease control implies a long term commitment. Any control programme must be cost effective and should reduce the target disease to a level at which costs are sustainable by the local community (or by public or private healthcare systems). Control seeks to bring the problems to a level at which the disease is no longer of public health importance with morbidity at an acceptable level within the community, an absence of mortality and, if appropriate, greatly reduced levels of disability. To translate the level of control achieved to eradication or elimination status requires a vastly increased cost per case treated or prevented which, for financial and ecological reasons, may never be feasible.

3 COMPONENTS OF CONTROL

Components of control are listed under the following headings: (1) situation analysis; (2) definition of objective and definition of strategy; (3) options and responsibilities at different levels of health system; (4) planning and resourcing; (5) evaluation; and (6) implementation and integration of selected methods of control.

3.1   Situation analysis

1   Desk study of published and unpublished reports to assess problems in the context of country, region and district.
2   Acquisition of information on prevalence and incidence.
3   Appraisal of the validity of information.
4   Evaluation of current epidemiological situations by passive surveillance at health centres.
5   Observation of changes over time and prediction of future change.
6   Definition of the structure of health services and their existing capacity, human resources available and needs for training and capacity building.
7   The priority afforded to the disease by the government, the MOH and the communities themselves.
8   Establishment of linkages to other sectors or organizations in planning for control (e.g. other ministries, development organizations, NGOs).
9   The influence of other activities such as development projects on planned programmes.
10 Spot surveillance of local prevalence, vectors and, if applicable, animal reservoirs.

3.2   Definition of objective and definition of strategy; options and responsibilities at different levels of health system

1   Selection of appropriate methodology and definition of control requirements.
2   Establishment of an inventory of personnel and facilities (including estimation of training needs and requirements for equipment and drug).
3   Analysis of cost effectiveness of different control approaches.
4   Establishment of feasibility in the context of other health needs.
5   Contrasting epidemic ('firefighting') problems for which vertical, rapid intervention is necessary with endemic situations for which a long term approach and integration are required (Table 5.2).

3.3   Planning and resourcing

1   Defining the expected contribution from the government.
2   Evaluating target approaches to donors in the context of donor priorities.
3   Defining appropriate timeframes for implementation of plans.
4   Defining the relationship of the action to overall health plans and budgets.

5   Establishment of linkages with appropriate international reference centres for technical support; control of an epidemic may merit application for emergency status to provide rapid funding (e.g. requests for therapeutic drugs and insecticides from international aid agencies).
6   Establishment of drug supply lines.
7   Definition of the role of the non-government sector (e.g. private providers, NGOs) in control policy.
8   Ensuring adequate information exchange about control policy between different bodies and individuals involved in healthcare provision.
9   Training through courses, instruction of trainers, educational materials and health education programmes.
10 Assessment of community acceptability and the perceived priority of any involvement that will require resource input from the lowest levels (e.g. role and views of village health workers (VHWs), volunteers, traditional birth attendants (TBAs), community leaders, school teachers).
11 Definition of the management structure of the programme and its relationship with existing management structures.

3.4   Evaluation

1   Assessment of progress towards objectives (prevalence distribution, vector status).
2   Definition of appropriate methods for epidemiological evaluation, e.g. parasitological, serological and vector sampling methods.
3   Longitudinal surveys or spot surveys at indicator villages.
4   Adjustment of the programme in the light of results.

3.5   Implementation and integration of selected methods of control

CHEMOTHERAPY AND CHEMOPROPHYLAXIS

1   Assessment of the availability and quality of drugs and the distribution system.
2   Assessment of, or monitoring for, resistance.
3   Assessment of the role of private providers and control of quality and price.
4   Utilization of other systems for distribution (e.g. schools, other health or government workers, NGOs, committees).

VECTOR AND RESERVOIR CONTROL

1   Availability, cost and appropriateness of insecticides.
2   Availability of skills to monitor resistance.
3   Availability and effectiveness of alternative chemicals.
4   Capacity for management of the control programme.
5   Relationship to other sectors in providing support for environmental control measures.

Table 5.2 Role of different levels of the health system in parasitic disease control

Community	— Identification of suspects
	— Follow-up of patients
	— Coordination of any vector control activities
	— Facilitation of cooperation
	— Communication by Village Health Committees
District	— Passive detection
	— Parasitological/serological diagnosis
	— Treatment and minimum clinical care
	— Follow-up of microscopy
Regional	— Active surveillance
	— Confirmatory diagnosis
	— Data collection
	— Technical supervision of vector control
	— Distribution of reagents and materials for vector control
Ministry and country level	— Situation analysis
	— National strategy and plan
	— Financing
	— Training needs and responsibility
	— Health education
	— Distribution of technical information, equipment, drugs, materials
	— Purchase of equipment and supplies
	— Human resource management

6   Acceptability of reservoir control.
7   Environmental acceptability of compounds.
8   Personal protection, e.g. bednets, sustainability of a bednet programme.

ENVIRONMENTAL MANAGEMENT

1   Ensuring effective linkages between health and other sectors.
2   Assessment of potential impact on other diseases.

IMMUNOPROPHYLAXIS

1   Availability of vaccines.
2   Capacity to manage the programme.
3   Linkage to existing programmes, e.g. expanded programme of immunization (EPI) to utilize the cold chain.

HEALTH EDUCATION

1   Media resources, including radio, television and videos.
2   Posters and drama sessions oriented around the local environment and traditions.
3   Participation of teachers, local leaders, health workers, local medical practitioners, religious leaders.

4 STRATIFICATION OF PARASITIC DISEASES IN RELATION TO ERADICATION AND CONTROL

Vertical control programmes involve specific approaches to arrest the transmission of infection (e.g. via vector control) or to prevent or cure a disease. Although such programmes have been successful in the past, integrated approaches are now recognized as being more appropriate for reducing prevalence and incidence. This is important if the strategy is aimed at alleviation of a disease problem in a community or population rather than in an individual. Integrated control is based on coordinated planning and detailed knowledge from many different areas: scientific, technical, inter-sectoral and managerial. An approach termed 'stratification' has been used in malaria control; this means that the strategy is modified according to different epidemiological situations (WHO 1993a). Malaria stratification has been taken a step further by those with particular interests in different environments, a process known as 'micro-stratification'. Whilst stratification has been most widely discussed with reference to malaria (Table 5.3), the process is equally applicable to other parasitic diseases although the term stratification has not been used (Tables 5.4–5.8). This is true of leishmaniasis (WHO 1990) and filariasis (WHO 1992a). Stratification can also be applied to schistosomiasis, onchocerciasis and African trypanosomiasis although with these diseases only a relatively small number of epidemiological situations exist. Tables 5.3–5.8 illustrate the concept of stratification in the planning of control in selected parasitic diseases.

5 APPROACHES TO CONTROL

Control of a parasitic infection can be focused on the individual, with a view to alleviating pain, reducing disability or avoiding death, whilst at the same time reducing the parasite load within a community. Such an approach will be less cost effective than larger scale

Table 5.3 Stratification of malaria epidemiology in relation to approaches to control (after WHO, 1993)

Malaria type	CHARACTERISTICS		ACTION REQUIRED	
	Epidemiological	Operational	Disease management	Prevention
Savanna malaria. Sub-saharan Africa, Papua New Guinea.	• *Plasmodium falciparum* dominant parasite. Perennial transmission but varying seasonality depending on distance from equator. Mortality and morbidity in young children and pregnant women. Drug resistance increasing problem.	Limited coverage by Health Services. Malaria control programme inadequate. Lack of appropriate capacity.	Increase interest through both government, NGO and private sector in malaria disease. Strengthen capacity for management of severe and complicated malaria.	Evaluate impregnated bednets and curtains. Chemoprophylaxis for pregnant women unless precluded by drug resistance.
Malaria of highland or desert fringe (Africa, South East Asia highland; Sahel, South Africa and South Pacific).	Risks of epidemics due to climate, conflict, changing agriculture practice or migration patterns.	Health services not available or limited. Terrain and distance present obstacles to control. Preparation poor for management of malaria where not historically a problem.	Establish facilities with effective drugs in case of epidemic. Active case detection and treatment of fever may be justified. Health services must be made aware of risk potential.	Vector control might reduce or eliminate transmission.
Malaria of plains and valleys outside Africa (Central America, China, Indian sub-continent)	Variable mainly moderate transmission. *P. vivax* may dominate. Strong seasonal variation. Drug resistance established.	Vector control not effective. Inadequate disease management. Health services inadequate; private services available.	Give responsibility of malaria control to General Health Services. Strengthen epidemiological systems.	Improve vector control if cost-effective. Environmental management might have impact hence intersectoral links necessary. Bednets can be useful (China).

Agricultural development projects. All malarious areas.	Increased transmission sometimes associated with irrigation. Seasonal malaria outbreaks in non-immune immigrant workers.	Insecticide resistance in cotton growing areas. Finance for malaria control more likely to be available.	Establish services for treatment or strengthen existing ones.	Environmental management should be considered. Site and construct habitation appropriately. Use of impregnated bednets for labour force. Larvivorous fish in rice growing areas. House spraying and chemoprophylaxis appropriate for work force. Larval control sometimes by chemical larviciding. Personal protection.
Urban and periurban malaria (Africa, South America, South Asia).	Transmission and immunity variable over short distance. Epidemics caused by specially adapted vector in South Asia.	Relatively good access to health services. Antimalarials available from different sources. High human population density. Breeding sites identifiable.	Standardise and harmonise treatment practices. Introduce drug quality and control systems. Facilities specific for malaria treatment required.	Larval control sometimes by chemical larviciding. Personal protection. Personal prevention. Impregnated bednets.
Malaria of forest and forest fringes South East Asia, South America.	Focally intense transmission. Occupational risk groups (e.g. mining) Severe multi-drug resistance. Non-immune migrant labour at high risk.	Health services inadequate or absent. No or limited social organisation in communities. Variety of drugs sold via different outlets. Vector control efficacy doubtful.	Treatment needs to be continually adjusted dependent on experience of response to drug regimes. Establish communication between medical staff involved in treatment.	
War zone malaria. Conflict/refugee emergency malaria.	Displacement of parasite carrying population or non-immunes. Environmental degradation increases mosquito breeding.	Disruption of vector control. No curative services available. Drug distribution only via humanitarian assistance. Drugs provided may be inappropriate.	Awareness by responsible authorities of malaria risk. Drugs for treatment available via emergency programmes must be appropriate to drug resistance prevailing. Establish treatment facilities.	Refugees and soldiers may be protected by personal protection/chemoprophylaxis for vulnerable groups. Environmental measures in refugee camps. Space spraying in emergency outbreaks in camps.

Table 5.4   Stratification of epidemiology of African and S. American trypanosomiasis in relation to control

Geographical locality	CHARACTERISTICS			
	Epidemiological	Operational	Disease management	Required prevention
Rhodesiense Sleeping Sickness East and Central Africa *T.b. rhodesiense* Vector *Glossina morsitans*, *S. pallidipes* *G. fuscipes* in Uganda and Kenya epidemics	Usually zoonosis with range of game and domestic animal reservoirs. Transmission associated with entry into areas where savanna flies feeding on game animals. Vector control inappropriate, occupation associated e.g. honey gatherers, fishermen, poachers. Epidemic associated with human to human transmission by *G. fuscipes* in Uganda/Kenya with domestic animal reservoir hosts.	Acute disease. Passive case detection in PHC, district health facilities by routine diagnostic techniques. Need for active case detection in epidemics.	Accurate disease stage diagnosis; availability of drugs and recognition of toxicity of arsenicals.	Avoidance of high risk areas. No vectors or reservoir control directly targeted but animal tryp control by vector control may have impact. Treatment of domestic livestock with trypanocides may reduce human cases. Epidemics stemmed by active case detection and vector control to reduce transmission.
West and Central Africa. *T.b. gambiense* Vector Riverine flies *G. palpalis* group	Person to person transmission via riverine flies. Limited importance of animal reservoirs. Site associated transmission around high humidity areas.	Active case detection followed by treatment. Diagnosis less easy and serological tests of value for screening. Vector control to arrest epidemic and halt transmission.	Provide diagnostic facilities at PHC and district level. Ensure drug availability. Maintain surveillance to detect early cases facilitating easier treatment. Provide adequate medical support for treatment and resuscitation.	Vector control can be employed by community (traps); residual spraying of resting sites. Maintain surveillance to reduce epidemic risk. Prophylaxis with pentamidine no longer employed.
South and Central America American Trypanosomiasis Chagas Disease *T. cruzi* Vectors: Triatomine bugs *Triatoma infestans* in Southern Cone	Zoonosis transmitted by intradomiciliary bugs. High vector infection rate. Many reservoir hosts. Acute disease in children but chronic in adults.	Diagnosis of chronic disease difficult and no effective remedy if diagnosed. Acute disease treatable but drugs expensive and toxic.	Limited efficacy of chemotherapy provides poor prognosis with death through cardiomyopathy. Transfusion disease averted by control of blood via trypanocidal additives (gentian violet).	Vector control by indoor house spraying or other insecticides approaches – paints, fumigant cans. Improved housing provides beneficial long term effect.

Table 5.5 Stratification of epidemiology and control of leishmaniasis

Geographical locality	Epidemiological	Operational	Disease management	Prevention
Old World visceral leishmaniasis Indian sub-continent *L. donovani.* Vector *P. argentipes.*	Anthroponotic sub-clinical cases frequent. No animal reservoir. Endemic with periodic epidemics.	Capacity to diagnose is limited. Antileishmanial drugs expensive, toxic and not easily available. Inadequate reporting and case follow-up. Parasitological diagnosis to be available at district level with serological examination at PHC level if serodiagnostic capacity exists.	Improve diagnostics. Active case detection to reduce human reservoir.	Possible use of impregnated materials or residual insecticide application in epidemics to reduce transmission by sandflies
East Africa *L. donovani.*	Reservoir hosts (rodents carnivores) likely though importance unknown. Suggested association with termite hills in Kenya. Epidemic in S. Sudan associated with movement of population and development of *Acacia/Balanites* woodland.	Passive case detection and treatment. Annual incidence requires to be checked by active surveillance. S. Sudan epidemic places major demands on availability of Pentostam worldwide.	Improved diagnostics and drug availability.	Reservoir or vector control not feasible.
Visceral leishmaniasis with canine reservoir or assumed canine reservoir. *L. infantum* and *L. chagasi* widely distributed throughout China, North Africa, Middle East and Central and South America. Vectors are *Larroussius* subgenus; *P. perfiliewi, perniciosus, P. ariasi.* New World *Lutzomyia longipalpis.*	Zoonotic disease – foxes and dogs reservoirs. Endemic over wide area; epidemics are infrequent. Sporadic cases over wide area with sub-clinical cases likely to be common. Usually found in children more frequently.	Limited knowledge of disease; difficult to diagnose; HIV associated increase in cases. Vector control not usually an option; diagnosis and treatment of dogs in endemic areas of Mediterranean. However, reservoir control while useful has limited impact where wild or feral reservoirs exist.	Ensure a minimum capacity for passive case detection and treatment.	Serological monitoring and treatment of dogs in Mediterranean.

Table 5.5   Continued

Geographical locality	Epidemiological	Operational	Disease management	Prevention
Anthroponotic cutaneous leishmaniasis. Old World urban centres *L. tropica.* Vector *P. sergenti.*	Predominantly found in densely populated settlements. Person–person transmission by *P. sergenti.* Reservoir host not important. Transmission seasonal at sandfly peak.	Passive case detection as a minimum to reduce human reservoir. Integrate any vector control activities (house spraying, impregnated nets and targets) with malaria control.	Ensure awareness of disease; transmission, diagnosis and treatment. Ensure drug availability.	Human reservoir control by active case detection. Vector control by residual insecticides of houses where cases found. Check susceptibility of vector to insecticide. Malaria control by house spraying has impact as do bednets; use of impregnated materials feasible.
Zoonotic cutaneous leishmaniasis caused by *L. major* widely distributed in arid rural areas of Old World. Vectors *P. papatasi, P. dubosqi.*	Arid rural habitats. Reservoir (rodent)/sandfly transmission systems; *Rhombomys/ P. papatasi* (Asia). *Psammomys/ P. papatasi* (Middle East/N. Africa). *Arvicanthis/ P. dubosqi* (sub-Saharan Africa). Settlements around rodent colonies at risk as are workers who penetrate into arid environment and disturb rodent colonies e.g. construction workers.	Passive case detection and treatment with drugs. Live vaccines used in military situations. Rodent control/ environmental control highly effective. Self healing lesions with total immunity, but high level of disfigurement.	Awareness at health facilities. Availability of drugs. Skin testing to determine status of disease.	Leishmanisation has been used but 2.5% have large non-healing lesions. Vector control not a cost-effective option. Environmental measures to prevent rodent establishment–ploughing, poisons, flooding.
Zoonotic cutaneous leishmaniasis East African highland *L. aethiopica.* Vectors *P. longipes, P. pedifer.*	Association with hyraxes. Human cases associated with the proximity to hyrax colonies.	Case detection. Epidemiological knowledge of high risk areas by health services.	Awareness at PHC level of clinical presentation; availability of antileishmanials.	Hyrax eradication possible locally. Vector control ineffective.
'Uta' Cutaneous leishmaniasis of Andean highlands/western Cordilleras *L. peruviana.* Vector *L. peruensis.*	Putative reservoirs are rodents (*Akodon* and *Phyllotis*) and dogs. Seasonal transmission. Lesions predominantly in children below school age.	Passive surveillance. Case monitoring.	PHC awareness and case reporting. Skin testing in young age groups.	Value of vector control is unknown except where proven peridomestic transmission.

Cutaneous leishmaniasis caused by *Leishmania guyanensis* Northern South America. Vector *Lu. umbratilis* (possibly *Lu. whitmani* and *Lu. anduzae*).	Forest edentates (Sloths *Choloepus* and anteater *Tamandua*). Reservoirs have high infection rate. *Didelphis* (oppossum) secondary peridomestic reservoir where ecology has altered.	Humans infected by encroaching into forest or by establishment of habitation at forest edge.	Case detection and treatment. Availability of antileishmanials.	Vector control of limited impact, clearing of forest up to 300m from habitation reduces incidence.
Cutaneous leishmaniasis caused by *L. panamensis* Central America/Northern South America. Vectors *Lu. trapidoi, gomezi, ylephiletor, panamensis*.	As above associated with forest penetration or association with secondary forest. Variety of reservoir hosts. Edentates, primates, dogs and rodents.	Passive case detection; awareness of risk for those entering or living in forest.	Case detection and treatment. Availability of anti-leishmanials.	Clearing of forest around villages will reduce transmission. Vector and/or reservoir control not practicable.
Cutaneous and mucocutaneous leishmaniasis. Central and South America caused by *L. braziliensis*. Vector *Lu. wellcomei, Lu. intermedia, Lu. whitmani*.	Infection associated with forest activities and clearing land. Perennial transmission with high incidence in at-risk groups. Reservoir not proven and many suspected vectors. In urban/peri-urban environment dogs, horses and pigs have been incriminated as reservoirs.	Espundia (Mucocutaneous lesions) develop after varying periods following self healing primary lesions.	Passive case detection; availability of drugs. Essential care of espundia cases to reduce sequelae of lesions.	No vector or reservoir control applicable in forest but vector control possible in periurban situations, personal protection might help if affordable.
Cutaneous leishmaniasis caused by *L. mexicana* complex. South and Central America. *Lu. olmeca, Lu. flaviscutellata*.	Variety of different ecological situations – wet forest, Igapo Brazil; dry Yucatan, fringe forest, Dominican Republic. Rodent and marsupial reservoir hosts, highly dispersed and diverse.	Associated with penetration into forest environments.	Passive case detection, PHC, awareness and availability of drugs.	Reservoir and vector control not possible. Personal protection in forest; reduce risk by not sleeping in forest. Health education.

Table 5.6 Stratification of epidemiology and control of onchocerciasis

Geographical locality	Epidemiological	Operational	Disease management	Prevention
Africa South of Sahara. Onchocerciasis Control Programme countries (OCP). 1. Original areas – Benin, Burkina Faso, Cote d'Ivoire, Ghana, Mali, Niger, Togo. 2. Extension areas. Southern areas of Ghana, Togo, Benin, western extension, Guinea, Guinea Bissau, Sierra Leone, Senegal. 3. Non-OCP countries: East of Benin to Sudan. 4. West and Equatorial Africa, Guinea-Bissau to Gabon. Rain forest. 5. Zaire Basin. 6. East Africa highlands. Ethiopia to Southern Malawi.	1. Savannah woodland of northern tropics. Hyper-endemic villages close to rivers. Historically associated with high blindness rate resulting in depopulation. Major migratory vectors in savanna *S. damnosum* and *S. sirbanum*. Annual transmission potential or more than 100 associated with blindness risk. 2. In forest areas less blinding form of *O. volvulus* transmitted by forest vectors *S. soubrense, S. yahense, S. sanctipauli, S. squamosam, S. leonense* (Sierra Leone) which are less efficient and non or less migratory.	1. Vector control by weekly aerial larviciding for 14 years eliminates adult worms in human reservoir. Ivermectin for foci with inadequate vector control 2. Combined vector control and Ivermectin for 12 years projected to reduce disease to non-significant level. Ivermectin alone in areas of low CMFL (<10) where no invasion of *Simulium* threatens original OCP area. 3– 5. Ivermectin through community based distribution systems. 6. Focal vector control could achieve eradication of *S. damnosum* or *S. neavei*. Ivermectin as in 5.	1. Vector control applied due to lack of availability of community-based drug until 1986. Thereafter ivermectin for morbidity control to reduce CMFL and arrest development of ocular lesions. 2. Ivermectin throughout for extended periods up to 20 years as ivermectin does not interrupt transmission. 3. Impact of ivermectin on skin disease and other manifestations of *O. volvulus* infection to be assessed.	Maintain surveillance system for recrudescence using tests for early detection of transmission. Institute ivermectin if appropriate. Establish appropriate surveillance via integration into public health systems. Possible detection of early transmission by detection of infective larvae in black flies. Maintenance of ivermectin distribution. Ensure high coverage cost-effectiveness and sustainable delivery via community directed treatment assisted by NGOs.
Central America Guatemala; Mexico in well defined foci. Cross border movement of migrant workers may spread the disease.	Anthrophilic *S. ochraceum* in highland foci; *S. metallicum* more zoophilic also involved. Inefficient as vector due to buccal armature complicated by abundance.	Control by ivermectin distribution via national programmes through twice yearly distribution.	Ivermectin based.	Ivermectin distribution over many years will reduce morbidity
South America 1. Brazil, S. Venezuela 2. N. Venezuela 3. Ecuador, Columbia.	1. Primary vectors. *S. oyapockense* and *S. guianense*. 2. Primary vector *S. metallicum*. 3. Primary vector *S. exiguum*. 1,2. Secondary vector. *S. exiguum*.	Vector control not feasible. Integration of ivermectin with other programmes.	Ivermectin based.	As above.
Yemen Distributed along Wadis.	A member of the *S. damnosum* complex	Control initiated.	Ivermectin based.	Ivermectin control embarked upon.

Table 5.7 Stratification of epidemiology and control of lymphatic filariasis

Geographical locality	Epidemiological characteristics	Operational approach	Disease management	Prevention
Tropical America N. E. Brazil, Guyana, Surinam, French Guyana, Haiti, Dominican Republic, Costa Rica, Trinidad and Tobago.	Focal transmission by *Culex quinquefasciatus*. Varying levels of endemicity; no recent surveys in Caribbean and Costa Rica, Guyana and Surinam.	Limited control programmes organised through Ministry of Health (in Brazil SUCAM). Urban mosquito control difficult.	Opportunities for introduction of new approaches. Treatment using topical antibiotics, hygiene of infected limbs. Single annual dose DEC and/or ivermectin.	Very limited control implemented except in Recife. Potential for all appropriate measures to reduce transmission by single annual treatment of DEC and ivermectin and/or DEC salt.
Tropical Africa Broad transmission zone in sub-saharan Africa.	Urban filariasis *Culex quinquefasciatus* transmitted. Coastal filariasis transmitted by *A. gambiae* complex in E. Africa, West Africa (Ghana, Nigeria, Liberia) and Madagascar. Extent of problem needs better definition.	Limited control programmes. DEC used in some control programmes. DEC salt in Tanzania in operational research stage.	As above but not recognised as significant public health problem in African environment due to low priority status and absence of appropriate data. Pilot project underway in Ghana. Hydrocoele predominant clinical feature.	Pilot projects in Zanzibar using polystyrene beads for larval *Culex* control; impregnated bednets and, in urban areas, *Bacillus sphaericus* larval toxins. Cost-effectiveness unknown.
Middle-East Egypt	Urban and peri-urban transmission in Cairo and Nile delta. Resurgence since control relaxed in 1965 resulting in prevalence of c. 20%. *Culex molestus* and *C. quinquefasciatus* transmitted.	Vector control by classical and new approaches. Standard courses of DEC currently used.	No current defined policy. New approaches to be implemented in accordance with WHO recommendations (see above).	Mosquito control and transmission reduction strategy, using chemotherapy including DEC-fortified salt.

Table 5.7 Continued

Geographical locality	Epidemiological characteristics	Operational approach	Disease management	Prevention
Indian sub-continent. South Asia, India, Sri Lanka, Bangladesh, Nepal, Vietnam, Thailand, Myanmar.	*C. quinquefasciatus, Anopheles* species. Urban and semi-urban with high clinical morbidity particularly in India.	Variable depending on country and resources available. Chemotherapy via DEC + ivermectin or DEC fortified salt mosquito control.	As above. Surgery of serious deformities widely practised in India, especially for hydrocoele, to reduce morbidity. Heavy cost burden on surgical services.	Variety of mosquito control measures + DEC/ivermectin and DEC salt.
Pacific rim + islands	*Aedes* transmitted on Pacific islands. *Anopheles puncitulatus* in Papua New Guinea. *C. quinquefasciatus* in China.	Ivermectin + DEC and DEC salt.	As above.	Vector control difficult although some success in trials with *B. sphaericus* biocides. DEC salt. DEC + ivermectin.
Brugia malayi, Brugia timori South Asia, India, Malaysia, Indonesia, China, Philippines, Vietnam.	*Mansonia, Anopheles.* In some areas animal reservoirs exist.	Community participation in assisting environmental vector (deweeding and fish culture) control and chemotherapeutic control in India; use of DEC and ivermectin and DEC salt in same manner as for *Wuchereria bancrofti* filariasis.	As above. Treatment using topical antibiotics, hygiene of infected limbs in Kerala, India to ameliorate acute episodes.	Chemical control against *Mansonia* difficult due to variable adult behaviour and larval association with weeds hence dependence on environmental control.

Table 5.8 Stratification of epidemiology and control of schistosomiasis

Geographical locality	Epidemiological features	Operational	Disease and management	Prevention
Africa *Schistosoma mansoni* and *S. haematobium* widespread. *S. intercalatum* is limited in West and Central Africa. **South America and Caribbean** *S. mansoni*	*S. mansoni/Biomphalaria* transmitted. *S. haematobium/Bulinus* transmitted. *S. mansoni* has peak prevalence in 10–24 year olds; heaviest parasite loads 10–14 age group. *S. haematobium* peak prevalence and intensity 10–14 years.	Linkage to other sectors in planning prevention and control via appropriate water resource management. Population movement to be monitored in context of potential disease impact after exposure to new water related development. Development of link to School for chemotherapeutic control and for health education. Assessment of potential for molluscicing.	Can result in significant morbidity and mortality, placing considerable burden on curative services. Severity of symptoms generally dependent on intensity of infection. *S. mansoni* symptoms associated with hepatic, splenic and intestinal systems. *S. haematobium* pathology concentrated in genital urinary systems and lower intestine. Use of haematuria as rapid assessment tool for intervention priority.	Primary prevention is to reduce access to contaminated water via improved management of water resources; involvement of other sectors in planning development projects. Chemotherapy assists in reducing infection reservoir; snail control may supplement control operations and be planned into irrigation schemes or impoundments. Health education via schools and community health providers. Maintenance of drug availability.
Middle East/North Africa *S. mansoni* and *S. haematobium.* Very small Indian focus of *S. haematobium.*			Praziquantel can reverse symptoms of severe disease. Carcinomas associated with Schistosomal disease but precise aetiology not established.	
South East Asia, China, Philippines, Thailand *S. japonicum,* *S. mekongi* in Kampuchea Laos.	*S. japonicum* transmitted by amphibious *Oncomelania* with many animal hosts (dogs, rats, pigs). *S. japonicum* has no typical age prevalence or intensity; variable depending on epidemiology. *S. mekongi* transmitted by *Tricula* snails (dog reservoir host).	National programmes in China developed via communist structures in integrating chemotherapy and snail control. In Philippines approaches to control through snail control case detection and treatment, environmental sanitation and health education. Redirection with increased emphasis with availability of praziquantel. Operational phases of control operations. Phase 1. planning data gathering; planning; resource allocation. Phase 2. attack/intervention. Phase 3. maintenance.	*S. japonicum* disease similar to *Mansoni* with most severe disease between 2–40. Praziquantel effective in treatment.	

control programmes that employ methods such as vector control, reservoir host control or mass drug distribution. Large scale measures have a public health objective that, whilst reducing individual suffering, also reduce the community morbidity and mortality. This provides socioeconomic benefits through the following: improved agricultural productivity; improved cognitive function; better nutrition as a result of a more varied diet; and enhanced population mobility, allowing for additional earning opportunities. Control of animal parasitic diseases also has benefits for human populations through increased protein availability and higher income from the sale of higher quality livestock, and this enhances both local and national economies. Parasitic disease control programmes vary in scale, but they have generally been targeted at 2 different types of disease situations (1) the alleviation of an endemic disease in which long term chronic infections have persisted in communities, e.g. river blindness (onchocerciasis), hydatid disease (*Echinococcus* infection), schistosomiasis, Guinea worm (dracunculiasis) and filariasis; and (2) the contrasting epidemic situation in which rapid intervention is required to prevent widespread morbidity and mortality. Epidemics are frequently predictable, but if health facilities are ill equipped or non-existent, high mortality may occur before control can be instigated. Examples of parasitic disease epidemics that have occurred in recent times are described in Table 5.9.

The following changes frequently result in epidemics of parasitic disease:

1 Movements of non-immune populations in areas where transmission occurs; such movements may be of an organized nature, e.g. mobilization of the workforce in Brazil to exploit forest resources has resulted in malaria epidemics. Alternatively, they may occur without formal organization, e.g. movements of workers involved in mining for gold or gems in the Amazon and South East Asia.
2 Climatic changes, e.g. temperature change is considered to be a cause of highland malaria in Kenya and Ethiopia.
3 Change in vegetation such as the development of thickets of the plant *Lantana* in Uganda, which provided a habitat for *Glossina fuscipes*, provoking epidemics of Rhodesian sleeping sickness. Another example is deforestation, which has resulted in exposure to leishmaniasis in the Amazon (Walsh, Molyneux and Birley 1993).
4 Development projects themselves frequently exacerbate the health problems of the local or incoming population (Birley 1995, Hunter et al. 1993).

5.1 Control of animal reservoir hosts

Many parasitic diseases are zoonoses, defined as 'those diseases and infections (the agents of) which are naturally transmitted between (other) vertebrate animals and man' (WHO 1979). A list of recognized parasitic zoonoses is provided by the WHO (1979). There are only certain situations in which it is appropriate to control human disease by controlling or treating the animal reservoir host. The list of zoonoses is extensive but most are of limited public health importance, despite having an impact on individual patients. The important zoonoses for which reservoir control can have a cost effective impact are discussed below. The presence of an animal reservoir host may be a major impediment to control of a disease, particularly if the habits and habitats of the animal hosts prevent intervention.

LEISHMANIASIS

The most important examples are the control programmes targeted against the great gerbil *Rhombomys opimus*, the reservoir host of *Leishmania major* in the former Soviet Union; a variety of techniques have been employed to eliminate this rodent in the central Asian republics of Uzbekistan, Kazakhstan and Turkmenia. Burrow systems were identified by aerial or ground surveys, then destroyed by deep ploughing. Alternatively, poisonous baits of zinc phosphide mixed with wheat and vegetable oil were introduced into every 3rd or 4th hole. The effects of the zinc phosphide were enhanced by prior application of the anticoagulant dicoumarol, 5–7 days earlier. Because of its high toxicity, zinc phosphide had to be inserted directly into the rodent burrows. Elimination of *R. opimus* can also be achieved by irrigation schemes. Reinvasion can be prevented by canal construction and agricultural development.

The fat sand rat *Psammomys obesus* (the reservoir of *L. major* in the Near East and North Africa) has not been effectively controlled as it is not granivorous and because anticoagulants are too expensive for large scale use. The other reservoir hosts of *L. major* (*Meriones* spp. and *Tatera* spp.) are not easily controlled. Large scale control of hyraxes (the reservoirs of *L. aethiopica*) needs to be organized at a local level using the methods of shooting and trapping.

The animal reservoirs of visceral leishmaniasis (*L. infantum* and *L. chagasi*) are domestic and wild canids. The instigation of dog control for other purposes, e.g. rabies control in China, has reportedly reduced the incidence of visceral leishmaniasis to almost zero. Elimination of stray dogs is justified for many reasons and although shooting and poisoning are effective they are not acceptable to some communities. In some countries (e.g. France) screening of domestic dogs for *Leishmania* spp. by serological examination, in parallel with clinical examination, permits infected animals to be identified and either destroyed or treated. Treatment is not, however, entirely effective and an alternative approach is to administer a single prophylactic treatment shortly before the peak transmission season. Control of canine leishmaniasis could be integrated with rabies control by: (1) registration of dogs; (2) regular evaluation and surveillance; (3) availability of serological diagnosis; and (4) mobilization and motivation of the dog owning community. The importance of controlling the canine population to limit leish-

Table 5.9 Recent epidemics of parasitic diseases, causes, impact and control

Malaria	Putative cause	Epidemiological impact	Control problems and approaches
1. Madagascar, Highland malaria – Ethiopia, Kenya. 2. Forest fringe malaria. South East Asia, South America. 3. Refugee camps.	1. Change in agricultural patterns, interruption of control, environmental degradation, resettlement schemes and possible temperature change. Non-immune population. 2. Penetration into forest for gem/gold mining. Non-immune population exposed. 3. New breeding sites; non-immune populations move to lower altitudes e.g. Rwanda.	1. Over 25 000 deaths in Madagascar in 1988.	1. Availability of appropriate drugs. Vector control difficult as vector biology changing. 2. Drug resistance severe; population uncontrolled. 3. Drug availability and efficacy. Vector control possible.
Leishmaniasis 1. Visceral leishmaniasis in South Sudan. 2. Cutaneous leishmaniasis in Khartoum. 3. Cutaneous leishmaniasis in Afghanistan.	1. Ecological changes provide enhanced breeding sites for *P. orientalis* in *Acacia/Balanites* woodland. 2. Not well documented. 3. Population movement.	1. 5000 cases/year; 100 000 at risk–75% mortality in children reported. 2. Outbreaks of CL in Khartoum with 100 000 cases due to *L. major.* 3. New urban foci of transmission in *P. sergenti.* 4000 cases in urban areas and 6000 from provinces.	1. NGO initiated treatment centres. Provision of emergency drugs. Limited diagnostic facilities. High incidence of post kala azar dermal leishmanoid PKDL. Treatment established. Availability of drugs problematic. 2. Chemotherapy; vector control; rodent control. 3. Active case detection and treatment; insecticide treatment of houses in cities; health education units.
Trypanosomiasis *T.b. rhodesiense* epidemic Busoga, Uganda.	Change in ecology due to encroachment of *Lantana* following civil disturbance and change agricultural practices.	Up to 8000 cases/year in 1980.	Surveillance and treatment. Establishment of treatment centres. Vector control via impregnated traps.
T.b. gambiense Zaire.	Breakdown of surveillance through disruption of health services.	Increased incidence.	Increase surveillance and treatment but coverage limited, drugs not available.
Schistosomiasis *S. haematobium* and *S. mansoni* epidemics increase associated with water impoundment and rice irrigation throughout Africa.	Non-immune migrant population exposed for first time. *Bulinus senegalensis* breeds in irrigation systems; increase in snail populations. *Biomphalaria* increases. Major dam projects (Aswan, Egypt; Diama, Senegal and Akosombo, Ghana). Well recognised cause but micro dams in West Africa provide additional and extensive new problems. War and refugee migration.	Increased incidence, high morbidity in non-immune populations.	Increase availability of chemotherapy. Target if possible through schools. Snail control or environmental management if feasible. Health education.

Table 5.10 Widely used diagnostic tools recommended by WHO

Disease	Personal diagnostic test (direct)	Personal diagnostic test (indirect)	Community assessment
American trypanosomiasis		serodiagnostic test using synthetic peptides	agglutination test for blood bank screening
Dracunculiasis	direct observation of worm		
Foodborne trematode infections	Kato technique (i.e. cellophane-faecal thick smear)	for Paragonimiasis: intradermal screening	
Leishmaniasis	• <u>CL</u>: parasitological diagnosis by smear, culture • <u>VL</u>: parasitological diagnosis by bone marrow puncture, spleen aspiration	• <u>VL</u>: direct agglutination test (DAT) • <u>CL</u>: ELISA immunofluorescence	
Lymphatic filariasis		• assays to detect Circulating filarial antigen (CFA) • ultrasound	hydrocoele survey
Malaria	light-microscopic examination of Giemsa-stained blood films		
Onchocerciasis			rapid assessment of nodule prevalence
Schistosomiasis	• Kato technique for: *S. intercalatum*, *S. japonicum* and *S. mansoni*	quantitative urine filtration technique for *S. haematobium*	• direct observation for gross haematuria, indicative of heavy *S. haematobium* infection in children in endemic areas • detection of microhaematuria by reagent strips (*S. haematobium*)
Sleeping sickness	• blood film • CSF examination • bone marrow aspiration	• lymph gland palpation • card agglutination test for trypanosomiasis (CATT) • Capillary tube centrifugation (CTC)	

Disease	Treatment tools
American trypanosomiasis	<u>acute phase</u>: nifurtimox crystal violet/sodium ascorbate to kill parasites in infected blood in blood banks (i.e. blood bank transmission control)
Dracunculiasis	treatment aimed only at superinfections
Foodborne trematode infections	praziquantel

Disease				
Leishmaniasis	pentavalent antimonials	amphotericin B		
Lymphatic filariasis	DEC-fortified salt	DEC (single dose mass administration once a year)	ivermectin plus DEC (single dose mass administration once a year)	pentamidine
Malaria	chloroquine	sulfadoxine/ pyrimethamine or sulfalene/ pyrimethamine; mefloquine	severe disease: quinine (+tetracycline where needed) where quinine resistance: artemether	radical treatment *P. vivax, P. ovale*: primaquine
Onchocerciasis	ivermectin (single dose mass administration once a year)			
Schistosomiasis	praziquantel	metrifonate	oxamniquine	
Sleeping sickness	early stage: pentamidine (*T.b. gambiense*) suramin (*T.b. rhodesiense*)	advanced stage: melarsoprol (for both forms)	mainly for arsenical resistant cases of *T.b. gambiense*: eflornithine	

Vector control tools

Disease				
American trypanosomiasis	indoor residual spraying with pyrethroids	pyrethroid paint	fumigant cannisters with pyrethroids	housing improvement
Dracunculiasis	temephos			
Foodborne trematode infections	environmental management, including land reclamation and drainage	niclosamide (molluscicide)	biological control (natural predators)	Hazard analysis critical control point (HACCP) and fish farm quality management program
Leishmaniasis	residual insecticide spraying (DDT, pyrethroids) *Bacillus sphaericus*			
Lymphatic filariasis	pyrethroid-impregnated bednets and curtains	polystyrene beads	pyrethroid-impregnated bednets and curtains	
Malaria	pyrethroid-impregnated bednets and curtains	indoor residual spraying (DDT, organophosphates, carbamates, pyrethroids)	environmental management	biological control (larvivorous fish)
Onchocerciasis	larviciding though aerial spraying (in rotational use: *B.t* H-14, temephos, pyraclofos, pyrethroids)			
Schistosomiasis	niclosamide (molluscicide) pyrethroid-impregnated screens	environmental management pyrethroid-impregnated traps; pyrethroid-impregnated and non-impregnated		
Sleeping sickness				

By courtesy of the Division of Control of Tropical Diseases of the WHO.

maniasis in humans is underlined by the finding that human *L. infantum* infection is more widespread in southern Europe than was previously thought and by the fact that visceral leishmaniasis is an HIV associated disease. In South America, and to a lesser extent in Europe, the presence of wild canid reservoirs necessitate a continuous commitment to control.

There is limited opportunity to control the wide range of reservoir hosts of New World cutaneous leishmaniasis. The WHO (1990) suggests that control of the opossum (*Didelphis marsupialis*) could be achieved by using baited pitfall traps in urban and peri-urban environments or in disturbed primary forest; this would result in control of *L. guyanensis*. *T. cruzi* might also be tackled by the same measure in peri-urban situations, but the cost effectiveness of such measures remains to be validated. The WHO suggests an environmental management approach combining primary forest clearance with insecticide application, in order to create a vector- and reservoir-free zone around villages. The transmission of *L. guyanensis* has been greatly reduced by these measures in French Guyana.

HYDATID DISEASE

Dogs and other canids are the definitive hosts of *Echinococcus granulosus*. Several countries have instigated dog control and surveillance and chemotherapeutic treatment (with praziquantel) to eliminate adult worms or to reduce access of dogs to larval stages in offal. Major hydatid control campaigns have been introduced in a number of countries including Australia, Iceland, New Zealand, Cyprus, Argentina and Uruguay. The major measures applied are (1) preventing dogs from gaining access to raw offal at abattoirs and farms or to dead animals in the field and (2) reducing parasite loads by culling dog populations in combination with mass treatment. The application of such measures resulted in a rapid reduction of cystic infections in livestock in Cyprus, where over 30 000 dogs were eliminated over a 2 year period. A parallel health programme was also introduced to inform the public about appropriate practices for feeding dogs and for slaughtering animals. A particular problem in hydatid control is that dog faeces are used for specific purposes in some areas of the world, for instance the Turkana people of northern Kenya use them to lubricate necklaces and they are used for leather curing in Lebanon. Further problems arise from the inappropriate disposal of animal corpses, or even human corpses, and from close relationships between humans and dogs (e.g. 'nurse dogs' in Kenya, or family pets in England). In such cultures the elimination of dogs cannot be envisaged.

Alveolar hydatid disease (caused by *E. multilocularis*) is a problem in mountainous areas of Europe, the northern USA, Siberia and China, where the fox is the main definitive host and larval (cystic) stages are found in microtine rodents. Health education campaigns in Europe have successfully discouraged the consumption of wild fruits, particularly blueberries, which can be contaminated with fox faeces. In China,

reduction of the canine population has resulted in reduced transmission to humans.

5.2 Community participation in parasitic disease control

The drive towards primary healthcare following the Alma-Ata declaration of 1978 provoked a greater degree of involvement of communities in healthcare through (1) the use of community leaders to support various programmes; (2) the identification of personnel to undertake health activities on a voluntary basis; and (3) emphasising the importance of such activities in community well being. The topic of community participation has been reviewed by Curtis (1991) who provides a series of examples of vector-borne diseases. MacCormack (1991) provides an insight into the underlying principles of sustainable vector control in a community context and reviews the factors that influence success and failure. She emphasizes that much of the success achieved in small pilot programmes has depended on particular characteristics such as leadership; a responsive, well motivated, well educated community; incentives from agencies and insecticide manufacturers; and ease of communication. Following initial success, there is a danger that a 'hot' project will fall into a steady state as enthusiasm and donor support wane while the project life-cycle faces inevitable problems. The scaling up of pilot projects to national ones within a primary healthcare context presents additional challenges. For instance, the community may be affected by the replacement of local leaders with national bureaucracy. In establishing a functional link between the communities and the health systems, each group must be trained to understand the social role on the one hand and technical skills on the other. Communities' local knowledge about insects should be exploited to aid in vector control. Appropriate control methods, and the importance of maintaining them, must then be clearly explained to all those involved at the local level.

It must also be established whether unpaid community labour can be sustained over time; although it has been achieved in pilot programmes, doubts exist about longer term sustainability (Walt 1988). Much is likely to depend on the community structure and its relationship with those in authority, who are perceived as those most likely to benefit. If, for example, a cost recovery system operates, the volunteers are less able to collect fees from their social superiors. Professional interaction between technicians and volunteers can also fuel conflicts based on perceptions about status.

The outcome of community participation in any project will depend on the numerous complex social interactions existing within the community environment. The interaction between weak and strong groups, and the impact of participation on such group relationships, are of critical importance (Antia 1988). It is valuable to define the boundaries of the community involved, as individuals tend to identify with a particular locale; this is despite the inherent social instability of most villages, resulting from factors such as migration, schooling and marriage. For practical reasons the community is usually defined by a geographical boundary such as an urban neighbourhood or an agricultural village whilst nomadic groups themselves represent a mobile community.

Communities differ in how they function and are stratified; for example, they may be democratic, autocratic or under military control. In a democratic environment, obtaining consensus may be a slow process, but the likelihood of sustainability will be high. MacCormack concludes that community participation in vector control will be sustainable only if the assessment of the costs to benefits ratio takes account of 'opportunity costs' (the value of activities people would undertake if they had not committed themselves to a particular control activity). Sustainability will be enhanced if the following apply: activities are linked to the communities' priorities; skills training enhances the communities' well being; and preventative work links to curative or care outcomes in the primary healthcare setting, or can produce income (Rajagopalan, Paniker and Das 1987).

Dedicated control programmes often achieve good results, but they are usually part of a research project. Therefore, coverage of the population in need is relatively small, but delivery costs are high, as are recurrent costs as a proportion of overall costs. This leaves little financial input for operational expenses. In situations in which the frequency of the intervention is limited (e.g. once a year) the commitment of dedicated resources is difficult to justify.

Community based treatments are usually better targeted and tend to involve volunteers, TBAs and primary healthcare workers. Increasingly, other types of groups are also becoming involved, such as women's groups, churches and other NGOs. Treatment can be given on specific days organized by governments such as independence days, Head of State's birthday, local festivals (e.g. to celebrate harvest or onset of rain). The use of such occasions may reduce the need for intense monitoring to ensure high coverage and compliance. There are no dedicated staff costs, administrative costs are absorbed by the system, transport costs are minimal, compliance is high and costs of monitoring and evaluation are low. These arguments have been developed to justify such approaches to lymphatic filariasis control in Papua New Guinea. Treatment with diethylcarbamazine (DEC) was simplified by creating ready made tablets based on a calculation of the average weight of adults and children; the appropriate amount of drug was formulated into one blue tablet for adults and one red tablet for children. This eliminated the need for scales for weighing, allowed the treatment to be administered by untrained personnel and improved compliance (by using a single tablet). The cost per treatment is US$0.8 per child and US$1.2 per adult (not including costs for transportation, health promotion materials, monitoring and coordination). In seeking to develop community treatment of any disease, certain problems (e.g. devising reporting forms for illiterate

communities) need to be addressed through locally organized operational research.

Because of the pressures on health systems, it is necessary to use personnel resources at the level of the community to participate in various phases of control activities. This is particularly relevant in the maintenance phase of programmes when the community has seen benefits from intervention phases; this promotes confidence between the programme participants and the communities themselves. Parasitic disease control programmes are increasingly becoming dependent on the involvement of human resources without specific technical knowledge or with only limited training.

With reference to a Chagas disease control programme, Garcia, Zapata and Marsden (1986) have described the value of community involvement in establishing vigilance over the presence of vector bugs following the attack phase. Bug information posts were linked to schools as it was recognized that children were sensitive to the renewed presence of triatomine bugs. Reappearance of bugs is the basis for initiating selective spraying at the local level. If given adequate information, local isolated farmers could also act as notifiers of bug presence. Simple devices for bug monitoring have been developed in Argentina.

CONTROL OF BRUGIAN FILARIASIS

A focus of filariasis caused by *Brugia malayi* existed in the Indian coastal state of Kerala, in the Cherthala region of Alleppey. There was a high prevalence of the disease with serious clinical manifestations of elephantiasis. The vectors in the area were *Mansonia* mosquitoes that breed on certain water plants (*Pistia*, *Eichhornia* and *Salvinia*), to which their larvae attach for respiration. The local people believed that vegetation in ponds improved the quality of the water, which was used for domestic purposes. Also, the water plants are used as green manure on coconut plantations (Rajagopalan, Paniker and Das 1987) and therefore the community were reluctant to use chemical larvicides or herbicides.

An extensive education and awareness programme was initiated via the media, targeting various levels of the community. A group of sociologists was used to pass on the necessary technology and to create interest. The Filariasis Patients' Association, headed by a former school teacher, developed a school health education programme. This campaign was targeted towards the female population of Cherthala, who were often not chosen as brides because of filariasis; the effectiveness of the campaign was enhanced by a high level of literacy among the local women. The main control measure was the removal of water plants; the community first had to be persuaded that alternative green manure fertilizers were adequate and that ponds could be cleared without financial loss. As no government organization was available to supervise the weed removal, this had to be done by the people themselves. To provide motivation, the community was encouraged to culture fish that could be sustained only in weed-free ponds. Species of fast growing edible fish were purchased from the State Fisheries Department and distributed free to those who agreed to remove weed from their ponds. The economic benefits derived from the fish motivated the community to keep the ponds free of weed, thereby removing the vector habitat. The programme is organized by the peoples' Filariasis Control Movement (FILCO) which supports a variety of approaches, ensuring that the whole community is involved:

1 In 6 secondary schools, Student Filariasis Control Clubs run programmes to detect and treat filariasis.

2 All educational institutions contribute voluntary labour to improve the environment.

3 The National Cadet Corps and National Service Scheme provide services for filariasis control.

4 The interns of Medical Colleges are involved in clinical and diagnostic night camps.

5 The Departments of Fisheries and Agriculture popularize fish culture and alternative fertilisers.

To publicize the message, hoardings depicting filariasis patients were erected in areas where they would have most impact (markets, hospitals, bus stations, railway stations). The slogan employed was 'Remove weeds and protect yourselves and your future generations from filariasis'. These messages were reinforced by the distribution of films depicting the suffering of a filariasis patients.

In parallel with environmental measures to reduce vector levels, screening and treatment of cases, previously under government control, are now undertaken by voluntary organizations. For instance, 75 Filariasis Detection and Treatment Centres are now screening the endemic area and positive individuals are being treated with DEC.

Guinea worm eradication

Guinea worm (dracunculiasis) has been the subject of a global eradication campaign, initiated in 1980 and involving a consortium of donors. The disease affects 16 African countries as well as India and Pakistan, its impact being concentrated at harvest and planting times when infected individuals are incapacitated and are unable to farm or to attend school for up to 3 months at a time. The infection is painful and secondary infections often result when the worms emerge through the skin of the extremities. As there are no effective drugs or vaccines, Guinea worm must be eradicated through a series of other measures some of which require community involvement, for instance filtering water; treatment of bodies of water with the insecticide temephos; provision of safe water; and case isolation to prevent contamination of water sources.

The eradication strategy is based on the establishment of a national programme in each affected country to survey every affected village, to estimate numbers of cases and to initiate plans. It is then necessary to establish village based surveillance, using VHWs to report cases on a monthly basis. Health education encourages the use of cloth filters and the prevention of contamination of water sources. Some villages can also be targeted for provision of safe water whilst the establishment of a community based surveillance system (with monthly supervision) might broaden to cover other major endemic conditions. Dracunculus-free certification can be issued to clear areas. To date, there has been considerable success with this approach, as incidence has decreased dramatically. VHWs are directly involved in measures that benefit health and increase agricultural productivity and school attendance. Such success increases confidence within communities and motivates them to become involved in other self-sustaining health interventions.

Community surveillance methods for eradication require the establishment of village development committees whose members are responsible for case notification, health education, distribution and maintenance of filters and patient care. In Mauritania this role has been assigned to females, who undertake the roles of water gathering and distribution. A potential weakness is that village eradication activities are dependent on monthly supervision from the health personnel at a sub-district level. Each village requires monthly visits, usually integrated with the extended vaccination programme or other health programmes. Dracunculiasis can be eradicated but only with considerable community commitment from village workers; in Burkina Faso and Mali these workers are rewarded by distribution of cloth in recognition of their contribution to the eradication programme.

Community malaria control in Pondicherry, India

In the coastal areas of Pondicherry, South India, malaria has been controlled by a combination of approaches organized by the Vector Control Research Centre (VCRC). These have achieved good control of the vector *A. subpictus* and also produced income for the local population. Vector control was achieved by removing the algae *Enteromorpha* from coastal lagoons, where it sheltered mosquito larvae from fish and other predators. The algae were collected in the pre-monsoon season and provided the raw material for producing paper to be sold by villagers. The lagoon became a focus of mosquito breeding during the dry season and the villagers were persuaded to deepen one of the ponds in order to allow the other to drain into it, the mud from the deepened pond being used to fill low lying areas. The deeper pond was then used for prawn culture, which provided extra income for the village.

Control of vectors was also necessary in other breeding sites, particularly the earthenware pots in which coconut husks are retted to make coir. Control was achieved by introducing larvae of the mosquito *Toxorhynchites* which predate larvae of vector mosquitoes. The water filled pits where *Casuarina* trees are grown also act as breeding sites and so these were stocked with the larvivorous fish *Gambusia*. This action was encouraged by using 'Science Clubs' in schools to stock the pits.

These achievements in involving the community initially faced resistance from villagers who were divided amongst themselves and inherently suspicious of officialdom. These communities placed a higher priority on services such as water, electricity and roads rather than vector control, except in situations in which malaria epidemics occurred. Only after the VCRC had intervened and asked government departments to provide electricity and a water supply did the villagers have enough confidence to allow vector control projects to commence. Success of this programme, as with that of filariasis, was largely due to the initiative of active locally based indigenous scientists (VCRC 1992).

CONTROL OF PARASITIC INFECTIONS THROUGH SCHOOL-AGE CHILDREN

Population increases and investments in education have increased the global population of school-age children. This group is a particularly important entry point for improving health status, using education to create norms of health behaviour and life-styles. The school also provides access to a population with a high prevalence of helminth infection in whom mass drug distribution can rapidly reduce morbidity, enhance nutritional status and improve cognition and hence school performance. Urbanization has increased enrolment into schools, but also promotes conditions such as lack of adequate waste disposal, overcrowding and the absence of clean water, that may encourage increased transmission of helminth diseases.

A WHO pamphlet from 1995 (WHO 1995a) estimated that of a global total of 1.2 billion school-age children, 700 million were registered in school with 400 million attending each day, and enrolment still increasing. The target parasitic diseases susceptible to control are schistosomiasis, *Ascaris lumbricoides*, *Trichuris trichiura*, hookworm (*Necator americanus* and *Ancylostoma duodenale*) and the food-borne trematodes, *Clonorchis*, *Opisthorchis* and *Paragonimus*. Many school-age children have mixed infections, providing justification for mass interventions based on effective single doses of drugs such as the benzimidazoles (mebendazole and albendazole) and praziquantel; these eliminate intestinal helminths and schistosomes.

The epidemiological characteristics of each particular situation require investigation; prevalence and intensity vary even in adjacent areas, as do the pattern and rate of reinfection. It is assumed that reinfection will occur and require retreatment, although emphasising the importance of personal hygiene should reduce the rate of reinfection. There is thus a need for field studies to ascertain whether intervention for schistosomiasis and intestinal helminths is warranted. Rapid assessment of haematuria is used to evaluate levels of morbidity due to *S. haematobium* whilst other approaches are being tested for *S. mansoni* and intestinal helminths.

Drugs for the treatment of intestinal helminths and schistosomes, and their treatment schedules and efficacy, can be found in a publication produced by the WHO (WHO 1995b). Albendazole and praziquantel have now been used in combination; combined drug delivery offers advantages in terms of lower cost and simplification of therapy. This results in improved compliance and improved drug efficacy by potentiation of the therapeutic effort. Trials have provided no evidence for adverse effects of combined treatment with praziquantel and albendazole. Phase I clinical trials showed a four-fold increase in the bioavailability of albendazole in the presence of praziquantel, whilst the bioavailability of praziquantel was unaffected by the administration of albendazole. Phase II studies on the safety and efficacy of combined treatment have shown no increase in adverse effects and no reduction in efficacy.

The WHO emphasizes the importance of targeting chemotherapy for intestinal helminths at school-age children, as they harbour the most intense infections of *Ascaris*, *Trichiuris* and *Schistosoma* although intensities of the different worm infections vary considerably between individuals. Treatment of this group achieves the maximum return in terms of reducing morbidity and schools provide the most accessible entry point for maximum coverage. The WHO also stresses the value of targeting schoolchildren for oral anti-schistosomal drugs; programmes should seek to provide complete coverage of the school-age population. Such approaches could be combined with other helminth control and also with other health oriented activities such as immunization, nutritional programmes, maternal and child health activities and general health education as part of the school curriculum. Retreatment should not be undertaken for schistosomiasis more than once a year and the WHO (1993b) suggests a 5 yearly interval. Epidemiological studies need to be established to evaluate the criteria for retreatment frequency in each area.

The integration of helminth control into the education sector not only fulfils the immediate objective of infection control, but also brings broader health issues to the attention of a group who can strongly influence the behaviour of future generations. WHO policy promotes school health programmes, with deworming as an entry point and with an emphasis on personal hygiene. The integration of school and community based chemotherapy into the primary healthcare system will improve coverage and promote optimal retreatment schedules. Another potential benefit may be gained through training personnel at the periphery, who will develop activities based on disease-specific interventions to reduce prevalence and intensity of infection; this will reduce morbidity through coverage of schools and other entry points. Whilst this approach to infection control will undoubtedly improve the health of schoolchildren and, to some extent, contribute to lower transmission rates over time, greater impact will be achieved if health education, improved water supplies, sanitation and environmental management are integrated into the activities involved in community development.

5.3 Role of vector control in disease control

INSECT CONTROL

The role of insects in the transmission of parasitic infections has been recognized since Manson discovered that filaria parasites were transmitted by mosquitoes. From the latter half of the last century onwards, recognition followed that numerous other diseases, including sleeping sickness, malaria, Chagas disease and onchocerciasis were also insect-borne. Knowledge of insect biology (particularly of breeding sites, habitat of pre-adult stages, adult resting sites, biting behaviour and host preferences, migration capacity and longevity) represents a key factor in assessing whether or not appropriate control can be directed at the vector. Early attempts to target malaria by controlling mosquitoes depended on knowledge of larval stages and breeding sites. The removal of breeding sites ('source reduction') was the only approach available to reduce vector populations and was achieved by applying oil and copper compounds and by rigorous removal or destruction of larval habitats by mechanical methods (WHO 1995c). Vectors such as tsetse flies were controlled by destroying savanna and riverine habitats of *G. morsitans* and *palpalis* group flies, respectively. In some countries game animals (the favoured hosts of *Glossina*) were eliminated by shooting prior to the introduction of cattle. Removal of game animals rapidly reduced the tsetse population in large areas of South Africa, Uganda and Zimbabwe, providing additional land for ranching.

The advent of chemical insecticides in the 1940s provided new tools for vector control that became incorporated into programmes designed to control, if not eradicate, numerous diseases. DDT, the most widely used of these insecticides, was one of the major tools in the campaign for malaria eradication (together with chloroquine) launched by the World Health Organization in 1955. In parallel, DDT was being utilized in tsetse control programmes for both human and animal trypanosomiasis, for the control of *Simulium* (black fly) larvae to control river blindness and for the successful eradication of *S. damnosum* in Uganda. Meanwhile, another chlorinated hydrocarbon, benzene hexachloride (BHC), or lindane, was successfully used against triatomine bugs in Chagas disease control.

Recognition of the environmental side effects of chlorinated hydrocarbons, both direct toxicity on non-target insects and bio-accumulation, led to a suspension of their widespread use and a drive to utilize other chemical classes of insecticide. This was accelerated by the realization that resistance of mosquitoes to DDT was creating problems for malaria control, particularly indoor house spraying programmes. Whilst DDT is still used in some public health control programmes for indoor house spraying there is evidence of adverse effects on humans which emphasizes the need for caution in any widespread future use (Curtis 1994). There is an increasing trend towards the use of synthetic pyrethroids for indoor house spraying for malaria control.

There are, however, many examples where vector control has had a profound public health impact. Outside the domain of parasitic disease, the eradication of yellow fever by source reduction of *Aedes aegypti* in Central America illustrates what can be achieved through intensive and well organized campaigns of vector control. The eradication of *A. gambiae* from Brazil, following its importation from West Africa in the 1930s, represented not only an important public health achievement but also a major contribution to the development of Brazil, given the efficiency of *A. gambiae* as a vector of malaria in Africa.

Currently, intensive programmes are underway to eliminate *Triatoma infestans* (the vector of *Trypanosoma cruzi*) by domiciliary spraying using the synthetic pyrethroids (deltamethrin and lambacyhalothrin) in the South Cone countries of South America. This has had a major impact on transmission, as determined by standardized serological procedures and community based bug monitoring systems in Brazil, Argentina, Paraguay, Chile and Uruguay. The initiative has been consolidated over recent years by increased coordination at the level of the MOH. Applied research has been geared towards providing additional methodologies to support government organized control schemes such as fumigant canisters, insecticidal paints and simple bug monitoring devices for surveillance of reinvasion. The Chagas disease control programmes do not benefit from the additional tool of an effective chemotherapeutic agent. This has extended the anticipated time for reducing Chagas disease as a public health problem, given that no drug or vaccine is likely to become available in the foreseeable future. Hence, the current approach of intensive vector control supported by national governments is the only feasible one (WHO 1991).

To achieve the objectives of the Onchocerciasis Control Programme (OCP), vector control has been the core strategy in 11 countries in West Africa. The programme, initiated in 1974, was based on larviciding the breeding sites of *S. damnosum* complex black flies, initially in 6 West African countries. The strategy was based on the need to break the life cycle for the lifetime of the adult *Onchocerca volvulus* which, in 1974, was considered to be 18–20 years. At that time only one insecticide (the organophosphate temephos) had the appropriate chemical characteristics to satisfy the environmental prerequisite of avoiding long term damage to the riverine ecology. Two major problems faced the programme early in its existence: migration of savanna black flies from outside the programme area and resistance of some black fly populations to temephos. These problems were solved by extending the area of the programme westwards and southwards and by engaging in a research programme that rapidly developed alternative insecticides. The extensive activities of the OCP and its management and structures are described by Samba (1994) and Molyneux (1995). At present, 7 larvicides from different chemical classes are in operational use They are used on a rotational basis in accordance with parameters such as cost effectiveness, environmental side effects, river discharge rates, carry distance of insecticide and risk of resistance development. The 7 insecticides in current use are *Bacillus thuringiensis israeliensis* H–14 serotype toxin (Bti); temephos, phoxim and pyraclofos (all organophosphates); carbosulfan (a carbamate); permethrin (a pyrethroid) and etofenprox, or vectron, (a pseudopyrethroid) (Hougard et al. 1993).

Whilst vector control has clearly been successful in breaking the onchocerciasis transmission cycle, the necessary duration of vector control has been reduced by the widespread use of the drug ivermectin; this became available for use as a microfilaricide suitable for use in communities in 1986 (Remme 1995). Epidemiological studies clearly indicate that the duration of adult worm life is 14 years and that distribution of ivermectin in hyperendemic areas on an annual basis rapidly reduces microfilarial loads and also has a rapid impact on ocular morbidity. Hence combined vector control and chemotherapy will reduce the duration of control to a 12 year period although ivermectin alone, at least in the African endemic areas, cannot prevent transmission (WHO 1995d).

Increasing numbers of displaced persons and refugees pose special problems for organizations responsible for management of disease. Intervention through vector control is an important component, as there is great potential for rapid disease outbreak in crowded, insanitary environments that contain traumatized, malnourished, displaced individuals who are exposed to vector-borne infection or ectoparasites. Epidemics are sometimes most effectively controlled through vector control. Thomson (1995) provides details of how such epidemics should be controlled, with specific reference to relief organizations.

SNAIL CONTROL

The elimination of snails for the control of schistosomiasis remains an important component of control activities and 3 approaches have been used: chemical, environmental and biological. Projects in several countries have shown that chemical control using molluscicides (e.g. niclosamide) in combination with other methods can reduce or eliminate transmission. Chemical molluscicides must be environmentally acceptable and must not produce adverse side effects if they enter the food chain. In addition, they must be cost effective, snail specific and easily applied. During the 1970s snail control, either by chemical methods or through environmental management (deweeding, irrigation canal construction and maintenance), was a key component for control. The advent of safe and effective chemotherapy for schistosomiasis (oxamniquine, praziquantel and metrifonate) capable of reducing morbidity through population based campaigns has shifted emphasis away from mollusciciding. Snail control is now considered as one of several approaches in integrated morbidity control, contributing to reduction in transmission at times of peak transmission. Target levels of reduction of snail populations should exceed 95% and must be maintained throughout the main season of transmission. Molluscides can be used to destroy snails in breeding sites in transmission foci, reducing transmission in recreational areas such as lakes. They are also useful for the following: as a means of reinforcing community involvement; to reduce transmission in areas where there is a special risk (e.g. fishing villages in the Volta Lake, Ghana); to eliminate newly introduced snail populations; for total elimination of snails in isolated focal transmission sites (e.g. oases in North Africa); and to prevent the establishment of dense populations in irrigation schemes (McCullough 1992).

Biological control of snail hosts of schistosomes has been attempted, by introducing other snail genera or species that out-compete the natural hosts, but the impact of this approach on schistosomiasis morbidity is likely to be limited.

Population based chemotherapy, combined with local and seasonal use of molluscicides, will be the central features of future schistosomiasis control in high priority foci. Mollusciciding must be planned effectively and better strategies and delivery systems are required to improve cost effectiveness. New inexpensive effective synthetic molluscicides are also needed, in addition to bayluscide, the only compound currently commercially available (WHO 1993b).

5.4   Role of chemotherapy and chemoprophylaxis

Drugs are the mainstay for controlling many diseases, but antiparasitic drugs present a considerable challenge for researchers interested in rational drug development. Investment by multinational drug companies into new agents for use in the tropics and the developing world is limited, as market forces tend to determine the research and investment strategies of the pharmaceutical industry.

Parasite infections pose a variety of other problems for chemotherapeutic control, as follows: (1) the organisms rapidly develop drug resistance; (2) effective compounds have a narrow therapeutic index and hence side effects are common; (3) parasites can invade specific sites of the body making drug delivery difficult; (4) helminth parasites can be relatively large and hence require proportionally more drug than microscopic organisms; (5) compounds may be difficult to obtain when required and may be manufactured only infrequently, particularly those compounds used for treatment of diseases that affect relatively small numbers of individuals; (6) some currently used compounds contain toxic elements such as arsenic and antimony; and (7) many compounds must be administered under medical supervision, require extensive hospitalization and are not affordable by individuals.

Despite these problems some compounds are highly effective for controlling parasitic infections and for the treatment of individuals. New drugs for human diseases have also originated from alternative sources over the last decade. For instance, veterinary research has produced ivermectin, used for treating onchocerciasis, lymphatic filariasis and scabies; ivermectin was originally marketed for the treatment of helminth infections of animals. Eflornithine, a drug that can cure late stage chronic sleeping sickness (albeit at very high cost), was originally developed as an anti-tumour drug. The artemisine derivative *qinghaosu*, produced from the Chinese herb *Artemisia* and used as a cure for fever in China for 2000 years, is now widely available in South East Asia and Africa for malaria treatment. Its availability is largely uncontrolled in China and this may encourage rapid development of resistance. This is of concern because the drug has valuable curative properties and thus should only be introduced in appropriate circumstances, in relation to the current drug resistance spectrum of malaria parasites in each region. New formulations of existing drugs have been developed, such as encapsulated liposomes that provide slow release of a drug; a slow release formulation of amphotericin B has been developed to reduce toxicity and enhance efficacy in leishmaniasis treatment.

A distinction must be made between drug treatment initiated to alleviate individual suffering, and mass treatment strategies that seek not only to improve the well being of individuals, but also that of communities. This latter objective is achieved by ensuring that no parasites can be transmitted by vectors, or that no parasites remain to reinfect the population. Drugs must therefore be regarded as having several functions in control. Gutteridge (1993) provides a summary of the drugs available for parasitic diseases and the rationale for their use.

A major problem in many parasitic diseases is that drug resistance frequently arises. Management of drug resistance in parasitic disease is difficult as there are few compounds available. Strategies for reducing the likelihood of development of drug resistance in malaria and helminth diseases are well documented and include the following: appropriate dosage regimes; control of drug quality and distribution (in malaria); and incorporation of vector control to reduce the development or spread of resistance. Mechanisms responsible for development of resistance include: the ability of the organism to metabolize the drug to an inactive form; changes in the permeability of the organism so that the drug is no longer taken up; development of alternative biochemical pathways; increased levels of target enzyme production; and a change in the biochemical target so that the drug cannot bind as well as it did to the original compound (Gutteridge 1993). The ability of micro-organisms to change and adapt rapidly will clearly represent a continuing problem and drug resistance is unlikely to be avoidable. Hence, any disease control strategy based on chemotherapy should anticipate such a problem and should seek to reduce the rate at which resistance develops, whilst also promoting strategies for management of resistance if it occurs.

In many developing countries drugs are available through many sources. From the perspective of the consumer the availability of drugs at a health facility is a major indicator of quality of care. In the household environment up to 50% of expenditure on health is on drugs. In the developing world pharmaceutical expenditure comprises 20–30% of recurrent costs, second only to personnel costs (World Bank 1994). Supply of drugs for the control of parasites is usually organized in the public sector through government formulated essential drug lists. The WHO *Essential*

Drug List (WHO 1992b) and programme includes drugs for the treatment of infection with parasites. The concept of an essential drug list is that such drugs should be available at all times, in adequate amounts and in the appropriate dosage forms (WHO 1992b). Several important drugs used for parasite disease control are often unavailable, despite being specified on essential drug lists.

Whilst governments have a responsibility to provide essential drugs to different levels of the health service, private providers play a major role in many countries where private expenditure on drugs considerably exceeds public expenditure. In Africa, c. 70% of the population has no regular access to essential drugs and drug stocks often run out as a result of problems with management, logistics or finances. This is particularly true in peri-urban and urban centres, even to the extent that hospitals may run out of drugs. Drug shortages are less frequent in commercial facilities and such supplies are more readily available in urban centres, but the perception of higher quality product availability in the private sector allows for prices to be inflated. Private suppliers are also frequently not subject to quality control. In the case of antimalarials, which are amongst the most frequently required drugs, there is over-pricing and supply is irregular. Furthermore, they are often supplied without diagnostic confirmation.

The problems of drug supply, cost (generic versus brand name), quality control, distribution, irrational prescribing, non-compliance and availability have been highlighted by the World Bank (1993, 1994). These problems potentially apply to all drugs and awareness of them and ways to circumvent them must be addressed if chemotherapy or chemoprophylaxis is to be an integral part of disease control. Other problems may arise if vertical programmes involving drug distribution are developed, for example, the free distribution of ivermectin for onchocerciasis. Such an approach may conflict with the development of revolving funds to sustain drug supplies at primary healthcare centres, as might drug distribution for control of schistosomiasis or intestinal helminths targeted through school health programmes. In the increasing number of emergency situations, the agencies involved should be aware of the potential needs of the affected populations as part of their response planning. In this context a predictive approach to supplying drugs and insecticides is necessary and must be based on a knowledge of the ecology of the area and the likely disease problems.

The use of reliable, systematic reviews of evidence of effectiveness to inform policy is becoming recognized as a vital contribution to enable resources to be used appropriately. A scientific approach is being developed by a process of systematic reviews of randomized control trials, that provide reliable assessment of the effectiveness of various healthcare interventions. This approach has been promoted, as traditional reviews are unsystematic and do not respect scientific principles or control for biases and random errors. The Cochrane Collaboration approach involves world-wide partners, designed to build on enthusiasm for the process, to minimize duplication, to avoid bias, to maintain an electronic database and to ensure wide access, in order to make the information available to decision makers.

The Parasitic Diseases Group is currently conducting a register of published and unpublished trials in parasitic diseases, identified by hand searching relevant journals, using editors in China, Chile, the USA and the UK. The review topics include malaria chemoprophylaxis in pregnancy, the use of artemisine derivatives in malaria, chemotherapy of filariasis and the treatment of neurocysticercosis and giardiasis.

5.5 Role of diagnosis in control

Diagnosis of an infection or disease is a fundamental concept of curative medicine. In some parasitic infections, identification of the presence of the organism is essential if the appropriate treatment is to be given. For example, in sleeping sickness it is important to confirm the stage of the disease, as well as the presence of the parasite; this is because the drug based treatment for late stage disease (melarsoprol) can be fatal. Hence treatment is not initiated without confirmation of central nervous system involvement. In areas of high prevalence in which mass treatment campaigns are in operation, diagnosis of the individual is not important.

In some diseases, such as schistosomiasis, onchocerciasis and lymphatic filariasis, for which the overall prevalence is high, it is important that available resources are concentrated on those populations most in need. The concept has therefore developed of rapid appraisal of disease burdens in communities so that interventions can be better targeted. Ngoumou, Walsh and Mace (1994) described such an approach to the rapid mapping of hyperendemic onchocerciasis using nodule frequency, which correlates closely with community microfilarial load, as a means of targeting ivermectin distribution. Similarly the frequency of haematuria can be used as an indicator for the prevalence of schistosomiasis in school children.

There is therefore a trend away from 'gold standard' parasitiological diagnostic techniques when disease control programmes are underway. This does not diminish the importance of diagnosis of the individual infection in need of specific treatment. The need to maintain diagnostic parasitological skills remains and is particularly relevant in the provision of diagnostic staff for microscopic diagnosis of malaria. Identification of parasites and differential diagnosis of *Plasmodium* species are important not only in determining treatment but also in saving unnecessary expenditure on drugs by defining whether or not a fever is of malarial origin. Despite the continuing need for skilled microscopists for malaria diagnosis, the amount of training provided is often inadequate, as are the quality of microscopes and staining materials available.

Serological diagnosis for screening populations has been used for surveillance of sleeping sickness. An antibody detection test, card agglutination test for trypanosomiasis (CATT), and antigen detection tests are used to screen populations. In those suspected of infection, parasites are detected by examination of blood or lymph by direct or concentration techniques. Similarly a direct agglutination test (DAT) has been developed to identify suspected cases of visceral leishmaniasis; this should be followed by a parasitological diagnosis, usually by the examination of bone marrow aspirate or splenic biopsy. These techniques are painful and risky, respectively, and not applicable to large numbers of cases.

Diagnostic developments include attempts to use single tests to detect antigens in urine; dip stick techniques based on enzyme-linked immunosorbent assay (ELISA) systems have been developed, using colour change as an indicator of the presence of antigens. In the case of urinary schistosomiasis, a colour test is used to indicate the presence of blood.

Lymphatic filariasis due to *Wuchereria bancrofti* poses particular problems for diagnosis as the parasites appear in the blood only at night-time, when it is not socially acceptable to take blood assays. Modern systems for detection of parasite antigen or DNA represent more effective ways of obtaining information about the endemic status of filariasis and for monitoring the impact of control. Nevertheless, while such testing is being evaluated, parallel night-time blood samples also need to be taken. There is also a need to develop an alternative diagnostic test to detect onchocerciasis in areas where the disease has been controlled, skin snipping is no longer acceptable, and prevalence and microfilarial load are low. Here, it is important to determine whether transmission is occurring and, although this could be undertaken by examining black flies, this may not be feasible. The ideal requirement for onchocerciasis serological diagnosis is for a test in humans that will detect the pre-patent developing adult worm stage of the infection, when few if any microfilaria will have reached the skin.

The role of diagnosis in the control of parasites varies considerably depending on the levels at which the question is approached, for instance the following factors may need to be compared: treatment at the level of the individual or the community; safe drug versus toxic drug; expensive versus cost effective interventions; cheap drug versus free drug; monitoring control versus obtaining baseline data on prevalence pre-intervention. The appropriate diagnostic approach is dependent on the particular situation.

5.6 Control of intestinal parasites

The impact on morbidity of intestinal helminths and, to a lesser extent, protozoal infections due to *Entamoeba* and *Giardia,* has been highlighted by the recognition that their public health impact was previously grossly underestimated (Table 5.1). There is now an accumulated body of evidence suggesting that intestinal helminths (*Ascaris, Trichuris* and hookworms) have significant effects on growth, nutritional status and school performance in children. The opportunity to provide alleviation of worm burdens through single dose, effective, inexpensive drugs (albendazole, mebendazole) is currently being exploited. This approach provides direct benefits as the worm burden is removed, reducing morbidity and also possibly reduces the rate of transmission. Repeat treatment ensures that burdens are maintained below levels associated with morbidity, preventing protein energy malnutrition and iron deficiency anaemia.

It is recommended that treatment for intestinal helminth infections is administered without prior screening as prevalence is high. The school based approach is one of a range of strategies that can be used for helminth control at the community level; it can be integrated into existing systems such as maternal and child healthcare, family planning, water supply and sanitation, and should be reinforced through health education. In areas where schistosomiasis is endemic,

control approaches can be combined, reducing costs, improving compliance and facilitating the logistics of control. In the longer term, health education, improved environmental sanitation and safe water supplies are the components essential for the reduction of morbidity caused by intestinal parasites transmitted by the orofaecal route or through the skin. In school based programmes it is vital to train teachers about prevention and control, and these topics should be included in the curriculum.

There are continuing plans in some countries for major parasitic disease control programmes. China has commenced a national de-worming programme for a population of 200 million children, whilst in Mauritius the World Food Programme is including de-worming in a school meals initiative.

REFERENCES

Antia NH, 1988, The Mandwa Project: an experiment in community participation, *Int J Health Serv*, **18:** 153–64.

Benton B, Skinner E, 1990, Cost benefits of onchocerciasis control, *Acta Leiden*, **59:** 405–11.

Birley MH, 1995, *The Health Impact Assessment of Development Projects*, HMSO, London.

Curtis CF (ed), 1991, *Control of Disease Vectors in the Community*, Wolfe, London, 233.

Curtis CF, 1994, Should DDT continue to be recommended for malaria vector control?, *Med Vet Entomol*, **8:** 107–12.

Garcia-Zapata MTA, Marsden PD, 1986, Chagas Disease, *Clinics in Tropical Medicine and Communicable Diseases*, WB Saunders, 557–85.

Gutteridge WE, 1993, Chemotherapy, *Modern Parasitology*, ed Cox FEG, Blackwell, Oxford, 219–42.

Hougard J–M, Poudiougo P et al., 1993, Criteria for the selection of larvicides by the Onchocerciasis Control Programme in West Africa, *Ann Trop Med Parasitol*, **5:** 435–42.

Hunter HJ, Rey L et al, 1993, *Parasitic Diseases in Water Resources Development. The Need for Intersectoral Negotiations*, World Health Organization, Geneva.

MacCormack CP, 1991, Appropriate Vector Control in Primary Health Care, *Control of Disease Vectors in the Community*, Wolfe, London, 221–227.

McCullough FS, 1992, The Use of Mollusciciding in Schistosomiasis Control, World Health Organization, Geneva.

Molyneux DH, Control, 1993, *Modern Parasitology*, ed Cox FEG, Blackwell, Oxford, 243–63.

Molyneux DH, 1995, Onchocerciasis control in West Africa: Current status and future of Onchocerciasis Control Programme, *Parasitol Today*, **11:** 399–402.

Murray CJL, Lopez AD, 1994, *Global Comparative Assessments in the Health Sector. Disease Burden, Expenditures, and Intervention Packages*, World Health Organization, Geneva.

Ngoumou P, Walsh JF, Mace J–M, 1994, A rapid mapping technique for the prevalence and distribution of onchocerciasis: a Cameroon case study, *Ann Trop Med Parasitol*, **88:** 463–74.

Rajagopalan PK, Paniker KN, Das PK, 1987, Control of malaria and filariasis in South India, *Parasitol Today*, **3:** 233–41.

Remme JHF, 1995, The African Programme for Onchocerciasis Control: Preparing to launch, *Parasitol Today*, **11:** 403–6.

Samba EM, 1994, *The Onchocerciasis Control Programme in West Africa. An Example of Effective Public Health Management*, World Health Organization, Geneva.

Thomson M, 1995, *Disease Prevention through Vector Control. Guidelines for Relief Organisations*, Oxfam, UK and Ireland.

Vector Control Research Centre, 1992, *Control of Brugian Filariasis*, Misc Publ VCRC, Pondicherry.

Walsh JF, Molyneux DH, Birley MH, 1993, Deforestation: effects on vector borne disease, *Parasitology*, **106:** 855–75.

Walt G, 1988, CHWs: are national programmes in crisis? *Health Policy and Planning*, **3:** 1–21.

World Bank, 1994, *Development in Practice. Better Health in Africa*, The World Bank, Washington.

World Bank, 1993, *World Development Report. Investing in Health*, Oxford University Press, Oxford.

World Health Organization, 1979, Parasitic zoonoses, *W H O Tech Rep Ser*, **637.**

World Health Organization, 1990, Control of the leishmaniases, *W H O Tech Rep Ser*, **793.**

World Health Organization, 1991, Control of Chagas diseases, *W H O Tech Rep Ser*, **811.**

World Health Organization, 1992a, Lymphatic filariasis. The disease and its control, *W H O Tech Rep Ser*, **721.**

World Health Organization, 1992b, The use of essential drugs. Model list of essential drugs, *W H O Tech Rep Ser*, **825.**

World Health Organization, 1993a, *A Global Strategy for Malaria Control*, World Health Organization, Geneva.

World Health Organization, 1993b, The control of schistosomiasis, *W H O Tech Rep Ser*, **830.**

World Health Organization, 1994, Lymphatic Filariasis Infection and Disease Control Strategies. Report of a consultative meeting. Penang Malaysia. World Health Organization. Division of Control of Tropical Diseases (CTD) and UNDP/World Bank/WHO Special programme for Research and Training in Tropical Diseases (TDR). TDR/CTD/FIL/PENANG, World Health Organization, Geneva.

World Health Organization, 1995a, Health of school children. Treatment of Intestinal Helminths and Schistosomiasis. Mimeographed document WHO/SCHISTO/95.112, World Health Organization, Geneva.

World Health Organization, 1995b, *WHO Model Prescribing Information. Drugs Used in Parasitic Diseases*, 2, World Health Organization, Geneva.

World Health Organization, 1995c, Vector control for malaria and other mosquito-borne diseases, *W H O Tech Rep Ser*, **857.**

World Health Organization, 1995d, Onchocerciasis and its control, *W H O Tech Rep Ser*, **852.**

Part II

PROTOZOA

CELLULAR ORGANIZATION OF PARASITIC PROTOZOA

H Mehlhorn

1 **Definition of the cell**	4 **Modes of reproduction**
2 **Unicellular eukaryotes**	5 **Concluding statement**
3 **The general morphology of parasitic protozoa**	

1 DEFINITION OF THE CELL

The organic elements on earth exist in the following forms: various types of cells; short sequences of stable proteins (prions); extracellular genomes (viroids, or naked RNA molecules); and protein capsules, or capsids, containing relatively short molecules of DNA or RNA often surrounded by an additional membrane (bacteriophages and viruses). Prions, viroids, phages and viruses lack their own metabolism and the ability to reproduce independently, whereas all types of cells are true living systems with metabolic ability and the capacity for independent reproduction. All cells share the following common attributes:

1 They are enclosed by a cell membrane.
2 Their systems of reproduction use DNA for information storage and RNA for directing cellular organization.
3 Their genomes may undergo accidental change (i.e. mutate).
4 They can use chemical bond energy or light energy to run their metabolic systems.
5 They can detect and respond to environmental signals and can receive, recognize and transmit signals and impulses.

They may also be motile and, in the case of eukaryotes, may have flowing cytoplasm (Mehlhorn and Ruthmann 1992).

Two basic types of true cells are distinguishable: prokaryotes and eukaryotes. There are no transitional forms in existence today and thus these 2 forms are quite distinct. Prokaryotes always occur as functionally single cells with no specialization, whereas eukaryotes may consist of a single cell (e.g. protozoa) or they may be multicellular organisms made up of differentiated (specialized) cells. If prokaryotic organisms such as mycoplasma and bacteria do aggregate, they occur as chains or clusters of unspecialized cells. In contrast, eukaryotes can consist of many cells functioning in a highly integrated fashion. Some significant differences between the cellular components of eukaryotes and prokaryotes are listed in Table 6.1.

Prokaryotic and eukaryotic cells represent the units of life. It was recognized by Virchow in 1855 that they are the smallest units capable of maintaining the continuity of life or, as he expressed it, 'Omnis cellula e cellula' (every cell derives from a cell).

2 UNICELLULAR EUKARYOTES

Within the kingdom of the protists, the higher protists (those that resemble plants and animals) are all composed of eukaryotic cells. Eukaryotes may be unicellular in all their developmental stages, as are the protists, or unicellularity may be limited to certain developmental stages, such as the generative forms (the oocytes and spermatids) of plants and animals. Protists have followed many evolutionary paths in the development towards multicellularity and the following protists represent intermediate steps in this process: (1) protist forms with many nuclei per cell; (2) stable, double nucleated forms, such as *Giardia*; (3) forms with cell aggregation including some green algae, like *Volvox*; (4) forms with chains of dividing organisms, e.g. Microspora; and (5) forms that have multicellular stages, e.g. Myxozoa. It may be preferable to group the Myxozoa with the Metazoa, rather than with the protists. Even highly differentiated Metazoa retain vestiges of their unicellular origin, as shown by their development from unicellular eggs, some of which

Table 6.1 Differences between prokaryotes and eukaryotes

Attribute	Prokaryote	Eukaryote
Cell nucleus		+
DNA		
Amount	Low	High
	(up to 1.4×10^{-2} pg/cell)	(1.6×10^{-2} – 96 pg/nucleus)
		(in haploidity)
Organization	Circular	Linear (chromosomes) plus
		circular elements
Recombination	Conjugation	Meiosis and syngamy
Introns		+
Cell division		
Speed	Quick (20 min)	Slow (hours)
Mode	By formation of septa	By mitosis and cytokinesis
Ribosome type (subunits)	70S (30S + 50S)	80S (40S + 60S)
Membrane bound organelles (mitochondria, plastids, Golgi, etc.)		+
Microtubules		+
Membrane bound flagella ($9 \times 2 \times 2$ pattern)		+
Use of actomyosin for movement		+
Endo- and exocytotic activity (i.e., movement)		+

+Present.

may develop even if they are not fertilized. They also have the ability to reconstruct their whole bodies from a single cell, as do the sponges.

The group termed 'protists' is comprised exclusively of unicellular eukaryotic organisms that may be phototrophic, autotrophic or heterotrophic. The protozoa are named after the Greek for 'first' (proto) and 'animal (zoön). They are heterotrophic, lacking the ability to use light and inorganic materials to obtain energy and to synthesize structural components. Therefore they must obtain pre-formed organic compounds and on this basis may be considered to be animals. Apart from a few sedentary species, most protozoa are motile. Because they have difficulty in retaining water, due in part to their small size, most live in aquatic (or at least moist) environments. Although the majority of protozoa are free living, many species are mutualists, commensals or true parasites. Some are highly pathogenic to their plant or vertebrate hosts and hence are relevant to veterinary and human medicine and agriculture (Mehlhorn et al. 1995).

3 THE GENERAL MORPHOLOGY OF PARASITIC PROTOZOA

Classification of the protozoa remains in flux, as new data continue to be obtained (see Chapter 7 and Mehlhorn 1988). Some of the attributes of the protozoa are, however, beyond dispute. For example, they are all organized according to the basic pattern of the eukaryotic cell (Fig. 6.1), the same type being found in all metazoan cells.

Eukaryotic cells consist of a membrane-bound cytoplasm containing one or more nuclei and various organelles that are also often membrane bound, their compartments and membranes acting as sites where reaction processes can occur (Kleinig and Sitte 1984).

3.1 The cell membrane

The parasitic protozoa are surrounded by a membrane 4–10 nm thick (the unit membrane or plasmalemma) (Figs. 6.2, 6.3). In living cells this membrane always forms a closed sac or vesicle.

The membrane is composed of species-specific amounts of various proteins and a double layer of lipids (Fig. 6.2). It is physiologically and morphologically asymmetric, presenting a 'p face' (directed towards the cytoplasm) and an external 'e face'. High magnification electron microscopy reveals that it is composed of 3 layers (trilaminar) (Fig. 6.3). It is semipermeable, i.e. only certain types of molecules may cross it (Gennis 1989).

Several models have been created to explain how this biomembrane functions. The most widely accepted is the fluid mosaic model of Singer and Nicolson (1972) in which it is proposed that the membrane consists of a relatively stable double layer of lipid molecules within which proteins float like icebergs. At least some of the proteins may be structured to form pores (Fig. 6.2). The membranes expand by

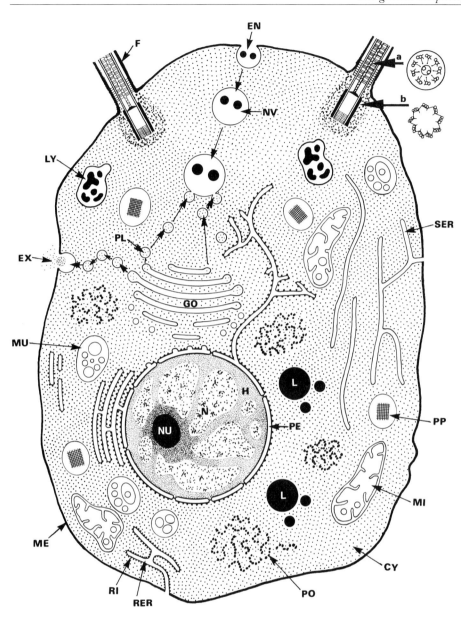

Fig. 6.1 Diagrammatic representation of the fine structure of a typical eukaryotic cell, (a) cross-section of the free flagellum; (b) cross-section of the basal body. B, basal body; CT, cytoplasm; EN, endocytosis; EX, exocytosis; F, flagellum; GO, Golgi apparatus; H, heterochromatin; L, lipid; LY, secondary lysosome (phagolysosome); ME, cell membrane (plus surface coat); MI, mitochondrion; MU, multivesicular body; N, nucleus; NU, nucleolus; NV, food vacuole (endocytotic vacuole); PE, perinuclear space; PL, primary lysosomes; PO, polyribosomes (chains); PP, peroxisome with protein crystal; RER, rough endoplasmic reticulum; RI, ribosome; SER, smooth endoplasmic reticulum.

additive inclusion of vesicles formed inside the cytoplasm and shrink by formation of endocytotic vesicles (Fig. 6.1) (Neupert and Lill 1992).

There are several systems for transporting substances through the cell membrane into the cytoplasm. Passage may occur by permeation (non-mediated transport), a process that is dependent upon concentration gradients. Active transport (mediated transport) using motile carriers may also occur. In this system a protein binds the molecule to be transported and then the complex moves actively from one side of the membrane to the other. Movement depends on changes in the electric charge that are linked with the binding and release of the transported molecule. The fixed pore (Fig. 6.2) is a protein structure that stretches through the membrane. The molecules to be transported pass through the space, or channel, formed between the subunits of the pore. All forms of active transport require energy, which is derived from various metabolic reactions.

In addition to the direct transport of molecules through the cell membrane, other mechanisms exist for internalization of materials by cells. For example, relatively large organic materials may be internalized by formation of endocytotic vesicles (Fig. 6.2), a process termed 'pinocytosis' for the uptake of liquids and 'phagocytosis' for the uptake of solid particles. Within the vacuoles the material is degraded and then transported into the cytoplasm by mechanisms similar to those used by the cell membrane. Alternatively, it may be released by dissolution of the membrane. Some protozoa have developed special places for the uptake of food, called 'cytostomes'. Many cells contain clathrin-coated pits that are involved in the receptor-mediated endocytosis of macromolecules, but our knowledge of coated pits in protozoa remains limited.

The cell membranes of both protozoa and metazoa are involved in many other tasks apart from transport functions, for example cell recognition. When cells come into contact with each other, recognition occurs

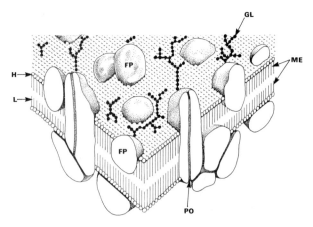

Fig. 6.2 Diagrammatic representation of the cell membrane of a typical eukaryotic cell following the fluid mosaic model of Singer and Nicolson (1972). Proteins (FP) float in a membrane that consists of a double layer of lipid molecules each with a hydrophilic component (H) and 2 lipophilic layers (L). The proteins, which may form pores (PO), often anchor glycoproteins, and together form the glycocalyx (GL).

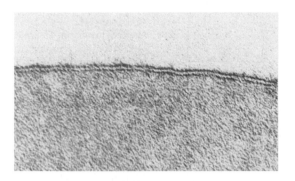

Fig. 6.3 Transmission electron micrograph of a section through the membrane of an erythrocyte showing the 3 layers of the membrane (×100 000).

via special receptors in the membranes that perceive chemical signals given off by other cells. Cell membranes also participate in excretion and secretion, these processes occurring by mechanisms similar to those for the intake of materials. Membrane-bound structures exist that mediate the joining of cells. These are needed for fusion of gametes and similar structures and are also found at places where flagella are attached to the surfaces of protozoa. The undulating membranes and recurrent flagella of trypanosomes and trichomonads are joined to the cell by means of such cell junctions (Figs. 6.4, 6.29a). Cell junctions also play a role in attachment of many parasites to the surfaces of host cells. For example, trypanosomes use junctions for attachment to the vector's intestine.

3.2 The pellicle and cytostomes

Many protozoa have more than one limiting membrane for at least some of their developmental stages (Table 6.2). In some groups the main cell membrane is underlined by one or more 'inner' membranes that are often derived from the endoplasmic reticulum (Table 6.2, Fig. 6.5).

Like the outer membranes, these inner membranes are species-specific and possess distinct inner and outer surfaces. The characteristics of the inner membranes have been revealed by the methods of freeze fracture and negative staining (Fig. 6.6). The single outer membrane and the membranous complexes often have subpellicular microtubules (c. 25 nm in diameter) underneath them.

These shape-stabilizing cell boundary complexes are called 'pellicles' (Figs. 6.4, 6.5). The motile stages of trypanosomes and *Leishmania* form a pellicle that consists of one membrane plus underlying microtubules (Fig. 6.7), whereas the motile stages of coccidia (sporozoites, merozoites, ookinetes, kinetes) have a pellicle consisting of 3 membranes plus underlying microtubules (Fig. 6.6).

In ciliates the pellicle is composed of an outer membrane, a system of alveolar sacs, longitudinal microtubules and kinetodesmal fibres. This complex pellicle produces a stable base to hold rows of cilia (Fig. 6.18).

In the free living euglenids the plasmalemma is reinforced by longitudinal microtubules and by a dense underlying epiplasm. The number of subpellicular microtubules is often stable within a species and may thus be used for species definition. For example, the merozoites of the tissue cyst-forming coccidia (e.g. *Sarcocystis, Toxoplasma, Besnoitia, Frenkelia*) always have 22 microtubules and various *Eimeria* species have 24, 26, 28, 30 or 32 microtubules. In some parasites, such as the trypanosomatids, the number of subpellicular microtubules varies with the size of the individual parasite form, i.e. a long slender form with a small diameter has fewer microtubules than a form of the same species with a larger diameter (Fig. 6.7).

The subpellicular microtubules may run from one pole to the other, as they do in gregarines and trypanosomes, or they may be restricted to limited portions of the pellicle. In ciliates, for example, they are restricted to the front half of the cell and in the coccidian motile stages they are localized to the front two-thirds of the cell (Fig. 6.8).

In the motile stages of the coccidia the microtubules are anchored to an anterior polar ring. At the attachment point there is an interruption of the 2 inner membranes (Fig. 6.9). If 2 or more polar rings are present, it is the outer one that is connected to the microtubules. The subpellicular microtubules are usually kept in contact with the inner surface of the pellicular membrane by means of side arms. The exact role of the microtubules in movement has not been identified.

As noted on p. 117, the membrane of the eukaryotic cell can take up material by various methods including permeation, active transport and endocytosis. Endocytosis (see Fig. 6.1) may occur at any point on the cell membrane or may occur only at predisposed places. For example, in *Giardia* trophozoites, endocytosis occurs only in the dorsal region, the region opposite the ventral sucker; in trypanosomes, endocytosis occurs in the flagellar pocket; and in

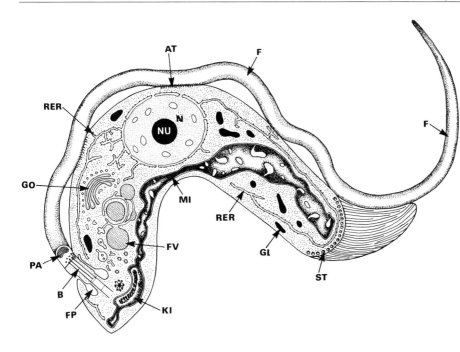

Fig. 6.4 Diagrammatic representation of a longitudinal section through a trypomastigote of *Trypanosoma* sp. AT, attaching zone of the flagellum; B, basal body; F, flagellum; FP, flagellar pocket (with cytostomal activity); FV, food vacuole; GL, glycosomes; GO, Golgi apparatus; KI, kinetoplast (containing DNA filaments); MI, mitochondrion; N, nucleus; NU, nucleolus; PA, paraxial rod; RER, rough endoplasmic reticulum; ST, subpellicular microtubules.

Table 6.2 Types of limiting membranes of some parasitic protozoa

Species	Stage	Single membrane	Two or more membranes	Pellicle with sub-pellicular microtubules	Cyst wall
Trichomonas vaginalis	Trophozoite	+			
Giardia lamblia	Trophozoite	+		Ventral	
	Cyst	+			+
Trypanosoma brucei group	Epi- and trypo-mastigotes			+	
Leishmania species	A-, pro-mastigotes			+	
Entamoeba histolytica	Magna-form	+			
	Minuta-form	+			
	Cyst	+			+
Pneumocystis carinii	Trophozoite	+			
	Cyst	+			+
Eimeria species	Sporozoites			+	
	Merozoites			+	
	Oocysts				+
	Sporocysts	+			+
	Meronts	+			
	Male gametes	+			
	Female gametes of some species		+		
Toxoplasma gondii	Sporozoites			+	
	Merozoites			+	
	Oocysts	+			+
	Sporocysts	+			+
	Meronts	+			
	Male gametes	+			
	Gamonts	+			
	Female gametes		+		

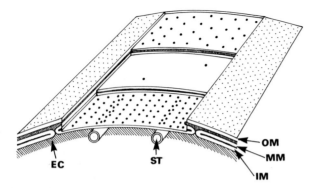

Fig. 6.5 Diagrammatic representation of the 3-layered pellicle of the invasive stage of a sporozoan as revealed by freeze etching. Note that each of the membranes has unique intramembranous particles. EC, ectoplasm; IM, inner membrane; MM, middle membrane; OM, outer membrane; ST, subpellicular microtubules.

sporozoans it is found at small cytostomes called 'micropores' (Fig. 6.10).

Large endocytic elements ('cytostomes' or 'cell mouths') are characteristic of many ciliates (Fig. 6.31e).

Cytostomes are reinforced by various structures (Fig. 6.10), for instance by bundles of microtubules in trypanosomes and ciliates. After the phagosomes enter the cytoplasm the contents are digested and resorption of the necessary molecules occurs. The residue may be voided to the outside or stored as an inclusion. The process of excretion, called 'exocytosis', may occur anywhere on the surface or, as in ciliates, at a specialized place called the 'cell anus' or 'cytopyge'. Exocytosis is a process similar to endocytosis but in reverse.

3.3 Cyst wall

Many parasitic protozoa (Table 6.2) are capable of undergoing encystation, which involves formation of a cyst wall either outside or inside the cell membrane. This cyst wall may be single layered or multilayered.

Walls formed outside the plasmalemma are produced by exocytosis of materials. Cyst walls have 2 main tasks: to protect the organism against unfavourable environmental conditions when passing from one host to another and to create spaces for reorganization and nuclear division. Cyst walls may also aid the parasite in transmission from one host to another by facilitating attachment to host cell surfaces.

The cyst wall has one layer in cysts of *Entamoeba histolytica*, *Giardia* and some ciliates, such as the fish parasite *Ichthyophthirius multifiliis* and the human parasite *Balantidium coli*. There are usually 2 types of cysts in the stages of coccidia in faeces: the oocysts and the sporocysts. The oocyst wall is usually 2-layered but in a few species it may have 4 layers. It is formed by 2 types of cyst wall-forming bodies. The sporocyst wall usually has only a single layer (Fig. 6.11).

The chemical composition of cyst walls varies according to the species, although proteins are usually the basic component. The cyst walls of *E. histolytica* and *G. lamblia* contain proteins which are keratin-like or elastin-like albuminoids composed of lysine, histidine, arginine, tyrosine, glutamic acid and glycine. The 2-layered oocyst wall of the sporozoans is 'periodic acid–Schiff-positive' (PAS–positive). The outermost layer of these oocysts consists mainly of fatty alcohols (e.g. hexacosanol), some phospholipids and fatty acids. It has no carbohydrates or proteins. The inner layer is composed of glycoproteins and contains most of the carbohydrates found in the oocyst wall. These carbohydrates are composed of mannose, galactose, glucose and hexosamine. The oocyst wall is highly resistant to the passage of potassium dichromate, sodium hypochloride, sulphuric acid and sodium hydroxide and these chemicals are therefore used in storage and cleaning of oocysts. It is permeable to O_2, CO_2, NH_3, methylbromide, carbon disulphide and various organic solvents. The oocyst wall is highly susceptible to mechanical pressure and therefore may be ruptured easily by shearing forces. Thus mechanical rupture of oocysts in the gizzard of the avian host is likely to be the normal method of excystation of avian cocci-

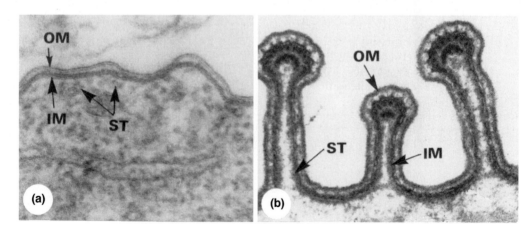

Fig. 6.6 Transmission electron micrographs of sections through the 3-layered pellicle of a coccidian (a) and a gregarine (b). Note that the 2 inner membranes appear mainly as a thick layer. IM, 2 inner membranes; OM, outer membrane; ST, subpellicular microtubule (× 70 000).

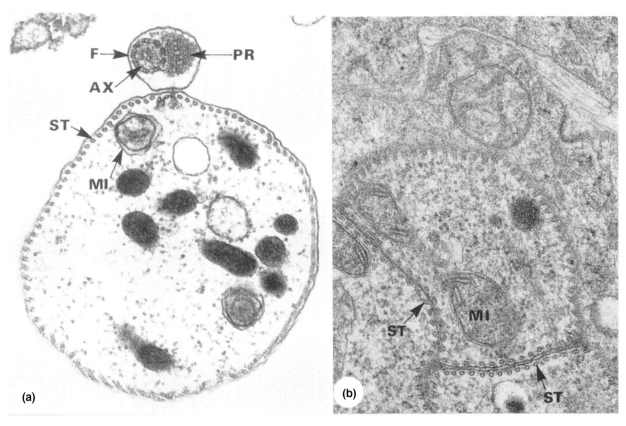

Fig. 6.7 Transmission electron micrographs of cross-sections through a trypomastigote of *Trypanosoma vivax* (a) and an amastigote of *Leishmania donovani* (b). Note that in both cases the pellicle consists of a single cell membrane plus subpellicular microtubules (ST). AX, axoneme; F, flagellum; MI, mitochondrion; PR, paraxial rod (× 35 000).

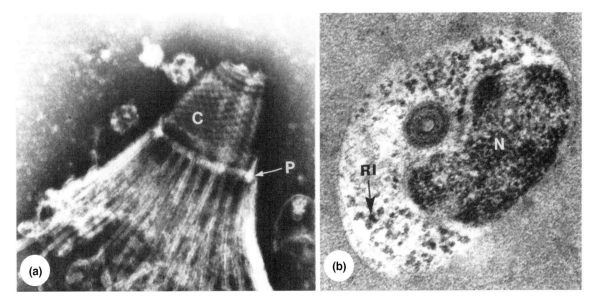

Fig. 6.8 Transmission electron micrographs. (a) Negatively stained apical pole of a merozoite of *Sarcocystis*. Note the protruded conoid (C), and the polar ring (P), to which the subpellicular microtubules are attached (× 50 000). (b) Cross-section of a micropore (in an erythrocytic stage of *Theileria annulata*, the agent of Mediterranean coast fever of cattle). N, nucleus; RI, ribosome (× 35 000).

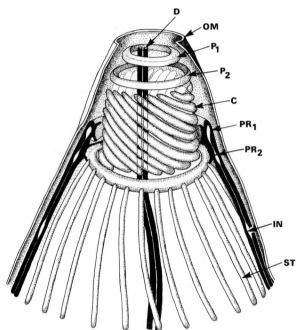

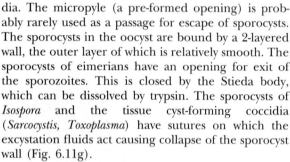

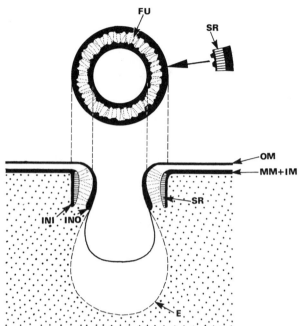

Fig. 6.9 Diagrammatic representation of a coccidian mero-zoite showing the apical pole and its protruded conoid. This structure is not present in haemosporidians and piroplasms. C, conoid consisting of microtubules; D, ductules of the rhoptries; IN, inclusion between the 2 inner membranes of the pellicle; OM, outer membrane of the 3-layered pellicle; P1, P2, preconoidal rings; PR1, PR2, polar rings (the pos-terior one is connected with the subpellicular microtubules); ST, subpellicular microtubule.

Fig. 6.10 Diagrammatic representation of a sporozoan micropore in longitudinal and tangential sections. E, enlargement during food uptake; FU, filamentous elements; IM, inner membrane of the pellicle; INI, interruption of the inner membrane (forms of the outer ring in tangential section); INO, dense material along the inner ring (invaginated outer membrane); MM, middle membrane; OM, outer membrane of the pellicle; SR, dense material between the inner and middle membranes.

dia. The micropyle (a pre-formed opening) is prob-ably rarely used as a passage for escape of sporocysts. The sporocysts in the oocyst are bound by a 2-layered wall, the outer layer of which is relatively smooth. The sporocysts of eimerians have an opening for exit of the sporozoites. This is closed by the Stieda body, which can be dissolved by trypsin. The sporocysts of *Isospora* and the tissue cyst-forming coccidia (*Sarcocystis*, *Toxoplasma*) have sutures on which the excystation fluids act causing collapse of the sporocyst wall (Fig. 6.11g).

The cyst walls of Myxozoa and Microspora are at least double-walled in most species (Fig. 6.12) and the layers can be resolved by electron microscopy. In Myxozoa the wall consists of valves that open at pre-formed sites to release the infectious sporoplasm. The Microspora have developed a hollow tube that is pro-truded from the surface of the wall. It penetrates into a host cell and the infectious sporoplasm is passed through it. The exospore layer in Microspora is pro-teinaceous and is 15–100 nm thick depending on the species. The endospore layer is chitinous and c. 150–200 nm thick. The spores are Gram-positive (i.e. stain reddish purple with the Gram stain), a fact that is of diagnostic value. They are also stained light blue by Giemsa.

3.4 Surface coat

The plasma membrane of eukaryotic cells is strikingly asymmetric (Fig. 6.2). The outer and inner layers are clearly delineated and the polypeptides on each sur-face (Figs. 6.13, 6.14) are distinct. Glycolipids and glycoproteins are present only on the external surface. The peripheral layer is rich in carbohydrate and is called the 'glycocalyx', or 'surface coat'. The thickness of this layer varies with the species and with the devel-opmental stage of the organism. Not only is the sur-face coat composed of glycoproteins and glycolipids, but various glycoproteins and proteoglycans (acid mucopolysaccharides) may also be adsorbed to it (Fig. 6.13).

The surface coat may be a rather delicate coating, a mass of delicate filaments or a thick mat. Whatever its structure, it has several functions in the life of the organism: (1) it acts as a mechanical or chemical bar-rier; (2) it plays a role in recognition and adhesion to other cells; (3) it contains enzymes that act on sub-stances in the environment; and (4) it contains mol-ecules that can act as antigens and thus plays an important role in immunological processes.

The surface coat may change its composition as the parasite develops from stage to stage. In addition many parasitic protozoa, in particular the trypano-somes, have developed sophisticated methods of anti-genic variation. This may be achieved by selective acti-

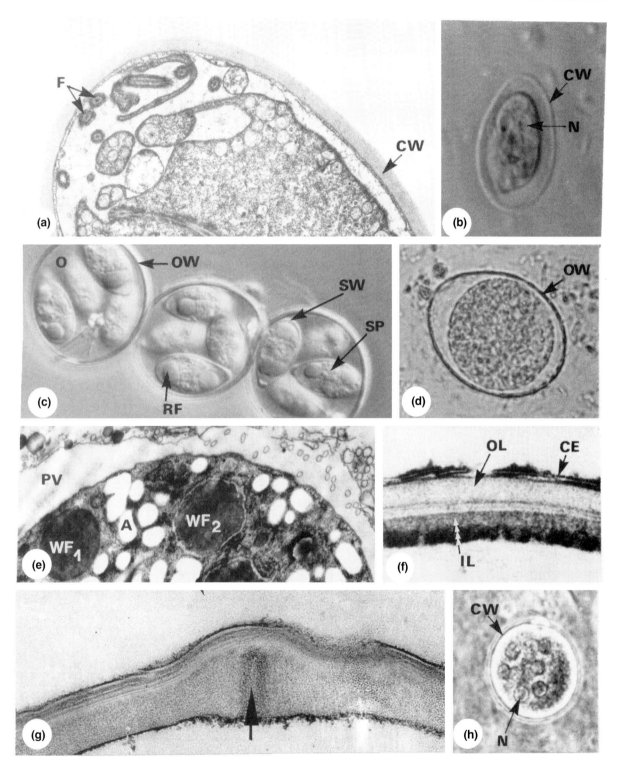

Fig. 6.11   Light (b, c, d, h) and electron micrographs (a, e, f, g) of cysts and cyst walls. (a, b) *Giardia lamblia*. CW, cyst wall; F, flagellum; N, nucleus. (c) *Eimeria* oocysts (O) containing sporocysts (SP). OW, oocyst wall; RF, refractile body of sporozoites; SW, sporocyst wall. (d) *Isospora* sp., unsporulated oocysts. OW, oocyst wall. (e) *Eimeria maxima*; macrogamete with wall forming bodies 1 and 2 (WF1, WF2). A, amylopectin; PV, parasitophorous vacuole. (f) Oocyst wall of *Eimeria* and *Isospora* spp. CE, cell membrane; IL, OL, inner and outer layer of oocyst wall. (g) Sporocyst wall in *Toxoplasma* and *Sarcocystis* spp., with the pre-formed suture (arrow) that ruptures during the excystation process. (h) *Entamoeba coli*; 8-nucleated cyst. CW, cyst wall; N nucleus.

vation of different genes at different times. Organisms of the *Trypanosoma brucei* group have up to 1000 genes that may become activated during the production of variant surface glycoproteins (VSGs). This selective activation results in changes in the variable antigen types (VATs) displayed and hinders the host defence against these blood-inhabiting flagellates. *Plasmodium* may also display variant antigen types, but there are fewer variants than those displayed by trypanosomes. The action of these genes results in antigenic variation and the production of immunologically different strains of protozoa; this explains why most antiprotozoal vaccines provide only limited protection, restricted to certain localities. The development of potent vaccines against protozoan parasites depends on the discovery of species-specific antigens with invariant epitopes that are accessible to the immune system during the parasite's life. In addition, they must be essential to the parasite's survival, possibly playing an important role in cell recognition, adhesion, immune evasion, metabolism, or cell invasion. Whether such antigens exist remains to be determined (Mehlhorn et al. 1995).

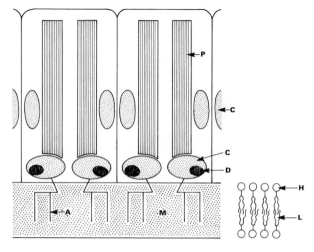

Fig. 6.13 Diagrammatic representation of the arrangement of the components of the surface coat along the surface of a trypanosome. A, anchor of a variant surface glycoprotein molecule; C, carbohydrate; D, cross-reacting determinant; H, hydrophilic component of the VSG molecule; L, lipophilic component; M, membrane consisting of 2 layers of lipid molecules; P, protein.

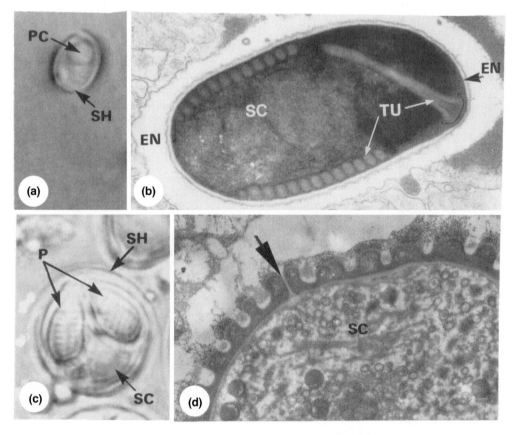

Fig. 6.12 Light (a, c) and electron micrographs (b, d) of Microspora (a, b) and Myxozoa (c, d). Note that the microsporidian wall (*Nosema* sp.) is entirely closed, while that of Myxozoa (d) (*Myxosoma* sp.) has 2 valves that leave a small opening (arrow). EN, endospore; EX, exospore; P, polar capsule with solid filaments; PC, polar capsule with a hollow tubule; SH, shell; SC, sporoplasm; TU, tubule.

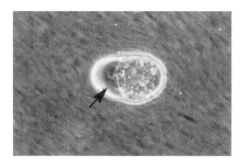

Fig. 6.15 Light micrograph of a trophozoite of *Entamoeba histolytica*. Note the presence of hyaline ectoplasm in the pseudopodium (arrow) and along the outer surface (× 1000).

3.5 Cytoplasm

The cytoplasm in protozoa is generally divided into 2 zones: the peripheral, electron-lucent ectoplasm (hyaloplasm); and the denser central endoplasm. The endoplasm contains the cell organelles and the nucleus. This differentiation is particularly prominent in the amoebae and in the gregarines (Figs. 6.15, 6.16) but is not apparent in all species.

In some species, endoplasm and ectoplasm cannot even be distinguished by electron microscopy. Microgametes of most sporozoans, apart from those of the piroplasms, have a very reduced cytoplasm. They are comprised mainly of flagella, a mitochondrion and a nucleus (Fig. 6.17).

The cytoplasm of most cells has a high viscosity and stability and a prominent cytoskeleton. Contractile elements of this cytoskeleton are responsible for the cytoplasmic flow and these include actin filaments with a diameter of c. 6 nm. These filaments are composed of a double chain of globular bodies. Cytoskeletons may also contain 10 nm filaments or intermediate filaments which, to date, have been found only in the cells of higher vertebrates. The various types of filaments are organized into the microtubules of the cytoskeleton. The tubules have an outer diameter of 25 nm and an inner diameter of 15 nm. They are composed of protofilaments that are visible in cross-sections. The protofilaments consist of α and ß tubulin elements in a helical arrangement. The microtubules are polymerized at particular points called 'microtubule organizing centres' (MTOCs). These centres exist at centromeres, centrioles and at certain places in membranes. They also occur as constituents of flagella and cilia (see Figs. 6.28, 6.29).

The processes that bring about motility of the cytoplasm are well documented for metazoan cells, but for protozoa these processes are still poorly understood (Fig. 6.17). In all cases, it is probably the aggregation of actin with myosin and tropomyosin to form an acto-myosin complex that leads to movement, as proposed in the sliding filament model of Huxley and Hanson (1954). This ATP-dependent system may produce relatively rapid movements, as occur in amoeba (20 μm × s^{-1}) and in the sporozoites and merozoites of sporozoans. In addition to the cytoskeletal system, most parasitic protozoa have developed unique skeletal elements composed of combinations of the usual cytoskeleton elements. These structures include the following:

1   The subpellicular microtubules of trypanosomes and the motile stages of the coccidia (see Figs. 6.4, 6.5).

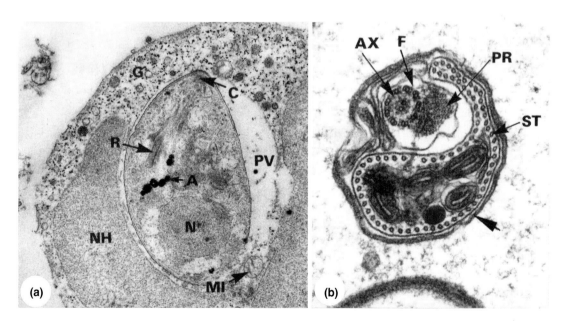

Fig. 6.14 Transmission electron micrographs of the surface coat. (a) *Toxoplasma gondii*; the zoite within a host cell vacuole (PV) shows a slight positive Thièry reaction along its surface (arrow). Note the presence of amylopectin (A) granules in the parasite and of glycogen (G) in the host cell. C, conoid; MI, mitochondrion; N, nucleus; NH, nucleus of the host cell; R, rhoptry (× 7000). (b) *Trypanosoma vivax*. Cross-section through a trypomastigote stage showing the discharge of the surface coat (arrow). AX, axoneme; F, flagellum; PR, paraxial rod; ST, subpellicular microtubule (× 25 000).

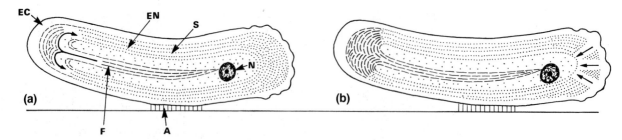

Fig. 6.16 Diagrammatic representation of amoebic movement, which is brought about by a steady forward flux of the central liquid endoplasm and its transformation into a more stable form as it moves posteriorly and laterally. The origin of the forces needed for such movement is explained by either apical (a) or posterior (b) contractions (arrows). A, zone of adhesion to the surface; EC, hyalinic ectoplasm; EN, dense, granulomatous endoplasm; F, fluid portion of endoplasm; N, nucleus; S, stable, non-fluid portion of endoplasm.

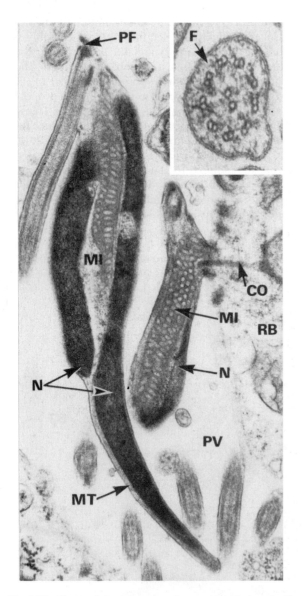

Fig. 6.17 Transmission electron micrographs of a longitudinal section through a coccidian microgamete (*Sarcocystis* sp.) and a cross-section through a flagellum (inset). CO, connection of the nucleus to the microgamont; F, flagellum; MI, mitochondrion; MT, microtubule; N, nucleus; PF, perforatorium (apical pole); PV, parasitophorous vacuole; RB, residual body (× 25 000; inset × 100 000).

2   The kinetodesmal fibrils of ciliates (Fig. 6.18a).

3   The bundles of cytoplasmic microtubules in gamonts of piroplasms (Fig. 6.18b).

4   The combined microtubules and filaments observed in the ventral disc of the diplomonadids (Fig. 6.18c).

5   The crystalloid protein densifications that occur below the membrane of giardial trophozoites and also at the apex of eimerian microgametes (Fig. 6.18d) and in the gamonts of piroplasms (Fig. 6.18b).

6   The axostyles and pelta, occurring prominently in the trichomonads and consisting of one or more parallel rows of microtubules (Fig. 6.19).

7   The costa and parabasal filaments, the filamentous, sometimes striated elements (Fig. 6.19) that line the recurrent flagellum or the Golgi apparatus in trichomonads.

8   The paraxial rods, which consist of a network of microfilaments that run along the axonemal microtubules of the flagella of Kinetoplastida (Figs. 6.4, 6.7, 6.29a).

9   The conoids, which are found in the motile stages of some coccidia, such as *Eimeria*, *Sarcocystis* and *Toxoplasma* (see Figs. 6.8, 6.9a), but which are always absent from the haemosporidians (e.g. *Plasmodium*, piroplasms).

The conoid (Fig. 6.9a) is a hollow truncated cone composed of spiralling microtubules 25 nm in diameter. Two accessory structures, the conoidal or preconoidal rings, form an integral part of the conoid and they are connected with each other by a canopy-like membrane. During cell penetration the conoid protrudes through the anterior polar ring system. The conoid is apparently involved in penetration of host cells.

3.6   Cytoplasmic inclusions

The endoplasm contains a variety of organelles and other structures within which metabolic processes occur.

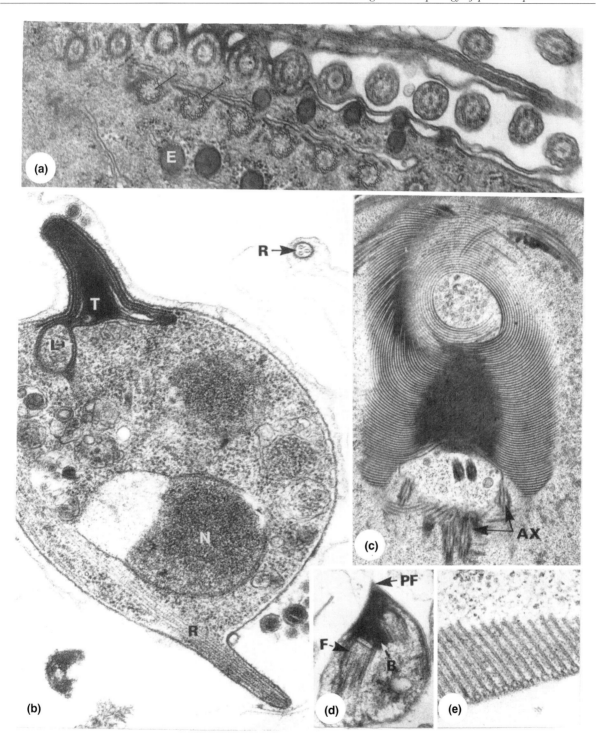

Fig. 6.18 Transmission electron micrographs. (a) Cross-section through the base of a cilium of *Ichthyophthirius multifiliis* showing interconnecting microtubules (arrows). E, extrusomes (× 30 000). (b) *Babesia canis*, longitudinal section through a microgamont. Note the thorn-like dense apex (A), the microtubule-containing ray (R), and the labyrinthine structure (L) at the base of the thorn (T). N, nucleus (× 25 000). (c) Tangential section through the ventral disc of *Giardia lamblia*. Note the helically arranged rows of material. AX, axoneme (× 20 000). (d) Perforatorium of the microgamete of eimerians, a structure needed for entering the macrogamete. B, basal body; F, flagellum; PF, perforatorium. (e) Cross section through the disc of *Giardia lamblia*, showing microtubules attached to filaments (× 95 000).

NUCLEUS

Protozoa possess at least one well developed nucleus that is usually spherical to ovoid (Fig. 6.20) and enclosed by a double-layered membrane containing pores (Fig. 6.1, 6.21). The pores are c. 50–70 nm in diameter with a central opening formed of 8 subunits.

When viewed by light microscopy, the nuclei may appear vesicular or compact. The karyoplasm is composed of structural and enzymatic proteins; the

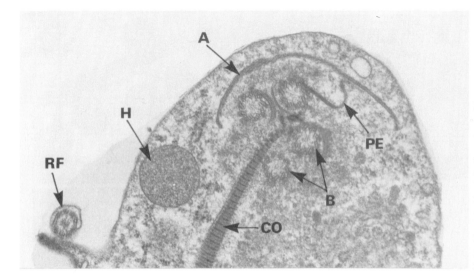

Fig. 6.19 Transmission electron micrographs of the apical pole of *Trichomonas vaginalis* showing the line of microtubules making up the axostyle (a), the basal bodies of the 4 anterior free flagella (b) and the costa (c) (× 15 000). H, hydrogenosome; PE, pelta; RF, recurrent flagellum running along a surface fold.

chromatin (DNA) which may be organized into chromosomes; and the nucleolus. No membranes exist within the nucleus. There is usually only one nucleolus but there may be several in some species and in certain developmental stages of other species. The nucleolus is the site of synthesis of the large RNAs (28S, 18S and 5.8S) and of the precursors of the ribosomes. It has 2 zones; one is composed of filaments measuring 5–8 nm wide and the other is composed of granules measuring 15 nm wide. The granular zone is situated at the periphery of the nucleolus. During nuclear division the nucleoli are often dissolved and the chromosomes may condense and become visible

(e.g. in ciliates) or they may remain stretched out and invisible (e.g. in the eimerians, the haemosporidians and the piroplasms). The nuclear membranes are retained in the protozoa during division and separation of the chromosomes is carried out by a spindle apparatus, the appearance, arrangement and placement of which is species-specific. The apparatus always consists of microtubules and filaments.

In ciliates, 2 morphologically distinct nuclei occur: a generative micronucleus and a somatic macronucleus (Fig. 6.31e). In other parasitic species and in some specific stages such as the meronts, sporonts and gamonts of the coccidia and haemosporidia, there

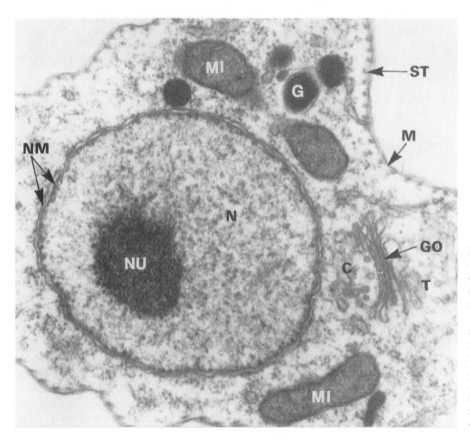

Fig. 6.20 Transmission electron micrograph of a developing stage of *Crithidia* sp. The section is in the region of the nucleus (× 25 000). GO, Golgi apparatus; M, cell membrane; MI, mitochondrion; N, nucleus; NM, nuclear membrane; NP, nuclear pore; NU, nucleolus; ST, subpellicular microtubules; T, trans side of the Golgi apparatus.

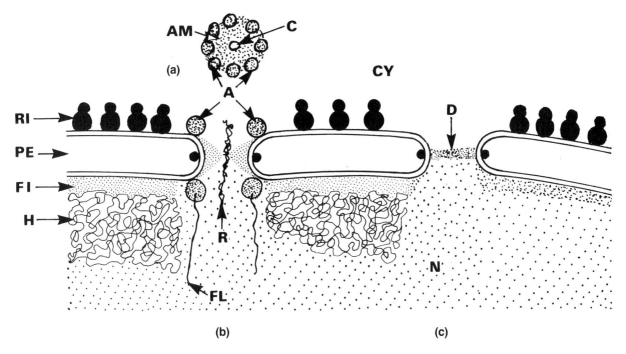

Fig. 6.21 Diagrammatic representation of nuclear pores (diameter c. 80 nm). (a) Surface view showing the 8 outer peripheral annuli. (b) Longitudinal section of an active pore. (c) Longitudinal section of an inactive pore. A, annular element; AM, amorphous material; C, central channel (diameter 15–20 nm) also called central granulum when RNA passes through; CY, cytoplasm; D, diaphragm; FI, filamentous layer; FL, filaments connected at inner annular elements; H, heterochromatin; N, nucleoplasm (karyoplasm); PE, perinuclear spore; R, RNA; RI, ribosome (with subunits).

may be many nuclei, all of which may have similar appearance. Morphologically similar nuclei may have similar functions or they may have different functions, as in the Myxosporea. During binary division the karyoplasm is usually completely distributed between the 2 daughter nuclei. In some cases, e.g. during the formation of microgametes in some coccidia, only one functional nucleus is produced and a part of the nucleus is left behind (Fig. 6.32c, e).

MITOCHONDRIA AND RELATED STRUCTURES

Mitochondria contain the enzymes for oxidative phosphorylation and the tricarboxylic acid cycle and are bound by 2 membranes. Most parasitic protozoa have one of 3 basic types of mitochondria, distinguished by characteristic infoldings of the inner membrane, which may be tubular, sack-like, or cristae-like (Fig. 6.22).

Mitochondria reproduce by division and are therefore termed 'semi-autonomous organelles'. This form of reproduction is possible because mitochondria have their own DNA. In most mitochondria this DNA is composed of 2 circular strands arranged in a supercoil. Some species have a single, large mitochondrion that contains more DNA, e.g. species of *Trypanosoma* and *Leishmania*. These organisms have 5% of their DNA in a single structure called the 'kinetoplast' (Figs. 6.4, 6.22a) which is located close to the basal body of the flagellum. Kinetoplastid flagellates have no infoldings in this region of the mitochondria, providing space for the thousands of minicircles (0.3–0.8 μm in length) and the few maxicircles (9–11 μm in length) that make up their mitochondrial DNA; this region stains with Giemsa solution and is visible as a deep purple dot. The DNA of only the maxicircles seems to be transcribed. During cell division the kinetoplast is always reproduced before nuclear division occurs. Trichomonads, some amoeba and Microspora have no mitochondria, but some amoeba contain symbiotic bacteria that may function as mitochondria. The trichomonads, which are anaerobic, have microbodies called 'hydrogenosomes'. These have a single membrane surrounding a granular matrix (Fig. 6.19). The enzyme system of these bodies differs from that of mitochondria, as they metabolize pyruvate from glycolysis into acetate, CO_2 and H_2. In ciliates, hydrogenosomes with double membranes are present, as well as mitochondria

The motile stages of sporozoans (i.e. merozoites and sporozoites, Figs. 6.23, 6.24a) have a Golgi-adjunct body (also called a 'double-walled organelle') close to the nucleus (Scholtyseck and Mehlhorn 1972).

In several species and genera (i.e. *T. gondii*, *Sarcocystis* and *Plasmodium*) this organelle contains genes of the photosystem II and resembles a plastid, or a remnant thereof, in terms of shape and activity (Hackstein et al. 1995).

ENDOPLASMIC RETICULUM, RIBOSOMES AND GOLGI APPARATUS

The endoplasmic reticulum (ER) is a large system of tubes and sacs that runs throughout the cell. It connects the nuclear space with the cell interior and with

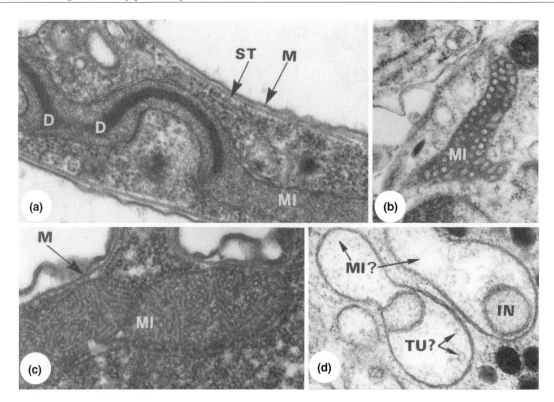

Fig. 6.22 Transmission electron micrographs of mitochondria or similar structures. (a) *Trypanosoma vivax*, kinetoplast in division (mitochondrion with cristae) (× 25 000). (b) *Sarcocystis* microgamont with a mitochondrion of the sacculus type (x 25 000). (c) *Ichthyophthirius multifiliis*; a trophozoite with a mitochondrion of the tubular type (x 40 000). (d) *Theileria* sp.; mitochondria-like structures within kinetes. D, DNA filaments; IN, invagination; M, cell membrane; MI, mitochondrion; ST, subpellicular microtubule; TU, tubule (× 30 000).

the cell surface (Figs. 6.1, 6.25). There are 2 types of ER: rough ER (rER) and smooth ER (sER).

The rER is characterized by the presence of ribosomes (Figs. 6.1, 6.25) along its outer surface, whereas these are lacking in the sER. The rER and the sER may be interconnected.

The ribosomes consist of RNA and protein. The ribosomal RNA represents about four-fifths of the total cellular RNA. There are several types of ribosomes, depending on the nature of their subunits (Table 6.1; Fig. 6.20); these subunits can be released by appropriate treatment of the ribosomal proteins. Several ribosomes often align in a chain to form 'polyribosomes', or 'polysomes' (Figs. 6.1, 6.25), where they are collectively active in protein synthesis. Ribosomes occur along the surface of the rER, either as single forms or as polysomes. They also occur in the cytoplasm and inside the mitochondria. In protozoa, ribosomes have a diameter of c. 30 nm and are composed of 2 subunits with sedimentation characteristics of 60S and 40S. The intact ribosome is of the 80S type. Mitochondrial ribosomes are of the 70S type or, in ciliates, 80S. The mitochondrial ribosomes are similar to those of prokaryotes (Bielka 1982) (see Table 6.1).

The Golgi apparatus is a flat sac with swollen regions (Fig. 6.1, 6.26), from which vesicles are formed (Farquhar and Palade 1981).

Several Golgi apparatuses together form dictyosomes. These organelles are always situated close to

the rER and the 2 organelles act together as functional units in the production and transport of membrane and in the formation and transport of all types of macromolecular proteins and lipids (Gal and Raikhel 1993). The Golgi apparatus is never covered by ribosomes. Although many parasitic protozoa have prominent dictyosomes, certain developmental stages of protozoa have only a single Golgi apparatus that is difficult to detect in electron micrographs. The principal function of the Golgi apparatus is the transport of secretions and excretions formed on the rER. These reach the Golgi apparatus at its 'cis' side and are transported within vacuoles that are cut off at its periphery (the 'trans' region) (Fig. 6.26). Endocytotic vesicles such as food vacuoles also come into contact with the Golgi apparatus and the rER system at points where they fuse with enzyme-containing vacuoles produced by the Golgi apparatus; this is how digestive enzymes and other products enter the endocytotic vacuoles.

LYSOSOMES

Lysosomes are vesicles measuring 0.2–0.5 μm and bound by a single membrane. They are derived from the sER and are formed and released from the secretion side of the Golgi apparatus (the 'trans' side). They contain enzymes such as phosphatases, proteinases, lipases, nucleases, etc. and have an internal pH of 4–5. When first released they are called 'primary' lysosomes. After fusion with the endocytotic vesicles

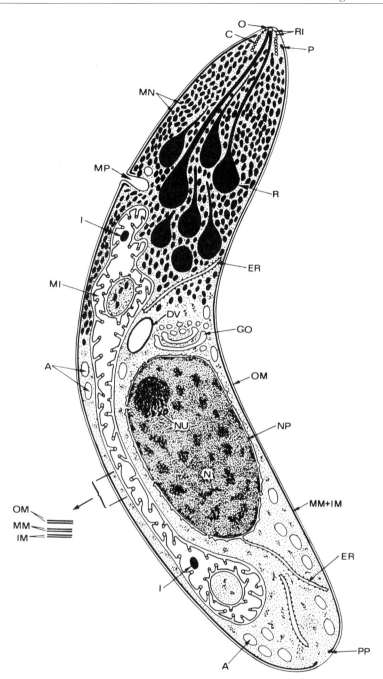

Fig. 6.23 Diagrammatic representation of a longitudinal section through a typical coccidian merozoite. A, amylopectin; C, conoid; D, dense, spherical bodies; DV, double-walled vesicle; ER, endoplasmic reticulum; GO, Golgi apparatus; I, dense inclusion; IM, inner membrane; MI, mitochondrion; MM, middle membrane; MN, micronemes; MP, micropore; N, nucleus; NP, nuclear pore; NU, nucleolus (karyosome); O, opening of the conoid; OM, outer membrane of pellicle; P, anterior polar ring; PP, posterior polar ring; R, rhoptries; RI ring-like elements of the conoidal canopy.

their enzymes become active and the vesicle is then called a 'secondary' lysosome. In these secondary lysosomes, or phagolysosomes, the ingested food is dispersed (Figs. 6.1, 6.26). Another type of secondary lysosome is the 'autolysosome', which is involved in the disintegration of cellular waste material, thus providing the function of disposal of debris.

MICROBODIES

Microbodies are ubiquitous in eukaryotic cells; they are bound by a single membrane and some have a catalase-containing matrix that breaks down H_2O_2. The microbodies are probably pinched off from the ER at sites where the enzymes contained in the microbodies accumulate (see Fig. 6.1). The 4 general types of microbodies are: the hydrogenosomes, the peroxisomes, the glyoxisomes and the glycosomes (Tolbert 1981).

The microbodies may attain diameters of 0.2–1.7 μm, depending on their type, and they have the following functions: the hydrogenosomes of trichomonads produce ATP; the peroxisomes break down toxic H_2O_2; the glycosomes of trypanosomes (diameter 0.2–0.3 μm) perform glycolysis; and the glyoxisomes of many protozoa process lipids for energy production. The so-called 'reservosomes' of *Trypanosoma cruzi* probably belong to this last group. It is not clear whether the dense bodies of the motile stages of sporozoans (Fig. 6.24a) are microbodies. Some of the dense bodies of coccidia are apparently excreted into

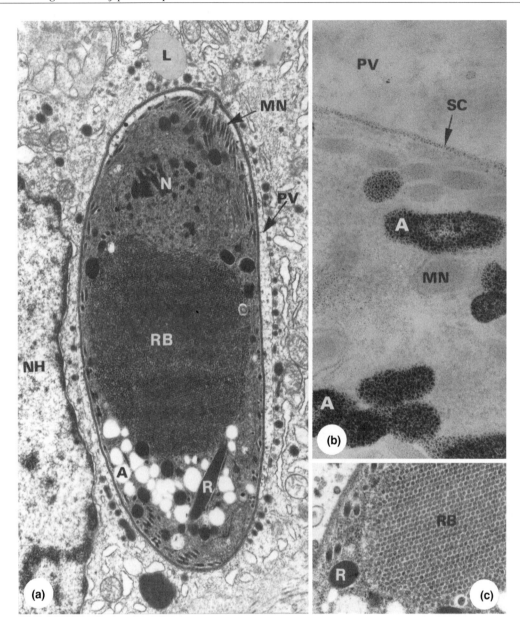

Fig. 6.24 Transmission electron micrograph of storage materials in coccidians. (a) Longitudinal section of a sporozoite of *Cystoisospora felis.* A, amylopectin; L, lipid; MN, micronemes; N, nucleus; NH, nucleus of the host cell; PV, parasitophorous vacuole; RB, refractile body (consisting of protein granules); RH, rhoptry; SC, surface coat (× 12 000). (b) The Thièry reaction shows polysaccharides (e.g. amylopectin) within granules (A) and along the surface (SC) of a merozoite (× 65 000). (c) Cross-section of *C. felis* showing structure of refractile body. RB, refractile body; R, rhoptry (× 30 000).

the parasitophorous vacuole by exocytosis. Most of the developmental stages of coccidia are surrounded by a parasitophorous vacuole while they are inside their host cell (Figs. 6.25, 6.24).

RHOPTRIES AND MICRONEMES

The osmiophilic rhoptries and micronemes are characteristic of the motile stages of sporozoans. They are usually located in the area between the nucleus and the apical pole. Rhoptries vary considerably in number (2–20) and in shape, appearing club shaped (*Eimeria*), teardrop shaped (*Plasmodium*) or elongated (*Sarcocystis, Toxoplasma*). The anterior neck portions of rhoptries are narrow and duct-like and are found at the extreme tip of the cell running through the conoid if one is present (Figs. 6.8, 6.24). Rhoptries release enzymes during the penetration process, after which they appear partly empty with a sponge-like interior. Micronemes are small rod-like structures 50–90 × 300–600 nm with rounded ends. These structures usually occupy the anterior regions of the motile stages of the sporozoans and are often arranged in bundles (Figs. 6.24, 6.27). The function of micronemes is not clear. They disappear during the reproductive process in meronts, macrogamonts and microgamonts.

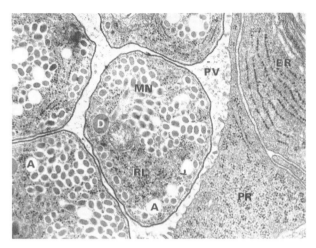

Fig. 6.25 Transmission electron micrograph of a cross-section through a mass of merozoites of *Eimeria*. The cytoplasm of the host cell adjacent to the parasitophorous vacuole (PV) shows the rough endoplasmic reticulum (ER) and many polyribosomes (PR). A, amylopectin; D, dense body; MN, micronemes; RI, ribosomes (× 30 000).

Wall-forming bodies

Parasites that produce walled cysts, such as amoebae, *Giardia*, coccidia, *Balantidium*, Myxozoa and Microspora, develop wall-forming bodies of various types (see Figs. 6.11E, 6.12). In amoebae, diplomonadids, Microspora and Myxozoa, the contents of the wall-forming bodies fuse outside the cell after being excreted by exocytosis. This fused material forms an external cyst wall (see Fig. 6.12). In macrogametes of coccidia the wall-forming bodies fuse in the region immediately below the cell membrane, thus producing an internal cyst wall (see Fig. 6.11).

One or 2 different types of wall-forming body may occur in coccidia of the various genera. For example, in *Eimeria* and *Isospora* the macrogametes have 2 types of wall-forming bodies: (1) electron-dense bodies that give rise to the outer layer of the oocyst wall; and (2) sponge-like bodies that fuse to produce the inner layer of the oocyst wall. The entire oocyst wall is produced inside the cell membrane (see Fig. 6.11e). The oocysts of *Sarcocystis* and the sporocysts of all coccidia are bound by a smooth wall that is formed by fusion of a single type of electron-dense wall-forming body (Fig.

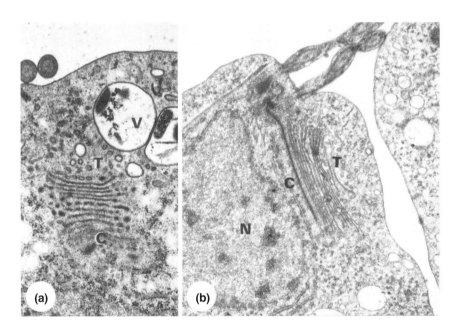

Fig. 6.26 Transmission electron micrograph of the Golgi apparatus in *Trichomonas vaginalis*. Note the active forms (a) and the inactive ones (b) (× 20 000). C, cis side of Golgi; N, nucleus; T, trans side of Golgi; V, food vacuole.

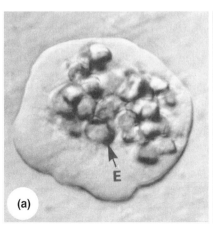
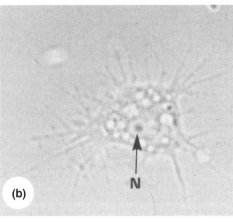

Fig. 6.27 Light micrographs showing amoebae with lobopodia (a) and filopodia (b). (a) *Entamoeba histolytica*, magna form. E, erythrocyte (× 2000). (b) *Acanthamoeba castellanii*. N, nucleus (× 1200).

6.11g). The cyst walls of all stages of coccidia provide good protection against adverse environmental conditions. Whether they are single- or double-walled, the oocysts and sporocysts of all *Eimeria* have openings, whereas the sporocysts of *Isospora* and of the tissue cyst-forming coccidia have sutures in their walls (Fig. 6.12d).

VACUOLES AND STORAGE ELEMENTS

All parasitic protozoa have various types of vacuoles, the largest of which are the food vacuoles (see Fig. 6.1); these disintegrate during digestion. Vacuoles that serve as storage elements contain crystalloid proteins (Fig. 6.24a), lipids or carbohydrates (Fig. 6.24c). Lipid-containing vacuoles appear slightly grey in electron micrographs and are present mainly in resting stages such as cysts. Large amounts of protein are found in the refractile bodies of sporozoan sporozoites (Fig. 6.24a) and in haemosporidian ookinetes. Carbohydrates are generally stored in the form of granules of glycogen or amylopectin (Figs. 6.24a, 6.25). Amylopectin-containing granules appear as brilliant white areas in electron micrographs of gregarines, coccidia and some endoparasitic ciliates. These granules are scattered throughout the cytoplasm of sporozoans of all developmental stages except microgametes, and are particularly numerous in the cytoplasm of macrogametes and oocysts (see Fig. 6.11e). Glycogen (see Fig. 6.14a) is present as small randomly distributed granules in the cytoplasm of *Tritrichomonas foetus* and as a large mass in the cytoplasm near the nucleus in *Entamoeba* or *Iodamoeba* cysts.

3.7 Locomotory systems

All protozoa are motile in at least one stage of their life cycles. The different species have developed distinct locomotory systems during their evolution.

Some protozoa use pseudopodia as locomotory organs. These structures, which may occur as thick lobopodia or as fine filopodia (Fig. 6.27), are produced by the cytoplasmic movement mediated by the activity of the Ca^{2+} regulated actin–myosin complexes. The contraction of filaments of actin–myosin causes pressure on the cytoplasm at the posterior pole and this initiates a forward flow of cytoplasm at the apical pole. At the apical pole the amoeboid movement is enhanced by a transformation of the local cytoplasm from a stable 'gel' form to a more liquid 'sol' form (see Fig. 6.16). Pseudopodia are most prominent in the various types of amoeba but may also be found in motile metazoan cells such as leucocytes.

Many protozoa use flagella or cilia as locomotory organs (Gibbons 1981). These structures are constructed according to a common plan. Whilst flagella are longer and generally less numerous than cilia, their basic structures are similar (Figs. 6.1, 6.28, 6.29).

Both types of organelle are c. 0.2–0.4 μm in diameter and both possess an axoneme (an arrangement of 9 pairs of outer microtubules and a single pair of central microtubules) that is anchored to a basal body (kinetosome) that resides inside the cortical cytoplasm

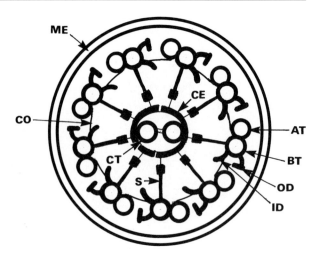

Fig. 6.28 Diagrammatic representation of a cross-section through a flagellum or cilium. AT, A tubules (consisting of 13 subunits); BT, B tubules; CF, central sheath; CO, connection between the outer pairs of microtubules; CT, central tubule; ID, inner dynein arm; ME, cell membrane; OD, outer dynein arm; S, spike.

of the cell (Figs. 6.1, 6.29d). The basal bodies are similar to centrioles in having 9 sets of 3 microtubules arranged in a ring-like pattern. The basal bodies may be connected to filamentous elements such as the kinetodesmal filaments of cilia. Several species of protozoa have a rod-like structure consisting of a network of protein filaments inside the flagellum (Figs. 6.4, 6.7, 6.29a). These rods lie beside the axoneme, probably adding to the thickness and stability of the flagellum. This enhancement may be particularly important for protozoa living in viscous media such as blood or intestinal fluids. Although flagella and cilia are constructed according to a general blueprint, in different protozoa the paired outer microtubules in the flagella and cilia may differ in shape (Fig. 6.28). The 'A tubule', which is furnished with 2 dynein arms, typically possesses 13 protofilaments, whereas the 'B tubule' has only 9 protofilaments and shares 3–4 of the protofilaments of the A tubule. The dynein arms act as enzymes for breaking down ATP and are proposed to represent the motor system in the 'gliding filament' theory. This theory postulates that the movement of flagella and cilia is initiated by the gliding of microtubules along each other using the dynein arms as linking elements. The central regions of flagella are stabilized by spike-like elements (Fig. 6.28) in addition to the rod mentioned on pp. 125 and 135. In the trichomonads and in the trypomastigote stages of trypanosomes, a flagellum may be connected to the cell surface by desmosomes (Fig. 6.29). The recurrent flagella are attached in this manner and when the attached flagellum pulls the plasmalemma away from the body, the undulating membrane is created. The recurrent flagella never run inside the cytoplasm, but the axonemes of *Giardia* trophozoites run inside the cytoplasm for several micrometres (Fig. 6.18c).

The invasive stages of sporozoans, i.e. the merozoites and sporozoites, have 3 types of movement: glid-

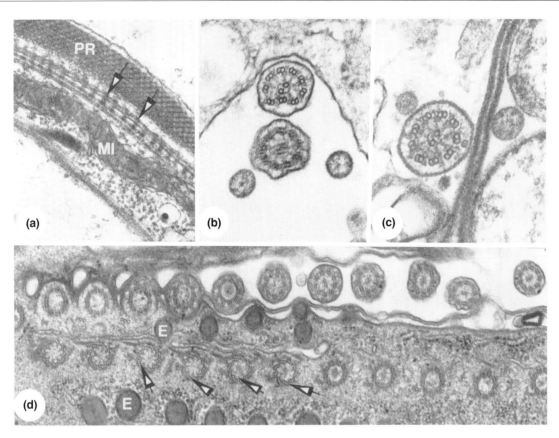

Fig. 6.29 Transmission electron micrographs of flagella (a–c) and cilia (d). (a) *Trypanosoma vivax*; longitudinal section of a flagellum, attached to the surface by semidesmosomes (arrows) ($\times$ 25 000). (b, c) Cross-section through the flagella of the gametes of *Eimeria* and *Sarcocystis* species showing the typical $9 \times 2 + 2$ pattern (b, $\times$ 25 000; c, $\times$ 40 000). (d) Cross-section through the basal bodies of cilia showing the typical 9×3 tubule arrangement (arrows). E, extrusomes; MI, mitochondrion; PR, paraxial rod of the flagellum.

ing, twisting and bending. Only the first of these leads to active displacement of the organisms; the other 2 only change the direction of movement. The gliding form of movement is extremely rare in eukaryotic cells. It is temperature sensitive and cytochalasin B sensitive, the latter property suggesting the participation of actin in the process. The gliding movement may be related to the capping phenomenon in sporozoans. In capping, the organisms aggregate materials on their surfaces and move them towards the posterior pole, from where they release them into the surroundings. A parasite floating in a liquid could move forward using this type of action. The most studied of the capping phenomena is the circumsporozoite reaction of *P. falciparum* sporozoites.

3.8   Surface interactions and penetration

Parasites living inside host cells use a variety of means, either active or passive, to enter the host cell. In active processes the parasite's motility mechanisms play a role, whereas in passive processes the host cell internalizes the parasite by a phagocytic mechanism in the same way that food particles are ingested. In all cases, however, entry occurs after an initial recognition step in which some structure on the parasite

surface reacts with and binds to some structure on the host cell surface.

Different types of invasion processes are used by different intracellular pathogens. Some, such as the Microspora, penetrate the host cell plasmalemma to enter the host cell cytoplasm whereas *Mycoplasma* and viruses invade by membrane fusion. Many parasites enter their host cells by phagocytosis. After entry by phagocytosis, different parasites follow different paths: the *Leishmania* develop in phagolysosomes; the mycobacteria inhibit fusion of the lysosomes with the phagosomes; and *T. cruzi* and some species of *Leishmania* and all schizonts of *Theileria* (Piroplasmea) escape from the phagosome into the host cell cytoplasm.

Some of the phagocytic processes are quite complex. Some organisms, such as malaria parasites, *Eimeria*, *Sarcocystis* and *Toxoplasma*, actively invade by forming a moving junction between the host membrane and the parasite. After completion of the process, the parasite rests in a parasitophorous vacuole bound by the invaginated host cell membrane. This parasitophorous vacuole membrane may disintegrate after the parasite has penetrated; for instance *Babesia* and *Theileria* are located directly in the cytoplasm of their host cells (red blood cells) shortly after invasion is completed (Fig. 6.30a, b.).

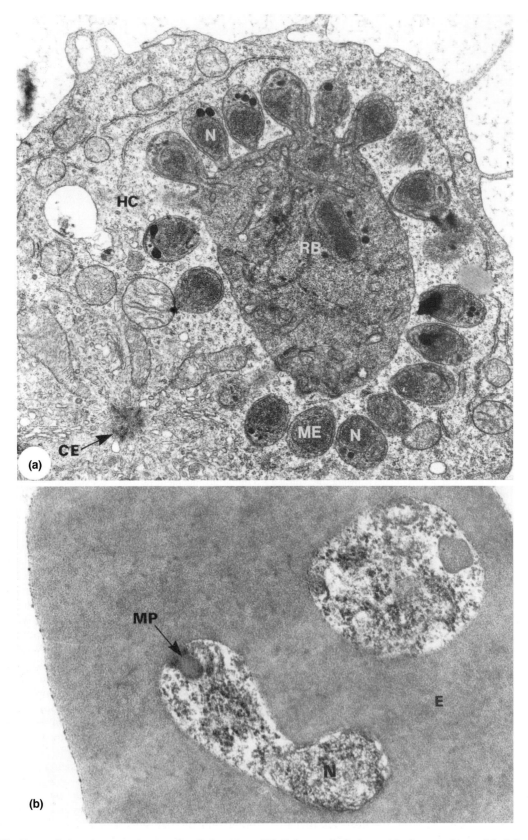

Fig. 6.30 Transmission electron micrographs of piroplasms (*Theileria annulata*) situated in the cytoplasm of their host cells. (a) A meront within a lymphocyte. The host cell was in the process of dividing; note the centriole (CE) and the spindle (× 12 000). (b) A slender trophozoite and a spherical gamont in a bovine erythrocyte. CE, centriole; E, erythrocyte; HC, host cell cytoplasm; ME, merozoite, MP, micropore; N, nucleus; RB, residual body (× 40 000).

4 MODES OF REPRODUCTION

In parasitic protozoa, cell division occurs during both vegetative and sexual development (in which it occurs during the formation of gametes). Cell division may occur in production of gametes of both sexes, as in the gregarines, or only during production of the male gamonts, as in the coccidia.

4.1 Binary fission

The most basic type of multiplication is binary fission (Fig. 6.31). This process produces 2 daughter cells, following duplication of the organelles of the mother cell. The axis of cell division is a characteristic feature of the various groups within the protozoa and different types of division can be distinguished: irregular, amoeba-like, longitudinal, oblique and transverse. In microsporideans (e.g. *Nosema*) binary fissions occur after nuclear divisions in an irregular fashion, the cytoplasm being divided irregularly and different sizes of daughter cells being formed. After freeing, however, the daughter cells all develop a similar shape. In rhizopods such as *Entamoeba* and *Acanthamoeba* cell division is irregular with respect to the cytoplasm but the constriction always occurs perpendicular to the spindle axis; this is called 'amoeba-like division' (Fig. 6.31a).

In flagellates such as the diplomonads, trichomonads and trypanosomatids and in sporozoans such as the coccidia, the axis of cell division runs longitudinally and the process is therefore called 'longitudinal division'. In flagellates the polarity of the division axis is determined by the initial axis of duplication of the basal bodies of the flagella (Fig. 6.31b). Unusual binary fissions occur in a few species of sporozoans. For instance, the process by which the merozoites of piroplasms bud from the parent cell, one at a time, could be considered to be an irregular form of binary fission. The processes of endodyogeny in those coccidia that form tissue cysts is a very peculiar form of longitudinal division (Fig. 6.31d). In this process, 2 daughter cells are formed within a mother cell, arching over and parallel to the axis of the dividing nucleus. The daughter cells produce the inner 2 pellicular membranes *de novo* from the membranes of the endoplasmic reticulum and take over the outer membrane of the mother cell's pellicle. The 2 inner membranes of the mother cell disintegrate. In trichomonads the axis (Fig. 6.31c) of cell division is longitudinal at the beginning of the process when the flagellar basal bodies and the nucleus are reduplicated. Later the divided nuclei move into positions opposite each other and as a result an oblique, or even a transverse, cytoplasmic division occurs.

In opalinid flagellates, which are characterized by oblique rows of 'cilia', binary fission occurs during the sexual and asexual developmental phases (Fig. 6.31f). The axis of the cytoplasmic division initially runs longitudinally, but soon becomes parallel to the oblique rows of cilia. This process is called 'oblique division'. It is intermediate between the longitudinal fission of flagellates and the transverse division of ciliates.

In ciliates such as *Balantidium* and *Ichthyophthirius* binary fission starts with the duplication of the cytostomal kinetosomes (basal bodies) and is followed by the division of the macronuclei and micronuclei. The axis of cytoplasmic division runs perpendicular to the axis of the nuclear spindles. Cell constriction may occur simultaneously with nuclear division or there may be a time lag. The process is called 'oblique division' or, as this division proceeds across the rows of the cilia, it is also described as 'homothetogenic fission' (Fig. 6.31e).

4.2 Rosette-like multiplication

If division of the cytoplasm is incomplete or delayed after nuclear division, the pair of newly formed nuclei may divide again before cytoplasmic division occurs. This may result in the simultaneous development of more than 2 offspring. In some cases the offspring remain attached at their posterior poles for some time, forming a mass that may appear as a rosette in stained preparations. Studies of this process by light microscopy were originally misinterpreted and the process was considered to be a multiple division. Rosettes of this type are frequently found in cultures of trichomonads and trypanosomes. They are also relatively common in preparations of *T. gondii* collected during the acute phase of infection, when endodyogenies are often repeated inside parasitophorous vacuoles of macrophages and reticuloendothelial cells.

4.3 Multiple divisions

Multiple divisions are characteristic of amoebae, sporozoans and Microspora, but are rarely observed in the other groups of parasitic protozoa. The formation of daughter cells by multiple division may be initiated by 3 main types of mother cells (Fig. 6.32a–f).

A multinuclear type of mother cell may initiate multiple divisions. In this case daughter cell formation starts at the end of a phase of repeated nuclear division in the mother cell. In this way multinucleate plasmodia are produced before cytoplasmic division starts and the occurrence of such multinucleate forms led to the naming of the genus *Plasmodium*. Multinucleate stages are also found in the life cycles of *E. histolytica*, in meronts and sporonts of gregarines and in some stages of some coccidia. They occur in all gamonts of gregarines, but only in the microgamonts of some coccidia and in some developmental stages of Myxozoa. The cytoplasm of the plasmodia may be divided or not, but when divided the pattern is always species-specific. In eimerian and theilerian meronts and in the sporonts of haemosporidia and of some piroplasms, daughter cell formation closely follows the last nuclear division. In eimerian microgamonts a microgamete is formed around each nucleus and an electron-lucent remnant of the mother cell's karyoplasm is left behind. Only occasionally do the nuclei

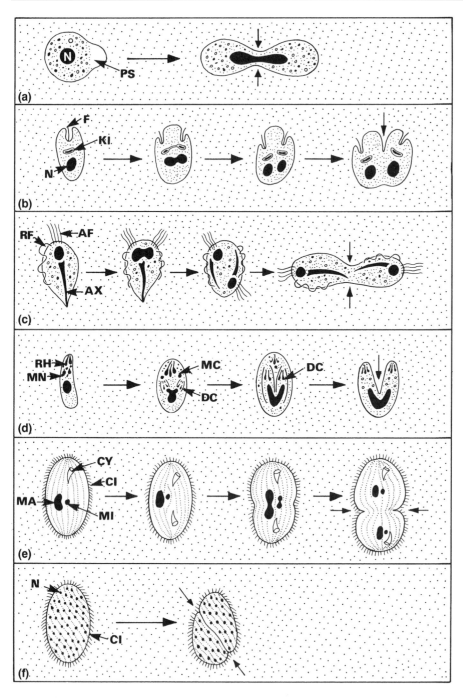

Fig. 6.31 Diagrammatic representation of different types of binary fission (invaginations are shown by small arrows). (a) Amoeba type; division without fixed axis. (b) Trypanosomatid type (here *Leishmania*): longitudinal division. (c) Trichomonad type (here *T. vaginalis*): note that there is a longitudinal division only at the beginning. (d) Endodyogeny of tissue cyst forming coccidia (e.g., *Toxoplasma, Sarcocystis*): inner development of daughter cells. (e) Ciliata type (e.g. *Balantidium*): cross-division. (f) Opalinata type: oblique division. AF, anterior free flagellum; AX, axostyle; B, basal body of flagellum; CI, cilium; CY, cytopharynx; DC, daughter cell; F, short flagellum in a pocket; KI, kinetoplast; MA, macronucleus; MC, mother cell; MI, micronucleus; MN, micronemes; N, nucleus; PS, pale pseudopodium; RF, recurrent flagellum; RH, rhoptries.

of the mother cell divide after cytoplasmic division starts and therefore it is rare for 2 microgametes to originate from a single nucleus of the microgamont.

A uninuclear type of mother cell may initiate multiple division. In this case daughter cell formation starts without a preceding phase of nuclear division but the nucleus of the parasite has generally grown considerably and developed a lobulate surface before daughter cell formation occurs. When division of this giant nucleus begins, daughter cell formation occurs simultaneously. The daughter cells incorporate portions of the giant nucleus, the chromosomal components of which have been increased by a preceding endomitosis. This process of nuclear splitting occurs

during the merogony of some cyst-forming coccidians and has been described as 'endopolygeny'. The microgamonts of some species of *Sarcocystis* and of *Plasmodium* produce their microgametes in this way. A similar process of simultaneous nuclear splitting and daughter cell formation is found in sporonts of some piroplasms during the production of sporozoites.

There is another type of multiple division that is intermediate between these 2 types. In these cases a large mother cell with a lobated giant nucleus is divided into numerous uninuclear cytomeres. The single limiting membrane of these cytomeres originates from the surface membrane of the original cell or from the endoplasmic reticulum of the mother cell. Such

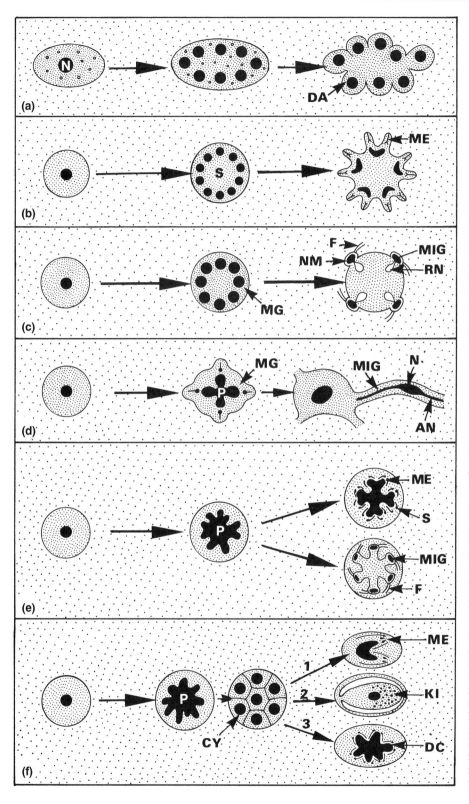

Fig. 6.32 Diagrammatic representation of multiple division. (a) *Amoeba* sp.: formation of vegetative stages after excystation. (b) Formation of merozoites by meronts of species of *Eimeria, Plasmodium, Theileria,* etc. (c) Formation of microgametes, e.g. *Eimeria* spp. (d) Formation of microgametes of *Plasmodium* spp. and other haemosporidia (e.g., exflagellation). (e) *Sarcocystis* sp.: formation of merozoites by meronts (1) and of microgametes by microgamonts (2). (f) Formation of cytomeres. These may each develop: (1) 2 merozoites (some *Eimeria* spp.); (2) a single kinete (*Babesia* spp.); (3) many parasitic stages in the life cycle of various coccidians, i.e. merozoites of *Globidium* spp. or sporozoites of species of *Plasmodium, Babesia* and *Theileria.* AN, axoneme (flagellum of microgamete); CT, cytomere; DA, daughter amoeba; DC, daughter cell; F, flagellum; KI, kinete; ME, merozoite anlage; MG, microgamont; MIG, microgamete; N, nucleus; NM, nucleus of microgamete (dense part); PN, polymorphous, multilobulated nucleus; RN, residual nucleus (light part); S, schizont.

cytomeres are regularly formed in meronts of some species of *Eimeria* such as *E. tenella,* in some species of *Globidium* and in sporonts of all species of *Babesia, Theileria, Plasmodium* and *Hepatozoon.* The uninuclear cytomeres ultimately produce the daughter cells. They give rise to 2 merozoites in *Eimeria,* to a single kinete in *Babesia* and *Theileria,* to many merozoites in *Globid-*

ium and to sporozoites in *Plasmodium, Babesia* and *Theileria.* Cytomeres merge in Myxozoa.

Additional information concerning the composition, metabolism, genetics and molecular biology of the cell can be found in Puytorac et al. (1987), Alberts et al. (1994), Darnell et al. (1994) and Hausmann and Hülsmann (1996).

5 CONCLUDING STATEMENT

This chapter illustrates that the protozoa are a heterogeneous group, with wide variations in morphology and life cycle. The parasitic protozoa are probably polyphyletic in origin and this is also probably true of the eukaryota (see Chapter 7). There is no good reason to assume that the eukaryota are of a single evolutionary line but rather they may have arisen by mutation and probably symbiosis from various prokaryotic predecessors at more than one time.

There are only a few features that are shared by all parasitic protozoa; they are all basically unicellular organisms and they are all eukaryotic. Based on their common unicellular eukaryotic plan, a vast array of forms has developed producing a wide variety of organisms. These organisms have successfully inhabited a great range of ecological niches, some of which, to our detriment, are located in the human body (Mehlhorn and Pierkarski 1994).

REFERENCES

Alberts B, Bray D et al., 1994, *Molecular Biology of the Cell*, 3rd edn, Garland, New York.

Bielka H, ed, 1982, *The Eukaryotic Ribosome*, Springer, Heidelberg.

Darnell J, Lodish H, Baltimore D, 1994, *Molekulare Zellbiologie*, De Gruyter, Berlin.

Farquhar MG, Palade GE, 1981, The golgi apparatus – from artifact to center stage, *J Cell Biol*, **91:** 775–1035.

Gal S, Raikhel VV, 1993, Protein sorting in the endomembrane system of plant cells, *Curr Opin Cell Biol*, **5:** 636–40.

Gennis RB, 1989, *Biomembranes: Molecular Structure and Function*, Springer, New York.

Gibbons JR, 1981, Cilia and flagella of eukaryotes, *J Cell Biol*, **91:** 1075–215.

Hackstein JHP, Mehlhorn H et al., 1995, Parasitic apicompleans harbor a chlorophyll–D1 complex, *Parasitol Res*, **81:** 207–16.

Hausmann K, Hülsmann N, 1996, *Protozoology*, Thieme, Stuttgart.

Huxley HE, Hanson J, 1954, Changes in the cross striations of muscle during contraction and stretch and their structural interpretation, *Nature (London)*, **173:** 873–6.

Kleinig H, Sitte P, 1984, *Zellbiologie*, Fischer, Stuttgart.

Mehlhorn H, ed, 1988, *Parasitology in Focus*, Springer, Heidelberg.

Mehlhorn H, Pierkarski G, 1994, *Grundriß der Parasitenkunde*, 4th edn, Fischer, Stuttgart.

Mehlhorn H, Ruthmann A, 1992, *Allgemeine Protozoologie*, Fischer, Jena.

Mehlhorn H, Eichenlaub D et al., 1995, *Diagnose und Therapie der Parasitosen des Menschen*, 2nd edn, Fischer, Stuttgart.

Neupert W, Lill R, 1992, *New Comprehensive Biochemistry: Membrane Biogenesis and Protein Targeting*, **22:** Elsevier, Amsterdam.

De Puytorac P, Grain J, Mignot JP, 1987, *Précis de Protistologie*, Ed Boubée, Paris.

Scholtyseck E, Mehlhorn H, 1970, Elektronenmikroskopische befunde ändern das system der einzeller, *Naturwiss Rundschau*, **10:** 420–7.

Singer SJ, Nicolson GL, 1972, The fluid mosaic model of the structure of cell membranes, *Science*, **175:** 720–31.

Tolbert NE, 1981, Metabolic pathways in peroxisomes and glyoxysomes, *Annu Rev Biochem*, **50:** 133–52.

CLASSIFICATION OF THE PARASITIC PROTOZOA

F E G Cox

1 INTRODUCTION

There are >200 000 named species of protozoa of which nearly 10 000 are parasitic in invertebrates and in almost every species of vertebrate. It is, therefore, not surprising that humans should act as hosts to protozoa, but what is surprising is that we should harbour so many; >50 species belonging to >20 genera (see the appendix to this chapter, p. 153). These range from forms that are never pathogenic to those that cause some of the major diseases of tropical countries: malaria, sleeping sickness, Chagas disease and leishmaniasis, which together threaten over one-quarter of the population of the world. In addition, many occur commonly in temperate regions and others are increasingly being implicated as major pathogens in immunosuppressed patients, particularly those suffering from HIV infections.

It is convenient to regard the protozoa as organisms that lie somewhere between the prokaryotic and higher eukaryotic organisms, sharing some of the characteristics of each. They are small, have short generation times, high rates of reproduction and a tendency to induce immunity to reinfection in those hosts that survive. These are features of infections with microparasites such as bacteria. On the other hand, protozoa are undoubtedly eukaryotic cells with organelles and metabolic pathways similar to those of their hosts.

Protozoa are unicellular eukaryotic cells, most of which measure 1–150 μm, the parasitic forms tending towards the lower end of this range. Structurally, each protozoan is the equivalent of a single metazoan cell with its plasma membrane, nucleus, nuclear membrane, chromosomes, endoplasmic reticulum and, in most cases, mitochondria, Golgi body, ribosomes and various specialized structures adapted to meet particular needs. Parasitic protozoa are not simple or degenerate forms and their particular adaptations frequently include complex life-cycles and specialized ways of entering their hosts and maintaining themselves once they have gained access. Their nutrition, physiology and biochemistry are largely geared to the parasitic habit and are specialized rather than degenerate. Sexual reproduction also occurs in some protozoa and, in the parasitic forms, is particularly important in the sporozoans in which it provides for apparently limitless variation and adaptability.

2 PARASITIC PROTOZOA AND PARASITIC INFECTIONS

Before attempting to classify the parasitic protozoa, it is necessary to introduce them and to comment briefly on the infections they cause. Traditionally, the parasitic protozoa of humans are listed in what used to be regarded as their taxonomic order but, as will be explained later, this is no longer possible. Nevertheless, listing them according to their normally accepted groupings is a convenient and familiar starting place.

2.1 Parasitic amoebae

Several species of amoebae are common in humans in most parts of the world but only one, *Entamoeba histolytica*, is an important pathogen, invading the small intestine and colon of humans, apes, monkeys, dogs, cats and rats. Sometimes the amoebae invade the mucosa and submucosa and may be carried via the portal vein to the liver and other parts of the body causing damage to the wall of the bowel or the liver but, in most people, there is no tissue invasion and the parasite causes no harm. The symptoms are variable but usually include diarrhoea or dysentery with the loss of blood (amoebic dysentery). Four other intestinal amoebae are commonly found all over the world: *E. dispar*, once regarded as a non-pathogenic race of *E. histolytica*, resembles the pathogenic form; *Entamoeba coli*, the most common amoeba of humans, is a harmless commensal; *Endolimax nana*, also a harmless commensal, which inhabits the upper part of the colon and has 4-nucleate cysts; and *Iodamoeba butschlii* which has cysts with a single nucleus. None of these 4 parasites causes any disease. A sixth amoeba, *Entamoeba gingivalis*, occurs in the mouth and is often associated with infected gums.

2.2 Facultative amoebae and flagellates of humans

There have been occasional reports of free-living amoebae infecting humans, sometimes with fatal results. Several species of *Acanthamoeba* can cause upper respiratory tract infections in immunocompromised individuals. *Acanthamoeba* spp. also act as reservoirs for *Legionella pneumophila*, the causative agent of legionellosis. *Balamuthia mandrillaris*, described relatively recently in humans, has been found in the brain. *Naegleria fowleri* and other *Naegleria* species, which are strictly speaking flagellates, have been implicated in primary meningoencephalitis in otherwise healthy individuals.

2.3 Intestinal and related flagellates

A number of flagellates occur in the alimentary canals of humans. In most cases, the life-cycles are very simple and involve the ingestion of food or water contaminated with encysted forms which excyst in the intestine where multiplication by binary fission takes place. Large infestations can build up but the infections are seldom harmful although some may cause gastrointestinal disorders. Flagellates similar to those in the intestine can occur in other parts of the body, such as the urogenital system, and these may cause more serious infections. Eight species of flagellate are ubiquitous and common parasites of the human gastrointestinal tract or urogenital system. Few do any real harm but some occasionally give rise to unpleasant symptoms which can usually be easily treated. The most important by far is *Giardia duodenalis*, also known as *G. lamblia*, *G. intestinalis* or *Lamblia intestinalis*, which invades the upper part of the

small intestine, where large infestations may cause malabsorption particularly in children. Giardiasis is one of the 10 major parasitic infections of humans, causing as many deaths as the large roundworm *Ascaris lumbricoides* in the developing world, and is the most common intestinal parasite in more developed countries world wide. Three species of *Trichomonas* are common in all parts of the world: *T. hominis* occurs in the caecum and large intestine; *T. tenax* invades the mouth; and *T. vaginalis* occurs in the vagina and urethra of women and in the urethra, seminal vesicles and prostate of men. *T. vaginalis* may cause inflammation and discharge and is an increasingly important venereal disease, especially in women. *Enteromonas hominis* is cosmopolitan and harmless. *Chilomastix mesnili* is rare and harmless. *Dientamoeba fragilis* is transmitted through the eggs of the pinworm *Enterobius vermicularis* and may cause diarrhoea.

2.4 Trypanosomes of humans in South America

Trypanosoma cruzi infects 16–18 million people in South and Central America and is infective to c. 100–150 species of wild and domesticated mammals. The vectors are bugs belonging to the family Reduviidae. In the human host, the trypanosomes enter various cells, particularly macrophages, muscle cells and nerve cells, where they round up and multiply as amastigote forms which develop into trypomastigotes that either enter new cells or are taken up when a vector feeds. The disease, which can last for the lifetime of the host, is called 'Chagas disease' and takes various forms depending on where the amastigotes develop, the most serious consequences being cardiac failure due to parasites in the heart muscles or the loss of nervous control of the alimentary canal due to parasites in the nervous system. *T. rangeli*, which is usually harmless, occurs in humans, primates, cats and dogs in Central and South America where it is transmitted by bugs and, although the parasite is quite different from *T. cruzi*, the 2 are occasionally confused.

2.5 Trypanosomes of humans in Africa

The African trypanosomes typically develop in the mid-gut of tsetse flies belonging to the genus *Glossina*. Two forms (subspecies) infect humans; *Trypanosoma brucei gambiense* and *T.b. rhodesiense*, the former in West and Central Africa where it causes chronic sleeping sickness and the latter in the savannah of East Africa where it causes acute sleeping sickness.

2.6 *Leishmania* parasites

Leishmania species, which are transmitted by sandflies, cause serious diseases in humans. The typical infection is a long-lasting or non-healing cutaneous lesion but in many species, and in particular individuals, the parasites may invade subcutaneous or deeper tissues causing hideous and permanent disfiguration. The most serious disease, kala azar, involves the macrophages of organs such as the liver and can result in multi-organ system failure. Leishmaniasis is now known to be caused by a complex of at least 19 species. As the morphology of all these parasites is similar, identification tends to be based on isoenzyme and DNA techniques. In the Old World, the main species causing cutaneous leishmaniasis are *L. tropica* and *L. major* and the species causing visceral leishmaniasis is *L. donovani*. In the New World, *L. chagasi* causes visceral leishmaniasis and cutaneous and mucocutaneous leishmaniasis are caused by at least 12 distinct species of *Leishmania*.

2.7 Coccidia: *Toxoplasma* and related coccidia

Coccidia are common parasites of the epithelial cells of the gut of vertebrates. The majority of this group of parasites cause little harm to their hosts, the most important exception being *Toxoplasma gondii*, a parasite of felids with a very wide range of intermediate hosts, including humans. In cats, and other felids, the life-cycle is confined to the gut but if the infective cysts passed in the faeces are ingested by other warm blooded animals, multiplication occurs in various cells of the body and eventually cysts are formed. Infections are normally symptomless, but in the foetus or immunosuppressed patients they may be very serious and they may occasionally cause ocular damage in healthy individuals.

2.8 *Cryptosporidium*

Coccidians belonging to the genus *Cryptosporidium* are relatively common parasites in the intestinal and respiratory tracts of mammals, birds and reptiles. *C. parvum* causes gastrointestinal disorders in cattle, sheep and humans. The infection is unpleasant but not normally dangerous except in immunocompromised individuals, such as AIDS sufferers, in whom it can be fatal.

2.9 *Cyclospora*

The most recently described widespread protozoal infection of humans is *Cyclospora cayetanensis;* since it was first recorded in 1986 it has been noted in both immunologically competent and immunologically compromised patients in many parts of the world including the UK and the USA (for a review see Chiodini 1994). *C. cayetanensis* is an intestinal coccidian that causes a self-limiting infection with diarrhoea and malabsorption. The actual route of infection is unknown, although water and meat have been implicated. It is also not clear whether or not there is any other host apart from humans (Chiodini 1994).

2.10 Malaria parasites

The malaria parasites belong to the same phylum as the coccidians but to a different group, the haemosporidians, members of which, as the name implies, are parasitic in the blood of vertebrates. The malaria parasites of mammals all belong to the genus *Plasmodium* and are transmitted by female mosquitoes belonging to the genus *Anopheles*. Human malaria, one of the most important diseases in the world with >500 million people at risk in tropical and subtropical parts of the world especially Africa, is caused by 4 species of *Plasmodium*: *P. falciparum*, *P. vivax*, *P. ovale* and *P. malariae*. The disease is characterized by periodic fevers. *P. falciparum* causes malignant tertian malaria and is the most common and serious of all the forms of malaria, often causing vascular blockage and cerebral damage resulting in death.

2.11 Piroplasms

The piroplasms are parasites of the erythrocytes of vertebrates and the vectors are ticks. *Babesia* species live in the blood of vertebrates and are transmitted by ticks and cause serious disease, babesiosis, in domesticated animals. *B. microti*, which is common in wild rodents, occasionally infects humans in North America and sporadically elsewhere but the infections are not usually fatal. In Europe, splenectomized humans are sometimes infected with *B. bovis*, a cattle species, and the infection is frequently fatal.

2.12 Microsporidians

There are some 700 species of microsporidians in nearly all groups of vertebrates and invertebrates, particularly fish and arthropods. All microsporidians possess an inherent ability to multiply in their vertebrate hosts but this seems to be curtailed in humans, except in those individuals whose immune system is compromised. The first human case of microsporidiosis was recorded in 1959 and since then several new species have been recorded mainly in AIDS sufferers and others undergoing immunosuppressive therapy (see Canning and Hollister 1992, Curry and Canning 1993 and Chapter 21). Microsporidiosis in humans is extremely rare but, relatively, the most common species is *Encephalitozoon cuniculi*, a parasite of peritoneal macrophages that also spreads to other parts of the body including the brain; this species occurs in rodents, rabbits, dogs and other carnivores and primates and there are increasing numbers of records from humans. None of the other species has yet been recorded from any animals although these must almost certainly be the sources of infection. *Encephalitozoon hellem* parasitises the cornea and conjunctiva and has been recorded in the viscera. *Septata intestinalis*, which some authorities consider should be called *Encephalitozoon intestinalis*, is an intestinal form that also occurs in a variety of cells in different parts of the body. *Enterocytozoon bieneusi* is also an intestinal form associated with chronic diarrhoea in AIDS patients. *Nosema corneum* infects the cornea and *N. connori* has been recorded as a disseminated infection in an athymic child. The most recently recorded species is *Trachipleistophora hominis* from the cornea and skeletal muscle of an AIDS patient. The taxonomy of the microsporidians is in a state of flux and there are indications of a number of species that have not yet been formally identified and are currently recorded as *Nosema* spp. or *Microsporidium* spp., a genus that has no real validity, for example *M. ceylonensis* and *M. africanum*.

2.13 Ciliophora

Parasitic ciliates occur in most groups of vertebrates and invertebrates but few are of any economic importance. *Balantidium coli* is a common parasite of pigs in all parts of the world and has also been recorded in rats, dogs, monkeys, apes and c.1000 humans. The ciliate lives in the lumen of the large intestine and may invade the gut wall, where it produces ulcers resembling those caused by *Entamoeba histolytica*, although the majority of cases are asymptomatic.

2.14 *Pneumocystis*

The taxonomic position of *Pneumocystis* is uncertain but it is almost certainly a fungus. However, as it has been long regarded as a protozoan, it is mentioned in passing here. *Pneumocystis carinii* is normally a harmless parasite in the lungs but in immunocompromised individuals parasite numbers increase until they fill the alveolar spaces causing pneumonia, which may be fatal. Pneumocystosis is a common complication in people suffering from HIV infection.

3 NATURE OF THE PARASITIC PROTOZOA

Protozoa are usually defined as single celled eukaryotic organisms but this definition is very simplistic and the group has always been an enigmatic one, largely because of the small size of the cells, the relative lack of morphological features and the absence of any meaningful evolutionary history. In this chapter the term Protozoa has been retained largely for convenience as it is widely used by parasitologists, even though it has been virtually abandoned by protozoologists. In order to understand the background to the currently used classifications it is necessary to consider briefly the history of the subject, the changes that have occurred and the reasons for these changes. The early history of protozoology has been described many times, for example by Cole (1926) and Hyman (1940). Although the shells of foraminiferans had often been seen before (for example the illustrations in Robert Hooke's *Micrographia* published in 1665) it is generally agreed that the single celled organisms that we now know to be protozoa were first recognized as such in 1676 by Antony van Leeuwenhoek, who described them as 'little animals' or 'animalcula' (Dobell 1960).

The word Protozoa, meaning 'first animals', was introduced by Goldfuss in 1818 (Goldfuss 1818) and has been in use in a modified form ever since. Unfortunately, Goldfuss included a number of metazoans such as sponges and bryozoans within the group and it was not until 1838, after the botanist Matthias Jacob Schleiden and the zoologist Theodor Schwann had elucidated their cell theory, that the phrase 'single celled animals' came into common usage by scientists. For instance, Barry wrote in 1843 that 'Monas and similar flagellates are single cells, and have a nucleus which corresponds to the cell nucleus in higher forms' (see Cole 1926). It was, however, Theodor von Siebold who formally established the doctrine of the unicellular nature of the protozoa; he was the first to use the word protozoa in its current sense for organisms which he described as 'animals in which the various systems of organs cannot be distinguished and whose irregular form and simple organization are represented by a single cell' (von Siebold 1848 and Coles' translation). von Siebold, like Goldfuss, regarded the protozoa as primitive invertebrates and divided the protozoa between 2 classes, the Infusoria and the Rhizopoda, roughly equivalent to the ciliates and amoebae. By the middle of the nineteenth century, a number of biologists had realized that single celled organisms included some that had greater affinities with plants than with animals and, in order to avoid the preconceptions inherent in the use of the word Protozoa, Hogg introduced the term 'Protoctista' (Hogg 1860) to embrace those forms that had plant, animal or no clear affinities. Haeckel, who considered that all these forms represented a coherent group, used the term 'Protista' (Haeckel 1876). Haeckel's ideas were translated into a system of classification that divided the animal kingdom into the single celled organisms, Protozoa, and multicellular organisms, Metazoa. This system has remained virtually unchanged in zoological textbooks until the present time and its basic concepts are clearly and unambiguously set out by Craig (1926) who wrote 'The Protozoa are animals composed of a single cell. They form one of the 2 great divisions of the Animal kingdom, the other being the Metazoa, or multicellular animals.' In 1938, Copeland grouped together all those single celled organisms that did not have obvious animal or plant affinities and used Haeckel's term Protista, which he later changed to Hogg's Protoctista on grounds of priority (Copeland 1938). Thus, 3 terms are currently widely used: Protozoa, Protista and Protoctista. This is not an appropriate place to discuss or to comment on the validity of these terms, the background of which is discussed in more detail by Lipscomb (1991) and Corliss (1994). However, parasitologists tend to be very conservative and the term Protozoa is now almost universally used by scientists working with those parasitic unicellular organisms that infect humans and domesticated animals.

4 KINGDOMS IN DISPUTE

In his 1758 classification of all living things, Carl Linnaeus recognized 2 kingdoms, Animalia and Plantae but, as mentioned on p. 144, by the middle of the nineteenth century, scientists had begun looking for a third category in which to classify organisms like the single celled ones, which were then being discovered with increasing frequency. Several scientists, including Hogg (1860) and Haeckel (1876), argued for the creation of an additional kingdom to accommodate these forms. Haeckel attempted to apply evolutionary trends to the classification of single celled organisms and he is often credited with the concept of 3 kingdoms of living things: Animalia, Plantae and Protista, (animals, plants and protozoa) which was expanded to 4 kingdoms, Animalia, Plantae, Protoctista and Mychota (prokaryote organisms) by Copeland (1938). With the removal of the fungi from the plant kingdom the erection of a fifth kingdom, Fungi, was necessary and a sixth was added by Jahn and Jahn (1949). Jahn and Jahn's kingdoms were the Archetista (viruses), Monera (bacteria and blue green algae), Metazoa (multicellular animals), Metaphyta (multicellular plants), Fungi and Protista. This classification did not recognize the fact that the single celled eukaryotic organisms were not a homogeneous assemblage and that there were unicellular members in the animal and plant kingdoms that could not logically be separated from the metazoa and metaphyta. In other words, there was an argument for the creation of groupings such as protozoa and protophyta within the animal and plant kingdoms. Nevertheless, Jahn and Jahn's classification became widely adopted and forms the basis of what is now known as Whittaker's 5 kingdom classification: Monera (prokaryotes), Animalia, Plantae, Fungi, and Protista (Whittaker 1969). Essentially, what this did was to remove the viruses (regarded as non-living) and to make minor readjustments between the fungi and plants.

Although there have been a number of major and minor modifications to this overall classification, as far as higher organisms are concerned Whittaker's 5 kingdom scheme has stood the test of time fairly well. However, studies at the biochemical and molecular levels have thrown up a number of problems and it has become necessary to adopt a rather more radical approach such as that set out by Cavalier-Smith (1993) and adopted by Corliss (1994). Corliss' classification has to be taken seriously for a number of reasons not least of which is his authority in the field and, as he says

'At the present time we are taxonomically in a state of flux. We are frustratingly trapped between existing classifications of protists that are recognized to be faulty and some future scheme(s) not yet available. The latter, hopefully closer to the ideal natural system long awaited, probably will not be ready for at least several years, perhaps not until the turn of the century' (Corliss 1994).

As far as the protozoa are concerned, Corliss goes on to say

'...there is a pressing need *now* for a useful/usable interim system treating the protists overall in a manner understandable to the general proto-zoologist/phycologist/mycologist and the myriads of cell and evolutionary biologists, biochemists and general biologists ...' (Corliss 1994).

As has already been pointed out, there is some confusion at the highest taxonomic level because 3 terms are in existence that can be applied to the unicellular eukaryotic organisms: Protozoa, Protista and Protoctista. Each has its own supporters; parasitologists tend to favour Protozoa (Cox 1993) whereas many proto-zoologists tend to use Protista (Corliss 1984) or, less frequently, Protoctista (Margulis et al. 1990). In this chapter, Protozoa will be used but, as any differences of opinion should disappear if Corliss' classification is used, this requires some further discussion.

Conventionally, since the time of Linnaeus, the term 'kingdom' has been used as the highest category in the taxonomic hierarchy but Corliss, echoing the views of most protistologists (or protozoologists), accepts that the 'lower' eukaryotes can no longer be accommodated within a single kingdom. He recognizes 6 kingdoms in what he calls the empire 'Eukaryota': the kingdoms Archezoa, Protozoa, Chromista, Plantae, Fungi and Animalia. The first 3 contain only single celled organisms but a number of single celled organisms occur in the kingdom Plantae and a few in the kingdom Fungi. None occur in the kingdom Animalia. There are 2 important consequences of this classification; the first is that the concept of a single kingdom, Protozoa, Protista or Protoctista, disappears; and the second is that the new kingdom Protozoa is not equivalent to any previous grouping with that name (Table 7.1). For parasitologists, this is a mixed blessing; a well liked and familiar name is retained but it now means something completely different. Nevertheless, in this chapter the traditional approach will be adopted and the word protozoa (with a small initial letter) will be used when writing about the single celled organisms that infect humans, which should be properly classified with either the Archezoa or Protozoa. This reflects the tradition of parasitology and, in any case, any other alternative is so cumbersome as to be confusing, if not useless.

5 INSTABILITY IN THE PHYLA AND CLASSES

When the Animalia was recognized as a kingdom, the Protozoa could be classified as a phylum and the subordinate groups as classes (Hyman 1940). However, with the creation of 3 kingdoms, the status of the protozoa was raised to that of a kingdom and the subordinate groups automatically became phyla. Now that the protozoa have been divided between 3 kingdoms, certain groups that previously enjoyed ordinal status have now been elevated to classes or even phyla. This causes a great deal of confusion and requires some explanation. Goldfuss (1818) established the concept of 3 great groups of protozoa (amoebae, flagellates and ciliates) on the basis of their mode of locomotion and this number was increased to 4 by the addition of the sporozoans by Butschli (1883). These 4 groups persisted in various guises until comparatively recently, as the Rhizopoda or Sarcodina (amoebae, protozoa that move by means of pseudopodia), Mastigophora (flagellates, protozoa that move by means of flagella), Ciliophora or Ciliata (ciliates, protozoa that move by means of cilia) and Sporozoa (sporozoans, protozoa that do not have any obvious means of locomotion). This will be referred to here as the traditional classification as used in classical works by Calkins (1901), Craig (1926), Wenyon (1926), Kudo (1954) and Manwell (1961). By the beginning of the 1960s, with the availability of increasingly sophisticated ways of studying protozoa, it was becoming clear that this classification was unworkable and in 1964 the Society of Protozoologists published a revised classification (Honigberg et al. 1964). This grouped the Sarcodina and Mastigophora together as the Sarcomastigophora and removed the myxosporidians and microsporidians from the Sporozoa, with which they had been traditionally classified. One particularly controversial action was to remove the piroplasms from the Sporozoa and to place them among the Sarcomastigophora, something that was resented and ignored by most protozoologists and virtually all parasitologists. The Society of Protozoologists' 1964 classification, with slight modifications (e.g. the replacement of the piroplasms among the Sporozoa) was widely accepted and appeared in standard textbooks such as those by Baker (1969) and Levine (1973). Subsequent changes involving *Toxoplasma* and related organisms were gradually incorporated into the 1964 scheme and a consensus classification, such as that of Baker, (1977) gradually emerged.

This consensus did not last long and rapid and major developments in our understanding of the protozoa necessitated a new classification and, in 1980, the Society of Protozoologists published its second classification (Levine et al. 1980). The working party responsible for this classification recognized that the protozoa did not represent an assemblage of primitive organisms but embraced a number of diverse and distinct groups. The 1980 classification recognized 7 phyla: Sarcomastigophora, Apicomplexa (essentially equivalent to the Sporozoa), Ciliophora, Microspora, Myxozoa, Ascetospora and Labyrinthomorpha. Nevertheless, the affinities with the traditional classification remained clear and a modification which took into account only the parasitic forms was described by Cox (1981) and used in information retrieval systems and parasitology textbooks such as Cox (1982), Kreier and Baker (1987) and Mehlhorn (1988). Like its predecessors, this scheme failed to keep up with developments and by 1985 the time was ripe for another look at the classification of the protozoa (Lee, Hutner and Bovee 1985). By the beginning of this decade, Sleigh (1991) had decided to ignore the concept of phyla and to simply recognize 4 'groups': the flagellated protozoa, the amoeboid protozoa, the ciliated protozoa and the sporozoans.

This approach, also adopted by Cox (1991, 1993), has the merit of simplicity and clear links with the traditional classification but is merely a classification of convenience and does not stand up to rigorous analysis at either the evolutionary or molecular level. Therefore, the classification suggested by Corliss will be adopted as a basis for a more rational classification of the parasitic protozoa.

6 TRADITIONAL CLASSIFICATIONS

Below is an outline version of the traditional classification typical of the ones still in use such as that outlined by Orihel and Ash (1995) based on Lee, Hutner and Bovee (1985). Here, this classification is provided simply as background for further discussion and to focus on the central problem of protozoan classification; the need to satisfy protozoologists on one hand and the need to be useful to parasitologists, especially medical parasitologists, on the other.

Subkingdom Protozoa
Phylum Sarcomastigophora (The amoebae and flagellates)
Subphylum Mastigophora. Intestinal, tissue and blood dwelling flagellates e.g. *Giardia, Chilomastix, Trichomonas, Dientamoeba, Leishmania, Trypanosoma*
Subphylum Sarcodina. Obligate and facultative amoebae e.g. *Entamoeba, Iodamoeba, Endolimax, Acanthamoeba, Balamuthia, Naegleria*

Phylum Apicomplexa (the sporozoans)
Class Sporozoea
Subclass Coccidia
Order Eucoccidiida
Suborder Eimeriina e.g. *Isospora, Sarcocystis, Toxoplasma, Cryptosporidium, Cyclospora*
Suborder Haemosporina e.g. *Plasmodium*
Subclass Piroplasmea e.g. *Babesia*

Phylum Microspora
Enterocytozoon, Encephalitozoon, Septata
Phylum Ciliophora (the ciliates) *Balantidium*

7 A UTILITARIAN CLASSIFICATION OF THE PARASITIC PROTOZOA OF HUMANS

There is, at present, no entirely satisfactory and universally accepted scheme for the classification of the protozoa, nor is there likely to be for some time to come. In recent years, the availability of a number of molecular markers has made it possible to analyze relationships between protozoans and to draw conclusions that would not have been possible using morphological characters alone. So far, there has been remarkable agreement between the different approaches and, in most cases, molecular techniques have confirmed the more traditional findings; in other cases they have clarified long standing controversies. In the long run, it is likely that molecular classifications of the protozoa will be the norm but until these can be applied to more than a handful of species there is a need for an interim workable categorization. Corliss (1994) has produced such an outline classification of the 200 000 or more free-living and parasitic protozoa, designed to fill the gap between the existing, unsatisfactory schemes and some perfect scheme yet to be devised. In his scheme he has used both traditional and contemporary approaches and has attempted to retain familiar names as far as possible. This laudable approach should be welcomed by the majority of parasitologists whose needs and habits do not necessarily involve them in the minutiae of systematics or the precise arguments of nomenclature. What most parasitologists require is a convenient, familiar and stable framework within which to work and communicate. Parasitologists in general are concerned with only relatively few species of protozoa and those interested in the parasitic protozoa of humans need to be familiar with only c. 20 genera and 50 species. It is therefore important that any classification should reflect modern thinking about the classification of the protozoa as a whole, while retaining sufficient traditional material to permit easy reference to past papers, textbooks and information retrieval systems. Such a classification must, of necessity, be a compromise and therefore the one outlined below is based on that of Corliss (1994) and is the one likely to be used most widely by the majority of protozoologists. However, this classification is not entirely satisfactory for parasitologists and the main points of controversy are discussed after the outline classification.

7.1   An outline classification of the parasitic protozoa of humans

Empire Eukaryota

Kingdom Archezoa Haeckel, 1894

Single celled eukaryotic organisms lacking plastids, mitochondria, hydrogenosomes, peroxisomes and Golgi bodies and exhibiting various prokaryotic features in their ribosomes and tRNA. Three phyla, comprising several classes and orders, of which 2 contain parasites of humans.

Phylum Metamonada
Possess 2, 4 or 8 (occasionally more) flagella.
Class Trepomonadea
1 or 2 karyomastigonts each with 1–4 flagella; no contractile axostyle; few cell surface cortical microtubules.
Order Diplomonadida. Genus *Giardia*
Order Enteromonadida. Genus *Enteromonas*
Class Retortamonadea
Cortical microtubules over entire body surface.
Order Retortamonadida. Genera *Chilomastix, Retortamonas*
Phylum Microspora
No flagellated stage in life-cycle; resistant spores containing extrusion apparatus and infective body.
Class Microsporea
Complex extrusion apparatus with coiled polar tube.
Order Microsporida. Genera *Encephalitozoon, Enterocytozoon, Nosema, Septata, Trachipleistophora*

Kingdom Protozoa Goldfuss 1818
Unicellular, plasmodial or colonial colourless phagotrophic organisms that typically possess tubular cristate mitochondria, Golgi bodies and peroxisomes. Fourteen phyla, comprising numerous classes and orders, of which 6 contain parasites of humans.

Phylum Percolozoa
Unicellular, non-pigmented organisms typically possessing 1–4 flagella, mitochondria and peroxisomes but lacking Golgi bodies.
Class Heterolobosea
The amoeboflagellates; trophic form amoeboid and temporary flagellated phase in life-cycle.
Order Schizopyrenida. Genus *Naegleria*
Phylum Parabasala
Unicellular flagellates with numerous flagella and one or more nuclei. 70S ribosomes, characteristic complex parabasal body equivalent of Golgi body, no mitochondria.
Class Trichomonadea
Typically 4–6 flagella and non-contractile axostyle.
Order Trichomonadida. Genera *Dientamoeba, Trichomonas*

Phylum Euglenozoa
Unicellular flagellates with 1–4 flagella, Golgi body and mitochondria.
Class Kinetoplastidea
Unicellular flagellates with 1–2 flagella, prominent kinetoplast (DNA-containing body) within a single mitochondrion.
Order Trypanosomatida. Genera *Leishmania, Trypanosoma*

Phylum Ciliophora
Unicellular organisms typically with rows of cilia; one or more polyploid macronuclei and diploid micronuclei.
Class Litostomatea
Inconspicuous oral ciliature.
Order Vestibuliferida. Genus *Balantidium*
Phylum Apicomplexa (Sporozoa)
Unicellular organisms possessing at some stage an apical complex composed of polar rings, rhoptries, micronemes and typically a conoid; elaborate life-cycles involving a sexual process; all parasites.
Class Coccidea
Sexual stages small and intracellular usually in epithelial cells of vertebrate host; resistant oocyst.
Order Eimeriida. Genera *Cryptosporidium, Cyclospora, Isospora, Sarcocystis, Toxoplasma*
Class Haematozoea
Sexual stages in blood of vertebrate host and in blood sucking arthropod.
Order Haemosporida. Genus *Plasmodium*
Order Piroplasmida. Genus *Babesia*

Phylum Rhizopoda
Unicellular non-flagellated organisms using pseudopodia for both feeding and locomotion.
Class Lobosea
Lobose or filiform pseudopodia
Order Acanthopodida. Genera *Acanthamoeba, Balamuthia*
Class Entamoebidea
Lobose pseudopodia; no mitochondria, peroxisomes or hydrogenosomes.
Order Euamoebida. Genera *Endolimax, Entamoeba, Iodamoeba*

Kingdom Chromista Cavalier-Smith, 1981
Unicellular filamentous or colonial phototrophic organisms

Kingdom Plantae Linnaeus 1753
The plant kingdom *sensu strictu*

Kingdom Fungi Linnaeus 1753
The fungi *sensu strictu*

Kingdom Animalia Linnaeus 1753
The animal kingdom *sensu strictu*

7.2 Comments on the outline classification

This classification retains many of the familiar features of more recent traditional classifications such as that of Cox (1991, 1993) but there are a number of differences that require some comment.

Kingdom Archezoa

It is now clear that the flagellated protozoa do not constitute a coherent group and all the evidence available suggests that a number of amitochondrial flagellates and amoebae, together with the microsporidians, represent a distinct primitive kingdom, the affinities of which are obscure.

The flagellated archezoans: *Giardia, Enteromonas, Chilomastix* and *Retortamonas*

These genera, which contain the flagellated species *Giardia duodenalis Enteromonas hominis, Chilomastix mesnili* and *Retortamonas intestinalis* (parasites of the human intestine) have been traditionally classified with a number of other flagellates within the phylum or subphylum Mastigophora. They have now been placed in a separate kingdom, Archezoa, in the phylum, Metamodada. Most protozoologists, largely basing their evidence on rRNA, now regard *Giardia* as very primitive and consider that it represents a very early stage of eukaryote evolution and that in any overall evolutionarily sound scheme it should be placed in some basal, pivotal position. Parallels between *Giardia* and the other genera listed suggest that they should all be grouped together in the same phylum and that *Giardia* and *Enteromonas* should be in one class and *Chilomastix* and *Retortamonas* in another. This classification clearly separates these flagellates from members of the Trichomonadida, containing the genera *Trichomonas* and *Dientamoeba*, with which they have traditionally been loosely grouped. This should present no problems for parasitologists, except that it might be confusing to find that these familiar parasites are no longer classified with the Protozoa *sensu stricto*. However, Corliss (1994) comments that some protozoologists believe that the whole of the phylum Parabasala, which contains the Trichomonadida, should be classified with the Archezoa and this would bring all these flagellated protozoa of humans closer together again.

The microsporidians: *Encephalitozoon, Enterocytozoon, Nosema, Trachipleistophora* and *Septata*

These tissue-inhabiting parasites have had a chequered history, first being classified with the Sporozoa, later in a group with the myxosporidians and now in a phylum of their own. This new classification seems eminently sensible and, as these species are becoming increasingly recognized as significant concomitants of HIV infections, it is important that they are not neglected on some classificatory sideline. However, microsporidians do possess spores with clearly recognizable characteristics and those working with these organisms have developed classifications in parallel with other single celled organisms (see, for example, Sprague, Becnel and Hazard 1992).

Kingdom Protozoa

The amoeboflagellates: *Naegleria*

These freshwater forms are occasional accidental parasites of humans. In previous classifications they have been placed either in the phylum Rhizopoda with the obligate parasitic amoebae, such as *Entamoeba*, and the other facultative organisms such as *Acanthamoeba*, or with the flagellated protozoa. There is now no doubt that these organisms should be classified with a number of other free-living protozoa in a separate class from the other amoebae, with which they share only superficial similarities.

The intestinal and related flagellates: *Dientamoeba* and *Trichomonas*

There is nothing new here except that *Dientamoeba fragilis* (parasitic in the intestine) and 3 species of *Trichomonas, T. vaginalis, T. tenax* and *T. gingivalis* (parasitic respectively in the urogenital system, intestine and mouth) are no longer classified with the other intestinal flagellates. *Dientamoeba* has no flagellum and is permanently amoeboid and was thus once classified with the amoebae; there is now no doubt that it is a flagellate and should be classified with *Trichomonas*.

The blood and tissue flagellates: *Leishmania* and *Trypanosoma*

These important genera include *Trypanosoma brucei gambiense, T.b. rhodesiense*, the causative agents of sleeping sickness in Africa, *T. cruzi*, which causes Chagas disease in South America and several species of *Leishmania* which cause a variety of diseases from oriental sore to kala azar. They have long been recognized as comprising a distinct assemblage which has been given several names, ranging from the order Kinetoplastida to the phylum Kinetoplasta. In the new classification, they are placed close to their free-living relatives, which should be satisfactory for both parasitologists and protozoologists.

The ciliated protozoa: *Balantidium*

The phylum Ciliophora contains ciliated protozoa that all possess distinctive patterns of ciliary distribution and can thus be classified satisfactorily on morphological grounds. *Balantidium coli* is the only ciliate that infects humans and, although in the past its taxonomic position has been uncertain, it is now accepted by most protozoologists that it is now correctly classified in the phylum Ciliophora, class Litostomatea and order Vestibuliferida. *Balantidium coli* is not an important parasite and is readily recognized so its classification is of little interest to most parasitologists.

The sporozoans

This group originally contained a heterogeneous collection of spore-forming single celled organisms including, at one time, the microsporidians, now classified in the kingdom Archezoa. The phylum Apicomplexa, with the exception of the class Perkinsea, an enigmatic group containing 2 genera, is identical with the Sporozoa established by Leuckart (1879). Few parasitiologists like or accept the phylum name Apicomplexa and many will be bitterly disappointed that it has not been replaced by the phylum Sporozoa, which has both priority and common usage. The traditional sporozoans (that is, all except the members of the class Perkinsea) possess sufficient common morphological features and life-cycles to justify this position, which is supported by studies at the molecular level. In the classification advocated here, Sporozoa will be adopted as an alternative to the phylum Apicomplexa as it has been elsewhere (Cox 1991).

The coccidians: *Isospora, Sarcocystis* and *Toxoplasma*

Members of this group are either parasites that undergo the whole of their life-cycle in a single host, typically in the epithelial cells of the gut, or divide a similar cycle between 2 hosts. Until the early 1970s these parasites were known only from miscellaneous stages in their hosts but since then they have been classified as a tight assemblage on the grounds of morphology, life-cycle and molecular similarities. Currently, the species recognized are *Isospora belli, Sarcocystis hominis, S. bovihominis, S. suihominis* and *Toxoplasma gondii*. Although there may be some controversy about their exact identity and relationships, there is no doubt that they are satisfactorily accommodated in the phylum Sporozoa, Class Coccidea and Order Eimeriida.

The haemosporidans: *Plasmodium* and *Babesia*

These parasites occur in the blood of their vertebrate hosts and they have been extensively studied, largely because members of the genus *Plasmodium* cause malaria and members of the genus *Babesia* cause red water fever and other important diseases in cattle. Corliss' class Haematozoa contains 2 orders; Haemosporida, containing the genus *Plasmodium*, and Piroplasmida, containing members of the genus *Babesia* which are rare and accidental parasites of humans. There can be little dispute about the classification of the Haemosporida which is conventional and well accepted. The piroplasms have had a more chequered history, originally being described as sporozoans as long ago as 1889 (Smith and Kilbourne 1893),

regarded as a suborder by Wenyon (1926), transferred to the amoebae (Honigberg et al. 1964), elevated to the level of a subclass of the class Sporozoa (Levine et al. 1980) and a class (Cox 1991). The proposed classification serves one specifically important purpose in that it does bring the malaria parasites and piroplasms close together in the same class, but superficial similarities are outweighed by fundamental differences and these are sufficient to justify further separation of the 2 groups, either as subclasses or classes.

The amoebae: *Acanthamoeba, Endolimax, Entamoeba* and *Iodamoeba*

The arguments for keeping all these amoebae together in one phylum, Rhizopoda, are very sound, as are the arguments for placing *Acanthamoeba* spp. (accidental parasites of humans) in one class, Lobosea, and the obligate species, *Entamoeba histolytica*, in another, Entamoebidea. This classification is essentially a traditional one and is likely to be acceptable to parasitologists. Although it is currently accepted that *Entamoeba* belongs to the phylum Rhizopoda there is some doubt about its relationship with the other genera, *Endolimax* and *Iodamoeba*, which have not been properly characterized. None has mitochondria, peroxisomes or hydrogenosomes, suggesting that they are very primitive, and Corliss (1994) comments that some protozoologists consider that these genera really belong to the Archezoa. The confusingly named flagella-less flagellate, *Dientamoeba*, is now classified in the class Trichomonadea in the phylum Parabasala.

In summary, the proposed utilitarian classification (Corliss 1994) can accommodate the parasitic protozoa of humans without creating any undue confusion.

8 GENERA AND SPECIES: OASES OF STABILITY

The names of the genera and species of protozoa that infect humans have been remarkably consistent throughout the upheavals that have characterized the classification of the protozoa over the past few years and many can be traced back to their original descriptions. The main changes have been the omission of the enigmatic species *Blastocystis hominis* and *Pneumocystis carinii*, now usually classified among the fungi, and the addition of species of the coccidians *Cryptosporidium* and *Cyclospora* and the microsporidians *Encephalitozoon, Enterocytozoon* and *Septata*, largely as concomitants of HIV infections, and *Balamuthia* as an accidental infection. In addition, previously unidentified tissue parasites have now been identified as *Sarcocystis* spp. The other main change has been the growth in the number of species in the genus *Leishmania*.

The increase in the number of parasitic protozoa recorded from humans and the accumulation of knowledge about their biology has resulted in the creation of taxonomic and other groupings at the subgenus and subspecies levels, largely as a result of an unwillingness to tamper with well established genera and species. As all the protozoa parasitic in humans have traditionally been classified with the animal kingdom, the International Code of Zoological Nomenclature applies to the naming of the subordinate groups subgenera and subspecies. However, as the rules have not been applied rigorously group by group, several apparent anomalies have arisen and the use of subgenera, species and subspecies across the whole of the parasitic protozoa has not been uniform.

Among the amoebae, the only controversy relates to the most important parasite, *Entamoeba histolytica*. For many years it has been known that this parasite exists in 2 forms, one pathogenic and one non-pathogenic. This has resulted in some workers suggesting that the pathogenic form *sensu strictu* should be called *E. histolytica* and the non-pathogenic form something different, for example *E. dispar* as suggested by Brumpt (1925). Previously, most people were content to use one name, *E. histolytica*, but isoenzyme and other biochemical and molecular studies have confirmed the differences between the pathogenic and non-pathogenic forms and have led a number of workers to suggest the reintroduction of *E. dispar* for the non-pathogenic form. Unfortunately, things are not that simple and there have been reports that some of the biochemical criteria used are not stable (Spice and Ackers 1992). Nevertheless, it seems sensible to use the 2 specific names for which there is some precedence.

The genus *Leishmania* has received the most attention. Originally there were 2 Old World species; the cutaneous form *L. tropica* and the visceral form *L. donovani*. *L. tropica* was subsequently differentiated as 2 varieties, *L. tropica* var. *minor* and *L. tropica* var. *major*, and later subspecies, *L. t. minor* and *L. t. major*, which have now been raised to species level as *L. tropica* and *L. major*. Two subspecies of *L. donovani*, *L. d. donovani* and *L. d. infantum*, have now been raised to species level, as *L. donovani* and *L. infantum*, as has *L. donovani* var. *archibaldi*. In the New World, it was originally thought that the leishmanias there were varieties of the Old World forms and the cutaneous form was called *L. tropica* var. *mexicana*, later changed to *L. mexicana*, and the mucocutaneous form was called *L. tropica* var. *braziliensis*, subsequently *L. braziliensis*. The New World visceral form of *L. donovani* subsequently became *L. d. chagasi* and then *L. chagasi*. The cutaneous forms have undergone massive revisions as more and more subspecies or species have been discovered. Initially, each new discovery was assigned either to *L. mexicana* or *L. braziliensis* as a subspecies, for example *L. b. braziliensis*, a practice that is occasionally still adopted, although current opinion favours the use of species. Recognition of the fact that these species could and should be grouped as the 'mexicana complex' and the 'braziliensis complex' led to the creation of 2 subgenera; *Leishmania*, which embraces all the Old World species and members of the 'mexicana complex' and *Viannia*, which includes the 'braziliensis' complex. A detailed account of this classification and its background is given by Lainson and Shaw (1987). It should be pointed out here that the classification of the leishmanias is now based on morpho-

logical, behavioural, geographical, clinical, biochemical and molecular criteria, and this will be returned to later (see also Chapter 13).

Subgenera and subspecies have also been used for the classification of the trypanosomes, *Trypanosoma* spp. Large numbers of trypanosomes parasitise all groups of vertebrates and, in an attempt to put some kind of order into what was becoming an increasingly heterogeneous genus, Hoare, in 1966, proposed the creation of a number of subgenera as a framework within which to classify the trypanosomes of mammals (see Hoare 1972). These subgenera were placed in 2 major groups; Stercoraria, containing *Megatrypanum*, *Herpetosoma*, and *Schizotrypanum*, and Salivaria, containing *Duttonella*, *Nannomonas*, *Pycnomonas* and *Trypanozoon*. The New World trypanosome of humans, *T. cruzi*, is classified in the subgenus *Schizotrypanum* and *T. rangeli* is placed in the subgenus *Herpetosoma*, whereas both the Old World forms, *T. brucei gambiense* and *T. b. rhodesiense*, are placed in the subclass *Trypanozoon*. This system both clarified the existing situation and also confused it. Most observers agree that *T. cruzi* is very different from *T. brucei* and its subspecies and the opportunity to emphasize the differences was welcomed. The use of the subgeneric name *Schizotrypanum* was quickly adopted, as was the use of *Trypanozoon* (see, for example, Lumsden and Evans 1976). However, the use of *Trypanosoma (Schizotrypanum) cruzi* and *Trypanosoma (Trypanozoon) brucei* was clumsy and the practice has now all but been abandoned.

The use of subspecific names is another matter. Human sleeping sickness in Africa is caused by 2 different trypanosomes both closely related to a natural parasite of equines and game, *Trypanosoma brucei*. The 2 human forms have sometimes been recognized as species, *T. gambiense* and *T. rhodesiense* (Levine 1973), but using all the available morphological, clinical, epidemiological, biochemical and molecular criteria there can be no doubt of the close relationship between the 2 human forms and between the human forms and the animal forms; the only logical conclusion is that they should be classified as *T. brucei gambiense* and *T. brucei rhodesiense*, whereas the animal form is *T. brucei brucei*. This approach has been adopted by the majority of workers in the field and by information retrieval services. The widespread use of these subspecies was partly responsible for the demise of the use of subgenera because most authors and editors did not want to be bothered with names like *Trypanosoma (Trypanozoon) brucei gambiense*.

The classification and nomenclature of the human trypanosomes is still not entirely satisfactory at the level of genus and species. There are real differences between *T. brucei* and its subspecies and *T. cruzi* and it would seem logical to classify them as separate genera. However, this cannot be done in isolation as there would be serious consequences for the classification of all the other trypanosomes of vertebrates and great disruption to the information retrieval systems if one of the 2 generic names were to change. At a subspecific level, there is increasing evidence that different strains of *T. cruzi* are so divergent that the creation of subspecies might be both necessary and helpful (see also Chapter 15).

The malaria parasites belonging to the genus *Plasmodium* have also been classified into subgenera largely on the same grounds as the trypanosomes; the numbers recorded in all groups of higher vertebrates and a perceived need to bring some order into the increasingly complex situation. Nine subgenera were proposed: *Plasmodium*, *Vinckeia*, *Laverania*, *Haemamoeba*, *Giovannolaia*, *Noyella*, *Huffia*, *Sauramoeba* and *Carinia*, of which 3 occur in mammals, 4 in birds and 2 in lizards (Garnham 1966). The human species, *Plasmodium falciparum*, was placed in the subgenus *Laverania* whereas the others, *P. malariae*, *P. ovale* and *P. vivax*, were placed in the subgenus *Plasmodium*. As far as human parasites are concerned, the use of subgenera served very little purpose and has fallen into disuse.

9 CLASSIFICATION BELOW THE SPECIES LEVEL

It has already been pointed out that the use of subspecies has been relatively common among protozoologists but in the genus *Leishmania*, in which it was most widely used, this practice has fallen into disuse. The only remaining consistent use of subspecies is in the case of the African trypanosomes, *T. brucei gambiense* and *T. brucei rhodesiense*. Nevertheless, there is a perceived need for some sort of category below that of species to differentiate between genetically distinct forms of parasites that produce markedly different diseases in humans. This has been formalized in the case of the leishmanias, in which there has been an incremental drift upwards towards separate species status. This tendency has been resisted by those working with the African trypanosomes. *Trypanosoma cruzi*, the causative agent of Chagas disease in South America, is an interesting case. There is no doubt that there are many different forms of *T. cruzi* and that their epidemiology and the diseases they produce are significantly different. Thus there seems to be a *de facto* case for the consideration of subspecies, but there has been little enthusiasm for such a move.

For many years it has been clear that amoebiasis manifests itself in 2 quite distinct ways; either as an asymptomatic infection or one that is accompanied by quite severe dysentery, ulceration and sometimes liver involvement. It has been suggested that the extremes of infection may caused by 2 species, by 2 races of the same species or by one species that produces different outcomes in different individuals. Current opinion favours the acknowledgement of the fact that there are 2 genetically distinct forms of *Entamoeba histolytica*, suggesting 2 species; *E. histolytica*, the pathogenic form, and *E. dispar* the non-pathogenic form, or 2 races of the same species. Because pathogenicity does not seem to be a stable characteristic the situation remains unresolved.

Giardia duodenalis is another intestinal parasite that causes a range of symptoms and what actually constitutes this species remains to be resolved, mainly because of the genetic variability that exists even within cloned lines (Thompson, Reynoldson and Lymbery 1993). There is little agreement about what the species name should actually be and *G. intestinalis* and *G. duodenalis* tend to be used interchangeably in western Europe and Australia, *G. lamblia* is used in the USA and *Lamblia intestinalis* is used in eastern Europe. Electrophoretic analysis suggests that the species in humans is morphologically *G. duodenalis*, which parasitises a number of mammals, but that it could be afforded specific status as *G. intestinalis* on grounds of host specificity (Mayrhofer et al. 1995). Whether or not there is a case for subspecific categories for the *Giardia* species in humans is still debatable.

Toxoplasma gondii is another parasite that seems to exist in 2 forms, a virulent one and an avirulent one, and it is also very interesting to note that a single strain of *T. gondii* probably accounts for all the virulent forms world wide (Sibley and Boothroyd 1992). Sibley and Boothroyd examined 28 strains of *T. gondii* from a variety of hosts from 5 continents and, using molecular and biochemical techniques, found that all the virulent strains were identical; thus all such infections must represent a single clonal lineage that has remained homogeneous despite the parasite's ability to reproduce sexually and its dispersal in a range of intermediate hosts world wide. Interestingly, non-virulent stains are polymorphic (Sibley and Boothroyd 1992) suggesting that the genetic potential of *T. gondii* is still considerable.

10 MOLECULAR AND BIOCHEMICAL APPROACHES TO THE CLASSIFICATION OF THE PARASITIC PROTOZOA

Fortunately there are alternative approaches to the classification of protozoa and they are more susceptible than metazoa to analysis using the techniques of molecular biology. Such techniques are increasingly being used to resolve phylogenetic, and consequently taxonomic, questions.

The first, most widely used and probably the most useful technique, has been the use of **isoenzyme profiles** which have proved to be extremely useful tools for distinguishing between apparently identical parasites. Isoenzymes are enzymes that perform the same functions but have different mobilities in electric fields and can thus be distinguished very easily. The technique involves using a number of characteristic enzymes to type different populations of parasite isolates in parallel and to compare them with previously characterized standard controls. Populations of parasites with identical isoenzyme patterns are called 'zymodemes'. This technique has been successfully used to distinguish the various species of *Leishmania* and the results obtained have correlated well with epidemiological and clinical findings. Isoenzymes have also been used to distinguish between: the subspecies of African trypanosomes; pathogenic and non-pathogenic forms of *Entamoeba histolytica;* and pathogenic and non-pathogenic forms of *T. gondii*. They have also indicated considerable diversity in isolates of *G. duodenalis* (Tibayrenc 1993). Isoenzyme studies on *Cryptosporidium parvum* suggest that separate cycles of transmission exist between animal and human hosts (Awad-el-Kaeiem et al. 1995) and this may have some relevance to the classification of members of this genus. Isoenzyme studies on *Giardia* species have shown that there are a number of assemblages that might well be separated into distinct species. Currently the form that parasitises humans is called either *G. intestinalis* or *G. duodenalis*, on the basis of presumed host specificity, but isoenzyme studies indicate that there is as much variability within *G. intestinalis* isolates as there is between *G. intestinalis* and *G. duodenalis* (Mayrhofer et al. 1995).

Isoenzyme techniques do have the major disadvantage of being reliable only for distinguishing between organisms that are closely related (Richardson, Adams and Baverstock 1986) and **DNA and RNA technology** is increasingly being used both for the diagnosis of parasitic infections and for resolving taxonomic and phylogenetic problems. Briefly, both DNA and RNA can be used to determine evolutionary distances, as nucleotide sequences tend to diverge over time and to evolve at a more regular rate than do morphological characters. Differences in nucleotide sequences can, therefore, be compared and the more similar the sequences in 2 organisms the more likely it is that they are related; large numbers of such studies can be used to create realistic phylogenetic trees. Different kinds of RNA, particularly small nuclear RNA (16S and 18S snRNA) and small subunit ribosomal RNA (srRNA) have been extensively used for taxonomic and phylogenetic investigations and, although data are currently based on very few taxa, these techniques have been very useful. Johnson and Baverstock (1989) were the first to attempt to produce a comprehensive phylogenetic tree of the protozoa with special reference to the parasitic forms, using data derived from srRNA. They concluded that, although the protozoa as whole did not form a monophyletic assemblage, the trypanosomes and sporozoans *sensu strictu* were monophyletic. These authors also state that

'...the rapid sequencing of the srRNA gene...is a useful method for testing current hypotheses concerning the evolutionary relationships and hence classification of the protozoa.'

This prediction has stood the test of time and RNA sequences have confirmed the differences between pathogenic and non-pathogenic strains of *E. histolytica* determined by isoenzyme studies (Petri et al. 1993). They have also identified similarities between the Old World trypanosome *T. cruzi* and New World *T. brucei* and have distanced both from *Leishmania* species, thus confirming the current classification of the kinetoplastid flagellates (Maslov and Simpson 1995). Even with protozoa with well characterized morphological characteristics, albeit at the electron microscope level, srRNA studies can be useful and have shown that the microsporidians *Encephalitozoon cuniculi* and *E. hellem* are so similar to *Septata intestinalis* as to suggest that

the latter should be classified as *Encephalitozoon* (Hartskeerl et al. 1995). Ribosomal RNA studies using 18S rRNA have also shown that *Toxoplasma* and *Sarcocystis* are monophyletic and thus derived from a common ancestor (Ellis et al. 1995).

DNA methodology has also proved to be very useful. DNA probes have been extensively used for studies on *Leishmania* species both for diagnosis and for determining relationships. Initial studies that distinguished between the New World forms *L. mexicana* and *L. braziliensis* have now been extended to all species and, coupled with isoenzyme studies, have been largely responsible for the present classification of the genus. The development of the polymerase chain reaction (PCR) has revolutionized the use of DNA techniques in parasitology and has been used to confirm the existence of virulent and avirulent strains of *T. gondii* (Guo and Johnson 1995).

Another technique that is being used is **molecular karyotyping**, which involves measuring size differences between chromosomes; this has now been applied to New World *Leishmania* species and has confirmed conventional geographical groupings (Dujardin et al. 1995)

Increasingly, biochemical and molecular criteria are being used for the identification of new species and it is now unlikely that any future descriptions of protozoa lacking good morphological characteristics will be published and accepted unless the descriptions are soundly based at the genetic level.

No matter how carefully any one particular species is characterized, this is of little use to any overall classification, which needs to take into account the characteristics of a diversity of organisms. One of the most powerful tools available for the study of evolution is parsimony analysis (Sober 1988, Stewart 1993). Essentially what this means is that the simplest explanation consistent with the available data should be used to reach conclusions about phylogenetic relationships. The concept is not a new one and many biologists are familiar with it in another guise, that of Occam's razor, which holds that entities should not be multiplied beyond necessity, i.e. where there is a simple explanation there is no need to look for a complex one. Parsimony analysis relies on the availability of raw data and, in the phylogenetic studies with which we are concerned here, these include morphology, lifecycles and molecular data. The ideal is to create taxa that can be ranked in a hierarchical order that reflects the underlying phylogeny. This approach has obvious advantages but also less obvious disadvantages: 2 taxa may possess characters that are only superficially similar; too much emphasis may be placed on too few examples; and the rates of morphological or molecular change may not be the same in the different groups under consideration. The most satisfactory examples of parsimony analysis are where traditional and molecular approaches produce the same overall pattern, but these may present the greatest difficulties if the various criteria used (e.g. morphological and molecular) are both based on the same invalid assumptions. On the other hand, where different approaches produce conflicting results it is possible that in seeking an explanation for the discrepancies, a better understanding of the relationships will emerge.

11 FUTURE TRENDS

Even as this chapter is being written the Society of Protozoologists is contemplating yet another classification of the protozoa. A 2 tier system is proposed, in which the lower levels (the infrastructure) are to be the responsibility of the authors of the *Illustrated Guide* (Lee, Hutner and Bovee 1985), following conventional taxonomic procedures, each contribution contained within the rank of 'Phylum'. The superstructure is to be the responsibility of the Society's Committee on the Systematics and Evolution and is to adopt an innovative rankless hierarchy using vernacular terminology. What the outcome will be and how it will affect parasitologists remains to be seen, but as the literature on parasitic protozoa vastly outweighs that on the free-living protozoa it is likely that parasitologists will continue along the conservative pathway outlined in this chapter.

12 APPENDIX. A CHECK LIST OF THE PARASITIC PROTOZOA OF HUMANS

Intestinal amoebae
  Endolimax nana
  Entamoeba coli
  Entamoeba histolytica
  Entamoeba dispar
  Entamoeba gingivalis
  Iodamoeba butschlii

Facultative amoebae and flagellates
  Acanthamoeba spp
  Balamuthia mandrillaris
  Naegleria fowleri

Intestinal and tissue flagellates
  Chilomastix mesnili
  Dientamoeba fragilis
  Giardia duodenalis (G. intestinalis)
  Trichomonas gingivalis
  Trichomonas hominis
  Trichomonas vaginalis

Blood and related flagellates
Old World *Leishmania* species
  Leishmania (Leishmania) tropica
  Leishmania (Leishmania) major
  Leishmania (Leishmania) aethiopica
  Leishmania (Leishmania) donovani
  Leishmania (Leishmania) archibaldi

Leishmania (Leishmania) infantum

New World *Leishmania* species
  Leishmania (Leishmania) mexicana
  Leishmania (Leishmania) amazonensis
  Leishmania (Leishmania) pifanoi
  Leishmania (Leishmania) garnhami
  Leishmania (Leishmania) venezuelensis
  Leishmania (Leishmania) chagasi

  Leishmania (Viannia) braziliensis
  Leishmania (Viannia) colombiensis
  Leishmania (Viannia) guyanensis
  Leishmania (Viannia) lainsoni
  Leishmania (Viannia) naiffi
  Leishmania (Viannia) panamensis
  Leishmania (Viannia) peruviana
  Leishmania (Viannia) shawi

Old World trypanosomes
  Trypanosoma brucei gambiense
  Trypanosoma brucei rhodesiense

New World trypanosomes
  Trypanosoma cruzi
  Trypanosoma rangeli

Coccidians
  Cyclospora cayetanensis
  Cryptosporidium parvum
  Isospora belli
  Sarcocystis hominis
  Sarcocystis suihominis
  Sarcocystis bovihominis
  Toxoplasma gondii

Malaria parasites
  Plasmodium falciparum
  Plasmodium malariae
  Plasmodium ovale
  Plasmodium vivax

Piroplasms
  Babesia bovis
  Babesia microti

Microsporidians
  Encephalitozoon cuniculi
  Encephalitozoon hellem
  Enterocytozoon bieneusi
  Nosema connori
  Nosema corneum (Vittaforma corneae)
  Nosema ocularum
  Septata intestinalis (Encephalitozoon intestinalis)
  Trachipleistophora hominis

Ciliate
  Balantidium coli

REFERENCES

Awad-el-Kariem FM, Robinson HA, Dyson DA et al., 1995, Differentiation between human and animal strains of *Cryptosporidium parvum* using isoenzyme typing, *Parasitology*, **110**: 129–32.

Baker JR, 1969, *Parasitic Protozoa*, Hutchinson, London.

Baker JR, 1977, Systematics of parasitic protozoa, *Parasitic Protozoa*, 1st edn, vol. 1, ed Kreier JP, *Parasitic Protozoa*, Academic Press, New York, 35–56.

Brumpt E, 1925, Etude sommaire de l' *Entamoeba dispar* n.sp. Amibe et kystes quadrinuclées parasite de l'homme, *Bull Acad Méd (Paris)*, **94**: 943–52.

Butschli O, 1883, Protozoa, *Klassen und Ordnungen des Thier-ReichsBronn*, vol 1, ed Bronn HG, C F Winter, Liepzig.

Calkins GN, 1901, *The Protozoa*, Macmillan, London.

Canning EU, Hollister WS, 1992, Human infections with microsporidia, *Rev Med Microbiol*, **3**: 35–42.

Cavalier-Smith T, 1993, Kingdom Protozoa and its 18 phyla, *Microbiol Rev*, **57**: 953–94.

Chiodini P, 1994, A 'new' parasite: human infection with *Cyclospora cayetanensis*, *Trans R Soc Trop Med Hyg*, **57**: 369–71.

Cole FJ, 1926, *The History of Protozoology*, University of London Press, London.

Copeland HF, 1938, The kingdoms of organisms, *Quart Rev Biol*, **13**: 383–420.

Corliss JO, 1984, The Kingdom Protozoa and its 45 phyla, *BioSystems*, **17**: 87–126.

Corliss JO, 1994, An interim utilitarian ('user-friendly') hierarchical classification and characterization of the protists, *Acta Protozoologica*, **33**: 1–51.

Cox FEG, 1981, A new classification of parasitic protozoa, *Protozoological Abs*, **5**: 9–14.

Cox FEG (ed), 1982, *Modern Parasitology*, 1st edn, Blackwell Scientific Publications, Oxford, 3–4.

Cox FEG, 1991, Systematics of parasitic protozoa, *Parasitic Protozoa*, 2nd edn, vol 1, eds Kreier JP, Baker JR, Academic Press, San Diego, 55–80.

Cox FEG (ed), 1993, *Modern Parasitology*, 2nd edn, Blackwell Scientific Publications, Oxford, 1–2.

Craig CF, 1926, *A Manual of the Parasitic Protozoa of Man*, JP Lippincott, London, 1–2.

Curry A, Canning EU, 1993, Human microsporidiosis, *J Inf*, **27**: 229–36.

Dobell C, 1960, *Antony van Leeuwenhoek and his 'Little Animals'*, Dover edition, Dover, New York, 112–3.

Dujardin JC, Dujardin JP et al., 1995, Karyotype plasticity in neotropical *Leishmania*: an index for measuring genomic distance among *L.(V.) peruviana* and *L.(V.) braziliensis* populations, *Parasitology*, **110**: 21–30.

Ellis JT, Luton K et al., 1995, Phylogenetic relationships between *Toxoplasma* and *Sarcocystis* deduced from a comparison of 18S rDNA sequences, *Parasitology*, **110**: 521–8.

Garnham PCC, 1966, *Malaria Parasites and other Haemosporidia*, Blackwell Scientific Publications, Oxford.

Goldfuss GA, 1818, *Uber die Entwicklungsstufen des Thieres*, Nurenberg, 18, 21.

Guo Z-G, Johnson AM, 1995, Genetic characterization of *Toxoplasma gondii* strains by random amplified polymorphic DNA polymerase chain reaction, *Parasitology*, **111**: 127–32.

Haeckel E, 1876, *The History of Creation: or the Development of the Earth and its Inhabitants by the Action of Natural Causes*, Appleton, New York.

Hartskeerl RA, van Gool T et al., 1995, Genetic and immunological characterization of the microsporidian *Septata intestinalis* Cali, Kotler and Orenstein, 1993: reclassification to *Encephalitozoon intestinalis*, *Parasitology*, **110**: 277–85.

Hoare CA, 1972, *The Trypanosomes of Mammals*, Blackwell Scientific Publications.

Hogg J, 1860, On the distinctions of a plant and an animal and on a fourth kingdom of nature, *Edinburgh New Phil J*, **12**: 216–2.

Honigberg BM, Balamuth W et al., 1964, A revised classification of the phylum Protozoa, *J Protozool*, **11**: 7–20.

Hyman L, 1940, *The Invertebrates: Protozoa through Ctenophora*, McGraw-Hill, New York, 46–8.

Jahn TL, Jahn FF, 1949, *How to know the Protozoa*, William Brown, Dubuque Iowa.

Johnson AM, Baverstock PR, 1989, Rapid ribosomal RNA sequencing and the phylogenetic analysis of protists, *Parasitol Today*, **5**: 102–5.

Kreier JP, Baker JR, 1987, *Parasitic Protozoa*, Allen and Unwin, Boston.

Kudo RR, 1954, *Protozoology*, 4th edn, Charles C Thomas, Springfield, Illinois.

Lainson R, Shaw JJ, 1987, Evolution, classification and geographical distribution, *The Leishmaniases in Biology and Medicine*, vol 1, eds Peters W, Killick-Kendrick R, Academic Press, London, 1–120.

Lee JJ, Hutner SH, Bovee EC, 1985, *An Illustrated Guide to the Protozoa*, Society of Protozoologists, Lawrence, Kansas.

Leuckart K, 1879, *Allgemeine Naturgeschichter der Parasiten*, CF Winter, Leipsig.

Levine ND, 1973, *Protozoan Parasites of Domestic Animals and of Man*, 2nd edn, Burgess, Minneapolis.

Levine ND, Corliss JO et al., 1980, A newly revised classification of the Protozoa, *J Protozool*, **27**: 37–58.

Lipscomb D, 1991, Broad classification: The Kingdoms and the Protozoa, *Parasitic Protozoa*, 2nd edn, eds Kreier JP, Baker JR, Academic Press, San Diego, 81–127.

Lumsden WHR, Evans DA (eds), 1976, *Biology of the Kinetoplastida*, vol 1, Academic Press, London.

Manwell RD, 1961, *Introduction to Protozoology*, Edward Arnold, London.

Margulis L, Corliss JO et al. (eds), 1990, *Handbook of Protoctista*, Jones and Bartlett, Boston.

Maslov DA, Simpson L, 1995, Evolution of parasitism in kinetoplastic protozoa, *Parasitol Today*, **11**: 30–2.

Mayrhofer G, Andrews RH et al., 1995, Division of *Giardia* isolates from humans into two genetically distinct assemblages by electrophoretic analysis of enzymes encoded at 27 loci and comparison with *Giardia muris*, *Parasitology*, **111**: 11–17.

Mehlhorn H (ed), 1988, *Parasitology in Focus: Facts and Trends*, Springer-Verlag, Berlin.

Orihel TC, Ash LR, 1995, *Parasites in Human Tissues*, American Society of Clinical Pathologists, Chicago.

Petri WA, Clark CG et al., 1993, International seminar on amebiasis, *Parasitol Today*, **9**: 73–6.

Richardson BJ, Adams M, Baverstock PR, 1986, *Allozyme Electrophoresis*, Academic Press, New York.

Siebold CTE von, 1848, *Lehrbuch der vergleichenden Anatomie der wirbellosen Thiere*, Theil, Berlin.

Sibley LD, Boothroyd JC, 1992, Virulent strains of *Toxoplasma gondii* comprise a single clonal lineage, *Nature (London)*, **359**: 82–5.

Sleigh MA, 1991, The nature of protozoa, *Parasitic Protozoa*, 2nd edn, vol 1, eds Kreier JP, Baker JR, Academic Press, San Diego, 1–53.

Smith T, Kilborne FL, 1893, Investigations into the nature, causation and prevention of Texas or Southern cattle fever, *Bull Bureau Anim Indust*, **1**: 177–304.

Sober E, 1988, *Reconstructing the Past. Parsimony, Evolution and Inference*, MIT Press, Cambridge, Maryland.

Spice WM, Ackers JP, 1992, The amoeba enigma, *Parasitol Today*, **8**: 402–6.

Sprague V, Becnel JJ, Hazard EI, 1992, Taxonomy of phylum Microspora, *Crit Rev Microbiol*, **18**: 285–395.

Stewart CB, 1993, The powers and pitfalls of parsimony, *Nature (London)*, **361**: 603–7.

Thompson RCA, Reynoldson JA, Lymbery AJ, 1993, *Giardia -*

from molecules to disease and beyond, *Parasitol Today*, **9:** 313–5.

Tibayrenc M, 1993, *Entamoeba, Giardia* and *Toxoplasma*: clones or cryptic species?, *Parasitol Today*, **9:** 102–5.

Wenyon CM, 1926, *Protozoology. A Manual for Medical Men, Veterin-* *arians and Zoologists*, vols 1 and 2, Ballière Tindall and Cox, London.

Whittaker RH, 1969, New concepts of kingdoms of organisms, *Science*, **163:** 150– 60.

Chapter 8

Intestinal Amoebae

A Martínez-Palomo and M Espinosa Cantellano

1 INTRODUCTION

Six species of amoebae are commonly found in the human gastrointestinal tract, including 4 that belong to the genus *Entamoeba*: *E. histolytica*, *E. hartmanni*, *E. coli* and *E. dispar*, and 2 that do not: *Endolimax nana* and *Iodamoeba buetschlii*. *Dientamoeba fragilis*, long considered to be another intestinal amoebae, is now known to be an aberrant trichomonad. Only *E. histolytica* is of medical importance. It is the causative agent of amoebiasis, a potentially fatal disease. Other amoebae are of interest mainly because their trophozoites may be difficult to distinguish from those of *E. histolytica* by light microscopy. *E. dispar* deserves special mention as it is morphologically indistinguishable from *E. histolytica* and accounts for most of the asymptomatic infections that were previously assigned to *E. histolytica*.

Because of its clinical importance, most of this chapter will be devoted to *E. histolytica* although reference to the non-pathogenic *E. dispar* will necessarily be included in those sections where differentiation between these species is relevant. At the end of the chapter, brief consideration will be given to the other intestinal amoebae of humans, as well as to *E. moshkovskii* (the 'Laredo type' of which can be found in humans), *E. polecki* from pigs, *E. invadens* from reptiles and *E. chattoni* from monkeys. Additional information may be obtained from Martínez-Palomo (1982, 1986, 1993), Ravdin (1988) and Kretschmer (1990).

For the last 70 years, 2 of the most puzzling aspects of the biology of *E. histolytica* have been the unexplained variability of its pathogenic potential and the restriction of human invasive amoebiasis to certain geographical areas despite world-wide distribution of the parasite. The main debate has centred on the question of whether there are one or 2 species of *E. histolytica*. In 1925 the French parasitologist Brumpt proposed that invasive amoebiasis is produced by a species of amoeba with world-wide distribution that is biologically distinct, but morphologically similar, to non-pathogenic amoebae (Brumpt 1925). Apart from some isolated studies by Simic, there was nothing to refute or confirm this hypothesis for almost 50 years (Simic 1931). In the 1970s, differences in surface properties were found between strains of *E. histolytica* isolated from carriers and those obtained from patients with invasive amoebiasis (Martínez-Palomo, González-Robles and de la Torre 1973, Trissl et al. 1977, Trissl et al. 1978). Starting in 1978, Sargeaunt and colleagues applied an isoenzyme technique to thousands of isolates of amoebae obtained from several continents (Sargeaunt, Jackson and Simjee 1982). This technique is based on the analysis of band patterns obtained after gel electrophoresis of the enzymes hexokinase and phosphoglucomutase. It revealed that invasive amoebiasis is produced by strains that have characteristic isoenzyme patterns (zymodemes) distinct from those obtained from amoebae harboured by most carriers. Moreover, monoclonal antibodies specifically recognized amoebae belonging to pathogenic zymodemes (Strachan et al. 1988, Petri et al. 1990, Tachibana et al. 1990). Results obtained in 3 independent laboratories demonstrated conversion of isolates with non-pathogenic zymodemes to pathogenic ones during the process of axenization; this reopened the debate as to whether there are one or 2 species, the former normally existing as a commensal in the human intestine and, under conditions not understood, becoming pathogenic to the host (Mirelman et al. 1986, Andrews, Mentzoni and Bjorvatn 1990, Orozco 1992). The application of molecular biology to the field seems to have finally resolved the problem and it is now widely accepted that there are 2 species: *E. histolytica*, previously known as 'pathogenic' or 'invasive' *E. histolytica* and *E. dispar* formerly designated 'non-pathogenic' or 'non-invasive' *E. histolytica*. For a comprehensive review of the history of the debate, as well as the scientific evidence that supports the conclusion of the distinct natures of *E. histolytica* and *E. dispar*, the reader is referred to Spice and Ackers (1992), Diamond and Clark (1993) and Clark and Diamond (1993).

2 CLASSIFICATION

The most recent generally accepted taxonomic scheme for the Protozoa was adopted 15 years ago; in it, according to the Committee on Systematics and Evolution of the Society of Protozoologists, all the true amoebae in humans are grouped in the family Endamoebidae, order Amoebida, subclass Gymnamoebia, class Lobosea, superclass Rhizopoda, subphylum Sarcodina, phylum Sarcomastigophora (Levine et al. 1980). Since then, new data on the ultrastructure and the molecular biology of numerous species have rendered this classification of the Protozoa obsolete and a revision of this taxonomic scheme is needed (Cox 1992, Corliss 1994, and see Chapter 7 of this volume). In Corliss's proposed classification, the amoebae are all placed in the phylum Rhizopoda, class Entamoebidea. Within this class, they are classified in the order Endamoebida and the family Endamoebidae. *Dientamoeba* is now considered to be a flagellate.

The factors currently considered to be useful for differentiating *Entamoeba* from other amoebae have been summarized by Neal (1988) and include intrinsic characteristics such as morphology, type of nuclear division, type of movement, type of physiology, antigenic nature, nature of DNA, variability of isoenzymes and susceptibility to drugs. They also include extrinsic characteristics such as host specificity, virulence factors, behaviour in laboratory hosts and clinical effects.

3 STRUCTURE AND LIFE-CYCLE

3.1 The trophozoite

The motile form of *E. histolytica*, the trophozoite (Fig. 8.1), is a highly dynamic and pleomorphic cell whose form and motility are strongly affected by changes in temperature, pH, osmolarity and redox potential. Actively motile amoebae are elongated, with protruding lobopodia and a trailing uroid, whereas resting trophozoites tend to be spherical. The diameter of the cell varies between 10 and 60 μm, not only due to the pleomorphism of the parasite, but also to the feeding conditions: amoebae obtained directly from intestinal or liver lesions are generally larger (20–40 μm) than those found in non-dysenteric stools or in cultures (10–30 μm). The cell surface has numerous circular

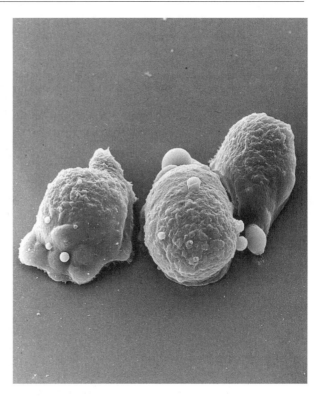

Fig. 8.1 Scanning electron micrograph of cultured trophozoites of *E. histolytica*. Note the rough appearance of the cell surface except in the regions of pseudopod extension. The parasite on the left shows a trailing uroid opposite to the pseudopod formations and abundant filopodia at the site of membrane attachment. A phagocytic opening of the membrane is clearly evident in the trophozoite located at the centre of the micrograph.

openings 0.2–0.4 μm in diameter that correspond to the mouths of micropinocytic vesicles. These openings are absent from the large protruding stomas of macropinocytic channels (2–6 μm in diameter) and from lobopodia. The uroid, when present, appears as a tail formed of irregular folds of the membrane and filiform processes called filopodia. Filopodia can also be found in other regions of the cell surface and are frequently observed in amoebae in monoxenic cultures or in contact with epithelial tissues (Martínez-Palomo 1982).

THE PLASMA MEMBRANE

The plasma membrane of *E. histolytica* is c. 10 nm thick and is covered by a uniform surface coat mainly composed of glycoproteins (Fig. 8.2). The binding of the lectin concanavalin A to the surface of the trophozoite suggests a high content of sugar residues (i.e., mannose, glucose). In actively motile trophozoites, a thin layer of material is deposited on the substrate, leaving a trail of microexudate with cytochemical properties similar to those of the surface coat (Martínez-Palomo 1982).

Interaction of the trophozoite plasma membrane with specific ligands induces a dramatic redistribution of surface components that accumulate at the uroid and are later released into the medium. This capping

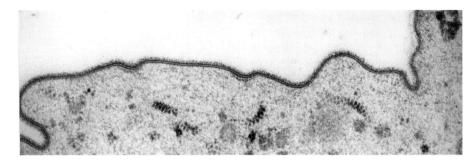

Fig. 8.2 Plasma membrane of a trophozoite of *E. histolytica* seen in a transmission electron micrograph of a cryofixed, cryosubstituted sample. A thick surface coat made of fibrilar material is clearly revealed with these techniques. The surface components shown here are usually lost during fixation and embedding by ordinary techniques. The section was counterstained with uranyl acetate and lead citrate only.

of surface molecules, suggested as a mechanism of evasion of the humoral immune response, occurs through a sliding mechanism that involves both actin and myosin and is regulated by calmodulin and a myosin light chain kinase (Espinosa-Cantellano and Martínez-Palomo 1994).

THE CYTOPLASM

The cytoplasm of *E. histolytica* trophozoites is characterized by the absence of most of the differentiated organelles found in other eukaryotic cells, i.e. mitochondria, Golgi apparatus, rough endoplasmic reticulum, centrioles and microtubules. Instead, the cytoplasm contains abundant vacuoles extremely variable in size, with diameters of 0.5–9.0 μm (Fig. 8.3). Some of these vacuoles have been identified using biochemical and ultrastructural techniques. They include phagocytic vacuoles, macropinocytic and micropinocytic vacuoles, lysosomes, residual bodies and autophagic vacuoles. Food vacuoles can be observed filled with starch or bacteria in amoebae in xenic and monoxenic cultures. Amoebae recovered from dysenteric stools usually contain ingested red blood cells; ingestion of red blood cells has traditionally been considered the best evidence of the invasive nature of the parasite. The lysosomes of amoebae differ from those of other eukaryotes in that the contained enzymes are bound to the lysosomal membrane rather than being free in the vacuolar compartment (Martínez-Palomo 1986). Our knowledge of this complex vacuolar system is mainly of the vacuoles involved in endocytic processes. The nature and functions of other vacuoles remain to be determined.

A lattice of tubules and vesicles superficially resembling smooth endoplasmic reticulum can very occasionally be found in the cytoplasm of *E. histolytica* trophozoites. The lattice is made up of extremely thin tubules of c. 20 nm in diameter forming irregular whorls or parallel arrays. In contrast to the 10 nm thick plasma and vacuolar membranes, the membrane enclosing these tubules is only 6 nm thick (Martínez-Palomo 1982).

Ribosomes appear to be mostly ordered in helical arrays c. 300 nm in length and 40 nm in diameter. In cysts and resting cultured trophozoites the helices aggregate in large crystalline inclusions that can be

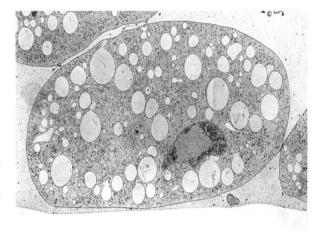

Fig. 8.3 Transmission electron micrograph of an *E. histolytica* trophozoite in culture. The ultrastructural appearance of the trophozoite is mainly characterized by the lack of mitochondria, a Golgi system, endoplasmic reticulum and cytoplasmic microtubules. Cryofixation and cryosubstitution of the sample provide a better preservation of cytoplasmic components than do standard procedures.

several micrometers in length, forming the classical chromatoid body with an hexagonal packing pattern. Whether ribosomes in helices and in chromatoid bodies are functionally mature ribosomes or ribosomal precursors remains to be established.

Despite the striking motility and plasticity of the trophozoite, little is known about the structural organization of its cytoskeleton. Prior to improvements in microscopy, only scarce microfilaments resembling actin (7 nm in diameter) were visible by transmission electron microscopy. They were located immediately below the plasma membrane. Regions known to concentrate actin contained a fibrogranular material with no evidence of structured filaments. The development of cryofixation and cryosubstitution allows much better preservation of biological materials and produces fewer artefacts than are induced by chemical fixation. This has improved the visualization of fine structure and has made it possible to observe more detail than through conventional techniques. Filaments with the appearance and size of actin have been visualized not only massed below the plasma membrane but also in pseudopodial extensions and phagocytic stoma. Moreover, filaments with the size and appearance of myosin, which were previously observed only in immunofluorescence preparations, have now been observed with transmission electron microscopy using these techniques. These studies have confirmed the absence of microtubules in both the cytoplasm and nuclei of non-dividing amoebae. Microtubules are known to be present in the nuclei of dividing trophozoites (González-Robles and Martínez-Palomo 1992).

The finding of cylindrical particles in the cytoplasm of *E. histolytica* has generated considerable interest. They are found in trophozoites obtained from such diverse sources as colonic exudates from patients with acute amoebic colitis, human liver lesions and axenic and polyxenic cultures. These particles are commonly arranged in rosettes and in thin sections of amoebae one or 2 rosette conglomerates are usually found surrounding a finely granular specialized area of the cytoplasm. Each conglomerate is c. 1 μm in diameter and is composed of 9–30 cylindrical bodies. The bodies vary in size and may be up to 250 nm in length and 90 nm in width, surrounded by a 7 nm thick membrane. They tend to be bullet shaped, although ocassionally they appear rounded at both ends. The morphological similarity of the cylindrical particles to rhabdoviruses and the cytochemical detection of a dense RNA-containing core in the rosette arrangements have led to speculation about their possible viral nature. There is, however, no conclusive evidence to date about their nature and biological significance.

THE NUCLEUS

The nucleus of *E. histolytica* is 4–7 μm in diameter. The nuclear membrane appears to be a double membrane, interrupted by numerous nuclear pores c. 65 nm in diameter, and lined by a thin uniform layer of granules, which gives the nucleus the appearance of a ring in optical section. Chromatin clumps are usually uniform in size and evenly distributed inside the nuclear membrane although in some cells the chromatin appears concentrated on one side as a crescentic mass. The karyosome or endosome is a small spherical mass, c. 0.5 μm in diameter, located in the central part of the nucleus. Intranuclear bodies 0.2–1.0 μm in diameter are frequently observed but their nature and function are unknown. Nuclear division proceeds without dissolution of the nuclear membrane and involves the participation of thick microtubule spindles, but the precise mechanism is unknown. Fluorescent dyes that bind to DNA reveal 6 DNA-containing plaques in dividing nuclei, probably corresponding to 6 chromosomes (Argüello, Valenzuela and Rangel 1992).

3.2   **The cyst**

Cysts have been studied far less extensively than trophozoites, mainly due to our inability to induce encystation in axenic cultures. Thus, most studies on *Entamoeba* cysts have been done on *E. invadens*, a parasite of reptiles that can be made to encyst in culture. *E. histolytica* cysts are round or slightly oval hyaline bodies

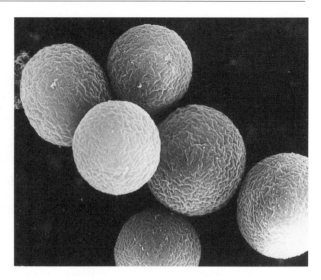

Fig. 8.4   Scanning electron micrograph of *E. histolytica* cysts recovered from faeces of a human carrier. The cyst wall allows the parasite to survive in a relatively hostile environment outside the host.

8–20 μm in diameter. They are surrounded by a refractile wall, 125–150 nm thick, apparently composed of fibrillar material. This forms a tight mesh and may give rise to several lamellae (Fig. 8.4). In *E. invadens* the cyst wall has been shown to contain chitin. The plasma membrane frequently has deep invaginations; polyribosomes and vacuoles containing dense fibrogranular material can be observed close to its cytoplasmic face. Food vacuoles tend to disappear as the cyst matures. Staining with iron-haematoxylin makes the cytoplasm appear vacuolated with numerous glycogen deposits that decrease in size and number as the cyst matures. Chromatoid bodies, which are aggregated ribosomes, can be identified inside the cytoplasm as rod shaped structures with blunt or rounded ends. Iodine stains allow the clear visualization of one to 4 small nuclei.

3.3   **The life-cycle**

Trophozoites dwell in the colon, where they multiply and encyst typically producing four-nucleated cysts. These appear in the formed stools of carriers as round or slightly oval hyaline bodies with a refractive wall. When a cyst is ingested, the cyst wall is dissolved in the upper gastrointestinal tract and the parasite excysts in the terminal ileum eventually giving rise to 8 uninucleated trophozoites. Cysts do not develop within tissues, but the invasive form of the parasite, the trophozoite, can penetrate the intestinal mucosa and disseminate to other organs. Trophozoites are short-lived outside the body and do not survive passage through the upper gastrointestinal tract. In contrast, cysts may remain viable in a humid environment and stay infective for several days.

4 BIOCHEMISTRY, MOLECULAR BIOLOGY AND GENETICS

4.1 Biochemistry

METABOLISM

The metabolism of *E. histolytica* is puzzling as it is a facultative aerobe with peculiar glycolytic enzymes of types also found in other amitochondriate eukaryotes like *Naegleria* and in certain bacteria. Glucose and, to a lesser extent, galactose are the main sources of energy. The uptake of glucose occurs via a specific transport system that provides c. 100 times the amount incorporated by endocytosis (Serrano and Reeves 1974). This transport system is the rate limiting step in glucose consumption. Glycogen is the main form of glucose storage.

Glucose-6-phosphate is degraded to pyruvate via the Embden-Meyerhof pathway. A unique aspect of glycolysis in *Entamoeba* is the utilization of inorganic pyrophosphate (PPi), generally considered an end product of metabolism, as an energy source in several glycolytic reactions (Mertens 1993). The genes coding for 2 of these enzymes, the third and last of the glycolytic pathway, have been cloned; pyrophosphate-dependent phosphofructokinase (PPi-PFK) (Huang et al. 1995) and pyruvate phosphate dikinase (PPDK) (Bruchhaus and Tannich 1993, Saavedra-Lira and Pérez-Montfort 1994). In addition, the primary structure of enolase, which catalyzes the conversion of 2-phosphoglycerate to phosphoenol pyruvate, has also been reported (Beanan and Bailey 1995).

The end products of pyruvate degradation depend on the degree of anaerobiosis; under aerobic conditions (5% oxygen concentration) acetate, ethanol and CO_2 are formed, whereas in an anaerobic environment only ethanol and CO_2 are produced. The enzymatic activities involved in this process include a pyruvate synthase, aldehyde dehydrogenase (ALDH) and both NAD^+ and $NADP^+$-linked alcohol dehydrogenases (ADH). The presence of a multifunctional NAD^+-dependent acetaldehyde–alcohol dehydrogenase, previously found only in anaerobic and facultative anaerobic bacteria, has now been reported (Bruchhaus and Tannich 1994, Yang et al. 1994). It has been suggested that during aerobiosis electrons are transferred from reduced substrates via a succession of carriers, including flavins, ferredoxin, other FeS proteins and ubiquinone, to molecular oxygen, which is reduced to water (Weinbach 1981, Ellis, Setchell and Kaneshiro 1994). The final electron acceptor under anaerobic conditions is not known.

Little is known about protein and nucleic acid metabolism in *Entamoeba* and even less about lipid synthesis and turnover (Reeves 1984, McLaughlin and Aley 1985, Avron and Chayen 1988).

E. histolytica is thought to be unique among eukaryotes in that it does not contain glutathione or glutathione-dependent enzymes (Fahey et al. 1984). In other organisms, the primary function of glutathione is to protect against oxygen toxicity. High concentrations of cysteine and other thiols have been identified in *Entamoeba*; these could carry out the functions of glutathione and its dependent enzymes (Fairlamb 1989). In addition, the presence of a disulphide oxidoreductase that binds FAD as a cofactor and can reduce alkyl hydroperoxides and H_2O_2 through NADH or NADPH has been suggested as a means of protection against damage by active oxidizing agents (Bruchhaus and Tannich 1995).

PLASMA MEMBRANE AND SURFACE MOLECULES

The biochemical characterization of cellular membranes and particularly of the plasma membrane is important for understanding host–parasite interactions. Progress in this field has been hampered by the presence of potent proteases, the unavailability of suitable enzyme markers in the parasite and the continuous turnover of surface membranes by endocytosis.

Membrane lipids have been studied both in whole extracts of trophozoites (Cerbón and Flores 1981) and in isolated plasma and internal membrane fractions (Aley, Scott and Cohn 1980). Cholesterol is enriched with phospholipid in the plasma membrane fraction to a molar ratio of 0.87, a finding consistent with previous reports in other types of cells. Phosphatidylethanolamine predominates over phosphatidylcholine in the plasma membrane, although the latter is the most abundant lipid in internal vesicles. An unusual phospholipid, ceramide aminoethyl phosphonate (CAEP) has been demonstrated in internal vesicles, but is mostly concentrated in the plasma membrane, where it accounts for 35% of the total lipid content (Aley, Scott and Cohn 1980). This may have biological importance as this compound is resistant to hydrolysis and may protect the parasite against the action of its own phospholipase.

Several surface molecules that mediate adhesion to cells or intestinal mucus are recognized by sera from patients cured of invasive amoebiasis. These include (1) a 260 kDa N-acetyl-D-galactosamine inhibitable lectin formed of 2 subunits, one of 170 and one of 35 kDa (Petri et al. 1989); (2) an N-acetylglucosamine inhibitable lectin of 220 kDa (Rosales-Encina et al. 1987); and (3) a 112 kDa surface adhesin (Arroyo and Orozco 1987). Antibodies raised against these proteins partially inhibit adhesion and phagocytosis of target cells in vitro, suggesting that the proteins participate in amoebic adherence. Other surface antigens identified by sera from patients include peptides of 30, 96 and 125 kDa, a serine rich *E. histolytica* protein and a lipopeptidophosphoglycan (reviewed in Espinosa-Cantellano and Martínez-Palomo 1991).

Among the enzymes identified in the plasma membrane of *E. histolytica* are Ca^{2+}–ATPase, phospholipase A, neuraminidase and a metallocollagenase thought to play an important role during parasite invasion (reviewed in Espinosa-Cantellano and Martínez-Palomo 1991). Cysteine proteases are the most abundant proteases present and have also been implicated in the pathogenicity of *E. histolytica* trophozoites (Keene et al. 1990). Four major cysteine proteases have been reported; (1) a 56 kDa cysteine protease (Keene et al. 1986); (2) a 26–29 kDa histolysin (Luaces and Barret 1988); (3) a 22–27 kDa amoebapain (Scholze et al. 1992) and (4) a 16 kDa cathepsin B-like protease (Lushbaugh, Hofbauer and Pittman 1985). The amoebic cysteine proteases are secreted enzymes and are thus mainly located in the internal vesicles, but some have been identified on the surface of the trophozoite.

Lytic factors

E. histolytica derives its name from its ability to lyse virtually every tissue in the human body and in the bodies of experimental animals (Fig. 8.5). Lysis of target cells involves contact-dependent as well as contact-independent mechanisms. Initial attachment of the trophozoite occurs via the amoebic adhesins described on p. 161. Once attached, it has been suggested that the parasite releases an active peptide, the amoeba-pore, that is capable of inserting ion channels into liposomes and that possesses cytolytic and bactericidal activities (Leippe et al. 1994). During the process of tissue invasion, degradation of extracellular matrix components (ECM) possibly involves specific receptors. A receptor common for fibronectin and laminin has been identified in trophozoites of *E. histolytica* (Talamás-Rohana, Hernández and Rosales-Encina

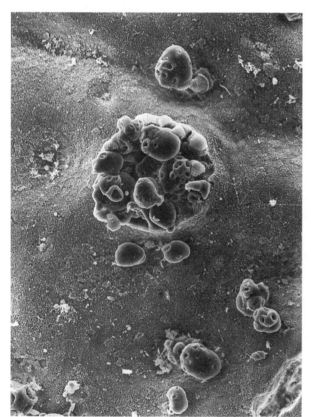

Fig. 8.5 Scanning electron micrograph of guinea pig caecal mucosa. A microulceration has been experimentally produced by administration of trophozoites of *E. histolytica*. This lesion exemplifies the earliest stage in the development of invasive intestinal amoebiasis.

1994). The actual degradation of ECM occurs as a result of action by the collagenase and secreted cysteine proteases that have been shown to be active against a wide variety of ECM proteins, including collagen, fibronectin, laminin and some proteoglycans. Interestingly, the expression of cysteine protease genes is 10- to 100-fold higher in pathogenic *E. histolytica* than in non-pathogenic *E. dispar* strains (Tannich et al. 1991b).

4.2 Molecular biology and genetics

The total DNA content is c. 0.5 pg DNA per cell, all of which concentrated in the nucleus; there are no DNA-containing organelles (Byers 1986). Cytological observations with fluorescent dyes that bind DNA demonstrate 6 areas of nuclear condensation that may correspond to chromatin organized as chromosomes (Argüello, Valenzuela and Rangel 1992). Molecular analysis indicates that there is a complex karyotype, 11–20 families of DNA molecules being noted in different studies (Orozco et al. 1993a, Petter et al. 1993) and differences in the numbers and sizes of these families have been identified not only among strains and species, but in different DNA preparations from the same strain. It has been suggested that these variations may be the result of massive DNA rearrangements.

In most other unicellular eukaryotes, rDNA is present intrachromosomally. In contrast, rDNA in *Entamoeba* seems to exist exclusively as extrachromosomal circular molecules (Bhattacharya et al. 1989, Huber et al. 1989). This peculiar characteristic is also shared by *Naegleria*.

Various circular DNA molecules that are not circular rDNA have been detected by Southern blot analysis (Dhar et al. 1995). The fact that such circular DNA exists in the nucleus is supported by the identification (through hybridization with various cDNA clones) of protein-coding regions in exonuclease resistant DNA (Lioutas, Schmetz and Tannich 1995). The origin and function of these circular DNA elements remains to be established but their presence could explain, at least partially, the large variations in number and size of the karyotype of the parasite.

The first *E. histolytica* gene was cloned in 1987 (Edman, Meza and Agabian 1987, Huber et al. 1987) and since then, numerous genes have been identified, their sequences analysed and their products characterized (Table 8.1).

Despite impressive advances in our understanding of the molecular biology of *Entamoeba*, many questions in the field are far from being resolved. *E. histolytica* has now been successfully transfected and this will allow studies on gene regulation, on the biological significance of various molecules for the survival of the parasite and on the mechanisms by which it produces disease (Nickel and Tannich 1994, Purdy et al. 1994).

Table 8.1   *E. histolytica* genes cloned

Cytoskeleton proteins	
Actin	(Edman, Meza and Agabian 1987, Huber et al. 1987)
Myosin II	(Raymond-Denise, Sansonetti and Guillén 1993)
Tubulin	(Katiyar et al. 1994, Sanchez et al. 1994)
Antigens	
29 kDa antigen	(Torian et al. 1990, Reed et al. 1992)
30 kDa antigen	(Tachibana et al. 1991, Bracha, Nuchamowitz and Mirelman 1995)
39 kDa antigen	(Plaimauer et al. 1994)
125 kDa antigen	(Edman et al. 1990)
Serine-rich antigen	(Stanley et al. 1990, Li, Kunz-Jenkins, and Stanley 1992)
Adhesion molecules	
170 surface lectin	(Petri et al. 1989, Mann et al. 1991, Tannich, Ebert and Horstmann 1992, McCoy et al. 1993a, McCoy et al. 1993b)
Lytic factors	
Amoebapore	(Leippe et al. 1992, Leippe et al. 1993, Leippe et al. 1994)
Cysteine proteases	(Eakin et al. 1990, Tannich et al. 1991b, Tannich et al. 1992, Reed et al. 1993)
Membrane/cytoplasmic components	
Elongation factors	(De Meester et al. 1991, Plaimauer et al. 1993, Shirakura et al. 1994)
Calcium-binding protein	(Prasad, Bhattaharya and Bhattacharya 1992)
20 kDa protein	(Zhang and Samuelson 1993a)
Proton-translocating ATPases	(Descoteaux, Yu and Samuelson 1994, Yi and Samuelson 1994)
Nuclear components	
Ribosomal genes	(Huber et al. 1989, Burch et al. 1991, Clark and Diamond 1991b, Mittal et al. 1991, Que and Reed 1991, Cruz-Reyes et al. 1992, Mittal, Bhattacharya, and Bhattacharya 1992, Mittal et al. 1992, Petter et al. 1992, Zurita et al. 1992, Cevallos et al. 1993, Orozco et al. 1993b, Ramachandran, Bhattacharya, and Bhattacharya 1993, Sehgal, Bhattacharya and Bhattacharya 1993, Jansson et al. 1994, Mittal, Bhattacharya and Bhattacharya 1994, Sehgal et al. 1994)
Histones	(Födinger et al. 1992, Födinger et al. 1993, Binder et al. 1995)
Zincprotein	(Stanley and Li 1992)
Multidrug resistance glycoproteins	
P-glycoprotein 1	(Descoteaux et al. 1992a)
P-glycoprotein 2	(Descoteaux et al. 1992b)
Other	
ABC-family transporter	(Zhang and Samuelson 1993b)

5   CLINICAL ASPECTS

5.1   Introduction

The term 'amoebiasis' includes all cases of human infection with *E. histolytica*, but only a proportion of cyst-releasing individuals experience symptoms caused by the penetration of the parasite into the tissues, a condition known as 'invasive amoebiasis'. The large group of infected asymptomatic individuals, previously described as having 'luminal amoebiasis', is now thought to be composed mainly of *E. dispar* carriers, as discussed in section 1, p. 157.

Invasive amoebiasis is a potentially fatal condition and there is a relatively high mortality among patients with severe forms of the disease. It ranks third on a global scale after malaria and schistosomiasis as a cause of death among people with parasitic infections produced by protozoa (Walsh 1984).

5.2   Clinical manifestations

An epidemic of amoebic dysentery that occurred in Chicago in 1933 provided an opportunity for studying the incubation period of the disease. Contamination of the water supply of 2 large hotels in the area was responsible for this outbreak, which resulted in c. 1400 cases. Although the complete history could not be obtained from all patients, reliable data were available from 391 cases. In these, the incubation periods ranged from 1 to 19 weeks, divided as follows: <1 week (6.7%); 1–4 weeks (59%); 4–8 weeks (24.7%); 9–13 weeks (7.4%); and >13 weeks (2.2%). Severe infections tended to have a shorter incubation period, most of them being reported within 1–6 weeks after initial exposure (US Treasury Department 1936).

Depending on the affected organ, the clinical manifestations of amoebiasis are intestinal or extra-intestinal. Both localizations can occur at the same time, but they are usually manifested separately.

Intestinal amoebiasis

There are 4 clinical forms of invasive intestinal amoebiasis, all of which are generally acute; (1) dysentery, or bloody diarrhoea; (2) fulminating colitis; (3) amoebic appendicitis; and (4) amoeboma of the colon. The first of these is considered to be relatively benign, but the other 3 are severe forms of the disease and require prompt medical attention.

Amoebic dysentery

Dysenteric and diarrhoeic syndromes account for 90% of cases of invasive intestinal amoebiasis. Their various clinical manifestations depend on where the lesions are located within the rectosigmoid or higher regions of the colon. In people with this form of the disease rectosigmoidoscopy may reveal superficial ulcerations extending over limited areas of the terminal portion of the large intestine. Patients with dysentery have an average of 3–5 mucosanguineous evacuations per day, with moderate colic pain preceding discharge and they have rectal tenesmus. In patients with bloody diarrhoea, evacuations are also few, but the stools are composed of liquid faecal material stained with blood and, although there is moderate colic pain, there is no rectal tenesmus. Fever and systemic manifestations are generally absent. These syndromes constitute classic ambulatory dysentery and can easily be distinguished from diseases of bacterial origin. The clinical course is moderate and symptoms disappear rapidly with treatment; spontaneous remissions are occasionally observed after several days (Sepúlveda and Treviño-García Manzo 1986, Martínez-Palomo and Ruíz-Palacios 1990).

Fulminating amoebic colitis

In contrast to the dysenteric syndrome, fulminating amoebic colitis is an extremely severe, rapidly evolving clinical condition with necrotic ulcerous lesions extending over large areas, even the entire colon. These can affect all layers of the intestinal wall. Evacuations, preceded by intense colic pain, are frequent (20 or more in 24h) and consist of faecal material mixed with blood or occasionally blood alone. Rectal tenesmus tends to be constant and acute. Systemic manifestations include abdominal discomfort, anorexia and nausea. High fever (39–40°C) is usually present, accompanied by a weak, rapid pulse and low blood pressure. The patient suffers from dehydration and prostration and may even develop shock. Peritonitis is a common complication due to the perforation of the intestinal wall (Sepúlveda and Treviño-García Manzo 1986, Martínez-Palomo and Ruíz-Palacios 1990).

Amoebic appendicitis

The symptoms of this condition are similar to those of bacterial appendicitis: acute pain and rigidity in the lower right quadrant of the abdomen, fever, tachycardia and nausea. In more than two-thirds of cases of amoebic appendicitis, patients have ulcerous lesions of the caecum. In these cases diarrhoea, often bloody, is also present (Sepúlveda and Treviño-García Manzo 1986, Martínez-Palomo and Ruíz-Palacios 1990).

Amoeboma

Amoebomas are pseudotumoural lesions, whose formation is associated with necrosis, inflammation and oedema of the mucosa and submucosa of the colon. Amoebomas always co-exist with amoebic ulcerations. These are generally single, but occasionally multiple, masses usually found in the vertical segments of the large intestine: the caecum, the rectosigmoid region of the colon, the ascending colon and the hepatic and splenic angles of the colon. The condition is usually acute, with dysentery or bloody diarrhoea, abdominal pain and a palpable mass in the corresponding area of the abdomen. If the lesion is located in the rectosigmoid region, it can be identified by endoscopy (Sepúlveda and Treviño-García Manzo 1986, Martínez-Palomo and Ruíz-Palacios 1990).

Extraintestinal amoebiasis

E. histolytica can infect almost every organ of the body, including the liver, brain, lung and skin. By far the most frequent form of extra-intestinal amoebiasis is the amoebic liver abscess which, due to its great clinical and epidemiological importance, will be the most extensively discussed.

Thoracic complications of amoebiasis, including pleuropulmonary, pericardial and mediastinal manifestations, are secondary to liver abscess. Involvement of the central nervous system is rare and lesions are single or multiple small areas of softening in the left cerebral hemisphere. Cutaneous amoebiasis is usually a complication of intestinal amoebiasis with dysentery. It may occur in the perianal region, or it may appear in the skin surrounding a fistula in cases of liver abscesses that involve the abdominal wall.

Amoebic liver abscess

This condition results from the migration of *E. histolytica* trophozoites from the colon to the liver via the portal circulation. The time lapse between penetration of the mucosa of the large intestine and damage to the hepatic parenchyma is unknown. It has been observed clinically and confirmed in a large series of autopsies that amoebic colitis is found in only one-third of cases of hepatic abscess. Amoebic liver abscesses have been reported in patients of all ages, but predominate in adults aged 20–60 years. It has a marked preference for the right lobe of the liver and it is at least 3 times more frequent in males than in females. Interestingly, it is 10 times more common in adults than in children (Sepúlveda and Treviño-García Manzo 1986).

The signs and symptoms of amoebic hepatic abscess vary, but in general the onset is abrupt, with pain in the right hypochondrium radiating towards the right shoulder and scapular area. The pain usually increases with deep breathing, coughing and while stepping on the right foot during walking. When the abscess is localized to the right lobe, symptoms include irritative cough, sometimes productive, and a pleuritic type of pain. Abscesses in the upper left lobe can cause epigastric, sometimes dyspneic pain, at times spreading to the base of the neck and to one or both shoulders. A sharp pain centred in the precordial region strongly suggests that the abscess has penetrated into the pericardial space. This complication is nearly always fatal due to cardiac tamponade. Localization of the abscess in the vicinity of the diaphragm can lead to perforation of the pleura, causing pleurisy or empyema. If the bronchi become involved pus may be vomited leading to clinical improvement. If the lung is involved there may be pulmonary consolidation and abscess formation. When located in the inferior part of the liver, the abscess can penetrate into the peritoneal cavity and into neighbouring organs (Sepúlveda 1970).

Fever between 38 and 40°C is found in all patients with amoebic liver abscess. The patient commonly has chills and profuse sweating in the afternoon and at night. Other symptoms include anorexia, nausea, vomiting and, of course, diarrhoea (with or without blood) and dysentery. On physical examination, the cardinal sign of amoebic liver abscess is painful hepatomegaly. Digital pressure and fist percussion often produce intense pain in the liver region. On pal-

pation, the liver is soft and smooth, in contrast to the rough hard irregular character of the liver in patients with cirrhosis and hepatocarcinoma. Jaundice is present in 8% of the patients that respond well to treatment. When jaundice is severe, multiple abscesses should be suspected (Fig. 8.6). Ascites and hepatic coma occur rarely, but prognosis is poor in these patients (Sepúlveda 1970).

6 IMMUNOLOGY

6.1 Humoral immune response

The time between infection with *E. histolytica* and the appearance of local antibody responses remains unknown. Coproantibodies have been found by indirect haemagglutination (IHA) in c. 80% of patients with amoebic dysentery, compared with 2% of healthy controls and 4% of patients with non-amoebic intestinal parasitic infections; this figure was obtained at the time when patients came in for treatment, but 3 weeks later it fell to 55%. This coincided with an increase in serum antibodies suggesting that the humoral immune reaction in people with invasive intestinal amoebiasis is initiated by a short and transient local secretory response, followed by an increase in systemic antibodies (reviewed in Pérez-Montfort and Kretschmer 1990). IgA type anti-*E. histolytica* antibodies have been found in human milk, colostrum and saliva and in the bile of intracaecally immunized rats. The protective role of secretory IgA (and IgE) in amoebiasis has not been established. In fact, *E. histolytica* trophozoites have been shown to degrade secretory IgA (Kelsall and Ravdin 1993).

Circulating antibodies to *E. histolytica* can be detected as early as one week after the onset of symptoms in humans and experimental animals. All immunoglobulin classes are involved, but there seems to be a predominance of IgG. In contrast to findings in animals, the levels of circulating antibodies in humans do not necessarily correlate with the severity of the disease. High titres of antibodies tend to appear early in the disease and to persist after invasive amoebiasis is cured and in patients whose subclinical amoebic infection is controlled (Knobloch and Mannweiler 1983). Antibody levels fall in different people at different rates following treatment. The detection of antibody in a patient depends on the sensitivity of the test used. Thus, if antibodies are measured by the sensitive techniques of IHA or by enzyme-linked immunosorbent assays (ELISA), antibodies can be detected more than 3 years after an invasive amoebic episode in the absence of any recurrent infection (reviewed in Kretschmer 1986, Trissl 1982).

Complement may also be involved in limiting amoebiasis, a role supported by the observation that experimental animals decomplemented with cobra venom factor are significantly more susceptible to development of amoebic liver abscesses than are normal animals (Capín et al. 1980). Also, the addition of cobra venom factor to normal human serum decreases the

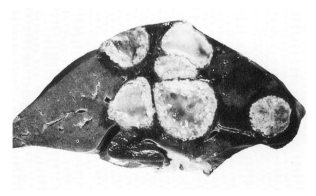

Fig. 8.6 Macroscopic appearance of amoebic liver abscesses. When viewed microscopically these lesions are areas of liquefactive necrosis, rather than true abscesses.

lysis of complement sensitive strains (Reed and Gigli 1990). Moreover, amoebae are capable of activating complement through the classical and alternative pathways, even in the absence of antibody (Calderón and Schreiber 1985). This activation is lethal in vitro to the non-pathogenic *E. dispar* and to *E. histolytica* strains that have been axenized and have partially lost their virulence. However, fresh isolates from patients with colitis or amoebic liver abscesses are resistant to complement mediated lysis (Reed, Sargeaunt and Braude 1983) and repetitive treatment with human serum may induce complement resistance of axenic *E. histolytica* in culture (Calderón and Tovar 1986) suggesting that some amoebae have developed a mechanism not yet understood for evasion of complement lysis. These observations may explain conflicting reports of complement levels in humans and in experimental animals with invasive amoebiasis; some suggest decreased levels of complement whereas others suggest elevated levels.

The deleterious effects of anti-amoebic antibodies on in vitro cultured trophozoites have been studied extensively. Immune sera can inhibit both erythrophagocytosis by *E. histolytica* and the cytotoxic effect of amoebae upon cells of cultured lines. At high concentrations, immune serum produces rapid lysis of trophozoites (reviewed in Kretschmer 1986). In apparent contrast to these observations, amoebae may survive exposure to antibody in some circumstances. Incubation of amoebae with immune serum induces the rapid redistribution of surface bound antigens to the uroid of the cell and the caps thus formed can be either released or endocytosed. This process is temperature and pH dependent, occurs through a sliding mechanism that involves both actin and myosin, and is regulated by calmodulin and a myosin light chain kinase (Espinosa-Cantellano and Martínez-Palomo 1994). The parasite, which has thus shed the antibody antigen complexes, apparently emerges undamaged and free of potentially harmful antibodies.

Taken together, these observations suggest that although a rapid humoral immune response is mounted by the host upon invasion by *E. histolytica*, the parasite has developed efficient evasion mechanisms that include resistance to complement and a mechanism for capping and shedding of surface antigens. It is therefore considered that humoral antibodies are not protective against *E. histolytica*, a conclusion further supported by the observation of high rates of reinfection in persons with elevated antibody titres and by the detection of high levels of antibodies in patients with symptomatic amoebiasis.

6.2 Cellular immune response

Even though the basic components of a local cellular immune response, such as mononuclear phagocytes and lymphocytes, are regularly present in early intestinal amoebic lesions, their role in the establishment or prevention of invasive infection is not well understood. Evidence of systemic cell mediated immunity has been confirmed (1) in vivo through delayed hypersensitivity skin reactions and (2) in vitro through lymphokine (macrophage inhibition factor, MIF), blastogenic response, leucocyte adherence inhibition and lymphocytotoxic assays. Many patients however fail to react to delayed skin tests with amoebic antigens during the early stages of the disease, apparently due to a state of specific unresponsiveness. Such unresponsiveness has been detected by in vitro assays, which show a transient failure to produce MIF, and by a reduction of lymphocyte cytotoxicity in patients in early stages of untreated hepatic amoebiasis (reviewed in Kretschmer 1986). Thus tissue invasion by *E. histolytica* may be preceded by, and is associated with, some degree of T cell suppression as a result of either selection or induction of suppressor T cells. Supporting the selective mechanism is the observation of increased susceptibility to invasive amoebiasis of patients and experimental animals immunosuppressed by mechanisms mediated by suppressor T cells. The coincidence of malnutrition and amoebic liver abscess in over 90% of clinical and autopsy cases and the significantly increased HLA–DR3 antigen levels found in Mexican patients with amoebic liver abscess also suggest that T cell mediated suppression is a factor in invasive amoebiasis. The inductive proposal, on the other hand, is based on the observation that cell-free extracts of the parasite can exhaust and thus suppress the cellular immune response of the host (Martínez-Palomo 1993).

The existence of an early transient anergy state does not necessarily preclude a protective role for cell mediated immunity against invasive amoebiasis. In fact, a state of cell mediated immunity may be responsible for the rarity of recurrences of amoebic liver abscesses in humans; 0.04% recurrences versus 0.20% amoebic liver abscess per initial infection per year was calculated in Mexico City (Kretschmer 1986). Furthermore, the following all support the existence of an effective cellular, rather than humoral, immunity against extraintestinal amoebiasis: (1) immunization studies and studies of the effect of immunosuppression of experimental animals on infection; (2) the results of a few studies of passive transfer of immunity with cells and (3) the cytolytic effect of activated lymphocytes and macrophages (irrespective of the presence of antibodies or complement) against *E. histolytica*. This conclusion is further supported by studies on severe combined immunodeficient (SCID) mice, in which 100% developed liver abscesses when challenged intrahepatically with *E. histolytica* trophozoites (Cieslak, Virgin and Stanley 1992). The actual defence strategy seems to depend heavily on macrophages; depressing macrophage function with silica or anti-macrophage serum increases the development of experimental amoebiasis, whereas enhancing their functions with BCG decreases it. Moreover, congenitally athymic nu–nu mice (devoid of T lymphocytes) develop amoebic liver abscesses or intestinal amoebic disease only after macrophage blockade with silica. *E. histolytica* may possess mechanisms to evade or modify the action of macrophages. The parasite has been found to release a small molecular weight factor that can inhibit the locomotion of monocytes, but not of polymorphonuclear cells (reviewed in Kretschmer 1986).

7 Pathology

A detailed description of the pathological changes in amoebiasis is beyond the objectives of this chapter, but a brief summary of the main characteristics of intestinal and hepatic lesions will be given. For a comprehensive review of the pathology of the disease, the reader is referred to Pérez-Tamayo (1986).

Invasion of the colonic and caecal mucosa begins in the interglandular epithelium. Cell infiltration around invading amoebae leads to rapid lysis of inflammatory cells and tissue necrosis (Fig. 8.7); thus, acute inflammatory cells are seldom found in biopsy samples or in scrapings of rectal mucosal lesions. Ulcerations may deepen and progress under the mucosa to form typical flask ulcers. These extend into the submucosa producing abundant microhaemorrhages, the presence of which explains the finding of haematophagous amoebae in stool specimens and in rectal scrapings. Such amoebae are the best indication of the amoebic nature of a case of dysentery or bloody diarrhoea. The ulcers are initially superficial, with hyperemic borders, a necrotic base and normal mucosa between the sites of invasion. Further progression causes the loss of mucosa and submucosa; the lesion can extend into the muscle layers and eventually cause rupture of the serosa (Martínez-Palomo 1993).

Complications of intestinal amoebiasis include perforation, direct extension to the skin and haematogenous dissemination, mainly to the liver. The presence and extent of liver involvement bears no relationship to the degree of intestinal amoebiasis, and these conditions do not necessarily coincide. The early stages of hepatic amoebic invasion have not been studied in humans. In experimental animals, inoculation of *E. histolytica* trophozoites into the portal vein produces multiple foci of infection in the liver with neutrophil accumulation around the parasites, followed by focal necrosis and granulomatous infiltration. As the lesions grow in size, the granulomas gradually become necrotic and coalesce, necrotic tissue occupying progressively larger portions of the liver. Hepatocytes close to the early lesions degenerate and become necrotic, but direct contact of hepatocytes with amoebae is rarely observed. The lesion can eventually consist of large areas of liquefied necrotic material surrounded by a thin capsule of fibrous appearance (Tsutsumi, Mena and Martínez-Palomo 1984).

8 Diagnosis

The diagnosis of invasive intestinal amoebiasis is based on the microscopic identification of *E. histolytica* trophozoites in rectal smears or recently evacuated stools and on the results of rectosigmoidoscopy. Trophozoites are most likely to be found in material obtained during rectosygmoidoscopy such as the bloody mucus

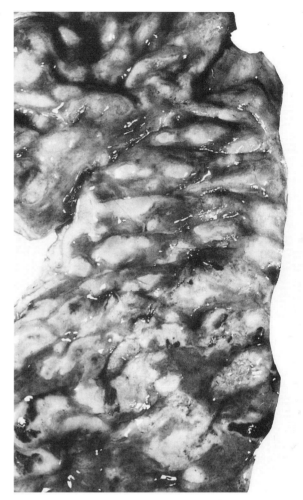

Fig. 8.7 Surface view of the mucosa of the colon in a person who died of amoebic colitis. Large and confluent ulcerations have destroyed most of the mucosal layers of the large intestine.

and in the yellowish exudate covering the mucosal ulcerations obtained during rectosigmoidoscopy. The finding of motile trophozoites containing ingested red blood cells confirms the diagnosis of amoebic infection in patients with the clinical gastrointestinal symptoms (described on p. 164). Problems arise when cysts alone are identified in stools of healthy or diarrhoeic individuals, as the cysts may be those of the non-pathogenic *E. dispar* which are morphologically indistinguishable from the cysts of the pathogenic *E. histolytica* (Martínez-Palomo 1993).

Diagnosis based on the detection of amoebae has several drawbacks. The procedure is tedious and time consuming; it requires a skilled technician; the sensitivity is relatively low; several samples must be taken to detect cyst passers; and fresh samples are needed for the detection of trophozoites. On the other hand, the standard for the differentiation of *E. histolytica* from *E. dispar* has been the determination of their isoenzyme pattern by gel electrophoresis. This procedure is expensive, slow and requires the cultivation of amoebae from faeces, which is not routinely applicable. Therefore, a simple, inexpensive method for the detection of the parasite in faeces and for discrimination between pathogenic and non-pathogenic amoeba is badly needed for the realization of large clinical and epidemiological studies.

Attempts to develop new diagnostic methods have used monoclonal antibodies in ELISA and in immunofluorescence assays of faecal samples. Although ELISA was reported to have high sensitivity and specificity in one study of 701 samples, it could not discriminate between pathogenic *E. histolytica* and non-pathogenic *E. dispar* (del Muro et al. 1987). The immunofluorescence test, on the other hand, proved to be much faster than isoenzyme determination, but still required cultivation of the organism and detected only the motile form of the parasite (Strachan et al. 1988). An ELISA based on monoclonal antibodies directed against cross-reactive and specific *E. histolytica* epitopes of the amoebic galactose adhesin was used to test single stool specimens from 82 patients with diarrhoea. The authors reported that the test gave 93% specificity and 96% sensitivity in the detection of infection with pathogenic *E. histolytica* (Haque et al. 1994).

Molecular probes provide another approach for the detection of the parasite directly in stools. A study with a specific probe of 123 stool samples from patients in Mexico City revealed a 93% specificity and 100% sensitivity for detection of amoeba, although it could not distinguish between amoeba with pathogenic and non-pathogenic isoenzyme patterns (Samuelson et al. 1989). A study carried out in the south-eastern state of Chiapas in Mexico, using the polymerase chain reaction (PCR) to amplify specific pathogenic and non-pathogenic sequences, resulted in 98% specificity and 96% sensitivity for the identification of *E. histolytica* in stools of 201 randomly selected individuals (Acuña-Soto et al. 1993). Several research groups are currently working to improve these techniques, to increase their sensitivity and specificity and to avoid the use of radioactive probes. It is hoped that this will result in development of simple, reproducible tests that will aid in the clinical and epidemiological diagnosis of amoebiasis (Katzwinkel-Wladarsch, Loscher and Rinder 1994).

The diagnosis of invasive intestinal amoebiasis may be confirmed by endoscopy. In patients with benign dysentery, examination by rectosigmoidoscopy reveals small superficial ulcerations of a linear or oval shape, covered by a yellowish exudate and surrounded by a normal or hyperemic mucosa. In patients with fulminating colitis, the ulcers are large and tend to be confluent, often with a necrotic appearance. The intervening mucosa shows intense inflammation and signs of haemorrhage. Endoscopy should be carried out with great care in these cases, as there is risk of intestinal perforation. If an amoeboma is situated in the terminal portion of the colon, it can be visualized by rectosigmoidoscopy. If it is located elsewhere, it is necessary to use colonoscopy or radiography and a barium enema to identify the pseudotumoural mass, which is often surrounded by ulcerations (Sepúlveda 1970).

The diagnosis of amoebic liver abscess is sometimes difficult. In endemic areas, or when there is a history of travel to such places, amoebic abscess should always be suspected in patients with spiking fever, weight loss and abdominal pain in the upper right quadrant or epigastrium, as well as in patients with tenderness in the liver area. The presence of leucocytosis, a high alkaline phosphatase level and an elevated right diaphragm (visible in a chest x-ray) suggests the presence of an hepatic abscess. The diagnosis is confirmed by ultrasonography or by computerized axial tomography (CAT) scans. The latter is the most precise method for identifying hepatic abscesses, particularly when they are small, and it is of great value in the differential diagnosis of other focal lesions of the liver (Sepúlveda and Treviño-García Manzo 1986).

Serological tests for anti-amoebic antibodies are positive in c. 75% of patients with invasive colonic amoebiasis and in >90% of patients with amoebic liver abscesses. Circulating antibodies have been detected by virtually all known serological tests, including tests based on immunofluorescent antibodies (IFA), IHA, radioimmunoassay (RIA), counterimmunoelectrophoresis (CIE) and ELISA. The latter is the most sensitive (it produces no false negatives in cases of amoebic liver abscess), it is reasonably specific (3.6% false positives in controls living in endemic areas) and remains positive longest (>3 years in the absence of recurrent infection). The IFA test also deserves special mention because it is much simpler than all other tests and when performed in conjunction with IHA gives a 100% positivity in cases of amoebic liver abscess. The Center for Disease Control in Atlanta, Georgia, has chosen the IHA as its standard serologic reference test for amoebiasis. Titres below 1:256 are considered non-specific. Because of its relative simplicity and efficiency, the CIE is particularly well suited for epidemiological surveys.

Although serological techniques are useful in the diagnosis of invasive intestinal amoebiasis and amoebic liver abscess and as a tool for epidemiological studies of the disease, they do not aid in the diagnosis of simple intestinal infection. In endemic areas the high prevalence of anti-amoebic antibodies in the general population reduces the usefulness of serologic tests for diagnosis and other tests must be performed before establishing the diagnosis of invasive amoebiasis. Attempts have been made to discriminate serologically between present and past invasive amoebiasis, using antibodies to specific antigens in sera of (1) patients with active or cured amoebic liver abscesses and (2) individuals who are asymptomatic cyst carriers (Ximénez et al. 1993). The development of serological techniques that distinguish between *E. dispar* and *E. histolytica* infection will redefine the epidemiology of invasive amoebiasis.

9 EPIDEMIOLOGY AND CONTROL

9.1 Introduction

Infection by *E. histolytica* is ubiquitous, but the highest incidence is usually found in communities with poor socioeconomic conditions and inadequate sanitation. In such communities the infection is typically endemic. According to the World Health Organization, c. 500 million people (not including those in the People's Republic of China) are infected, with a 10% annual morbidity index (Walsh 1986) and up to 110 000 deaths annually can be attributed to complications of the disease (WHO 1985). The actual frequency of amoebiasis due to *E. histolytica* has been difficult to establish as there is a tendency to overestimate it in endemic areas, where many cases of dysentery or bloody diarrhoea are often misdiagnosed as amoebiasis. In non-endemic areas with a low incidence of the disease there is a tendency to overlook the presence of *E. histolytica* in stools (Walsh 1986). So far, no seroepidemiological study has distinguished between infections with *E. dispar* or *E. histolytica*.

In areas with high levels of poverty, illiteracy, overcrowding, with inadequate and contaminated water supplies and poor sanitation, direct faecal-oral transmission occurs frequently and thus the endemic character of the disease is maintained. Although difficult to implement, programmes for the control of the disease require the improvement of environmental sanitation, health education and early detection and treatment of infected people.

9.2 Epidemiology

SEROLOGICAL SURVEYS

Anti-amoebic antibodies are relatively long-lasting in the serum of recovered patients and although antibodies cannot be used to discriminate between persons with recent and past infection, or between those infected with *E. histolytica* and *E. dispar*, detection of antibodies in the population has proven a valuable tool in epidemiological prevalence studies. A national seroepidemiological survey was undertaken throughout all 32 states of Mexico, with a probability based sampling of almost 68 000 individuals representative of the population in terms of age, socioeconomic status and urban or rural origin. Antibodies to *E. histolytica* were detected by IHA assays in 8.41% of the population, ranging from 9.80% in the South Pacific region to 6.26% in the north-eastern parts, with a higher prevalence in rural (9.89%) than in urban (7.93%) areas. Frequency of presence of antibodies increased during the first decade of life, peaking between 5 and 9 years. Antibody was detected more frequently in women (9.34%) than in men (7.09%). There was a clear correlation between high seroprevalence, low socioeconomic and educational levels and inadequate housing conditions, although some positive samples were found in all groups (Caballero-Salcedo et al. 1994).

A previous national serological survey of nearly 20 000 serum samples from 46 Mexican urban regions detected an average frequency of amoebic seropositivity of 5.95% (Gutiérrez et al. 1976). The differences between these studies do not necessarily reflect an increase in seroprevalence in the Mexican population, but may be due to differences in the populations studied (the latter including only urban areas) and the methodology applied (IHA versus CIE).

HUMAN SUSCEPTIBILITY

The main reservoirs of *E. histolytica* are humans, although morphologically similar amoebae may be found in primates, dogs and cats. The parasite has been transmitted to various mammalian species but it is doubtful whether these serve as significant reservoirs of the parasite. Human susceptibility to infection seems to be widespread, but most individuals harbouring the parasite do not develop disease. Most of these asymptomatic carriers are infected with the non-pathogenic *E. dispar* although *E. histolytica* has been positively identified in some asymptomatic persons. In a semi-rural area south of Durban, South Africa, 1% of apparently healthy individuals were carriers of pathogenic *E. histolytica* and a one year follow up revealed that 90% of these carriers remained asymptomatic and underwent spontaneous cure, the remaining 10% developed amoebic colitis (Ghadirian and Jackson 1987). The factors involved in the development of the disease are unknown, but probably include host as well as parasite characteristics.

A major increase in frequency of luminal amoebic infection has occurred in male homosexual populations in North America, northern Europe and Japan, the spread being associated with specific sexual practices. Prevalence rates are as high as 32% and most reported cases are asymptomatic or present diffuse symptoms. *E. dispar* is most frequently identified, except in Japan, where pathogenic *E. histolytica* is not uncommon (Takeuchi et al. 1990).

INCIDENCE OF INVASIVE AMOEBIASIS

There are a few epidemiological reports of invasive intestinal amoebiasis that are accompanied by microscopic identification of *E. histolytica* trophozoites and rectosigmoidoscopy studies showing intestinal ulcerative lesions; these reports provide divergent data. The frequency of invasive intestinal amoebiasis has been reported to range from 2.2% to 16.2% in patients with acute diarrhoea or dysentery and the case-fatality rate ranges from 0.5% in uncomplicated cases to 40.2% in patients with amoebic dysentery complicated by peritonitis (these figures are drawn from Mexico, Nigeria, Venezuela and South Africa) (reviewed in Muñoz 1986). Although a large number of cases were included in these studies, the populations sampled were biased by including only those admitted to hospitals and healthcare centres.

The frequency of amoebic liver abscess is a reliable measure of rates of liver infection, as liver lesions can be identified clinically, in the laboratory, or through post-mortem studies. Liver abscess occurs in c. 2% of adult amoebiasis patients in endemic areas (Sepúlveda 1982). Elsdon-Dew tabulated the geographical distribution of patients with amoebic liver abscesses and concluded that the condition is prevalent in West and South East Africa, South East Asia, Mexico and the western portion of South America (Elsdon-Dew 1968).

Amoebic hepatic abscess is at least 10 times more common in adults than in children. It predominates in adults between 20 and 60 years of age and within this group, 3 times as many men suffer from the condition as women. The reason for the notable differences in the frequency and severity of invasive amoebiasis according to age and sex are unknown.

10 CHEMOTHERAPY

The use of amoebicides in the treatment of patients with amoebiasis has contributed greatly to reducing the morbidity and mortality of the disease. Anti-amoebic drugs may be classified into 3 groups: luminal, tissue and mixed amoebicides. The most frequently used amoebicides with luminal action are diiodohydroxyquin (650 mg orally 3 times daily for 20 days), diloxanide furoate (500 mg orally 3 times daily for 10 days) and paromomycin (500 mg orally 3 times daily for 5–10 days). The amoebicides effective in tissues are emetine and dehydroemetine, which act in the liver, intestinal wall and other tissues and chloroquine, which acts only in the liver. Emetine and dehydroemetine given intramuscularly may be toxic to the myocardium and are currently seldom used.

Amoebicides effective in both tissues and the intestinal lumen include metronidazole and the nitroimidazole derivatives tinidazole and ornidazole. In addition to being active both in tissues and the intestinal lumen, these drugs have the advantage that they are given orally and are most effective therapeutically. They are reasonably well tolerated and despite their reported carcinogenic effect in rodents and their mutagenic potential in bacteria, no such effect has been detected in humans. They are therefore the drugs of choice in the treatment of invasive amoebiasis in spite of some unpleasant, but not serious, side effects. Metrodinazole is given orally 500–800 mg 3 times a day for 5 days to persons with invasive intestinal amoebiasis and for 5–10 days to persons with liver abscesses. Tinidazole or ornidazole are administered orally, 2 g once a day for 1–3 days. For further details on the chemotherapy of amoebiasis, the reader is referred to Martínez-Palomo and Ruíz-Palacios (1990).

There is no drug resistance in amoebiasis. Those few reports of failed treatment refer to advanced cases in which most of the liver parenchyma was replaced by the amoebic abscess and treatment was administered too late. In vitro studies performed with fresh isolates from symptomatic patients and asymptomatic carriers, as well as axenically cultured pathogenic amoebae, confirmed drug sensitivity in all cases (Burchard and Mirelman 1988). A drug resistant clone could be obtained only by chemically induced mutagenesis and culture in the presence of emetine; several multidrug resistant (MDR) genes have been isolated that show 38–41% identity to mammalian P-glycoprotein aminoacid predicted sequences (reviewed in Orozco et al. 1995). In the absence of drug resistance in the parasite, the functional role of these genes is yet to be established.

Two severe forms of invasive intestinal amoebiasis require surgery in addition to chemotherapy; these are toxic megacolon and amoebic appendicitis. Amoebic liver abscesses should be treated by chemotherapy; percutaneous or surgical drainage is indicated only in cases of imminent rupture.

One of the most striking features of invasive amoebiasis, whether intestinal, hepatic, cutaneous, or other, is that the amoebic lesions heal without scarring once adequate treatment has been initiated. There is no apparent explanation for this peculiar aspect of the pathology of the disease.

11 VACCINATION

Evidence for the existence of acquired immunity against amoebiasis is based essentially on 2 sets of observations. The first is the widely accepted knowledge that recurrence of amoebic liver abscess is exceedingly rare. Although no recent data are available, estimates in the early 1970s in Mexico City indicated that 0.04% of patients who had recovered from an amoebic liver abscess had recurrences during a 7 year follow up period (versus a prevalence of 0.1–0.2% of amoebic liver abscesses per year in the general population) (reviewed in Kretschmer 1986). The second set of observations supporting acquired immunity are from studies on experimental animals that are refractory to amoebic hepatic reinvasion after spontaneous or induced recovery. Severe combined immunodeficient (SCID) mice can be partially protected by passive immunization procedures (Cieslak, Virgin and Stanley 1992) and partial protection of intact mice has also been obtained through immunization with crude and fractionated preparations of *E. histolytica* and with live trophozoites. Local and systemic antibody responses have been reported to occur in experimental animals after immunization with fixed trophozoites and with an immunogenic peptide fused to the cholera toxin B subunit (Moreno-Fierros, Domínguez-Robles and Enríquez-Rincón 1995, Zhang, Li and Stanley 1995).

There is also evidence against the development of immunity to invasive amoebiasis. The rise in morbidity and mortality due to *E. histolytica* with increasing age, for example, casts some doubt on the concept of effective acquired protective immunity. In addition, it has been observed that not all antibodies are protective, as passive immunization with purified anti-amoebic immunoglobulins fails to protect hamsters against intrahepatic challenge with *E. histolytica* (Campos-Rodríguez et al. 1995). It has therefore been suggested that induction of protective immunity depends on the recognition by antibody of specific molecules. Recombinant peptides of 3 *E. histolytica* antigens show promise for prevention of experimental amoebic liver abscess: the serine-rich *E. histolytica* protein (SREHP), the 170 kDa subunit of the N-acetyl-D-galactosamine inhibitable lectin and the 29 kDa cysteine-rich antigen (reviewed in Stanley 1996). Much work still needs to be undertaken before an anti-amoebic vaccine is produced.

12 INTEGRATED CONTROL

Transmission of amoebiasis may be accomplished through a variety of mechanisms. Asymptomatic carriers passing large numbers of cysts in their stools are important sources of infection, particularly if they are engaged in the preparation and handling of food. The cysts may remain viable and infective for a few days in faeces, but are killed by desiccation and temperatures >68°C, so boiled water is safe. The amount of chlorine normally used to purify water is insufficient to kill cysts; higher levels of chlorine are effective, but the water thus treated must be dechlorinated before use. Houseflies and cockroaches ingest cysts present in faeces and can pass them from their guts after periods as long as 24h.

Faecal contamination of springs, unprotected shallow wells and streams may occur as a result of surface runoff. Contamination may also result from discharge of sewage into rivers. Occasionally, siphonage of sewage into the water supply system has been responsible for outbreaks of infection. Freshening of vegetables and fruits with contaminated water and using human excreta as fertilizer may produce heavy contamination, a particularly serious problem with vegetables and fruits that are usually eaten raw (Walsh and Martínez-Palomo 1986).

The basic means of preventing amoebic infection is the improvement of living conditions and education in countries where invasive amoebiasis is prevalent. The main targets should be improvements in sanitation of the environment, detection and treatment of infected persons and health education.

The most effective preventive measure is the adequate disposal of human faeces through proper drainage systems or the use of septic tanks. Purified water should be distributed through pipelines to avoid contamination. In areas where amoebic infection is common, drinking water should be boiled for several minutes, or filtered or chlorinated with higher levels of chlorine than those used to eliminate bacterial contamination. Freshening of vegetables and fruits with contaminated water and the use of excrement as fertilizer should be avoided. People should be instructed to clean vegetables carefully with uncontaminated running water, because treatment with iodine, chlorine, or silver solutions gives unreliable results. Food handlers should be periodically checked for intestinal infection and treated if found positive. Houseflies and cockroaches should be controlled and food should be adequately protected from them.

Cases of invasive amoebiasis require prompt chemotherapy and it was previously recommended that all asymptomatic carriers of *Entamoeba* should be treated. With the development of methods to differentiate between *E. histolytica* and *E. dispar*, *E. histolytica* carriers may be identified and should be treated, whereas *E. dispar* carriers should be monitored closely for the possibility of superinfection with *E. histolytica*. Whether such a course of action will be practicable for general control of amoebiasis remains to be seen.

As part of health education of the population, hygienic practices such as hand washing after defecation and before eating, boiling of drinking water and avoiding the consumption of raw vegetables and exposed food should be constantly reiterated in schools and healthcare units and through periodic campaigns in the mass media.

Healthcare personnel should be given training to improve the accuracy of their examination of stools. Doctors should be constantly reminded of the problem of amoebiasis and informed of advances in diagnostic and therapeutic procedures; their active participation in prevention programmes should be encouraged.

13 OTHER INTESTINAL AMOEBAE

The genus *Entamoeba* includes several species of human parasites: *E. histolytica* Schaudinn, 1903; *E. hartmanni* von Prowazek, 1912; *E. coli* (Grassi 1879) Casagrandi and Barbagallo, 1895; *E. gingivalis* (Gros 1849) Smith and Barrett, 1914; and *E. dispar* Brumpt, 1925. Other species that are not usually found in humans, but are present in various animals, include *E. polecki* von Prowazek, 1912; *E. invadens* Rodhain, 1934; *E. chattoni* Swellengrebel, 1914; and *E. moshkovskii* Tshalaia, 1941, which is a free living amoebae. Except for *E. gingivalis*, for which no cyst form is known, classification of the species of *Entamoeba* is based on the number of nuclei in the mature cyst; 8, 4 or one. *E. coli* belongs to the octonucleate cyst group. The quadrinucleate cyst group includes *E. histolytica*, *E. dispar*, *E. hartmanni*, *E. moshkovskii* and *E. invadens*. Uninucleate cysts are characteristic of *E. polecki* and *E. chattoni*. In addition, *Endolimax nana* and *Iodamoeba buetschlii*, although not belonging to the genera *Entamoeba*, are other intestinal amoebae of man.

An indication of the relative frequency of the various parasitic amoebae in the human large intestine can be found in a survey carried out by Sargeaunt et al. (1983) in a population of 470 unselected male homosexuals residing in London. *E. dispar* was found in 11%, *E. coli* in 18%, *E. hartmanni* in 9%, *E. nana* in 16% and *I. buetschlii* in 4%. In a comparative group of heterosexuals living in London, the incidence of *E. histolytica* was only 0.5%.

13.1 *E. coli* (Grassi, 1879); Casagrandi and Barbagallo, 1895

E. coli is the amoeba most commonly found in humans and it is surprising how little is known about it. Study has been hindered by the lack of axenic or monoxenic cultures. Its isoenzyme profiles are clearly different from those of *E. histolytica*, which it closely resembles in other ways (Sargeaunt and Williams 1979). Although *E. coli* is a harmless commensal, it is essential that it be distinguished from *E. histolytica*. Accurate differential diagnosis is required in order to avoid unnecessary treatment as both species are commonly found in the same individual.

Living trophozoites of *E. coli* are 20–30 μm in diameter and cysts range from 15 to 22 μm. Trophozoites move in a sluggish manner using short, broad pseudopodia. Numerous food vacuoles, frequently containing ingested bacteria, occur in the cytoplasm. Red blood cells are very rarely ingested by *E. coli;* their presence should cause the examiner to suspect that the amoeba is *E. histolytica*. In parasitological practice, *E. coli* is distinguished from *E. histolytica* by the possession of cysts with 8 nuclei and chromatoid bodies with irregular splintered ends. Most other microscopical differences reported between these species are of little practical use.

13.2 *E. hartmanni* von Prowazek, 1912

In the quadrinucleate cyst group, *E. histolytica* can be differentiated from *E. hartmanni* on the basis of the diameter of the cysts, which are <10 μm in the latter. In addition, *E. hartmanni* has some distinct morphological features and is not pathogenic (Burrows 1957). The introduction of molecular markers to the study of amoebae has provided additional data to support the status of *E. hartmanni* as a species distinct from *E. histolytica* (Neal 1966). Although *E. histolytica* and *E. hartmanni* are distinguishable by measuring the diameter of the cysts, *E. hartmanni* is usually not differentiated from *E. histolytica* in most clinical laboratories, as cysts are not routinely measured.

13.3 *E. polecki* von Prowazek, 1912

E. polecki is commonly found in the intestines of pigs, but it also parasitizes monkeys, cattle, goats, sheep and dogs. It has only rarely been identified infecting humans, in whom it does not produce symptoms (Chacín-Bonilla 1992). The clinical importance of this amoeba centres solely in the possibility of its being confused with *E. histolytica*. Trophozoites of both species are very similar microscopically. The cysts are 10–18 μm in diameter, uninucleated and many contain an inclusion that stains uniformly with iron hematoxylin.

13.4 *E. chattoni* Swellengrebel, 1914

E. chattoni is the amoeba most commonly found in monkeys and has occasionally been identified in humans, usually after close contact with monkeys (Sargeaunt, Patrick and O'Keefe 1992). Trophozoites, when found, are seen to have a vacuolated endoplasm containing food bodies, bacteria and broad pseudopodia, only slightly extended. Uninucleated cysts are 11–13 μm in diameter and contain an average of 40–60 chromatoid bodies, which can be small and rounded or irregularly angular. A glycogen vacuole, smaller than the one found in *E. histolytica,* is frequently present. *E. chattoni* is non-pathogenic to monkeys (Salis 1941).

13.5 *E. invadens* Rodhain, 1934

E. invadens is a parasite of reptiles. Turtles that harbour this amoeba are not harmed by it and serve as carriers. For lizards and snakes it is pathogenic and produces destructive lesions in the intestine and liver (Geiman and Ratcliffe 1936). Trophozoites are 10–38 μm in diameter and cysts are 11–20 μm. *E. invadens* has distinctive isoenzyme profiles (Sargeaunt and Williams 1979) and has been extensively used for biochemical studies because it can grow at room temperature. Rapid and effective encystation can be induced experimentally in cultures, facilitating study of the encystation process in *Entamoeba*.

13.6 *E. moshkovskii* Tshalaia, 1941

E. moshkovskii is a free-living amoeba that has been recovered from sewage in the Americas and Europe and its clinical importance is due to its 'Laredo strain', which has been infrequently isolated from humans. This strain was formerly known as '*E. histolytica*-like Laredo amoeba' although the isoenzyme profile resembled that of *E. moshkovskii* (Sargeaunt, Williams and Neal 1980). Molecular biological techniques have now positively identified the strain as a type of *E. moshkovskii* (Clark and Diamond 1991a). The Laredo strain is morphologically similar to *E. histolytica* but differs mainly in its abilities to multiply at room temperature and to withstand suspension in hypotonic solutions (Richards, Goldman and Cannon 1966). It also has a distinct antigenic profile, a very low level of infectivity to humans and laboratory animals and is resistant to emetine and various antibiotics (De Carneri 1959).

13.7 *Endolimax nana* (Wenyon and O'Connor 1917); Brug, 1918

Endolimax nana is a non-pathogenic, cosmopolitan and common intestinal amoeba of humans, primates and pigs; it can be confused with *E. histolytica*. The trophozoites are small (6–15 μm in diameter with an average of 10 μm). The cysts measure 8–10 μm in diameter. Details of the nuclear structure and the appearance of the cytoplasm closely resemble those of *I. buetschlii*. Usually there is only one nucleus in trophozoites and 4 nuclei in mature cysts. *E. nana* has no chromatoid body in stained samples and the nuclear membrane appears devoid of peripheral chromatin.

13.8 *Iodamoeba buetschlii* (von Prowazek, 1911); Dobell, 1919

Iodamoeba buetschlii is the most common amoeba of the pig, which was probably its original host, but is also frequently found in humans and monkeys. Trophozoites vary greatly in size, from 6 to 20 μm in diameter. The cytoplasm contains one or more glycogen masses, which are visualized by iodine staining, as well as bacteria, yeasts and debris. Cysts of *I. buetschlii* are commonly ovoid or irregularly pyriform in shape and are

8–15 μm in diameter. These amoebae are distinctive in preparations stained with iodine because of the presence of the large, sharply outlined and dense glycogen-containing vacuoles. Only one nucleus is found in most cysts.

I. buetschlii is non-pathogenic in humans and its presence has only rarely been linked to symptomatic infections. As with other amoebae commonly found in the large intestine of man, *I. buetschlii* has a distinct isoenzyme profile (Sargeaunt and Williams 1979).

13.9 *D. fragilis* Jepps and Dobell, 1918

Although no longer considered an amoeba, but a

trichomonad flagellate, *D. fragilis* is included here because it is frequently identified in human stool samples. It is a small (6–12 μm) cosmopolitan parasite. Only the trophozoite stage has been identified and this is easily differentiated from intestinal amoebae as it generally contains 2 nuclei. There have been reports of infections with *D. fragilis* associated with gastrointestinal symptoms, but in most cases, the parasite is non-pathogenic and can be differentiated by its distinct isoenzyme profile (Sargeaunt and Williams 1979).

REFERENCES

Acuña-Soto R, Samuelson J et al., 1993, Application of the polymerase chain reaction to the epidemiology of pathogenic and nonpathogenic *Entamoeba histolytica*, *Am J Trop Med Hyg*, **48:** 58–70.

Aley SB, Scott WA, Cohn ZA, 1980, Plasma membrane of *Entamoeba histolytica*, *J Exp Med*, **152:** 391–404.

Andrews BJ, Mentzoni L, Bjorvatn B, 1990, Zymodeme conversion of isolates of *Entamoeba histolytica*, *Trans R Soc Trop Med Hyg*, **84:** 63–5.

Argüello C, Valenzuela B, Rangel E, 1992, Structural organization of chromatin during the cell cycle of *Entamoeba histolytica* trophozoites, *Arch Med Res*, **23:** 77–80.

Arroyo R, Orozco E, 1987, Localization and identification of *Entamoeba histolytica* adhesin, *Mol Biochem Parasitol*, **23:** 151–8.

Avron B, Chayen A, 1988, Biochemistry of *Entamoeba*: a review, *Cell Biochem Funct*, **6:** 71–86.

Beanan MJ, Bailey GB, 1995, The primary structure of an *Entamoeba histolytica* enolase, *Mol Biochem Parasitol*, **69:** 119–21.

Bhattacharya S, Bhattacharya A et al., 1989, Circular DNA of *Entamoeba histolytica* encodes ribosomal RNA, *J Protozool*, **36:** 455–9.

Binder M, Ortner S et al., 1995, Sequence and organization of an unusual histone H4 gene in the human parasite *Entamoeba histolytica*, *Mol Biochem Parasitol*, **71:** 243–7.

Bracha R, Nuchamowitz Y, Mirelman D, 1995, Molecular cloning of a 30-kilodalton lysine-rich surface antigen from a non-pathogenic *Entamoeba histolytica* strain and its expression in a pathogenic strain, *Infect Immun*, **63:** 917–25.

Bruchhaus I, Tannich E, 1993, Primary structure of the pyruvate phosphate dikinase in *Entamoeba histolytica*, *Mol Biochem Parasitol*, **62:** 153–6.

Bruchhaus I, Tannich E, 1994, Purification and molecular characterization of the NAD⁺-dependent acetaldehyde/alcohol dehydrogenase from *Entamoeba histolytica*, *Biochem J*, **303:** 743–8.

Bruchhaus I, Tannich E, 1995, Identification of an *Entamoeba histolytica* gene encoding a protein homologous to prokaryotic disulphide oxidoreductases, *Mol Biochem Parasitol*, **70:** 187–91.

Brumpt E, 1925, Étude sommaire de l'"Entamoeba dispar' n sp Amibe à kystes quadrinucléés, parasite de l'homme, *Bull Acad Méd (Paris)*, **94:** 943–52.

Burch DJ, Li E et al., 1991, Isolation of a strain-specific *Entamoeba histolytica* cDNA clone, *J Clin Microbiol*, **29:** 696–701.

Burchard GD, Mirelman D, 1988, *Entamoeba histolytica*: virulence potential and sensitivity to metronidazole and emetine of four isolates possessing nonpathogenic zymodemes, *Exp Parasitol*, **66:** 231–42.

Burrows RR, 1957, *Entamoeba hartmanni*, *Am J Hyg*, **65:** 172–88.

Byers TJ, 1986, Molecular biology of DNA in *Acanthamoeba, Amoeba, Entamoeba* and *Naegleria*, *Int Rev Cytol*, **99:** 311–41.

Caballero-Salcedo A, Viveros-Rogel M et al., 1994, Seroepidemiology of amebiasis in Mexico, *Am J Trop Med Hyg*, **50:** 412–19.

Calderón J, Schreiber RD, 1985, Activation of the alternative and classical complement pathways by *Entamoeba histolytica*, *Infect Immun*, **50:** 560–5.

Calderón J, Tovar R, 1986, Loss of susceptibility to complement lysis in *Entamoeba histolytica* HM1 by treatment with human sera, *Immunology*, **58:** 467–71.

Campos-Rodríguez R, Shibayama-Salas M et al., 1995, Passive immunization during experimental amebic liver abscess development, *Parasitol Res*, **81:** 86–8.

Capín R, Capín NR et al., 1980, Effect of complement depletion on the induction of amebic liver abscess in the hamster, *Arch Invest Med (Mex)*, **11 (Suppl 1):** 173–80.

Cerbón J, Flores J, 1981, Phospholipid composition and turnover of pathogenic amebas, *Comp Biochem Physiol*, **69B:** 487–92.

Cevallos MA, Porta H et al., 1993, Sequence of the 5.8S ribosomal gene of pathogenic and non-pathogenic isolates of *Entamoeba histolytica*, *Nucleic Acids Res*, **21:** 355.

Chacín-Bonilla L, 1992, *Entamoeba polecki*: human infections in Venezuela, *Trans R Soc Trop Med Hyg*, **86:** 634.

Cieslak PR, Virgin HW, Stanley SL, 1992, A severe combined immunodeficient (SCID) mouse model for infection with *Entamoeba histolytica*, *J Exp Med*, **176:** 1605–9.

Clark CG, Diamond LS, 1991a, The Laredo strain and other *Entamoeba histolytica*–like amoebae are *Entamoeba moshkovskii*, *Mol Biochem Parasitol*, **46:** 11–18.

Clark CG, Diamond LS, 1991b, Ribosomal RNA genes of 'pathogenic' and 'nonpathogenic' *Entamoeba histolytica* are distinct, *Mol Biochem Parasitol*, **49:** 297–302.

Clark CG, Diamond LS, 1993, *Entamoeba histolytica*: an explanation for the reported conversion of 'nonpathogenic' amebae to the 'pathogenic' form, *Exp Parasitol*, **77:** 456–60.

Clark CG, Roger AJ, 1995, Direct evidence for secondary loss of mitochondria in *Entamoeba histolytica*, *Proc Natl Acad Sci USA*, **92:** 6518–21.

Corliss JO, 1994, An interim utilitarian ('user friendly') hierarchical classification and characterization of the protists, *Acta Protozool*, **33:** 1–51.

Cox FEG, 1992, Systematics of parasitic protozoa, *Parasitic Protozoa*, vol 1, eds Kreier JP, Baker JR, Academic Press, San Diego, 55–80.

Cruz-Reyes JA, Spice WM et al., 1992, Ribosomal DNA sequences in the differentiation of pathogenic and non-pathogenic isolates of *Entamoeba histolytica*, *Parasitology*, **104:** 239–46.

De Carneri I, 1959, The use of specific anti-amoebic drugs for comparative taxonomic studies, *Trans R Soc Trop Med Hyg*, **53:** 120–1.

De Meester F, Bracha R et al., 1991, Cloning and characterization of an unusual elongation factor-1 alpha cDNA from *Entamoeba histolytica*, *Mol Biochem Parasitol*, **44:** 23–32.

Del Muro R, Oliva A et al., 1987, Diagnosis of *Entamoeba histolytica* in feces by ELISA, *J Clin Lab Anal*, **1**: 322–5.

Descoteaux S, Yu Y, Samuelson J, 1994, Cloning of Entamoeba genes encoding proteolipids of putative vacuolar proton-translocating ATPases, *Infect Immun*, **62**: 3572–5.

Descoteaux S, Ayala P et al., 1992a, Primary sequences of 2 P-glycoprotein genes of *Entamoeba histolytica*, *Mol Biochem Parasitol*, **54**: 201–12.

Descoteaux S, Shen PS et al., 1992b, P-glycoprotein genes of *Entamoeba histolytica*, *Arch Med Res*, **23**: 23–5.

Dhar SK, Choudhury NR et al., 1995, A multitude of circular DNAs exist in the nucleus of *Entamoeba histolytica*, *Mol Biochem Parasitol*, **70**: 203–6.

Diamond LS, Clark CG, 1993, A redescription of *Entamoeba histolytica* Schaudinn, 1903 (emended Walker, 1911) separating it from *Entamoeba dispar* Brumpt, 1925, *J Euk Microbiol*, **40**: 340–4.

Eakin AE, Bouvier J et al., 1990, Amplification and sequencing of genomic DNA fragments encoding cysteine proteases from protozoan parasites, *Mol Biochem Parasitol*, **39**: 1–8.

Edman U, Meza I, Agabian N, 1987, Genomic and cDNA actin sequences from a virulent strain of *Entamoeba histolytica*, *Proc Natl Acad Sci USA*, **84**: 3024–8.

Edman U, Meraz MA et al., 1990, Charaterization of an immunodominant variable surface antigen from pathogenic and non-pathogenic *Entamoeba histolytica*, *J Exp Med*, **172**: 879–88.

Ellis JE, Setchell KDR, Kaneshiro ES, 1994, Detection of ubiquinone in parasitic and free-living protozoa, including species devoid of mitochondria, *Mol Biochem Parasitol*, **65**: 213–24.

Elsdon-Dew R, 1968, The epidemiology of amoebiasis, *Adv Parasitol*, **6**: 1–62.

Espinosa-Cantellano M, Martínez-Palomo A, 1991, The plasma membrane of *Entamoeba histolytica*: structure and dynamics, *Biol Cell*, **72**: 189–200.

Espinosa-Cantellano M, Martínez-Palomo A, 1994, *Entamoeba histolytica*: Mechanism of surface receptor capping, *Exp Parasitol*, **79**: 424–35.

Fahey RC, Newton GL et al., 1984, *Entamoeba histolytica*: a eukaryote without glutathione metabolism, *Science*, **224**: 70–2.

Fairlamb AH, 1989, Novel biochemical pathways in parasitic protozoa, *Parasitology*, **99**: S93–112.

Födinger M, Ortner S et al., 1992, cDNA cloning of *Entamoeba histolytica* histone H3, *Arch Med Res*, **23**: 19–21.

Födinger M, Ortner S et al., 1993, Pathogenic *Entamoeba histolytica*: cDNA cloning of a histone H3 with a divergent primary structure, *Mol Biochem Parasitol*, **59**: 315–22.

Geiman QM, Ratcliffe HL, 1936, Morphology and life-cycle of an amoeba producing amoebiasis in reptiles, *Parasitology*, **28**: 208–28.

Ghadirian V, Jackson TFHG, 1987, A longitudinal study of asymptomatic carriers of pathogenic zymodemes of *Entamoeba histolytica*, *S Afr Med J*, **72**: 669–72.

González-Robles A, Martínez-Palomo A, 1992, The fine structure of *Entamoeba histolytica* processed by cryo-fixation and cryo-substitution, *Arch Med Res*, **23**: 73–6.

Gutiérrez G, Ludlow A et al., 1976, Encuesta serológica nacional II Investigación de anticuerpos contra *Entamoeba histolytica* en la República Mexicana, *Proceedings of the International Conference on Amebiasis*, eds Sepúlveda B, Diamond LS, Instituto Mexicano del Seguro Social, Mexico, 599–608.

Haque R, Neville LM et al., 1994, Detection of *Entamoeba histolytica* and *E. dispar* directly in stool, *Am J Trop Med Hyg*, **50**: 595–6.

Huang M, Albach RA et al., 1995, Cloning and sequencing a putative pyrophosphate-dependent phosphofructokinase gene from *Entamoeba histolytica*, *Biochim Biophys Acta*, **1260**: 215–17.

Huber M, Garfinkel L et al., 1987, *Entamoeba histolytica*: cloning and characterization of actin cDNA, *Mol Biochem Parasitol*, **24**: 227–35.

Huber M, Garfinkel L et al., 1988, Nucleotide sequence analysis of an *Entamoeba histolytica* ferredoxin gene, *Mol Biochem Parasitol*, **31**: 27–34.

Huber M, Koller B et al., 1989, *Entamoeba histolytica* ribosomal RNA genes are carried on palindromic circular DNA molecules, *Mol Biochem Parasitol*, **32**: 285–96.

Jansson A, Gillin F et al., 1994, Coding of hemolysins within the ribosomal RNA repeat on a plasmid in *Entamoeba histolytica*, *Science*, **263**: 1440–3.

Katiyar SK, Gordon VR et al., 1994, Antiprotozoal activities of benzimidazoles and correlations with b tubulin sequence, *Antimicrob Agents Chemother*, **38**: 2086–90.

Katzwinkel-Wladarsch S, Loscher T, Rinder H, 1994, Direct amplification and differentiation of pathogenic and non-pathogenic *Entamoeba histolytica* DNA from stool specimens, *Am J Trop Med Hyg*, **51**: 115–18.

Keene WE, Petitt MG et al., 1986, The major neutral proteinase of *Entamoeba histolytica*, *J Exp Med*, **163**: 536–49.

Keene WE, Hidalgo ME et al., 1990, *Entamoeba histolytica*: correlation of the cytopathic effect of virulent trophozoites with secretion of a cysteine proteinase, *Exp Parasitol*, **71**: 199–206.

Kelsall BL, Ravdin JI, 1993, Degradation of human IgA by *Entamoeba histolytica*, *J Infect Dis*, **168**: 1319–22.

Knobloch J, Mannweiler E, 1983, Development and persistence of antibodies to *Entamoeba histolytica* in patients with amebic liver abscess, *Am J Trop Med Hyg*, **32**: 727–32.

Kretschmer RR, 1986, Immunology of amebiasis, *Amebiasis*, ed Martínez-Palomo A, Elsevier Science Publishers, Amsterdam, 95–167.

Kretschmer RR, 1990, *Amebiasis: Infection and Disease by* Entamoeba histolytica, ed Kretschmer RR, CRC Press, Boca Raton.

Kumar A, Shen PS et al., 1992, Cloning and expression of an NADP$^+$-dependent alcohol dehydrogenase gene of *Entamoeba histolytica*, *Proc Natl Acad Sci USA*, **89**: 10188–92.

Leippe M, Tannich E et al., 1992, Primary and secondary structure of the pore-forming peptide of pathogenic *Entamoeba histolytica*, *EMBO J*, **11**: 3501–6.

Leippe M, Bahr E et al., 1993, Comparison of pore-forming peptides from pathogenic and nonpathogenic *Entamoeba histolytica*, *Mol Biochem Parasitol*, **59**: 101–10.

Leippe M, Andrae J et al., 1994, Amoebapores, a family of membranolytic peptides from cytoplasmic granules of *Entamoeba histolytica*: Isolation, primary structure, and pore formation in bacterial cytoplasmic membranes, *Mol Microbiol*, **14**: 895–904.

Levine ND, Corliss JO et al., 1980, A newly revised classification of the protozoa, *J Protozool*, **27**: 37–58.

Li E, Kunz-Jenkins C, Stanley SL, Jr, 1992, Isolation and characterization of genomic clones encoding a serine-rich *Entamoeba histolytica* protein, *Mol Biochem Parasitol*, **50**: 355–7.

Lioutas C, Schmetz C, Tannich E, 1995, Identification of various circular DNA molecules in *Entamoeba histolytica*, *Exp Parasitol*, **80**: 349–52.

Lohia A, Samuelson J, 1993a, Cloning of the Eh cdc2 gene from *Entamoeba histolytica* encoding a protein kinase p34^{cdc2} homologue, *Gene*, **127 (2)**: 203–7.

Lohia A, Samuelson J, 1993b, Molecular cloning of a *rho* family gene of *Entamoeba histolytica*, *Mol Biochem Parasitol*, **58**: 177–80.

Lohia A, Samuelson J, 1994, Molecular cloning of an *Entamoeba histolytica* gene encoding a putative *mos* family serine/threonine-kinase, *Biochim Biophys Acta*, **1222**: 122–4.

Luaces AL, Barret AJ, 1988, Affinity purification and biochemical characterization of histolysin, the major cysteine protease of *Entamoeba histolytica*, *Biochem J*, **250**: 903–9.

Lushbaugh WB, Hofbauer AF, Pittman FE, 1985, *Entamoeba histolytica*: purification of cathepsin B, *Exp Parasitol*, **59**: 328–36.

Mann BJ, Torian BE, Vedvick TS, 1991, Sequence of a cysteine-rich galactose-specific lectin of *Entamoeba histolytica*, *Proc Natl Acad Sci USA*, **88**: 3248–52.

Martínez-Palomo, A, 1982, The biology of *Entamoeba histolytica*, *Tropical Medicine Research Studies Series*, John Wiley and Sons, Chichester.

Martínez-Palomo A, 1986, Biology of *Entamoeba histolytica*, *Amebiasis*, ed Martínez-Palomo A, Elsevier, Amsterdam, 11–43.

Martínez-Palomo A, 1993, Parasitic amebas of the intestinal tract, *Parasitic Protozoa*, eds Kreier JP, Baker JR, Academic Press, San Diego, 65–141.

Martínez-Palomo A, González-Robles A, de la Torre M, 1973, Selective agglutination of pathogenic strains of *Entamoeba histolytica* induced by Concanavalin A, *Nature (London) New Biol*, **245**: 186–7.

Martínez-Palomo A, Ruíz-Palacios G, 1990, Amebiasis, *Tropical and Geographical Medicine*, eds Warren KS, Mahmoud AAF, McGraw Hill, New York, 327–44.

McCoy JJ, Mann BJ et al., 1993a, Structural analysis of the light subunit of the *Entamoeba histolytica* galactose-specific adherence lectin, *J Biol Chem*, **268**: 24223–31.

McCoy JJ, Mann BJ et al., 1993b, Sequence analysis of genes encoding the light subunit of the *Entamoeba histolytica* galactose-specific adhesin, *Mol Biochem Parasit*, **61**: 325–8.

McLaughlin J, Aley S, 1985, The biochemistry and functional morphology of the *Entamoeba*, *J Protozool*, **32**: 221–40.

Mertens E, 1993, ATP versus pyrophosphate: glycolysis revisited in parasitic protists, *Parasitol Today*, **9**: 122–6.

Mirelman D, Bracha R et al., 1986, Changes in isoenzyme patterns of a cloned culture of nonpathogenic *Entamoeba histolytica* during axenization, *Infect Immun*, **54**: 827–32.

Mittal V, Bhattacharya A, Bhattacharya S, 1992, Organization of repeated sequences in the region downstream to rRNA genes in the rDNA episome of *Entamoeba histolytica*, *Arch Med Res*, **23**: 17–18.

Mittal V, Bhattacharya A, Bhattacharya S, 1994, Isolation and characterization of a species-specific multicopy DNA sequence from *Entamoeba histolytica*, *Parasitology*, **108**: 237–44.

Mittal V, Ramachandran S et al., 1991, Sequence analysis of a DNA fragment with yeast autonomously replicating sequence activity from the extrachromosomal ribosomal DNA circle of *Entamoeba histolytica*, *Nucleic Acids Res*, **19**: 2777.

Mittal V, Sehgal D et al., 1992, A second short repeat sequence detected downstream of rRNA genes in the *Entamoeba histolytica* rDNA episome, *Mol Biochem Parasitol*, **54**: 97–100.

Moreno-Fierros L, Domínguez-Robles MC, Enríquez-Rincón F, 1995, *Entamoeba histolytica*: Induction and isotype analysis of antibody producing cell responses in Peyer's patches and spleen after local and systemic immunization in male and female mice, *Exp Parasitol*, **80**: 541–9.

Muñoz O, 1986, Epidemiology of amebiasis, *Amebiasis*, ed Martínez-Palomo A, Elsevier, Amsterdam, 213–39.

Neal RA, 1966, Experimental studies on *Entamoeba* with reference to speciation, *Adv Parasitol*, **4**: 1–51.

Neal RA, 1988, Phylogeny: The relationship of *Entamoeba histolytica* to morphologically similar amebae of the four-nucleate cyst group, *Amebiasis: Human Infection by* Entamoeba histolytica, ed Ravdin JI, John Wiley and Sons, New York, 13–26.

Nickel R, Tannich E, 1994, Transfection and transient expression of chloramphenicol acetyltransferase gene in the protozoan parasite *Entamoeba histolytica*, *Proc Natl Acad Sci USA*, **91**: 7095–8.

Orozco, E, 1992, Pathogenesis in amebiasis, *Infect Agents Dis*, **1**: 19–21.

Orozco E, Báez-Camargo M et al., 1993a, Molecular karyotype of related clones of *Entamoeba histolytica*, *Mol Biochem Parasitol*, **59**: 29–40.

Orozco E, Lazard D et al., 1993b, A variable DNA region of *Entamoeba histolytica* is expressed in several transcripts which differ in genetically related clones, *Mol Gen Genet*, **241**: 271–9.

Orozco E, Pérez DG et al., 1995, Multidrug resistance in *Entamoeba histolytica*, *Parasitol Today*, **11**: 473–5.

Ortner S, Plaimauer B et al., 1992, Humoral immune response against a 70-kilodalton heat shock protein of *Entamoeba histolytica* in a group of patients with invasive amoebiasis, *Mol Biochem Parasitol*, **54**: 175–84.

Pérez-Montfort R, Kretschmer RR, 1990, Humoral immune responses, *Amebiasis: Infection and Disease by* Entamoeba histolytica, ed Kretschmer RR, CRC Press, Boca Raton, 91–103.

Pérez-Tamayo R, 1986, Pathology of amebiasis, *Amebiasis*, ed Martínez-Palomo A, Elsevier, Amsterdam, 45–94.

Petri WA, Chapman MD et al., 1989, Subunit structure of the galactose and N-acetyl-D-galactosamine-inhibitable adherence lectin of *Entamoeba histolytica*, *J Biol Chem*, **264**: 3007–12.

Petri WA Jr, Jackson TFHG et al., 1990, Pathogenic and nonpathogenic strains of *Entamoeba histolytica* can be differentiated by monoclonal antibodies to the galactose-specific adherence lectin, *Infect Immun*, **58**: 1802–6.

Petter R, Rozenblatt S et al., 1992, Linkage between actin and ribosomal protein L21 genes in *Entamoeba histolytica*, *Mol Biochem Parasitol*, **56**: 329–34.

Petter R, Rozenblatt S et al., 1993, Electrophoretic karyotype and chromosome assignments for a pathogenic and a nonpathogenic strain of *Entamoeba histolytica*, *Infect Immun*, **61**: 3574–7.

Plaimauer B, Ortner S et al., 1993, Molecular characterization of the cDNA coding for translation elongation factor-2 of pathogenic *Entamoeba histolytica* DNA, *Cell Biol*, **12**: 89–96.

Plaimauer B, Ortner S et al., 1994, An intron-containing gene coding for a novel 39-kilodalton antigen of *Entamoeba histolytica*, *Mol Biochem Parasitol*, **66**: 181–5.

Prasad J, Bhattaharya S, Bhattacharya A, 1992, Cloning and sequence analysis of a calcium-binding protein gene from a pathogenic strain of *Entamoeba histolytica*, *Mol Biochem Parasitol*, **52**: 137–40.

Purdy, JE, Mann BJ et al., 1994, Transient transfection of the enteric parasite *Entamoeba histolytica* and expression of firefly luciferase, *Proc Natl Acad Sci USA*, **91**: 7099–103.

Que X, Reed SL, 1991, Nucleotide sequence of a small subunit ribosomal RNA (16S-like rRNA) gene from *Entamoeba histolytica*: differentiation of pathogenic from nonpathogenic isolates, *Nucleic Acids Res*, **19**: 5438.

Que X, Samuelson J, Reed S, 1993, Molecular cloning of a *rac* family protein kinase and identification of a serine/threonine protein kinase gene family of *Entamoeba histolytica*, *Mol Biochem Parasitol*, **60**: 161–70.

Ramachandran S, Bhattacharya A, Bhattacharya S, 1993, Nucleotide sequence analysis of the rRNA transcription unit of a pathogenic *Entamoeba histolytica* strain HM-1:IMSS, *Nucleic Acids Res*, **21**: 2011.

Ravdin JI, 1988, *Amebiasis: Human Infection by* Entamoeba histolytica, John Wiley and Sons, New York.

Raymond-Denise A, Sansonetti P, Guillén N, 1993, Identification and characterization of a myosin heavy chain gene (mhc A) from the human parasitic pathogen *Entamoeba histolytica*, *Mol Biochem Parasitol*, **59**: 123–32.

Reed SL, Gigli I, 1990, Lysis of complement-sensitive *Entamoeba histolytica* by activated terminal complement components, *J Clin Invest*, **86**: 1815–22.

Reed SL, Sargeaunt PG, Braude AI, 1983, Resistance to lysis by human serum of pathogenic *Entamoeba histolytica*, *Trans R Soc Trop Med Hyg*, **77**: 248–53.

Reed SL, Flores BM et al., 1992, Molecular and cellular characterization of the 29-kilodalton peripheral membrane protein of *Entamoeba histolytica*: Differentiation between pathogenic and nonpathogenic isolates, *Infect Immun*, **60**: 542–9.

Reed S, Bouvier J et al., 1993, Cloning of a virulence factor of *Entamoeba histolytica* . Pathogenic strains possess a unique cysteine proteinase gene, *J Clin Invest*, **91**: 1532–40.

Reeves RE, 1984, Metabolism of *Entamoeba histolytica* Schaudinn, 1903, *Advances in Parasitology*, eds Baker JR, Muller R, Academic Press, London, 105–142.

Richards CS, Goldman M, Cannon LT, 1966, Cultivation of *Entamoeba histolytica* and *Entamoeba histolytica*-like strains at reduced temperature and behavior of the amebae in diluted media, *Am J Trop Med Hyg*, **15**: 648–55.

Rosales-Encina JL, Meza I et al., 1987, Isolation of a 220 kDa protein with lectin properties from a virulent strain of *Entamoeba histolytica*, *J Infect Dis*, **156**: 790–7.

Saavedra-Lira E, Pérez-Montfort R, 1994, Cloning and sequence determination of the gene coding for the pyruvate phosphate dikinase of *Entamoeba histolytica*, *Gene*, **142:** 249–51.

Saavedra-Lira E, Robinson O, Pérez Montfort R, 1992, Partial nucleotide sequence of the enzyme pyruvate, orthophosphate dikinase of *Entamoeba histolytica* HM-1:IMSS, *Arch Med Res*, **23:** 39–40.

Salis H, 1941, Studies on the morphology of the *E histolytica*-like amoebae found in monkeys, *J Parasitol*, **27:** 327–39.

Samuelson J, Acuña-Soto R et al., 1989, DNA hybridization probe for clinical diagnosis of *Entamoeba histolytica*, *J Clin Microbiol*, **27:** 671–6.

Sanchez MA, Peattie DA et al., 1994, Cloning, genomic organization and transcription of the *Entamoeba histolytica* α-tubulin gene, *Gene*, **146:** 239–44.

Sargeaunt PG, Jackson TFHG, Simjee A, 1982, Biochemical homogeneity of *Entamoeba histolytica* isolates, especially those from liver abscess, *Lancet*, **1:** 1386–8.

Sargeaunt PG, Patrick S, O'Keefe D, 1992, Human infections of *Entamoeba chattoni* masquerade as *Entamoeba histolytica*, *Trans R Soc Trop Med Hyg*, **86:** 633–4.

Sargeaunt PG, Williams JE, 1979, Electrophoretic isoenzyme patterns of the pathogenic and nonpathogenic amoebae of man, *Trans R Soc Trop Med Hyg*, **73:** 225–7.

Sargeaunt PG, Williams JE, Neal RA, 1980, A comparative study of *Entamoeba histolytica* (NIH:200, HK9, etc), '*Entamoeba histolytica*-like' and other morphologically identical amoebae using isozyme electrophoresis, *Trans R Soc Trop Med Hyg*, **74:** 469–74.

Sargeaunt PG, Oates JK et al., 1983, *Entamoeba histolytica* in male homosexuals, *Br J Venereal Dis*, **59:** 193–5.

Scholze H, Löhden-Bendinger U et al., 1992, Subcellular distribution of amebapain, the major cysteine proteinase of *Entamoeba histolytica*, *Arch Med Res*, **23:** 105–8.

Sehgal D, Bhattacharya A, Bhattacharya S, 1993, Analysis of a polymorphic locus present upstream of rDNA transcription units in the extrachromosomal circle of *Entamoeba histolytica*, *Mol Biochem Parasitol*, **62:** 129–30.

Sehgal D, Mittal V et al., 1994, Nucleotide sequence organization and analysis of the nuclear ribosomal DNA circle of the protozoan parasite *Entamoeba histolytica*, *Mol Biochem Parasitol*, **67:** 205–14.

Sepúlveda B, 1970, La amibiasis invasora por *Entamoeba histolytica*, *Gaceta Médica de México*, **100:** 201–54.

Sepúlveda B, 1982, Amebiasis: host-pathogen biology, *Rev Infect Dis*, **4:** 836–42.

Sepúlveda B, Treviño-García Manzo N, 1986, Clinical manifestations and diagnosis of amebiasis, *Amebiasis*, ed Martínez-Palomo A, Elsevier, Amsterdam, 169–88.

Serrano R, Reeves RE, 1974, Glucose transport in *Entamoeba histolytica*, *Biochem J*, **144:** 43–8.

Shen P-S, Lohia A, Samuelson J, 1994, Molecular cloning of ras and rap genes from *Entamoeba histolytica*, *Mol Biochem Parasitol*, **64:** 111–20.

Shirakura T, Hashimoto T et al., 1994, Phylogenetic place of a mitochondria-lacking protozoan, *Entamoeba histolytica*, inferred from amino acid sequences of elongation factor II, *Jpn J Genet*, **69:** 119–35.

Simic T, 1931, Infection expérimentale de l'homme par *Entamoeba dispar* Brumpt, *Ann Parasitol Hum Compar*, **9:** 385–91.

Spice WM, Ackers JP, 1992, The amoeba enigma, *Parasitol Today*, **8:** 402–6.

Stanley Jr SL, 1996, Progress towards an amebiasis vaccine, *Parasitol Today*, **12:** 7–14.

Stanley Jr SL, Li E, 1992, Isolation of an *Entamoeba histolytica* cDNA clone encoding a protein with a putative zinc finger domain, *Mol Biochem Parasitol*, **50:** 185–7.

Stanley Jr SL, Becker A et al., 1990, Cloning and expression of a membrane antigen of *Entamoeba histolytica* possessing multiple tandem repeats, *Proc Natl Acad Sci USA*, **87:** 4976–80.

Strachan WD, Spice WM et al., 1988, Immunological differentiation of pathogenic and non-pathogenic isolates of *Entamoeba histolytica*, *Lancet*, **1:** 561–3.

Tachibana H, Kobayashi S et al., 1990, Identification of a pathogenic isolate-specific 30,000-M$_r$ antigen of *Entamoeba histolytica* by using a monoclonal antibody, *Infect Immun*, **58:** 955–60.

Tachibana H, Ihara S et al., 1991, Differences in genomic DNA sequences between pathogenic and nonpathogenic isolates of *Entamoeba histolytica* identified by polymerase chain reaction, *J Clin Microbiol*, **29:** 2234–9.

Takeuchi T, Miyahira Y et al., 1990, High seropositivity for *Entamoeba histolytica* infection in Japanese homosexual men, *Trans R Soc Trop Med Hyg*, **84:** 250–1.

Talamás-Rohana P, Hernández VI, Rosales-Encina JL, 1994, A β1 integrin-like molecule in *Entamoeba histolytica*, *Trans R Soc Trop Med Hyg*, **88:** 596–9.

Tannich E, Ebert F, Horstmann RD, 1992, Molecular cloning of cDNA and genomic sequences coding for the 35-kilodalton subunit of the galactose-inhibitable lectin of pathogenic *Entamoeba histolytica*, *Mol Biochem Parasitol*, **55:** 225–8.

Tannich E, Bruchhaus I et al., 1991a, Pathogenic and nonpathogenic *Entamoeba histolytica*: identification and molecular cloning of an iron-containing superoxide dismutase, *Mol Biochem Parasitol*, **49:** 61–72.

Tannich E, Scholze H et al., 1991b, Homologous cysteine proteinases of pathogenic and nonpathogenic *Entamoeba histolytica*, *J Biol Chem*, **266:** 4798–803.

Tannich E, Nickel R et al., 1992, Mapping and partial sequencing of the genes coding for two different cysteine proteinases in pathogenic *Entamoeba histolytica*, *Mol Biochem Parasitol*, **54:** 109–11.

Torian BE, Lukehart SA, Stamm WE, 1987, Use of monoclonal antibodies to identify, characterize, and purify a 96,000-Dalton surface antigen of pathogenic *Entamoeba histolytica*, *J Infect Dis*, **156:** 334–43.

Torian BE, Flores BM et al., 1990, cDNA sequence analysis of a 29-kDa cysteine-rich surface antigen of pathogenic *Entamoeba histolytica*, *Proc Natl Acad Sci USA*, **87:** 6358–62.

Trissl D, 1982, Immunology of *Entamoeba histolytica* in human and animal hosts, *Rev Infect Dis*, **4:** 1154–84.

Trissl D, Martínez-Palomo A et al., 1977, Surface properties related to concanavalin A-induced agglutination A comparative study of several *Entamoeba* strains, *J Exp Med*, **145:** 652–65.

Trissl D, Martínez-Palomo A et al., 1978, Surface properties of *Entamoeba*: increased rates of human erythrocyte phagocytosis in pathogenic strains, *J Exp Med*, **148:** 1137–45.

Tsutsumi V, Mena R, Martínez-Palomo A, 1984, Cellular bases of experimental liver abscess formation, *Am J Pathol*, **130:** 112–19.

US Treasury Department and Public Health Service, 1936, Epidemic Amebic Dysentery. The Chicago Outbreak of 1933, *Bulletin 166, National Institutes of Health*.

Walsh JA, 1984, Estimating the burden of illness in the Tropics, *Tropical and Geographical Medicine*, ed Warren KS, Mahmoud A, McGraw-Hill, New York, 1073–85.

Walsh JA, 1986, Problems in recognition and diagnosis of amebiasis: Estimation of the global magnitude of morbidity and mortality, *Rev Infect Dis*, **8:** 228–38.

Walsh J, Martínez-Palomo A, 1986, Control of amebiasis, *Amebiasis*, ed Martínez-Palomo A, Elsevier, Amsterdam, 241–60.

Weinbach EC, 1981, Biochemistry of enteric parasitic protozoa, *Trends Biochem Sci*, **6:** 254–7.

W H O, 1985, Amoebiasis and its control, *Bull W H O*, **63:** 417–26.

Wostmann C, Tannich E, Bakker-Grunwald T, 1992, Ubiquitin of *Entamoeba histolytica* deviates in 6 amino acid residues from the consensus of all other known ubiquitins, *FEBS Lett*, **308:** 54–8.

Ximénez C, Leyva O et al., 1993, *Entamoeba histolytica*: antibody response to recent and past invasive events, *Ann Trop Med Parasitol*, **87:** 31–9.

Yang W, Li E et al., 1994, *Entamoeba histolytica* has an alcohol dehydrogenase homologous to the multifunctional adhE gene product of *Escherichia coli*, *Mol Biochem Parasitol*, **64:** 253–60.

Yi Y, Samuelson J, 1994, Primary structure of the *Entamoeba histolytica* gene (Ehvma1) encoding the catalytic peptide of a putative vacuolar membrane proton-translocating ATPase (V-ATPase), *Mol Biochem Parasitol*, **66:** 165–9.

Yu Y, Samuelson J, 1994, Primary structure of an *Entamoeba histolytica* nicotinamide nucleotide transhydrogenase, *Mol Biochem Parasitol*, **68:** 323–8.

Zhang T, Li E, Stanley SL, Jr, 1995, Oral immunization with the dodecapeptide repeat of the serine-rich *Entamoeba histolytica* protein (SREHP) fused to the cholera toxin B subunit induces a mucosal and systemic anti-SREHP antibody response, *Infect Immun*, **63:** 1349–55.

Zhang W-W, Samuelson J, 1993a, The cDNA sequence of an abundant *Entamoeba histolytica* 20-kilodalton protein containing four repetitive domains, *Mol Biochem Parasitol*, **60:** 323–6.

Zhang W-W, Samuelson J, 1993b, Molecular cloning of the gene for a novel ABC superfamily transporter of *Entamoeba histolytica*, *Mol Biochem Parasitol*, **62:** 131–4.

Zhang W-W, Shen P-S et al., 1994, Cloning and expression of an NADP$^+$-dependent aldehyde dehydrogenase of *Entamoeba histolytica*, *Mol Biochem Parasitol*, **63:** 157–61.

Zurita M, Lizardi PM et al., 1992, Characterization of a repetitive DNA element from *Entamoeba histolytica*, *Mol Biochem Parasitol*, **51:** 165–8.

Chapter 9

OPPORTUNISTIC AMOEBAE

D T John

1 INTRODUCTION

Free-living amoebae of the genera *Naegleria*, *Acanthamoeba* and *Balamuthia* can cause disease in humans and other animals (reviewed by John 1993). Normally they live as phagotrophs in aquatic habitats where they feed on bacteria, but as opportunists, they may produce serious infection of the central nervous system (CNS) and the eye. The term 'amphizoic', Gr. *amphi* = on both sides, has been proposed to describe the ability of these amoebae to live in 2 worlds, as free-living organisms and as endoparasites.

Naegleria fowleri is responsible for a rapidly fatal infection involving the CNS, called 'primary amoebic meningoencephalitis' (PAM). Infection occurs most often in healthy young people who have a recent history of swimming in freshwater. Several species of *Acanthamoeba* cause disease. *Acanthamoeba* may produce a chronic CNS infection known as 'granulomatous amoebic encephalitis' (GAE) or an eye infection referred to as '*Acanthamoeba* keratitis'. Human infections originally attributed to *Hartmannella*, another free-living amoeba, were actually caused by *Acanthamoeba*. *Balamuthia mandrillaris*, a newly described leptomyxid amoeba (Visvesvara, Schuster and Martinez 1993), causes a chronic CNS infection similar to that produced by *Acanthamoeba*, also termed GAE.

2 CLASSIFICATION

The classification of the Protozoa is in a state of flux and, following the precedents set out elsewhere in this volume (Chapter 7, Classification of the Protozoa), the scheme proposed by Corliss (1994) and widely adopted by scientists working with free-living protozoa will be used. On the basis of the traditional classification published by the Society of Protozoologists (Lee, Hutner and Bovee 1985), all the opportunistic amoebae were classified in the phylum Sarcomastigophora, subphylum Sarcodina, in 2 classes: (1) Lobosea, containing 2 orders, Amoebida (family Acanthamoebidae, e.g. *Acanthamoeba*) and Schizopyrenida (family Valkampfidae, e.g. *Naegleria*); and (2) Acarpomyxea containing the order Leptomyxida (family Leptomyxidae, e.g. *Balamuthia*). In Corliss' classification both *Acanthamoeba* and *Balamuthia* are classified in the phylum Rhizopoda, class Lobosea, and *Naegleria* has been removed to the phylum Percolozoa and placed in the class Heterolobosea and order Schizopyrenida.

3 STRUCTURE AND LIFE-CYCLES

3.1 Morphology

The nuclei of the opportunistic amoebae are characterized by a large central nucleolus, or karyosome, and a nuclear membrane without chromatin granules. These features are especially useful for identification when examining histological sections and readily distinguish these organisms from *Entamoeba histolytica*, the most important parasitic amoeba of humans.

NAEGLERIA

The trophozoites of *N. fowleri* are known as 'limax amoebae', from the Latin word meaning slug. These amoebae are elongate and move in a directional manner by eruptive, blunt pseudopodia called lobopodia. Actively moving amoebae average c. 22 μm in length (range 15–30 μm); inactive, rounded forms range from 9 to 15 μm in diameter (Carter 1970).

Trophozoites of pathogenic *Naegleria* have distinctive phagocytic structures known as 'amoebostomes' (Fig. 9.1) (John, Cole and Bruner 1985). Amoebostomes are used for engulfment and vary in number, depending on the strain. By transmission electron microscopy, amoebostomes appear to be densely granular in contrast to the highly vacuolated body of the amoeba. Amoebostomes are visible by light microscopy but appear as thick-walled vacuoles. Similar food cups or phagocytic stomata occur on *E. histolytica* (Gonzalez-Robles and Martinez-Palomo 1983).

Reproduction in *Naegleria* is by simple binary fission of the trophozoite. Nuclear division is promitotic, which means that the nucleolus and the nuclear membrane persist during nuclear division (karyokinesis). The nucleolus elongates, forming a dumbbell-shaped structure, and divides into 2 polar masses, or nucleoli. During this process the nuclear membrane remains intact (Page 1988).

When *Naegleria* are suspended in distilled water or non-nutrient buffer, they transform into temporary flagellated forms. The typical *N. fowleri* flagellate is a bluntly elongate cigar- or pear-shaped cell with 2 flagella emerging from beneath the anterior rostrum (Fig. 9.2). Of the different species of *Naegleria*, *N. fowleri* flagellates are the most uniform, generally having 2 flagella (John, Cole and John 1991).

The cysts of *N. fowleri* (Fig. 9.3) are spherical, often clumped closely together, and are 7–15 μm in diameter (Carter 1970, Page 1988). Examination of cysts by electron microscopy reveals an average of <2 mucoid-plugged pores, or ostioles, per cyst and a relatively thin cyst wall (Schuster 1975), a feature that makes *N. fowleri* cysts susceptible to desiccation.

ACANTHAMOEBA

A feature that readily distinguishes the amoebae of *Acanthamoeba* from those of *Naegleria* is the presence of acanthopodia (Gr. *acanth* = spine or thorn), tapering spike-like pseudopodia (Fig. 9.4); hence the name *Acanthamoeba*. In contrast to *Naegleria*, which has rapid, directional locomotion, *Acanthamoeba* moves slowly on

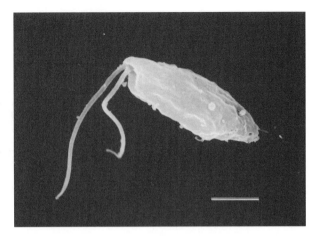

Fig. 9.2 SEM of a *Naegleria fowleri* flagellate with 2 flagella emerging from beneath the anterior rostrum. Bar = 3 μm.

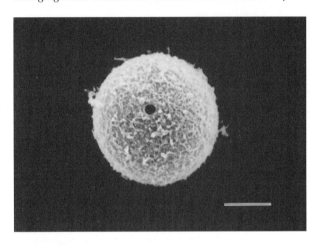

Fig. 9.3 SEM of a *Naegleria fowleri* cyst having a single pore or ostiole. Bar = 3 μm.

a broad front without direction. Trophozoites of *Acanthamoeba* are larger than those of *Naegleria* and average c. 24–56 μm in length (Lewis and Sawyer 1979). Nuclear division in *Acanthamoeba* is metamitotic, whereby the nucleolus and the nuclear membrane disintegrate during early karyokinesis, a pattern similar to that of dividing metazoan cells (Page 1988).

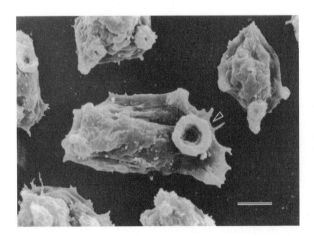

Fig. 9.1 Scanning electron micrograph (SEM) of a *Naegleria fowleri* amoeba with a single amoebostome (arrowhead). Bar = 5 μm.

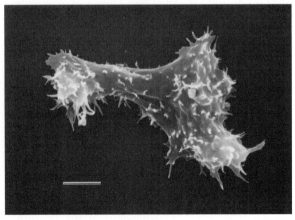

Fig. 9.4 SEM of a pathogenic *Acanthamoeba castellanii* amoeba displaying numerous acanthopodia. Bar = 5 μm.

Considerable variation in cyst morphology occurs among the different species of *Acanthamoeba*, resulting in the naming of new species. Page (1967) recognized 4 species of *Acanthamoeba*; by 1976 he had recorded 7. On the basis of morphology and isoenzyme analysis, De Jonckheere (1987) identified 17 species of *Acanthamoeba*, of which 7 have been associated with human infection. The cysts of *Acanthamoeba* are double-walled and, therefore, quite resistant in the environment. The cyst wall is made up of an outer wrinkled, or rippled, ectocyst and an inner endocyst. The encysted amoeba conforms to the shape of the endocyst. The characteristic wrinkled appearance of *Acanthamoeba* cysts is readily seen in culture (Fig. 9.5) and in histological sections (see Fig. 9.11).

BALAMUTHIA

The trophozoites of *B. mandrillaris* are mostly irregular or branching in shape (Fig. 9.6),with some limax forms. Their length ranges from 12 to 60 μm (mean c. 30 μm) (Visvesvara, Schuster and Martinez 1993). These amoebae exhibit little directional motility, although a spider-like walking movement may be seen with amoebae grown in Vero cell culture. Nuclear division is metamitotic, as in *Acanthamoeba*. Cysts are irregularly round and are 6–30 μm in diameter (mean 15 μm) with 2 walls. The inner cyst wall is thin and spherical and the outer cyst wall is thick and wavy or wrinkled (Fig. 9.6), much like the cysts of *Acanthamoeba* (Visvesvara, Schuster and Martinez 1993).

3.2 Life-cycles

Naegleria, Acanthamoeba and leptomyxid amoebae are distributed worldwide in freshwater and soil. *Acanthamoeba* and some leptomyxids are found in marine environments as well. Life-cycles are simple; a feeding trophozoite, or amoeba, a resting cyst and, in *Naegleria*, a transient flagellate.

NAEGLERIA

The life-cycle of *N. fowleri* is illustrated in Fig. 9.7. The term 'amoeboflagellate' is used to describe amoebae

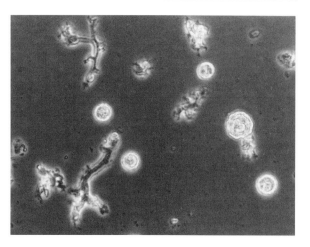

Fig. 9.6 Phase-contrast micrograph of *Balamuthia mandrillaris* amoebae and cysts. (Courtesy Dr. Govinda S. Visvesvara, Centers for Disease Control and Prevention, Atlanta, Georgia).

that can transform into flagellates. When *Naegleria* amoebae are placed in a non-nutrient medium, such as distilled water or buffer, they differentiate into transient, non-feeding, non-dividing flagellates that, after a time, will revert back to amoebae. Amoebae will also encyst when conditions are appropriate and, later, excyst in a favourable environment.

The invasive stage of *N. fowleri* is the amoeba and infection is acquired by intranasal absorption of amoebae in fresh water, which then invade the nasal mucosa, cribriform plate and olfactory bulbs of the brain. It is likely that flagellates or cysts of *N. fowleri* could enter the nose of a swimmer as readily as amoebae. However, flagellates would revert quickly to amoebae or the amoebae could escape from cysts, the point being that amoebae are the invading organisms. Flagellates or cysts of *N. fowleri* have never been found in tissue or cerebrospinal fluid.

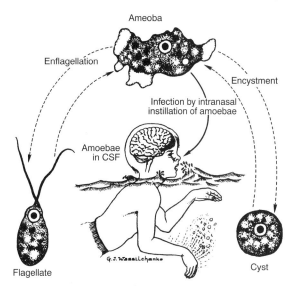

Fig. 9.7 Life-cycle of *Naegleria fowleri* and human infection.

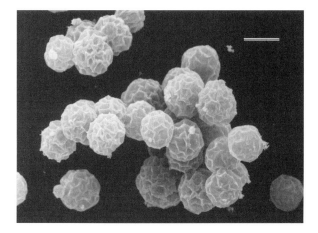

Fig. 9.5 SEM of pathogenic *Acanthamoeba polyphaga* cysts. Bar = 10 μm.

ACANTHAMOEBA AND BALAMUTHIA

Fig. 9.8 illustrates the life-cycle of *Acanthamoeba* and shows human involvement. The free-living cycle of the amoeba and cyst is also reflected in human infection, in which both amoebae and cysts are seen in tissue, in contrast to naeglerial infection in which only amoebae occur. *Acanthamoeba* seems to be truly amphizoic in all respects. Amoebae and cysts of *Balamuthia* are also found in tissue.

Human infection by *Acanthamoeba* involves the CNS, the eye and other organs. Although amoebae of pathogenic *Acanthamoeba* are able to invade the nasal mucosa and cause fatal CNS disease in experimental animals, this is not thought to be the usual route of invasion in human infection. Invasion of the CNS seems to be by way of the circulation, the amoebae originating from a primary focus elsewhere in the body, possibly the lower respiratory tract, ulcers of the skin or mucosa or other wounds. The modes of invasion by leptomyxid amoebae are thought to be the same. GAE tends to occur in persons who are debilitated, chronically ill or immunocompromised. In contrast, *Acanthamoeba* keratitis usually occurs in healthy individuals and infection is by direct invasion of the cornea through trauma to the eye or the wearing of contaminated contact lenses.

4 BIOCHEMISTRY, MOLECULAR BIOLOGY AND GENETICS

Most research on the cell and molecular biology of free-living amoebae has been with non-pathogenic rather than pathogenic species. Nonetheless, some observations can be made and comparisons drawn between the 2 groups.

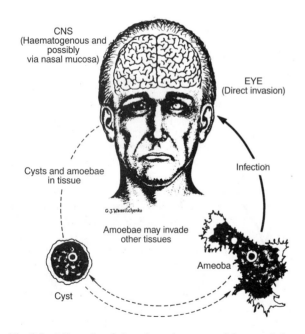

Fig. 9.8 Life-cycle of *Acanthamoeba* spp. and human infection.

4.1 Cell differentiation

Cell differentiation is the process by which amoebae become cysts or flagellates and, of course, become amoebae again. *Acanthamoeba*, *Balamuthia* and *Naegleria* all produce cysts, but only *Naegleria* produces flagellates. Thus, free-living amoebae provide useful models for studying the developmental biology and molecular mechanisms controlling morphogenesis and differentiation in eukaryotic cells.

ENCYSTMENT

Most of what is known about encystment in *Naegleria* and *Acanthamoeba* has come from studies involving the non-pathogenic species. Encystment is an adaptive mechanism that enables the organism to survive conditions that would kill the amoeba. Factors thought to induce cyst formation include starvation, drying and various chemicals. Excystment is the process by which amoebae exit from their protective cysts. It is generally held that unfavourable conditions induce encystment and that favourable conditions stimulate excystment.

There are no definitive studies that describe the conditions for encystment and excystment in *N. fowleri*. Chemical factors that induce encystment in *A. castellanii* include the inhibitors of DNA synthesis, fluorodeoxyuridine, mitomycin C, Trenimon (Neff and Neff 1972) and hydroxyurea (Rudick 1971); the mitochondrial inhibitors, diminazine (Berenil), ethidium bromide, erythromycin and chloramphenicol (Akins and Byers 1980); and acetate and glucose starvation (Byers et al. 1980). Medium from encysting cultures of *A. castellanii* contains an extracellular encystment-enhancing activity that stimulates cyst formation in early log phase cultures (Akins and Byers 1980). Encystment-enhancing activity is required for encystment in cultures induced by diminazine and by glucose starvation, but not when it is induced by total deprivation of nutrients (Akins, Gozs and Byers 1985).

ENFLAGELLATION

Although spontaneous enflagellation occurs in cultures of *Naegleria*, especially exponential phase cultures of *N. fowleri*, synchronized enflagellation may be achieved by suspending amoebae in distilled water or non-nutrient buffer. Enflagellation in *Naegleria* apparently occurs not as an obligatory phase in the life-cycle but as a response to changes in the environment. Factors affecting enflagellation in *N. fowleri* include: nutrient depletion, temperature, phase of growth and culture agitation. Maximum enflagellation in axenically grown *N. fowleri* occurs 4–5 h after suspension in buffer (Cable and John 1986). For axenically grown non-pathogenic *N. gruberi*, maximum enflagellation occurs somewhat sooner, c. 1.5 h after suspension in buffer (Fulton 1977).

Cyclohexamide and actinomycin D completely prevent enflagellation in *N. fowleri* when added before enflagellation commences but, when added after initiation of enflagellation, both prevent further differentiation and cause existing flagellates to revert to amoebae (Woodworth, Keefe and Bradley 1982b). The ultrastructure of *N. fowleri* flagellates is that of a typical eukaryotic protist. There is a distinct nuclear membrane and a prominent nucleolus, numerous vacuoles and cytoplasmic inclusions, pleomorphic mitochondria and some rough endoplasmic reticulum. Basal bodies, rootlets and flagella are formed quickly after an initial lag of 90 min (Patterson et al. 1981).

4.2 Macromolecular composition

Changes in cell composition of *N. fowleri* are related to culture age. For shaken axenic cultures, average cell mass remains constant during logarithmic growth at 150 pg/amoeba but decreases by 30% during the stationary phase at 96 h. During logarithmic growth, 80–85% of the cell dry mass is protein (120 pg/amoeba) (Weik and John 1978). Cell dry mass and protein of *N. fowleri* are c. 70% of values reported for *N. gruberi* (Weik and John 1977). The majority of *N. fowleri* polypeptides have molecular masses within the range of 20-60 kDa (Woodworth, Keefe and Bradley 1982b). During logarithmic and stationary phases of growth of *N. fowleri*, carbohydrate content averages 15 pg/amoeba and RNA is c. 18 pg/amoeba (Weik and John 1978). By comparison, *N. gruberi* carbohydrate averages c. 35 pg/amoeba and the RNA content is 8 pg/amoeba (Weik and John 1977). The more than 2-fold higher RNA value for the smaller pathogenic *N. fowleri* reflects different biosynthetic capabilities and maintenance of a larger ribosome complement. Total DNA in *N. fowleri* is 0.2 pg/amoeba during logarithmic growth; it doubles during transition from exponential phase to stationary phase and then gradually decreases almost to initial levels. The peak in DNA content corresponds to an increase in the average number of nuclei per amoeba; nuclear number then decreases as cells enter the stationary phase (Weik and John 1978). In *N. gruberi*, the total DNA content of 0.2 pg/cell increases by 50% during exponential growth (Weik and John 1977).

4.3 Respiratory metabolism

As an opportunistic pathogen, *N. fowleri* lives in the brain, an oxygen-rich environment, and would thus be expected to have an aerobic metabolism. The use of the synonym '*N. aerobia*' (Singh and Das 1970) recognized the aerobic nature of the organism, in contrast to the anaerobic nature of strictly parasitic amoebae. Unlike *E. histolytica*, an anaerobic parasite that lacks mitochondria, *N. fowleri* lives in aerobic aqueous environments and has many mitochondria.

Whole-cell respiration rates were measured polarographically throughout the growth cycle of *N. fowleri* (Weik and John 1979a). In agitated cultures, amoebae consume 30 ng atoms O/min/mg of cell protein during logarithmic growth. Under similar conditions, *N. gruberi* amoebae consume 80 ng atoms O/min/mg of cell protein (Weik and John 1979b). The lower oxygen consumption, and presumably oxygen requirement, of *N. fowleri* probably explains the presence of the pathogen in heated waters in which dissolved oxygen concentrations are substantially reduced. The respiratory rate gradually declines during the stationary phase. The reduction in respiratory rate may involve respiratory control as increases in respiratory rate did not occur despite the addition of oxygen (Weik and John 1979a). The respiratory process of isolated *N. fowleri* mitochondria is similar to that of classic mammalian cell mitochondria. Oxidation is coupled to phosphorylation (ATP formation) as shown by the 2–3-fold increase in respiration on addition of a phosphate acceptor or an uncoupling agent. The spectra of oxidized and dithionite-reduced mitochondria show distinct absorption bands of flavins and *c*-type, *b*-type and *a*-type cytochromes (Weik and John 1979a).

4.4 Genetics

It has generally been assumed that reproduction in *Acanthamoeba* and *Naegleria* is asexual and that sexuality, or genetic exchange, does not occur. In the past, genetic studies have been hampered because of difficulty in visualizing the very small, numerous chromosomes of these amoebae, which may number 16 for *Naegleria* (De Jonckheere 1989) and 80 for *Acanthamoeba* (Volkonsky 1931). Fulton (1970) reported that one strain of *N. gruberi* had twice the ploidy of another strain, based on cell and nuclear volume and DNA content. Cariou and Pernin (1987) and Pernin, Ataya and Cariou (1992) provided evidence for diploidy and genetic recombination in *N. lovaniensis*. De Jonckheere (1989) compared the electrophoretic karyotypes of all the species of *Naegleria* and concluded that, although karyotype analysis cannot be used to identify *Naegleria* species, it is useful for studying gene localization and genetic exchange. No genetic studies on the opportunistic amoebae have been published. Clark and Cross (1987) described a self-replicating ribosomal DNA plasmid in *N. gruberi*, making it the third eukaryotic genus to have a nuclear plasmid DNA. Additionally, they sequenced the small-subunit ribosomal RNA (rRNA) gene of *N. gruberi* and showed that circular rRNA genes are a general feature of schizopyrenid (amoeboflagellate) amoebae, including, presumably, *N. fowleri* (Clark and Cross 1988).

5 CLINICAL ASPECTS

5.1 Introduction

N. fowleri causes a rapidly fatal infection involving the CNS known as 'primary amoebic meningoencephalitis' (PAM). A number of *Acanthamoeba* species may produce a chronic CNS infection called 'granulomatous amoebic encephalitis' (GAE), or an eye infection referred to as '*Acanthamoeba* keratitis'. *B. mandrillaris* also causes GAE.

5.2 Clinical manifestations

PRIMARY AMOEBIC MENINGOENCEPHALITIS (PAM)

PAM typically occurs in healthy children or young adults with a recent history of swimming in freshwater. The disease is rapidly fatal, usually resulting in death within 72 h of the onset of symptoms. Infection follows entry of water containing amoebae or flagellates into the nose. It has been suggested that inhalation of cysts, e.g. during dust storms, could lead to infection (Lawande et al. 1979). Amoebae penetrate the nasal mucosa and the cribriform plate and travel along the olfactory nerves to the brain. Amoebae first invade the olfactory bulbs and then spread to the more posterior regions of the brain. Within the brain they provoke inflammation and cause extensive destruction of tissue (Carter 1970, Martinez 1985).

The clinical course is dramatic. Symptoms begin with severe frontal headache, fever (39–40°C) and anorexia followed by nausea, vomiting and signs of meningeal irritation, frequently evidenced by a positive Kernig's sign. Involvement of the olfactory lobes may cause disturbances in smell or taste and may be noted early in the course of the disease. Visual disturbance may occur. The patient may experience confusion, irritability and restlessness and may become irrational before lapsing into a coma. Generalized seizures may also occur. In order of frequency of occurrence, the more important symptoms include headache, anorexia, nausea, vomiting, fever and neck stiffness (Carter 1970, Martinez 1985).

GRANULOMATOUS AMOEBIC ENCEPHALITIS (GAE)

GAE usually occurs in debilitated or chronically ill persons, some of whom may be undergoing immunosuppressive therapy. The underlying conditions reported in GAE are Hodgkin's disease, systemic lupus erythematosus, diabetes mellitus, G6PD deficiency, alcoholism and acquired immunodeficiency syndrome (AIDS). Some of the victims of GAE are not debilitated or immunocompromised, but are otherwise healthy individuals. GAE is a disease not as well defined as that caused by *N. fowleri*. The course of infection is subacute or chronic, lasting weeks, months or even years, and is characterized by focal granulomatous lesions of the brain. The onset of GAE, unlike that of PAM, is insidious with a prolonged clinical course (Carter et al. 1981, Martinez 1987).

Acanthamoeba infection probably occurs through the lower respiratory tract or through ulcers of the skin or mucosa. Invasion into the CNS is by hematogenous spread from the primary focus of infection. As there are no lymphatic channels in the brain, invasion of the brain must be via the bloodstream (Martinez 1987). Even though some *Acanthamoeba* isolates are able to produce a CNS infection after intranasal instillation in mice, there is no proof that similar invasion occurs in the human disease. The portal of entry and spread in *Balamuthia* infection is believed to be the same as for *Acanthamoeba*. The incubation period is not known, but probably lasts weeks or months, and during the prolonged clinical course single or multiple space-occupying lesions develop. An altered mental state is a prominent feature in GAE. Headache, seizures and neck stiffness occur in about half of the cases. Nausea and vomiting may also be noted (Martinez 1987).

ACANTHAMOEBA KERATITIS

Acanthamoeba keratitis is a chronic infection of the cornea caused by several species of *Acanthamoeba* including *A. castellanii*, *A. culbertsoni*, *A. hatchetti*, *A. polyphaga* and *A. rhysodes* and infections are being diagnosed with increasing frequency (Stehr-Green, Bailey and Visvesvara 1989). Infection is by direct contact of the cornea with amoebae, which may be introduced through minor corneal trauma or by exposure to contaminated water or contact lenses. The wearing of contact lenses and the use of home made saline solutions are important risk factors. Saline solutions contaminated with protein residues from contact lenses promote the growth of bacteria and yeast which, in turn, are a source of food for the amoebae. Amoebae attach to the contact lenses stored in contaminated solutions and are transferred to the eye when lenses are placed over the cornea. Amoebae become established as part of the conjunctival flora and may invade the corneal stroma through a break in the epithelium or through the intact epithelium. They produce an infection that progresses to *Acanthamoeba* keratitis, which usually develops over a period of weeks to months, and is characterized by the following: severe ocular pain (often out of proportion to the degree of inflammation); affected vision; and a stromal infiltrate that is frequently ring shaped and composed predominantly of neutrophils. *Acanthamoeba* keratitis is a serious ocular infection which, if not properly managed, can lead to loss of vision and even loss of the eye.

6 IMMUNOLOGY

The factors responsible for susceptibility and innate resistance to infection by pathogenic free-living amoebae are undefined. Relatively few human infections have occurred, even though large numbers of individuals must have been exposed to amoebae. Most cases of PAM occur in otherwise healthy children or young adults. *Acanthamoeba* keratitis also generally occurs in healthy individuals. In contrast, GAE usually occurs in persons who are chronically ill, debilitated or immunosuppressed.

Antibodies to opportunistic amoebae have been detected in human sera including agglutinating antibodies against pathogenic and non-pathogenic *Naegleria* (Marciano-Cabral, Cline and Bradley 1987, Reilly et al. 1983). The agglutinating activity was specific for each species, indicating exposure to each of the *Naegleria* species. Antibodies to both pathogenic and non-pathogenic *Acanthamoeba* and *Naegleria* were detected in normal human sera by indirect fluorescent antibody testing of 93 serum samples, all of which were positive with titres ranging from 1:5 to 1:80 (Cursons et al. 1980). An avidin-biotin horseradish peroxidase assay has been used to detect antibodies to pathogenic and non-pathogenic *Naegleria* in samples of human serum (Dubray, Wilhelm and Jennings 1987). Antibodies were detected in 88% of sera from 115 hospital patients. Antibodies were identified as IgG and IgM, with IgG antibody titres ranging from 1:20 to 1:640. Radioimmunoassay detected antibody to *N. fowleri* in a pool of normal human sera (Tew et al. 1977). Antibody titres were nearly 9 times greater against intracellular antigens than against cell surface antigens. The apparent widespread occurrence of antibodies to pathogenic free-living amoebae in human sera may reflect the global distribution of these organisms. Alternatively, it may represent cross-reacting antibodies to antigens that have yet to be identified.

Serum from a victim of PAM in New Zealand was reported to have a low level of serum IgA, although IgG and IgM levels were normal (Cursons et al. 1979). In contrast, normal serum levels of IgA were found in a child who died of naeglerial infection in England (Cain, Mann and Warhurst 1979). Because serum IgA levels may not be an accurate reflection of secretory IgA concentrations, both patients may have had deficient levels of secretory IgA. As *N. fowleri* invades the nasal mucosa, it seems reasonable to suggest that secretory IgA may play a role in protection. Except for the serological surveys described above, all other information on immune responses to pathogenic free-living amoebae has come from experimental laboratory studies, mostly with animals (reviewed by John 1993).

7 PATHOLOGY

7.1 Pathogenicity

Pathogenicity is the ability of a micro-organism to produce disease, whereas cytopathogenicity is the ability to produce pathologic change in cells or a cytopathic effect in vitro in cultured cells. The proposed mechanisms of cytopathogenicity for *N. fowleri* include phagocytosis, release of cytolytic substances and the presence of a biologically active component, NACM (*Naegleria* amoeba cytopathogenic material).

Phagocytosis is a basic function of amoebae and one that causes the destruction of cells, whether in cell culture or in human tissue, and is therefore intimately involved in pathogenesis. Brown (1979) named the piecemeal engulfment of mouse embryo cells by *N. fowleri* as 'trogocytosis', from the Greek meaning 'to nibble'. It is now known that trogocytosis is accomplished by amoebostomes (John, Cole and Bruner 1985) that the amoebae use to engulf particles of various sizes, including cultivated mammalian cells. In addition to phagocytosis and trogocytosis, *N. fowleri* seems to injure cultivated mammalian cells by another contact-mediated means. Marciano-Cabral, Zoghby and Bradley (1990) reported cytolytic factors on the membranes of amoebae that lyse B103 rat nerve cells on contact. Lysis is followed by engulfment of cellular debris. Cytopathic activity was enhanced by the divalent cations calcium or magnesium.

Various phospholipases (phospholipase A, lysophospholipase, sphingomyelinase) have been identified in culture media in which *N. fowleri* is grown (Cursons, Brown and Keys 1978, Hysmith and Franson 1982). The phospholipase activities from cultures of pathogenic *Naegleria* are much greater than from cultures of non-pathogenic *Naegleria*. Phospholipases have also been reported to be present in media in which *A. culbertsoni* is grown. The amounts are greater in pathogenic *A. culbertsoni* cultures than in those of non-pathogenic *A. castellanii* (Cursons, Brown and Keys 1978). Other enzymes, some with a possible role in pathogenesis, occur in *N. fowleri* extracts. These are various hydrolases, including acid phosphatase, several glycosidases and elastase.

A cytopathic effect has been attributed to an agent known as '*Naegleria* amoeba cytopathogenic material' (NACM) obtained from lysed amoebae (Dunnebacke and Dixon 1989). NACM is isolated from lysates of *Naegleria* by centrifugation, filtration and lyophilization and has been obtained from *N. fowleri*, *N. gruberi*, and *N. jadini* but not from *Acanthamoeba*. NACM kills cells of a variety of avian and mammalian cell lines. After cultures are inoculated, there is a long latent period (4–10 days) followed by a short period (<24 h) during which the monolayer is destroyed. The cytopathic effect has been maintained in cell cultures through 9 serial passages. NACM is a protein with a molecular mass

of 36 000 kDa and an isoelectric point of pH 4.2. Monoclonal antibodies to NACM prevent its cytopathic activity. Fluorescent staining shows NACM to be located at the tips of the amoeba's pseudopodia and in the peripheral cytoplasm. It forms ring-shaped structures resembling amoebostomes (Dunnebacke and Dixon 1989).

PRIMARY AMOEBIC MENINGOENCEPHALITIS

The gross pathologic findings in PAM are remarkably constant. The cerebral hemispheres are usually oedematous and swollen, meninges are diffusely hyperaemic with a slight purulent exudate and the cortex contains many focal superficial haemorrhages. There is severe involvement of the olfactory bulbs, with haemorrhage, necrosis and purulent exudate (Carter 1972, Martinez 1985).

Microscopic examination reveals many amoebae in the subarachnoid and perivascular spaces. Presumably, the perivascular spaces provide a path of migration for the amoebae, and the blood vessels supply the oxygen needed by these aerobic organisms. Small numbers of amoebae are found clustered within the brain tissue and in the purulent exudate of the meninges and brain substance. Within the exudate some amoebae may be seen engulfed by macrophages. Many amoebae contain phagocytosed cellular debris and erythrocytes. The purulent exudate contains numerous polymorphonuclear and mononuclear leucocytes (Carter 1972, Martinez 1985). Fig. 9.9 shows *N. fowleri* amoebae with engulfed erythrocytes in brain tissue; cysts do not occur in tissue.

The cortical grey matter is a preferred site for the amoeba's development; consequently severe involvement occurs in the cerebral hemispheres, cerebellum, brain stem and upper portions of the spinal cord. Encephalitis may be a result of light amoebic invasion and inflammation or massive invasion with purulent, haemorrhagic necrosis. Typically, the olfactory bulbs are extensively invaded, with haemorrhage and an inflammatory exudate; the involvement here is greater than in other areas of the brain. Infection of the central nervous system with *N. fowleri* may be described best as an acute, haemorrhagic, necrotizing meningo-

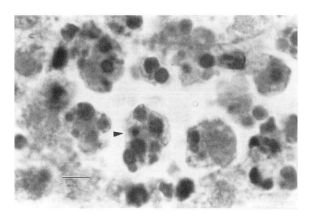

Fig. 9.9 Histological section of brain with *Naegleria fowleri* amoebae containing engulfed erythrocytes (H & E stain). Prominent nucleolus visible within nucleus of one amoeba (arrowhead). Bar = 10 μm.

encephalitis (Carter 1972, Martinez 1985). Focal demyelination in the white matter of the brain and spinal cord may occur (Chang 1979, Duma et al. 1971). Curiously, demyelination may occur in the absence of amoebae or cellular infiltrate. Chang (1979) suggests that demyelination may be caused by a phospholipolytic enzyme or enzyme-like substance produced by actively growing amoebae present in the adjacent grey matter.

Granulomatous amoebic encephalitis

In contrast to naeglerial infection, which is characterized by a diffuse meningoencephalitis, *Acanthamoeba* and *Balamuthia* CNS disease is a focal granulomatous encephalitis. Martinez (1980) gave a summary of the neuropathological features for 15 patients with GAE. In affected areas, the leptomeninges contain a moderate amount of purulent exudate. The cerebral hemispheres show moderate or severe oedema with foci of softened tissue and associated haemorrhagic necrosis. Lesions are usually multifocal and more posterior, including the upper portion of the spinal cord. The olfactory bulbs are not usually involved. Lesions of the CNS in GAE are characterized by necrosis with haemorrhagic foci and localized leptomeningitis. The chronic inflammatory exudate over the cortex comprises mostly mononuclear cells with a few polymorphonuclear leucocytes. The brain substance may have a prominent granulomatous reaction with foreign body giant cells, which are never seen in naeglerial infection. The multinucleated giant cells may not be present in immunosuppressed patients (Carter et al. 1981, Martinez 1987).

Amoebae reach the brain via the bloodstream, invasion of the CNS is thus centrifugal, from the deeper tissues toward the brain surface. Trophozoites and cysts (Figs. 9.10 and 9.11) occur in most infected tissues and around blood vessels. *Acanthamoeba* and *Balamuthia* reach the CNS by haematogenous spread from a primary focus of infection elsewhere in the body, most probably the skin, mucosa or lungs. Within the infected primary tissues, there occurs a chronic granulomatous reaction like that seen in the brain, with multinucleated giant cells, trophozoites and cysts. Similar lesions have been described from other tissues including prostate, thyroid, uterus and pancreas, probably resulting from hematogenous dissemination of amoebae from the primary focus in the skin or lungs, or possibly even a secondary CNS lesion (Martinez 1987).

Acanthamoeba keratitis

Ocular infections with *Acanthamoeba* are characterized by chronic progressive ulcerative keratitis (Cohen et al. 1985). During early corneal infection there may be pseudodendritic figures in the epithelium or just beneath the epithelium in the anterior stroma (Johns et al. 1987). In advanced cases of *Acanthamoeba* keratitis there may be a marked stromal infiltrate and necrosis. The whitish inflammatory infiltrate, often appearing ring-shaped around the corneal ulcer, consists mainly of polymorphonuclear leucocytes and

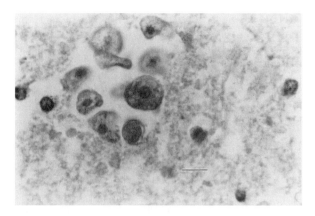

Fig. 9.10 Histological section of brain with *Acanthamoeba castellanii* amoebae (H & E stain). Bar = 10 μm.

macrophages, with a few lymphocytes (Mathers et al. 1987). Although granulomatous inflammation has been described in *Acanthamoeba* keratitis, in most of the reports, neutrophils (not lymphocytes) are the predominant infiltrating cells. Corneal ulceration may progress to perforation (Lindquist, Sher and Doughman 1988).

8 Diagnosis

8.1 Introduction

The laboratory diagnosis of infection by the opportunistic amoebae depends on the recovery and identification of amoebae in CSF, brain tissue or corneal scrapings. Amoebae in a clinical specimen may also be cultivated on non-nutrient agar spread with gram-negative bacteria and later transferred to liquid medium with antibiotics for axenic growth.

Primary amoebic meningoencephalitis

The diagnosis of PAM is made by microscopic identification of living or stained amoebae in CSF and motile amoebae are readily seen in simple wet-mount preparations. Amoebae can be distinguished from

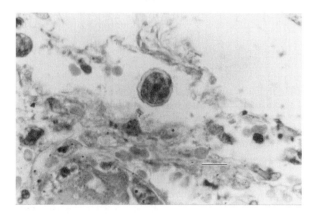

Fig. 9.11 Histological section of brain with *Acanthamoeba castellanii* cyst exhibiting typical wrinkled ectocyst (H & E stain). Bar = 10 μm.

other cells by their limax (slug-like) shape and progressive movement. It is not necessary to warm the slide as amoebae remain fully active at room temperature. Refrigeration of the spinal fluid is not recommended because this may kill the amoebae.

Spinal fluid smears may be stained with Wright or Giemsa stains. The bacterial Gram stain is of little value because heat fixing destroys the amoebae and causes them to stain poorly and appear as degenerating cells. Giemsa- or Wright-stained amoebae have considerable amounts of sky-blue cytoplasm and relatively small, delicate, pink nuclei. Mononuclear leucocytes, on the other hand, have large purplish nuclei with only a small amount of sky-blue cytoplasm. In cytospin preparations of CSF, the amoebae tend to be rounded and flattened, without pseudopodia. Occasionally, enlarged teardrop-shaped food vacuoles appear to radiate from the nucleus but this is an artefact induced by the cytospin procedure (Benson et al. 1985). Amoebae may be cultivated by placing some of the CSF on non-nutrient agar (1.5%) spread with a 'lawn' of washed *Esherichia coli* or *Enterobacter aerogenes* and incubated at 37°C. The amoebae will grow on the moist agar surface and will use the bacteria as food, producing plaques as they clear the bacteria.

Clinically, PAM very closely resembles fulminating bacterial meningitis, and the laboratory findings are also similar. The CSF is purulent or sanguinopurulent, with leucocyte counts (predominantly neutrophils) ranging from a few hundred to >20 000 cells mm^{-3}. Spinal fluid glucose levels are low and protein content is generally increased. Typically, Gram-stained smears and cultures of spinal fluid are negative for bacteria (Carter 1972, Martinez 1985).

GRANULOMATOUS AMOEBIC ENCEPHALITIS

The laboratory diagnosis of GAE is made by identifying amoebic forms of *Acanthamoeba* or *Balamuthia* in the CSF or amoebae and cysts in brain tissue. Whereas *N. fowleri* is readily cultured from CSF, *Acanthamoeba* and *Balamuthia* are not. *Acanthamoeba* has only rarely been isolated from patients with GAE. *A. culbertsoni* and *A. rhysodes* have been cultured from CSF, and *Acanthamoeba* sp. and *A. palestinensis* have been cultured from aspirated and biopsied brain material, respectively. Leptomyxid amoebae have been cultivated twice from biopsy material (Visvesvara et al. 1990, Gordon et al. 1992).

As with *N. fowleri*, *Acanthamoeba* may be cultured on non-nutrient agar spread with washed *E. coli* or *E. aerogenes*. *Balamuthia* must be grown in tissue culture, preferably Vero cell (Visvesvara, Schuster and Martinez 1993). *Acanthamoeba* and *Balamuthia* do not have a flagellate stage but amoebae are identified by their small spiky acanthopodia or branching shape, respectively, and cysts are readily identified by their distinctive double-walled wrinkled appearance. Species identification may be made by using the indirect fluorescent antibody technique (IFAT) and specific antisera against *Acanthamoeba* species or *B. mandrillaris*. The species of *Acanthamoeba* identified most fre-

quently from cases of GAE have been *A. castellanii* and *A. culbertsoni*.

ACANTHAMOEBA KERATITIS

Acanthamoeba keratitis is diagnosed by identifying amoebae cultured from corneal scrapings or by histological examination of infected corneal tissue. As in GAE, *Acanthamoeba* may be cultured from corneal scrapings on non-nutrient agar spread with gram-negative bacteria. Cultures of corneal material should be incubated at 30°C rather than 37°C. Of the 5 species of *Acanthamoeba* identified as capable of causing eye infections, only *A. hatchetti* has not been cultured from clinical material. Species identification is based on indirect immunofluorescent antibody staining. The 2 species most frequently identified in *Acanthamoeba* keratitis have been *A. castellanii* and *A. polyphaga*. *A. castellanii* is the species that has most often been identified in cases of *Acanthamoeba* GAE and ocular infection.

Rapid diagnosis of *Acanthamoeba* keratitis may be made by identifying amoebae or cysts in corneal scrapings using procedures for Giemsa staining, calcofluor white staining (Wilhelmus et al. 1986) and IFAT (Epstein et al. 1986). The calcofluor white procedure and IFAT both require the use of fluorescence microscopy and IFAT also requires an antiserum to *Acanthamoeba*.

Histopathological preparations of corneal tissue may be stained using the conventional haematoxylin and eosin procedure or by the more specialized staining procedures of Heidenhain's haematoxylin, Gomori's chromium haematoxylin, periodic acid-Schiff, Bauer chromic acid-Schiff and silver methenamine (McClellan et al. 1988). The special staining techniques are useful for demonstrating the presence of cysts in corneal tissue. IFAT and calcofluor white staining also may be used (Silvany, Luckenbach and Moore 1987).

Herpes simplex keratitis is the disease most commonly mistaken for *Acanthamoeba* keratitis (Johns et al. 1987, Mannis et al. 1986, Moore and McCulley 1989). The single most consistent clinical symptom of *Acanthamoeba* keratitis is severe ocular pain, which is not characteristic of an infection limited to the cornea and generally not present in persons with herpes simplex keratitis. Additional distinguishing features of *Acanthamoeba* keratitis include a history of direct exposure to soil or water, wearing contact lenses, scleritis and failure of cultures from the inflamed eye to reveal bacteria, fungi or viruses (Mannis et al. 1986).

9 EPIDEMIOLOGY AND CONTROL

9.1 Introduction

Human infection by *Naegleria* and *Acanthamoeba* has been reported world wide, as has the environmental isolation of these opportunistic amoebae (reviewed by John 1993). Although leptomyxid amoebae have been identified as a cause of human disease (Visvesvara et al. 1990, Lowichik et al. 1995) and have been cultivated twice from tissue (Visvesvara et al. 1990, Gordon et al. 1992), the environmental isolation of pathogenic leptomyxid amoebae has been reported only once (John and Howard 1995).

9.2 Epidemiology

PRIMARY AMOEBIC MENINGOENCEPHALITIS

Most of the reports of PAM have been from the developed rather than the developing nations, probably because of greater awareness rather than greater incidence. Australia, Czechoslovakia and the USA have reported 75% of all cases of PAM. In the USA, most reported cases have been from the coastal states of Virginia, Florida and Texas, accounting for 67% of the cases.

The majority of patients with naeglerial infection have had a history of recent swimming in freshwater during hot summer weather. In Richmond, Virginia, infection in 14 of 16 cases was probably acquired in 2 man-made lakes located within a few miles of each other (Callicott 1968, Duma et al. 1971, dos Santos 1970). Over a 3 year period, 16 young people died in Czechoslovakia after swimming in the same heated, chlorinated, indoor swimming pool (Červa, Novak and Culbertson 1968). Similar fatal cases have been reported following swimming in the following: swimming pools in Belgium, England and New Zealand; hot springs in California and New Zealand; lakes in Arkansas, Florida, Missouri, Nevada, South Carolina and Texas; streams in Belgium, Mississippi and New Zealand; and in an irrigation ditch in Mexico. Individual references for the above cases may be found in John (1993).

Infection has not always been acquired by swimming. The South Australian and northern Nigerian cases occurred in arid regions where swimming is unusual; the proposed means of infection were bathing and face washing (Anderson and Jamieson 1972, Lawande et al. 1980) and inhalation of dust-borne cysts (Lawande et al. 1979).

N. fowleri has been isolated from a variety of environmental sources world wide in Africa, Asia, Australia, New Zealand, Europe and North and South America, with 33 references describing 211 isolates (see John 1993 and John and Howard 1995 for specific references). *N. fowleri* is more readily isolated from warm, clean water than from warm, organically enriched water. The average water temperature has been c. 30°C (range 15–45°C). Although laboratory animals may succumb to naeglerial infection, there is no evidence for an animal reservoir of *N. fowleri*.

GRANULOMATOUS AMOEBIC ENCEPHALITIS

There have been even fewer cases of *Acanthamoeba* CNS infection than of *Naegleria* infection. More than half of these have been reported from the USA. Unlike naeglerial infection, GAE is not associated with swimming. Infections often occur in persons who are debilitated or immunosuppressed including patients with AIDS. In one of the AIDS patients, the clinical

features were more like those of PAM than of GAE, presumably because of immunosuppression (Wiley et al. 1987). With the current increase in the number of immunosuppressed persons, it is likely that there will be a corresponding increase in disseminated *Acanthamoeba* infections.

GAE caused by the leptomyxid, *B. mandrillaris*, was first described in a pregnant mandrill baboon that died of meningoencephalitis at the San Diego Zoo (Visvesvara et al. 1990). Amoebae were cultivated from brain tissue and used to prepare immune serum for indirect immunofluorescence assays; these revealed 16 human cases of leptomyxid infection originally identified as *Acanthamoeba* infections. Leptomyxid infections were also identified in a sheep and a gorilla. Since the original description, leptomyxid infections continue to be reported in humans, including patients with AIDS.

At the time of writing, the world literature contains 26 references that describe the environmental isolation of 144 pathogenic *Acanthamoeba* isolates (see John 1993 and John and Howard 1995 for specific references). These have been recovered from a variety of sources at somewhat lower average temperatures than for the isolation of *N. fowleri* (in the low 20s°C). Only one report describes the environmental recovery of pathogenic leptomyxid isolates and these do not appear to be *Balamuthia* (John and Howard 1995). As with *N. fowleri*, there is no evidence for an animal reservoir of pathogenic *Acanthamoeba* or *Balamuthia*.

ACANTHAMOEBA KERATITIS

The first cases of *Acanthamoeba* keratitis were reported from the UK in 1974 (Nagington et al. 1974) and the USA in 1975 (Jones, Visvesvara and Robinson 1975) and were associated with trauma to the eye or exposure to contaminated water. Since 1985 there has been a dramatic increase in the number of cases associated with the wearing of contact lenses; the greatest increase occurred in wearers of soft contact lenses (Stehr-Green, Bailey and Visvesvara 1989). The continued increase in the number of contact lens wearers, and of those not properly caring for them, will undoubtedly result in an increase in the incidence of *Acanthamoeba* keratitis, mainly in the developed nations where the wearing of contact lenses is widespread.

10 CHEMOTHERAPY

10.1 Introduction

Although *Acanthamoeba* keratitis may be treated with antimicrobial agents, virtually all cases of PAM and GAE have been fatal because there is not an effective treatment.

PRIMARY AMOEBIC MENINGOENCEPHALITIS

At present there exists no satisfactory treatment for PAM. The antibiotics used to treat bacterial meningitis are ineffective in naeglerial infection, as are the anti-amoebic drugs. Amphotericin B, a drug of considerable toxicity, is the antinaeglerial agent for which there is evidence of clinical effectiveness. The 4 known survivors of PAM, children from Australia (Anderson and Jamieson 1972), the UK (Apley et al. 1970), India (Pan and Ghosh 1971) and the USA (Seidel et al. 1982), were treated with amphotericin B, given intravenously and intrathecally. The patient in the USA was also given parenteral miconazole and oral rifampicin (Seidel et al. 1982). In experimental infections, tetracycline acts synergistically with amphotericin B to protect mice (Thong, Rowan-Kelly and Ferrante 1979).

Amphotericin B is administered intravenously at high doses; 1–15 mg kg^{-1} of body weight daily for 3 days and then 1 mg kg^{-1} per day for 6 days. Additionally, amphotericin B may be given intrathecally and miconazole is administered intravenously (Carter 1972, Seidel et al. 1982). Amphotericin B is a polyene compound that acts on the plasma membrane, disrupting its selective permeability and causing leakage of cellular components. On exposure to amphotericin B, amoebae round up and fail to form pseudopodia. Membrane-related changes, evident by electron microscopy, include enhanced nuclear plasticity, increased amounts of smooth and rough endoplasmic reticulum, decreased food vacuole formation and production of blebs on the plasma membrane (Schuster and Rechthand 1975).

Granulomatous amoebic encephalitis

As with naeglerial infection, there is no satisfactory treatment for GAE, partly because most cases have been diagnosed after death and there has not been adequate opportunity to evaluate therapeutic regimens. There are 3 reports of persons having recovered from *Acanthamoeba* CNS infection. A 7-year-old girl with a single *Acanthamoeba*-induced granulomatous brain tumour recovered following total excision of the mass and treatment with ketoconazole. *A. palestinensis* was cultured from the brain biopsy material (Ofori-Kwakye et al. 1986). The second report involved a 40-year-old man with *Acanthamoeba* meningitis who recovered following treatment with penicillin and chloramphenicol. *A. culbertsoni* was repeatedly cultured from the patient's CSF (Lalitha et al. 1985). The third case, for whom complete recovery cannot be claimed because the patient returned home and was not followed-up, was a 30-year-old man with chronic meningoencephalitis who was treated with sulfamethazine and from whose CSF *A. rhysodes* was cultured (Cleland et al. 1982).

Because the cysts of *Acanthamoeba* and *Balamuthia* form in tissues, a potentially effective drug for GAE must be able to destroy cysts as well as amoebae. Otherwise, a possible relapse could occur after the course of treatment has ended.

Acanthamoeba keratitis

Most of the earlier cases of *Acanthamoeba* keratitis required corneal transplants in order to manage the disease. Even so, there were reported instances of surgical enucleation. With present therapies, *Acanth-*

amoeba keratitis can be managed by medical treatment alone if infection is identified soon enough (Moore and McCulley 1989). The first successful medical cure of *Acanthamoeba* keratitis was reported by Wright, Warhurst and Jones (1985) and involved the use of a combination of dibromopropamidine and propamidine isethionate ointment and drops and neomycin drops. The success of this treatment has been confirmed by others. Signs of toxicity of propamidine and dibromopropamidine have been reported in one patient (Yeoh, Warhurst and Falcon 1987), but when treatment was discontinued, there seemed to be a recurrence of the *Acanthamoeba* keratitis.

In addition to topical propamidine, other successful treatment regimens have used the following: topical miconazole and systemic ketoconazole (Wilhelmus et al. 1986); topical miconazole and neosporin with epithelial debridement (Lindquist, Sher and Doughman 1988); topical clotrimazole (Driebe et al. 1988); oral itraconazole with topical miconazole and surgical debridement (Ishibashi et al. 1990); and topical polyhexamethylene biguanide (Larkin, Kilvington and Dart 1992).

11 Vaccination

There is no vaccine to protect against infection by the opportunistic amoebae. Numerous attempts have been made to immunize mice against infection by *N. fowleri* or *Acanthamoeba*, without producing solid immunity (see John 1993 for details of the studies).

12 Integrated control

Because of the relationship of swimming to naeglerial infection, many swimming areas have been subjected to intense investigation. Although *N. fowleri* has been isolated from many such areas, not all sampling efforts have yielded *N. fowleri*. Obviously, there are factors that favour the development of *N. fowleri* in swimming areas, including a warm temperature, the presence of an adequate food supply, insufficient residual free chlorine, minimal competition from other protozoans and probably optimal pH and oxygen levels. With the present limited understanding of the ecology of *N. fowleri*, practical measures for the prevention and control of the infection include education of the public, awareness within the medical community and adequate chlorination of public water supplies, including swimming facilities. Adequate chlorination requires a continuous free residual chlorine level of 0.5 mg l^{-1} of water (Derreumaux et al. 1974) and remains the single most effective disinfectant system for controlling opportunistic amoebae in public waters. This level of chlorination has effectively controlled the *N. fowleri* problem in the public water supplies of South Australia (Dorsch, Cameron and Robinson 1983). The risk of acquiring naeglerial infection through swimming in Florida's freshwater lakes is estimated at c. 1 in 2.6 million exposures (Wellings 1977). Considering the millions of persons who swim outdoors each summer, it is truly remarkable that there are not more cases of PAM.

Factors that have been associated with *Acanthamoeba* keratitis in contact lens wearers have been (1) using non-sterile, home made saline; (2) disinfecting lenses less frequently than recommended and (3) wearing lenses while swimming (Stehr-Green et al. 1987). Contact lens wearers should closely follow the manufacturer's recommendations for wear, care and disinfection of the lenses. Home made saline solutions remain an important risk factor associated with *Acanthamoeba* keratitis. Contamination of the contact lens care system with bacteria or fungi encourages the survival and growth of *Acanthamoeba*. Amoebae, including *A. polyphaga* and *A. hatchetti*, have been isolated from laboratory eyewash stations, especially stations contain-

ing reservoirs (Bier and Sawyer 1990, Tyndall, Lyle and Ironside 1987). Eyewash stations with reservoirs should be flushed weekly, otherwise they present a potential health hazard to users, particularly to those wearing contact lenses.

With the expected increase in the number of contact lens wearers, there will undoubtedly be a corresponding increase in the number of cases of *Acanthamoeba* keratitis. As immunosuppression becomes more widespread (not just because of AIDS but because of organ transplantation, cancer chemotherapy, congenitally acquired immunodeficiency and suppression resulting from the indiscriminate release of toxic chemicals and carcinogens into the environment) the possibility of more CNS and disseminated *Acanthamoeba* infections also increases.

REFERENCES

Akins RA, Byers TJ, 1980, Differentiation promoting factors induced in *Acanthamoeba* by inhibitors of mitochondrial macromolecule synthesis, *Dev Biol*, **78**: 126–40.

Akins RA, Gozs SM, Byers TJ, 1985, Factors regulating the encystment enhancing activity (EEA) of *Acanthamoeba castellanii*, *J Gen Microbiol*, **131**: 2609–17.

Anderson K, Jamieson A, 1972, Primary amoebic meningoencephalitis, *Lancet*, **1**: 902–3.

Apley J, Clarke SKR et al., 1970, Primary amoebic meningoencephalitis in Britain, *Br Med J*, **1**: 596–9.

Benson RL, Ansbacher L et al, 1985, Cerebrospinal fluid centrifuge analysis in primary amebic meningoencephalitis due to *Naegleria fowleri*, *Arch Pathol Lab Med*, **109**: 668–71.

Bier JW, Sawyer TK, 1990, Amoebae isolated from laboratory eyewash stations, *Curr Microbiol*, **20**: 349–50.

Brown T, 1979, Observations by immunofluorescence microscopy and electron microscopy on the cytopathogenicity of *Naegleria fowleri* in mouse embryo-cell cultures, *J Med Microbiol*, **12**: 363–71.

Byers TJ, Akins RA et al., 1980, Rapid growth of *Acanthamoeba* in defined media; induction of encystment by glucose-acetate starvation, *J Protozool*, **27**: 216–19.

Cable BL, John DT, 1986, Conditions for maximum enflagellation in *Naegleria fowleri*, *J Protozool*, **33**: 467–72.

Cain ARR, Mann PG, Warhurst DC, 1979, IgA and primary amoebic meningoencephalitis, *Lancet*, **1**: 441.

Callicott JH Jr, 1968, Amoebic meningoencephalitis due to free-living amebas of the *Hartmannella* (*Acanthamoeba*)-*Naegleria* group, *Am J Clin Pathol*, **49**: 84–91.

Cariou ML, Pernin P, 1987, First evidence for diploidy and genetic recombination in free-living amoebae of the genus *Naegleria* on the basis of electrophoretic variation, *Genetics*, **115**: 265–70.

Carter RF, 1970, Description of a *Naegleria* sp. isolated from two cases of primary amoebic meningo-encephalitis, and of the experimental pathological changes induced by it, *J Pathol*, **100**: 217–44.

Carter RF, 1972, Primary amoebic meningo-encephalitis. An appraisal of present knowledge, *Trans R Soc Trop Med Hyg*, **66**: 193–213.

Carter RF, Cullity GJ et al., 1981, A fatal case of meningoencephalitis due to a free-living amoeba of uncertain identity – probably *Acanthamoeba* sp., *Pathology*, **13**: 51–68.

Červa L, Novak K, Culbertson CG, 1968, An outbreak of acute, fatal amebic meningoencephalitis, *Am J Epidemiol*, **88**: 436–44.

Chang SL, 1979, Pathogenesis of pathogenic *Naegleria* amoeba, *Folia Parasitol (Praha)*, **26**: 195–200.

Clark CG, Cross GAM, 1987, rRNA genes of *Naegleria gruberi* are carried exclusively on a 14-kilobase-pair plasmid, *Mol Cell Biol*, **7**: 3027–31.

Clark CG, Cross GAM, 1988, Circular ribosomal RNA genes are a general feature of schizopyrenid amoebae, *J Protozool*, **35**: 326–9.

Cleland PG, Lawande RV et al., 1982, Chronic amebic meningoencephalitis, *Arch Neurol*, **39**: 56–7.

Cohen EJ, Buchanan HW et al., 1985, Diagnosis and management of *Acanthamoeba* keratitis, *Am J Ophthalmol*, **100**: 389–95.

Corliss JO, 1994, An interim 'user-friendly' hierarchical classification and characterization of the protists, *Acta Protozool*, **33**: 1–51.

Cursons RTM, Brown TJ, Keys EA, 1978, Virulence of pathogenic free-living amebae, *J Parasitol*, **64**: 744–5.

Cursons RTM, Keys EA et al., 1979, IgA and primary amoebic meningoencephalitis, *Lancet*, **1**: 223–4.

Cursons RTM, Brown TJ et al., 1980, Immunity to pathogenic free-living amoebae: role of humoral antibody, *Infect Immun*, **29**: 401–7.

DeJonckheere JF, 1987, Taxonomy, *Amphizoic Amoebae: Human Pathology*, ed Rondanelli EG, Piccin, Padua, Italy, 25–48.

DeJonckheere JF, 1989, Variation of electrophoretic karyotypes among *Naegleria* spp., *Parasitol Res*, **76**: 55–62.

Derreumaux AL, Jadin JB et al., 1974, Action du chlore sur les amibes de l'eau, *Ann Soc Belge Med Trop*, **54**: 415–28.

Dorsch MM, Cameron AS, Robinson BS, 1983, The epidemiology and control of primary amoebic meningoencephalitis with particular reference to South Australia, *Trans R Soc Trop Med Hyg*, **77**: 372–7.

Driebe WT Jr, Stern GA et al., 1988, *Acanthamoeba* keratitis. Potential role for topical clotrimazole in combination therapy, *Arch Ophthalmol*, **106**: 1196–201.

Dubray BL, Wilhelm WE, Jennings BR, 1987, Serology of *Naegleria fowleri* and *Naegleria lovaniensis* in a hospital survey, *J Protozool*, **34**: 322–7.

Duma RJ, Rosenblum WI et al., 1971, Primary amoebic meningoencephalitis caused by *Naegleria*. Two new cases, response to amphotericin B, and a review, *Ann Intern Med*, **74**: 923–31.

Dunnebacke TH, Dixon JS, 1989, NACM, a cytopathogen from *Naegleria* ameba: purification, production of monoclonal antibody, and immunoreactive material in NACM-treated vertebrate cell cultures, *J Cell Sci*, **93**: 391–401.

Epstein RJ, Wilson LA et al., 1986, Rapid diagnosis of *Acanthamoeba* keratitis from corneal scraping using indirect fluorescent antibody staining, *Arch Ophthalmol*, **104**: 1318–21.

Fulton C, 1970, Amebo-flagellates as research partners: the laboratory biology of *Naegleria* and *Tetramitus*, *Methods Cell Physiol*, **4**: 341–476.

Fulton C, 1977, Cell differentiation in *Naegleria gruberi*, *Annu Rev Microbiol*, **31**: 597–629.

Gonzalez-Robles A, Martinez-Palomo A, 1983, Scanning electron microscopy of attached trophozoites of pathogenic *Entamoeba histolytica, 1983*, **30:** 692–700.

Gordon SM, Steinberg JP et al., 1992, Culture isolation of *Acanthamoeba* species and leptomyxid amebas from patients with amebic meningoencephalitis; including two patients with AIDS, *Clin Infect Dis*, **15:** 1024–30.

Hysmith RM, Franson RC, 1982, Degradation of human myelin phospholipids by phospholipase-enriched culture media of pathogenic *Naegleria fowleri, Biochem Biophys Acta*, **712:** 698–701.

Ishibashi Y, Matsumoto Y et al., 1990, Oral itraconazole and topical miconzaole with debridement for *Acanthamoeba* keratitis, *Am J Ophthalmol*, **109:** 121–6.

John DT, 1993, Opportunistically pathogenic free-living amebae, *Parasitic Protozoa*, 2nd edn, vol 3, eds Kreier JP, Baker JR, Academic Press, San Diego, 143–246.

John DT, Cole TB Jr, Bruner RA, 1985, Amebostomes of *Naegleria fowleri, J Protozool*, **32:** 12–19.

John DT, Cole TB Jr, John RA, 1991, Flagella number among *Naegleria* flagellates, *Folia Parasitol (Praha)*, **38:** 289–95.

John DT, Howard MJ, 1995, Seasonal distribution of pathogenic free-living amebae in Oklahoma waters, *Parasitol Res*, **81:** 193–201.

Johns KJ, O'Day DM et al., 1987, Herpes simplex masquerade syndrome: *Acanthamoeba* keratitis, *Curr Eye Res*, **6:** 207–12.

Jones DB, Visvesvara GS, Robinson NM, 1975, *Acanthamoeba polyphaga* keratitis and *Acanthamoeba* uveitis associated with fatal meningoencephalitis, *Trans Ophthalmol Soc UK*, **95:** 221–32.

Lalitha MK, Anandi V et al., 1985, Isolation of *Acanthamoeba culbertsoni* from a patient with meningitis, *J Clin Microbiol*, **21:** 666–7.

Larkin DFP, Kilvington S, Dart JKG, 1992, Treatment of *Acanthamoeba* keratitis with polyhexamethylene biguanide, *Ophthalmology*, **99:** 185–92.

Lawande RV, Abraham SN et al., 1979, Recovery of soil amebas from the nasal passages of children during the dusty harmattan period in Zaria, *Am J Clin Pathol*, **71:** 201–3.

Lawande RV, MacFarlane et al., 1980, A case of primary amebic meningoencephalitis in a Nigerian farmer, *Am J Trop Med Hyg*, **29:** 21–5.

Lee JJ, Hutner SH, Bovee EC, 1985, *An Illustrated Guide to the Protozoa*, Allen Press, Lawrence, Kansas, 1–629.

Lewis EJ, Sawyer TK, 1979, *Acanthamoeba tubiashi* n. sp., a new species of fresh-water Amoebida (Acanthamoebidae), *Trans Am Micros Soc*, **98:** 543–9.

Lindquist TD, Sher NA, Doughman DJ, 1988, Clinical signs and medical therapy of early *Acanthamoeba* keratitis, *Arch Ophthalmol*, **106:** 73–7.

Lowichik A, Rollins N et al., 1995, Leptomyxid amebic meningoencephalitis mimicking brain stem glioma, *Am J Neuroradiol*, **16:** 926–9.

Mannis MJ, Tamaru R et al., 1986, *Acanthamoeba* sclerokeratitis, *Arch Ophthalmol*, **104:** 1313–17.

Marciano-Cabral F, Cline ML, Bradley SG, 1987, Specificity of antibodies from human sera for *Naegleria* species, *J Clin Microbiol*, **25:** 692–7.

Marciano-Cabral F, Zoghby KL, Bradley SG, 1990, Cytopathic action of *Naegleria fowleri* amoebae on rat neuroblastoma target cells, *J Protozool*, **37:** 138–44.

Martinez AJ, 1980, Is *Acanthamoeba* encephalitis an opportunistic infection?, *Neurology*, **30:** 567–74.

Martinez AJ, 1985, *Free-living Amebas: Natural History, Prevention, Diagnosis, Pathology, and Treatment of Disease*, CRC Press, Boca Raton, Florida, 1–156.

Martinez AJ, 1987, Clinical manifestations of free-living amebic infections, *Amphizoic Amoebae: Human Pathology*, ed Rondanelli EG, Piccin, Padua, Italy, 161–77.

Mathers W, Stevens G Jr et al., 1987, Immunopathology and electron microscopy of *Acanthamoeba* keratitis, *Am J Ophthalmol*, **103:** 626–35.

McClellan KA, Kappagoda NK et al., 1988, Microbiological and histopathological confirmation of acanthamebic keratitis, *Pathology*, **20:** 70–3.

Moore MB, McCulley JP, 1989, *Acanthamoeba* keratitis associated with contact lenses: six consecutive cases of successful management, *Br J Ophthalmol*, **73:** 271–5.

Nagington J, Watson PF, 1974, Amoebic infection of the eye, *Lancet*, **2:** 1537–40.

Neff RJ, Neff RH, 1972, Induction of differentiation in *Acanthamoeba* by inhibitors, *CR Trav Lab Carlsberg*, **39:** 111–68.

Ofori-Kwakye SK, Sidebottom DG et al., 1986, Granulomatous brain tumor caused by *Acanthamoeba, J Neurosurg*, **64:** 505–9.

Page FC, 1967, Re-definition of the genus *Acanthamoeba* with description of three species, *J Protozool*, **14:** 709–24.

Page FC, 1974, *Rosculus ithacus* Hawes, 1963 (Amoebida, Flabellulidae) and the amphizoic tendency in amoebae, *Acta Protozool*, **13:** 143–54.

Page FC, 1976, *An Illustrated Key to Freshwater and Soil Amoebae*, Freshwater Biol Assoc, Ambleside, Cumbria, England, 1–122.

Page FC, 1988, *A New Key to Freshwater and Soil Gymnamoebae*, Freshwater Biol Assoc, Ambleside, Cumbria, England, 122 pp.

Pan NR, Ghosh TN, 1971, Primary amoebic meningoencephalitis in two Indian children, *J Indian Med Assoc*, **56:** 134–7.

Patterson M, Woodworth TW et al., 1981, Ultrastructure of *Naegleria fowleri* enflagellation, *J Bacteriol*, **147:** 217–26.

Pernin P, Ataya A, Cariou ML, 1992, Genetic structure of natural populations of the free-living amoeba, *Naegleria lovaniensis*. Evidence for sexual reproduction, *Heredity*, **68:** 173–81.

Reilly MF, Marciano-Cabral F et al., 1983, Agglutination of *Naegleria fowleri* and *Naegleria gruberi* by antibodies in human serum, *J Clin Microbiol*, **17:** 576–81.

Rudick VL, 1971, Relationships between nucleic acid synthetic patterns and encystment in aging unagitated cultures of *Acanthamoeba castellanii, J Cell Biol*, **49:** 498–506.

dos Santos JG, 1970, Fatal primary amebic meningoencephalitis: a retrospective study in Richmond, Virginia, *Am J Clin Pathol*, **54:** 737–42.

Schuster FL, 1975, Ultrastructure of cysts of *Naegleria* spp: a comparative study, *J Protozool*, **22:** 352–9.

Schuster FL, Rechthand E, 1975, In vitro effects of amphotericin B on growth and ultrastructure of the amoeboflagellates *Naegleria gruberi* and *Naegleria fowleri, Antimicrob Agents Chemother*, **8:** 591–605.

Seidel JS, Harmatz P et al., 1982, Successful treatment of primary amebic meningoencephalitis, *N Engl J Med*, **306:** 346–8.

Silvany RE, Luckenbach MA, Moore MB, 1987, The rapid detection of *Acanthamoeba* in paraffin-embedded sections of corneal tissue with calcofluor white, *Arch Ophthalmol*, **105:** 1366–7.

Singh BN, Das SR, 1970, Studies on pathogenic and non-pathogenic small free-living amoebae and the bearing of nuclear division on the classification of the order Amoebida, *Philos Trans R Soc Lond [Biol]*, **259:** 435–76.

Stehr-Green JK, Bailey TM, Visvesvara GS, 1989, The epidemiology of *Acanthamoeba* keratitis in the United States, *Am J Ophthalmol*, **107:** 331–6.

Stehr-Green JK, Bailey TM et al., 1987, *Acanthamoeba* keratitis in soft contact lens wearers, *J Am Med Assoc*, **258:** 57–60.

Tew JG, Burmeister J et al., 1977, A radioimmunoassay for human antibody specific for microbial antigens, *J Immunol Methods*, **14:** 231–41.

Thong YH, Rowan-Kelly B, Ferrante A, 1979, Delayed treatment of experimental amoebic meningo-encephalitis with amphotericin B and tetracycline, *Trans R Soc Trop Med Hyg*, **73:** 336–7.

Tyndall RL, Lyle MM, Ironside KS, 1987, The presence of free-living amoebae in portable and stationary eye wash stations, *Am Ind Hyg Assoc J*, **48:** 933–4.

Visvesvara GS, Schuster FL, Martinez AJ, 1993, *Balamuthia mandrillaris*, n.g., n.sp., agent of amebic meningoencephalitis in humans and other animals, *J Euk Microbiol*, **40:** 504–14.

Visvesvara GS, Martinez AJ et al., 1990, Leptomyxid ameba, a new agent of amebic meningoencephalitis in humans and animals, *J Clin Microbiol*, **28:** 2750–6.

Volkonsky M, 1931, *Hartmannella castellanii* Douglas et classification des Hartmannelles (Hartmanelliane nov. subfam., *Acanthamoeba* nov. gen., *Glaeseria* nov. gen.), *Arch Zool Exp Gén*, **72:** 317–39.

Weik RR, John DT, 1977, Cell size, macromolecular composition, and O_2 consumption during agitated cultivation of *Naegleria gruberi*, *J Protozool*, **24:** 196–200.

Weik RR, John DT, 1978, Macromolecular composition and nuclear number during growth of *Naegleria fowleri*, *J Parasitol*, **64:** 746–7.

Weik RR, John DT, 1979a, Cell and mitochondria respiration of *Naegleria fowleri*, *J Parasitol*, **65:** 700–8.

Weik RR, John DT, 1979b, Preparation and properties of mitochondria from *Naegleria gruberi*, *J Protozool*, **26:** 311–8.

Wellings FM, 1977, Amoebic meningoencephalitis, *J Fla Med Assoc*, **64:** 327–8.

Wiley CA, Safrin RE et al., 1987, *Acanthamoeba* meningoencephalitis in a patient with AIDS, *J Infect Dis*, **155:** 130–3.

Wilhelmus KR, Osato MS et al., 1986, Rapid diagnosis of *Acanthamoeba* keratitis using calcofluor white, *Arch Ophthalmol*, **104:** 1309–12.

Woodworth TW, Keefe WE, Bradley SG, 1982a, Characterization of proteins in flagellates and growing amebae of *Naegleria fowleri*, *J Bacteriol*, **150:** 1366–74.

Woodworth TW, Keefe WE, Bradley SG, 1982b, Characterization of the proteins of *Naegleria fowleri*: relationships between subunit size and charge, *J Protozool*, **29:** 246–51.

Wright P, Warhurst D, Jones BR, 1985, *Acanthamoeba* keratitis successfully treated medically, *Br J Ophthalmol*, **69:** 778–82.

Yeoh R, Warhurst DC, Falcon MG, 1987, *Acanthamoeba* keratitis, *Br J Ophthalmol*, **71:** 500–3.

Chapter 10

GIARDIASIS

L S Garcia

1 INTRODUCTION

Giardia was first discovered by Leeuwenhoek in 1681 in his own stool specimens, but was not described until 1859 by Lambl. In the early 1930s, Clifford Dobell also demonstrated his interest in Leeuwenhoek; not only did he teach himself modern Dutch and then 17th century Dutch, but translated a number of Leeuwenhoek's works from Dutch and Latin. In the account of his own giardiasis infection, Leeuwenhoek writes

> 'All the particles aforesaid (description of stool debris) lay in a clear transparent medium, wherein I have sometimes also seen animalcules a-moving very prettily (trophozoites); some of 'em a bit bigger, others a bit less, than a blood-globule, but all of one and the same make. Their bodies were somewhat longer than broad, and their belly which was flatlike, furnisht with sundry little paws, wherewith they made such a stir in the clear medium and among the globules, that you might e'en fancy you saw a pissabed (woodlouse or sow-bug) running up against a wall; and albeit they made a quick motion with their paws, yet for all that they made but slow progress.' (Dobell 1920)

However, there is no evidence that either Leeuwenhoek or Lambl saw or recognized the cyst forms of the organism; they were first noted by Grassi in 1879 and were thought to be coccidia. Only later did Grassi associate the cyst form with the flagellated trophozoite form (Meyer 1990). The history of giardiasis is given in Chapter 1.

Giardia lamblia is world wide in distribution, apparently more prevalent in children than in adults and more common in warm climates than in cool ones. It is the most commonly diagnosed flagellate in the intestinal tract, and it may be the most commonly diagnosed intestinal protozoan in some areas of the world (Meyer and Jarroll 1980).

2 CLASSIFICATION

Although various criteria have been used to differentiate species of *Giardia*, including host specificity, various body dimensions, and variations in structure, there is still considerable debate over the appropriate classification and nomenclature of this group of organisms. Based on work by Filice on structural variations, 3 groups have been proposed: amphibian *Giardia* (represented by *G. agilis*), the 'muris' group from rodents and birds (represented by *G. muris*), and the 'intestinalis' group from a variety of mammals (including humans), as well as birds and reptiles (represented by *G. duodenalis*) (Filice 1952). Despite disagreement concerning the names *intestinalis* and *lamblia*, both continue to be used to describe this organism. Meyer prefers to use *Giardia duodenalis*, which is often followed by the name of the animal from which the organism was obtained (Meyer 1990).

Ten strains from human- and animal-source *G. duodenalis* were evaluated using an isoelectric focusing technique. Banding patterns obtained from trophozoite total cell proteins demonstrated both similarities and differences. These findings confirm the heterogeneity of this group of *Giardia* spp., from animal and human hosts and from hosts within the same geographical area (Isaac-Renton, Byrne and Prameya 1988, Ey et al. 1996).

Within the USA, the term *Giardia lamblia* has been commonly used for many years and refers to those organisms found in humans, as well as other mammals; in some geographic areas, this designation tends to eliminate any confusion, since the majority of health workers are used to this name and continue to report the presence of the organism using '*Giardia lamblia*'. Others feel the designation *G. duodenalis* is taxonomically correct and refers to the many 'species' containing the 'duodenalis' double medial bodies. As long as the same species designation is used by both laboratory staff and physicians, the choice is optional. Chemotaxonomic studies may also provide key information related to species designations.

3 STRUCTURE AND LIFE CYCLE

The life cycle is seen in Figure 10.1 and is similar to the simple, direct life cycle of most intestinal protozoa. Both the trophozoite and cyst are included in the life cycle of *G. lamblia*. Trophozoites divide by means of longitudinal binary fission producing 2 daughter trophozoites. The trophozoites are the intestinal dwelling stages and attach to the epithelium of the host villi by means of the ventral disc. The attachment is substantial and results in disc 'impression prints' when the organism detaches from the surface of the epithelium. Trophozoites may remain attached or may detach from the mucosal surface. Since the epithelial surface sloughs off the tip of the villus every 72 h the trophozoites apparently detach at that time.

There are several theories on possible mechanisms for attachment by the ventral disk including microtubule mediation, hydrodynamic action, contractile protein activity and the interaction of lectins with surface bound sugars. Based on conflicting information, the attachment process probably depends on multiple mechanisms. A study by Katelaris and colleagues indicates that attachment to enterocyte-like differentiated Caco-2 cells is primarily by cytoskeletal mechanisms that can be inhibited by interfering with contractile filaments and microtubules; attachment by mannose binding lectin also seems to mediate binding (Katelaris, Naeem and Farthing 1995).

The most common location of the organisms is in the crypts within the duodenum. Again, for reasons that are not known, cyst formation takes place as the organisms move down through the colon. Based on results by Halliday, Inge and Farthing (1995). *Giardia*

appears to take up conjugated bile salts by active and passive transport mechanisms like the mammalian ileum. As conjugated bile salts are known to promote encystation, these uptake mechanisms may play an important role in the survival of the cyst stage and ultimate completion of the life cycle of the parasite (Healy 1990). Cholesterol starvation may also play a role in stimulating encystation (Lujan et al. 1996). The trophozoites retract the flagella into the axonemes, the cytoplasm becomes condensed and the cyst wall is secreted (Erlandsen et al. 1996). As the cyst matures, the internal structures are doubled, so that when excystation occurs the cytoplasm divides, thus producing 2 trophozoites. Excystation would normally occur in the duodenum or appropriate culture medium (Figure 10.1) (Bingham and Meyer 1979). If kept cool and moist, cysts can remain viable for several months, but they cannot survive if moisture is lacking.

At the light microscopic level and seen on permanent stained faecal smears stained with trichrome or iron-hematoxylin stains, the trophozoite is usually described as being teardrop-shaped from the front with the posterior end being pointed (Figures 10.2, 10.3). If one examines the trophozoite from the side, it resembles the curved portion of a spoon. The concave portion is the area of the sucking disc (Figure 10.2). There are 4 pairs of flagella, 2 nuclei, 2 axonemes, and 2 slightly curved bodies called the median bodies. The trophozoites usually measure 10–20 μm in length and 5–15 μm in width (Figure 10.3) (Table 10.1)

The cysts may be either round or oval and contain 4 nuclei, axonemes, and median bodies (Figure 10.3). Often some cysts appear to be shrunk or distorted and one may see 2 halos, one around the cyst wall itself and one inside the cyst wall around the shrunken

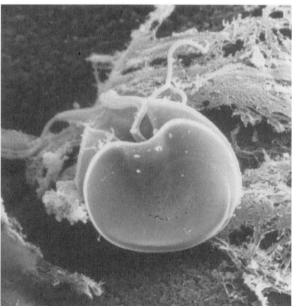

Fig. 10.2 *Giardia lamblia* trophozoite on the mucosal surface. (Scanning electron micrograph courtesy of Marietta Voge) From Garcia and Bruckner 1997.

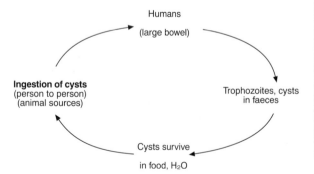

Fig. 10.1 Life cycle of *Giardia lamblia*. Adapted from Garcia and Bruckner 1997.

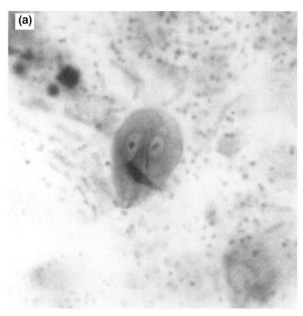

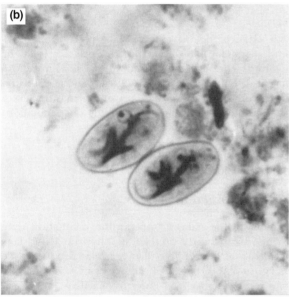

Fig. 10.3 *Giardia lamblia* (a) trophozoite, (b) cysts from permanent stained faecal smears.

organism. The halo effect around the outside of the cyst is particularly visible on permanent stained smears. Cysts normally measure 11–14 μm in length and 7–10 μm in width (Figure 10.3) (Table 10.2).

4 BIOCHEMISTRY, MOLECULAR BIOLOGY AND GENETICS

Organisms in the genus *Giardia* are described as being aerotolerant anaerobes that use substrate level phosphorylation, iron-sulphur protein and flavoprotein mediated electron transport for the production of energy (Jarroll and Lindmark 1990). *Giardia* lacks mitochondria and microbodies, but contains lysosome-like organelles that accumulate ferritin and stain positively for acid phosphatase and aryl sulphatase.

In the presence of exogenous glucose, intact *Giardia* trophozoites produce ethanol and acetate as organic end products; aerobically 6 times more acetate than ethanol is produced and anaerobically, twice as much ethanol as acetate is produced. In both situations, CO_2 is the only gaseous end product that has been detected. Based on the pattern of CO_2 production, glucose is metabolized using the Embden-Meyerhof-Parnas (EMP) and the hexose monophosphate (HM) pathways. A number of energy metabolism enzymes have been identified and are reviewed by Jarroll and Lindmark (1990).

Carbohydrate and energy metabolism studies have also been conducted using the cyst stage; enzyme data confirm that specific activities occur, regardless of the life cycle stage involved. Studies also show that the cyst stage respires at c. 10–20% of that observed in trophozoites; respiration is not stimulated by exogenous glucose, but is stimulated by exogenous ethanol. It is also interesting to note that cyst respiration decreases as water temperature decreases, findings that may explain increased cyst viability with decreased storage temperature.

In summary, a proposed energy metabolic pathway for *Giardia* indicates oxidation of endogenous and exogenous glucose incompletely to ethanol, acetate, and CO_2. Energy is produced through substrate-level phosphorylation; iron-sulphur proteins and flavins are involved in electron transport. There is no evidence

Table 10.1 *Giardia lamblia* trophozoite morphology

Organism stage	Shape and size	Motility	Nuclei	Flagella	Other features
Giardia lamblia Trophozoite	Pear-shaped, 10–20 μm; width 5–15 μm	'Falling leaf' motility may be difficult to see if organism in mucus	2 nuclei Not visible in unstained mounts	4 lateral, 2 ventral, 2 caudal	Sucking disc occupying $\frac{1}{2}$–$\frac{3}{4}$ of ventral surface pear-shaped front view; spoon-shaped side view

Table 10.2 *Giardia lamblia* cyst morphology

Organism stage	Shape and size	Motility	Nuclei	Flagella	Other features
Giardia lamblia Cyst	Oval, ellipsoidal or may appear round 8–19 μm; usual range 11–14 μm; width, 7–10 μm	Non-motile	4 nuclei Not distinct in unstained preparations; usually located at one end	Flagella not visible	Longitudinal fibres in cysts may be visible in unstained preparations; deep staining median bodies usually lie across the longitudinal fibres; there is often shrinkage and the cytoplasm pulls away from the cyst wall; there may also be a 'halo' effect around the outside of the cyst wall due to shrinkage caused by dehydrating reagents

for oxidative phosphorylation or a cytochrome-mediated electron transport system. (Jarroll and Lindmark 1990).

Culture studies indicate that *Giardia* trophozoites have the capacity to de novo synthesize isoprenoid lipids, as well as incorporate preformed lipids; also, steryl esters are abundant and increase during encystation, while triglycerides are low (Ellis et al. 1996). Phospholipids include phosphatidylcholine, phosphatidylethanolamine, phosphatidylglycerol, phosphatidylinositol, phosphatidylserine and sphingomyelin. Neutral lipids include sterols, mono-, di-, and triacylglycerides. Fatty acids can be incorporated into phospho- and neutral lipids (Jarroll and Lindmark 1990). Increased fatty acid unsaturation and the accumulation of storage lipids are consistent with the parasite differentiation into a cyst stage that can survive outside the host.

In the trophozoite, nucleic acid requirements are met by the salvage of pyrimidines, purines and their nucleosides. Various carrier mediated mechanisms have been proposed.

In contrast to trophozoites of *Entamoeba* and the trichomonads, *Giardia* has very few carbohydrate-splitting hydrolases. It has also been found that *Giardia* trophozoites exhibit increased levels of chitin synthetase activity during encystment (Jarroll and Lindmark 1990).

Although antigenic analysis shows promise in helping to identify and classify *Giardia*, both common and different antigens have been recovered in axenic cultures. The use of monoclonal antibodies in the study of antigens has proven to be useful; technical methods also involve quantitation, an important requirement in this type of analysis. Another potential problem involves antigenic variation; a single *Giardia* trophozoite can give rise in vivo, as well as in vitro, to trophozoites with varying surface antigens. Immune pressure may play a role in antigenic variation, but the speed with which antigenic changes take place after infection suggests that other mechanisms may also be involved. The antigenic profile of *Giardia* in culture may also change if the trophozoites harbour endosymbionts; the presence of these organisms may influence both antigenic and chemotaxonomic determinations (Meyer 1990).

5 CLINICAL ASPECTS

5.1 Introduction

From available data, it appears the incubation time for giardiasis is c. 12–20 days. Because the acute stage usually lasts only a few days, giardiasis may not be recognized as the cause of the symptoms observed, but may mimic acute viral enteritis, bacillary dysentery, bacterial or other food poisonings, acute intestinal amoebiasis or 'traveller's diarrhoea' (toxigenic *E. coli*). However, the type of diarrhoea plus the lack of blood, mucus and cellular exudate is consistent with giardiasis.

5.2 Clinical manifestations

Onset may be accompanied by nausea, anorexia, malaise, low grade fever and chills. There may be a sudden onset of explosive, watery, foul-smelling diarrhoea with flatulence and abdominal distention. Other symptoms include epigastric pain and cramping. There is increased fat and mucus in the stool, but no blood. Weight loss often accompanies these symptoms. The acute infection usually resolves spontaneously, although in some patients, particularly children, the acute symptoms may last for months. Acute giardiasis must be differentiated from other acute viral, bacterial, and protozoal agents.

The acute phase is often followed by a subacute or

chronic phase. Symptoms in these patients include recurrent, brief episodes of loose, foul stools; there may be increased distention and foul flatus. Between mushy stools, the patient may have normal stools or may be constipated. Abdominal discomfort continues to include marked distention and belching with a rotten egg taste. Chronic disease must be differentiated from amoebiasis and other intestinal parasites such as *Dientamoeba fragilis, Cryptosporidium parvum, Cyclospora cayetanensis, Isospora belli,* microsporidia *Strongyloides stercoralis* and from inflammatory bowel disease and irritable colon (see also Chapters 17, 18 and 30). Based on symptoms such as upper intestinal discomfort, heartburn and belching, giardiasis must also be differentiated from duodenal ulcer, hiatal hernia and gallbladder and pancreatic disease.

Various types of malabsorption have been described including steatorrhoea, disaccharidase (lactose, xylose) deficiency, Vitamin B_{12} malabsorption, hypocarotenemia, low serum folate and protein-losing enteropathy. Lactose intolerance may persist after effective therapy, particularly in patients from ethnic groups with a predisposition for lactose deficiency. This should be considered prior to retreatment, especially if the patient continues to have diarrhoea, but post-treatment negative stool specimens.

Although there is speculation that the organisms coating the mucosal lining may act to prevent fat absorption, this does not completely explain why the uptake of other substances normally absorbed at other intestinal levels is prevented (Tandon et al. 1977). Occasionally the gallbladder may also be involved, causing gallbladder colic and jaundice. *G. lamblia* has also been identified from bronchoalveolar lavage fluid (Stevens and Vermeire 1981) and the urinary tract (Meyers, Kuharic and Holmes 1977). Reasons for such a dramatic variation in host susceptibility are not well delineated. Host factors such as nutritional status and both systemic and mucosal immunity may also play a role.

6 IMMUNOLOGY

Recent studies document antigenic variation with surface antigen changes during human infections with *Giardia,* and although the biological importance of this work is not clear, it suggests that this may provide a mechanism enabling the organism to escape the host's immune response (Nash et al. 1990). Also one would suspect that the more rapid the rate of change, the more likely that a chronic infection would be seen. Certain surface antigens may allow the organisms to survive better in the intestinal tract and might not be immunologically selected.

Although patients with symptomatic giardiasis usually have no underlying abnormality of serum immunoglobulins, a high incidence of giardiasis has been shown to occur in patients with immunodeficiency syndromes, particularly in common variable hypogammaglobulinemia (Ament, Ochs and David 1973). Giardiasis was found to be the most common

cause of diarrhoea in these patients and was associated with mild to severe villus atrophy. Successful treatment of giardiasis led to symptomatic cure and improvement in mucosal abnormalities, with the exception of nodular lymphoid hyperplasia.

Acute (polymorphonuclear leucocyte and eosinophils) and chronic inflammatory cells have been found in the lamina propria together with increased epithelial mitoses, findings which revert to normal after therapy. The presence of these inflammatory cells has been linked to epithelial cell damage. The range of patient response is from normal to almost complete villous atrophy. Crypt mitosis is also increased based on the degree of villous damage but, it has also been reported that mucosal changes return to normal within several days of treatment and that patients with giardiasis have reduced surface area compared with uninfected individuals.

Although no definitive pattern has been identified, it appears that lamina propria plasma cells producing IgM and IgE increase, whereas local production of IgA seems to be suppressed. More severe villous damage has also been reported in patients with diminished gammaglobulins.

7 PATHOLOGY

Although the organisms in the crypts of the duodenal mucosa may reach very high densities, they may not cause any pathology. The organisms feed on the mucous secretions and do not penetrate the mucosa as *G. muris* does in mice where trophozoites have been recovered in the deeper tissues (Owen, Allen and Stevens 1981). Although some organisms have been seen in biopsy material inside the intestinal mucosa, others have been seen attached only to the epithelium. In one in vitro study using cultured epithelial cells, the organisms showed no toxic or invasive effect (Chavez et al. 1986). Another study by Chen and colleagues has demonstrated a *G. duodenalis* cysteine-rich surface protein (CRP136) that shares 57% homology with the gene encoding the precursor of the sarafotoxins, a group of snake toxins from the burrowing adder known to cause symptoms similar to those of humans acutely infected with *Giardia* (Chen, Upcroft and Upcroft 1995). Thus, CRP136 represents the first evidence for a potential *Giardia* toxin. In symptomatic cases, there may also be irritation of the mucosal lining, increased mucus secretion, and dehydration (Erlandsen 1974, Peterson 1957).

With the advent of AIDS, there was speculation that *G. lamblia* might be an important pathogen in this group, but clinical findings to date do not seem to confirm this possibility (Meyer 1990, Smith et al. 1988). Although giardiasis has certainly been reported in AIDS patients, clinical experience does not suggest a more pathogenic role for *G. lamblia* in these patients than in other non-AIDS individuals.

Isoenzyme studies, primarily designed to assist in organism identification and classification, have also provided additional information regarding pathogenicity, implication in waterborne outbreaks and human disease. In one study where isoenzyme patterns of 32 isolates of *Giardia* obtained from both humans and animals were examined, there was no obvious correlation between clinical symptoms and isoenzyme patterns. Isolates from asymptomatic individuals were found in the same zymodemes (isoenzyme groups) as isolates from symptomatic hosts. This study also confirmed previous observations regarding genetic heterogeneity and demonstrated significant differences between isolates from within a single region and other widely separated geographic locations (Proctor et al. 1989). A study from Australia provided data on 2 *Giardia* demes derived from children with similar chronic symptoms both of which appear to be pathogenic (Upcroft et al. 1995).

8 DIAGNOSIS

Generally, routine laboratory test results are normal, including haematology; eosinophilia is rare. Malabsorption of fat, glucose, lactose, xylose, carotene, folic acid and vitamin B_{12} is occasionally present in some patients. Diagnosis of giardiasis is usually based on identification of the organisms from stool or duodenal aspirate specimens (Table 10.3).

Routine stool examinations are normally recommended for the recovery and identification of intestinal protozoa. In the case of *G. lamblia*, because they are attached so securely to the mucosa by means of the sucking disc, a series of even 5 or 6 stools may be examined without recovering the organisms. These parasites also tend to be passed in the stool on a cyclical basis. The EnteroTest capsule may be helpful in recovering the organisms as can duodenal aspirates. Although cysts can often be identified on the wet stool preparation, many infections may be missed without the examination of a permanent stained smear (Collins, Keller and Brown 1978, Garcia and Bruckner 1997, National Committee for Clinical Laboratory Standards 1993). If material from the string test (EnteroTest) or mucus from a duodenal aspirate are submitted, they should be examined as a wet preparation for motility; motility may be represented by nothing more than a slight flutter of the flagella because the organism will be caught up in the mucus. After diagnosis, the rest of the positive material can be preserved and processed for permanent staining. Experience in the clinical laboratory setting has shown that the examination of duodenal fluid after a series of negative stool examinations rarely confirms a positive infection. This may be due to parasite location or small numbers. Because of these considerations, the examination of intestinal fluid should not replace routine stool examinations, all of which should include the use of permanent stained smears (Garcia and Bruckner 1997).

Procedures have also been developed using the enzyme-linked immunosorbent assay (ELISA) to detect *Giardia* antigen in faeces. The ELISA is at least as sensitive as microscopic wet examinations (Addis et al. 1991, Nash, Herrington and Levine 1987). A fluorescent method using monoclonal antibodies has also proven to be extremely sensitive and specific in detecting *Giardia* in faecal specimens (Garcia, Shum and Bruckner 1992). Many of these newer methods are being used to screen patients suspected of having giardiasis or those who may be involved in an outbreak situation.

Occasionally, after multiple stool examinations and examination of intestinal fluid have been negative, a small bowel biopsy may confirm the suspect diagnosis of giardiasis. It is recommended that the biopsy be taken from the area of the duodenojejunal junction; biopsies from multiple duodenal and jejunal sites are preferred. Fluid smears and touch preparations can be air dried, fixed in methanol, and stained with Giemsa stain. The organisms appear somewhat purple and the epithelial cells appear pink. Routine histological procedures should also be performed with very careful screening of the material; trophozoites are very difficult to see and may be present in very few of the sections. Normally, the trophozoites are more likely to be seen attached to the microvillous border within the crypts.

Radiological findings from the small intestine may be normal in giardiasis, but abnormalities can occur and are usually seen in the duodenum or jejunum. Findings may include thickened mucosal folds, increased secretions and a pattern of oedema and segmentation, none of which is diagnostic for giardiasis, but merely suggestive. Approximately 20% of patients with giardiasis may exhibit these findings after routine barium examination. It is always recommended that

Table 10.3 Laboratory diagnosis of giardiasis – key points

1.	Even if a series of 3 stool specimens (ova and parasite examinations) are submitted and examined correctly, the organisms may not be recovered and identified.
2.	Motility on wet preparations may be difficult to see because the organisms may be caught up in mucus.
3.	Any examination for parasites in stool specimens must include the use of a permanent stained smear (even on formed stool).
4.	Duodenal drainage either alone or in combination with the EnteroTest capsule may be very helpful in organism recovery. This technique does not take the place of the ova and parasite examination.
5.	Immunodiagnostic procedures have been found to be more sensitive than the routine stool methods (ova and parasite examination) and are now being routinely used by some laboratories. Other considerations such as cost, training, equipment availability, batching of tests, and number of requests will also play a role in test selection.

the stools be collected for routine examinations prior to the patient receiving barium; organisms may be difficult to identify in the stool for several days to more than a week after the patient has received barium. Because giardiasis may not produce any symptoms at all, demonstration of the organism in symptomatic patients may not rule out other possibilities such as peptic ulcer, coeliac disease of some other etiology, strongyloidiasis and possibly carcinoma. Refer to Fig. 10.4 for detailed information.

Unfortunately, serodiagnostic procedures for giardiasis do not yet fulfil the criteria necessary for wide clinical use, particularly since they may indicate either past or present infection. In contrast, the detection of antigen in a stool or visual identification of the organisms using immunodiagnostic reagents both indicate current infection. With the increase in numbers of *Giardia* infections and awareness of particular situations such as nursery school settings, perhaps additional detection assays will emerge as rapid and reliable immunodiagnostic procedures (Addis et al. 1992, Craft 1982, Keystone, Karjden and Warren 1978, Sealy and Schuman 1983).

9 EPIDEMIOLOGY AND CONTROL

9.1 Introduction

Giardiasis is one of the most common intestinal parasitic infections in humans and is distributed world wide in developed and developing countries. There are, however, differences in the numbers of infections, not only between countries, but within geographic regions. Infections seem to be more common in children than adults and other social, environmental, climatic and economic factors also play a role in disease prevalence. Susceptibility to infection with *Giardia* is influenced by sex, age, environmental conditions, socioeconomic conditions, occupation, nutritional status, gastric acidity and overall host immune status.

Transmission occurs through ingestion of as few as 10 viable cysts and can be acquired from food, water and person to person by the oro-faecal route. Often there are outbreaks due to poor sanitation facilities or breakdowns as evidenced by travellers and campers (Kettis and Magnius 1973, Knaus 1974, Lopez et al. 1978, Moore et al. 1969). There has also been an increase in the prevalence of giardiasis in the male homosexual population, probably due to anal and oral sexual practices (Phillips et al. 1981, Schmerin, Jones and Klein 1978).

9.2 Epidemiology

Geographical distribution varies considerably world wide with reported prevalence figures ranging from a low of 5% in Indonesia to 43% in the Seychelles; the United States figure is c. 7.4% (Islam 1990). When reviewing reported prevalence figures, it is always important to remember that data will vary considerably, depending on the sensitivity and specificity of the diagnostic methods used. In areas of the world in which *Giardia* is endemic, the majority of infections in children occur in those under 10 years of age. A decrease in infections seen in children older than 10 may reflect acquired immunity and behavioural changes that decrease potential environmental exposure to the organism. High population density and overcrowding probably contribute to higher prevalences of giardiasis.

Although seasonal patterns have been identified for some infectious diseases, limited information is available for giardiasis. Some data suggest an association with the cooler, wetter months of the year; this is not surprising if one considers the issue of environmental conditions advantageous to cyst survival.

It has been documented that certain occupations may place an individual at risk of infection and these include sewage and irrigation workers who may become exposed to infective cysts. In situations where young children are grouped together, such as nursery schools, there may be an increased incidence of exposure and subsequent infection of both children and staff.

The possible association between gastric acidity and giardiasis has been debated for some time; decreased gastric acid production may predispose people to infection with *Giardia*. It is thought that normal gastric acidity acts as a barrier to the establishment of an infection; patients who have had a gastrectomy are prone to infection with *Giardia*. Although achlorhydria is associated with blood group A and some evidence suggests that this group is more susceptible to giardiasis, subsequent evidence has not confirmed this information. Since reduction in gastric acid also occurs as a result of malnutrition, these factors may be linked and, as a group, increase the susceptibility to infection with this organism. This link between mal-

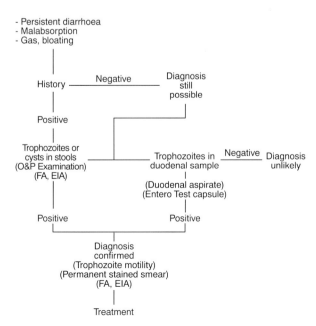

Fig. 10.4 Giardiasis.

nutrition and giardiasis may also be explained by the impairment of the host's immune system.

The issue of breast milk in modifying infection with *Giardia* has also been discussed (Islam 1990). Lower incidence of giardiasis in children ≤6 months of age may be related to an association with breast-feeding and some protection against infection through secretory IgA. However, lower incidence may also be related to decreased exposure to *Giardia* in breast-fed infants.

Giardiasis is one of the more common causes of traveller's diarrhoea and has been recorded from all parts of the world. It has also been speculated that visitors to areas endemic for *Giardia* are more likely to present with symptoms than individuals who live in the area; this difference is probably due to the development of immunity from prior, and possible continued, exposure to the organism.

There have been a number of outbreaks atttributed to either resort or municipal water supplies in Oregon, Colorado, Utah, Washington, New Hampshire and New York (Craun 1990, Kirner 1978, Shaw et al. 1977, Wright et al. 1977). Most waterborne outbreaks have occurred in water systems using surface water sources (Dykes et al. 1990). High rates of infection have also been reported from hikers and campers who drank stream water: because some of these areas were remote from human habitation, infected wild animals, especially beaver, are suspected as being a possible source of infection (Dykes et al. 1990). In addition to beavers and muskrats, *Giardia* infects a number of different animals, including dogs, cats, cattle, sheep, pigs, goats, gerbils, and rats; however, the role of some of these species in zoonotic giardiasis is relatively unknown (Halliday et al. 1995, Karanis et al. 1996).

During the past few years, giardiasis has received much publicity. With increased travel, there has been a definite increase in symptomatic giardiasis within the USA (Addis et al. 1992). Various surveys show infection rates of 2–15% in various parts of the world.

10 CHEMOTHERAPY

If giardiasis is diagnosed, the patient should be treated; however, the therapy is controversial, depending on geographical location throughout the world. In the majority of cases, giardiasis can be eliminated with the use of quinacrine, but its side effects include: nausea, vomiting, headache and dizziness. Vertigo, excessive sweating, fever, pruritis, corneal oedema, myalgias and insomnia have also been reported.

Metronidazole is also very effective and is approved by the WHO (WHO, 1995) but is listed as the second drug of choice by the Centers for Disease Control in the United States because of potential carcinogenicity in rats and mutagenic changes in bacteria. Although these changes have never been demonstrated in humans, and the issue is still debated, metronidazole is not recommended for pregnant women. The most frequent side effects are gastrointestinal and include: nausea, vomiting, diarrhoea and crampy abdominal pain. Additional complaints may include metallic taste, headache, dizziness, drowsiness, lassitude, paresthesias, urticaria and pruritis. Alcohol should be avoided when taking this medication.

Tinidazole has also been used and has proven more effective than metronidazole as a single dose (Jokipii and Jokipii 1979). Furazolidone is often used for treating children and paromomycin has been suggested for use in pregnancy (Davidson 1990).

In the absence of a parasitological diagnosis, the treatment of suspected giardiasis is a common question with no clear cut answer. The approach depends on the alternatives and the degree of suspicion of giardiasis, both of which will vary among patients and physicians. It is not recommended that treatment be given without good parasitological evidence particularly since relief of symptoms does not allow a retrospective diagnosis of giardiasis; the most commonly used drug, metronidazole, also targets other organisms besides *Giardia*.

The third question involves treatment of asymptomatic patients. Generally, it is recommended that all cases of proven giardiasis be treated because the infection may cause subclinical malabsorption, symptoms are often periodic and may appear later and a carrier is a potential source of infection for others. Certainly in areas of the world where infection rates are extremely high, as well as the prospect of reinfection, the benefit per cost ratio also has to be examined.

11 INTEGRATED CONTROL

Because of the potential for wild animal, and possibly other domestic animal, reservoir hosts, other measures as well as personal hygiene and improved sanitary measures have to be considered (Brightman and Slonka 1979, Hewlett et al. 1982). Iodine has been recommended as an effective disinfectant for drinking water, but it must be used according to the appropriate directions (Jarroll, Bingham and Meyer 1980, Jarroll, Bingham and Meyer 1981, Zemlyn, Wilson and Hillweg 1981). Filtration systems have also been recommended, although they have certain drawbacks, such as clogging. Water treatment systems tend to be unavailable in developing countries, many of which do not have piped water available to the general population. Boiling the water is effective, but carries with it the cost of fuel, another consideration in many parts of the world. Improved personal hygiene, routine hand-washing, better preparation and storage of food and water, control of insects which may come in contact with infected stools and then contaminate food or water and treatment of symptomatic and asymptomatic individuals would all lead to a decrease in the overall numbers of infections with this parasite.

Although the potential for a vaccine has been discussed, prospects are poor for the development of actual vaccine reagents in the near future. Control measures will continue to be centered on environmental and personal hygiene issues.

REFERENCES

Addis DG, Davis JP et al., 1992, Epidemiology of giardiasis in Wisconsin: increasing incidence of reported cases and unexplained seasonal trends. *Am J Trop Med Hyg,* **47:** 13–19.

Addis DG, Mathews HM et al., 1991, Evaluation of a commercially available enzyme-linked immunosorbent assay for *Giardia lamblia* antigen in stool, *J Clin Microbiol,* **29:** 1137–42.

Ament ME, Ochs HD, David SD, 1973, Structure and function of the gastrointestinal tract in primary immunodeficiency syndromes: a study of 39 patients, *Medicine (Baltimore),* **52:** 224–48.

Bingham AK, Meyer EA, 1979, *Giardia* encystation can be induced in vitro in acidic solutions, *Nature* (London), **277:** 301–2.

Brightman II, AH, Slonka GF, 1979, A review of five clinical cases of giardiasis in cats, *J Am Anim Hosp Assoc,* **12:** 492–7.

Chavez B, Knaippe F et al., 1986, *Giardia lamblia:* Electrophysiology and ultrastructure of cytopathology in cultured epithelial cells, *Exp Parasitol,* **61:** 379–89.

Chen N, Upcroft JA, Upcroft P, 1995, A *Giardia duodenalis* gene encoding a protein with multiple repeats of a toxin homologue, *Parasitology,* **111:** 423–31.

Collins JP, Keller KF, Brown L, 1978, 'Ghost' forms of *Giardia lamblia* cysts initially misdiagnosed as *Isospora, Am J Trop Med Hyg,* **27:** 334–5.

Craft JC, 1982, *Giardia* and giardiasis in children, *Pediatr Infect Dis,* **1:** 196–211.

Craun GF, 1990, Waterborne giardiasis. In: *Giardiasis,* ed. Meyer EA, Elsevier, Amsterdam, 267–93.

Davidson RA, 1990, Treatment of giardiais: the North American perspective. In: *Giardiasis,* ed. Meyer EA, Elsevier, Amsterdam, 325–53.

Dobell C, 1920, The discovery of the intestinal protozoa of man, *Proc R Soc Med,* **13:** 1–15.

Dykes AC, Juranek DD et al., 1980, Municipal waterborne giardiasis. An epidemiologic investigation, *Ann Intern Med,* **93:** 165–70.

Ellis JE, Wyder MA et al., 1996, Changes in lipid composition during in vitro encystation and fatty acid desaturase activity of *Giardia lamblia, Mol Biochem Parasitol,* **81:** 13–25.

Erlandsen SL, 1974, Scanning electron microscopy of intestinal giardiasis: Lesions of the microvillous border of villus epithelial cells produced by trophozoites of *Giardia.* In: *Scanning Electron Microscopy,* ed. Johari O, IIT Research Institute, Chicago, 775–82.

Erlandsen SL, Macechko PT et al., 1996, Formation of the *Giardia* cyst wall: Studies on extracellular assembly using immunogold labeling and high resolution field emission SEM, *J Eukaryotic Microbiol,* **43:** 416–29.

Ey PL, Bruderer T et al., 1996, Comparison of genetic groups determined by molecular and immunological analyses of *Giardia* isolated from animals and humans in Switzerland and Australia, *Parasitol Res,* **82:** 52–60.

Filice FP, 1952, Studies on the cytology and life history of a *Giardia* from the laboratory rat, *Univ Calif Publ Zool,* **47:** 53–146.

Garcia LS, Bruckner DA, 1997, *Diagnostic Medical Parasitology,* 3rd edn, American Society for Microbiology, ASM Press, Washington, D.C.

Garcia LS, Shum AC, Bruckner DA, 1992, Evaluation of a new monoclonal antibody combination reagent for direct fluorescence detection of *Giardia* cysts and *Cryptosporidium* oocysts in human fecal specimens, *J Clin Microbiol,* **30:** 3255–7.

Halliday CEW, Inge PMG, Farthing MJG, 1995, Characterization of bile salt uptake by *Gardia lamblia, Int J Parasitol,* **25:** 1089–97.

Healy GR, 1990, Giardiasis in perspective: the evidence of animals as a source of human *Giardia* infections. In: *Giardiasis,* ed. Meyer EA, Elsevier, Amsterdam, 305–13.

Hewlett EL, Andrews JS et al., 1982, Experimental infection in mongrel dogs with *Giardia lamblia* cysts and cultured trophozoites, *J Infect Dis,* **145:** 89–93.

Isaac-Renton JL, Byrne SK, Prameya R, 1988, Isoelectric focusing of ten strains of *Giardia duodenalis, J Parasitol,* **74:** 1054–6.

Islam A, 1990, Giardiasis in developing countries. In: *Gardiasis,* ed. Meyer EA, Elsevier, Amsterdam, 235–66.

Jarroll Jr EL, Bingham AK, Meyer EA, 1980, *Giardia* cyst destruction: Effectiveness of six small-quantity water disinfection methods, *Am J Trop Med Hyg,* **29:** 8–11.

Jarroll Jr EL, Bingham AK, Meyer EA, 1981, Effect of chlorine on *Giardia lamblia* cyst viability, *Appl Environ Microbiol,* **41:** 483–7.

Jarroll EL, Lindmark DG, 1990, Giardia metabolism. In: *Giardiasis,* ed. Meyer EA, Elsevier, Amsterdam, 61–76.

Jokipii L, Jokipii AMM, 1979, Single-dose metronidazole and tinidazole as therapy for giardiasis: success rates, side effects, and drug absorption and elimination, *J Infect Dis,* **140:** 984–8.

Karanis P, Opiela K et al., 1996, Possible contamination of surface waters with *Giardia* spp. through muskrats, *Zentralblatt Fur Bakteriologie – Int J Med Microbiol Virol Parasitol Infect Dis,* **284:** 302–6.

Katelaris PH, Naeem A, Farthing MJG, 1995, Attachment of *Giardia lamblia* trophozoites to a cultured human intestinal cell line, *Gut,* **37:** 512–18.

Kettis AA, Magnius L, 1973, *Giardia lamblia* infection in a group of students after a visit to Leningrad in March 1970, *Scand J Infect Dis,* **5:** 289–92.

Keystone JS, Karjden S, Warren MR, 1978, Person-to-person transmission of *Giardia lamblia* in day-care nurseries, *Can Med Assoc J,* **119:** 242–4.

Kirner JC, 1978, Waterborne outbreak of giardiasis in Camas, Washington, *J Am Waterworks Assoc,* **January:** 35–40.

Knaus WA, 1974, Reassurance about Russian giardiasis, *N Engl J Med,* **291:** 156.

Lopez CE, Juranek DD et al., 1978, Giardiasis in American travelers to Madeira Island, Portugal, *Am J Trop Med Hyg,* **27:** 1128–32.

Lujan HD, Mowatt MR et al., 1996, Cholesterol starvation induces differentiation of the intestinal parasite *Giardia lamblia, Proc Nat Acad Sci USA,* **93:** 7628–33.

Meyer EA, 1990, Taxonomy and nomenclature. In: *Giardiasis,* ed. Meyer EA, Elsevier, Amsterdam, 51–60.

Meyer EA, Jarroll EL, 1980, Giardiasis, *Am J Epidemiol,* **111:** 1–12.

Meyers JD, Kuharic HA, Holmes KK, 1977, *Giardia lamblia* infection in homosexual men, *Br J Vener,* **53:** 54–5.

Moore GT, Cross WM et al., 1969, Epidemic giardiasis at a ski resort, *N Engl J Med,* **281:** 402–7.

Nash TE, Herrington DA, Levine MM, 1987, Usefulness of an enzyme-linked immunosorbent assay for detection of *Giardia* antigen in feces, *J Clin Microbiol,* **25:** 1169–71.

Nash TE, Herrington DA et al., 1990, Antigenic variation of *Giardia lamblia* in experimental human infections, *J Immunol,* **144:** 4362–9.

National Committee for Clinical Laboratory Standards, 1993, Procedures for the recovery and identification of parasites from the intestinal tract, Proposed Guideline, M28-P, National Committee for Clinical Laboratory Standards, Villanova, PA.

Owen RL, Allen CL, Stevens DP, 1981, Phagocytosis of *Giardia muris* by macrophages in Peyer's patch epithelium in mice, *Infect Immun,* **33:** 591–601.

Peterson JM, 1957, Intestinal changes in *Giardia lamblia* infestation, *Am J Roentgenol,* **77:** 670–7.

Phillips SC, Mildran D et al., 1981, Sexual transmission of enteric protozoa and helminths in a venereal-disease-clinic population, *N Engl J Med,* **305:** 603–6.

Proctor EM et al., 1989, Isoenzyme analysis of human and animal isolates of *Giardia duodenalis* from British Columbia, Canada, *Am J Trop Med Hyg,* **41:** 411–5.

Schmerin MJ, Jones TC, Klein H, 1978, Giardiasis: Association with homosexuality, *Ann Intern Med,* **88:** 801–3.

Sealy DP, Schuman SH, 1983, Endemic giardiasis and day care, *Pediatrics,* **72:** 154–8.

Shaw PK, Brodsky RE et al., 1977, A community wide outbreak of giardiasis with evidence of transmission by a municipal water supply, *Ann Intern Med,* **87:** 426–32.

Smith PD, Lane HC et al., 1988, Intestinal infections in patients with the acquired immunodeficiency syndrome (AIDS), *Ann Intern Med,* **108:** 328–33.

Stevens WJ, Vermeire PA, 1981, *Giardia lamblia* in bronchoalveolar lavage fluid, *Thorax,* **36:** 875.

Tandon BN, Tandon RK et al., 1977, Mechanism of malabsorption in giardiasis: A study of bacterial flora and bile salt deconjugation in upper jejunum, *Gut,* **18:** 176–81.

Upcroft JA, Boreham PFL et al., 1995, Biological and genetic analysis of a longitudinal collection of *Giardia* samples derived from humans, *Acta Tropica,* **60:** 35–46.

WHO, 1995, Drugs used in Parasitic Diseases, 2nd edn, WHO, Geneva.

Wright RA, Spencer HC et al., 1977, Giardiasis in Colorado: An epidemiologic study, *Am J Epidemiol,* **105:** 330–6.

Zemlyn S, Wilson WW, Hillweg PA, 1981, A caution on iodine water purification, *West J Med,* **135:** 166–7.

Chapter 11

TRICHOMONADS AND INTESTINAL FLAGELLATES

D E Burgess

1 INTRODUCTION

Of the 3–5 trichomonad species found in humans, only *Trichomonas vaginalis* regularly displays the capacity for producing disease. Human trichomoniasis persists and is essentially cosmopolitan in its occurrence despite the availability of effective chemotherapeutic agents and little evidence of the development of significant drug resistance. A sexually transmitted disease, trichomoniasis caused by *T. vaginalis* ranges from a mild or inapparent infection to one causing a chronic and substantial level of inflammation in the reproductive tract of women and significant urethritis in men (Krieger et al. 1993). Rare cases of perinatal infection of females born to infected mothers (Sobel 1992) and respiratory trichomonad infections (Walzer, Rutherford and East 1978) have been reported, the latter possibly attributable to trichomonads other than *T. vaginalis*.

2 CLASSIFICATION

T. vaginalis is a parasitic protozoan and is classified as follows (see also Chapter 7):

Class Trichomonadea, Kirby, 1947

Order Trichomonadida, Kirby, 1947 emend. Honigberg, 1974. There are typically 4–6 flagella, which may be recurved, free or attached to an undulating membrane (when present). There are usually no true cysts.

Family Trichomonadidae, Wenyon, 1926. Characterized by possession of: a cytostome; 3–5 free flagella (one flagellum on the margin of an undulating membrane); and an axostyle protruding through the posterior of the cell.

Genus *Trichomonas*, Donné, 1837. Trophozoites that typically possess: 4 free flagella (one along the outer margin of the undulating membrane); a costa at the base of the undulating membrane; and an axostyle. No cysts are present.

3 STRUCTURE AND LIFE-CYCLE

The shape of *T. vaginalis* is typically pyriform in culture, although amoeboid shapes are evident in parasites adhering to mammalian cells (Nielsen and Nielsen 1975). Light- and electron-microscopic studies (Honigberg and King 1964; Nielsen 1975), summarized previously (Honigberg and Burgess 1994), indicate that *T. vaginalis* is c. 9.7×7 μm and that non-dividing organisms have 4 anterior flagella. In addition to the flagella (4 anterior and one recurrent) the undulating membrane and the costa also originate in the kinetosomal complex at the anterior of the parasite. Internal organelles include a prominent nucleus and a rigid structure, the 'axostyle', that runs through the cell from the anterior to posterior ends (Fig. 11.1).

A respiratory organelle, the 'hydrogenosome' (Lindmark and Müller 1973), is present and appears by light microscopy as a paraxostylar and paracostal chromatic granule. The hydrogenosome is seen as an osmiophilic, dense granule by electron microscopy (Nielsen 1975, Nielsen 1976; Fig. 11.2).

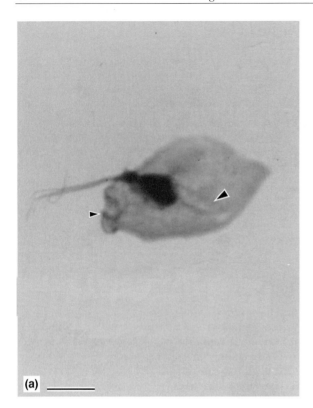 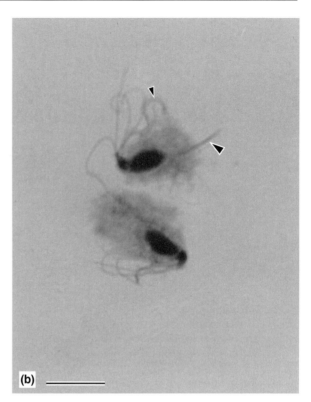

Fig. 11.1 *Trichomonas vaginalis* from culture, stained with Giemsa's stain and showing the undulating membrane and recurrent flagellum (small arrows) and the axostyle (large arrows). (a) Cells show characteristic colour. (b) Four distinct anterior flagella are visible. Bar = 10 μm. (Micrographs kindly provided by Jovanka Voyich, VMBL.)

The life-cycle of *T. vaginalis* is simple in that the trophozoite is transmitted through coitus and no cyst form is known. The trophozoite divides by binary fission giving rise to a population in the urogenital tract of humans.

4 BIOCHEMISTRY, MOLECULAR BIOLOGY AND GENETICS

Anaerobic metabolism produces most of the parasite's energy. Earlier work on the biochemistry of *T. vaginalis* (reviewed in Shorb 1964, von Brand 1973 and Honigberg 1978) indicated that several sugars (e.g. maltose, glucose) are fermented by the parasite through a glycolytic pathway. Subsequent studies revealed that transport of glucose across the cell membrane occurred by facilitated diffusion (ter Kuile and Müller 1992). The metabolism of *T. vaginalis* differs from that of eukaryotic cells with mitochondria in 3 major areas: the importance of inorganic pyrophosphates in carbohydrate catabolism; the importance of sulphur proteins in metabolism; and the disposal of electrons by H_2 formation (Searle and Müller 1991, Müller 1992). Trichomonads lack both cytochrome-mediated electron transport and the associated electron transport-linked phosphorylation, as well as the familiar mitochondrion that houses this system in other eukaryotic cells. Instead, the site of fermentative

carbohydrate metabolism is the hydrogenosome (Lindemark and Müller 1973), an organelle thought to have arisen by endosymbiosis with an anaerobic bacterium or conversion of mitochondria (Lahti, D'Oliveira and Johnson 1992). Hydrogenosomes isolated from *T. vaginalis* have an NADH/ferredoxin oxidoreductase activity and these organelles ferment pyruvate to acetate, malate, H_2 and CO_2. This fermentation is dependent on ADP, P_i, Mg_2 and succinate and CO_2-dependent carboxylation of pyruvate to malate by malate dehydrogenase. Detergent disruption (Triton X100) stops pyruvate-dependent H_2 formation (this effect is overcome by adding exogenous ferredoxin), indicating that the structural integrity of the hydrogenosome is crucial to its effective functioning (Steinbuchel and Müller 1986).

Further progress in delineation of the components of the metabolic machinery of the hydrogenosome is being made by the cloning of genes coding for enzymes associated with this organelle. The structural gene for succinyl-coenzyme A synthetase from hydrogenosomes of *T. vaginalis* has been cloned and has an amino acid sequence 65% similar to the same enzyme from *Escherichia coli* (Lahti, d'Oliveira and Johnson 1992). Hydrogenosomes contain a single copy gene, devoid of introns, that codes for an iron-sulphur ferredoxin containing 93 amino acids and that is similar to the [2Fe–2S]putidaredoxin of *Pseudomonas putida* (Johnson et al. 1990).

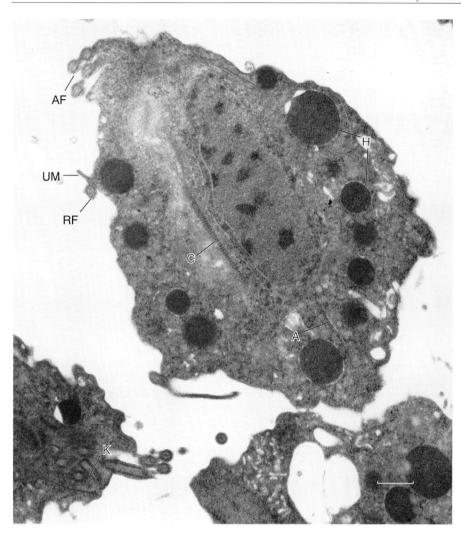

Fig. 11.2 Transmission electron micrograph of *Trichomonas vaginalis* from culture. A, axostyle; C, costa; H, hydrogenosome; K, kinetosome; N, nucleus; AF, anterior flagella; RF, recurrent flagellum; UM, undulating membrane. Bar = 1 μm. (Micrograph kindly provided by Andy Blixt, VMBL.)

4.1 Hydrolytic enzymes

Proteinases of *T. vaginalis* have been known since the 1970s and detailed investigations of these enzymes have been made during the last 10 years. Cysteine proteinases seem to be particularly prevalent, as dithiothreital stimulates the activity of several proteinases from *T. vaginalis*. These range from 20 to 110 kDa (Lockwood et al. 1987), the lower molecular weight proteinases being released from the cell (Lockwood, North and Coombs 1984, 1988, Lockwood et al. 1987, North, Robertson and Coombs 1990). The release of proteinases from *T. vaginalis* is of interest in the context of its ability to elicit varying degrees of inflammation and the possible role of these enzymes in pathogenesis. There are reports of cell detaching factors released by the parasite into the growth medium (Garber, Lemchuk-Favel and Bowie 1989, Lushbaugh et al. 1989) some of which are reported to have trypsin-like activity. These factors are active on human and hamster cells, causing them to detach and round up. Release of cell detaching factors and proteinases from *T. vaginalis* clearly implies that these

parasite products could degrade proteins such as laminin, vitronectin and other components of the extracellular matrix, thus effecting the release of host cells from tissue.

The substrate specificity and structure of some of the proteinases of *T. vaginalis* are now being determined. Parasite proteinases were not inhibited by pepstatin, phenyl methyl sulphonyl fluoride or EDTA, but they were inhibited by iodoacetic acid, antipain, leupeptin and N-α-ρ-tosyl-L-lysine chloromethyl ketone. Lower molecular sizes of proteinases were released from the parasite; proteinases of 25, 27 and 34 kDa specifically hydrolyzed synthetic substrates with arginine–arginine residues whereas other proteinases had activity over a wide substrate range (North, Robertson and Coombs 1990). Recent cloning studies of cysteine proteinase genes of *T. vaginalis* indicate that at least 4 distinct genes are present and that they have considerable homology (up to 45% identity) with cysteine proteinase genes of *Dictyostelium discoideum*. Three of the proteinase genes were present as single copies, whereas the other was present as a multiple copy gene. The amino acid sequence data indicated that these proteinases were of the L/cathepsin H/papain type (Mallinson et al. 1994).

4.2 Nucleic acids

Nucleic acid synthesis in trichomonads differs markedly from that in mammalian cells, as trichomonads do not synthesize either purines or pyrimidines *de novo*. *T. vaginalis* does not incorporate purine ring precursors into nucleic acids but rather directly salvages purine nucleosides through adenosine and guanosine kinases. Neither inosine nor hypoxanthine are incorporated and no interconversion between adenylate and guanylate occurs (Heyworth, Gutteridge and Ginger 1982).

Trichomonads are also unable to synthesize pyrimidines from aspartate, orotate and bicarbonate, the typical *de novo* pathway. Neither thymidylate synthetase nor dihydrofolate reductase activity has been found. Conversion of cytidine by cytidine phosphotransferase and nucleotide kinases to cytidine monophosphate (CMP), cytidine diphosphate (CDT) and cytidine triphosphate (CTP) allows *T. vaginalis* to salvage exogenous cytidine, uridine, uracil and, to some extent, thymidine into its nucleotide pool (Wang and Cheng 1984). Cytidine is converted to uridine by cytidine deaminase whereas uracil is converted to uridine by uridine phosphorylase before conversion into nucleotides.

Nucleosides (but not nucleotides) are transported across the cell membrane of *T. vaginalis*. The nucleosides adenosine, guanosine and uridine are transported across the cell membrane by a 2-carrier, facilitated transport mechanism at a rate apparently sufficient to sustain growth (Harris et al. 1988). Intracellularly, nucleosides are rapidly converted to nucleotides so that transport is not affected by any appreciable build up of nucleosides. Neither bases nor D-ribose affect uptake of nucleosides, suggesting that the carriers operating in *T. vaginalis* are similar to those in other parasitic protozoa such as *Plasmodium berghei* (Hansen, Sleeman and Pappas 1980) and *Leishmania donovani* (Aronow et al. 1987).

5 CLINICAL ASPECTS

5.1 Introduction

T. vaginalis is site-specific, usually surviving in only the urogenital tract of humans. Approximately 10% of vulvovaginitis is due to infection with *T. vaginalis* (Sobel 1992). In men, clinical features of the infection may include urethral discharge and inflammation of the tissues lining the reproductive/urinary tract (Krieger, Jenny et al. 1993a), but it is more usual for men to display no symptoms or clinical disease.

5.2 Clinical manifestations

A female patient infected with *T. vaginalis* may have no obvious clinical signs yet may still suffer vaginitis of varying severity. Asymptomatic patients can also carry the infection and remain at risk of developing symptomatic disease at a later date (Krieger et al.

1988). Clinical features that may develop in 50 –90% of infected women include: purulent vaginal discharge, pruritus and dyspareunia. Leukorrhea and dysuria are occasionally seen. Vaginal discharge is observed in 50–75% of diagnosed women and is considered malodorous in only c. 10% of these patients. Although the discharge has often been described as 'yellow-green' and 'frothy', only c. 8% of patients produce a discharge characterized as frothy and c. 59% produce a discharge characterized as purulent. Diffuse vulvar erythema and copious vaginal discharge are often present. Punctate haemorrhages of the cervix may result in a strawberry-like appearance, apparent by inspection in only 1–2% of patients but apparent in 45% of patients examined by colposcopy (Wolner-Hanssen et al. 1989). Pruritus, particularly vulvar itching, is a frequent symptom (25–50% of patients) and may be severe (Sobel 1992).

6 IMMUNOLOGY

Some of the earliest investigations into immunity centred on reports that sera obtained from a variety of mammals can lyse *T. vaginalis* and agglutinate the parasite. Although earlier investigators considered lysis to be dependent on antibody action, *T. vaginalis* is now known to activate complement by the alternative pathway (Gillin and Sher 1981). An extensive study of the agglutinating and lytic activities of normal human, bovine, sheep, horse, swine and dog sera against *T. vaginalis* (Reisenhofer 1963, summarized by Honigberg 1970) showed that these sera had agglutination titres of 1:32 to 1:64.

Early experimental studies on acquired immune responses to *T. vaginalis* examined various immunizations of laboratory animals and evaluated antibody from patients with *T. vaginalis* infection. Guinea pigs given intraperitoneal inoculations of vaginal material containing trichomonads produced antibody responses, as did rabbits given formalin-killed parasites (Riedmüller 1932, Tokura 1935). In mice, intramuscular inoculation induced protection against challenge infection that lasted at least 15 weeks (Kelly and Schnitzer 1952, Schnitzer and Kelly 1953). Intramuscular injection of *T. vaginalis* protected up to 100% of mice against an intraperitoneal challenge, but much less protection was afforded against a subcutaneous challenge (Kelly, Schumacher and Schnitzer 1954).

The protective effect of sera from infected humans was shown in experiments in which human sera were transferred to mice inoculated intraperitoneally with *T. vaginalis* (Teras and Nigesen 1969, reviewed in Honigberg 1970). Similar mouse inoculation experiments with human sera (Nigesen 1966) or rabbit hyperimmune sera (Teras 1963) indicated that these antibodies were both protective. Levels of protective antibodies in the sera of patients quickly diminish following elimination of infection (Nigesen 1964, 1966, Teras and Nigesen 1969). The conclusion from these and subsequent observations (Sobel 1992) is that although an immune response to *T. vaginalis* occurs in infected patients and produces circulating antibody against the parasite, the response is short-lived and does not provide protection against reinfection.

Antibody responses during infection with *T. vaginalis* have been evaluated in numerous surveys by several immunoassays (summarized in Honigberg and Burgess 1994). Although some infected patients do not have detectable anti-*T. vaginalis* antibodies, most display secreted and circulating (serum) antibodies. Secretory antibody levels in the reproductive tract seem to increase in women infected with *T. vaginalis* and parasite-specific antibodies occur in the urogenital tract of persons harbouring *T. vaginalis*. IgA antibody, specific for *T. vaginalis,* was present in vaginal secretions of 76% of 29 infected women and 42% of 19 apparently uninfected women with higher levels in the infected patients (Ackers et al. 1975). Subsequent reports have verified the presence of parasite-specific antibody in vaginal secretions. Street et al. (1982) reported that 73.2% of infected women had anti-*T. vaginalis* IgG or IgA antibodies, compared to 41% of uninfected women. Additional studies on women with proven *T. vaginalis* trichomoniasis have confirmed these findings (Romia and Othman 1991, Alderete et al. 1991a).

6.1 Cellular immune responses

Both macrophages and polymorphonuclear neutrophils (PMNs) have been shown to be capable of killing *T. vaginalis* in vitro (Rein, Sullivan and Mandell 1980) and PMNs have been reported to be attracted to a factor(s) secreted by live *T. vaginalis* (Mason and Forman 1980). Leucocytic vaginal discharge was previously considered to be an important clinical finding expected in women infected with *T. vaginalis*, but more recent studies indicate no significant difference between the numbers of infected and uninfected women with vaginal discharge (Fouts and Kraus 1980). Even so, recruitment of macrophages and PMNs to the site of infection (by the sensitized T lymphocytes and the lymphokines they produce, or by parasite-derived factors that are directly chemotactic for PMNs) could be important elements in protective immunity and the pathological changes present in persons with trichomoniasis.

Other evidence that a cellular immune response is elicited in patients infected with *T. vaginalis* comes from the observation that such patients develop positive delayed-type hypersensitivity (DTH) reactions to whole parasite antigen preparations (Adler and Sadowskiy 1947, Aburel et al. 1963, Sinelnikova 1961). Peripheral blood lymphocytes from individuals with active infections proliferated in vitro when stimulated with whole cell antigen preparations; lymphocytes from uninfected persons gave minimal responses (Yano et al. 1983, Mason and Patterson 1985). Similar results have been obtained in studies of DTH reactions (Michel 1971, Michel and Westphal 1969, Michel et al. 1968) and lymphocyte proliferation responses in mice (Mason and Gwanzura 1988). These results,

together with the findings in patients, indicate that systemic sensitization of T lymphocytes occurs during infection.

6.2 Immunoassays

Extensive discussions have been published of the earlier reports on the use of enzyme immunoassays, complement fixation, agglutination (including microagglutination), haemagglutination and fluorescent antibody techniques in the study of trichomoniasis (Jírovec and Petru 1968, Honigberg 1970). The collective findings of these studies indicate that *T. vaginalis* contains some antigens whose expression levels are rather constant over time, whereas the expression levels of other antigens fluctuates (see section 6.3).

Several types of enzyme-linked immunosorbent assay (ELISA, Engvall and Pearlman 1971) have been developed for *T. vaginalis*, either to measure patient antibodies or to detect antigens of *T. vaginalis* in clinical samples. In one example, whole-cell antigen preparations of *T. vaginalis* (Street et al. 1982) together with aqueous extracts (Alderete 1984) were used as antigens to detect antibodies in serum and vaginal secretions of patients. Affinity-purified, rabbit antibodies to *T. vaginalis* have been used as both capture and detection antibodies in a 'sandwich' ELISA to detect antigens of *T. vaginalis* (Watt et al. 1986). This assay had a sensitivity of 77%, a specificity of 100% and was more sensitive than microscopic examination of wet mounts, but less sensitive than culture methods for detection of infection.

Detection of *T. vaginalis* antigens in fluids on vaginal swabs by ELISA had a sensitivity of 93.2% and a specificity of 97.5% in a study of 44 culture-positive patients in a study group of 482 (Yule et al. 1987). Employing a monoclonal anti-*T. vaginalis* antibody as a capture and detection antibody, a sensitivity of 89% and a specificity of 97% have been achieved (Lisi et al. 1988).

6.3 Antigens

Early immunological studies of *T. vaginalis* indicated that there were antigenic differences between geographically distinct strains of this parasite. In a series of studies in the 1960s, 4 serotypes (TLR, TN, TRT and TR) were described by the use of cross-agglutination and complement fixation methods. These serotypes had common and unique antigens and were present in a large geographical area of central and eastern Europe (reviewed by Honigberg 1970). In another study, agglutination, complement fixation and fluorescent antibody methods were used to demonstrate 3 serotypes of *T. vaginalis* in one geographical area of the former USSR (Andreeva and Mihov 1976). This report was among the first to describe molecular differences between strains of *T. vaginalis* and to attempt to correlate these with serological type; on the basis of the electrophoretic patterns of 10 strains of *T. vaginalis*, 5 different antigenic groups were detectable.

Since this initial work, numerous antigens of *T.vaginalis* have been described, some being shared between strains and others being strain-specific.

Several antigens of *T. vaginalis* have been at least partially characterized and for a few some limited information about function is available (Table 11.1).

Using rabbit antisera, Alderete (1983) detected at least 20 immunogenic polypeptides, ranging from 20 to 200 kDa, in distinct strains of *T. vaginalis*; although there were differences between strains, many common antigens were also recognized. In a separate study of one strain of *T. vaginalis*, by immunoprecipitation of iodinated antigens, the gel profiles obtained were remarkably similar although again there were some differences in patterns (Alderete et al. 1985). These results indicate that some surface antigens of the trichomonads are similar, whereas others are different. Torian and colleagues, using monoclonal antibodies prepared against one clone of *T. vaginalis*, showed that these mAbs reacted with surface epitopes on 4 of 9 distinct parasite clones (Torian et al. 1984, Connely, Torian and Stibbs 1985). Further analysis of antigens by affinity chromatography and Western blots revealed that these mAbs recognized epitopes on a 115 kDa polypeptide. A 58 kDa and a 64 kDa antigen also bound the same mAb as the 115 kDa polypeptide (Torian et al. 1988). These results indicate that *T. vaginalis* has conserved antigens as well as antigen heterogeneity (and epitope heterogeneity on certain antigens).

Some isolates of *T. vaginalis* possess a 270 kDa surface antigen, P270, that is strongly expressed, whereas other isolates express little P270 on their surface (Alderete, Suprun-Brown and Kasmal 1986, Alderete et al. 1986). Expression of higher amounts of P270 correlates with lower *T. vaginalis* cytotoxicity toward HeLa cells, suggesting that the degree of expression of P270 may be a useful virulence marker. A 6 amino acid epitope of P270, DREGRD, binds mAbs specific for P270, as well as a high percentage of the antibody in serum from infected patients, suggesting that P270 could be an immunodominant antigen (Alderete and Neale 1989, Dailey and Alderete 1991). Additional *T. vaginalis* antigens have been detected, including a 230 kDa surface antigen that binds to vaginal antibodies present in infected patients (Alderete et al. 1987, Ald-

erete et al. 1991a) and proteinases that elicit serum and secreted antibodies (Alderete et al. 1991b, Bosner et al. 1992). Four antigenic surface molecules have also been implicated in the adhesion of *T. vaginalis* to vaginal epithelial cells, their expression being upregulated during attachment to host cells (Arroyo et al. 1993). Antibodies to these molecules protect target cells from parasite-mediated cytotoxicity (Engbring and Alderete 1992) suggesting that anti-adhesion immune responses could be important in protecting against the pathogenic effects of *T. vaginalis*.

Current understanding of immunity to *T.vaginalis* is unsatisfactory and it is not clear whether induced immunity is protective and if so, how. Although there is evidence that protection may be achieved by immunization of laboratory animals, strong protective immunity does not seem to follow natural infection in humans. Immunosuppressed persons, such as those with AIDS, do not develop fulminating *T. vaginalis* infections despite the high prevalence of the parasite in the general population. These observations may indicate that systems of 'natural' or constitutive immunity (reliant on mechanisms such as chemotaxis and subsequent influx of neutrophils or activation of the alternative pathway of complement) are much more important than acquired immunity in controlling infections with *T. vaginalis*. In fact, neutrophils are often reported as the most numerous leucocyte present in sites of infection (see Section 7).

7 PATHOLOGY

Although *T. vaginalis* was first described by Donné in 1836 its role as a cause of vaginitis was not recognized for another 80 years (Höhne 1916). The early report of Hogue (1943) on the pathogenic effects of *T. vaginalis* on cells in cultures suggested that the parasite could directly damage host cells. The clinical features, including pathogenicity, of human urogenital trichomonads have been reviewed (Jírovec and Petru 1968, Brown 1972, Catterall 1972, Honigberg 1990, Honigberg and Burgess 1994).

Trichomoniasis is a frequently encountered, sexually transmitted disease (Lossick and Kent 1991) and a common cause of vaginitis and exocervicitis (Heine

Table 11.1 Antigens of *Trichomonas vaginalis* and their characteristics

Reference	Molecular size[1]	Chemical composition	Function
Torian et al. 1984; Connely et al. 1985	115, 64, 58	CHO; polypeptide	surface antigen
Alderete et al. 1986	270	polypeptide; 50% composed of repeating DREGRO sequence	expression inversely correlates with level of cytotoxicity; possible virulence marker
Alderete et al. 1987	230	polypeptide	binds vaginal antibody
Arroyo et al. 1993	65, 51, 33, 23	polypeptides	allow parasite adhesion to host cells

[1]Molecular size in kDa.

and McGregor 1993, Sobel 1992). Children born to women with trichomoniasis may suffer from low birth weight (discussed by Heine and McGregor 1993, Gibbs et al. 1992, Cotch et al. 1991), probably as a result of tissue damage from the cytopathic effect of this parasite on mammalian cells (Alderete and Perlman 1983, Krieger, Ravdin and Rein 1985).

7.1 Histological findings

Histological findings in women with trichomonad cervicitis have been described (Koss and Wolinska 1959); up to one-third of biopsies of female patients infected with *T. vaginalis* show no histological changes. Patients displaying changes had increased vascularity of the squamous epithelium and the presence of the trichomonads was often accompanied by distension of blood vessels within papillae. The 'strawberry cervix' (Lang and Ludmir 1961, Fouts and Kraus 1980) appearance of the exocervix is due to the local extravasation of blood resulting in petechiae (rather than to ulceration) and is not usually due to inflammation. There is much less pronounced dilation of epithelial vessels in patients with non-trichomonad cervicitis than in those with trichomonad-induced cervicitis.

Oedema of the squamous epithelium is accompanied by separation of epithelial cells from each other, inflammation of the squamous epithelium and desquamation. Perinuclear haloes may develop that can be confused with the koilocytotic atypia caused by human papilloma virus infection (Quinn and Holmes 1984); these are often confined to the basal layers of the epithelium. A proportion of epithelial cells display a variety of other abnormalities including enlarged nuclei, hyperchromasia and binucleation. Pycnotic nuclei are evident in the damaged epithelium indicating necrosis and a purulent exudate often coats the epithelial surface; this is a rare condition in non-trichomonad cervicitis.

Biopsy material from 11 women infected with *T. vaginalis* was examined by Nielsen and Nielsen (1975) in an electron microscope study. Generally there was evidence of chronic non-specific inflammation with subepithelial infiltration by neutrophils and lymphocytes. Three of the patients had cervical erosion; the lumens of the glands were packed with neutrophils. In cases of more severe inflammation, neutrophils were present in deeper layers of the epithelium, the neutrophils near the surface being arranged in lacunae. *T. vaginalis* was occasionally found on the surface of the stratified squamous epithelium in clusters situated in areas of shallow depression in the epithelial surface. The trichomonads were often seen on the vaginal surface in a dense mantle, but were not attached to the epithelium in observations in 7 patients. Amoeboid trichomonads attached only to necrotic epithelial cells with the undulating membrane on the surface away from the substrate. In the areas of contact between parasites and epithelial cells there was interdigitation of cytoplasmic projections from the parasite and host

cell, which is evidence for intimate contact between the parasite and host during human infection.

In women with florid vaginitis, the secretion typically contains numerous motile trichomonads, thus rendering diagnosis reasonably easy. In women with latent trichomoniasis, in which the parasite has retreated into the cervical region and in which bizarre and atypically hyperplastic cells may be present in smears, the trichomonads are more difficult to find. In the diffuse or patchy inflammatory secretion, the trichomonads may not be motile. *T. vaginalis* is often difficult to recognize in routinely fixed and stained smears (such as those stained with haemotoxylin and eosin). Antibody-based immunohistochemical procedures have been developed that compare favourably with wet mount methods (Kreiger et al. 1988).

7.2 Mechanism of pathogenicity

Studies of the cytopathic effects of *T. vaginalis* on a variety of cell lines in vitro provide support for a cytopathic mechanism in which both parasite-host cell contact and soluble factors play a role. It was previously known that efficient killing of several target cell lines by *T. vaginalis* required close approximation or contact between parasite and target (Krieger, Ravdin and Rein 1985, Alderete and Garza 1985, 1988). Evidence that parasite adhesion to target cells is important for induction of damage of targets has come from experiments in which various treatments lowered adhesion of parasites to targets. For example treatment of parasites with the following all inhibited adhesion of *T. vaginalis* to target cells: trypsin (Alderete and Garza 1985), cysteine proteinase inhibitors (Arroyo and Alderete 1989), low temperature (4°C) (Alderete and Garza 1985) or cytochalasin D (Krieger, Ravdin and Rein 1985). This suggests that proteinaceous surface structures synthesized by the parasite play a role in adhesion. Four antigenic surface molecules have been implicated in the adhesion of *T. vaginalis* to host cells (Enbring and Alderete 1992) and parasites in contact with HeLa cells or vaginal epithelial cells increase their expression of these adhesion molecules (Arroyo et al. 1993).

Although these reports indicate that intimate association of *T. vaginalis* to targets leads to efficient killing in these experimental systems, they do not prove the absence of one (or more) soluble mediators responsible for host cell damage. There are several reports of soluble factors produced by *T. vaginalis* that are active against nucleated host cells (Garber, Lemchuk-Favel and Bowie 1989, Lushbaugh et al. 1989, Pindak, Gardiner and Pindak 1986). Most of the 'cell detachment factors' that have been described vary in potency and remain uncharacterized in terms of their molecular components and precise modes of action. When homogeneous preparations of such molecules become available, the precise structure and function of such 'factors' will be established and a better understanding of the mechanisms of pathogenesis of trichomoniasis at the molecular level will be possible.

8 DIAGNOSIS

Microscopy and culture procedures are the most widely used methods for the detection of *T. vaginalis* in men and women. The most commonly employed procedures are:

1 direct microscopic examination of fresh (stained or unstained) material in wet mounts, accomplished with the aid of bright-field, dark-field, or phase-contrast microscopy
2 microscopic examination of fixed and stained preparations, usually smears, stained with Giemsa's stain
3 cultivation employing a variety of media.

A combination of the wet mount and culture procedures is both efficient and cost-effective in detection of *T. vaginalis*-positive cases among both women and men. Early reports of an improved culture device, InPouch TV® (BioMed Diagnostics Inc.), indicate that it compares favourably with standard culture procedures in a clinical setting (Draper et al. 1993).

Immunological methods have not been used widely for diagnosis of *T. vaginalis* infection although the relative specificity and sensitivity of individual techniques has been improved recently. In a comparison of several methods, direct detection of *T. vaginalis* using fluorescein-labelled monoclonal antibody compared favourably with wet mounts, staining of fixed material and culture (Krieger et al. 1988). Immuno-histochemical methods detected the related trichomonad, *Tritrichomonas foetus*, in sections of formalin-fixed tissue from the reproductive tract of infected cattle more easily than standard microscopic methods (Burgess and Knoblock 1988, Rhyan et al. 1995).

Nucleic acid hybridization methods for detection of *T. vaginalis* (Rubino et al. 1991) have sensitivity and specificity as good as culture methods. Riley et al. (1992) developed a polymerase chain reaction (PCR) method, using primers that produced a 102 bp product, termed 'A6p'. They used the method to test 24 isolates of *T. vaginalis*, all of which reacted positively. A PCR method based on conserved sequences within a 2000 bp segment of repetitive DNA has also been described; this yielded a 450 bp product in all strains of *T. vaginalis* tested (Kengne et al. 1994). In both cases, PCR procedures produced no false positive reactions with template DNA from sources such as human cells, other parasitic protozoa and viruses. These results suggest that DNA methodology may soon prove to be an efficient, sensitive and accurate approach to the detection of this parasite and an attractive alternative to microscopic methods.

9 EPIDEMIOLOGY AND CONTROL

9.1 Introduction

Trichomoniasis persists throughout the world, despite the availability of effective chemotherapeutic agents and seemingly adequate awareness of the disease on the part of physicians, public health workers and the general population. In recent years, there has been a focus on *T. vaginalis*, due partly to heightened awareness of sexually transmitted diseases generally, as well as the fact that people with *T. vaginalis* infections seem to be at higher risk of HIV infection than are non-infected persons.

9.2 Epidemiology

Infections with *T. vaginalis* are quite common; the prevalence of *T. vaginalis* in non-selected female populations is probably 5–20%. Most estimates of prevalence are based on data from selected patient populations, e.g. those attending sexually transmitted disease clinics; such estimates are unlikely to be representative of the population at large Even so, the data indicate that there has been a slow decline in the prevalence of *T. vaginalis* infections over the past 20 years. In 1972, >180 million women and men were estimated to be infected with *T. vaginalis* world wide (Brown 1972), including c. 2.5 million women in the USA and 1 million women in the UK (Catterall 1972). *T. vaginalis* infection prevalence in American women is estimated at 3 million cases annually (Rein 1990) and some investigators consider trichomoniasis to be the most common sexually transmitted protozoan disease (Levine 1991) and perhaps even the most common sexually transmitted disease (Hammill 1989).

Although estimates in non-selected male populations are not as certain as for women, the prevalence in men is probably c. 50–60% of that in women (Rein and Müller 1989). One study noted a prevalence of 11% in men attending an STD clinic (Krieger et al. 1993b).

10 CHEMOTHERAPY

Treatment of vaginal trichomoniasis relies on the 5-nitroimidazole compounds: metronidazole, tinidazole and ornidazole. Metronidazole is the only one of these currently recommended by the WHO (WHO 1995). Tinidazole with metronidazole have comparable efficacies when used in a single dose regimen (Gabriel, Robertson and Thin 1982). Metronidazole acts by interfering with DNA synthesis, apparently as the result of the production of a transient cytotoxic intermediate form (Lossick 1990). Daily treatment for 7 days or treatment by a single 2 g dose gave equivalently high cure rates (>90%) (Lossick 1982). The daily treatment regimen consists of oral administration of 250 mg of metronidazole 3 times daily for 7 days, producing a cure rate of c. 95% (Lossick 1990, Sobel 1992). Although the multiple dose regimen is efficacious for the patient even without treatment of the sexual partner, it suffers from a degree of non-compliance. The single dose regimen is particularly effective if used with simultaneous treatment of sexual partners, but it does not protect against the relatively frequent event of prompt reinfection by untreated sexual partners. Because of the multifocal nature of infection with *T. vaginalis,* systemic (rather than local) treatment is preferred. In fact, endogenous reinfection by parasites harboured in the urethra and periurethral glands is known to occur when local treatment is attempted (Rein and Müller 1989).

11 VACCINATION

There is no vaccine currently available for use against *T. vaginalis.* The search for vaccines against protozoa is complicated by their ability to evade and modulate host immune responses. *T. vaginalis* may be able to evade the immune response as it exists largely outside the host in the lumen of the reproductive tract. Effector mechanisms such as secretory antibody (sIgA) may prove to be crucial in protection against the cytotoxic effects of this parasite on host cells.

Many basic questions concerning the immune response to *T. vaginalis* remain unanswered and lack of knowledge about the immune response to the organism impedes vaccine development. For example, we do not know the mechanisms by which natural infections are eliminated, nor which target antigens elicit protective immunity. We do not even know if an effective protective immunity develops during natural infection. The absence of an appropriate laboratory animal model for trichomoniasis has delayed progress in answering these questions.

The natural history of infection by *T. vaginalis* in humans suggests that adaptive immune responses during infection do not play a significant role in controlling infections. Indeed, the most prevalent leucocyte response in the reproductive tract during infection is by neutrophils and chemotaxis of neutrophils by components of *T. vaginalis* has been reported (Mason and Forman 1980). These findings, together with the pattern of frequent reinfection, suggest that effective immunological memory may not be established in most infected persons. Other explanations for the absence of protective immunity after infection are the presence of a considerable number of distinct antigenic types of *T. vaginalis* (Krieger et al. 1985), or the occurrence of some form of antigenic drift over time, as has been observed with certain surface antigens (Alderete et al. 1986). A combination of

these phenomena could produce a reinfection pattern similar to that seen with the rhinoviruses that cause the common cold. If such drifts occur, new antigenic profiles in the parasite population would occur so rapidly that the host could not effectively respond to the ever-changing epitopes being displayed.

12 INTEGRATED CONTROL

Control of trichomoniasis due to *T. vaginalis* should include:

1 thorough examination to determine infection status of the patient
2 appropriate treatment of the patient and sexual partner(s)
3 continued surveillance by public health agencies to provide updated prevalence estimates.

Current knowledge of the immune response to *T. vaginalis* is insufficient to predict whether the development of a vaccine represents a realistic goal. A rational vaccine development strategy should include research toward understanding the roles of certain surface antigens and secreted antigenic molecules (e.g. proteinases) and identification of new target antigens.

13 INTESTINAL FLAGELLATES

Two intestinal flagellates (other than *Giardia lamblia,* or *G. intestinalis,* discussed in Chapter 10) are encountered in the human intestinal tract with some frequency: *Chilomastix mesnili* and *Dientamoeba fragilis.* The former has been discussed elsewhere (Beaver, Jung, Cupp 1984, Garcia and Bruckner 1993) and is not considered pathogenic in humans.

D. fragilis was initially thought to be an amoeba (Jepps and Dobell 1918) but was later determined to be a flagellate related to *Histomonas* (Camp, Mattern and Honigberg 1974, Honigberg 1974). The life-cycle and transmission of *D. fragilis* are not completely understood as no cyst stage has been described. The trophozoite form is seen in the faeces and typically contains 2 nuclei although up to 4 may be seen. Although symptoms such as intermittent diarrhoea, abdominal pain, nausea, anorexia and malaise have been associated with *D. fragilis* infections, the organism's pathogenic capacity remains controversial.

REFERENCES

Aburel E, Zervos G et al., 1963, Immunological and therapeutic investigations in vaginal trichomoniasis, *Rum Med Rev,* **7:** 13–19.

Ackers JP, Lumsden WHR et al., 1975, Anti-trichomonal antibody in the vaginal secretions of women infected with *T. vaginalis, Br J Vener Dis,* **51:** 319–23.

Adler S, Sadowsky A, 1947, Intradermal reaction in trichomonad infection, *Lancet,* **252:** 867–8.

Alderete JF, 1983, Identification of immunogenic and antibody-binding membrane proteins of pathogenic *Trichomonas vaginalis, Infect Immun,* **40:** 284–91.

Alderete JF, 1984, Enzyme-linked immunosorbent asay for detection of antibody to *Trichomonas vaginalis*: Use of whole cells and aqueous extracts as antigens, *Br J Vener Dis,* **60:** 164–70.

Alderete JF, Garza GE, 1985, Specific nature of *Trichomonas vaginalis* parasitism of host cell surfaces, *Infect Immun,* **50:** 701–8.

Alderete JF, Garza GE, 1988, Identification and properties of *Trichomonas vaginalis* proteins involved in cytadherence, *Infect Immun,* **56:** 28–33.

Alderete JF, Neale KA, 1989, Relatedness of a major immunogen in *Trichomonas vaginalis* isolates, *Infect Immun,* **57:** 1849–53.

Alderete JF, Perlman E, 1983, Pathogenic *Trichomonas vaginalis* cytotoxicity to cell culture monolayers, *Br J Vener Dis,* **60:** 99–105.

Alderete JF, Suprun-Brown L, Kasmala L, 1986, Monoclonal antibody to a major surface glycoprotein immunogen differentiates isolates and subpopulations of *Trichomonas vaginalis, Infect Immun,* **52:** 70–5.

Alderete JF, Suprun-Brown L et al., 1985, Heterogeneity of *Trichomonas vaginalis* and supopulations with sera of patients and experimentally infected mice, *Infect Immun*, **49**: 463–8.

Alderete JF, Kasmala L et al., 1986, Phenotypic variation and diversity among *Trichomonas vaginalis* isolates and correlation of phenotype with trichomonal virulence determinants, *Infect Immun*, **53**: 285–93.

Alderete JF, Demes P et al., 1987, Phenotypes and protein-epitope phenotypic variation among fresh isolates of *Trichomonas vaginalis*, *Infect Immun*, **55**: 1037–41.

Alderete JF, Newton E et al., 1991a, Vaginal antibody of patients with trichomoniasis is to a prominent surface immunogen of *Trichomonas vaginalis*, *Genitourin Med*, **67**: 220–5.

Alderete JF, Newton E et al., 1991b, Antibody in sera of patients infected with *Trichomonas vaginalis* is to trichomonad proteinases, *Genitourin Med*, **67**: 331–4.

Andreeva N, Mihov L, 1976, Electrophoretic studies of the water soluble proteins from ten local strains of *Trichomonas vaginalis*, *Folia Med (Prague)*, **18**: 67–73.

Aronow B, Kaur K et al., 1987, Two high affinity nucleoside transporters in *Leishmania donovani*, *Mol Biochem Parasitol*, **22**: 29–37.

Arroyo R, Alderete JF, 1989, *Trichomonas vaginalis* surface proteinase activity is necessary for parasite adherence to epithelial cells, *Infect Immun*, **57**: 2991–7.

Arroyo R, Gonzalez-Robles A et al., 1993, Signaling of *Trichomonas vaginalis* for amoeboid transformation and adhesion synthesis follows cytoadherence, *Mol Microbiol*, **7**: 299–309.

Beaver CH, Jung RC, Cupp EW, 1984, *Clinical Parasitology*, 9th edn, Lea and Febiger, Philadelphia, Pennsylvania, 42–3.

Bosner P, Gonbosova A et al., 1992, Proteinases of *Trichomonas vaginalis*:antibody response in patients with urogenital trichomoniasis, *Parasitology*, **105**: 387–91.

von Brand T, 1973, *Biochemistry of Parasites*, 2nd edn, Academic Press, New York.

Brown MT, 1972, Trichomoniasis, *Practitioner*, **209**: 639–44.

Burgess DE, Knoblock KF, 1988, Identification of *Tritrichomonas foetus* in sections of bovine placental tissue with monoclonal antibodies, *J Parasitol*, **75**: 977–80.

Camp RR, Mattern CFT, Honigberg BM, 1974, Study of *Dientamoeba fragilis* Jepps and Dobell. I. Electronmicroscopic observations of the binucleate stages, *J Protozool*, **21**: 69–79.

Catterall RD, 1972, Trichomonal infections of the genital tract, *Med Clin North Am*, **56**: 1203–9.

Connely RJ, Torian BE, and Stibbs HH, 1985, Identification of a surface antigen of *Trichomonas vaginalis*, *Infect Immun*, **49**: 270–4.

Cotch MF, Pastorek JG et al., 1991, Demographic and behavioral predictors of *Trichomonas vaginalis* infection among pregnant women, *Obstet Gynecol*, **78**: 1087–92.

Dailey DC, Alderete JF, 1991, The phenotypically variable surface protein of *Trichomonas vaginalis* has a single, tandemly repeated immunodominant epitope, *Infect Immun*, **59**: 2083–8.

Donné A, 1836, Animalcules observés dans les matières purulents et le produit des sécrétions des organes genitaux de l'homme et de la femme, *C R Acad Sci*, **3**: 385–6.

Draper D, Parker R et al., 1993, Detection of *Trichomonas vaginalis* in pregnant women with the InPouch TV culture system, *J Clin Microbiol*, **31**: 1016–18.

Enbring J, Alderete JF, 1992, Molecular basis of host epithelial cell recognition by *Trichomonas vaginalis*, *Mol Microbiol*, **6**: 853–62.

Engvall E, Perlmann P, 1971, Enzyme-linked immunosorbent assay (ELISA) quatantitative assay of immunoglobulin G, *Immunochemistry*, **8**: 871–9.

Fouts AC, Kraus SJ, 1980, *Trichomonas vaginalis*: Reevaluation of its clinical presentation and laboratory diagnosis, *J Infect Dis*, **141**: 137–43.

Gabriel G, Robertson E, Thin RNT, 1982, Single dose treatment of trichomoniasis, *J Int Med Res*, **10**: 129–30.

Garber GE, Lemchuk-Favel LT, Bowie WR, 1989, Isolation of a cell-detaching factor of *Trichomonas vaginalis*, *J Clin Microbiol*, **27**: 1548–53.

Garcia LS, Bruckner DA, 1993, *Diagnostic Medical Parasitology*, 2 edn, American Society for Microbiology, Washington DC, 42–3.

Gibbs RS, Romero R et al., 1992, A review of premature birth and subclininical infection, *Am J Obstet Gynecol*, **166**: 1515–28.

Gillin FD, Sher A, 1981, Activation of the alternative complement pathway by *Trichomonas vaginalis*, *Infect Immun*, **34**: 268–73.

Hammill HA, 1989, *Trichomonas vaginalis*, *Obstet Gynecol Clin North Am*, **16**: 531–40.

Hansen BE, Sleeman HK, Pappas PW, 1980, Purine base and nucleoside uptake in *Plasmodium berghei* and host erythrocytes, *J Parasitol*, **66**: 205–12.

Harris DI, Beechey RB et al., 1988, Nucleoside uptake by *Trichomonas vaginalis*, *Mol Biochem Parasitol*, **29**: 105–16.

Heine P, McGregor JA, 1993, *Trichomonas vaginalis*: A reemerging pathogen, *Clin Obstet Gynecol*, **36**: 137–44.

Heyworth PG, Gutteridge WE, Ginger CD, 1982, Purine metabolism in *Trichomonas vaginalis*, *FEBS Lett*, **141**: 106–10.

Hogue MJ, 1943, The effect of *Trichomonas vaginalis* on tissue-culture cells, *Am J Hyg*, **37**: 142–52.

Höhne O, 1916, *Trichomonas vaginalis* als häufiger Erreger einer typischen colpitis purulenta, *Centralbaltt Gynaekol*, **40**: 4–15.

Honigberg BM, 1970, Trichomonads, *Immunity to Parasitic Animals*, vol 2, eds Jackson GJ, Herman R, Singer L, Appleton, New York, 469–550.

Honigberg BM, 1974, Study of *Dientamoeba fragilis*: II Taxonomic position and revision of the genus, *J Protozool*, **21**: 79–82.

Honigberg BM, 1978, Trichomonads of importance in human medicine, *Parasitic Protozoa*, vol 2, ed Kreier JP, Academic Press, New York, 275–454.

Honigberg BM, ed, 1990, *Trichomonads Parasitic in Humans*, Springer-Verlag, New York.

Honigberg BM, Burgess DE, 1994, Trichomonads of importance in human medicine including *Dientamoeba fragilis*, *Parasitic Protozoa*, 2nd edn, vol 9, ed Kreier JP, Academic Press, New York, 1–109.

Honigberg BM, King VM, 1964, Structure of *Trichomonas vaginalis* Donné, *J Parasitol*, **50**: 345–364.

Jepps MW, Dobell C, 1918, *Dientamoeba fragilis*, n.g., n. sp. a new intestinal amoeba from man, *Parasitology*, **10**: 352–67.

Jírovec O, Petru M, 1968, *Trichomonas vaginalis* and Trichomoniasis, *Adv Parasitol*, **6**: 117–88.

Johnson PJ, d'Oliveira CE et al., 1990, Molecular analysis of the hydrogenosomal ferredoxin of the anaerobic protist *Trichomonas vaginalis*, *Proc Natl Acad Sci USA*, **87**: 6097–101.

Kelly DR, Schnitzer RJ, 1952, Experimental studies on trichomoniasis. II. Immunity to reinfection in *T. vaginalis* infections of mice, *J Immunol*, **69**: 337–42.

Kelly DR, Schumacher A, Schnitzer RJ, 1954, Experimental studies in trichomoniasis. III. Influence of the site of the immunizing infection with *Trichomonas vaginalis* on the immunity of mice to homologous reinfection by different routes, *J Immunol*, **73**: 40–3.

Kengne P, Veas F et al., 1994, *Trichomonas vaginalis*: repeated DNA target for highly sensitive and specific polymerase chain reaction diagnosis, *Cell Mol Biol*, **40**: 819–31.

Koss LG, Wolinska WH, 1959, *Trichomonas vaginalis* cervicitis and its relationship to cervical cancer, *Cancer*, **12**: 117–19.

Krieger JN, Ravdin JI, Rein MF, 1985, Contact-dependent cytopathogenic mechanisms of *Trichomonas vaginalis*, *Infect Immun*, **50**: 778–86.

Krieger JN, Holmes KK et al., 1985, Geographic variation among isolates of *Trichomonas vaginalis*: Demonstration of antigen heterogeneity by using monoclonal antibodies and the indirect immunofluorescence technique, *J Infect Dis*, **152**: 979–84.

Krieger JN, Tam MR et al., 1988, Diagnosis of trichomoniasis.

Comparison of conventional wet-mount examination with cytologic studies, cultures, and monoclonal antibody staining of direct specimens, *JAMA*, **259**: 1223–7.

Krieger JN, Jenny C et al., 1993a, Clinical manifestations of trichomoniasis in men, *Ann Intern Med*, **118**: 844–9.

Krieger JN, Verdon N et al., 1993b, Natural history of urogenital trichomoniasis in men, *J Urol*, **149**: 1455–8.

Lang WR, Ludmir A, 1961, A pathognomonic colposcopic sign of *Trichomonas vaginalis* vaginitis, *Acta Cytol*, **5**: 390–2.

Lahti CJ, d'Oliveira CE, Johnson PJ, 1992, Beta-succinyl-coenzyme A synthetase from *Trichomonas vaginalis* is a soluble hydrogenosomal protein with an amino-terminal sequence that resembles mitochondrial presequences, *J Bacteriol*, **174**: 6822–30.

Levine GI, 1991, Sexually transmitted parasitic diseases, *Prim Care*, **18**: 101–28.

Levine ND, Corliss JO et al., 1980, A newly revised classification of the Protozoa, *J Protozool*, **27**: 37–58.

Lindmark DG, Müller M, 1973, Hydrogenosome, a cytoplasmic organelle of the anaerobic flagellate *Tritrichomonas foetus*, and its role in pyruvate metabolism, *J Biol Chem*, **235**: 7724–8.

Lisi PJ, Dondero RS et al., 1988, Monoclonal-antibody-based enzyme-linked immunosorbent assay for *Trichomonas vaginalis*, *J Clin Microbiol*, **26**: 1684–6.

Lockwood BC, North MJ, Coombs GH, 1984, *Trichomonas vaginalis*, *Tritrichomonas foetus*, and *Trichomitus batrachorum*: Comparative proteolytic activity, *Exp Parasitol*, **58**: 245–53.

Lockwood BC, North MJ, Coombs GH, 1988, The release of hydrolases from *Trichomonas vaginalis* and *Tritrichomonas foetus*, *Mol Biochem Parasitol*, **30**: 135–42.

Lockwood BC, North MJ et al., 1987, The use of a highly sensitive electrophoretic method to compare the proteinases of trichomonads, *Mol Biochem Parasitol*, **24**: 89–95.

Lossick JG, 1982, Treatment of *Trichomonas vaginalis* infections, *Rev Infect Dis*, **4 (supp)**: S801–18.

Lossick JG, 1990, Treatment of sexually transmitted vaginosis/vaginitis, *Rev Infect Dis*, **12:(supp.)**: S665–89.

Lossick JG, Kent HL, 1991, Trichomoniasis: Trends in diagnosis and management, *Am J Obstet Gynecol*, **165**: 1217–22.

Lushbaugh WB, Turner AC et al., 1989, Characterization of a secreted cytoactive factor from *Trichomonas vaginalis*, *Am J Trop Med Hyg*, **41**: 18–28.

Mallinson DJ, Lockwood BC et al., 1994, Identification and molecular cloning of four cysteine proteinase genes from the pathogenic protozoan *Trichomonas vaginalis*, *Microbiology (reading)*, **140**: 2725–35.

Mason PR, Forman L, 1980, In vitro attraction of polymorphonuclear leukocytes by *Trichomonas vaginalis*, *J Parasitol*, **66**: 888–92.

Mason PR, Gwanzura L, 1988, Mouse spleen cell responses to trichomonal antigens in experimental *Trichomonas vaginalis* infection, *J Parasitol*, **74**: 93–7.

Mason PR, Patterson BA, 1985, Proliferative response of human lymphocytes to secretory and cellular antigens of *Trichomonas vaginalis*, *J Parasitol*, **71**: 265–8.

Michel R, 1971, Nachweis des allergischen Spätreaktionstyps bei Mäusen nach Sensibilisiergun mit *Trichomonas vaginalis* und ein weiterer Beitrag zur Spezifität der Peritonealzellreaktion, *Z Tropenmed Parasitol*, **22**: 91–7.

Michel R, Westphal A, 1969, Die Spezifität der Dermal- und Peritonealzellreaktion sowie der Eosinotaxes bei der durch *Trichomonas vaginalis* sensibilisier ten Maus, *Z Tropenmed Parasitol*, **20**: 151–61.

Michel R, Westphal A et al., 1968, Die pertionealzellreaktion mit *Trichomonas vaginalis* sensibilisierter mäuse, *Z Tropenmed Parasitol*, **19**: 355–70.

Müller M, 1992, Energy metabolism of ancestral eukaryotes: A hypothesis based on the biochemistry of amitochondrate parasitic protists, *Biosystems*, **28**: 33–40.

Nielsen MH, 1975, The ultrastructure of *Trichomonas vaginalis* Donné before and after transfer from vaginal secretion to Diamond's medium, *Acta Pathol Microbiol Scand Sect B*, **83**: 581–9.

Nielsen MH, 1976, In vitro effect of metronidazole on the ultrastructure of *Trichomonas vaginalis* Donné, *Acta Pathol Microbiol Scand Sect B*, **84**: 93–100.

Nielsen MH, Nielsen R, 1975, Electron microscopy of *Trichomonas vaginalis* Donné: interaction with vaginal epithelium in human trichomoniasis, *Acta Pathol Microbiol Scand Sect B*, **83**: 305–20.

Nigesen UK, 1964, Issledovaniia zashchitnogo deistviia syvorotki brovi bolynkh trichomonozom urogenitalnogo trakta (Investigations of protective activity of sera of patients suffering from urogenital trichomoniasis), *Materialy k tretiemu Nauchno-Koordiinatisionnomu Soveshchaniiu po Parasitalogicheskim Problemam Litovskoi SSR, Latviiskoi SSR i Estonskoi SSR*, Gazetno-Zhurnalnoe Izdatel'stvo, Vilnius, 99–101.

Nigesen UK, 1966, Reaktsia aggliutinatsii i test seroproteksii pri trichomonoze urogenitalnogo trakta (Agglutinationa reaction and seroprotection test in urogenital trichomoniasis), *Diss Cand Med Sci Acad Sci*, Estonian SSR, Tallinn.

North MJ, Robertson CD, Coombs GH, 1990, The specificity of trichomonad proteinases analysed using fluorogenic substrates and specific inhibitors, *Mol Biochem Parasitol*, **39**: 183–94.

Pindak FF, Gardiner WA, Pindak MM, 1986, Growth and cytopathogenicity of *Trichomonas vaginalis* in tissue cultures, *J Clin Microbiol*, **23**: 672–5.

Quinn TC, Holmes KK, 1984, Trichomoniasis, *Tropical and Geographical Medicine*, eds Warren KS, Mahmoud A, McGraw Hill, New York, 335–41.

Rein MF, 1990, *Manual of Clinical Problems in Obstetrics and Gynecology*, eds Rivlin ME, Morrison JC, Bates GW, Little, Brown and Co, Boston, 287–95.

Rein MF, Müller M, 1989, *Sexually Transmitted Diseases*, eds Holmes KK, Mardt DA, Starling AF et al, McGraw Hill, New York, 481–92.

Rein MF, Sullivan JA, Mandell GL, 1980, Trichomonacidal activity of human polymorphonuclear neutrophils: killing by disruption and fragmentation, *Infect Dis*, **142**: 575–85.

Reisenhofer U, 1963, Über die Beeinflussung von *Trichomonas vaginalis* durch verschiedene Sera, *Arch Hyg Bakteriol*, **146**: 628–35.

Rhyan JC, Wilson KL et al., 1995, Immunohistochemical detection of *Tritrichomonas foetus* in formalin-fixed, paraffin-embedded sections of bovine placenta and fetal lung, *J Vet Diagn Invest*, **7**: 98–101.

Riedmüller L, 1932, Zur Frage der ätiologischen Bedeutung der bei Pyometra und sporadischen Abortus des Rindes gefundenen Trichomonaden, *Schweiz Arch Tierheilkd*, **74**: 343–51.

Riley DE, Roberts MC et al., 1992, Development of a polymerase chain reaction-based diagnosis of *Trichomonas vaginalis*, *J Clin Microbiol*, **30**: 465–72.

Romia SA, Othman TA, 1991, Detection of antitrichomonal antibodies in sera and cervical secretions in trichomoniasis, *J Egypt Soc Parasitol*, **21**: 373–81.

Rubino S, Muresu R et al., 1991, Molecular probe for identification of *Trichomonas vaginalis* DNA, *J Clin Microbiol*, **29**: 702–6.

Schnitzer RJ, Kelly DR, 1953, Short persistence of *Trichomonas vaginalis* in reinfected immune mice, *Proc Soc Exp Biol Med*, **82**, 404–6.

Searle SM, Müller M, 1991, Inorganic pyrophosphatase of *Trichomonas vaginalis*, *Mol Biochem Parasitol*, **44**: 91–6.

Shorb MS, 1964, *Biochemistry and Physiology of Protozoa*, vol 3, eds Hutner SH, Lwoff A, Academic Press, New York, 383–457.

Sinelnikova NV, 1961, Kozhno-allergicheskaia veaktsiia pri urogenitaluon trichomoniaze cheloveka i eë diagnostitcheskoe znachenie, *Tr Odess Inst Epidemiol Mikrobiol Metchntidova*, **5**: 102–5.

Sobel JD, 1992, Vulvovaginitis, *Dermatol Clin*, **10**: 339–59.

Steinbuchel A, Müller M, 1986, Anaerobic pyruvate metabolism of *Tritrichomonas foetus* and *Trichomonas vaginalis* hydrogenosomes, *Mol Biochem Parasitol*, **20:** 57–65.

Street DA, Taylor-Robinson D et al., 1982, Evaluation of an enzyme-linked immunosorbent assay for the detection of antibody to *Trichomonas vaginalis* in sera and vaginal secretions, *Br J Vener Dis*, **58:** 330–3.

ter Kuile BH, Müller M, 1992, Interaction between facilitated diffusion of glucose across the plasma membrane and its metabolism in *Trichomonas vaginalis*, *FEMS Microbiol Lett*, **110:** 27–31.

Teras JK, 1963, Genito-Urinary Trichomoniasis (in Russian, English summary), *Collect Pap Acad Sci*, ed Klinskii KS, Estonian SSR, Tallinn, 33–42.

Teras JK, Nigesen U, 1969, On the protective effect of blood sera of persons infected with *Trichomonas vaginalis* Donné, *Wiad Parazytol*, **15:** 481–3.

Tokura N, 1935, Biologische und immunologische Untersuchungen über die memschenparasitären Trichomonaden, *Igaku Kenkyu*, **9:** 1–13.

Torian BE, Connelly RJ et al., 1984, Specific and common anti-

gens of *Trichomonas vaginalis* detected by monoclonal antibodies, *Infect Immun*, **43:** 270–5.

Torian BE, Connelly RJ et al., 1988, Antigenic heterogeneity in the 115,000 Mr major surface antigen of *Trichomonas vaginalis*, *J Protozool*, **35:** 273–80.

Walzer, PD, Rutherford I, East R, 1978, Empyema with *Trichomonas* species, *Am Rev Respir Dis*, **118:** 415–18.

Wang CC, Cheng H-W, 1984, Salvage of pyrimidine nucleosides by *Trichomonas vaginalis*, *Mol Biochem Parasitol*, **10:** 171–84.

Watt RM, Philip A et al., 1986, Rapid assay for immunological detection of *Trichomonas vaginalis*, *J Clin Microbiol*, **24:** 790–5.

Wolner-Hanssen P, Krieger JN et al., 1989, Clinical manifestations of vaginal trichomoniasis, *JAMA*, **264:** 571–6.

Yano A, Yui K et al., 1983, Immune response to *Trichomonas vaginalis* IV. Immunochemical and immunobiological analysis of *T. vaginalis* antigen, *Int Arch Allergy Appl Immunol*, **72:** 150–7.

Yule A, Gellan MC et al., 1987, Detection of *Trichomonas vaginalis* antigen in women by enzyme immunoassay, *J Clin Pathol*, **40:** 566–8.

Chapter 12

LEISHMANIASIS IN THE OLD WORLD

R W Ashford and P A Bates

1 Biology of the organisms	7 Pathology
2 Classification	8 Diagnosis
3 Structure and life-cycle	9 Epidemiology
4 Biochemistry, molecular biology and genetics	10 Chemotherapy and treatment
5 Clinical aspects	11 Vaccination
6 Immunology	12 Integrated control

1 BIOLOGY OF THE ORGANISMS

The leishmaniases are a group of human diseases that afflict people in many tropical and sub-tropical regions. They are caused by parasitic protozoa of the genus *Leishmania* and are transmitted to humans by the bite of female phlebotomine sandflies, small blood-feeding insects. Leishmaniasis is not a single entity but a collection of diseases, each with its own clinical manifestations and epidemiology. Fortunately for the microbiologist, the basic pattern of the life-cycle is well conserved among members of the genus, and each species of *Leishmania* tends to cause a certain type of disease within a specific epidemiological context. Therefore, *Leishmania spp.* are most conveniently studied by first considering their general properties before dealing with those specific to individual species; this is the approach adopted here. Five species of *Leishmania* are agents of Old World leishmaniasis: *L. major, L. tropica, L. aethiopica, L. donovani,* and *L. infantum* (Figs 12.1, 12.2). The first 3 of these are predominantly agents of cutaneous leishmaniasis, an infection which is limited to the skin. The last 2 are predominantly agents of visceral leishmaniasis, an infection of the liver and spleen that can be fatal. In addition to these 5 well established species a number of other named species can be found in the literature on Old World leishmaniasis. Some have subsequently turned out to be very close, if not identical, to known species; others have not been examined in sufficient detail to reach a firm conclusion with regard to their identity.

2 CLASSIFICATION

2.1 The genus *Leishmania*

Leishmania is one of several genera within the family Trypanosomatidae (class Kinetoplastidea, order Trypanosomatida) and, therefore, shares certain properties with other members of this family described elsewhere in this volume (see Chapter 14, African trypanosomiasis; Chapter 15, New World trypanosomiasis). These common properties include: the possession of a kinetoplast (a unique form of mitochondrial DNA, see p. 220); a single flagellum arising from a flagellar pocket; and an alternation between arthropod and mammalian hosts during the life-cycle.

The features that uniquely identify the genus *Leishmania* are the nature of its vertebrate and invertebrate hosts and the developmental cycles and morphological stages found within each. The vertebrate hosts are all mammals in which the parasites reside within the phagolysosomal system of mononuclear phagocytic cells, typically macrophages (reviewed by Alexander and Russell 1992). This is an unusual location for a eukaryotic parasite and is also used by a handful of prokaryotic parasites (Garcia-del Portillo and Finlay 1995). The parasite gains entry to this intracellular residence via host cell phagocytosis. The invertebrate hosts are all phlebotomine sandflies of 2 genera; *Phlebotomus* in the Old World and *Lutzomyia* in the New World (see Chapter 13). These are small, hairy, dipteran flies of the family Psychodidae, in which only the females bloodfeed and transmit disease. The parasites are extracellular, development occurs exclusively in the gut of the sandfly and transmission is via the mouthparts during bloodfeeding (reviewed by Schlein 1993, Walters 1993, Bates 1994a).

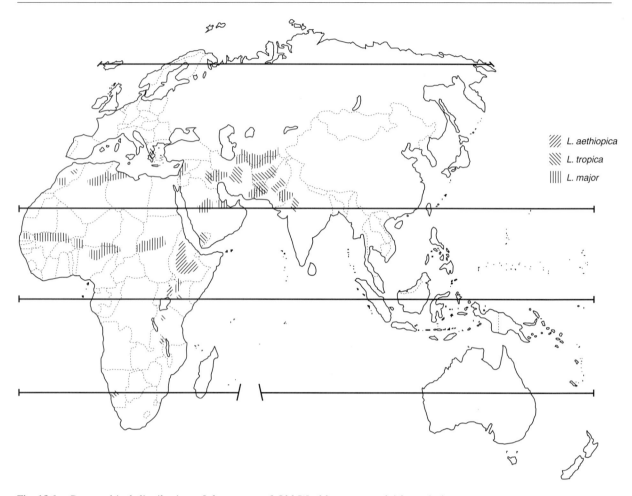

Fig. 12.1 Geographical distribution of the agents of Old World cutaneous leishmaniasis.

Various taxonomic distinctions have been proposed at the subgeneric, species and subspecies levels, but at present there is no generally accepted classification that incorporates all of these elements. Here we adopt a conservative pragmatic approach, essentially following Lainson and Shaw (1987), but without any subgeneric or subspecific qualifiers. In *Leishmania* the biological species concept of a population of potentially interbreeding individuals cannot be applied, as the genus seems to be largely, if not exclusively, asexual in its mode of reproduction. The ideal classification for an asexual organism at the level of the 'species' combines the maximum biological homogeneity within each species, but separates biologically different organisms. Among the techniques available for the classification of *Leishmania*, isoenzyme analysis has been found to describe strains at a level that allows the construction of phenograms and cladograms at an ideal resolution (Rioux et al. 1990). Using a panel of c. 12 enzymes it is possible to reliably identify and distinguish all of the currently accepted species. The group of strains that share a given pattern of electrophoretic mobilities are known as a 'zymodeme'. A given species may contain a number of zymodemes indicating subpopulations or subspecies, but zymodeme profiles do not cross between species. There has been an enormous accumulation of data

using this method; it has largely confirmed what was known or expected biologically but has also provided valuable new insights, such as the fact that cutaneous leishmaniasis in Europe is caused by *L. infantum*. An example of a cladogram constructed using isoenzyme data is shown in Fig. 12.3. The main disadvantage of isoenzyme analysis is the lack of standardization between laboratories; the importance of the strictest laboratory protocols to prevent mixing of cultures cannot be overemphasized.

Of the other techniques that have been used, the resolution of restriction fragment length polymorphisms and karyotype analysis has been found to be too fine, except for studies at the population genetic level. DNA and ribosomal RNA sequence information hold much promise and have given valuable results at the generic level and above, but have not been sufficiently widely used to contribute to classification at the species level. Monoclonal antibody and DNA probes, with or without PCR amplification, are of value in identification of stocks that have been well classified, but provide insufficient information to be of value in constructing a classification. A disadvantage of most current methods is the requirement to culture the parasite in question before identification can be made.

Of the 5 species considered in this chapter all are

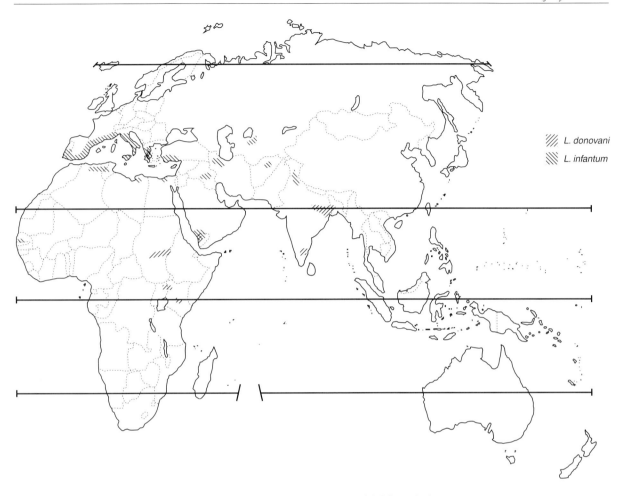

Fig. 12.2 Geographical distribution of the agents of Old World visceral leishmaniasis.

distinct from those found in the New World (see Chapter 13) with one important exception, *L. infantum*. Biochemically this is practically identical to *L. chagasi* found in the New World. We favour the explanation that '*L. chagasi*' is in fact *L. infantum* that was introduced into the New World in post-Columbian times via the domestic dog; both parasites should be referred to as *L. infantum* (Momen et al. 1993). Although others may disagree with this interpretation it is certain that these 2 parasites are very closely related. The remaining New World parasites have rather different biology, clinical manifestations and epidemiology to those of the Old World and are dealt with separately in Chapter 13. The main features of the Old World species are summarized in Table 12.1.

3 STRUCTURE AND LIFE-CYCLE

3.1 Life-cycle

The basic life-cycle of *Leishmania* is illustrated in Fig. 12.4 (reviewed by Molyneux and Killick-Kendrick 1987). The parasite exists in 2 main morphological forms, termed 'amastigotes' and 'promastigotes'. Amastigotes are ovoid, non-motile, largely intracellular stages; promastigotes are elongated, motile, largely

extracellular stages. The form introduced into the skin of the mammalian host is a promastigote, but this soon transforms into an amastigote. The precise kinetics of parasite transformation and uptake by skin macrophages is uncertain, but it is generally assumed that uptake occurs soon after inoculation and that the promastigote to amastigote transformation occurs mainly inside the host cell. In vitro studies indicate that this process can be completed in 12–24 hs. Thereafter the parasite remains in the amastigote form for the duration of the mammalian phase of the life-cycle. The amastigotes grow and divide within their host cells, intermittently bursting out and infecting new macrophages. This phase is chronic and can last from months to years, even a lifetime, depending on the host species involved. Furthermore, the duration and course of infection can vary widely between individuals, as there is a strong influence of host genetics on susceptibility to infection. The location of infected host cells varies with the type of disease. In cutaneous leishmaniasis the amastigotes remain confined to the skin. They are not generally distributed through the skin, but are present in skin lesions, commonly as raised papules or ulcers. In visceral leishmaniasis there may be an initial skin lesion, but usually the first symptoms of overt disease occur later with the onset

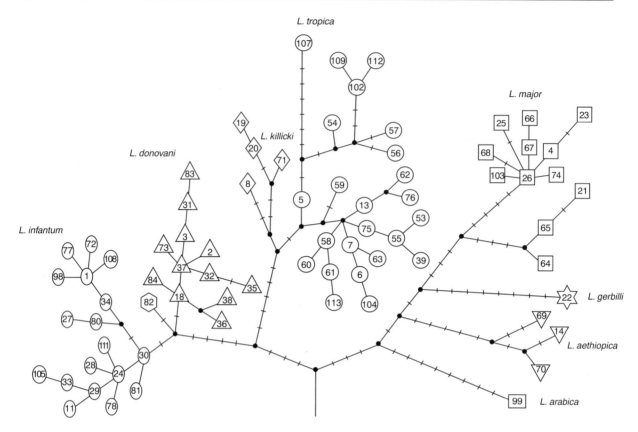

Fig. 12.3 Cladogram of Old World *Leishmania* zymodemes showing grouping into 'species'. *L. gerbilli* and *L. arabica* are not known from humans. Modified from Rioux et al. 1990.

Table 12.1

Species	Disease in humans	Geographical distribution	Important mammalian hosts	Important sandfly hosts
L. major	rural, zoonotic, cutaneous leishmaniasis, oriental sore	North Africa, Sahel of Africa, Central and West Asia	great gerbil *Rhombomys opimus,* fat sand rat *Psammomys obesus*	*Phlebotomus papatasi P. dubosqi, P. salehi*
L. tropica	urban, anthroponotic cutaneous leishmaniasis, oriental sore	Central and West Asia	humans	*Phlebotomus sergenti*
L. aethiopica	cutaneous leishmaniasis, diffuse cutaneous leishmaniasis	Ethiopia, Kenya	rock hyraxes *Heterohyrax brucei* and *Procavia* spp.	*Phlebotomus longipes, P. pedifer.*
L. donovani	visceral leishmaniasis, kala-azar, post kala-azar dermal leishmaniasis.	Indian subcontinent, East Africa	humans	*Phlebotomus argentipes P. orientalis, P. martini.*
L. infantum	infantile visceral leishmaniasis	Mediterranean basin, Central and West Asia	domestic dog	*Phlebotomus ariasi, P. perniciosus*

of fever and other clinical symptoms associated with visceral infection.

The opportunity for transmission from an infected mammalian host to a female sandfly occurs when the sandfly feeds. Sandflies are pool feeders, i.e. they possess cutting mouthparts that slice into the skin and they feed from the small pool of blood that seeps into the wound. Thus despite their small size, 2–3 mm, sandflies give a noticeable and sometimes painful bite. Parasites causing cutaneous disease are acquired by a sandfly along with the bloodmeal, if the fly happens to feed on a cutaneous lesion. Tissue damage from the bite releases infected macrophages or free amastigotes into the wound. Visceral parasites are probably acquired with the blood itself. Although the principal pathological events of visceral leishmaniasis occur in the spleen and liver where the host cells probably remain resident, another site of infection is the bone marrow. This is a major site of haemopoiesis and

blood monocytes infected with *Leishmania* amastigotes are released into the peripheral circulation and thus made available to feeding sandflies. It is also possible that infected monocytes leave the circulation and become resident in the skin to act as a source of parasites, especially in the case of post kala-azar dermal leishmaniasis. Nevertheless, in most endemic foci the acquisition of *Leishmania* parasites by individual flies is a rare event and the vast majority of flies are uninfected. The few infected flies are, however, efficient vectors.

The phase of the life-cycle in sandflies is relatively acute. Flies that acquire a *Leishmania* infection probably remain infected for life, but this is usually only a matter of weeks. In most parasite–vector combinations that have been studied experimentally, development of the parasite is sufficiently rapid that mammal-infective promastigotes are produced by the time the female is ready to take her next bloodmeal. This may be as short as 5–7 days under optimal conditions.

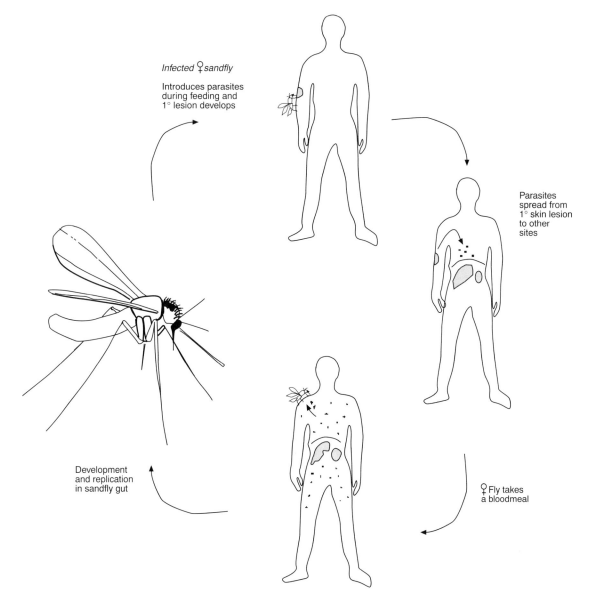

Fig. 12.4 General life-cycle of *Leishmania*.

Development occurs exclusively in the gut and begins with infected macrophages or free amastigotes in the bloodmeal. The macrophages disintegrate over a matter of hours and, as with the mammalian phase, the first event is transformation, in this case to the promastigote form, which takes 24–48 h. The promastigotes grow and divide in the sandfly gut. The ultimate products of the developmental cycle are the mammal-infective forms, termed 'metacyclic promastigotes', which accumulate in the anterior midgut and foregut of the sandfly.

The opportunity for transmission from an infected sandfly to a mammalian host occurs when the fly is ready to take another bloodmeal. There is debate concerning the precise mechanisms that aid transmission and the extent to which the parasites themselves contribute to this process; these may vary with the specific vector–parasite combination. For the parasites to become lodged in the skin of a mammal they must travel against the predominant flow of blood, which is into the gut of the fly.

In a sandfly containing a mature infection the majority of promastigotes are found in the anterior midgut, which is separated from a smaller population in the foregut by the stomodeal valve (Fig. 12.5). The number of promastigotes required to initiate a mammalian infection is unknown and likely to vary between hosts, but is generally believed to be in the range of 10–100, although theoretically a single infective promastigote could suffice.

Under experimental conditions, infected flies show differences in feeding behaviour in comparison with uninfected flies. Frequently they are seen to probe the skin an increased number of times and appear to find difficulty in taking a bloodmeal; this behaviour may enhance transmission (reviewed by Molyneux and Jeffries 1986, Molyneux and Killick-Kendrick 1987). Massive infections develop in the anterior midgut of both experimentally infected and wild-caught flies, with the promastigotes appearing to be embedded in a gel-like substance. It has been proposed that together these form a physical obstruction to feeding, resulting in multiple probing and failed attempts to engorge. Alternatively, infection in the foregut may interfere with mechanoreceptors that detect a bloodmeal, again producing multiple probing behaviour. Whether infected sandflies indulge in multiple probing or not, infective promastigotes may be carried out along with saliva during probing. It is known that sandfly saliva is introduced into the mammalian host during bloodfeeding and there is also evidence that sandfly saliva can enhance the subsequent infectivity of the promastigotes in the mammalian host (Titus and Ribeiro 1990). Nevertheless, for multiple or single probing to be useful in transmission there need to be infective forms present in the foregut. Much debate has centred on the position and the types of promastigote found in the foregut; it has not been fully resolved whether they are mammal-infective forms (Killick-Kendrick 1990a). A different idea comes from experimental observations that the stomodeal valve can be damaged and remain permanently open as a result of the parasite infection. This has been described with infections of *L. major* in *Phlebotomus papatasi* (Schlein, Jacobson and Messer 1992) but has not been reported in other parasite–vector combinations. In cases where such damage does occur, it may permit mixing of the contents of the anterior midgut with an incoming bloodmeal and therefore when the pharynx contracts to deposit blood in the midgut, there is also a forward surge of promastigote-contaminated blood into the wound.

3.2 Amastigote structure

Amastigotes are ovoid cells of 5–3 μm length on the main axis and, therefore, lie at the lower limit of size described for eukaryotic cells. Due to their small size, little internal structure can be discerned in stained preparations at the light microscope level beyond the central round or oval nucleus and adjacent but smaller round or rod-shaped kinetoplast. At the ultrastructural level more detail is revealed (Fig. 12.6). The surface membrane is a conventional unit membrane under which lies a corset of microtubules, serving as a form of cytoskeleton. These are closely spaced in parallel rows which, together with the small size, make the amastigote a very robust eukaryotic cell. One unfortunate consequence of this feature is that it has not proved possible to develop subcellular fractionation techniques for amastigotes that will disrupt the surface membrane without destroying the organelles contained within. On the positive side, fairly vigorous homogenization techniques can be employed for the isolation of amastigotes from infected tissue without destroying their viability or structural integrity.

An infolding of the surface membrane creates an internal space, termed the 'flagellar pocket'. This is so named because a flagellum emerges from the surface membrane and projects into the pocket. This flagellum is not functional in amastigotes and does not extend beyond the cell body. The flagellar pocket is thus topologically external to the cell although contained within it. In addition to anchoring the flagellum the main function of the pocket is as a site of endocytosis and exocytosis (Webster and Russell 1993). Microtubules do not underlie the surface of the flagellar pocket membrane thus allowing access of vesicular traffic. Immediately below the origin of the flagellum lies the kinetoplast, a dense mass of mitochondrial DNA. The kinetoplast DNA is composed of several thousand circular DNA molecules linked together in a catenated network (Shlomai 1994). The DNA circles are of 2 size classes: each kinetoplast contains 25–50 maxicircles of c. 30 kb, and 5 000–10 000 minicircles of c. 2 kb. Together these constitute the mitochondrial genome. Branches of the surrounding mitochondrion extend throughout the cell body and contain plate-like cristae.

The cytoplasm contains both rough and smooth endoplasmic reticulum. The Golgi complex is typically found in the vicinity of the flagellar pocket, which probably reflects the role of this organelle in the endocytic and exocytic pathways. Lysosomes are also found in the cytoplasm together with an organelle unique to kinetoplastids, the glycosome. This is so named because a number of glycolytic enzymes are specifically located in this organelle, together with some others (Opperdoes 1991).

Cell biology of amastigote development

The developmental cycle of *Leishmania* in the mammalian host is illustrated in Fig. 12.7. This is initiated by the interaction of metacyclic promastigotes with

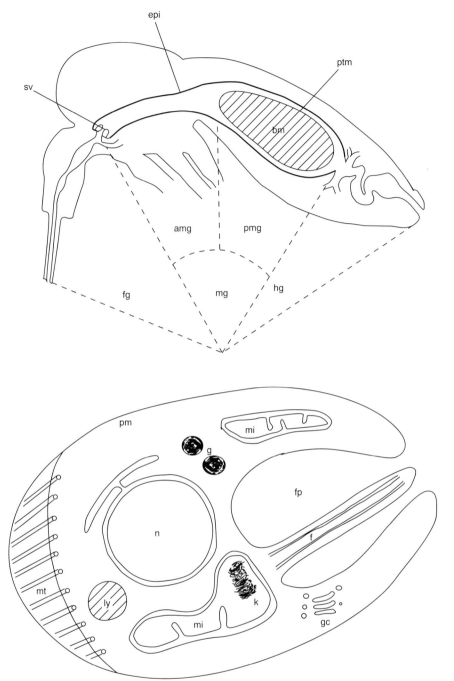

Fig. 12.5 Structure of the female sandfly gut. The gut can be subdivided into 3 sections: the foregut (fg), midgut (mg) and hindgut (hg). The midgut is lined by epithelial cells (epi) with microvilli that project into the lumen of the gut and is subdivided itself into the anterior or thoracic midgut (amg) and the posterior or abdominal midgut (pmg). The junction between the anterior midgut and the foregut is formed by the stomodeal valve (sv). The foregut, stomodeal valve and hindgut are lined by a chitinous cuticular layer. Initial development of the parasite occurs within the bloodmeal (bm) encased in a peritrophic membrane (ptm) in the posterior midgut.

Fig. 12.6 Ultrastructure of a *Leishmania* amastigote. Amastigotes possess a central nucleus (n) and adjacent kinetoplast (k) within a single branching mitochondrion (mi). The flagellum (f) arises from a flagellar pocket (fp) but does not extend beyond the cell body. Lysosomes (ly), glycosomes (gl) and Golgi complex (gc) are found in the cytoplasm. Rows of microtubules (mt) run just below the plasma membrane (pm).

skin macrophages. Direct studies on the binding and uptake of metacyclics by skin macrophages are not possible but this process has been modelled in vitro (Alexander and Russell 1992). Two important caveats must be attached to the published reports: the type of macrophage used is either a peritoneal exudate cell or a macrophage-like cell line (inappropriate host cells) and the parasites used are never sandfly-derived metacyclic promastigotes but cultured forms that are sometimes not properly characterized. Nevertheless, these studies have shown that complement fixation by metacyclic promastigotes is not only an inevitable consequence of exposure to mammalian blood and tissue fluids, but is an important adaptation for gain-

ing entry to the host cell. Metacyclic promastigotes are relatively resistant to complement-mediated lysis and use the surface-bound complement components as ligands for binding to macrophage complement receptors. This promotes phagocytosis by the macrophage. After uptake and internalization in a phagosome, fusion with lysosomes proceeds as normal and the parasite inhabits a secondary lysosome or phagolysosome. During this process the metacyclic promastigote transforms into an amastigote, a process that takes 12–24 h to complete. The amastigotes then continue to grow and divide within the phagolysosomal compartment of the host cell in a parasitophorous vacuole. Different species of parasite inhabit different sized vacuoles. The species causing Old World leishmaniasis all inhabit small vacuoles, in which the vacuole membrane is closely opposed to the surface of the parasite itself. As the parasite divides, so does the surrounding vacuole and, consequently, the host cell becomes occupied by multiple parasites and vacuoles. Division of the amastigote is by simple binary fission. Some of the New World parasites for example, *L. mexicana* (see Chapter 13) occupy larger vacuoles, and these presumably have a different effect on host cell endocytic traffic through their vacuoles. After division the parasites remain together in clusters within large vacuoles.

The phagolysosomal compartment presents 2 threats to amastigotes: the battery of lysosomal enzymes and low pH (4.5–5.5). Defence against the enzymes seems to be mainly passive and relies on the unusual structures of the surface glycolipids and lipophosphoglycans (see p. 226) rendering the amastigotes indigestible. Low pH is not a problem as amastigotes seem to be acidophiles: they have effective means of regulating their internal pH in an acidic environment; they are metabolically more active at low pH; and some species can only be cultured axenically in vitro as amastigotes at low pH (Bates 1993, Zilberstein and Shapira 1994). There does not seem to be a specific mechanism for escape from the host cell. The parasites simply multiply until the host cell bursts open making them available for uptake by other macrophages. Amastigotes are usually regarded as

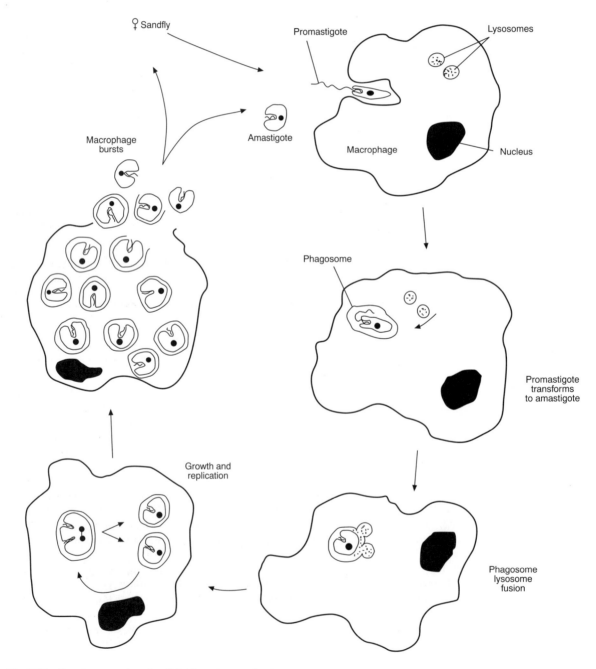

Fig. 12.7 Developmental cycle of *Leishmania* amastigotes.

obligate intracellular parasites but this may not be strictly true: it is now possible to culture certain species axenically and at least in experimental infections it is possible to find extracellular amastigotes in heavily parasitized tissues. Despite this, the vast majority have an intracellular existence. Different species infect macrophages at different sites in the body but it is not known whether amastigotes are able to specifically target subpopulations of mononuclear phagocytic cells or whether they simply do not have access to or do not survive in macrophages in the wrong site. All amastigotes appear to be equivalent and there is no evidence for functionally distinct subpopulations.

3.3 Promastigote structure

In the sandfly host the parasite is found mainly as a promastigote form (Fig. 12.8). The structural elements of promastigotes are the same as those described for amastigotes, although there may be variations in organelle numbers. The main difference with amastigotes is that the cell body is elongated, in the range of 8–15 μm, the flagellum emerges from the cell body, and is functional, making these motile cells. The flagellum is found at the anterior end of the cell, i.e. as they move the cell body is trailed behind the flagellum. Desmosomal plaques anchor the flagellum to the cell body as it emerges from the flagellar pocket. A further difference is that the promastigote flagellum has a paraxial rod, a paracrystalline structure running parallel to the microtubules of the axoneme. It is assumed that this structure plays some role in flagellar motility.

CELL BIOLOGY OF PROMASTIGOTE DEVELOPMENT

The developmental cycle of *Leishmania* in the sandfly host is illustrated in Fig. 12.9. Promastigote development has been studied using a variety of combinations of parasite and vector (Killick-Kendrick 1990a, Walters 1993, Bates 1994a) and 2 patterns have emerged for those species infective to mammals. Certain species normally include a phase of development in the hindgut of the sandfly, for example, *L. braziliensis*. They share certain other features and form a distinct cluster of species according to isoenzyme analysis. Consequently, it has been proposed that these be placed in a separate subgenus, *L. (Viannia)*. These are exclusively New World species and are described in detail in Chapter 13. The majority of *Leishmania* species, in which there is no hindgut development, are placed in the subgenus *L. (Leishmania)*, including all the Old World parasites.

There are a variety of different promastigote forms that can be separated on morphological grounds and various authors refer to these by different names, often interchanging cultured and sandfly-derived promastigotes. The evidence for functional distinction is less complete. Here, 5 developmental forms are recognized during development in the subgenus *L. (Leishmania)*, namely: procyclic promastigotes, nectomonad promastigotes, haptomonad promastigotes, paramastigotes and metacyclic promastigotes (Fig. 12.10). Other categories and subdivisions can be found in the literature, but at present there is little evidence for functional distinction between these.

The first developmental event in the sandfly is probably the transformation of amastigotes to procyclic promastigotes. Doubt exists because very few observations of the early events have been made. It is also possible that amastigotes may divide before transforming to promastigotes. Amastigote to promastigote transformation occurs readily in vitro and is completed in 24–48 h when a suitable culture medium and an appropriate temperature (usually c. 26°C) are used. The media used vary widely, but the optimal pH for promastigote growth (i.e. that used in culture media) is generally neutral to slightly alkaline (pH 7.0–7.5). In vitro transformation to promastigotes and cell division occur coincidentally, so that the majority of the first forms observed in division are partially transformed intermediates (Bates 1994b). The signals initiating both processes may be the same and they may be mechanistically linked.

These events occur in the posterior midgut in the bloodmeal that is itself encased in a peritrophic membrane (PM) secreted by the midgut epithelium. The PM is not a true membrane but a lattice of chitin fibrils, proteins and glycoproteins secreted by the midgut epithelium in response to a bloodmeal. In phlebotomine sandflies the PM is of the type that is produced at one time and encapsulates the whole bloodmeal. The procyclics are short ellipsoid promastigotes, generally c. 6–8 μm in body length. Multiplication of procyclic promastigotes occurs within the PM but gradually the promastigotes elongate and transform to nectomonad forms of 15–20 μm body length.

Approximately 3 days after bloodfeeding the PM usually begins to break down and promastigotes begin to make their escape, the infection spreading forward to the anterior midgut. There is an accelerated breakdown of the PM in

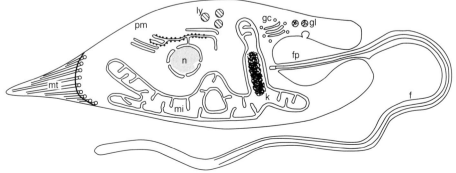

Fig. 12.8 Ultrastructure of a *Leishmania* promastigote. Many of the features found in the amastigote stage are also found in the promastigotes (see Fig. 12.6 for abbreviations). Some differences are that the cell body is elongated, the flagellum extends beyond the cell body and the kinetoplast has a more anterior location relative to the nucleus.

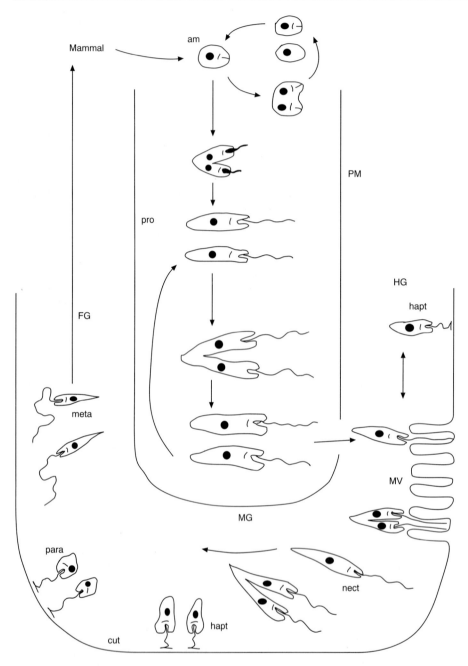

Fig. 12.9 Developmental cycle of *Leishmania* promastigotes. Amastigotes (am) are ingested by a female sandfly and transform to procyclic promastigotes (pro) in the bloodmeal, itself encased in a peritrophic membrane (PM) in the midgut (MG). Procyclic promastigotes are gradually replaced by nectomonad promastigotes (nect) that escape from the PM; some attach to the microvilli (MV) via their flagella. In some species haptomonad forms (hapt) attach to the cuticular lining (CUT) in the hindgut (HG), in others they attach in only the foregut (FG) and stomodeal valve. Paramastigotes (para) may also be found in the foregut. Metacyclic promastigotes (meta) complete the developmental cycle.

infections of *L. infantum* in *Lu. longipalpis* (Walters 1993) and *L. major* in *Phlebotomus papatasi* (Schlein, Jacobson and Shlomai 1991). One explanation for this phenomenon is the discovery of a chitinase secreted by promastigotes (Schlein, Jacobson and Shlomai 1991). This is of presumed survival value to the parasite as it would permit establishment of a midgut infection outside the PM earlier than otherwise. In some vectors it could be essential for escape from the PM before defaecation of the bloodmeal remnants by the sandfly.

The transformation from procyclics to nectomonads can be mimicked in vitro (Bates 1994b). In this study, lesion amastigotes were allowed to transform, procyclics appeared on day 2, and after 3 days of growth a population consisting predominantly of nectomonad forms was obtained. The timing of these events is strongly reminiscent of the situation in sandfly infections. This seems to be a function of the cell density rather than being due to a developmental clock within the organism. If promastigotes are kept in the log phase of growth by repeated subpassage then the appearance of nectomonads can be delayed until the density is permitted to increase. Thus it seems that the transformation to nectomonads is a density-dependent phenomenon and could be triggered, for example, by a factor such as nutrient depletion. This could be a useful adaptation in vivo as the initial source of nutrition, the bloodmeal, becomes exhausted. Charlab and Ribeiro (1993) found that inhibition of growth by exposure of promastigotes to salivary gland homogenate from *Lu. longipalpis* caused transformation to nectomonads in vitro. It is uncertain whether parasites are exposed to sandfly saliva during their development in the midgut, but is a possibility after escape from the PM. Flies continue to take sugar meals over the several days that the bloodmeal is being digested and as promastigote development occurs.

Some of the nectomonads attach to the midgut epi-

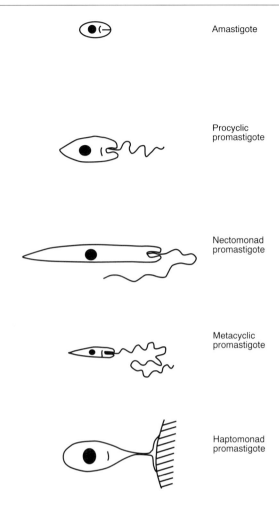

Fig. 12.10 Promastigote developmental forms. The 5 main morphological stages found in the life-cycle of *Leishmania* drawn to show their relative sizes and shapes.

thelium, inserting their flagella between the microvilli (Killick-Kendrick 1990a, Lang et al. 1991). The major surface glycolipid of promastigotes, termed 'lipophosphoglycan' (LPG), seems to mediate this attachment and this process is important for establishment of a mature infection, i.e. one that persists beyond the initial multiplicative phase in the bloodmeal (Lang et al. 1991, Pimenta et al. 1992, 1994). These authors showed that binding of promastigotes to dissected midguts in vitro can be inhibited by free LPG or its constituents. Most convincingly, there is a positive correlation between the binding of LPG isolated from a particular parasite to dissected midguts of sandflies, and the ability of the given vector to transmit that parasite (Pimenta et al. 1994, Sacks et al. 1994).

LPG covers the entire surface, including the flagellar membrane where it could mediate binding (Lang et al. 1991). One unexplained feature of midgut attachment is the striking feature of flagellar insertion. The reason may be that the juxtaposition of elongated flagella and microvilli provides a good fit that maximizes the number of binding sites and, hence, with time the promastigotes will adopt this orientation. It is premature to discount the possibility that other flagellar-specific molecules could be involved and provide additional specificity.

Usually by 5 days the infection has spread to the anterior midgut and the cuticular surface of the stomodeal valve (SV), at the junction with the foregut. Haptomonad promastigotes,

broad cells of 5–8 μm, are found attached to the SV via hemidesmosomes in expansions of their flagellar membranes (reviewed by Vickerman and Tetley 1990). Similarly attached paramastigotes (nucleus adjacent to kinetoplast) and haptomonads may be found in the foregut. At the ultrastructural level the flagellar membrane can be seen closely opposed to the surface, forming a junctional complex. An electron-dense plaque and associated filaments are located below the flagellar membrane; thus these attachment organelles bear a superficial resemblance to the hemidesmosomes found at the basal surfaces of vertebrate epithelial cells. The biochemical composition of these hemidesmosomes is unknown, as is the function of the haptomonads and paramastigotes. As the haptomonads form part of the blockage that possibly interferes with bloodfeeding (see p. 220) it has been suggested that these are 'altruistic' forms, whose function is to promote transmission of the metacyclic promastigotes.

From day 5 onwards, increasing numbers of small (5–8 μm), narrow, highly motile, metacyclic promastigotes, the mammal-infective forms, can be observed in the lumen of the anterior midgut or foregut, or both, in a position that facilitates their transmission upon subsequent bloodfeeding by the female sandfly. The progenitors of metacyclics in vivo still remain uncertain, but the metacyclics of *L. mexicana* can be induced in vitro by culture at low pH (Bates and Tetley 1993) and both metacyclogenesis and chitinase secretion by *L. major* can be inhibited by the inclusion of haemoglobin in the culture medium (Schlein and Jacobson 1994a). These reports give the first clues to the regulation of metacyclogenesis. Unlike the other transformations described so far, this is more properly described as a differentiation process, as the end product is in a non-dividing state. The results described by Schlein and Jacobson (1994a) are clearly of potential relevance in vivo, for despite our general ignorance of sandfly gut conditions, it is certain that promastigotes are exposed to haemoglobin. The role of a fall in gut pH in inducing metacyclogenesis is more speculative, but promastigotes are known to acidify their culture media during growth in vitro (Bates and Tetley 1993). Interestingly, both effects are again density-dependent: the inhibitory effect of haemoglobin will decrease with time as bloodmeal digestion proceeds and the inductive effect of a fall in pH, if it occurs, will simultaneously increase with promastigote numbers and their metabolic products.

4 BIOCHEMISTRY, MOLECULAR BIOLOGY AND GENETICS

4.1 Surface membrane structure

The surface membrane proteins of *Leishmania* can be subdivided into 2 groups. Those in the first group are present at high copy numbers per cell and are major structural components of the surface membrane. Members of the second group are present at low copy numbers per cell and have been identified using functional assays, for example, enzymes, transporters and ion pumps.

Three major surface components have been described: gp63 (or promastigote surface protease, PSP), lipophosphoglycan and glycosylphosphatidylinositols. gp63 is a major surface protein of c. 63 000 kDa that has been found on the surface of cultured promastigotes in all species of *Leishmania* that have been examined (reviewed by Chang, Chauduri and Fong 1990, Etges and Bouvier 1991). It has also been demonstrated on the surface of sandfly-derived promastigotes. gp63 is a zinc metalloprotease, the active site of which is exposed on the external face of the surface membrane (an ectoenzyme). There is some evidence for low level expression of gp63 by amastigotes in some species, but efforts to demonstrate active protease on the amastigote surface have revealed very low or no activity. Potential functions of gp63 in the life-cycle of *Leishmania* are not certain, but are likely to be most important in the sandfly or during the brief existence of metacyclic promastigotes in the mammalian host. In the sandfly, gp63 may fulfil a digestive function, helping to provide a supply of amino acids for the parasite. The most abundant substrate would be haemoglobin and by digesting this molecule gp63 could also help to provide pre-formed haem, an essential nutrient for *Leishmania*. It might also help the parasite to penetrate the peritrophic membrane, which is partially proteinaceous in nature.

After transmission to a mammalian host the proteolytic activity of gp63 may help metacyclic promastigotes to defend themselves against lysosomal enzymes whilst they are transforming to amastigotes in the macrophage. gp63 has also been identified as a significant site of complement fixation on the promastigote surface and, therefore, has been proposed to be involved in the binding of promastigotes to macrophages via complement receptors on the latter.

Lipophosphoglycan (LPG) is the major surface molecule found on the promastigotes of *Leishmania* species (Turco and Descoteaux 1992). LPG contains 4 covalently linked structural components: a phospholipid tail that anchors the molecule in the surface membrane; a glycan core of several saccharide residues that lies immediately above the surface membrane; a repeating phosphodisaccharide backbone comprising 15–30 phosphate-galactose-mannose units; and a cap of 2–3 saccharide residues. LPG has been most extensively studied in *L. major* but is assumed to fulfil similar functions in other species. The number of repeated phosphodisaccharide units varies between life-cycle stages, approximately doubling in number between *L. major* multiplicative and metacyclic promastigotes. Modelling suggests that the backbone projects away from the surface; it also carries a number of short saccharide side chains which, in *L. major*, terminate mainly in galactose or arabinose residues. LPG is either absent or expressed at low levels on the surface of amastigotes.

LPG has been proposed to fulfil a variety of functions in both the sandfly and mammalian hosts. The unusual structure of LPG may give the parasites general protection against hydrolytic enzymes in both the sandfly midgut and macrophage phagolysosome. One specific function has been described on p. 225, that of mediating attachment of promastigotes to microvilli on the sandfly midgut epithelium. Detachment from the midgut is correlated with developmental modification of the side chains of LPG in *L. major*. In procyclic promastigotes the side chains terminate in galactose residues which can bind to the midgut epithelium. Sub-

sequently these are replaced with LPG-carrying side chains that terminate with arabinose residues. These do not bind to the microvilli, allowing the promastigotes to detach, migrate forward to the anterior midgut and differentiate into metacyclic promastigotes (Pimenta et al. 1992). At the same time the number of repeat units increases. This latter change is believed to be responsible for the observed resistance to complement-mediated lysis shown by metacyclic promastigotes, a prerequisite for survival in the mammalian host. LPG is the major site of complement fixation on the metacyclic promastigote. Mechanistically it is proposed that elongated LPG interferes with complement lysis by steric hindrance, the components of a potential membrane attack complex being too far from and lacking access to the plasma membrane to enable insertion. LPG with bound complement components can be released from the surface, which may represent an additional defence mechanism.

LPG is also proposed to have functions in the establishment of the parasite in the macrophage (Descoteaux and Turco 1993). As with gp63, fixation of complement by LPG provides ligands that can be bound by macrophage complement receptors, stimulating phagocytic uptake of the metacyclic promastigote. LPG has a strong inhibitory effect on macrophage protein kinase C and consequently may have the effect of inhibiting signal transduction pathways that trigger microbicidal responses. It is also an efficient scavenger of toxic oxygen radicals.

Glycosylphosphatidylinositols (GIPLs) have been found on the surface of both promastigote and amastigotes stages; in the latter they are a major surface component. These glycolipids resemble the lipid anchor-glycan core moiety of LPG. The glycocalyx formed by these abundant molecules is assumed to help protect amastigotes against the potentially hostile environment of the phagolysosme.

4.2 Surface membrane biochemistry

In addition to gp63 a number of other ectoenzymes have been described on the surface membrane of promastigotes: acid phosphatase, 3′ and 5′ nucleotidases (Bates 1991). Promastigotes, and probably amastigotes, possess a surface membrane proton ATPase (Zilberstein and Shapira 1994). This serves an important function in pH regulation, extruding protons and preventing acidification, particularly in the phagolysosmal environment. Transporters for glucose, amino acids, ribose, nucleosides and folate have been described (Beck and Ullman 1991, Marr 1991, ter Kuile 1993, Zilberstein and Shapira 1994). The surface membrane has an unusual sterol composition with ergosterol as the major membrane sterol (Haughan and Goad 1991). Two enzymatically active secretory molecules have been described in promastigotes; acid phosphatase (Bates and Dwyer 1987) and chitinase (Schlein Jacobson and Shlomai 1991). In addition, promastigotes and amastigotes secrete various phosphoglycans whose functions are yet to be determined (Ilg et al. 1994).

4.3 Molecular biology

Leishmania spp., in common with other kinetoplastids, possesses several unusual features that differentiate them from other eukaryotes described to date, and thus merit brief mention here. The structure of kinetoplast DNA (kDNA) is unique for a mitochondrial genome (Shlomai 1994), but kDNA also exhibits a unique form of postranscriptional RNA processing termed 'RNA editing' (Seiwert 1995). The 25–50 identical maxicircle DNA molecules of each kinetoplast encode various mitochondrial proteins, but the primary RNA transcripts from these are not directly translatable. When compared to the final transcript the gene sequences are found to contain insertions and deletions of uridine residues. The maxicircle primary transcripts are corrected in an editing process using short sequences, called 'guide RNAs', that are themselves encoded by the other component of kDNA, the more numerous minicircles. This process is unique to kinetoplastids and is assumed to have been retained since the early divergence of the group from other eukaryotes.

Leishmania and kinetoplastids also exhibit several unusual features in the expression of their nuclear genes (Graham 1995). Such genes are usually grouped together in polycistronic transcription units, an arrangement more commonly found in prokaryotes. There is a single promoter for RNA polymerase which then proceeds to transcribe in turn the several individual genes of the array. Although transcription appears to be continuous, a giant transcript is not produced because as it is synthesized each gene is individually processed. A specific 39 nucleotide leader sequence is spliced in *trans* to the 5′ end and a poly(A) tail added to the 3′ end of each gene transcript. These 2 processes may be mechanistically linked. There are no intervening sequences in the coding regions of nuclear genes. Finally gene expression itself is rarely regulated at the transcriptional level (the general rule for eukaryotes), but additionally occurs at a number of post-transcriptional steps, depending on the specific gene concerned. These include mRNA stability, translational control and post-translational turnover of proteins.

4.4 Genetics

Leishmania appear to be diploid organisms (Bastien, Blaineau and Pagès 1992, Lighthall and Giannini 1992). This has been confirmed for a number of specific genes in which 2 rounds of gene disruption are required in order to generate null mutants. Chromosomes do not condense during mitosis but can be separated and enumerated by pulsed-field gel electrophoresis. Current estimates indicate 20–25 chromosomes in the genome, ranging in size from 200 to 4000 kb. There is circumstantial evidence for a sexual cycle in *Leishmania* (Bastien, Blaineau and Pagès 1992), but so far no-one has succeeding in performing a genetic cross (as in African trypanosomes, Chapter 14). Population genetic data indicate that *Leishmania*

has a predominantly clonal structure and reproduces asexually (Tibayrenc, Kjellberg and Ayala 1990). Therefore, sex, if present, may be more important on an evolutionary scale than in the routine life-cycle progression of the parasite.

5 CLINICAL ASPECTS

5.1 Clinical manifestations

One of the most remarkable features of the leishmaniases is the diversity of diseases caused by morphologically similar parasites living in a single series of cells (Fig. 12.11). This diversity is by no means fully explained by genetic diversity among the parasites. It is generated in part by the variety of host responses to the infection and in part by the (largely unexplained) restriction of the parasites to specific parts or organs of the body. One factor restricting parasites to the skin may simply be temperature, to which some species of *Leishmania* are particularly sensitive. In experimental animals, genetics has been shown to have a great effect on the host response to infection.

There is considerable evidence that even the most virulent *Leishmania* parasites may cause no detectable disease in certain individuals. Wherever transmission occurs, numerous people are found who have positive immunological reactions but no cutaneous scar or history of visceral disease. Sub-clinical infection must be particularly common in foci of *L. infantum*. Here, disease in adults is usually associated with underlying immunosuppressive disease and may then be very common; even among children overt disease may be extremely rare despite intense transmission.

CUTANEOUS LEISHMANIASIS OR ORIENTAL SORE

A single cutaneous lesion, or leishmanioma, at the site of each infective sandfly bite is characteristic of infection with *L. tropica*, *L. major*, *L. aethiopica*, certain strains of *L. infantum* and, rarely, *L. donovani*. Usually oriental sore is painless and self-curing, and is frequently passed off as a trivial matter. Although this may be true of a single lesion in a hidden place, multiple lesions of *L. major* or disfiguring facial lesions due to *L. tropica* may be physically or psychologically crippling.

Generally all lesions on any one patient have a similar appearance and progress synchronously. In *L. major* infection the centre of the 'wet' lesion becomes necrotic and exudative, forming a loose crust of congealed serum above a granulomatous base that eventually produces the characteristic scar. *L. major* lesions may number >100. With *L. tropica* the 'dry' lesion is more swollen and less necrotic; the exudate is less profuse and accumulates as a thicker crust. Numerous lesions are rare, the average number being around 2. These differences are by no means consistent and are certainly not diagnostic. *L. aethiopica* lesions are even more swollen and less necrotic that those of *L. tropica*; frequently they are barely exudative, with gradual sca-

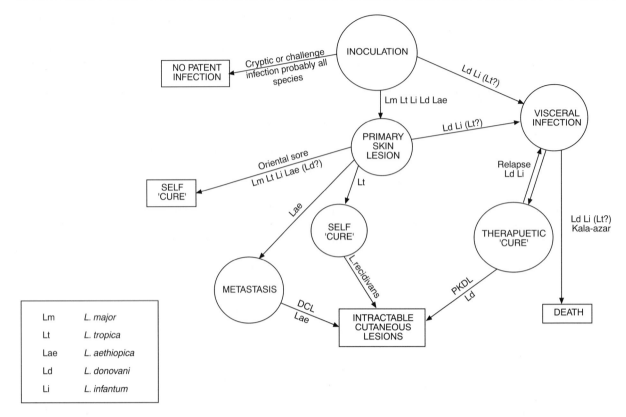

Fig. 12.11 The 'leishmaniasis spectrum', showing the potential progress and outcome of infection with Old World species. Modified from Molyneux and Ashford (1983).

ling or exfoliation of the dermis at the centre. These lesions often last for years before healing. Cutaneous lesions resulting from *L. infantum* resemble those of *L. tropica* but are generally smaller and more indolent.

Oriental sore is not usually associated with systemic manifestations, although there may be enlargement of the draining lymph nodes. The necrotic centres of lesions are heavily contaminated with bacteria but these are not usually invasive, so inflammation, suppuration and pain are atypical.

LEISHMANIASIS RECIDIVANS (LR)

LR is an unusual sequel of oriental sore caused by *L. tropica* infection. In this condition small, usually non-ulcerating lesions appear, mainly on the margin of an apparently healed scar of oriental sore. These may last indefinitely, gradually extending the limits of the initial scar, and causing severe disfigurement. LR is associated with a strong cell-mediated immune response; both superficially and histologically it closely resembles cutaneous tuberculosis, so the name 'lupoid leishmaniasis' is sometimes used.

DIFFUSE CUTANEOUS LEISHMANIASIS (DCL)

Diffuse (more correctly 'disseminated') CL is a rare form of disease, caused by *L. aethiopica* in the Old World; just over 100 cases have been recorded. The parasites are restricted to the skin, but become widely distributed over much of the surface, in large, swollen plaques and nodules. This condition resembles lepromatous leprosy, for which it was initially mistaken, but

the abundant parasites in the nodules provide easy distinction. This is an immunologically anergic condition in which neither humoral nor cell-mediated responses are activated; it is very difficult to treat and may last for the rest of the greatly disrupted life of the patient.

VISCERAL LEISHMANIASIS OR KALA-AZAR

Visceral leishmaniasis is characteristic of infection with *L. donovani* and *L. infantum*. There are also suggestions that occasional cases are caused by *L. tropica* (see p. 234). The 2 main viscerotropic species cause broadly similar diseases, although *L. infantum* mainly affects young children and has a greater tendency to cause lymph node enlargement. The general course of the disease is thought to be closely related to the health status of the patient at the time of infection and longitudinal studies have provided good evidence that malnutrition exacerbates *L. infantum* infection (Badaro et al. 1986).

The infection begins at the site of the infective sandfly bite, where there may be an initial ulcerating lesion. This has been best described in dogs, where its occurrence does not reflect the eventual outcome (Vidor et al. 1991). In humans a leishmanioma is rarely seen. If present, it may become a self-limiting lesion resembling oriental sore without producing visceral disease.

The clinical features are well described by Rees and Kager (1987). Typically, visceral disease develops after an incubation period of 2–6 months and is accompanied by a persistent, irregular low grade fever, but onset may be delayed for many years. Once established subsequent development of disease is quite variable; onset of severe symptoms may be very acute with rapid progression to life-threatening disease within 2 weeks, or progression may be insidious, almost unnoticed, probably passed off by the patient as a mere malaria attack, until the abdominal swelling becomes a major concern. Splenomegaly is the most consistent and noticeable sign. The spleen becomes enormously enlarged, extending well below the umbilicus, its size emphasized by an accompanying cachexia. Hepatomegaly is less consistent and less extreme, but is usually present in late cases. The haematological picture is greatly altered (see p. 231), with anaemia and leucopenia the most manifest changes. The outcome of untreated fully symptomatic visceral leishmaniasis is usually fatal.

POST KALA-AZAR DERMAL LEISHMANIASIS (PKDL)

PKDL is a relatively common consequence of therapeutic cure from visceral leishmaniasis caused by *L. donovani*. It is not associated with *L. infantum* infection. PKDL is occasionally seen in patients with no history of visceral disease, but only in places where *L. donovani* is transmitted; this is probably a sequel to subclinical infection. Sometimes PKDL develops before the visceral infection has cured, but its onset may be delayed for as much as 2 years. The extent to which chemotherapy actually causes PKDL is an interesting conundrum and one which is unlikely to be resolved soon, as visceral disease is always treated if drugs are available and untreated cases have a poor prognosis. PKDL was reported in some 20% of cured cases in India; it was said to be rare in Africa but a very high incidence has been seen in the current Sudanese epidemic (Zijlstra et al. 1994).

PKDL is a variable disease; it may start as a widespread punctate, progressive depigmentation giving the skin a mottled or freckled effect, or may first be noticed as discrete papules, mainly on surfaces exposed to light. It can progress to produce an extensive surface of coalescing papules, or large discrete nodules, which superficially resemble DCL or lepromatous leprosy. The lesions are delicate but do not ulcerate unless traumatized. The duration of the untreated condition, the numbers of parasites and the immune responses of patients with PKDL are very variable.

LEISHMANIA AND HUMAN IMMUNODEFICIENCY VIRUS (HIV) COINFECTION

Most of the information on coinfection relates to *L. infantum*; few coinfections with other *Leishmania* species have been described. Some 40% of visceral leishmaniasis cases presenting in France are coinfected with HIV (Dereure et al. 1995). The diversity of strains found is much greater than usual, and strains that are normally associated with cutaneous disease may visceralize in coinfection (Pratlong et al. 1995). Serological evidence suggests that HIV may either activate sub-

clinical leishmaniasis or make the patient susceptible to a new infection (Gradoni et al. 1993); serology is of little use in diagnosing coinfection. In a group of patients in Spain, the clinical presentation was characteristic of kala-azar, and most were at CDC HIV stage 4 with $<200 \times 10^6$ CD4+ lymphocytes 1^{-1}. Visceral leishmaniasis was the first reported severe infection in 10 of 47 cases (Medrano et al. 1992). Other workers have found a wider diversity of presentations, frequently with infection of the upper alimentary tract (Peters et al. 1990). Many authors have suggested that visceral leishmaniasis should be included in the list of opportunistic infections indicative of AIDS (e.g. Altes et al. 1991). The predominance of intravenous drug users among these patients suggests that syringe transmission may occur (Alvar and Jimenez 1994).

6 IMMUNOLOGY

6.1 Introduction

The responses of the immune system to *Leishmania* infection are highly complex (reviewed by Mauel and Behin 1987, Liew and O'Donnell 1993). They may accelerate cure or exacerbate the disease, depending on the particular circumstances. This is partly due to the effects of genetic variation in the mammalian host, partly due to genetic variation in the parasites between species and strains, and partly due to chance factors such as the location, inoculum size and number of infective bites received.

6.2 Host genetic variability

The evidence that genetic variation in humans contributes to variability in their immune responses and clinical outcome is mainly anecdotal, and essentially based on the wide clinical spectrum produced by apparently identical parasites. Hard evidence is difficult to obtain; even under circumstances in which individuals share the same environment and differences exist in incidence or severity of disease, it is impossible to be certain whether this reflects human genetic variation or, for example, different numbers of bites received. The main evidence supporting the importance of human genetic variation is indirect and comes from experimental studies conducted with inbred strains of mice (reviewed by Bradley 1987, Blackwell 1992). It is difficult to determine the extent to which these findings can be extrapolated to human patients. Nevertheless, this experimental approach has proved productive and several genetic loci have been identified in the mouse that are linked to resistance phenotypes. The genes encoding some of these have now been cloned and, although the functions of these are not fully resolved, this opens up the possibility of a search for homologues in the human genome. This should lead to progress in assessing the contribution of human genetic variability to the clinical spectrum of disease.

6.3 Human cutaneous leishmaniasis

Spontaneous cure of uncomplicated *L. major* and *L. tropica* infection usually results in a solid immunity. There is a marked development of cell-mediated reactions but a weak antibody response, although specific antibody can be detected. The cell mediated reactions are responsible for a marked delayed type hypersensitivity (DTH) response to the inoculation of leishmanin (washed promastigotes in 0.5% phenol saline) in active and cured cases. The DTH response can often be detected before healing. In *L. tropica* infections which persist and result in leishmaniasis recidivans there is still a strong DTH response, indicating that the parasite can survive despite the high immunological reactivity of the host. In contrast, diffuse cutaneous leishmaniasis (DCL) caused by *L. aethiopica* is characterized by a lack of DTH response but the presence of antibody response, thus tending more to resemble response to visceral leishmaniasis.

6.4 Human visceral leishmaniasis

Radical cure of *L. donovani* infection by chemotherapy can also generate protective immunity in some individuals. In contrast to cutaneous leishmaniasis, cell-mediated immunity is impaired in active kala-azar patients who consequently lack a DTH response, but this can be demonstrated after cure. There is, however, a marked humoral response to visceral leishmaniasis. Polyclonal B cell activation produces mainly IgG and IgM, most of which is non-specific antibody, but high titres of specific antibody can also be detected. In PKDL a curious situation arises in which there seems to be immunity in the viscera but not in the skin. Only a proportion of PKDL patients show a DTH response, antibody levels are elevated but are not as high as in active kala-azar.

6.5 Experimental leishmaniasis

The relative paucity of information on the immunology of human leishmaniasis is in contrast to an explosion in the literature relating to experimental infections in inbred strains of mice, particularly using *L. major* (Liew and O'Donnell 1993, Milon, Del Giudice and Louis 1995, Solbach and Laskay 1995). This explosion is not only due to the potential impact that such work may eventually have on human medicine, but also to the role that *Leishmania* has played in fundamental immunological research itself. The relatively recent nature of these findings, together with the difficulties of investigating human immunology, means that the extent to which they can be extrapolated to human leishmaniasis is difficult to predict at present. In all of these experimental studies it should be remembered that the infection occurs against a specific genetic background, usually in a highly susceptible strain of mouse, and that the interaction between innate genetic factors and specific immune responses is not well understood. Despite these caveats, some of the major findings are likely to

be borne out and thus merit brief discussion. The main effector cell in murine cutaneous leishmaniasis is the CD4+ T cell. The cell populations are not homogeneous, but can be separated into 2 functionally distinct subsets, termed Th1 and Th2, each of which is associated with a distinct cytokine profile. Resistance and healing in mice is associated with a Th1 type response, whereas susceptibility and disease progression is accompanied by a Th2 response. These polarized Th1 or Th2 responses have not been demonstrated in murine *L. donovani* infection, which instead is associated with an absence of a Th1 response in susceptible strains (Kaye 1995). Early events in the dermis and epidermis of the skin may play a crucial role influencing the development of resistance or susceptibility (Moll 1993, Solbach and Laskay 1995). A Th1/Th2-like dichotomy in CD4+ T cell clones can be demonstrated in human leishmaniasis (Kemp et al. 1993, 1994, Ghosh et al. 1995). The main effector cell in protective immunity is the macrophage host cell itself, in which the killing mechanism is a cytokine-induced production of nitric oxide (Liew and Cox 1991).

7 PATHOLOGY

In visceral leishmaniasis, parasites may be found in practically every organ, whereas they are largely limited to the skin in cutaneous leishmaniasis; nevertheless the histological spectrum of the different diseases is surprisingly uniform. Cells of the mononuclear phagocyte system are infected (Ridley 1987), particularly the more actively phagocytic members of the series. Further phagocytic cells are attracted to the site. These in turn become infected, so a colony of infected cells is produced. The parasites may be restricted to the initial cutaneous site, or may disseminate, after a variable delay, in the blood rather than the lymphatics, to establish metastatic colonies in almost any organ. The temperature dependence of each species may partly be responsible for the ultimate distribution of the lesions. Dissemination is also limited by the histological immune response.

In cutaneous leishmaniasis a spectrum of histological response to infection, somewhat analogous to that in leprosy, is based on the amount of lymphocyte, plasma cell and giant cell infiltration constituting the granulomatous inflammation. The minimal, anergic, Ridley's 'group I' response is best seen in DCL, with abundant, heavily infected macrophages, few other cells and no giant cells. There is little necrosis and no ulceration. The other extreme, the 'group V', hypersensitive response, is tuberculoid, with an epithelioid cell granuloma, large Langerhans cells, variable plasma cell numbers and scanty lymphocytes. Few parasites are present and, again, there is no necrosis. Langerhans cells may migrate to the draining lymph nodes where they present antigen to T cells, initiating the immune response (Moll 1993). Between these 2 histologically stable extremes, both of which produce long lasting lesions, intractable to treatment, are 3 less well defined categories, which to some extent represent a progression, associated with lymphocyte infiltration, variable amounts of necrosis, and healing. Necrosis is the main feature of an effective immune response and subsequent healing, whereas small numbers of parasites may be destroyed by macrophages and giant cells.

The histological pattern in deep tissues is less fully described, but seems to be similar; again, the main feature of healing is the presence of lymphocytic granulomata and necrotic centres. In contrast to cutaneous leishmaniasis, however, natural healing is not the rule and the lesions are more like the anergic, group I type described above, with widely disseminated proliferations of infected macrophages and little infiltration. Most of the pathology is caused by this hyperplasia and damage to the organs caused by associated congestion. According to El Hag and Hashim (1994), the liver shows infected Kupffer cells and macrophages, with chronic mononuclear cell infiltration of the portal tracts and lobules, ballooning degeneration of the hepatocytes and fibrosis of the terminal hepatic venules.

8 DIAGNOSIS

Relative unfamiliarity with the leishmaniases among practitioners in non-endemic areas occasionally leads to serious misdiagnosis and mistreatment. A good travel history may arouse suspicion in those versed in geographical medicine, but reference to a tropical specialist is usually required to confirm the diagnosis. In areas where the disease is better known, clinical diagnosis is frequently regarded as sufficient. Although this may be justified during epidemics, a number of alternative diagnoses will inevitably be missed if demonstration of the parasites is not attempted on all patients.

8.1 Clinical diagnosis

Clinical diagnosis of any of the leishmaniases depends primarily on awareness. None of the signs or symptoms is diagnostic but, when combined with a relevant travel history, or in an endemic area, a good presumptive diagnosis may be made clinically and can be confirmed parasitologically. 'Diagnosis' by therapeutic trial is commonly practised but unsatisfactory, particularly in view of the expense of the drugs.

Visceral leishmaniasis is often mistakenly recorded post-mortem as 'malaria which failed to respond to treatment' (and probably included in malaria mortality statistics). The typical patient presents at a late stage, with persistent but fluctuating low grade fever, weight loss giving the appearance of severe starvation, and spleno- or hepatosplenomegaly. The patient is usually alert and feels remarkably well, considering his or her condition. The skin is sometimes said to be 'muddy', 'pale' or 'dark', but these are not diagnostically useful descriptions. There is frequently persistent diarrhoea. Lymphadenopathy is an irregular feature.

Non-specific laboratory tests will show marked leucopenia (pancytopenia, mainly neutropenia), anaemia, raised serum proteins with reversal of the albumin/globulin ratio due to greatly raised IgG levels.

Manson-Bahr (1987) suggests the following differential diagnoses: malaria, relapsing fever, trypanosomiasis, brucellosis, liver abscess, tuberculosis, tropical splenomegaly, myeloid leukaemia, lymphoma, cirrhosis of the liver, schistosomiasis, thalassaemia, histoplasmosis and various gammopathies.

Diagnosis of visceral leishmaniasis in the presence of HIV infection is particularly difficult as the presentation may be very atypical and serological tests may be negative.

All forms of cutaneous leishmaniasis usually present without systemic disease. Typical lesions of oriental sore are readily recognized by the raised edges, necrotic, exudative centre with granulomatous base, long duration and painlessness. Less typical lesions take a bewildering array of forms and must be distinguished from basal cell carcinoma, tuberculosis, various mycoses, cheloid and lepromatous leprosy.

Leishmaniasis recidivans may be indicated by the presence of a scar and positive skin test (see p. 232), whereas diffuse cutaneous leishmaniasis shows no ulceration or scarring and has a negative skin test.

8.2 Parasitological diagnosis

A diagnosis of leishmaniasis can be formally confirmed only by the demonstration of the parasites. These are readily seen in smears or touch preparations of infected tissue stained with Giemsa's stain, preferably at pH 7.2 rather than the pH 6.8 normally used in haematology. Sections of tissue stained more conventionally, with H&E, are much more difficult to interpret, so the diagnosis must be suspected before material is prepared.

Preparations from cutaneous lesions may be made from punch biopsies, but it is usually sufficient to take a small quantity of material from the living, but diseased, tissue at the edge of the lesion, by a slit smear or other minimally invasive technique.

Deeper tissues may be sampled by needle biopsy. Material may be aspirated from lymph nodes following injection of a small quantity of physiological saline. Bone marrow smears are made using standard haematological techniques. Spleen aspirate is the most reliable material for demonstrating parasites in kala-azar. Although many practitioners are reluctant to take spleen aspirates, others have no hesitation, and even use this method to monitor treatment. It is vital to use the correct technique and equipment with confidence, so that the capsule of the spleen is penetrated by a fine needle for only a fraction of a second (see Bryceson (1987a) for precise instructions).

Parasites may be scanty and are mostly extracellular in slide preparations, so these may have to be examined for at least 15 min using oil immersion before the diagnosis can be confirmed. Amastigotes are identified by their size (3–5 μm) and the possession of a nucleus and kinetoplast; although smaller, the latter is often easier to detect because the DNA is very densely packed and produces a deep purple spot or rod upon staining. It may be possible to provisionally identify the parasites to species level by the circumstances and clinical features. *L. major* and *L. tropica* can be separated with some confidence by the abundance of parasites in the latter, their smaller size, and the presence of more numerous parasites in each infected histiocyte. Complete identification requires the isolation of parasites in culture.

Whatever material is collected, it is desirable to culture the parasites in blood-agar or insect tissue culture medium so that they can be identified at strain level by isoenzyme analysis. For special purposes, material can be inoculated into a hamster, generally the most susceptible experimental host. Monoclonal antibody and DNA probes, with or without PCR amplification, have been developed for identification of the parasites. These are not yet commercially available, but are of great use in epidemiological or ecological investigations.

8.3 Immunological diagnosis

Immunological diagnosis (reviewed by Kar 1995) is of value in screening suspected kala-azar patients, other than those coinfected with HIV, and in epidemiological studies.

In the formol-gel test, a drop of full strength formalin is added to 1 ml of serum. A positive result is indicated by the rapid and complete coagulation of the serum. This simple test merely indicates greatly increased serum proteins and thus is non-specific. Nevertheless it is still widely used; in order to be acceptable in peripheral clinics in endemic areas, this is the level of technology that any new test will have to approach.

More specific tests which become positive earlier in kala-azar include the indirect fluorescent antibody test (IFAT), the enzyme-linked immunosorbent assay (ELISA) and a direct agglutination test (DAT). This last technique requires minimal equipment, is robust in the most difficult conditions and is exquisitely sensitive. DAT is fast becoming available for use at peripheral level clinics and the development of freeze-dried antigen (Meredith et al. 1995) promises even wider availability of this test. For active case detection, numerous positive responses to serological tests are found in people who show no disease. To treat all these people as patients would be a mistake; probably the best thing is to examine them carefully, treat those with signs of disease and carefully monitor the others.

The specific reagents for the above serological tests are not readily available commercially, but they can be prepared relatively easily in the laboratory.

A delayed hypersensitivity reaction to intradermal crude *Leishmania* antigen is produced in healing or cured cases of both cutaneous and visceral leishmaniasis. This leishmanin, or Montenegro, skin test is of great value in epidemiological studies but is of little clinical use. The number of positive reactors is usually much greater than the number with a history of disease; either the test is non-specific or there is a lot of sub-clinical infection.

9 EPIDEMIOLOGY

9.1 Introduction

Knowledge of the epidemiology of the leishmaniases has benefited in recent years from our growing understanding of the taxonomy of the group and from the possibility of accurate identification of morphologically similar parasites derived from human cases, sandfly vectors or non-human mammalian hosts. Current taxonomy corresponds much better with ecology and epidemiology than it does with clinical manifestations (See Molyneux and Ashford 1983). Anomalies and questions remain and the 'spectral epidemiology' (different diseases caused by ostensibly similar organisms) is largely unexplained.

It has been conservatively estimated that in the Old World, 150 million people in 40 countries are at risk of infection with cutaneous leishmaniasis and 180 million people in 39 countries are at risk of visceral leishmaniasis. The total number of reported cases was estimated at 240 000 and 73 000 annually, for cutaneous and visceral leishmaniasis respectively, but this is doubtless a gross underestimate of the real numbers (Desjeux 1991, Ashford, Desjeux and deRaadt 1992). The figure of 12 million cases annually was estimated some time ago by Walsh and Warren (1979); this is sometimes misquoted as 1.2 million but W H O (1990) use the higher figure. It is hard to know how the figure of 12 million was derived.

Although transmission is possible by contagion, by transfusion or in utero, these routes have little, if any, known epidemiological significance. Effectively all transmission is by the bite of a phlebotomine sandfly (Diptera: Phlebotominae) (Reviewed by Killick-Kendrick 1990b). The leishmaniases illustrate the entire gamut of zoonotic patterns of transmission.

9.2 Epidemiology of *L. major* infection

L. major is widely distributed in the Palaearctic and Aethiopian zoogeographical regions along the northern and southern fringes of the Sahara, extending south into northern Kenya and through Arabia, southern Iraq and Iran, into the central Asian states of Turkmenistan, Uzbekistan and northern Afghanistan. It also ranges through Iranian and Pakistani Baluchistan to the Indian border in Rajasthan (see Fig. 12.1).

Throughout this wide range the parasite is restricted to arid and semi-arid zones. Its broad distribution seems to be determined by that of its vectors, and its detailed distribution is largely determined by that of its natural mammalian hosts.

The 3 known vectors belong to the subgenus *Phlebotomus* (*Phlebotomus*), of which *P. papatasi* is the most widespread and abundant. *P. papatasi* transmits *L.*

major in all but the sub-Saharan and Indian parts of its distribution; it is replaced by *P. duboscqi* in the former and *P. salehi* in the latter. *P. papatasi* has a much wider distribution than *L. major*, especially in northern India, but here it is largely synanthropic and has no access to suitable reservoir hosts. The efficiency of this species as a vector may be affected by the plant juices on which it feeds, some of which may inhibit growth of the parasites (Schlein and Jacobson 1994b).

The known reservoir hosts of *L. major* are rodents. In the central Asian deserts the great gerbil *Rhombomys opimus* lives in dense colonies with deep and complex burrow systems that provide shelter and possibly a breeding site for *P. papatasi*. The gerbils breed throughout the warmer months and by the end of the transmission season, in autumn when the rodent population is greatest, almost every animal may be infected. The infection is usually restricted to the ears, which become only slightly swollen and eroded, and there is no indication that the rodent is seriously affected.

Great gerbil colonies are best developed in areas where the soil is deep and of a consistency that allows permanent burrows to be constructed. These conditions are found on the alluvial fans in the valleys of the largest rivers draining the great central Asian loess deposits, such as the Amudarya.

The distribution of the rodent extends much further north in central Asia than that of the vector. In these zones they are infected with other parasites, *L. gerbilli* and *L. turanica*, which behave similarly in the rodent but do not infect humans and are transmitted by different sandfly vectors (Strelkova et al. 1993).

The other rodent reservoir host of *L. major*, which has very narrow habitat requirements, is the fat sand rat *Psammomys obesus*. This host maintains populations of the parasite in Algeria, Tunisia, Libya, north Sinai, the Jordan Valley, southern Syria and much of Arabia. This rodent is unique in being able to derive its entire nutrient and water requirements from the succulent, but highly saline, stems and leaves of halophilic plants of the family Chenopodiaceae. These plants dominate the internally draining salt pans, *sebchet* or playas of much of the desert fringes, and it is here that the sand rats are concentrated. *P. obesus* burrows are less deep or extensive than those of *R. opimus* and provide a less favourable habitat for *P. papatasi*. Furthermore, the rodents breed mainly in the winter when there is no transmission so the young are not exposed to infection until they are a few months old. Nevertheless all the evidence supports the conclusion that *P. obesus* is responsible for the maintenance of *L. major* in most of this part of its range.

Some foci of *L. major* in the Palaearctic occur in the absence of both *P. obesus* and *R. opimus* and have been attributed to various rodent hosts such as jirds *Meriones* spp. (Rioux et al. 1982), or the mole rat *Nesokia indica*. The structure of these foci, notably that on the Iraq–Iran border, remain to be fully understood.

In its Aethiopian range, where *L. major* is usually transmitted by *P. duboscqi*, various rodents have been found infected, notably the grass rats *Arvicanthis* spp and the multimammate rats *Mastomys* spp. In these hosts the parasites are found in the viscera but do not seem to cause serious pathology. Populations of these rodents fluctuate wildly and they do not have narrow habitat requirements, so they are not good candidates for the maintenance of vector-borne infections. Possibly there is no individual rodent species maintaining the parasite but a diversity of hosts may be required.

L. major infection in humans is most conspicuous in epidemics in groups of people entering sparsely inhabited zoonotic foci. Major outbreaks have occurred in military groups and in workers on development projects. Development frequently alters the environment sufficiently that following a brief epidemic period the infection disappears. This has been seen particularly in irrigation schemes. Residents in zoonotic foci usually become infected at an early age and, being familiar with the infection, are less concerned.

The dynamics of human infection are largely governed by the rate of exposure to infection and the almost complete resistance to reinfection. Beliaev and Lysenko (1977) have modelled the stable-state system, making minimal, realistic assumptions; they show that at low rates of exposure (<0.05 exposures per person per year), incidence is proportional to this rate. They term locations where these conditions prevail 'hypoendemic foci'. In contrast, hyperendemic foci are those where the exposure rate is >0.25 per person per year. In such foci, incidence is largely independent of the exposure rate, change in which alters only the mean age at which people become infected. As most people in such hyperendemic foci are infected when young and subsequently become immune, the incidence is dependent on the rate at which non-immune people are recruited into the population, whether by being born or by immigrating.

In sub-Saharan Africa outbreaks are much less frequent and human cases occur sporadically in both space and time. In some foci, in Ethiopia and Kenya for example, human infection is extremely rare even in places where infected rodents have been found.

Transmission between humans without a mammalian reservoir host has not been well established, although the possibility cannot be excluded. A series of epidemics in Khartoum and nearby towns in the late 1980s occurred in dense, stable human populations that had never previously known the infection (El Safi, Peters and Evans 1988). The best available explanation is that the parasite was introduced by displaced people from endemic areas to the west and that it was transmitted to residents by the abundant *P. papatasi* living close to the Nile.

9.3 Epidemiology of *L. tropica* infection

L. tropica is mainly found in the ancient cities of west and central Asia (see Fig. 12.1). Generally, *L. tropica* inhabits slightly wetter areas than *L. major*; the 2 species are geographically sympatric in places but are ecologically separated. Vernacular names for the infection frequently refer to endemic cities such as Balkh,

Baghdad, Aleppo, Delhi; this probably reflects the perception of visitors rather than indigenous people.

Urban cutaneous leishmaniasis is transmitted by *Phlebotomus* (*Paraphlebotomus*) *sergenti* throughout its range. This sandfly can reach high populations in crowded cities and suburbs but is not restricted to the peridomestic environment. Dogs have been found infected but it is generally thought that the main hosts are humans. Unlike *L. major*, the rate of exposure to infection depends on the number of active human lesions as well as other factors. The human lesion normally lasts around one year and people with cured lesions are immune. Therefore, in conditions of potentially high transmission most people are immune, few are susceptible, leaving even fewer actually infected. The maintenance of stable transmission in a stable human population has been estimated to require some 20 000 sandfly bites per person per year which, in the seasonal climates of central Asia, may mean 100 bites per person per night. Such conditions are rarely, if ever, met and the infection must rely either on movements of people (Ashford, Kohestany and Karimzad 1992) or on spatial heterogeneity in the immunity of the population, moving from place to place in localized epidemics (Ashford et al. 1993). In this way *L. tropica* resembles a viral infection such as measles rather than most other eukaryotic parasites.

There are reports of *L. tropica* infection occurring sporadically in rural settings that cannot easily be explained by the above patterns. Furthermore, the findings of *L. tropica* causing visceral leishmaniasis in American soldiers who served in Operation Desert Storm (Magill et al. 1993, 1994) and in Kenyan and Indian villagers (Mehbratu et al. 1989, Sacks et al. 1995) in the heart of areas of *L. donovani* transmission, pose intriguing epidemiological questions for which no sensible answer can yet be proposed.

It was previously thought that *L. tropica* did not occur in Africa. Parasites from an ostensibly zoonotic outbreak of cutaneous leishmaniasis in Tunisia were identified as a new species, *L. killicki* which, on the cladograms of Rioux et al. (1990) (see Fig. 12.3), is close to *L. tropica*. A wide variety of *L. tropica*-like strains are responsible for another apparently zoonotic focus in Morocco (Pratlong et al. 1991). Parasites from sporadic cutaneous cases, hyraxes *Procavia* spp. and from the sandflies *P. rossi* and *P. guggisbergi* in Namibia and Kenya were found to be intermediate between the original *L. killicki* and *L. tropica*. It is a matter of opinion whether these parasites should be included with *L. tropica* or not (Sang, Pratlong and Ashford 1992). Occasional aberrant cutaneous, visceral, or mixed infections have been reported elsewhere in Africa, notably in Tanzania, Zambia and Malawi (Pharoah et al. 1993). The parasites have not been isolated and their identity is unknown but presumably they originated in zoonotic foci that await discovery and description.

9.4 Epidemiology of *L. aethiopica* infection

L. aethiopica is restricted to the highlands of East Africa in Ethiopia and Kenya, between c. 1800 m and 2700 m above sea level, and within the 800 mm isohyet (see Fig. 12.1). In all known foci it is associated with hyraxes (Mammalia: Hyracoidea) which are the natural reservoir hosts (Ashford et al. 1973). These animals have very poor temperature regulation and live in deep clefts in rocks or trees in which they can find the shelter they require for the maintenance of their body temperature. Despite this restriction, they are found at all altitudes between below sea level in the Danakil desert and above 4000 m, where there is frost every night. Hyraxes are long-lived and live in colonies or family groups, so although their rate of reproduction is low, they are good candidate reservoir hosts. Parasites have been isolated from normal skin and external mucosa showing no sign of the infection, which presumably lasts a long time.

The vectors *P. longipes* and *P. pedifer* have less specific habitat requirements, being common in houses or associated with cattle, but they are restricted in altitude. The distribution of the parasite is, therefore, governed by the habitat of the reservoir host and the altitude range of the vectors. Wherever they have been adequately studied, human cases can be attributed to the nearby presence of infected hyraxes. Incidence of disease in humans is rarely high, and the rare cases of diffuse cutaneous leishmaniasis caused by this parasite have not been explained epidemiologically.

9.5 Epidemiology of *L. donovani* infection

L. donovani is surely one of the great scourges of mankind, having been responsible for a series of deadly epidemics, each causing depopulation of affected areas. The geographical distribution of *L. donovani* infection is somewhat labile (see Fig. 12.2). In the Indian subcontinent it occurs in the valleys of the Ganges and Brahmaputra Rivers, in Bihar, lowland Nepal, West Bengal, Bangladesh and Assam as well as further south, around Madras (reviewed by Sanyal 1985). It is often presumed that visceral leishmaniasis in south China was caused by *L. donovani* but this has not been confirmed. In Africa, the infection is largely restricted to Sudan, Ethiopia and Kenya.

The ecological distribution of *L. donovani* is quite well known but poorly understood. In Asia, where humans are the only known hosts, the infection occurs in heavily populated rural areas in the rich silty floodplains of the great rivers. Here the vector *P. argentipes* is abundant and strictly synanthropic, breeding in the organically rich material on the floors of cow byres (Ghosh and Bhattacharya 1991) (this is almost the only sandfly whose larval habitat is reasonably well described). Here, the only known reservoirs of infection are humans and persistent cases of PKDL may be particularly important in maintaining the parasite between epidemics (Addy and Nandy 1992).

In Africa there are 2 types of habitat, each associated with a specific vector. *P. orientalis* occurs in *Acacia seyal* woodland, which is the dominant natural vegetation of the light, alluvial, montmorillonite, silty clays of eastern Sudan between latitudes 9°N and 14°N, extending into the western Ethiopian lowlands. *P. martini* occurs in less well defined habitats but is commonly associated with eroded termitaria in the heavy laterite clays of the southern borders of Sudan and Ethiopia, northern Uganda and much of Kenya. *L. donovani* infection occurs either in fairly stable endemic conditions or as violent epidemics throughout the distribution of these 2 vectors. The Nile grass rat *Arvicanthis niloticus* has been found infected in good numbers in southern Sudan and may be an important reservoir host, but the shifting distribution of the epidemics and persistence of intensely endemic residual foci, too dangerous to even visit in the transmission season, remain largely unexplained.

Human *L. donovani* infection is endemic in parts of southern Ethiopia, Sudan and northern Kenya, where most people are exposed to infection at some time during their lives, but relatively few become sick (e.g. Zijlstra et al. 1994). An Ethiopian study indicated an exposure rate of c. 11% per year, but there were only 2% cases of overt disease per 100 non-immune individuals (Ali and Ashford 1994). Nearly all adult males and more than half the females showed evidence of previous exposure.

This apparent insusceptibility of most of the people cannot be true of the early epidemics in northwest India where the disease swept through the population like a plague killing a large proportion (and, incidentally, giving rise to the dreadful reputation of malaria: kala-azar was thought to be *the* malignant, lethal form of malaria [Rogers 1908]). The epidemic of the late 1980s in southern Sudan was equally virulent, and was estimated to have killed half of the affected population, some 100 000 people, in 5 years (Seaman et al. 1992).

Epidemics of kala-azar are often associated with natural disasters or social upheavals, although causal relationships are difficult to establish. The work of Sati (1962) documents the spread of an epidemic with famine-related displacement. The 1980s Sudan epidemic may have resulted from the introduction of the parasite by people coming from endemic areas on the Ethiopian border to settled areas with potential transmission. These movements were related to the civil war, as was the poor condition of the recipient people, but the precise interpretation is largely informed speculation.

Although epidemics in Africa occur in rural, largely pastoral environments, those in India are in towns and villages with settled agriculture. In the north Bihar epidemic, maximum incidence was estimated at 6 per 1000 per year, with more than 100 000 cases reported in some years. In 1992 there were 80 000 cases (Sacks et al. 1995). Reported cases are surely only a small fraction of the actual number occurring.

9.6 Epidemiology of *L. infantum* infection

L. infantum parasites are difficult to separate objectively from *L. donovani* and the distribution of the 2 forms is largely allopatric, so there is a good case for regarding them as subspecies. It is convenient to treat them separately, though, because they are very distinct in both in their ecology and epidemiology.

L. infantum is the only *Leishmania* species that occurs in both the Old and New Worlds (in the Americas it is sometimes called by its junior synonym *L. chagasi*; see chapter 13 for New World features). In the Old World it is distributed in much of the Mediterranean basin, both in Europe and North Africa (see Fig. 12.2). It extends erratically through Arabia, Turkey and Iran to the Central Asian republics, Pakistan and Kashmir (Rab and Evans 1995), as well as into northwest China. It is thought to have been much more widely distributed in China but visceral leishmaniasis has been almost eradicated throughout that country.

Throughout this range the main host is the domestic dog, which develops an acute or chronic disease. Though eventually fatal, canine visceral leishmaniasis presents abundant parasites in the skin, available for transmission. The distribution of foci of infection depends on the presence of vector sandflies, usually species of the subgenus *Phlebotomus* (*Larroussius*). Although we are ignorant of the mechanisms by which the distribution of sandflies is regulated, each species has clearly defined ecological preferences. *P. ariasi*, for example, is largely restricted to hillsides with mixed oak *Quercus* spp. woodland. A more important vector, *P. perniciosus*, occurs at lower altitudes, in drier, limestone country, where it is particularly abundant in gardens and suburbs with outcrops and dry-stone walls. These are the main vectors in the western Mediterranean; they are replaced further east by *P. major* and a wide variety of less well studied probable vectors.

In areas where transmission is intense, almost all dogs become infected and kennels become very difficult to keep. Individual dogs vary greatly in their response to infection and there is some evidence that regionally bred dogs are less susceptible than exotic breeds.

Human infection must be very much more common than overt disease. The latter is classically restricted to children, especially those below the age of 2 years. In post-war years the incidence in children, though not in dogs, in most of southern Europe has decreased greatly so the small number of adult cases have become a greater proportion of the total (Marty et al. 1994). In fact, adult cases have now actually increased owing to greater susceptibility to disease in association with the HIV virus and immunosuppression associated with transplant surgery.

10 CHEMOTHERAPY AND TREATMENT

Treatment of leishmaniasis has a chequered history. Few adequate clinical trials have been carried out, especially with cutaneous leishmaniasis; recommended dosages are frequently based on spurious information and definition of the state of the disease is rarely standardized. Patients frequently present at a late stage, having been treated informally with unknown remedies. Courses of treatment are usually prolonged and so are difficult to monitor or even achieve. Despite these misgivings, the various diseases can generally be cured quite effectively, albeit with drugs that come from archaic pharmacopoeia. In addition to healing the patient, treatment may also reduce the transmission of anthroponotic *L. tropica* or *L. infantum* infection.

10.1 Placebo and physical treatment

The first question is whether or not chemical treatment is justified or even required. Simple single lesions due to *L. major* will heal naturally in a few months and leave the patient immune for life. It is only with multiple or disfiguring lesions that chemotherapy is justified. The same may be said of lesions due to *L. tropica*, though these are of longer duration. With *L. donovani* infection, sick patients have a high risk of death if left untreated, but active case detection may reveal numerous sub-clinical infections. It may be preferable to keep these under observation if possible, especially if, as is frequently the case, resources are very limited.

Cutaneous lesions, whether or not to be treated, should be disinfected and covered, to prevent secondary infection and to avoid infecting sandflies. Heat treatment, with hot compresses or infra-red radiation may accelerate cure. Hot water, in the form of frequent baths or saunas, is beneficial in diffuse cutaneous leishmaniasis, which responds very poorly to chemotherapy. Removal of lesions by cryotherapy has been recommended but is controversial. For visceral leishmaniasis associated with massive splenomegaly and unresponsiveness to antimonial drugs, surgical removal of the spleen used to be practised occasionally and has also been undertaken relatively recently (Magill et al. 1994).

10.2 Pentavalent antimonials

Pentavalent antimony, currently used in the form of meglumine antimoniate or sodium stibogluconate, replaced tartar emetic many years ago and is still the first line drug of choice. Intralesional infiltration is used for simple single cutaneous lesions but intramuscular injection is required for all other cases. Despite the prolonged period of repeated treatment required for the cure of visceral leishmaniasis, these drugs are remarkably safe if administered in the correct doses; their reputation for toxicity is unjustified and relates rather to the trivalent antimonials used previously (Bryceson 1987b). Antimony is excreted rapidly from the body so doses are repeated daily and treatment is continuous throughout each course.

For visceral leishmaniasis, the W H O (1995) recommends intramuscular injection of 20 mg Sb^{5+} kg^{-1} daily (to a maximum of 850 mg) for a minimum of 20 days, and until no parasites can be seen in spleen or marrow biopsies taken 14 days apart. Doses may be divided to counteract rapid excretion. Relapsing patients should be treated similarly.

For cutaneous leishmaniasis, the W H O (1995) recommends 1–3 ml of either of the main antimony preparations, to be infiltrated into the base of the lesion, to be repeated once or twice, at intervals of 1–2 days. For parenteral treatment, 10–20mg Sb^{5+} kg^{-1} i.m. is given daily until a few days after clinical cure.

10.3 Aromatic diamidines

Pentamidine, as the isethionate or dimethylsulphonate, is used as a second choice in cases that are unresponsive to antimony. This product may, however, have serious toxic effects, due to sensitivity at the site of intramuscular injection, too rapid intravenous injection, accumulation, or overdosage. The drug may disrupt blood-sugar homeostasis and lead to intractable diabetes after prolonged use. The margin between therapeutic and toxic doses is narrow and the drug is only slowly excreted, so prolonged treatment at well spaced intervals is required.

The W H O (1995) recommends treatment with 4 mg kg^{-1} 3 times per week for 5–25 weeks, or even longer, for visceral leishmaniasis. For African diffuse cutaneous leishmaniasis, the only other likely use of this drug in Old World leishmaniasis, treatment is once weekly, but continued for at least 4 months.

10.4 Monomycin/paromomycin/aminosidine

The antibiotic monomycin was developed in Russia both for intralesional injection and as a topical treatment for cutaneous leishmaniasis. In the latter use, the active ingredient was contained in a collagen pad tightly applied to the lesion. Paromomycin and aminosidine are probably the same as monomycin, and show considerable promise in topical ointments but in current formulations, irritation and inflammation are too severe for these products to be more than experimental. This antibiotic shows promise as a synergist when used in combination with antimonials, in both visceral and diffuse cutaneous leishmaniasis (Seaman et al. 1993, Teklemariam et al. 1994).

10.5 Amphotericin B

This product is too toxic to be used except in cases where all else has failed; careful monitoring is required. It is administered very slowly, by intravenous route, and the early doses must be reduced in order to check for excessive side-effects. This drug is mainly used to treat cases of mucocutaneous leishmaniasis in South America (see Chapter 13) and is rarely indicated in Old World leishmaniasis. The recommended dose is 0.5–1 mg kg^{-1} on alternate days (WHO 1995).

10.6 Allopurinol

Allopurinol has the attraction that it is a widely used and well established drug. Furthermore, biochemical and in vitro studies indicate that it should be effective against *Leishmania*. Despite these factors, clinical trials have been disappointing, although there are suggestions that the drug may have a synergistic effect when used together with antimony.

10.7 Liposome preparations

Encapsulation of active ingredients in liposomes holds considerable promise for parasites of reticulo-endothelial cells. Trials with amphotericin B in this formulation show that dosage (and therefore toxicity) can be reduced enormously. As yet this treatment is only experimental and is very expensive.

11 VACCINATION

Two important factors suggest that vaccination or other immunological intervention holds promise for the protection of people from at least some of the leishmaniases. First, many individuals seem to be innately insusceptible. This is demonstrated by the survival of some people in even the most serious epidemics and by the finding that some individuals who have never been exposed produce a lymphocyte proliferation response to antigen (Akuffo and Britton 1992, Kurtzhals et al. 1995). Secondly, the immunity produced naturally in response to *L. major* infection is usually solid and there is no evidence that it is not sterile. There may even be a cross-immunity between *L. major* and other species. At present, no vaccine is available against Old World leishmaniasis, although a number are now undergoing Phase I, Phase II and Phase III trials, the results of which are expected in the next 1–2 years (Modabber 1995).

Immunization against cutaneous leishmaniasis by deliberate infection with virulent parasites is traditional in parts of west Asia and was carried out on a massive scale during the Iran–Iraq war (Nadim 1988). Both the Russian and Israeli armies abandoned this measure as there were an unacceptable number of serious side-effects. Trials are in progress using various crude antigen preparations with acceptable adjuvants and it is hoped that vaccination, at least against *L. major* infection, may become feasible soon.

12 INTEGRATED CONTROL

Control of infection depends greatly on local information which, in turn, depends on efficient passive case detection and epidemiological surveillance. These are the minimal activities recommended by the W H O (1990). Increased knowledge of the structure of foci of leishmaniasis has led to the proposal of numerous potential active control strategies, but few of these have been evaluated or even tried in practice.

Avoidance of areas of risk is the simplest method and could be applied to military or other activities involving entry into semi-arid areas where zoonotic *L. major* can be a serious risk. In north Africa and west Asia, barracks for soldiers or labourers should be situated well away from depressions with halophilic vegetation and *P. obesus* colonies. People infected with the HIV virus should avoid much of southern Europe in summer, although the coast itself is generally free of *L. infantum* infection. The few known residual foci of intense *L. donovani* transmission in Africa should be avoided. Some of the national parks of Sudan are particularly notorious and are rarely visited in the transmission season.

Environmental management, such as the destruction of desert rodent colonies in inhabited areas, has been attempted with great success in central Asian irrigation schemes, the design of which was modified to prevent reinvasion by *R. opimus*. The results of pilot schemes to clear land around affected towns in Tunisia (Ben Ismail 1994) and Jordan (Kamhawi et al. 1993) are eagerly awaited. In Ethiopia it has been suggested that villages affected by *L. aethiopica* infection could be protected by shooting the hyraxes in the vicinity, but this intervention has yet to be tried.

In areas where transmission is peridomestic, as with *L. tropica* and *L. donovani* in Asia, sandfly numbers can be greatly reduced by insecticides. In fact, antimalarial campaigns were credited with the near-eradication of kala-azar in India in the 1950s. Active case detection, treatment and insecticide spraying eliminated *L. tropica* in Azerbaijan in the 1960s. A mass campaign in China in the 1950s, using case detection and treatment, insecticides and elimination of dogs, reduced the number of cases from an estimated 500 000 in 1951 to almost zero (Wang Chao-Tsung 1985; Guan Lee-Ren 1991). Experiments with insecticide-impregnated bednets or curtains have given promising results (Maroli and Majori 1991).

Where transmission is sylvatic, as in the *L. donovani* epidemics in southern Sudan, the economic and political problems that prevent effective control elsewhere are compounded by technological problems. There is no realistic way to alter the environment, we know of no way to reduce sandfly numbers, and the reservoir hosts maintaining residual foci have not been identified. Little can be done other than the provision of active case detection and treatment or the promotion of impregnated bednets, with no guarantee that the latter will be effective. These measures are almost impracticable in such a poor, isolated and war-torn country. Much of northern Sudan has undergone massive environmental change with the replacement of woodland by mechanized agricultural projects. This elimination of much of the *P. orientalis* habitat has incidentally greatly reduced the area in which kala-azar epidemics can be expected to occur.

REFERENCES

Addy M, Nandy A, 1992, Ten years of kala azar in West Bengal Part 1. Did post kala azar dermal leishmaniasis initiate the outbreak in 24 Parganas?, *Bull W H O*, **70:** 341–6.

Akuffo HO, Britton SF, 1992, Contribution of non *Leishmania*-specific immunity to resistance to *Leishmania* infection in humans, *Clin Exp Immunol*, **87:** 58–64.

Alexander J, Russell DG, 1992, The interaction of *Leishmania* species with macrophages, *Adv Parasitol*, **31:** 175–254.

Ali A, Ashford RW, 1994, Visceral leishmaniasis in Ethiopia IV. Prevalence, incidence and relation of infection to disease in an endemic area, *Ann Trop Med Parasitol*, **88:** 289–93.

Altes J, Salas A et al., 1991, Visceral leishmaniasis: another HIV-associated opportunistic infection? Report of eight cases and review of the literature, *AIDS*, **5:** 201–7.

Alvar J, Jimenez M, 1994, Could infected drug users be potential *Leishmania* reservoirs?, *AIDS*, **8:** 854.

Ashford RW, Desjeux P, de Raadt P, 1992, Estimation of population at risk and numbers of cases of leishmaniasis, *Parasitol Today*, **8:** 104–5.

Ashford RW, Kohestany KA, Karimzad MA, 1992, Cutaneous leishmaniasis in Kabul, Afghanistan: observations on a 'prolonged epidemic', *Ann Trop Med Parasitol*, **86:** 361–71.

Ashford RW, Bray, RS et al., 1973, The epidemiology of cutaneous leishmaniasis in Ethiopia, *Trans R Soc Trop Med Hyg*, **67:** 568–601.

Ashford RW, Rioux JA et al., 1993, Evidence for a long term increase in the incidence of *Leishmania tropica* in Aleppo, Syria, *Trans R Soc Trop Med Hyg*, **87:** 247–9.

Badaro R, Jones TC et al., 1986, A prospective study of visceral leishmaniasis in an endemic area of Brazil, *J Infect Dis*, **154:** 639–49.

Bastien P, Blaineau C, Pagès M, 1992, *Leishmania*: sex, lies and karyotype, *Parasitol Today*, **8:** 174–7.

Bates PA, 1991, Phosphomonoesterases of parasitic protozoa, *Biochemical Protozoology*, eds Coombs GH, North MJ, Taylor and Francis, London, 537–53.

Bates PA, 1993, Axenic culture of *Leishmania* amastigotes, *Parasitol Today*, **9:** 143–6.

Bates PA, 1994a, The developmental biology of *Leishmania* promastigotes, *Exp Parasitol*, **79:** 215–18.

Bates PA, 1994b, Complete developmental cycle of *Leishmania mexicana* in axenic culture, *Parasitology*, **108:** 1–9.

Bates PA, Dwyer DM, 1987, Biosynthesis and secretion of acid phosphatase by *Leishmania donovani* promastigotes, *Molec Biochem Parasitol*, **26:** 289–95.

Bates PA, Tetley L, 1993, *Leishmania mexicana*: induction of metacyclogenesis by cultivation at acidic pH, *Exp Parasitol*, **76:** 412–23.

Beck JT, Ullman B, 1991, Genetic analysis of folate transport and metabolism in *Leishmania donovani*, *Biochemical Protozoology*, eds Coombs GH, North MJ, Taylor and Francis, London, 554–9.

Beliaev AE, Lysenko AJ, 1987, Measurements of endemicity of zoonotic cutaneous leishmaniasis, *Écologie des Leishmanioses*, CNRS, Paris, 271–8.

Ben Ismail R, 1994, Rapport de fonctionnement: Laboratoire d'Epidemiologie et d'Ecologie Medicale, *Arch Inst Pasteur Tunis*, **71:** 86–107.

Blackwell JM, 1992, Leishmaniasis epidemiology: all down to the DNA, *Parasitology*, **104:** S19–S34.

Bradley DJ, 1987, Genetics of susceptibility and resistance in the vertebrate host, *The Leishmaniases*, vol 2, eds Peters W, Killick-Kendrick R, Academic Press, London, 551–81.

Bryceson A, 1987a, Splenic aspiration procedure as performed at the Clinical Research Centre, Nairobi, 1982, *The Leishmaniases*, vol 2, eds Peters W, Killick-Kendrick R, Academic Press, London, 728–9.

Bryceson A, 1987b, Therapy in man, *The Leishmaniases*, vol 2,

eds Peters W, Killick-Kendrick R, Academic Press, London, 847–907.

Chang K–P, Chauduri G, Fong D, 1990, Molecular determinants of *Leishmania* virulence, *Annu Rev Microbiol*, **44:** 499–529.

Charlab R, Ribeiro JMC, 1993, Cytostatic effect of *Lutzomyia longipalpis* salivary gland homogenates on *Leishmania* parasites, *Am J Trop Med Hyg*, **48:** 831–8.

Dereure J, Reyes J et al., 1995, Visceral leishmaniasis in HIV-infected patients in the south of France, *Bull W H O*, **73:** 245–46.

Descoteaux A, Turco SJ, 1993, The lipophosphoglycan of *Leishmania* and macrophage protein kinase C, *Parasitol Today*, **9:** 468–71.

Desjeux P, 1991, Information on the epidemiology and control of the leishmaniases by country and territory, Report number WHO/Leish/91.30, 47 pp.

El Hag IA, Hashim FA, 1994, Liver morphology and function in visceral leishmaniasis (kala-azar), *J Clin Pathol*, **47:** 547–51.

El Safi SH, Peters W, Evans D, 1988, Current situation with regard to leishmaniasis in Sudan with particular reference to the recent outbreak of cutaneous leishmaniasis in Khartoum, *Research on Control Strategies for the Leishmaniases. Proceedings of an International Workshop, Ottawa, Canada, 1–4 June 1987*, I.D.R.C. Ottawa, 60–77.

Etges R, Bouvier J, 1991, The promastigote surface proteinase of *Leishmania*, *Biochemical Protozoology*, eds Coombs GH, North MJ, Taylor and Francis, London, 221–33.

Garcia-del Portillo F, Finlay BB, 1995, The varied lifestyles of intracellular pathogens within eukaryotic vacuolar compartments, *Trends Microbiol*, **3:** 373–80.

Ghosh KN, Bhattacharya A, 1991, Breeding places of Phlebotomus argentipes in West Bengal, India, *Parassitologia*, **33 supplement:** 267–72.

Ghosh MK, Nandy A et al., 1995, Subpopulations of T lymphocytes in the peripheral blood, dermal lesions and lymph nodes of post kala-azar dermal leishmaniasis patients, *Scand J Immunol*, 11–17.

Gradoni L, Scalone A, Gramiccia M, 1993, HIV–*Leishmania* coinfections in Italy: serological data as an indication of the sequence of acquisition of the two infections, *Trans R Soc Trop Med Hyg*, **87:** 94–6.

Graham SV, 1995, Mechanisms of stage-regulated gene expression in Kinetoplastida, *Parasitol Today*, **11:** 217–23.

Griffiths WAD, 1987, Old World cutaneous leishmaniasis, *The Leishmaniases*, vol 2, eds Peters W, Killick-Kendrick R, Academic Press, London, 617–36.

Guan Lee-Ren, 1991, Current status of kala-azar and vector control in China, *Bull W H O*, **69:** 595–601.

Haughan PA, Goad LJ, 1991, Lipid biochemistry of trypanosomatids, *Biochemical Protozoology*, eds Coombs GH and North MJ, Taylor and Francis, London, 312–28.

Ilg T, Stierhof Y-D et al., 1994, Characterization of phosphoglycan-containing secretory products of *Leishmania*, *Parasitology*, **108:** S63–S71.

Kamhawi S, Arbagi A et al., 1993, Environmental manipulation in the control of a zoonotic cutaneous leishmaniasis focus, *Arch Inst Pasteur Tunis*, **70:** 383–90.

Kar K, 1995, Serodiagnosis of leishmaniasis, *Crit Rev Microbiol*, **21:** 123–52.

Kaye PM, 1995, Costimulation and the regulation of antimicrobial immunity, *Immunol Today*, **16:** 423–7.

Kemp M, Kurtzhals JA et al., 1993, Interferon gamma and interleukin 4 in human *Leishmania donovani* infection, *Immunol Cell Biol*, **71:** 583–7.

Kemp M, Kurtzhals JA et al., 1994, Dichotomy in the human CD4+ T-cell response to *Leishmania* infection, *APMIS*, **102:** 81–8.

Killick-Kendrick, R, 1990a, The life-cycle of *Leishmania* in the sandfly with special reference to the form infective to the vertebrate host, *Ann Parasitol Hum Comp*, **65, Suppl.1:** 37–42.

Killick–Kendrick R, 1990b, Phlebotomine vectors of the leishmaniases: a review, *Med Vet Entomol*, **4:** 1–24.

Kurtzhals JA, Kemp M et al., 1995, Interleukin 4 and interferon gamma production by *Leishmania*-stimulated peripheral blood mononuclear cells from non-exposed individuals, *Scand J Immunol*, **41:** 343–9.

Lainson R, Shaw JJ, 1987, Evolution, classification and geographical distribution, *The Leishmaniases*, vol 1, eds Peters W, Killick-Kendrick R, Academic Press, London, 1–120.

Lang T, Warburg A et al., 1991, Transmission and scanning EM-immunogold labeling of *Leishmania major* lipophosphoglycan in the sandfly *Phlebotomus papatasi*, *Eur Journal Cell Biol*, **55:** 362–72.

Liew FY, Cox FEG, 1991, Nonspecific defence mechanisms: the role of nitric oxide, *Parasitol Today*, **7:** A17–A21.

Liew FY, O'Donnell CA, 1993, Immunology of leishmaniasis, *Adv Parasitol*, **32:** 161–259.

Lighthall GK, Giannini SH, 1992, The chromosomes of *Leishmania*, *Parasitol Today*, **8:** 192–9.

Magill AJ, Grogl M et al., 1993, Viscerotropic leishmaniasis caused by *Leishmania tropica* in veterans of Operation Desert Storm, *N Engl J Med*, **328:** 1383–7.

Magill AJ, Grogl M et al., 1994, Visceral leishmaniasis due to *L. tropica* in a veteran of Operation Desert Storm who presented two years after leaving Saudi Arabia, *Clin Infect Dis*, **19:** 805–6.

Manson-Bahr PEC, 1987, Diagnosis, *The Leishmaniases*, vol 2, eds Peters W, Killick-Kendrick R, Academic Press, London, 703–29.

Maroli M, Majori G, 1991, Permethrin impregnated curtains against phlebotomine sandflies: laboratory studies, *Parassitologia*, **33 Supplement:** 399–404.

Marr JJ, 1991, Purine metabolism in parasitic protozoa and its relationship to chemotherapy, *Biochemical Protozoology*, Taylor and Francis, London, 524–36.

Marty P, Le Fichoux et al., 1994, Human visceral leishmaniasis in Alpes Maritimes, France: epidemiological characteristics for the period 1985–1992, *Trans R Soc Trop Med Hyg*, **88:** 33–4.

Mauel J, Behin R, 1987, Immunity: clinical and experimental, *The Leishmaniases*, vol 2, eds Peters W, Killick–Kendrick R, Academic Press, London, 731–91.

Medrano FJ, Hernandez-Quero J et al., 1992, Visceral leishmaniasis in HIV 1 infected individuals: a common opportunistic infection in Spain?, *AIDS*, **6:** 1499–1503.

Mehbratu Y, Lawyer P et al., 1989, Visceral leishmaniasis unresponsive to Pentostam caused by *Leishmania tropica* in Kenya, *Am J Trop Med Hyg*, **41:** 289–94.

Meredith SE, Kroon NC et al., 1995, Leish–KIT, a stable direct agglutination test based on freeze-dried antigen for serodiagnosis of visceral leishmaniasis, *J Clin Microbiol*, **33:** 1742–5.

Milon G, Del Giudice G, Louis JA, 1995, Immunobiology of experimental cutaneous leishmaniasis, *Parasitol Today*, **11:** 244–7.

Moll H, 1993, Epidermal Langerhans cells are critical for immunoregulation of cutaneous leishmaniasis, *Immunol Today*, **14:** 383–7.

Molyneux DH, Ashford RW, 1983, *The Biology of* Trypanosoma *and* Leishmania *Parasites of Man and Domestic Animals*, Taylor and Francis, London, 1–294.

Molyneux DH, Jeffries D, 1986, Feeding behaviour of pathogen-infected vectors, *Parasitology*, **92:** 721–36.

Molyneux DH, Killick-Kendrick R, 1987, Morphology, ultrastructure and life cycles, *The Leishmaniases*, vol 1, eds Peters W, Killick-Kendrick R, Academic Press, London, 121–76.

Momen H, Pacheco RS et al., 1993, Molecular evidence for the importation of Old World *Leishmania* into the Americas, *Biol Res*, **26:** 249–55.

Nadim A, 1988, Leishmanization in the Islamic Republic of Iran, *Research on Control Strategies for the Leishmaniases. Proceedings of an International Workshop, Ottawa, Canada, 1–4 June 1987*, IDRC, Ottawa, 336–339.

Opperdoes FR, 1991, Glycosomes, *Biochemical Protozoology*, eds Coombs GH, North MJ, Taylor and Francis, London, 134–44.

Peters BS, Fish D et al., 1990, Visceral leishmaniasis in HIV infection and AIDS: clinical features and response to therapy, *Q J Med*, **77:** 1101–11.

Pharoah PD, Ponnighaus JM et al., 1993, Two cases of cutaneous leishmaniasis in Malawi, *Trans R Soc Trop Med Hyg*, **87:** 668–70.

Pimenta PFP, Turco SJ et al., 1992, Stage-specific adhesion of *Leishmania* promastigotes to the sandfly midgut, *Science*, **256:** 1812–15.

Pimenta PFP, Saraiva EMB et al., 1994, Evidence that the vectorial competence of phlebotomine sandflies for different species of *Leishmania* is controlled by structural polymorphisms in the surface lipophosphoglycan, *Proc Natl Acad Sci USA*, **91:** 9155–9.

Pratlong F, Rioux JA et al., 1991, *Leishmania tropica* in Morocco IV. Intrafocal enzyme diversity, *Ann Parasitol Hum Comp*, **66:** 100–104.

Pratlong F, Dedet JP et al., 1995, *Leishmania*-human immuno-deficiency virus coinfection in the Mediterranean basin: isoenzymatic characterization of 100 isolates of the *Leishmania infantum* complex, *J Infect Dis*, **172:** 323–7.

Rab MA, Evans DA, 1995, *Leishmania infantum* infection in the Himalayas, *Trans R Soc Trop Med Hyg*, **89:** 27–32.

Rees PH, Kager PA, 1987, Visceral leishmaniasis and post-kala-azar dermal leishmaniasis, *The Leishmaniases*, vol 2, eds Peters W, Killick-Kendrick R, Academic Press, London, 583–615.

Ridley DS, 1987, Pathology, *The Leishmaniases*, vol 2, eds Peters W, Killick-Kendrick, Academic Press, London, 665–701.

Rioux JA, Petter F et al., 1982, *Meriones shawi* reservoir de *Leishmania major* dans le sud maroccain, *C R Acad Sci*, **294:** 515–17.

Rioux JA, Lanotte G et al., 1990, Taxonomy of *Leishmania*. Use of isoenzymes. Suggestions for a new classification, *Ann Parasitol Hum Comp*, **65:** 111–25.

Rogers L, 1908, *Fevers in the Tropics*, Oxford University Press, London, 343pp.

Sacks, DL, Saraiva EM et al., 1994, The role of lipophosphoglycan of Leishmania in vector competence, *Parasitology*, **108:** S55–S62.

Sacks DL, Kenney RT et al., 1995, Indian kala azar caused by *Leishmania tropica*, *Lancet*, **345:** 959–61.

Sang DK, Pratlong F, Ashford RW, 1992, The identity of *Leishmania tropica* in Kenya, *Trans R Soc Trop Med Hyg*, **86:** 621–2.

Sanyal RK, 1985, Leishmaniasis in the Indian sub-continent, *Leishmaniasis*, eds Chang KP, Bray RS, Elsevier, Amsterdam, 443–67.

Sati MH, 1962, Early phases of an outbreak of kala azar in the southern Fung, *Sudan Med J*, **1:** 98–111.

Schlein Y, 1993, *Leishmania* and sandflies: interactions in the life cycle and transmission, *Parasitol Today*, **9:** 255–8.

Schlein Y, Jacobson RL, 1994a, Haemoglobin inhibits the development of infective promastigotes and chitinase secretion in *Leishmania major* cultures, *Parasitology*, **109:** 23–8.

Schlein Y, Jacobson RL, 1994b, Mortality of *Leishmania major* in *Phlebotomus papatasi* caused by plant feeding of sandflies, *Am J Trop Med Hyg*, **50:** 20–7.

Schlein Y, Jacobson RL, Messer G, 1992, *Leishmania* infections damage the feeding mechanism of the sandfly vector and implement parasite transmission by bite, *Proc Natl Acad Sci USA*, **89:** 9944–8.

Schlein Y, Jacobson RL, Shlomai J, 1991, Chitinase secreted by *Leishmania* functions in the sandfly vector, *Proc R Soc London (Ser B)*, **245:** 121–6.

Seaman J, Ashford RW et al., 1992, Visceral leishmaniasis in southern Sudan: status of healthy villagers in epidemic conditions, *Ann Trop Med Parasitol*, **86:** 481–6.

Seaman J, Pryce D et al., 1993, Epidemic visceral leishmaniasis in Sudan: a randomised trial of aminosidine plus sodium stibogluconate versus sodium stibogluconate alone, *J Infect Dis*, **168:** 715–20.

Seiwert SD, 1995, The ins and outs of editing RNA in kinetoplastids, *Parasitol Today*, **11:** 362–8.

Shlomai J, 1994, The assembly of kinetoplast DNA, *Parasitol Today*, **10:** 341–6.

Solbach W, Laskay T, 1995, *Leishmania major* infection: the overture, *Parasitol Today*, **11:** 394–7.

Strelkova MV, Eliseev LN et al., 1993, The isoenzyme identification of *Leishmania* isolates taken from great gerbils, sandflies and human patients in foci of zoonotic cutaneous leishmaniasis in Turkmenistan, *Med Parazitol Moscow*, **1993:** 34–37.

Teklemariam S, Hiwot AG et al., 1994, Aminosidine and its combination with sodium stibogluconate in the treatment of diffuse cutaneous leishmaniasis caused by *Leishmania aethiopica*, *Trans R Soc Trop Med Hyg*, **88:** 334–9.

ter Kuile, BH, 1993, Glucose and proline transport in kinetoplastids, *Parasitol Today*, **9:** 206–10.

Tibayrenc M, Kjellberg F, Ayala FJ, 1990, A clonal theory of parasitic protozoa: The population structures of *Entamoeba, Giardia, Leishmania, Naegleria, Plasmodium, Trichomonas,* and *Trypanosoma* and their medical and taxonomical consequences, *Proc Natl Acad Sci USA*, **87:** 2414–18.

Titus RG, Ribeiro JMC, 1990, The role of vector saliva in transmission of arthropod–borne disease, *Parasitol Today*, **6:** 157–60.

Turco SJ, Descoteaux A, 1992, The lipophosphoglycan of *Leishmania* parasites, *Annu Rev Microbiol*, **46:** 65–94.

Vickerman K, Tetley L, 1990, Flagellar surfaces of parasitic protozoa and their role in attachment, *Ciliary and Flagellar Membranes*, ed Bloodgood RA, Plenum, New York and London, 267–304.

Vidor E, Dereuse J et al., 1991, Le chancre d'inoculation dans la leishmaniose canine à *Leishmania infantum*. Etude d'une cohorte en région cérenole, *Prat Méd Chir Animal Compagnie*, **26:** 133–7.

Walsh JA, Warren KS, 1979, Selective primary health care. An interim strategy for disease control in developing countries, *N Engl J Med*, **301:** 967–74.

Walters LL, 1993, *Leishmania* differentiation in natural and unnatural sand fly hosts, *J Euk Microbiol*, **40:** 196–206.

Wang Chao-Tsung, 1985, Leishmaniasis in China: epidemiology and control programme, *Leishmaniasis*, eds Chang KP, Bray RS, Elsevier, Amsterdam, 469–78.

Webster P, Russell DG, 1993, The flagellar pocket of trypanosomatids, *Parasitol Today*, **9:** 201–206.

W H O, 1990, Control of the Leishmaniases, *W H O Tech Rep Ser*, **793:** 158.

W H O, 1995, *WHO Model Prescribing Information. Drugs Used in Parasitic Diseases*, 2nd edn, W H O, Geneva, 1–146.

Zijlstra EE, El Hassan AM et al., 1994, Endemic kala azar in eastern Sudan: a longitudinal study on the incidence of clinical and subclinical infection and post kala azar dermal leishmaniasis, *Am J Trop Med Hyg*, **51:** 826–36.

Zilberstein D, Shapira M, 1994, The role of pH and temperature in the development of Leishmania parasites, *Annu Rev Microbiol*, **48:** 449–70.

Chapter 13

New World leishmaniasis – the neotropical *Leishmania* species

R Lainson and J J Shaw

1 INTRODUCTION

Neotropical cutaneous leishmaniasis (NCL) seems to be of great antiquity. Pottery from Peru and Ecuador, dated c. AD 400–900, commonly depicted human faces with mutilations that are remarkably similar to those caused by present day cutaneous and mucosal leishmaniasis (Fig. 13.1) and, at the time of the 'conquistadores', Spanish historians wrote about ugly facial lesions that frequently afflicted the local Amerindians.

The earliest traceable clinical description of the disease is probably that of a certain Dr. L. Villar who, in 1859, wrote

'the disease (Peruvian 'uta') is very like the Aleppo button'

(i.e. 'oriental sore' due to *Leishmania tropica*) (vide Matta 1918). The first suspicions that phlebotomine sandflies might be involved in the transmission of NCL seem to have been those of Cosme Bueno who, in 1764, implicated these insects in 'uta' in endemic areas; uta is caused by *L. (Viannia) peruviana* in the Peruvian highlands (vide Herrer and Christensen 1975). Final proof that NCL was due to infection with *Leishmania* was to await publications by Lindenberg (1909) and Carini and Paranhos (1909), who independently demonstrated 'Leishman-Donovan bodies' in the skin lesions of patients from the State of São Paulo, Brazil. It was left to another Brazilian, Gaspar Vianna (1911) to give the name of *Leishmania brazilienses* to the parasite, later corrected to *L. braziliensis* by Matta (1916).

It is quite extraordinary that until 1972 all cases of NCL in Brazil and a number of neighbouring coun-

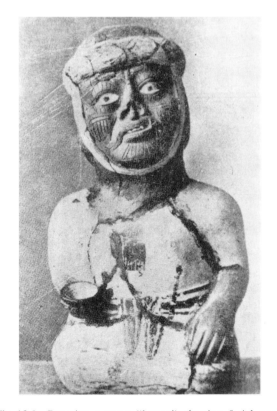

Fig. 13.1 Peruvian pottery ('huaco') showing facial mutilations thought to represent mucosal leishmaniasis. (From Pessôa and Barretto 1948).

tries were attributed solely to this parasite, although specific species names were attributed in different regions: Velez (1913) had given the name of *L. peruviana* to the causative agent of Peruvian 'uta'; Biagi

(1953) had named the parasite of Mexican 'chiclero's ulcer' as *L. tropica mexicana,* emended to *L. mexicana* by Garnham (1962); and Floch (1954) considered 'pianbois' in French Guyana to be due to *L. tropica guyanensis,* later emended to *L. braziliensis guyanensis* by the Brazilian parasitologist Pessôa (1961). During the past 30 years intensive ecological and epidemiological studies in the Americas have revolutionized previous ideas regarding the aetiology of NCL and the classification of its causative parasites. No less than 20 species of *Leishmania* are now recognized within the Neotropical Region, of which 14 are known to cause either cutaneous or mucocutaneous leishmaniasis in humans, or both. There is little doubt that others remain to be discovered and described, particularly in the rich sandfly and mammalian faunas of the great South American forests.

Cutaneous leishmaniasis is very widespread in Latin America; the only 2 countries that seem to be free of the disease are Chile and Uruguay: cases have even been recorded in the extreme south of the USA, in Texas. A reliable figure for its incidence is virtually impossible to obtain: it is not a notifiable disease in most of the countries where it occurs. Most of these countries also have poor facilities for unequivocal diagnosis so heavy reliance is placed on clinical aspects, which are often misleading. In Costa Rica, a small country, but with very good communications and medical assistance, the impressive figure has been given of >2000 cases a year in a population of 2 000 000 (Walton 1987). In Brazil, the Ministry of Health reported an increase in the number of cases from 2 856 in 1977 to 4 821 in 1982, (Walton 1987). Lacerda (1994) suggested the considerably higher figure of 154 103 recorded cases between the years 1980 and 1990, with an incidence of c. 5 persons in 1000 infected between the years 1980 and 1984, rising to 25 per 1000 during 1987–1990.

In all known instances NCL is a zoonosis: that is, the causative parasites are primarily those of wild animals. When the various sandfly vectors also feed on humans there may be transmission of a number of species of *Leishmania*; in this 'unnatural' host they will usually provoke an intense reaction and the eventual development of a skin lesion at the site of the bite. Some 7–10 days later a tiny papule appears which, although usually painless, may itch considerably. In most cases the papule eventually ulcerates, producing a steadily growing and crater-like lesion with a characteristically inflamed, elevated border (Fig. 13.2). A lesion may remain single, but in some cases infected macrophages may transport the parasites to other parts of the body and establish secondary lesions. One parasite in particular, *L. (V.) braziliensis,* tends to produce such metastatic lesions in the nasal, pharyngeal and laryngeal mucosae. These may arise within a few months of the original skin lesion, or years later when the patient has supposedly been cured of his initial infection; they may be extremely mutilating (Figs. 13.3, 13.4).

Other neotropical *Leishmania* species may produce an even more serious and incurable condition in individuals who fail to mount a fully functional cell-

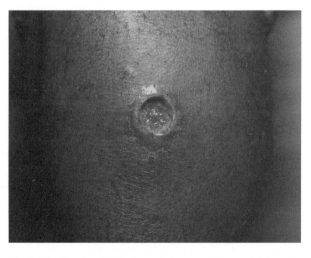

Fig. 13.2   Simple skin lesion of the arm, due to *Leishmania (Viannia) braziliensis.* Pará, Brazil. See Plate 13.2.

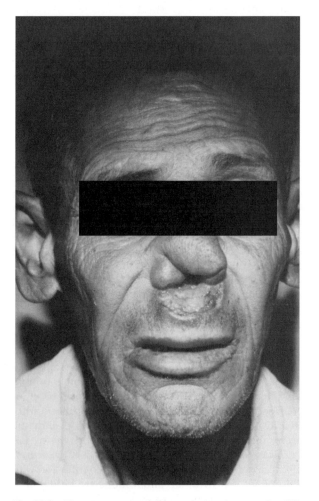

Fig. 13.3   Mucocutaneous leishmaniasis, due to *L. (V.) braziliensis.* Pará, Brazil. See Plate 13.3.

mediated immune reaction against the parasite. Such patients, who develop large numbers of nodular lesions scattered over almost the whole skin surface (Figs 13.5, 13.6), have been referred to as cases of 'diffuse cutaneous leishmaniasis' (DCL). This is a mis-

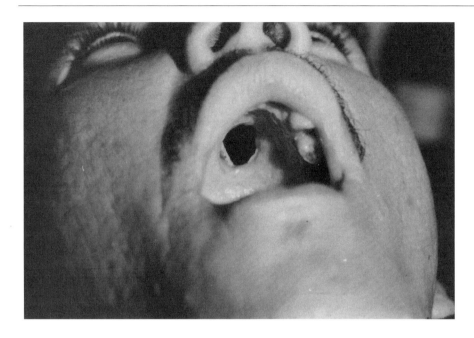

Fig. 13.4 Destruction of the palate, due to *L. (V.) braziliensis*. Pará, Brazil. See Plate 13.4.

leading term as other perfectly curable cases of cutaneous leishmaniasis in immunologically competent patients may have numerous lesions scattered over the body surface (Fig. 13.7 and see under *L. (V.) guyanensis*, p. 254); the term 'anergic diffuse cutaneous leishmaniasis' (ADCL) is more appropriate. In the Americas this condition has been found associated only with infection by members of the *mexicana* complex, e.g. *L. (Leishmania) mexicana*, *L. (L.) pifanoi* and *L. (L.) amazonensis*. In the Old World, another member of the subgenus *Leishmania*, *L. (L.) aethiopica*, causes a similar incurable disease in immunologically incompetent patients (see Chapter 12).

The fact that a number of *Leishmania* species cause disease in humans in the neotropics is reflected in variations in chemotherapeutic responses. Thus, drugs that work well in one region may not be so efficient in another because the species of the parasite infecting the patients are different. In Guatemala, for example, individuals infected with *L. (L.) mexicana* responded to treatment with ketoconazole better than those infected with *L. (V.) braziliensis* s.l., but the reverse applied when patients were treated with sodium stibogluconate (Navin et al. 1992).

Unlike humans, the natural sylvatic hosts of the various neotropical *Leishmania* species rarely suffer disease from the infection, which is usually of a benign, inapparent nature. Under certain circumstances (see *L. (V.) braziliensis*, p. 252) domestic animals such as dogs, mules and horses may be found with extensive skin ulcers due to *Leishmania*: an indication that they, like humans, are unnatural and unaccustomed hosts.

The known history of American visceral leishmaniasis (AVL), due to *L. (L.) chagasi*, is comparatively short compared with that of the Old World (Chapter 12). The first record was probably that of Migone (1913), who saw 'corpuscles', which he was convinced were amastigotes of *Leishmania*, in the blood of a sick man in Paraguay. The patient's symptoms were highly indicative of visceral leishmaniasis and, failing to respond to antimalarial treatment, he died. Prior to his illness the man had been working on the construction of the São Paulo–Corumbá railway in Brazil, where he most probably became infected. The first undoubted cases to be registered in Latin America were documented by Mazza and Cornejo (1926) in 2 Argentinian children.

In 1934, Penna used the viscerotome to examine liver samples from patients suspected to have died from yellow fever in various parts of Brazil. He diagnosed 41 of them as being cases of visceral leishmaniasis, the largest number coming from the north-east of that country. Sporadic cases began to be recorded in Bolivia, Colombia, Guatemala, Paraguay and El Salvador, but the full importance of the disease as a public health problem was not realized until as recently as 1953, when a dramatic outbreak was estimated to have been responsible for >100 deaths in the small country town of Sobral, in the State of Ceará, north-east Brazil (Deane 1956). Clearly, the history of AVL goes back much further than this (see pages 246 and 248) and deaths from this highly lethal infection must have long been attributed to other causes, including malaria and yellow fever. To this day AVL remains second in importance only to malaria among the Latin American tropical diseases, with the very conservative number of over 6000 cases recorded in Brazil alone, up to 1980 (Deane and Grimaldi 1985).

Although a wide variety of *Leishmania* species have been recorded in humans, the prevalence of each of these will clearly depend on just how anthropophilic their respective sandfly vectors are. Thus, by far the largest proportion of NCL cases in Brazil are due to *L. (V.) braziliensis* and *L. (V.) guyanensis*, both of which have sandfly vectors that feed avidly on humans. On the other hand, human infection with *L. (V.) lainsoni* and *L. (V.) naiffi* is relatively rare, as their vectors are disinclined to bite humans. Some neotropical *Leishmania* species, like *L. (L.) hertigi* and *L. (L.) deanei* of porcupines, are unknown in humans, possibly due to

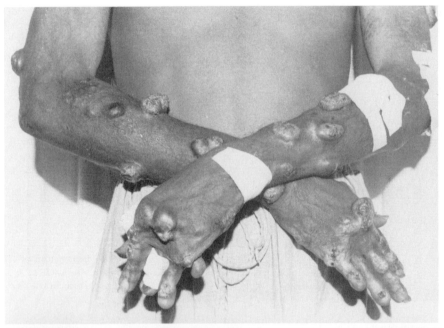

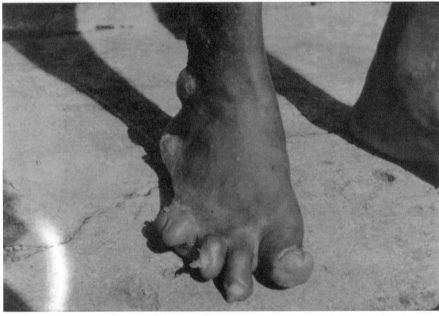

Fig. 13.5–6 Anergic diffuse cutaneous leishmaniasis (ADCL) due to *L. (L.) amazonensis*. Note the amputation of some fingers (Fig. 13.5) and toes (Fig. 13.6), simulating lepromatous leprosy, with which disease ADCL is often confused. Pará, Brazil. (Fig. 13.5 from Lainson 1982b).

their inability to survive in human tissues, but more probably because their sandfly vectors never feed on humans.

It is likely that all neotropical *Leishmania* species once shared a sylvatic ecology, as is still the case in the remaining areas of extensive primary and secondary forest in the Amazon Region. Following the Iberian colonization and ensuing destruction of the forests, some phlebotomine sandfly species adapted to a peridomestic habitat. The persistence of cutaneous leishmaniasis in such ecologically disturbed, although still essentially rural areas, has been taken to indicate the evolution of a secondary, peridomestic transmission of the causative parasite; the occurrence of leishmanial skin lesions in village dogs, mules and horses suggests that such domestic animals might have now become secondary reservoir hosts. Their development of

extensive skin lesions tends to suggest, however, that, like humans, these animals still remain unnatural and unaccustomed 'victim' hosts. Firm evidence is required to show that infected humans, dogs and equines are capable of infecting sandflies fed upon them and maintaining the parasite in the absence of another source of infection in wild animals, still existing in nearby, surviving pockets of woodland.

Although *Lutzomyia longipalpis*, the vector of AVL, is better known as a peridomestic or intra-domiciliary sandfly, its origin is sylvatic (Lainson 1989, Lainson et al. 1990a). In Amazonian Brazil, for example, it has been captured in primary rain forest far from human habitation and when crude roads are cut through such forest, newly constructed houses and animal sheds are soon invaded by this insect. It follows that whether the source of *L. (L.) chagasi* be local foxes (*Cerdocyon*

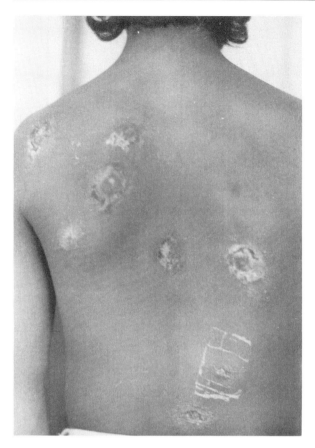

Fig. 13.7 Multiple skin lesions due to *L. (V.) guyanensis.* Similar lesions were present on this man's legs, arms and face. Pará, Brazil (from Lainson 1982b).

thous), in which the infection rate may be >50%, or infected dogs brought to the area from distant endemic foci of AVL, transmission of the parasite will ensue and a new focus of the canine and human disease will be established.

Studies on the ecology of the New World leishmanial parasites have strongly suggested the existence of environmental barriers that limit the different species of *Leishmania* to specific sandfly species that transmit to certain mammalian hosts in distinct ecotopes. Extreme care and considerable field research is needed, therefore, before conclusions can be reached as to the principal sandfly vectors of the different parasites. The mere presence of a *Leishmania* in a specimen of a given sandfly species does not necessarily mean that this insect is the vector of that parasite. Before such a conclusion can be reached the organism must be found with frequency in that particular sandfly and must show abundant proliferation in the alimentary tract, with migration to the foregut and mouthparts. Although transmission may be achieved by 2 different but very closely related sandflies, it remains unlikely that this capacity extends to those of different genera or subgenera in nature. Ideally, a definite association with the wild mammalian host should be shown to exist and, if the parasite is a cause of human leishmaniasis, the fly must be shown to bite humans.

Similarly, the efficiency of a given mammal in main-taining a *Leishmania* species in nature and in serving as a source of infection for the sandfly vector must be considered. Determining a significant infection rate in the mammalian host and providing experimental proof that the sandfly vector can be infected by feeding on it are prerequisites in labelling the animal as a reservoir host.

A number of the neotropical *Leishmania* species were first described in their wild mammalian or sandfly hosts, considerable time elapsing before they were incriminated as a cause of human leishmaniasis. For this reason the present chapter discusses all the known New World species, regardless of the fact that some have yet to be found in humans. Chapter 12 deals with the systematic position of the genus *Leishmania*, morphology and development of the organism in the mammalian and sandfly hosts, the application of biochemistry and molecular biology to identification of the different species of the parasite, genetics and immunology, clinical features and the treatment of human cutaneous and visceral leishmaniasis. Many features of these topics are common to both Old World and New World leishmanial parasites and the present chapter will only discuss those that seem to be peculiar to the American leishmaniases and their causative agents. Lengthy discussions on the evolution, ecology, epidemiology and classification of the parasites have been given elsewhere (Lainson and Shaw 1979, 1987, Lainson 1983, Lainson et al. 1994, Shaw and Lainson 1987, Shaw 1994). Reviews on the history of the neotropical leishmaniases have also been dealt with in other publications (Lainson and Shaw 1992, Lainson 1996). For methods in the laboratory diagnosis of these diseases, see Lainson and Shaw (1981).

2 CLASSIFICATION OF THE RECOGNIZED NEOTROPICAL *LEISHMANIA* SPECIES

The genus *Leishmania* has been subdivided into 2 subgenera, as follows:

2.1 The subgenus *Leishmania* Saf'yanova 1982

This subgenus possesses the characteristics of the genus (see Chapter 12). The life-cycle in the natural sandfly vector is limited to the midgut and foregut of the alimentary tract. Species occur in both the Old World and the New World (TYPE SPECIES *Leishmania (Leishmania) donovani* (Laveran and Mesnil 1903) Ross 1903, of the Old World). The recognized neotropical species are: (1) *Leishmania (Leishmania) chagasi** Cunha and Chagas 1937; (2) *L. (L.) enriettii* Muniz and Medina 1948; (3) *L. (L.) mexicana** Biagi 1953 *emend* Garnham 1962; (4) *L. (L.) pifanoi** Medina and Romero 1959 *emend* Medina and Romero 1962; (5) *L. (L.) hertigi* Herrer 1971; (6) *L. (L.) amazonensis** Lainson and Shaw 1972; (7) *L. (L.) deanei* Lainson and Shaw 1977; (8) *L. (L.) aristidesi* Lainson and Shaw 1979; (9) *L. (L.) garnhami** Scorza et al. 1979; (10) *L. (L.) venezuelensis** Bonfante-Garrido 1980; (11) *L. (L.) forattinii* Yoshida et al. 1993.

*Recorded from humans. For distribution, see Table 13.1.

2.2 The subgenus *Viannia* Lainson and Shaw 1987

This subgenus possesses the characteristics of the genus (see Chapter 12). The developmental cycle in the natural sandfly vector includes a prolific and prolonged phase of division of rounded or ovoid paramastigotes and promastigotes attached to the wall of the hindgut (pylorus and ileum, see Fig. 13.8) by flagellar hemidesmosomes, followed by migration of free promastigotes to the midgut and foregut. Members of this subgenus are known only in the Neotropical Region and the recognized species are as follows:

(1) *Leishmania (Viannia) braziliensis** Vianna 1911 *emend* Matta 1916. TYPE SPECIES; (2) *L. (V.) peruviana** Velez 1913; (3) *L. (V.) guyanensis** Floch 1954; (4) *L. (V.) panamensis** Lainson and Shaw 1972; (5) *L. (V.) lainsoni** Silveira et al. 1987; (6) *L. (V.) shawi** Lainson *et al.* 1989; (7) *L. (V.) naiffi** Lainson and Shaw 1989; (8) *L. (V.) colombiensis** Kreutzer et al. 1991; (9) *L. (V.) equatorensis* Grimaldi et al. 1992.

*Recorded from humans. For distribution, see Table 13.1.

2.3 Species within the subgenus *Leishmania* Saf'yanova 1982

LEISHMANIA (LEISHMANIA) CHAGASI CUNHA AND CHAGAS 1937

Known geographical distribution

Distribution has been noted throughout most of the Latin American continent: Argentina, Bolivia, Brazil, Colombia, Ecuador, Paraguay, Surinam, Venezuela, Guatemala, Guadeloupe, Honduras, Martinique, Mexico and El Salvador.

Known mammalian hosts

Known mammalian hosts include humans and the domestic dog, *Canis familiaris*. Among wild animals the foxes *Lycalopex vetulus* and *Cerdocyon thous* seem to be important natural reservoirs in north-east and north of Brazil (States of Ceará and Pará), respectively (Deane 1956, Lainson et al. 1987).There are reports of isolates of *L. (L.) chagasi* from domestic rats in Honduras (Walton, personal communication) and opossums of the genus *Didelphis* in Bahia, north-east Brazil (Sherlock et al. 1984) and Colombia (Corredor et al. 1989, Travi et al. 1994). Intensive study of these animals in foci of American visceral leishmaniasis in Amazonian Brazil has so far failed to incriminate them as hosts of *L. (L.) chagasi* (Lainson et al. 1987).

Recorded sandfly hosts

Lutzomyia (Lutzomyia) longipalpis is the vector of *L. (L.) chagasi* throughout its geographic range (Deane and Grimaldi 1985, Lainson 1989) and the parasite has been transmitted experimentally by the bite of this sandfly, using both laboratory-infected and naturally-infected flies (Lainson et al. 1977, 1985). There is, however, strong evidence indicating that *Lu. longipalpis* represents a species complex of at least 2 taxa (Ward et al. 1988), based on slight morphological differences (males with pale spots on tergites 3 and 4, versus others with a similar spotted pheromonal gland, on only the 4th tergum). Attempts to cross-breed the 2 forms failed, adding strong support to this suggestion (Ward et al. 1983).

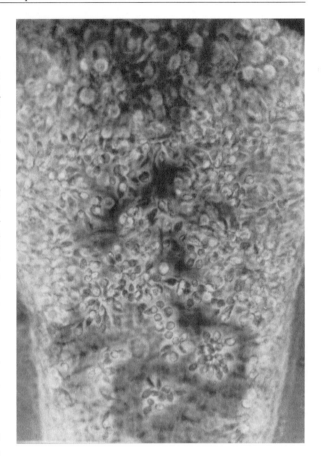

Fig. 13.8 The pylorus ('hindgut triangle') of a sandfly-infected with *L. (V.) braziliensis*. Prolific division of rounded or ovoid promastigotes and paramastigotes attached by flagellar hemidesmosomes to the gut wall, a characteristic of *Leishmania* species within the subgenus *Viannia*.

In one particular region endemic for visceral leishmaniasis, in the Córdoba Department of Colombia, 87% of the sandflies captured were found to be *Lutzomyia evansi* and one fly was infected with *L. (L.) chagasi* (Travi et al. 1990). The apparent absence of *Lu. longipalpis* in the area led to the suggestion that *Lu. evansi* may be an alternative vector of *L. (L.) chagasi* and, on purely circumstantial evidence, the same suggestion has been made in Costa Rica and Venezuela. Further long-term investigations are clearly needed to substantiate these claims.

Disease caused by the parasite in humans

The parasite causes visceral leishmaniasis, commonly with a fatal outcome unless treated (see Chapter 12). On rare occasions the visceral disease may be preceded by a cutaneous lesion. Common names include 'kala-azar' or 'calazar' but it is more appropriate to reserve these terms for Indian visceral leishmaniasis and to use the name American visceral leishmaniasis (AVL).

Opinions are divided as to whether *L. (L.) chagasi* is indigenous to the Americas or whether AVL is due to *L. (L.) infantum* which was introduced into the New World by immigrants from the Iberian peninsula in post-Columbian times (probably via infected dogs). Points in favour of the first hypothesis and retention of the name *L. (L.) chagasi* are as follows:

Table 13.1 A country by country list of the neotropical *Leishmania* species recorded in man and their resultant pathologies

Country	Species	Disease forms recorded[g]
Argentina	*L.(L.) chagasi*	VL
	L.(V.) braziliensis s.l.	CL
Belize	*L.(L.) mexicana*	CL
	L.(V.) braziliensis s.l.	CL
Bolivia	*L.(L.) amazonensis*	CL, ADCL
	L.(L.) chagasi	VL
	L.(L.) sp.	CL
	L.(V.) braziliensis s.l.	CL, MCL
Brazil	*L.(L.) amazonensis*	CL, ADCL, MCL[h], VL[i]
	L.(L.) chagasi	VL, (CL[j])
	L.(L.) sp.	CL[k]
	L.(V.) braziliensis	CL, MCL
	L.(V.) guyanensis	CL, MCL
	L.(V.) lainsoni	CL
	L.(V.) naiffi	CL
	L.(V) shawi	CL
Colombia	*L.(L.) amazonensis*	CL, ADCL
	L.(L.) chagasi	VL
	L.(L.) mexicana	CL, ADCL
	L.(V.) braziliensis s.l.	CL, MCL
	L.(V.) colombiensis	CL
	L.(V.) guyanensis	CL
	L.(V.) panamensis	CL, MCL
Costa Rica	*L.(L.) mexicana*	CL
	L.(V.) braziliensis s.l.	CL, MCL
	L.(V.) panamensis	CL
Dominican Republic	*L.(L.) mexicana-like*	ADCL
Ecuador	*L.(L.)* sp.[a]	CL
	L.(L.) mexicana[a]	CL
	L.(V.) braziliensis s.l.	CL, MCL
El Salvador	*L.(L.) chagasi*	VL
	L.(L.) mexicana	CL
French Guyana	*L.(L.) amazonensis*	CL, ADCL
	L.(V.) braziliensis s.l.[b]	CL, MCL
	L.(V.) guyanensis	CL
	L.(V.) naiffi[c]	CL
Guadeloupe	*L.(L.) chagasi*	VL
	Leishmania sp.	CL
Guatemala	*L.(L.) chagasi*	VL
	L.(L.) mexicana	CL
	L.(V.) braziliensis s.l.	CL
Guyana	*L.(V.) guyanensis*	CL
	Leishmania sp.	MCL
Honduras	*L.(L.) chagasi*	VL, CL[l]
	L.(L.) mexicana	CL, ADCL
	L.(V.) braziliensis s.l.	CL, MCL
	L.(V.) panamensis	CL, MCL
Martinique	*L.(L.)* sp.	CL
Mexico	*L.(L.) chagasi*	VL
	L.(L.) mexicana	CL, ADCL
	L.(L.) sp.	CL, ADCL[m]
Nicaragua	*L.(L.) chagasi*	VL
	L.(V.) braziliensis s.l.	CL, MCL
	L.(V.) panamensis	CL, MCL
	L.(V.) braziliensis/panamensis[d]	CL
Panama	*L.(L.) aristedesi*	CL
	L.(V.) braziliensis s.l.	CL
	L.(V.) panamensis	CL
	Leishmania sp.	MCL
Paraguay	*L.(L.) amazonensis*	CL, ADCL
	L.(L.) chagasi	VL

Table 13.1 Continued

Country	Species	Disease forms recorded[g]
Peru	*L.(V.) braziliensis* s.l.	CL, MCL
	L.(V.) peruviana	CL
	L.(V.) braziliensis/L.(V.) peruviana[e]	CL, MCL
Surinam	*Leishmania* sp.	CL
USA	*L.(L.) mexicana*	CL, ADCL[m]
Venezuela	*L.(L.) chagasi*	VL
	L.(L.) garnhami	CL
	L.(L.) pifanoi	CL, ADCL
	L.(L.) venezuelensis	CL
	L.(V.) braziliensis s.l.	CL, MCL
	L.(V.) colombiensis	VL[n]
	L.(V.) braziliensis/L.(V.) guyanensis[f]	CL

The majority of the data in this table are taken from the review articles of Lainson and Shaw, 1979, 1987, Shaw and Lainson 1987 and Grimaldi, Tesh and McMahon-Pratt 1989 except [a]Katakura et al., 1993, [b]Raccurt et al., 1995, [c]Darie et al., 1995, [d]Darce et al., 1991, [e]Dujardin et al., 1995, [f]Bonfante-Garrido 1992.
[g]CL = Cutaneous leishmaniasis, ADCL = Anergic diffuse cutaneous leishmaniasis, MCL = Mucocutaneous leishmaniasis, VL = Visceral leishmaniasis; [h]In cases of ADCL; [i]Only recorded in a small region of Bahia State, BR; [j]Only in Rio de Janeiro, BR; [k]Localized in Minas Gerais, BR; [l]Ponce et al., 1991; [m]In Texas on the Mexico/USA border; [n]bone marrow only.

1 There is a high incidence of infection in the native fox, *Cerdocyon thous,* in relatively remote areas of Amazonian Brazil and the benign and inapparent nature of these infections is indicative of an ancient host–parasite relationship.

2 Wild canids are considered to be the source from which members of the *L. (L.) donovani* complex originated (Lysenko 1971) and canids were present in the Americas as long ago as the Pleistocene era, some 2–3 million years ago.

3 *Lu. longipalpis* is the vector of *L. (L.) chagasi* throughout the entire geographic range of the parasite, but is not known to transmit any other neotropical species of *Leishmania*; the vectors of *L. (L.) infantum* belong to a different sandfly genus. The host specificity of *Leishmania* species in nature is most pronounced among their sandfly vectors, thus it seems unlikely that introduced *L. (L.) infantum* could have made the relatively sudden jump from one phlebotomine genus to another.

4 There are differences in both the kinetoplast DNA fragment patterns and the radio-respirometry profiles of *L. (L.) infantum* and *L. (L.) chagasi* (Jackson et al. 1982, 1984, Decker-Jackson and Tang 1982) and the 2 parasites are antigenically different (Santoro et al. 1986). The hypothesis that American visceral leishmaniasis is due to imported *L. (L.) infantum* is based largely on the similarity of those isoenzyme profiles of the 2 parasites that have been studied and the dual role of the dog as an amplification host in their respective epidemiologies (Rioux et al. 1990, Killick-Kendrick 1985).

LEISHMANIA (LEISHMANIA) ENRIETTII MUNIZ AND MEDINA 1948

Known geographical distribution

To date, this parasite has been found only in the States of Paraná and São Paulo, Brazil.

Known mammalian hosts

Natural infections have, until now, only been found in domestic guinea-pigs (*Cavia porcellus*). When this strange parasite was first discovered, producing large tumour-like lesions on the ears of 2 laboratory guinea-pigs (Medina 1946), the ori-

gin of the infected animals was obscure. As phlebotomine sandflies are the only known vectors of *Leishmania* species, however, it is difficult to imagine that domestic guinea-pigs are the principal natural hosts of *L. (L.) enriettii*, and it can only be assumed that the animals had spent some time in or near a rural area where transmission was occurring among the true, wild mammalian hosts. There have been 2 further spontaneous reappearances of the parasite in domestic guinea-pigs, again in Curitiba, Paraná (Luz et al. 1967) and more recently in a rural district of São Paulo State (Machado et al. 1994). Although the exact locality of the animals was on these occasions well documented, attempts to discover the wild animal source of the parasite were not made.

Recorded sandfly hosts

The natural vector of *L. (L.) enriettii* remains to be discovered. Luz et al. (1967) examined the sandfly population of neighbouring forest around the site of isolation, where *Lu. monticola* and *Lu. correalimai* were the only species encountered. *Lu. monticola* was caught on tree trunks, in the nests of opossums (*Didelphis*) and from human bait and 6/10 specimens fed on the lesions of guinea-pigs became heavily infected.

Absence of infection in humans

Human infection has not yet been reported. Muniz and Medina (1948) attempted to infect human volunteers, rhesus monkeys, dogs, mice and the wild guinea-pig ('preá') by the intradermal inoculation of promastigotes from in vitro cultures, without success. Out of 8 hamsters inoculated, only one developed an inconspicuous lesion containing scanty amastigotes. Failure to infect the closely related wild guinea-pig (*Cavia aperea*) at first seems surprising. Lainson and Shaw (1979) suggested, however, that if this animal is the natural host of *L. (L.) enriettii* the inoculated preá may well have developed an inapparent infection that went unnoticed.

LEISHMANIA (LEISHMANIA) MEXICANA BIAGI 1953 EMEND GARNHAM 1962

Known geographical distribution

The areas of known geographical distribution are Southern Texas, USA, Mexico, Belize, Guatemala,

Honduras amd Costa Rica. In view of extensive geographic separation from the type locality of *L. (L.) mexicana* and considerable differences in the mammalian and phlebotomine sandfly faunas, reports of this parasite in Panama and some South American countries must be viewed with caution.

Known mammalian hosts

The known mammalian hosts are humans and the forest rodents *Ototylomys phyllotis* (primary host), *Nyctomys sumichrasti*, *Heteromys desmarestianus* and *Sigmodon hispidus* (secondary hosts).

Recorded sandfly hosts

Lutzomyia olmeca olmeca is the only proven vector, but *Lu. (Lu.) diabolica* has been suspected as a vector in foci of cutaneous leishmaniasis due to *L. (L.) mexicana* in southern Texas and northern Mexico.

Disease caused by the parasite in humans

This parasite causes cutaneous leishmaniasis, with a pronounced tendency towards long-lasting and destructive lesions of the external ear (Fig. 13.9). Relatively rare cases of diffuse, anergic cutaneous leishmaniasis (ADCL) have been recorded, principally from southern Texas and northern Mexico. Local names include 'chiclero's ulcer', 'chiclero's ear' and 'Bay-sore'.

Parasites clearly related to *L. (L.) mexicana* have been reported from humans and wild animals in Panama, Colombia, Venezuela, Peru and parts of Brazil. In the absence of the vector, *Lu. olmeca olmeca*, it is unlikely that any of these are true *L. (L.) mexicana*. Sandflies of the *Lu. flaviscutellata* complex, to which subspecies of *Lu. olmeca* belong, range through these South American countries, however and are probably the vectors of a number of closely related parasites within the *mexicana* complex: at present this includes *L. (L.) pifanoi*, *L. (L.) amazonensis*, *L. (L.) aristidesi*, *L. (L.) garnhami*, *L. (L.) venezuelensis* and *L. (L.) forattinii* (see pages 249–252).

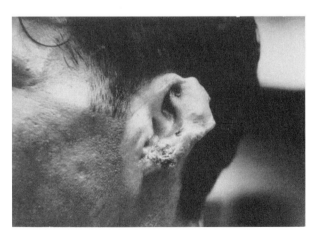

Fig. 13.9 'Chiclero's ulcer', due to *L. (L.) mexicana*. Almost total destruction of the the external ear in a chiclero from Belize with an infection of many years duration. (From Lainson and Strangways-Dixon 1963.)

LEISHMANIA (LEISHMANIA) PIFANOI MEDINA AND ROMERO 1959 EMEND MEDINA AND ROMERO 1962

Known geographical distribution

Known distribution is limited to Venezuela, specifically in the States of Yaracuy, Lara and Miranda.

Known mammalian hosts

Humans are the the the only known mammalian host: the wild mammalian hosts of the parasite have yet to be discovered. A parasite isolated from the forest rodent *Heteromys anomalus* was shown to behave in hamsters in the same way as *L. (L.) pifanoi* isolated from humans, but its conclusive identification remains in doubt.

Recorded sandfly hosts

A parasite with similar characteristics was also found in a specimen of *Lu. flaviscutellata* but, once again, has not been conclusively identified. This sandfly is the proven vector of *L. (L.) amazonensis*, another member of the *mexicana* complex often found in rodents in South American forests and it remains likely that the Venezuelan workers were dealing with this parasite (see p. 250).

Disease caused by the parasite in humans

All isolates found to date have been from cases of ADCL. It is most likely, however, that simple, curable lesions also occur in immunologically competent individuals. There has been much controversy regarding the validity of this member of the *mexicana* complex, some authors regarding it merely as an enzymic variant of either *L. (L.) amazonensis* (see p. 250) or *L. (L.) mexicana*. Much confusion has certainly resulted from the laboratory mix-up of parasites. Although there are relatively few isolates of *L. (L.) pifanoi*, interest in the clinical features of the human infection has resulted in a wide distribution of the parasite to laboratories throughout the world.

LEISHMANIA (LEISHMANIA) HERTIGI HERRER 1971

Known geographical distribution

Known distribution is limited to Panama and Costa Rica.

Known mammalian hosts

The tree-porcupine *Coendou rothschildi* is the only known mammalian host.

Recorded sandfly hosts

The sandfly vector of the parasite has still to be discovered. The remarkably high infection rate of 88% found in the porcupines studied suggests a close association of the vector with the mammalian host, possibly in the hollow trees where these animals live.

Absence of infection in humans

Human infection has not been recorded. *L. (L.) hertigi* seems to be specific to *Coendou rothschildi*, as the parasite has not been found in a wide variety of other forest mammals studied in the Panamanian forests. The apparent absence of human infection may be due to the failure of the parasite to survive in human tissues, or because the sandfly vector does not bite humans.

L. (L.) *hertigi* is included in the *hertigi* complex, together with another closely related parasite of porcupines, *L.(L.) deanei* (see pages 250 and 251).

LEISHMANIA (LEISHMANIA) AMAZONENSIS LAINSON AND SHAW 1972

Known geographical distribution

The parasite has been noted in Bolivia, Brazil, Colombia, French Guyana and Paraguay. It is also very likely to occur in other South American countries where the sandfly vector is found.

Known mammalian hosts

Known mammalian hosts are: the forest rodents *Proechimys* (principal host), *Oryzomys, Neacomys, Nectomys* and *Dasyprocta*; the marsupials *Marmosa, Metachirus, Didelphis* and *Philander*; and the fox *Cerdocyon*.

Recorded sandfly hosts

The principal vector of the parasite is *Lutzomyia (Nyssomyia) flaviscutellata*. Occasional infections have been found in the closely related flies *Lu. (N.) olmeca nociva* and *Lu.(N.) reducta* but, if these are capable of transmitting the parasite, they probably play a small role in its ecology and epidemiology.

Disease caused by the parasite in humans

The parasite causes cutaneous leishmaniasis, usually of the single sore type and ADCL in individuals with a defective cell-mediated immune system (Figs 13.5, 13.6, 13.10). If it does occur, classical mucocutaneous leishmaniasis following metastasis to the naso-pharyngeal mucosae from a simple cutaneous lesion is extremely rare. In advanced cases of ADCL, however, the disseminated infection may also include those tissues.

Typical visceral leishmaniasis in patients from one particular region of Bahia State Brazil, has been attributed to *L. (L.) amazonensis* (Barral et al. 1986). Conversely, no records exist to confirm this anywhere else in the geographical range of the parasite and cases of ADCL of very long duration show no signs or symptoms of visceral involvement, in spite of their defective immune system.

Silveira examined the tissues from a patient who suffered from ADCL due to *L. (L.) amazonensis* from the age of 5 y until his death at the age of 57 (Figs 13.5, 13.6) (F.T. Silveira, unpublished observations). At the time of his death, scarcely any of his body surface remained unaffected and the cutaneous lesions contained enormous numbers of parasites (Fig. 13.11). No macroscopic or microscopic pathological changes were seen in the viscera and no amastigotes were found in stained impression smears prepared from the spleen, liver and lungs and bone-marrow. Finally, hamsters inoculated intradermally with triturates of these visceral tissues failed to become infected.

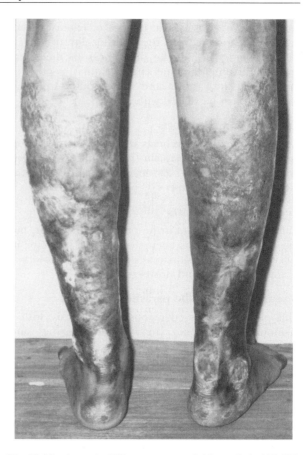

Fig. 13.10 Anergic diffuse cutaneous leishmaniasis (ADCL) due to *L. (L.) amazonensis* in a young girl from Pará, Brazil, showing active lesions and extensive scarring of the legs in an infection of some 15 years duration.

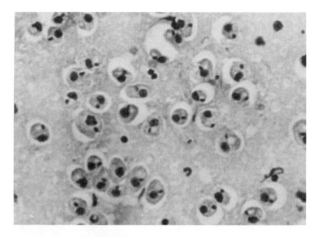

Fig. 13.11 Amastigotes of *L. (L.) amazonensis* in a Giemsa-stained smear from one of the nodular lesions of the patient with ADCL shown in Fig. 13.5.

LEISHMANIA (LEISHMANIA) DEANEI LAINSON AND SHAW 1977

Known geographical distribution

The parasite has been noted only in Amazonian Brazil.

Known mammalian hosts

Known mammalian hosts are the tree-porcupine *Coendou p. prehensilis* and another as yet unnamed species of *Coendou*.

Recorded sandfly hosts

The vector of *L. (L.) deanei* remains to be discovered. As with *L. (L.) hertigi*, the infection rate in Brazilian porcupines is very high, again suggesting a close association of the vector with the mammalian host, probably in the animal's home in hollow trees. A tree-inhabiting sandfly, *Lu. (Viannamyia) furcata*, taken from a tree-hole in which an infected porcupine was living, was shown to have promastigotes of *L. (L.) deanei* in its midgut (Miles et al. 1980). There was, however, no evidence of migration of the parasites to the anterior station of the gut; in subsequent experimental infections of this sandfly it was shown that the promastigotes disappeared following complete digestion of the bloodmeal (Lainson and Shaw 1987).

Absence of infection in humans

Human infection has not been recorded. As with *L. (L.) hertigi*, this could be because the sandfly vector is not attracted to humans or because the parasite cannot survive in human tissues.

L. (L.) deanei, like *L. (L.) hertigi*, seems to be restricted to species of the porcupine *Coendou* and an exhaustive examination of other animals in areas of forest where porcupines are commonly infected failed to indicate any other mammalian hosts (Lainson and Shaw, unpublished observations). Although both parasites seem to be peculiar to porcupines, they are readily distinguishable by their isoenzyme profiles and the morphology of their amastigote stages; those of *L. (L.) hertigi* are strangely elongated and measure from 3.5 × 1.2 to 4.8 × 2.5 μm. The amastigotes of *L. (L.) deanei* are the largest of all known species of *Leishmania*, measuring from 5.1 × 3.1 to 6.8 × 3.7 μm.

Working with 12 isolates of *L. (L.) deanei* from Pará, north Brazil, Miles et al. (1980) found that they were separable into 2 groups by the enzyme profiles of: malate dehydrogenase (oxaloacetate-decarboxylating) (NADP) E.C.1.1.1.40 (ME); phosphoglucomutase E.C.2.7.5.1. (PGM); and malate dehydrogenase E.C.1.1.1.37 (MDH). Whether or not this is indicative of a third species of *Leishmania* in the *hertigi* complex is debatable and further study is indicated on the biology, biochemistry and molecular biology of the 2 zymodemes.

Leishmania (Leishmania) aristidesi Lainson and Shaw 1979

Known geographical distribution

The parasite is known to occur in the Sasardi forest, San Blas Territory, Eastern Panama.

Known mammalian hosts

Known mammalian hosts are the rodents *Oryzomys capito*, *Proechimys semispinosus* and *Dasyprocta punctata*; and the marsupial *Marmosa robinsoni*.

Recorded sandfly hosts

The species most suspected is *Lutzomyia (Nyssomyia) olmeca bicolor*. Christensen et al. (1972) showed it to be the dominant fly on Disney-traps baited with rodents and opossums in the area where infected animals had been captured and the most common species collected among leaf litter on the forest floor.

Possibility of infection in humans

Human infection has not yet been reported. *Lu. olmeca bicolor* does bite humans on rare occasions and it is likely that the parasite may eventually be found infecting humans. In this respect it should be remembered that following the discovery of *L. (V.) naiffi* in armadillos in 1979, 11 years were to pass before cases of human cutaneous leishmaniasis due to this parasite were diagnosed (Lainson et al. 1979, 1990b, Naiff et al. 1989).

Leishmania (Leishmania) garnhami Scorza et al. 1979

Difference of opinion exists regarding the validity of *L. (L.) garnhami*, which is indistinguishable from *L. (L.) amazonensis* on isoenzyme profiles (Rioux et al. 1990). Guevera et al. (1992), however, noted clear differences between the non-transcribed rDNA intergenic spacer sequences of these 2 parasites and in our own laboratory they have been separated by monoclonal antibodies (Shaw, Ishikawa and Lainson, unpublished observations).

Known geographical distribution

The parasite has been found only in the Venezuelan Andes.

Known mammalian hosts

Man is a known host and a single infection has been recorded in the marsupial *Didelphis marsupialis*.

Recorded sandfly hosts

Experimental infections in the sandfly *Lu. youngi* (*verrucarum* group) in Venezuela have led some authors to suggest this species to be the vector (Grimaldi et al. 1989, Young and Duncan 1994, Killick–Kendrick 1990). In addition, Scorza (in Márquez and Scorza 1982) reported that he had found natural infections with flagellates in *Lu. youngi* (at the time identified as *Lu. townsendi*) that, on inoculation into the skin of hamsters, produced 'amastigotes de *Leishmania garnhami*'. Unfortunately the parasite was not specifically identified and the role of *Lu. youngi* as the vector still remains in doubt.

Disease caused by the parasite in humans

The parasite causes cutaneous leishmaniasis but there are no recorded cases of mucocutaneous leishmaniasis or ADCL.

Leishmania (Leishmania) venezuelensis Bonfante-Garrido 1980

Known geographic distribution

The parasite has been found in the Lara and Yaracuy States, Venezuela.

Known mammalian hosts

The known mammalian hosts are humans, equines and the domestic cat. These are best regarded as 'victim' hosts and the wild animal source of infection has yet to be ascertained.

Recorded sandfly hosts

Lu. olmeca bicolor is suspected as a possible vector.

Disease caused by the parasite in humans

The parasite causes single or multiple skin lesions, sometime of a disseminated, nodular type simulating ADCL but curable by the current method of antimonial treatment.

LEISHMANIA (LEISHMANIA) FORATTINII YOSHIDA ET AL. 1993

Known geographical distribution

The parasite has been found in São Paulo and Bahia States, Brazil.

Known mammalian hosts

The opossum *Didelphis marsupialis aurita* (São Paulo) and the rodent *Proechimys iheringi denigratus* (Bahia) are the known mammalian hosts.

Recorded sandfly hosts

The sandfly vector is unknown. Barretto et al. (1985) showed experimentally that the parasite was capable of development throughout the intestines of the sandflies *Psychodopygus ayrozai* and *Lutzomyia yuilli* from the Três Braços area, Bahia, where the 2 insects are very common.

Possibility of infection in humans

The parasite has not yet been reported to cause human disease. Both *Ps. ayrozai* and *Lu. yuilli* occasionally feed on humans and if one or other of these sandflies is indeed the vector among the wild animal hosts, human infection with *L. (L.) forattini* may well occur.

2.4 Species within the subgenus *Viannia* Lainson and Shaw 1987

LEISHMANIA (VIANNIA) BRAZILIENSIS VIANNA 1911 EMEND MATTA 1916

Known geographical distribution

The distribution of this important parasite is badly defined, due to inadequate methods of identification used in the past. Parasites variously described as '*L. braziliensis*', '*L. braziliensis braziliensis*' or '*L. braziliensis* sensu lato' have been reported from most Latin American countries, including Argentina, Belize, Bolivia, Brazil, Colombia, Costa Rica, Ecuador, French Guyana, Guatemala, Honduras, Nicaragua, Panama, Paraguay, Peru, Surinam and Venezuela.

Environmental factors seem to govern the combinations of sandfly vector and wild mammalian host in the natural history of the different species of *Leishmania*. It seems unlikely, therefore, that *L. (V.) braziliensis* sensu stricto can have such an enormous geographic range and the parasites recorded in many of these regions may represent related, but different, parasites of the *braziliensis* complex. The situation is aggravated by the fact that the type material of *L. (V.) braziliensis* Vianna 1911, from Além Paraiba, Minas Gerais, Brazil, is no longer available for comparison. It is further complicated by distinctly different ecological and epidemiological features of cutaneous and muco-

cutaneous leishmaniasis due to *L. (V.) braziliensis* s.l. in different regions, sometimes within the same country, due to human destruction of the sylvatic habitat.

Known mammalian hosts

Humans are known hosts. Among sylvatic mammals the parasite has been recorded from a number of rodent genera, including *Akodon, Proechimys, Rattus, Oryzomys* and *Rhipidomys* and the marsupial *Didelphis* but the strains from these animals are not available for identification using modern methods. Domestic animals such as dogs, mules, horses and (very rarely) cats have been found with skin lesions due to parasites regarded as *L. (V.) braziliensis* s.l. or simply recorded as leishmanias of the *braziliensis* complex. These reports, in areas of suspected peridomestic transmission of the parasite, come principally from localities of extensive deforestation in Argentina, southern Brazil, Bolivia, Colombia and Venezuela.

Recorded sandfly hosts

Uncertainties regarding the exact distribution of *L. (V.) braziliensis* make it difficult to indicate its vector (or vectors). An isolate of the parasite responsible for human cutaneous leishmaniasis in primary Amazonian rain forest in the Carajás highlands of Pará State, Brazil, has been used as a reference strain of *L. (V.) braziliensis* (MHOM/BR/75/M2903) and in this area the vector is undoubtedly *Psychodopygus wellcomei*. This sandfly, referred to by some as *Lutzomyia (Psychodopygus) wellcomei*, has been found heavily infected on numerous occasions. *Ps. wellcomei* is essentially sylvatic and avidly feeds on humans, not only at night but also in the daylight hours during overcast weather. It is extremely abundant in the rainy season (November–April), when it may represent c. 65% of the total catch of some 25 different species of sandflies taken off human bait. Captures of sandflies from humans stationed at different heights on tree-ladders have shown that *Ps. wellcomei* has a vertical flight range of only 1–2 metres above ground level: this and the insect's abundance (25.5%) in catches of different sandflies taken from rodent-baited traps suggest that the principal wild mammalian hosts of *L. (V.) braziliensis,* in the area in question, are likely to be terrestrial animals, probably rodents.

In the lowland regions of Pará State the vector is *Ps. complexus* (de Souza et al. 1996), also highly anthropophilic. The females of this species are morphologically indistinguishable from those of *Ps. wellcomei*, but the males of each species are quite distinct.

In the State of Amazonas another highly anthrophilic species, *Ps. carrerai*, has been found infected with *L. (V.) braziliensis* s.l. The strain was biochemically similar to *L. (V.) braziliensis* of humans from the same region but antigenically different from those from other areas of Brazil, including the lower Amazon region.

In other parts of Brazil, occasional isolates of *L. (V.) braziliensis* s.l. have been made from the sandfly *Lutzomyia (Nyssomyia) whitmani* sensu stricto, caught in and around houses in rural parts of Bahia and Ceará States (north-east Brazil). In the northern part of Paraná and in the States of São Paulo and Minas Gerais (south-east Brazil) it is again suspected as a vector due to its highly anthropophilic feeding habits and its high density in and around human dwelling places and animal sheds in the endemic areas of cutaneous leishmaniasis.

Lutzomyia (Nyssomyia) intermedia is another highly anthropophilic sandfly that although originally sylvatic has now adapted well to a peridomestic habitat in deforested, rural areas. It is, for similar reasons, suspected as a vector of *L. (V.) braziliensis* s.l. in the State of Rio de Janeiro and some parts of the State of São Paulo, Brazil and certain regions of Argentina. Flagellates thought to have been promastigotes of *Leishmania* were on one occasion seen in histological sections of the intestines of the sandflies *Lutzomyia migonei* and *Lu. (Pintomyia) pessoai* caught in endemic areas of cutaneous leishmaniasis in São Paulo State. Their true nature, however, remains obscure.

In Bolivia *L. (V.) braziliensis* s.l. has been isolated from *Ps. carrerai carrerai, Ps. llanosmartini* and *Ps. yucumensis,* whereas in Colombia and Venezuela similar parasites have been found in *Lu. spinicrassa.*

Disease caused by the parasite in humans

The parasite causes cutaneous leishmaniasis, usually with one or few lesions and also mucocutaneous and mucosal leishmaniasis (Figs. 13.2–4). Common names include: 'úlcera de Bauru', 'ferida brava', 'ferida sêca', 'bouba', 'buba', 'nariz de anta' ('tapir nose') and 'espundia'.

The various zymodemes of *L. (V.) braziliensis* s.l. are placed in the *braziliensis* complex, together with the closely related parasite *L. (V.) peruviana.*

LEISHMANIA (VIANNIA) PERUVIANA VELEZ 1913

Known geographical distribution

The parasite has been noted in Peru, on the western slopes of the Andes and in the inter-Andean valleys. Its range may possibly extend into the Argentinian highlands and it is probably more widely distributed in the Andean countries than previously suspected. This is apparently the rare exception of a neotropical *Leishmania* species with an original, non-sylvatic eco-epidemiology. Transmission seems to take place in relatively barren, mountainous areas with scant vegetation and a relatively restricted wild mammalian fauna.

Known mammalian hosts

The dog, *Canis familiaris,* is the only known mammalian host other than humans, but this animal's role in the epidemiology of the human disease remains obscure. It remains likely that a primitive reservoir of infection exists in local rodents or marsupials.

Recorded sandfly hosts

Lutzomyia (Helcocyrtomyia) peruensis and *Lutzomyia verrucarum* have long been suspected as probable vectors, in view of their anthropophilic feeding habits. Isolation of a parasite with the biological characteristics of *L. (V.) peruviana* from the former fly, captured in an endemic area, implies its involvement in transmission, but much research in the field is needed before significant evidence can be obtained.

Disease caused by the parasite in humans

The parasite causes simple cutaneous leishmaniasis, not associated with the mucocutaneous disease. It is particularly frequent in school children, commonly resulting in extensive facial scars. Ulcers are usually self-healing and a firm immunity to reinfection with the same parasite is usually imparted. Common names include 'uta', 'Tiacc-araña' and 'llaga'.

LEISHMANIA (VIANNIA) GUYANENSIS FLOCH 1954

Known geographical distribution

This is an essentially sylvatic species that is an extremely common cause of human cutaneous leishmaniasis, particularly in Brazil, north of the Amazon river and the Guyanas. Its range also extends into Ecuador, Venezuela and the lowland forests of Peru.

Known mammalian hosts

Known mammalian hosts include humans and in primary forest the major reservoir hosts are the sloth *Choloepus didactylus* and the lesser anteater *Tamandua tetradactyla* (Xenarthra) with occasional infections found in rodents (*Proechimys*) and opossums (*Didelphis*). The infection is always inapparent, with parasites located in apparently normal skin and in viscera such as the spleen and liver.

Recorded sandfly hosts

The principal vector among wild animals and to humans is the sandfly *Lutzomyia (Nyssomyia) umbratilis,* with infections relatively infrequently found in a closely related fly, *Lu. (N.) anduzei.* Records of the parasite in *Lu. (N.) whitmani* s.l., in Amazonian Brazil, probably refer to *Leishmania (V.) shawi* (see p. 254).

Lu. (N.) umbratilis is a sandfly that dwells in the forest canopy and tree trunks. During the early hours of daylight it may be found in large numbers, resting on the larger tree trunks, from which the flies will readily fly off and attack humans when disturbed. Although infection of this sandfly clearly takes place when it feeds on the reservoir hosts at night in the canopy, transmission to humans is principally during the day (early morning), when gangs of forest labourers are engaged in their work, particularly deforestation. Others at risk include the collectors of Brazil nuts and other fruits, topographers, visiting botanists and zoologists and even the occasional tourist.

The enzootic of *L. (V.) guyanensis,* as studied in primary rain forest, is unlikely to survive in secondary forests or man-made plantations of non-indigenous trees. The small girth of young trees provides a microhabitat that is unsuitable for resting sandflies due to the low surface humidity of the smooth trunks. In addition such immature trees are an equally unsuitable environment for relatively large and heavy animals such as sloths and anteaters. Finally, in monoculture plantations (e.g. pine and gmelina) sloths are deprived of their normal diet of indigenous fruits and foliage.

Cutaneous leishmaniasis due to *L. (V.) guyanensis* may reach high prevalence in human communities situated in or very near primary forest, leading to an erroneous impression that the sandfly vector, *Lu. (N.) umbratilis,* has adapted to a peridomestic habitat.

There is, as yet, no evidence that this occurs and peri-domestic acquisition of the disease is doubtless due to infected flies that have been attracted to the lights of houses at night, from nearby forest. Esterre et al. 1986 showed experimentally that clearing forest to c. 500 m from a village situated in primary forest in French Guyana completely interrupted the transmission of *L. (V.) guyanensis* among its inhabitants.

The marsupial *Didelphis* has rarely been found infected with *L. (V.) guyanensis* in primary forest where there is intensive transmission of the parasite among sloths and anteaters and to humans. Strangely, however, a high rate of infection has been recorded in the abnormally large populations of this opossum that are attracted to human refuse in villages on the borders of virgin forest (Arias and Naiff 1981). Reasons for this are not clear, nor is it certain whether opossums serve as a source of *L. (V.) guyanensis* for the sandfly vector, or if they merely represent 'dead-ends' in the life-cycle of the parasite.

Disease caused by the parasite in humans

The parasite causes cutaneous leishmaniasis, very frequently with multiple skin lesions (Fig. 13.7). Cases of mucocutaneous disease appear to be very rare. Common names for the disease include 'pian-bois', 'bosch-yaws' and 'forest-yaws'.

Multiplicity of the skin lesions arises in 2 very different ways. First, sloths are rather sedentary animals and an infected animal may remain in a given spot for a considerable period. The infection rate of *Lu. (N.) umbratilis* resting on neighbouring tree trunks will thus tend to rise to a high level, with levels as high as 25% found among many hundreds of specimens taken from a single tree. It follows that persons attacked by sandflies in the area may receive numerous infective bites at the same time on all exposed parts of the body. Forest workers tend to be shirtless and frequently use shorts: for this reason many patients present with lesions scattered over the face, trunk, arms and legs (Fig. 13.7). The developing multiple lesions of such individuals tend to be of a similar size and evolution. Secondly, there is abundant clinical evidence indicating the formation of metastatic lesions in persons originally presenting with a single skin lesion. These lesions tend to follow a distinct migratory course along the lymphatics and because of this evolution they are frequently nodular and, when ulcerated, of very unequal size

L. (V.) guyanensis gives its name to the *guyanensis* complex of closely related leishmanias including *L. (V.) panamensis* and *L. (V.) shawi* (see pages 254 and 255).

LEISHMANIA (VIANNIA) PANAMENSIS LAINSON AND SHAW 1972

Known geographical distribution

As the name suggests, most information on this parasite comes from Panama and the Canal Zone, where the very frequent acquisition of cutaneous leishmaniasis by American military personnel prompted intensive eco-epidemiological studies. It is also recorded in west and central Colombia, Ecuador, Venezuela, Costa Rica, Honduras and Nicaragua.

Known mammalian hosts

Humans are a host to the parasite. The eco-epidemiology of *L. (V.) panamensis* follows a very similar pattern to that of *L. (V.) guyanensis,* which is not surprising in view of the close biological and biochemical relationship of the 2 parasites. The major host is the 2-toed sloth *Choloepus hoffmanni*, with occasional infections reported in the 3-toed sloths *Bradypus infuscatus* and *B. griseus*. More rarely, infections have been registered in other sylvatic animals such as *Bassaricyon gabbi, Nasua nasua* and *Potos flavus* (Carnivora: Procyonidae), *Aotus trivirgatus* and *Saguinus geoffroyi* (Primates: Cebidae and Callitrichidae) and *Heteromys* (Rodentia). Hunting dogs occasionally develop skin lesions due to *L.(V.) panamensis*: like humans they are 'victim hosts' that rarely, if ever, serve as a source of parasites for the sandfly vector(s), or as a means of maintaining the enzootic.

Recorded sandfly hosts

The major sandfly vector is considered to be *Lu. (N.) trapidoi*, whereas *Lu. (N.) ylephiletor, Lu. (Lu.) gomezi* and *Psychodopygus panamensis* may act as secondary vectors.

Disease caused by the parasite in humans

The parasite usually causes single or a limited number of skin lesions. Rare cases of mucocutaneous leishmaniasis have been attributed to *L. (V.) panamensis*.

LEISHMANIA (VIANNIA) LAINSONI SILVEIRA ET AL. 1987

Known geographical distribution

This parasite has until now been encountered only in the Amazon Region of north Brazil, but it probably exists in other regions where the known mammalian and sandfly hosts coexist.

Known mammalian hosts

Humans are a known mammalian host. The only known reservoir host among wild animals is the rodent *Agouti paca* (Rodentia: Dasyproctidae).

Recorded sandfly hosts

Lu. (Trichophoromyia) ubiquitalis is a known host and the first representative of the subgenus *Trichophoromyia* to be incriminated as a vector of a *Leishmania* species.

L. (V.) lainsoni was isolated only from this sandfly, among many other species dissected in forested areas where patients had become infected with this parasite. The puzzling fact remained that *Lu. (T.) ubiquitalis* had not been caught biting humans in the forest. It was found, however, that this sandfly would feed avidly on humans if maintained for some hours in the laboratory after capture and this prompted the conclusion that under certain conditions it must also feed on humans in its natural habitat. Continuing field studies confirmed this, although the factors influencing the sandfly's biting habits remain obscure. *Lu. (T.) ubiquitalis* is clearly not particularly fond of human blood, which accounts for the relatively low rate of infection with *L. (V.) lainsoni* in humans, compared with other species of *Leishmania*, such as *L. (V.) braziliensis* and *L. (V.) guyanensi;* these have highly anthropophilic sandfly vectors.

Disease caused by the parasite in humans

The parasite causes cutaneous leishmaniasis, usually with a single ulcerating skin lesion. Cases of mucocutaneous leishmaniasis due to this parasite have not yet been encountered.

LEISHMANIA (V.) *SHAWI* LAINSON ET AL. 1989

Geographical distribution

The parasite is found in the Amazon Region of north Brazil, south of the Amazon river.

Known mammalian hosts

Humans are a known mammalian host. Reservoir hosts among the forest animals include: the monkeys *Cebus apella* and *Chiropotes satanas* (Cebidae); the sloths *Choloepus didactylus* and *Bradypus tridactylus* (Xenarthra); and the coatimundi *Nasua nasua* (Procyonidae). It remains likely that other arboreal animals may harbour the parasite.

Recorded sandfly hosts

Infections have so far been recorded in only one species of sandfly caught feeding on humans or monkeys and by other methods of capture. It was provisionally identified as *Lutzomyia* (*Nyssomyia*) *whitmani*, but morphometric differences between the vector and the type material of *Lu. (N.) whitmani* sensu stricto from other parts of Brazil have now been noted. This, and further separation by DNA probes, suggests the fly to be a 'cryptic' species (as yet unnamed) of a *Lu. (N.) whitmani* complex (Rangel et al. 1996). The 2 organisms are biologically and biochemically very similar and clearly closely related.

Disease caused by the parasite in humans

The parasite causes cutaneous leishmaniasis, usually with a single ulcerating skin lesion, but cases of multiple lesions of varying pathologies have been observed (Fig. 13.12). Cases of mucocutaneous leishmaniasis due to this parasite have not yet been encountered.

LEISHMANIA (*VIANNIA*) *NAIFFI* LAINSON AND SHAW 1989

Known geographical distribution

Isolates of the parasite from humans and the reservoir host and sandfly vector are registered in the Brazilian States of Pará and Amazonas. The range of this parasite will almost certainly extend into other parts of Brazil and neighbouring countries where the wild animal host and the sandfly vector coexist.

One case has been recorded from outside Brazil, in a French soldier who had visited French Guyana, Martinique and Guadeloupe (Darie et al. 1995). The authors felt that he could have become infected in any of these 3 places, but because there was an interval of 2 years between his visit to French Guyana and the appearance of the lesion, it was unlikely that he contracted the infection there. There are examples in the literature, however, of long pre-patent periods in other forms of cutaneous leishmaniasis, sometimes of several years and the fact that the reservoir host of *L. (V.) naiffi*, the 9-banded armadillo, does not exist in either Martinique or Guadeloupe makes it most likely that the man's infection was acquired in French Guyana.

Known mammalian hosts

Humans are a known mammalian host. To date the only known reservoir host is the 9-banded armadillo, *Dasypus novemcinctus* (Xenarthra: Dasypodidae), in which there is a high infection rate in apparently normal skin and viscera.

Recorded sandfly hosts

Most recorded sandfly infections involve the sandfly *Psychodopygus ayrozai* which is therefore most suspected as the vector among armadillos. This fly is not highly anthropophilic, which possibly accounts for the paucity of human infection with *L. (V.) naiffi*. On the other hand the parasite has, on rarer occasions, also been found in *Ps. paraensis* and *Ps. s. squamiventris*, both of which are highly anthropophilic and possibly involved in transmission to man. Further studies are clearly necessary to establish the respective roles of these 3 sandflies in the eco-epidemiology of *L. (V.) naiffi*.

Disease caused by the parasite in humans

The parasite causes cutaneous leishmaniasis, usually with single, small, ulcerating lesions. No case of mucocutaneous leishmaniasis has yet been attributed to this parasite.

Unlike most species of *Leishmania*, *L. (V.) naiffi* rarely produces a visible lesion when inoculated into the skin of hamsters, although the parasite may be reisolated following culture of skin from the inoculation site in blood-agar media after at least one year. For this reason human infection with this parasite may have remained undiagnosed in the past, when inoculation of hamsters has been the sole method of isolation attempted from human skin lesions. In addition, it may be that *L. (V.) naiffi* can also produce an occult, benign infection in the skin of humans, as it does in the hamster and that transmission to humans is more frequent than has been suspected.

LEISHMANIA (*VIANNIA*) *COLOMBIENSIS* KREUTZER ET AL. 1991

Known geographical distribution

The parasite exists in Colombia, Panama and Venezuela, probably extending into the neighbouring forests of Brazil, the Peruvian lowlands and other Latin American countries where the wild mammalian and sandfly hosts coexist.

Known mammalian hosts

Humans are a known mammalian host. To date, only one isolate has been made from a wild animal, the sloth *Choloepus hoffmanni*, in Panama.

Recorded sandfly hosts

In Colombia is *Lu.* (*Helcocyrtomyia*) *hartmanni* has been found infected, and in Panama the sandfly hosts are *Lu.* (*Lu.*) *gomezi* and *Psychodopygus panamensis*. It remains to be determined which of these sandflies acts as the vector.

Disease caused by the parasite in humans

The parasite causes single to multiple ulcerating skin lesions. Cases of mucocutaneous leishmaniasis caused by the parasite have not yet been seen. The strain identified from Venezuela by Delgado et al. (1993) was isolated from a bone marrow aspirate of a patient with visceral leishmaniasis. It is, however, uncertain whether or not this was the parasite responsible for the clinical symptoms observed.

LEISHMANIA (VIANNIA) EQUATORENSIS GRIMALDI ET AL. 1992

Known geographical distribution

The parasite is, so far, known only from sylvatic mammals from the forest of the Pacific coast of Ecuador.

Known mammalian hosts

Isolations were from the viscera of the sloth *Choloepus hoffmanni* and the squirrel *Sciurus granatensis* (Rodentia: Sciuridae).

Recorded sandfly hosts

Infected sandflies have not yet been located.

Absence of infection in humans

Human disease caused by this parasite has not yet been recorded.

2.5 'Hybrid' *Leishmania* of the subgenus *Viannia*

Strains with phenotypic and genotypic characters of 2 species have been recorded in different geographical areas of Latin America. There are 2 possible interpretations for such strains: either they represent strains that originated directly from a common ancestor or they are the result of genetic exchange.

L.(V.) BRAZILIENSIS/*L.(V.)* PANAMENSIS HYBRID

Known geographical distribution

The parasite has been found in northern Nicaragua (Darce et al. 1991) close to the border with Honduras. To the south, the strains are *L.* (*V.*) *panamensis* and to the north, *L.* (*V.*) *braziliensis*.

Known mammalian hosts

So far, the parasite is only known in humans.

Recorded sandfly hosts

No sandfly host has been recorded to date.

Disease caused by the parasite in humans

The parasite causes ulcerating skin lesions. Cases of mucocutaneous have not yet been seen.

*L. (V.)*BRAZILIENSIS/*L. (V.)* GUYANENSIS HYBRID

Known geographical distribution

The parasite has been found in Lara State, Venezuela (Bonfante-Garrido et al. 1992).

Known mammalian hosts

So far, the parasite has only been recorded from humans.

Recorded sandfly hosts

No sandfly hosts have yet been found.

Disease caused by the parasite in humans

The parasite causes ulcerating skin lesions. Cases of mucocutaneous leishmaniasis caused by this parasite have not yet been seen.

*L. (V.)*BRAZILIENSIS/*L. (V.)* PERUVIANA HYBRID

Known geographical distribution

To date, 4 strains have been isolated from patients in the Limapampa region of the Huanuco Valley, Peru (Dujardin et al. 1995).

Known mammalian hosts

Humans are the only known mammalian host to date.

Recorded sandfly hosts

No sandfly vectors have been recorded.

Disease caused by the parasite in humans

Ulcerating skin lesions were noted in all patients and one also had a mucosal lesion.

3 GENETICS

The New World *Leishmania* have 20–25 chromosomes that exhibit high degrees of intra and interspecies size polymorphism. This is thought to reflect a high level of genomic plasticity. Leishmanial genomic DNA is composed of repetitive, moderately repetitive and unique sequences that respectively form c. 25%, 13% and 60% of the total. Repeated sequences are useful for identification regardless of their distribution, function or copy numbers. Fernandes et al. (1994) found that the mini-exon repeat units of 4 *Viannia* species were different. Considerable genomic differences have been noted between the 2 subgenera, but they appear greater for species of *Viannia*. Mendoza-León, Havercroft and Barker (1995) found that the β-tubulin gene regions showed a much greater degree of heterogeneity within and between parasites of the *braziliensis* complex than those of the *mexicana* complex. This suggests that there are more random mutations in the former than in the latter. The same gene may be located in more than one chromosome. This may be the result of gene duplication and transposition to another chromosome or chromosomal duplication followed by size divergence (Spithill and Samaras 1985).

Genetic exchange between neotropical *Leishmania* has not been demonstrated experimentally, but the finding of hybrids (see p. 256) amongst *Viannia* species suggests that it may occur. Hybrids only occur in some localities and it is possible that ecological conditions may be important in determining the contact between the species involved. No hybrids have been noted amongst neotropical species of the subgenus *Leishmania*.

4 VIRAL INFECTIONS IN LEISHMANIA

Virus-like particles have been described in the cytoplasm of cultured promastigotes of 5 isolates of *L. (L.) hertigi* and 3 of *L. (L.) deanei* (Molyneux and Killick-Kendrick 1987). Although unidentified, they were shown to be associated with cytopathological changes in the mitochondrion of the promastigote. The number of virus-like particles was drastically reduced when *L. (L.) hertigi* was grown as amastigotes in mouse peritoneal macrophages and dog sarcoma cell lines incubated at 32°C. The particles were not transmissible to other *Leishmania* species, nor to cell lines susceptible to viruses.

RNA virus particles belonging to the family Totaviridae were described by Tarr et al. (1988) in cultured promastigotes of a strain of *L. (V.) guyanensis* from French Guyana. Subsequent studies revealed the presence of similar viruses in promastigotes of 11 *Leishmania* strains isolated from humans, including both *L. (V.) guyanensis* and *L. (V.) braziliensis* from the Amazonian region of Brazil and Peru (Guilbride, Myler and Stuart 1992). All the viral isolates are considered to be different and are classified within a single genus, *Leishmaniavirus*. None, however, has been given specific status within this genus. The virus-bearing promastigotes were those of *Leishmania* isolated from uncomplicated cases of cutaneous leishmaniasis, but so far the viral particles have not been demonstrated in amastigotes from the skin lesions. The effect that such viruses may have on the *Leishmania* is not known, but in experimental infections of *Leishmania major* in mice it was noted that an infected line was less pathogenic than an uninfected one.

5 CLINICAL FEATURES

5.1 American visceral leishmaniasis (AVL)

The clinical features of AVL closely resemble those of 'infantile visceral leishmaniasis' due to *L. (L.) infantum* of the Old World (see Chapter 12) and this similarity extends to the fact that the disease is seen mainly in children (Fig. 13.13).

On rare occasions, parasites considered to be *L. (L.) chagasi* have been isolated from cutaneous lesions of humans in endemic areas of AVL in southern Brazil (Oliveira et al. 1986) and reference has already been made to the strange situation in Honduras where cutaneous lesions have been attributed to this parasite in the apparent absence of the visceral disease (Ponce et al. 1991). Reasons for these unusual infections are not clear. There is evidence that *L. (L.) chagasi* may

produce a benign, inapparent infection in some individuals and that severity of the disease depends to some extent on the nutritional state of the infected person (Baderó et al. 1986). Differential diagnosis has to be made principally from malaria, schistosomiasis, cirrhosis of the liver, visceral syphilis and other causes of hepatosplenomegaly.

Although serological methods such as the indirect fluorescent antibody, dot-enzyme-linked immunosorbent assay (ELISA) and direct agglutination tests are useful indicators, unequivocal diagnosis of the disease depends on the demonstration of amastigotes in stained smears of aspirates from the spleen, bone-marrow or lymph glands. Usually such smears contain abundant parasites: if not, the material can be cultured in a suitable blood-agar medium (varieties of NNN), although some difficulty may be experienced in culturing the parasite, especially when the aspirates contain scanty amastigotes. The intraperitoneal inoculation of aspirates into hamsters is by far the most reliable method of isolating *L. (L.) chagasi* for further study, but the long delay before parasites are detectable in these animals makes the method impractical for quick diagnosis. The polymerase chain reaction (PCR) will probably be the future method of choice in the larger and better equipped hospitals and clinics, but the traditional methods of demonstrating the parasite will remain vitally important for many more years to come in the more remote rural areas where, after all, the majority of cases are concentrated.

5.2 Cutaneous leishmaniasis

Simple cutaneous lesions are produced by 12 of the 14 neotropical species of *Leishmania* known to infect humans. It is not possible, however, to diagnose the causative species by the appearance of these lesions, that are in many cases indistinguishable from the classical leishmanial lesion of the Old World, forming a rounded, crater-like ulcer with a raised border (see Chapter 12 and Fig. 13.2). In addition, the 'simple' lesion may vary greatly in appearance (Figs 13.12, 14–16), evoking such descriptions as 'framboesiform', 'lichenoid', 'lupoid', 'nodular', 'vegetative', 'verrucose', 'ulcerative' etc., from clinicians and dermatologists. All of these forms have one thing in common in that they are painless; unfortunately this means that the infected person often fails to seek medical advice until the lesion has reached large proportions. Differential diagnosis needs to consider tropical ulcer (painful and suppurative), sporotrichosis, cutaneous tuberculosis, yaws, blastomycosis, lupus and tertiary syphilis. Bacterial infection of insect bites or skin abrasions are frequently misdiagnosed as early lesions due to *Leishmania* and are particularly common in children living in rural areas with an abundance of biting flies such as *Simulium* and *Culicoides*.

Although patients under examination may show a positive Montenegro (leishmanin) skin-test, this may be due to a previous infection with *Leishmania*, subsequently eliminated and may be unrelated to present

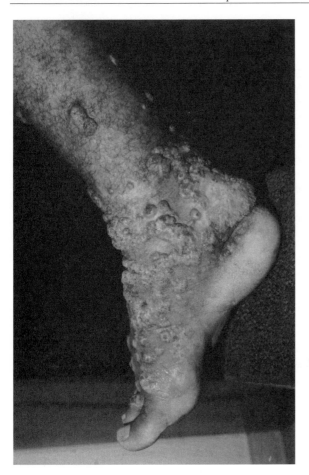

Fig. 13.12 Strange multiple nodules on the foot due to *L.* (*V.*) *shawi*, clinically resembling mycotic disease. See Plate 13.12.

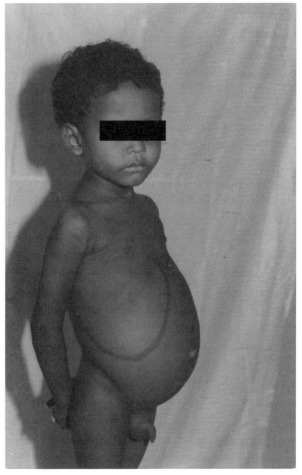

Fig. 13.13 American visceral leishmaniasis (AVL), due to *L.* (*L.*) *chagasi*, in a boy from Marajó island, Pará, Brazil. Note the greatly distended abdomen resulting from hepato-splenomegaly. See Plate 13.13.

skin lesions. The demonstration of amastigotes in stained smears prepared from the border of the lesions and isolation of the parasite in blood-agar culture medium are prerequisite for diagnosis.

5.3 Mucocutaneous and mucosal leishmaniasis

For excellent general reading on this unique form of leishmaniasis, reference should be made to Pessôa and Barretto (1948), Marsden (1986) and Walton (1987).

Although the disease has on rare occasions been attributed to *L.* (*V.*) *guyanensis* and *L.* (*V.*) *panamensis*, the great villain is undoubtedly *L.* (*V.*) *braziliensis* s.l.. The exact percentage of individuals infected with this parasite who develop mucosal lesions is difficult to calculate. In what was almost certainly a hospital series, in São Paulo State, southern Brazil, Pessôa (1941) produced figures indicating that among 171 patients with cutaneous lesions of less than one year's duration, 105 lacked mucosal lesions and 66 (38.5%) had mucosal involvement. Of 110 individuals with cutaneous lesions of more than one year's duration 21 had no mucosal lesions, and 89 (80.9%) had developed them. Marsden (1986), however, described Pessôa's figure of 80.9% as

'widely quoted out of text......giving the impression that the great majority (of cases) will proceed to mucosal metastasis'.

In field studies in an endemic area in Três Braços, Bahia State, north-east Brazil, Marsden and his colleagues found only 2.7% of 371 patients examined to have both cutaneous and mucosal lesions. Mucosal infection seems to be much more common in some Latin American countries (e.g. Bolivia and Ecuador) than in others, suggesting that certain parasites referred to as *L.* (*V.*) *braziliensis* have a greater propensity for producing mucosal lesions than others (these may, in fact, represent different subspecies, or even species, of the *braziliensis* complex).

In spite of its antiquity, the most detailed study of the mucosal lesions remains that of Klotz and Lindenberg (1923), but a wealth of clinical and pathological data is also available in the works mentioned on this page and that of Ridley (1987). It is generally agreed that involvement of the mouth, nose and throat is always the result of metastases from a simple skin lesion elsewhere on the body (Fig. 13.2). Appar-

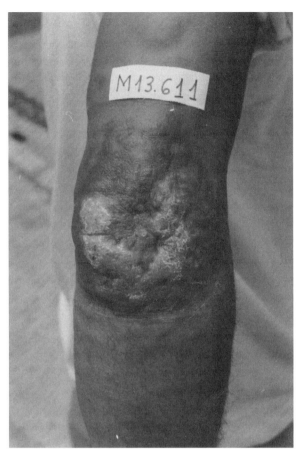

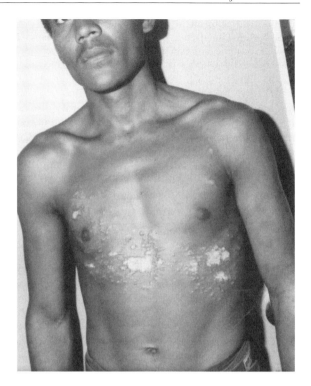

Fig. 13.14–15 A variety of skin lesions due to different neotropical *Leishmania* species (also see Figs. 9 and 12). Fig. 13.14. Infection with *L. (L.) amazonensis,* on the elbow. Fig. 13.15. A large number of small, papular satellite lesions surrounding the larger, primary lesions in a case of 'pian-bois' due to *L. (V.) guyanensis.* See Plate 13.14–15.

ently, migration of the parasites to the mucosae, by way of the lymphatics or the blood stream, may take place quite early in the infection, for amastigotes have been demonstrated in scrapings of the apparently normal nasal mucosae of 12 patients with skin lesions of only 1–11 months evolution (Villela, Pestana and Pessôa 1939). The nose is the major site of the metastases (Fig. 13.3) and it remains a mystery as to why this occurs in some individuals and not in others. From the observations of Villela et al. and the fact that years may elapse between the disappearance of the primary skin lesion and the onset of mucosal disease, it seems that the parasite remains dormant in the mucosae for a variable period. Exactly what triggers this occult infection into destructive activity is another mystery, although minor injury to the mucosae may be one cause. The following account of the developing pathology of the mucosal disease is summarized from Ridley (1987).

When a nasal lesion develops it is initiated in the deep mucosa of the nose, an accumulation of plasma cells and lymphocytes forming around the small blood vessels. A few amastigotes may appear in the endothelial cells. The major part of the lesion stays in the deep mucosa, accompanied by

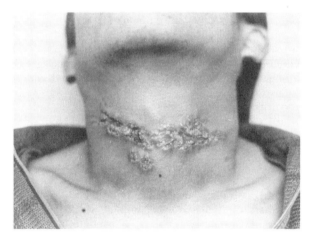

Fig. 13.16 Another atypical lesion, due to the same parasite. Figs 13.14–16 (and Fig. 12) all cases from Pará, Brazil.

congestion and oedema, a pronounced infiltration of plasma cells and a characteristic proliferation of the vascular endothelial cells, which contain variable numbers of amastigotes. Inflammatory foci proceed towards the mucosal surface, resulting in a patchy desquamation, followed by hyalinization and necrosis of the exposed tissue, accompanied by polymorph infiltration. It should be stressed that the ulcer is due to the desquamation resulting from the inflammatory process and not to the necrosis. In the area of deep inflammation the endothelial nodule, with its perivascular inflammatory cells, undergoes central necrosis or, in the case of large nodules, hyalinization. Scanty amastigotes may still be found, but they are absent in the necrotic area. Considerable endarteritis may be associated with thrombosis which, together with subsequent fibrosis, deforms and erodes the nasal septum. Liquefaction of cartilage continues, even some distance from the leishmanial nodule and the vascular supply is so reduced that only coarse fibrous tissue can survive.

Blockage of the nasal passages due to the developing lesion usually results in respiratory distress, mouth breathing and a high frequency of pulmonary infection that may lead to death. Palatal (Fig. 13.4), laryngeal and tracheal lesions are less common: for first-hand accounts of these, reference should be made to Marsden (1986) and Walton (1987).

Differential diagnosis of mucosal leishmaniasis must be made from nasal syphilis (no destruction of the septum), gangosa (ulcerating yaws), blastomycosis, rhinosporidiosis, midline granuloma, carcinoma and cancrum oris.

Sudanese and Ethiopian oro-nasal (mucosal) leishmaniasis bears a superficial resemblance to American 'espundia' (see El-Hassan et al. 1995 for review). Due largely to *L. (L.) donovani* s.l. and, more rarely, *L. (L.) major*, it is not preceded by a cutaneous lesion. In addition, unlike patients with the South American disease, advanced cases of Sudanese mucosal leishmaniasis respond readily to treatment with pentavalent antimonials and ketoconazole.

5.4   Anergic, diffuse cutaneous leishmaniasis (ADCL)

In Venezuela, Convit and Lapenta (1946) described a bizarre form of cutaneous leishmaniasis characterized by: nodular lesions scattered all over the body and containing vast numbers of rather large amastigotes; a negative Montenegro skin-test reaction; and almost total resistance to chemotherapy. Further cases were recorded in that country and subsequently in Bolivia, Brazil, Colombia, the Dominican Republic, Honduras, northern Mexico, Texas, USA and Peru. The causative parasites in Venezuela, Mexico and Texas and Brazil are *L. (L.) pifanoi*, *L. (L.) mexicana* and *L. (L.) amazonensis* respectively and it is likely that this form of leishmaniasis elsewhere in the Americas is also due to members of the *mexicana* complex within the subgenus *Leishmania*. The disease, as its name suggests, is the outcome of infection by this group of parasites in individuals with little or no cell-mediated immunity. Curiously, parasites of the subgenus *Viannia* do not seem to possess the potential to produce this strange disease.

At one time it appeared that ADCL was an irreversible condition and that the best treatment merely kept the disease in check, without eliminating the parasite. There is some evidence to suggest, however, that prognosis is not always so grim. One of the several ADCL patients studied in the authors' laboratory acquired her infection with *L. (L.) amazonensis* when she was <5 years of age and, in spite of constant chemotherapy, her condition had not improved greatly by the age of 28. However, the lesions faded away and the patient made a complete recovery following immunochemotherapy (p. 262). We had noted that,

unlike the lesions of other cases of ADCL, those of this girl had occasionally ulcerated and healed, leaving her with very unsightly scars on her face and legs (Fig. 13.10). This and the final recovery, suggests that there is a gradation in the degree of anergic condition, from total to partial. In many patients the nodular lesions remain unulcerated, whereas in others there may be ulceration and even amputation of fingers and toes, resembling that seen in leprosy (Figs 13.5, 13.6).

Whereas ADCL usually forms a minute proportion of the total number of cases of cutaneous leishmaniasis caused by parasites of the *mexicana* complex, an exception is found in the Dominican Republic, where ADCL occurs in the apparent absence of simple, curable cutaneous leishmaniasis. The causative parasite is clearly a member of the *mexicana* complex, but is as yet unnamed and its animal reservoir and sandfly vector are unknown. The occurrence of 3 cases in a single family in the Dominican Republic suggests involvement of an hereditary component (Walton 1987) and Peterson et al. (1982) demonstrated a population of specific suppressor cells in 4 other patients. The deficient immune response in ADCL in general is considered to be related to a thymus dependant system in both the New World and the Old World diseases (Convit, Pinardi and Rondón 1971, Bryceson 1970).The only other disease with which ADCL has frequently been confused is lepromatous leprosy; this mistake is unpardonable if Giemsa-stained smears of the skin lesions have been examined (Fig. 13.11).

6   TREATMENT

Of the various drugs discussed for the treatment of Old World leishmaniasis (see Chapter 12; Lainson 1982a), the pentavalent antimonials are likewise those of first choice in dealing with the neotropical leishmaniases. It is of historical interest that the first use of antimony to treat leishmaniasis was in Brazil. A young clinician, Gaspar Vianna, impressed by the effectiveness of tartar emetic (antimony potassium tartrate) in the treatment of African trypanosomiasis (see Chapter 14), realized its potential against the related organism *Leishmania* and, in 1912, published his spectacular results obtained with this drug in advanced cases of mucocutaneous leishmaniasis (Vianna 1912). There followed development of the somewhat less toxic trivalent antimonials which, nevertheless, still produced unpleasant side effects and then the much better tolerated pentavalents which, some 5 decades later, are still the clinician's principal armaments.

6.1   American visceral leishmaniasis

Treatment usually follows that given in Chapter 12. Unresponsiveness to the recommended antimonial dosage schedule, however, has been noted in some AVL patients from Bahia, Brazil. In such cases there is little alternative other than elevating the dosage or using second line drugs such as pentamidine. In this manner, Bryceson et al. (1985) cured 4 of 10 unresponsive patients with Kenyan kala azar, but all 10 suffered serious side effects from both stibogluconate and pentamidine at the dosage levels used.

6.2 Cutaneous leishmaniasis

Once again, the treatment is much the same as that for Old World cutaneous leishmaniasis, using the pentavalent antimonials. Many clinicians prefer, however, to use the intravenous route for both pentostam and glucantime, rather than intramuscular inoculation.

In general, lesions due to the neotropical leishmanias tend to much greater chronicity than those of the Old World and there is not such a ready response to treatment. There is no justification in delaying treatment in anticipation of an early spontaneous cure, as recommended with *L. (L.) major* or *L. (L.) tropica* infections, or limiting treatment to intra-lesional injection of drugs or the topical application of these in ointments. The following hazards must be considered: subsequent mucosal disease due to *L. (V.) braziliensis*; ADCL due to parasites of the *mexicana* complex; and multiple lesions following lymphatic or haematogenous spread on the part of *L. (V.) guyanensis*. Treatment should, therefore, be systemic and immediate and identification of the causative parasite is most important. If it proves to be *L. (V.) braziliensis* treatment should be particularly intensive.

Effectiveness of the pentavalents pentostam and glucantime may vary considerably, not only when dealing with different parasites, but in treating different patients infected with the same organism. Some patients with simple lesions due to *L. (V.) guyanensis*, for example, may be cured by a single course of treatment, whereas others may require 3 or 4. In some cases of poor response, recourse must be made to other drugs, or combinations of drugs, in spite of their greater toxicity. The most commonly used second line drug is pentamidine, which has been used routinely by French workers in treating cases due to *L. (V.) guyanensis* in French Guyana.

6.3 Mucocutaneous and mucosal leishmaniasis

Advanced cases are difficult to treat, with slow response to the pentavalent antimonials. The high dosage recommended (20 mg Sb^{5+} per kg body weight, given in a single daily injection for a mean of 30 days, or until no evidence of activity of the lesion has been noted for a week) may sometimes produce pronounced side effects, so that treatment has to be suspended (Marsden 1986). The considerably more toxic amphotericin B and pentamidine are used only when there is failure to respond to the pentavalent antimonials. In some patients the early treatment provokes a severe inflammation around the lesion, presumed to be caused by antigen released from killed parasites. Although this reaction is regarded as a favourable prognostic sign, it may prove highly dangerous in patients with laryngeal or tracheal lesions. It is recommended that corticoids be used as a prophylactic measure when treating such cases and that there should be a gradual elevation of the drug dose (Marsden 1986).

Another difficulty confronting the clinician is in evaluating the effectiveness of treatment. What are the criteria of cure? Serological monitoring has used the complement fixation and indirect fluorescent antibody tests and it has been suggested that cure is indicated by decline and disappearance of antibody titres (Walton 1987). This method is likely to prove the most useful, providing measurements of leishmanial antibody can be standardized. Both parasitological and histological examination entail biopsy trauma to the treated lesion and may reactivate a lesion that seems to be healed but still contains parasites.

Mutilation following the mucosal lesions may be so extreme that even after cure the patient is ostracized and unable to lead a normal life. Plastic surgery is helpful, but only when there is no doubt of cure: Walton (1987) cites the case of one patient, with apparently complete healing, who underwent cosmetic surgery to reconstruct his nose:

'The results were disastrous, with widespread reactivation along the surgical wounds and in the patient's words – the new nose fell off!'.

6.4 Anergic diffuse cutaneous leishmaniasis (ADCL)

A smooth, fleshy, unulcerated lesion containing very abundant, large amastigotes in a patient with a negative Montenegro skin-test reaction is a danger signal that should prompt immediate, high-dosage antimonial treatment. In the authors' laboratory in Amazonian Brazil, this is virtually diagnostic of an early lesion due to *L. (L.) amazonensis* which, in an individual with a defective cell-mediated immune response (suggested by his negative skin-test), will proceed to ADCL unless adequately treated. Fortunately, although simple, curable skin lesions due to this parasite are quite common, ADCL is rare.

Of all the forms of leishmaniasis this disease undoubtedly represents the clinician's greatest challenge, for the patient is unable to offer the all-important immunological collaboration necessary for successful drug treatment. Advanced cases of ADCL, with multiple nodular lesions, may respond dramatically to the first antimonial treatment, with complete disappearance of the lesions. Unfortunately this may be taken to indicate cure, but with the cessation of treatment the nodules reappear some time later, usually more abundantly. Repeated treatment with the same drug may again give good results, but the patient relapses once more and his response steadily diminishes until the treatment is virtually ineffective. Similar results may be obtained with a variety of other drugs, until the list is exhausted and the patient's situation becomes desperate.

In patients with ADCL due to *L.(L.) amazonensis*, very hot baths taken daily, together with periodic chemotherapy, have been found to reduce the size of the nodules substantially, giving the patient a much improved appearance over periods of many years (Lainson 1982a). More recently, immuno-chemotherapy has been used with considerable success in the treatment of persons suffering from ADCL in Venezuela (Convit et al. 1989). 'Marked clinical improvement' was observed in 9 out of 10 patients given intradermal injections of a mixture of heat-killed promastigotes of '*L. mexicana amazonensis*' (*L. (L.) pifanoi* ?) isolated from a Venezuelan case of ADCL, plus 'variable amounts' of BCG, together with the standard glucantime treatment. A similar treatment of Brazilian ADCL patients infected with *L. (L.) amazonensis*, however, has met with limited success (F. T. Silveira, unpublished observations).

7 PREVENTION AND CONTROL

7.1 Visceral leishmaniasis

Campaigns are of fundamental importance, with the distribution of illustrated pamphlets to alert the populations as to the early symptoms of the disease, the signs of infection in the dog and the appearance and habits of the sandfly vector. The staff of small, rural clinics must be trained to recognize visceral leishmaniasis and should have means of reporting suspected cases to centres where more conclusive diagnosis can be made. In view of the impecunious situation of many inhabitants of the rural districts of developing countries, the staff of such centres may need to travel to the patient's village, where the possibility of other cases must be investigated. Periodic surveillance of populations at risk may detect cases of early infection, either clinically or, more effectively, by serological methods that can easily be carried out under field conditions, such as the direct agglutination test (DAT) or the dot-ELISA.

In areas of high endemicity, such as the States of Ceará and Bahia in north east Brazil, past control measures (i.e. destroying infected dogs, regular insecticide spraying of houses and animal sheds and the early treatment of patients) resulted in a dramatic drop in the number of cases of AVL. A problem arises, however, in maintaining such a control programme, which is costly and inevitably meets with considerable opposition on the part of dog owners, who fail to understand why their apparently healthy (but serologically positive) animals must be killed. A more critical evaluation of the effectiveness of this dog slaughtering policy points out the vast amount of work and expense expended in surveying dog populations and destroying all (?) the positive animals and the great difficulty of including the very large number of strays. The apparent failure of this method in control programmes in some parts of Brazil has led to the question as to what extent the dog population needs to be reduced in order to eliminate AVL or to bring it under control. It has been suggested that it may be preferable to find improved methods of eliminating or controlling the sandfly vector.

7.2 Cutaneous and mucosal leishmaniasis

Most inhabitants of the endemic areas are very familiar with the dermal leishmaniases, under their wide variety of local names, but ignorance and negligence are all too frequently to blame for allowing these diseases to reach debilitating or mutilating proportions. The painless nature of the lesions makes them of no great inconvenience in their early stages and this encourages the tendency to wait and see if they will cure spontaneously. Again, as these diseases are predominantly zoonotic, most infections are acquired by those living in rural areas, often long distances from the simplest of medical attention. As a result, a high proportion of cases only seek help when the infection is well advanced and, in regions where the causal agent is frequently *L. (V.) braziliensis*, this may prove disastrous. As for visceral leishmaniasis, health education campaigns can help to indicate the importance of early treatment.

Personal avoidance of cutaneous leishmaniasis is at present limited to the use of insect repellents, protective clothing and the avoidance of danger areas, particularly at night when the sandfly vectors are most active. These are precautions that may be feasible for the visiting tourist, but they are not very practical for the shirtless forest-worker who can ill afford to be constantly purchasing insect repellents, who is most comfortable wearing shorts (far less expensive than trousers) and long-sleeved shirts and who has to eke out his living by hunting in the forest at night.

The prevention or control of sylvatic leishmaniasis among gangs of labourers, topographers and other forestry workers can be effective on a small scale by the following measures: placing the encampments of such men in adequate clearings; spraying the bases of the larger, nearby tree trunks with insecticides (e.g. in areas where the vectors are known to be arboreal: see pages 253 and 254 under *L. (V.) guyanensis*); and prohibiting night-time hunting. Destruction of the wild animal reservoirs of sylvatic leishmaniasis is clearly neither practical nor desirable. Finally, knowledge of the ecology of a vector can sometimes help in preventing acquisition of the disease under certain circumstances. Thus, *Psychodopygus wellcomei*, an important vector of *L. (V.) braziliensis* s.l. in the highland forests of Pará, north Brazil, is highly anthropophilic and attacks humans not only at night but also frequently during the day. Field studies have shown, however, that this sandfly is only active for c. 6 months of the year, during the rainy season (November–April) and that it enters into diapause in the dry season during the rest of the year, when adult flies are rarely seen. The area in question is one of intense human activity due to the mining of iron ore and other minerals and the incidence of cutaneous leishmaniasis has been very high among those clearing the primary forest. Planning such work for the dry season clearly avoids contact with the sandfly vector.

Although drastic ecological changes such as deforestation and the planting of non-indigenous pine, gmelina and eucalyptus trees might lead to unfavourable conditions for the enzootics of some species of *Leishmania*, it can actually encourage others. Thus, the creation of vast monoculture plantations of non-indigenous trees for paper pulp production in north Brazil has eliminated cutaneous leishmaniasis due to *L. (V.) guyanensis* in the immediate areas, as neither the major reservoir host (the 2-toed sloth) nor the sandfly vector (*Lu. umbratilis*) find this new environment suitable. On the other hand, the wild rodent and marsupial hosts of *L. (L.) amazonensis* and the sandfly vector, *Lu. flaviscutellata*, find it ideal.

In those parts of Latin America where vector species have adapted to a peridomestic or domiciliary habitat, the use of insecticides is clearly indicated. In the absence of firm evidence that domestic animals with leishmanial skin lesions offer a source of infection to sandflies, it would seem unwise to recommend their destruction, even in the unlikely event of their owners' consent. Equines respond well to antimonial treatment.

8 VACCINATION

As yet, there is no commercially available vaccine that is effective against any of the leishmaniases. Killed promastigote vaccines for use against both canine visceral leishmaniasis and human cutaneous leishmaniasis are still being tested in Brazil. So far, however, studies on their efficacy are encouraging but by no means conclusive.

9 CONCLUDING REMARKS

We have discussed the possible origin of the parasitic Kinetoplastida, the family Trypanosomatidae and the genus *Leishmania* elsewhere (Lainson and Shaw 1987). It is the general opinion that the trypanosomatids have their origin in monogenetic intestinal flagellates of invertebrates and that they subsequently adapted to spend a part of their life-cycle in vertebrates. Thus, it is more correct to consider the phlebotomine sandfly as the primary host of *Leishmania* species, rather than the vertebrate hosts that merely function as reservoirs of infection for the sandfly. The finding that promastigotes may undergo a form of conjugation (Lanotte and Rioux 1990), with possible exchange of nuclear material, supports this hypothesis on the reasonable assumption that such a process is more likely to take place in the definitive or primary host of a heteroxenous parasite.

It is difficult to assess the specificity of the *Leishmania* species in their sandfly hosts and unwise to base one's conclusions on the results of laboratory experiments, when unnaturally large numbers of amastigotes or promastigotes, fed to laboratory-bred flies, may well overwhelm the natural resistance of a non-vector species. In nature, however, there is considerable evidence suggesting the limitation of the life-cycle of most leishmanial parasites to specific sandfly vectors. Thus, *Lu. longipalpis* is the only proven vector of *L. (L.) chagasi* throughout the whole geographical range of this parasite; *Lu. olmeca olmeca* and *Lu. flaviscutellata* are the only confirmed vectors of *L. (L.) mexicana* and *L. (L.) amazonensis* respectively, in Central and South America, in spite of the presence of many other species of sandflies known to feed on rodents in the endemic areas of these 2 parasites. As far as is known, *Ps. wellcomei* is the sole vector of *L. (V.) braziliensis* sensu lato in the Carajás highlands of Pará and *Lu. umbratilis* is responsible for the transmission of *L. (V.) guyanensis* throughout its geographical distribution, again in spite of the presence of a large number of other species of sandflies. On the other hand, because some sandfly vectors feed on a variety of mammalian hosts in nature, the *Leishmania* of a given species of sandfly may sometimes be isolated from a variety of mammalian hosts sharing the same habitat. *Lu. flaviscutellata*, for example, is a low-flying sandfly and transmits *L. (L.) amazonensis* to a number of predominantly terrestrial rodents and marsupials; canopy and tree trunk dwelling sandflies such as *Lu. umbratilis* and an unnamed species of the *Lu. whitmani* complex transmit *L. (V.) guyanensis* and *L. (V.) shawi*, respectively, to arboreal animals such as sloths, anteaters, monkeys and procyonids.

The number of *Leishmania* species in a given locality will largely be governed by the number of sandfly species, although some sandflies seem to be resistant to infection with this parasite. The multiplicity of species within the genus is a relatively recent realization and much research is still needed to further our knowledge regarding the diversity, ecology and taxonomy of the neotropical leishmanias. For the clinician the continued isolation and characterization of parasites from cases of human leishmaniasis is sufficient to indicate the spectrum of *Leishmania* species commonly infecting humans in a given area. The parasitologist's interests, however, are much wider. He not only requires information on the wild mammalian reservoir and sandfly vector of those parasites infecting humans, but is interested in the possible existence of other *Leishmania* species that rarely, if ever, infect humans.

The number of *Leishmania* species in the neotropical region is anybody's guess and some idea of this will only be gained when sufficient numbers of mammalian and sandfly species have been examined. Clearly, it is easier and more economical to concentrate on the sandfly population, a truly gigantic task, nonetheless, considering that nearly 400 different species of these insects have been identified in the Americas (Young and Duncan 1994). The Amazon Region has already provided us with almost half of the recognized species of neotropical leishmanias and doubtless this great forest will continue to provide us with many more!

ACKNOWLEDGEMENTS

The authors are indebted to the Wellcome Trust, London, for the financial support of our studies on the ecology, epidemiology and taxonomy of *Leishmania* in the Amazon Region of Brazil over the past 30 years and to the Instituto Evandro Chagas, Belém, Pará, where this work was carried out.

REFERENCES

Arias JR, Naiff RD, 1981, The principal reservoir host of cutaneous leishmaniasis in the urban areas of Manaus, Central Amazon of Brazil, *Mem Inst Oswaldo Cruz*, **76:** 279–86.

Badaró R, Jones TC et al, 1986, A prospective study of visceral leishmaniasis in an endemic area of Brazil, *J Infect Dis*, **154:** 639–49.

Barral A, Badaró R et al, 1986, Isolation of *Leishmania mexicana amazonensis* from the bone marrow in a case of American visceral leishmaniasis, *Am J Trop Med Hyg*, **35:** 732–4.

Barreto AC, Peterson NE et al, 1985, *Leishmania mexicana* in *Proechimys iheringi denigratus* Moojen (Rodentia: Echimyidae) in a region endemic for American cutaneous leishmaniasis, *Rev Soc Bras Med Trop*, **18:** 243–6.

Biagi FF, 1953, Algunos comentarios sobre las leishmaniasis y sus agentes etiológicos, *Leishmania tropica mexicana*, nueva subespecie, *Medna Mexico*, **33:** 401–6.

Bonfante-Garrido R, 1980, New sub-species of leishmaniasis isolated in Venezuela, *Proc 10th Int Cong Trop Med Malar, Manila*, 203.

Bonfante-Garrido R, Meléndez E et al., 1992, Cutaneous leishmaniasis in Western Venezuela caused by infection with *Leishmania venezuelensis* and *L braziliensis* variants, *Trans R Soc Trop Med Hyg*, **86:** 141–8.

Bryceson ADM, 1970, Diffuse cutaneous leishmaniasis in Ethiopia III. Immunological studies, *Trans R Soc Trop Med Hyg*, **64:** 380–7.

Bryceson ADM, Chulay JD et al., 1985, Visceral leishmaniasis unresponsive to antimonial drugs 1. Clinical and immunological studies, *Trans R Soc Trop Med Hyg*, **79:** 700–4.

Carini A, Paranhos U, 1909, Identification de l'Úlcera de Bauru avec le bouton d'Orient, *Bull Soc Pathol Exot Filiales*, **2:** 225–6.

Christensen HA, Herrer A, Telford SR, 1972, Enzootic cutaneous leishmaniasis in eastern Panama. II. Entomological investigations, *Ann Trop Med Parasitol*, **66:** 55–66.

Convit J, Lapenta P, 1986, Sobre un caso de leishmaniose tegumentaria de forma disseminada, *Revta Policlin Caracas*, **18:** 153–8.

Convit J, Pinardi ME, Rondón AJ, 1971, Diffuse cutaneous leishmaniasis: a disease due to an immunological defect of the host, *Trans R Soc Trop Med Hyg*, **66:** 603–10.

Convit J, Castellanos PL et al., 1989, Immunotherapy of localized, intermediate and diffuse forms of American cutaneous leishmaniasis, *J Infect Dis*, **160:** 104–15.

Corredor A, Gallego JF et al., 1989, *Didelphis marsupialis*, an apparent wild reservoir of *Leishmania donovani chagasi* in Colombia, South America, *Trans R Soc Trop Med Hyg*, **83:** 195.

Cunha AM, Chagas E, 1937, Nova espécie de protozoário do gênero *Leishmania* pathogenico para o homem. *Leishmania chagasi*, n. sp. Nota Prévia, *Hospital (Rio de Janeiro)*, **11:** 3–9.

Darce M, Moran J et al., 1991, Etiology of human cutaneous leishmaniasis in Nicaragua, *Trans R Soc Trop Med Hyg*, **85:** 58–9.

Darie H, Deniau M et al., 1995, Cutaneous leishmaniasis of humans due to *Leishmania (Viannia) naiffi* outside Brazil, *Trans R Soc Trop Med Hyg*, **89:** 476–7.

Deane LM, 1956, *Leishmaniose Visceral no Brasil*, Serviço Nacional de Educação Sanitária, Rio de Janerio, 1–162.

Deane LM, Grimaldi G, 1985, Leishmaniasis in Brazil, *Leishmaniasis*, eds Chang KP, Bray RS, Elsevier, New York, USA, 247–75.

Decker-Jackson JE, Tang DB, 1982, Identification of *Leishmania* spp. by radiorespirometry II. A statistical method of data analysis to evaluate the reproducibility and sensitivity of the technique, Biochemical characterization of Leishmania. Proceedings of a Workshop held at the Pan American Health Organization. 9–11 December 1980, UNDP/WORLD BANK/WHO, Geneva, Switzerland, eds Chance ML, Walton BC, 205–45.

Delgado O, Castes M et al., 1993, *Leishmania colombiensis* in Venezuela, *Am J Trop Med Hyg*, **48:** 145–7.

de Souza A, Ishikawa E et al., 1996, *Pyschodopygus complexus*, a new vector of *Leishmania braziliensis* to humans in Pará State Brazil, *Trans R Soc Trop Med Hyg*, **90:** 112–3.

Dujardin JC, Bañuls AL et al., 1995, Putative *Leishmania* hybrids in the Eastern Andean valley of Huanuco, Peru, *Acta Trop (Basel)*, **59:** 293–307.

El-Hassan AM, Meredith SEO et al., 1995, Sudanese mucosal leishmaniasis: epidemiology, clinical features, diagnosis, immune responses and treatment, *Trans R Soc Trop Med Hyg*, **89:** 647–52.

Esterre P, Chippaux JP et al., 1986, Evaluation d'un programme de lutte contre la leishmaniose cutanée dans un village forestier de Guyane française, *Bull W H O*, **64:** 559–65.

Fernandes O, Murthy VK et al., 1994, Mini-exon gene variation in human pathogenic *Leishmania* species, *Mol Biochem Parasitol*, **66:** 261–77.

Floch H, 1954, *Leishmania tropica guyanensis* n,ssp., agent de la leishmaniose tégumentaire des Guyanas et de l'Amérique Centrale, *Arch Inst Pasteur Guyane fr*, **15:** 1–4.

Garnham PCC, 1962, Cutaneous leishmaniasis in the New World with special reference to *Leishmania mexicana*, *Sci Rep Inst Sup Sanit*, **2:** 76–82.

Grimaldi G, Tesh RB, McMahon-Pratt D, 1989, A review of the geographic distribution and epidemiology of leishmaniasis in the New World, *Am J Trop Med Hyg*, **41:** 687–725.

Grimaldi G, Kreutzer RD et al., 1992, Description of *Leishmania equatorensis* sp.n. (Kinetoplastida: Trypanosomatidae), a new parasite infecting arboreal mammals in Ecuador, *Mem Inst Oswaldo Cruz*, **87:** 221–8.

Guevara P, Alonso G et al., 1992, Identification of new world *Leishmania* using ribosomal gene spacer probes, *Mol Biochem Parasitol*, **56:** 15–26.

Guilbride L, Myler PJ, Stuart K, 1992, Distribution and sequence divergence of LRV1 viruses among different *Leishmania* species, *Mol Biochem Parasitol*, **54:** 101–4.

Herrer A, 1971, *Leishmania hertigi* sp. n., from the tropical porcupine, *Coendou rothschildi* Thomas, *J Parasitol*, **57:** 626–9.

Herrer A, Christensen HA, 1975, Implication of *Phlebotomus* sandflies as vectors of bartonellosis and leishmaniasis as early as 1764, *Science*, **190:** 154–5.

Jackson PR, Wohlhieter JA, Hockmeyer WT, 1982, *Leishmania* characterization by restriction endonuclease digestion of kinetoplastic DNA, Abstracts of the Vth International Congress of Parasitology, 7–14 August 1982: Toronto, Canada, 342.

Jackson PR, Stiteler JM et al., 1984, Characterization of *Leishmania* responsible for visceral disease in Brazil by restriction endonuclease digestion and hybridization of kinetoplast DNA, Proc 11th Int Cong Trop Med Malar, Calgary, 68.

Katakura K, Matsumoto Y et al., 1993, Molecular karyotype characterization of *Leishmania panamensis*, *Leishmania mexicana*, and *Leishmania major*-like parasites: agents of cutaneous leishmaniasis in Ecuador, *Am J Trop Med Hyg*, **48:** 707–15.

Killick-Kendrick R, 1985, Some epidemiological consequences of the evolutionary fit between leishmaniae and their phlebotomine vectors, *Bull Soc Pathol Exot Filiales*, **78:** 747–55.

Killick-Kendrick R, 1990, Phlebotomine vectors of the leishmaniases: a review, *Med Vet Ent*, **4:** 1–24.

Klotz O, Lindenberg H, 1923, The pathology of leishmaniasis of the nose, *Am J Trop Med Hyg*, **3:** 117–41.

Kreutzer RD, Corredor A et al., 1991, Characterization of *Leishmania colombiensis* sp.n. (Kinetoplastida: Trypanosomatidae), a new parasite infecting humans, animals, and phlebotomine sand flies in Colombia and Panama, *Am J Trop Med Hyg*, **44:** 662–75.

Lacerda MM, 1994, The Brazilian Leishmaniasis Control Program, *Mem Inst Oswaldo Cruz*, **89:** 489–95.

Lainson R, 1982a, Leishmaniasis, *Hand book Series in Zoonoses, Section C: Parasitic Zoonoses*, vol 1, ed Steele JH, CRC Press, Boca Raton, Florida, 41–103.

Lainson R, 1982b, Leishmanial parasites of mammals in relation to human disease, *Animal Disease in Relation to Animal Conservation*, eds Edwards MA, McDonnel U, Academic Press, London, 137–79.

Lainson R, 1983, The American leishmaniases: some observations on their ecology and epidemiology, *Trans R Soc Trop Med Hyg*, **77:** 569–96.

Lainson R, 1989, Demographic changes and their influence on the epidemiology of the American leishmaniases, *Demography and Vector-Borne Diseases*, Service MW, ed., CRC Press, Boca Raton, Florida, 85–106.

Lainson R, 1996, New World leishmaniasis, *The Wellcome History of Tropical Diseases*, ed Cox FEG, 218–29.

Lainson R, Ward RD, Shaw JJ, 1977, Experimental transmission of *Leishmania chagasi*, the causative agent of neotropical visceral leishmaniasis, by the sandfly *Lutzomyia longipalpis, Nature (London)*, **226:** 628–30.

Lainson R, Shaw JJ, 1972, Leishmaniasis of the New World: Taxonomic problems, *Br Med Bull*, **28:** 44–8.

Lainson R, Shaw JJ, 1977, Leishmanias of neotropical porcupines: *Leishmania hertigi deanei* nov.subsp, *Acta Amazonica*, **7:** 51–7.

Lainson R, Shaw JJ, 1979, The role of animals in the epidemiology of South American leishmaniasis, *Biology of the Kinetoplastida*, vol 2, eds Lumsden WHR, Evans DA, Academic Press, London, New York and San Francisco, 1–116.

Lainson R, Shaw JJ, 1981, The leishmanial parasites, *Medical Laboratory Manual for Tropical Countries*, ed Cheesbrough M, S Austin and Sons, Hertford, England, 206–17.

Lainson R, Shaw JJ, 1987, Evolution, classification and geographical distribution, *The Leishmaniases in Biology and Medicine*, vol 1, eds Peters W, Killick-Kendrick R, Academic Press, London, 1–120.

Lainson R, Shaw JJ, 1989, *Leishmania (Viannia) naiffi* sp.n., a parasite of the armadillo, *Dasypus novemcinctus* (L.) in Amazonian Brazil, *Ann Parasitol Hum Comp*, **64:** 3–9.

Lainson R, Shaw JJ, 1992, A brief history of the genus *Leishmania* (Protozoa: Kinetoplastida) in the Americas with particular reference to Amazonian Brazil, *Ciência e Cultura*, **44:** 94–106.

Lainson R, Strangways-Dixon J, 1963, *Leishmania mexicana*: The epidemiology of dermal leishmaniasis in British Honduras, *Trans R Soc Trop Med Hyg*, **57:** 242–65.

Lainson R, Shaw JJ et al., 1979, Leishmaniasis in Brazil: XIII. Isolation of *Leishmania* from armadillos (*Dasypus novemcinctus*), and observations on the epidemiology of cutaneous leishmaniasis in North Pará State, *Trans R Soc Trop Med Hyg*, **73:** 239–42.

Lainson R, Shaw JJ et al., 1985, Leishmaniasis in Brazil: XXI: Visceral leishmaniasis in the Amazon Region and further observations on the role of *Lutzomyia longipalpis* (Lutz and Neiva 1912) as the vector, *Trans R Soc Trop Med Hyg*, **79:** 223–6.

Lainson R, Shaw JJ et al., 1987, American visceral leishmaniasis: on the origin of *Leishmania (Leishmania) chagasi, Trans R Soc Trop Med Hyg*, **81:** 517.

Lainson R, Braga RR et al., 1989, *Leishmania (Viannia) shawi* n.sp., a parasite of monkeys, sloths and procyonids in Amazonian Brazil, *Ann Parasitol Hum Comp*, **64:** 200–7.

Lainson R, Dye C et al., 1990a, Amazonian visceral leishmaniasis – Distribution of the vector *Lutzomyia longipalpis* (Lutz and Neiva) in relation to the fox *Cerdocyon thous* (Linn.) and the efficiency of this reservoir host as a source of infection, *Mem Inst Oswaldo Cruz*, **85:** 135–7.

Lainson R, Shaw JJ et al., 1990b, Cutaneous leishmaniasis of humans due to *Leishmania (Viannia) naiffi* Lainson and Shaw 1989, *Ann Parasitol Hum Comp*, **65:** 282–4.

Lainson R, Shaw JJ et al., 1994, The dermal leishmaniases of Brazil, with special reference to the eco-epidemiology of the disease in Amazonia, *Mem Inst Oswaldo Cruz*, **89:** 435–43.

Lanotte G, Rioux J-A, 1990, Fusion cellulaire chez les *Leishmania* (Kinetoplastida, Trypanosomatidae), *C R Acad Sci*, **310:** 285–8.

Laveran A, Mesnil F, 1903, Sur un protozoaire nouveau (*Piroplasma donovani* Lav. et Mesn.).Parasite d'une fièvre de l'Inde, *C R Acad Sci*, **137:** 957–61.

Lindenberg A, 1909, A úlcera de Bauru e seu micróbio, *Revta Méd, S Paulo*, **12:** 116–20.

Luz E, Giovannoni M, Borba AM, 1967, Infecção de *Lutzomyia monticola* por *Leishmania enriettii*, *Anais Fac Med Univ Fed Paraná*, **9–10:** 121–8.

Lysenko AJ, 1971, Distribution of leishmaniasis in the Old World, *Bull W H O*, **44:** 515–20.

Machado MI, Milder RV et al., 1994, Naturally acquired infections of *Leishmania enriettii* Muniz and Medina 1948 in guinea-pigs from São Paulo, Brazil, *Parasitology*, **109:** 135–8.

Marsden PD, 1986, Mucosal leishmaniasis ('espundia' Escomel 1911), *Trans R Soc Trop Med Hyg*, **80:** 859–76.

Màrquez M, Scorza JV, 1982, Criterios de nuliparidad y paridad en *Lutzomyia townsendi* (Ortiz 1959) del occidente de Venezuela, *Mem Inst Oswaldo Cruz*, **77:** 229–46.

Matta A, 1916, Sur les leishmanioses tégumentaires. Classification générale des leishmanioses, *Bull Soc Pathol Exot Filiales*, **9:** 494–503.

Matta A, 1918, Notas para a historia das leishmanioses da pele e das mucosas, *Amaz Méd*, **1:** 11–7.

Mazza S, Cornejo AJ, 1926, Primeros casos autóctonos de kala-azar infantil comprobados en el norte de la República (Tabacal y Orán, Salta), *Bol Inst Clín Quir (Buenos Aires)*, **2:** 140–4.

Medina H, 1946, Estudos sôbre leishmaniose. I. Primeiros casos de leishmaniose espontânea observados em cobaias, *Arq Biol Tec, Curitiba*, **1:** 39–74.

Medina R, Romero J, 1959, Estudio clinico y parasitologico de una nueva cepa de leishmania, *Arch Ven Pat Trop Parasit Méd*, **3:** 298–326.

Medina R, Romero J, 1962, *Leishmania pifanoi* n.sp. El agente causal de la leishmaniasis tegumentaria difusa, *Arch Ven Pat Trop Parasit Méd*, **4:** 349–53.

Mendoza-León A, Havercroft JC, Barker DC, 1995, The RFLP analysis of the β-tubulin gene region in New World *Leishmania*, *Parasitology*, **111:** 1–9.

Migone LE, 1913, Un caso de kala-azar a Assuncion (Paraguay), *Bull Soc Pathol Exot Filiales*, **6:** 118–20.

Miles MA, Póvoa MM et al., 1980, Some methods for the enzymic characterization of Latin-American *Leishmania* with particular reference to *Leishmania mexicana amazonensis* and subspecies of *Leishmania hertigi*, *Trans R Soc Trop Med Hyg*, **74:** 243–52.

Molyneux DH, Killick-Kendrick R, 1987, Morphology, ultrastructure and life cycles, *The Leishmaniases in Biology and Medicine*, Vol 1, eds Peters W, Killick-Kendrick R, Academic Press, London, 121–76.

Muniz J, Medina H, 1948, Leishmaniose tegumentar do cobaio (*Leishmania enriettii* n. sp.), *Hospital (Rio de Janeiro)*, **33:** 7–25.

Naiff RD, Freitas RA et al., 1989, Aspectos epidemiológicos de uma *Leishmamia* de tatus (*Dasypus novemcinctus*), Resumos do XI Congresso Brasileira de Parasitologia, July-August 1989, Rio de Janeiro, 24.

Navin TR, Arana BA et al., 1992, Placebo-controlled clinical trial of sodium stibogluconate (Pentostam) versus Ketoconazole for treating cutaneous leishmaniasis in Guatemala, *J Infect Dis*, **165:** 528–34.

Oliveira MP, Marzochi MCA et al., 1986, Concurrent human infection with *Leishmania donovani* and *Leishmania braziliensis braziliensis*, *Ann Trop Med Parasitol*, **80:** 587–92.

Penna HA, 1934, Leishmaniose visceral no Brasil, *Bras-Méd*, **48:** 949–50.

Pessôa SB, 1941, Dados sobre a epidemiologia da leishmaniose tegumentar em São Paulo, *O Hospital*, **19:** 389–409.

Pessôa SB, 1961, Classificação das leishmanioses e das espécies do gênero *Leishmania*, *Arq Hig Saúde Púb*, **26:** 41–50.

Pessôa SB, Barretto MP, 1948, *Leishmaniose Tegumentar Americana*, Imprensa Nacional, Rio de Janeiro, Brasil, 1–527.

Peterson EA, Neva FA et al., 1982, Specific inhibition of lymphocyte-proliferation response by adherent suppressor cells in diffuse cutaneous leishmaniasis, *N Engl J Med*, **306:** 387–92.

Ponce C, Ponce E et al., 1991, *Leishmania donovani chagasi*: new clinical variant of cutaneous leishmaniasis in Honduras, *Lancet*, **337:** 67–70.

Raccurt CP, Pratlong F et al., 1995, French Guiana must be recognized as an endemic area of *Leishmania (Viannia) braziliensis* in South America, *Trans R Soc Trop Med Hyg*, **89:** 372.

Rangel EF, Lainson R et al., 1996, Variation between geographical populations of *Lutzomyia (Nyssomyia) whitmani* (Antunes and Coutinho 1939) *sensu lato* (Diptera: Psychodidae: Phlebotominae) in Brazil, *Mem Inst Oswaldo Cruz*, **91:** 43–50.

Ridley DS, 1987, Pathology, *The Leishmaniases in Biology and Medicine*, vol. 2, eds Peters W, Killick-Kendrick R, Academic Press, London, 665–701.

Rioux JA, Lanotte G et al., 1990, Taxonomy of *Leishmania*. Use of isoenzymes. Suggestions for a new classification, *Ann Parasitol Hum Comp*, **65:** 111–25.

Ross R, 1903, (1) Note on the bodies recently described by Leishman and Donovan and (2) further notes on Leishman's bodies *Br Med J*, **2:** 1261–2 and 1401.

Saf'yanova VM, 1982, [The problems of *Leishmania* taxonomy] In Russian, *Protozoologiya (Leishmanii) Leningrad*, **7:** 3–109.

Santoro F, Lemesre JL et al., 1986, Spécificité au niveau des protéines de surface des promastigotes de *Leishmania donovani* (Laveran et Mesnil 1903) *Leishmania infantum* Nicolle 1908 et *Leishmania chagasi* Cunha et Chagas 1937, Leishmania Taxonomie et phylogenèse. Applications éco-épidémiologiques. Colloque International. J-A Rioux, Ed., (2–6 July 1984), IMEEE, Montpellier, 71–5.

Scorza JV, Valera M et al., 1979, A new species of *Leishmania* parasite from the Venezuelan Andes region, *Trans R Soc Trop Med Hyg*, **73:** 293–8.

Shaw JJ, 1994, Taxonomy of the genus *Leishmania*: Present and future trends and their implications, *Mem Inst Oswaldo Cruz*, **89:** 471–8.

Shaw JJ, Lainson R, 1987, Ecology and epidemiology: New World, *The Leishmaniases in Biology and Medicine*, vol 1, eds Peters W, Killick-Kendrick R, Academic Press, London, 291–363.

Sherlock IA, Miranda JC et al., 1984, Natural infection of the opossum *Didelphis albiventris* (Marsupialia: Didelphidae) with *Leishmania donovani* in Brazil, *Mem Inst Oswaldo Cruz*, **79:** 511.

Silveira FT, Shaw JJ et al., 1987, Dermal leishmaniasis in the Amazon Region of Brazil: *Leishmania (Viannia) lainsoni* sp.n., a new parasite from the State of Pará, *Mem Inst Oswaldo Cruz*, **82:** 289–92.

Spithill TW, Samaras N, 1985, The molecular karyotype of *Leishmania major* and mapping of α and β tubulin gene families to multiple unlinked chromosomal loci, *Nucleic Acids Res*, **13:** 4155–69.

Tarr PI, Aline RF et al., 1988, LR1: a candidate RNA virus of *Leishmania*, *Proc Natl Acad Sci USA*, **85:** 9572–5.

Travi BL, Jaramillo C et al., 1994, *Didelphis marsupialis*, an important reservoir of *Trypanosoma (Schizotrypanum) cruzi* and *Leishmania (Leishmania) chagasi* in Colombia, *Am J Trop Med Hyg*, **50:** 557–65.

Travi BL, Vélez ID et al., 1990, *Lutzomyia evansi*, an alternate vector of *Leishmania chagasi* in a Colombian focus of visceral leishmaniasis, *Trans R Soc Trop Med Hyg*, **84:** 676–7.

Velez LR, 1913, Uta e espundia, *Bull Soc Pathol Exot Filiales*, **6:** 545.

Vianna G, 1911, Sôbre uma nova especie de *Leishmania* (Nota Preliminar), *Bras-Méd*, **25:** 411.

Vianna G, 1912, Tratamento da leishmaniose pelo tartaro emético, *Arch Venez Patol Trop Parasitol Méd*, **2:** 426–8.

Villela F, Pestana BR, Pessôa SB, 1939, Presença de *Leishmania braziliensis* na mucosa nasal sem lesão aparente em casos recentes de leishmaniose cutânea, *Hospital*, **16:** 953–60.

Walton BC, 1987, American cutaneous and mucocutaneous leishmaniasis, *The Leishmaniases in Biology and Medicine*, vol. 2, eds Peters W, Killick-Kendrick R, Academic Press, London, 637–64.

Ward RD, Ribeiro AL et al., 1983, Reproductive isolation between different forms of *Lutzomyia longipalpis* (Lutz and Neiva), (Diptera:Psychodidae), the vector of *Leishmania donovani chagasi* Cunha and Chagas and its significance to kala-azar distribution in South America, *Mem Inst Oswaldo Cruz*, **78:** 269–80.

Ward RD, Phillips A et al., 1988, The *Lutzomyia longipalpis* complex: reproduction and distribution, *Biosystematics of Haematophagus Insects*, vol 37, ed Service MW, Clarendon Press, Oxford, 257–69.

Yoshida ELA, Cuba Cuba CA et al., 1993, Description of *Leishmania (Leishmania) forattinii* sp. n., a new parasite infecting opossums and rodents in Brazil, *Mem Inst Oswaldo Cruz*, **88:** 397–406.

Young DG, Duncan MA, 1994, Guide to the identification and geographic distribution of *Lutzomyia* sand flies in Mexico, the West Indies, Central and South America (Diptera: Psychodidae), Memoirs of the American Entomological Institute no. 54. Associated Publishers, American Entomological Institute, Gainsville, Florida, 1–881.

Chapter 14

AFRICAN TRYPANOSOMIASIS

J R Seed

1	Classification	6	Diagnosis
2	Structure and life cycle	7	Epidemiology and control
3	Biochemistry, molecular biology and genetics	8	Chemotherapy
4	Clinical manifestations	9	Vaccination
5	Pathology and immunology	10	Conclusion

African trypanosomiasis has been known since the fifteenth century but only began to be actively studied after the start of European colonial expansion (Ford 1971). Various historical accounts of the early work on the epidemiology, the control measures and the social and economic consequences of trypanosomiasis are available (Duggan 1970, Ford 1971). These accounts record the great impact of trypanosomiasis on Africans during the early colonial period.

Unfortunately, African trypanosomiasis of humans is a serious public health problem in much of subsaharan Africa today. The reasons for this are many, but social disorder, the breakdown of public health programmes and, as a consequence, a reduction of surveillance and treatment, are key factors. The epidemics that have occurred in countries in which political unrest has disrupted the normal public health infrastructure are evidence for this analysis. In 1960 in Zaire, following a breakdown of surveillance, there was an increase in prevalence from 0.01% to 12%. In the 1970s, during the civil war in Uganda, there was a large increase in trypanosomiasis. In 1972 52 cases were reported; during the next 8-year period there were over 8000 cases. In 1987 there were over 7000 new cases, and some villages had over 25% infection rates (Abaru 1985, Kuzoe 1991, 1993). In the 1990s new outbreaks were reported in northwestern Uganda. These were imported with individuals migrating from areas of civil and political unrest in the Sudan (Kuzoe 1991). Other increases have been observed in the Cameroon, Chad, the Central African Republic and Côte d'Ivoire. It can be predicted that similar flareups will occur in Rwanda and Burundi as a result of the civil wars there.

1 CLASSIFICATION

Stephens and Fantham (1910) placed *Trypanosoma rhodesiense* into a separate species from *Trypanosoma gambiense* on the basis of its causing an acute rather than a chronic infection, its causing a high parasitaemia and its morphology in humans. Today, the species are not considered to be separate. There are now considered to be 3 subspecies of *T. brucei*: *Trypanosoma brucei brucei*, the closely related *T. b. rhodesiense* and the more distant *T. b. gambiense* (Table 14.1). Only *T. b. gambiense* and *T. b. rhodesiense* are generally considered to be infectious to humans. *Trypanosoma b. brucei* is generally considered to be restricted to animal hosts. However, recent experimental data indicate that infectivity to humans can develop in *T. b. brucei* during passage in animal hosts (Paindavoine et al. 1989). Currently the only way to distinguish isolates of *T. b. brucei* from *T. b. rhodesiense* is to test for their susceptibility to lysis by human serum; *T. b. brucei* is susceptible to lysis, *T. b. rhodesiense* is not. The trypanolytic factor in human serum is part of the high density lipoprotein fraction. It appears to act after it is taken into acidic lysosomal vacuoles by the trypanosomes (Hajduk, Hager and Esko 1994).

The members of the *Trypanosoma (Trypanozoon) brucei* complex, *T. b. brucei*, *T. b. rhodesiense*, and *T. b. gambiense*, share phenotypic characteristics including their morphology, life cycle and major biochemical features. However, based upon data from electrophoretic analysis of isoenzymes and analysis of restriction fragment length polymorphisms (RFLP) it would appear that the brucei group trypanosomes have significant intraspecific variation. By cluster analysis of data on isoenzyme variation the African trypanosomes can be placed into a number of different principal zymodeme groups. The data suggest that organisms of the *T. b.*

Table 14.1 Classification of the order Kinetoplastida

Order	Kinetoplastida				
Family	Trypanosomatidae				
Genus	*Trypanosoma*				
Section	Stercoraria		Salivaria		
Subgenus	*Schizotrypanum*	*Duttonella*	*Nannomonas*	*Trypanozoon*	*Pycnomonas*
Species	*T. (S.) cruzi*	*T. (D.) vivax*	*T. (N.) congolense*	*T. (T.) brucei*	*T. (P.) suis*
				T. (T.) b. brucei	
				T. (T.) b. rhodesiense	
				T. (T.) b. gambiense	
				T. (T.) equiperdum	
				T. (T.) evansi	

gambiense group are fairly homogenous by zymodeme analysis and can be distinguished by this method from organisms of the *T. b. rhodesiense* and *T. b. brucei* groups (Stevens and Godfrey 1992). In addition, it has also been shown that *T. b. brucei* can be distinguished from human serum resistant stocks of *T. b. rhodesiense* by RFLP analysis (Hide et al. 1994). However despite broad similarity among *T. b. gambiense* strains it would appear that they are microheterogenous by isoenzyme and RFLP analysis (Enyaru et al. 1993).

Many workers have concluded that the African trypanosomes are evolving rapidly with respect to their population genetics and epidemiology, and that is why quite complex variations in isoenzyme and RFLP patterns are found among various isolates from tsetse, from different host groups and from distinct geographical locations.

There are 2 other members of the subgenus *Trypanozoon*, *T. equiperdum* and *T. evansi*. These are important animal parasites but are not infective to humans. Both organisms are distinguished from *T. b. brucei* in their mode of transmission. Neither *T. equiperdum* nor *T. evansi* uses the tsetse vector, and they are therefore not restricted to the African continent.

2 STRUCTURE AND LIFE CYCLE

2.1 Structure

The African trypanosomes are single-celled flagellated protozoa that infect a wide variety of animal hosts including humans. Except for *T. b. evansi* and *T. b. equiperdum*, they are transmitted by flies of the genus *Glossina*, order Diptera.

All members of the subgenus *Trypanozoon* have a similar basic morphology which they share with other members of the order Kinetoplastida as well as with other protozoa and eukaryotic cells. The organelles within the cell, as observed by light and transmission electron microscopy, include a basal body and flagellar pocket from which the flagellum extends, a nucleus with peripheral chromatin and nucleolus, an endoplasmic reticulum, a Golgi apparatus, glycosomes and a kinetoplast–mitochondrion complex which shares many characteristics with the mitochondria of other eukaryotic cells. The trypanosomes also have a typical unit cell membrane which is covered by a surface coat. This coat contains the variant surface glycoprotein (VSG). Just below the cell membrane there is a complex of microtubules and microfilaments which are anchored to the cell membrane. These structures are shown diagrammatically in Fig. 14.1, and the literature on them has been reviewed by Seed and Hall (1992) and Vickerman and Barry (1982). The flagellar pocket is free of microtubules and of VSG. This area has receptors for transferrin, low density lipoprotein and possibly various proteins, and is involved in receptor-mediated endocytosis. By electron microscopy it has been possible to demonstrate the presence of large molecular weight molecules in a line of vacuoles extending from the flagellar pocket into the cytoplasm. Endocytosis apparently occurs both in the blood forms and in the procyclic stages of the parasite in the vector. The rate of endocytosis is much less in the procyclic form, and the process, to the extent it does occur, may differ from that observed in the metacyclic and blood stages.

The trypanosomes have an organelle called a **kinetoplast** which is unique to the Kinetoplastidia. In Giemsa stained preparations viewed by light microscopy the kinetoplast resembles a small nucleus. The morphology of the kinetoplast–mitochondrial complex differs considerably among the different

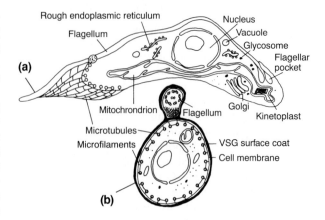

Fig. 14.1 Ultrastructure of an African trypanosome: (a) longitudinal section of an intermediate to short stumpy blood trypanosome; (b) cross-sectional view. (From Seed and Hall 1992, with permission of Academic Press.)

forms existing at the various stages of the trypanosomes life cycle. In the long slender (LS) stage in the vertebrate host (20–40 × 0.1 μm) the mitochondrion is non-functional. When viewed ultrastructurally this stage is seen to have a mitochondrion without cristae. In the forms in the vector the mitochondrion is functional and has cristae.

2.2 Life cycle

When an uninfected tsetse bites an infected vertebrate the development in the vector is initiated. The trypanosomes in the vector's bloodmeal pass through the oesophagus, the crop and the proventriculus until they finally reach the midgut. In the fly's midgut the short stumpy (SS) forms present in the vertebrate blood complete their morphological and biochemical differentiation into procyclic stages. They complete the development of their mitochondrion, change their surface coat and begin to divide. As the procyclic form has a fully functional mitochondrion it differs from the bloodstream forms in metabolic activity. The procyclic forms also differ from the bloodstream forms in the relative position of the kinetoplast and nucleus, as well as in their mode of motility. After a period of growth in the midgut, the trypanosomes undergo a further series of morphological changes, migrate from the midgut into the endoperitrophic space and finally into the tsetse's salivary glands where they develop into **epimastigotes**. The epimastigote form is not infective for the mammalian host. The epimastigotes attach to the cells of the gland. They divide repeatedly and then transform into non-dividing **metacyclic forms**, which are small, highly motile, short and stumpy (Fig. 14.2). They have a terminally located kinetoplast but no free flagellum. When mature the metacyclic forms detach from the salivary gland cells, synthesize a surface coat of the type found on the bloodstream forms and become infective to the vertebrate host (Vickerman et al. 1988, Vickerman 1989). The signals for these morphological and physiological changes in the trypanosome in its vector are not known. The time required for the trypanosomes ingested by the fly to complete their development in the tsetse and to regain infectivity is approximately 3–4 weeks. The length of time will vary depending upon the external environmental conditions of humidity and temperature and on the age, sex and other factors in the tsetse (Molyneux and Ashford 1983).

The infective metacyclic forms of the trypanosome are injected into the mammalian host by the biting fly. They transform in the vertebrate host into the LS trypanomastigote form and increase in number. Following an increase in the LS population a switch in trypanosome morphology occurs. The dividing LS form transforms into first an intermediate (I) stage and then into a non-dividing short stumpy (SS) form (15–25 × 3.5 μm). The SS stage has a terminal (posteriorly located) kinetoplast and no free flagellum. While this morphological transition occurs there are also morphological and biochemical changes in the kinetoplast–mitochondrion complex. These changes are initial steps in the development of a functional mitochondrion. The specific environmental signals and the molecular triggers which induce this switch are not known. It has been suggested that the SS stage (which no longer divides in the mammalian host) is the stage infective for the tsetse. The transition from the LS to SS form may therefore be critical for fly transmission and successful completion of the life cycle.

The trypanosomes have a complex life cycle and a low infection rate in their vectors. It is known that age, sex and genotype of the vector, the type of bloodmeal taken by the vector and many environmental factors can all influence the susceptibility of the tsetse to the trypanosomes (Maudlin and Ellis 1985, Molyneux and Ashford 1983, Otieno et al. 1983, Vickerman et al. 1988). It has also been suggested that a trypanosome infection influences the behaviour of flies, causing them to probe and feed more frequently (Jenni et al. 1980, Molyneux and Jefferies 1986). These factors make knowledge of the life cycle important in the epidemiology of African trypanosomiasis.

3 BIOCHEMISTRY, MOLECULAR BIOLOGY AND GENETICS

3.1 Cultivation

Since the 1980s significant progress has been made in the cultivation of trypanosomes, and it is now possible to grow all stages of the African trypanosomes in vitro. Excellent reviews of both old and recent work exist (Brun and Jenni 1985, Gray, Hirumi and Gardines 1987, Kaminsky, Beaudoin and Cunningham. 1988, Kaminsky and Zweyaath 1989). The early systems for the cultivation of the blood form required the co-cultivation of the trypanosomes with a layer of mammalian feeder cells. It is now possible to cultivate the trypanosomes in axenic cultures containing reducing agents such as cysteine, β-mercaptoethanol or monothioglycerol (Baltz et al. 1985, Duszenko et al. 1985, Hamm et al. 1990). The axenic system is especially attractive for use in research on the biochemistry of the organisms. The major problem with the use of all culture systems for the growth of the blood forms is the low yields obtained ($1–2 × 10^6$ organisms/ml). The loss in culture of pleomorphy and therefore the loss of the ability to differentiate into the SS and procyclic forms is also a problem for those wishing to produce trypanosomes in all their morphologic forms in culture.

3.2 Biochemistry

The blood stage trypanosomes have a high rate of glucose catabolism. The glycolytic enzymes carrying out this process are present in a unique microbody-like organelle called the **glycosome**. In the bloodstream form the 9 enzymes involved in the conversion of glucose into phosphoglycerate or glycerol account for more than 90% of the protein in the glycosome

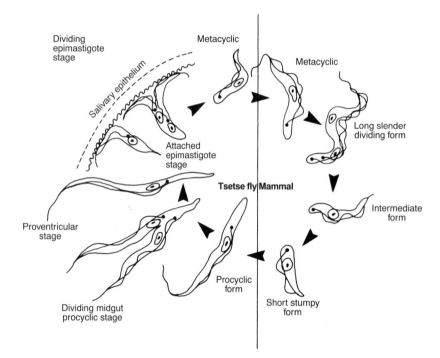

Fig. 14.2 Life cycle of trypanosomes of the *Trypanosoma brucei* group. (From Seed and Hall, 1992, with permission of Academic Press.)

(Hannaert and Michels 1994, Opperdoes 1987, Opperdoes et al. 1990). Various other enzymes, including those involved in pyrimidine and in ether lipid biosynthesis, and the enzymes malate dehydrogenase and phosphoenolpyruvate decarboxylase are also present in the glycosome. The activity levels of these enzymes differ in the blood and procyclic stages, reflecting the different metabolic states of the different forms of the parasite.

The compartmentation of the trypanosome's glycolytic enzymes in the glycosomes is a pattern different from that which occurs in other eukaryotic organisms where the enzymes involved in glycolysis are present in the cytoplasm. It has been suggested that the close physical association of the glycolytic enzymes in the glycosome and their high concentration there account for the very high rate of glucose catabolism by the blood stage parasites (Hannaert and Michels 1994, Sommer and Wang 1994). There is evidence to suggest that glucose uptake is the rate-limiting step of the pathway for glucose utilization. Once glucose is within the cell it must enter the glycosome where it is catabolized via the Embden–Meyerhof pathway under aerobic conditions to form pyruvate. The blood stage trypanosomes lack lactate dehydrogenase and pyruvate decarboxylase enzymes and therefore pyruvate is directly excreted into the blood and other tissue fluids. Pyruvate can also be transaminated to alanine and therefore alanine is also excreted. The reoxidation of the NADH formed during glycolysis is carried out in the African trypanosomes by a dihydroxyacetone phosphate:-glycerol-3-phosphate oxidase (Fig. 14.3). This oxidase uses molecular oxygen as its final acceptor, is cyanide insensitive, does not require pyridine nucleotide cofactors nor cytochromes, and does not generate ATP (Bowman and Flynn 1976, Fairlamb 1989, Fairlamb and Opperdoes 1986). ATP is produced primarily by substrate phosphorylation during glycolysis. Under anaerobic conditions the trypanosomes still metabolize glucose, and in the process equimolar amounts of pyruvate and glycerol are formed. Dehydroxyacetone phosphate acts as the electron acceptor for the reoxidation

of NADH directly by enzymes in the glycosome, and net ATP formation occurs during the formation of glycerol from glycerol-3-phosphate (Fig. 14.3).

The procyclic forms are adapted to the environment of the vector which is entirely different from the environment that the blood forms inhabit. In the procyclic forms, the mitochondrion becomes functional; it has cristae, and contains the tricarboxylic acid cycle enzymes, cytochromes and cytochrome-dependent respiratory chain enzymes, all of which are absent from the LS form. The procyclic form has a much lower rate of glucose catabolism than does the LS form. Phosphoenolpyruvate is carboxylated by procyclics to form oxaloacetic acid with subsequent conversion to malate, fumarate and succinate. The major end products of glucose

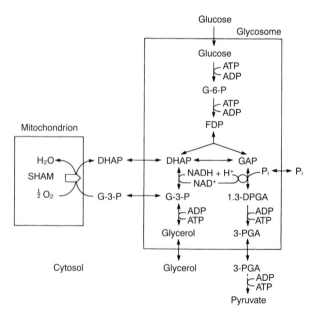

Fig. 14.3 Glucose metabolism in the bloodstream form of African trypanosomes (Opperdoes 1987).

utilization by the procyclic forms are succinate, acetate, carbon dioxide and alanine. ATP is generated primarily by oxidative phosphorylation. Amino acids, particularly proline, are the primary substrates used by the procyclics to obtain energy.

All the enzymes of the pentose phosphate pathway have been found in *T. b. brucei* (Cronin, Nolan and Voorheis 1989). These trypanosomes therefore possess the enzymes required to produce d-ribose-5-phosphate for nucleic acid synthesis and NADPH for other synthetic reactions. There are differences between the procyclic and blood forms in the enzymes of the non-oxidative segment of the pentose phosphate pathway. Both forms lack key enzymes necessary for classical glyconeogenesis, and both lack the enzymes of the Entner–Douderoff pathway (Cronin, Nolan and Voorheis 1989).

There has been relatively little study of amino acid synthesis and utilization by trypanosomes, but it appears that the organisms have limited ability to synthesize amino acids *de novo*. A majority of the amino acids required by trypanosomes must either be formed by a salvage pathway such as that bringing about the transamination of pyruvate, oxaloacetic and α-ketoglutarate to alanine, aspartic and glutamic acids, respectively, or be directly supplied by the host (Gutteridge and Coombs 1977).

Some amino acids are used for purposes other than protein synthesis. In the procyclic forms, proline is used as a respiratory substrate, and threonine may serve as the preferred substrate for formation of acetyl coenzyme A, which is required for the elongation of fatty acid chains. The only enzymes involved in amino acid metabolism which have received extensive study are those bringing about aromatic amino acid catabolism and those for the use of ornithine in the synthesis of polyamines. The polyamines are known to be important in the proliferation and differentiation of the blood stage trypanosomes. Inhibition of putrescine and spermidine synthesis blocks trypanosome division and causes changes in cellular morphology (Pegg and McCann 1988).

A novel low molecular weight dithiol called trypanothione is synthesized by the trypanosomes from the polyamine spermidine and the tripeptide glutathione (Fairlamb 1989, Fairlamb and Cerami 1992). Trypanothione appears to have a function in the trypanosomes similar to that of glutathione in other eukaryotes, acting as an intracellular antioxidant.

Neither the blood nor procyclic forms of the trypanosomes synthesize purines de novo; they require salvage mechanisms to obtain them (Hammond and Gutteridge 1984). Most of the enzymes of the salvage pathway are located in the cytoplasm, although hypoxanthine–guanine phosphoribosyl transferase is found in the glycosome. The trypanosomes can synthesize pyrimidine by a pathway which appears similar to that used by mammalian cells, although there are 2 differences in the pathway: (1) in mammals the enzyme dihydroorotate dehydrogenase is present in the mitochondria, but in the trypanosomes it is present in the cytosol; (2) in the trypanosomes the last 2 enzymes of the pathway (orotate phosphoribosyl transferase and orotidine 5-phosphate decarboxylase) are in the glycosomes rather than in their cytosol as in mammals (Fairlamb 1989).

Trypanosomes contain the usual lipids found in other eukaryotic cells. They have limited ability to synthesize lipids and generally depend on the host for fatty acids, choline and other lipids (reviewed in Mellors and Samad 1989). The trypanosomes contain large amounts of phospholipids similar to those found in mammals, much of it linked to glycerol. The trypanosomes can synthesize glycerol phospholipids. Interest in trypanosome lipid metabolism has recently increased because lipids are important in anchoring surface membrane proteins into the cell membrane.

3.3 Molecular biology and genetics

The nucleus of the African trypanosomes contains a limited number of large chromosomes and a large number of small chromosomes. The chromatin is organized into regularly spaced nucleosomes and the nucleus contains 4 histones analogous to those of other eukaryotic cells (Hecker et al. 1995). Recent work suggests that the trypanosome H-1 histone differs from the H-1 histone in other eukaryotic cells in its weak interaction with DNA at low salt concentrations (Hecker et al. 1995). This difference might help to explain why discrete chromosomes have not been observed in trypanosomes prepared by standard techniques.

In the African trypanosomes the nuclear membrane does not break down during cell division. During division the spindle apparatus is contained within the nuclear membrane.

There is considerable evidence that exchange of genetic information can occur in the African trypanosomes, and that this exchange occurs in the vector's salivary glands, not in the mammalian host (Gibson and Garside 1991, and Gibson and Whittington 1993). Although it is apparent from the analysis of isoenzyme patterns, as well as restriction fragment length polymorphisms (RFLP) among different stocks, that sexual recombination does occur among trypanosomes in the field, there is also considerable evidence that much of the genetic heterogeneity in field isolates is due to clonal reproduction and recombination during mitosis. Additions, deletions and point mutations must also contribute to trypanosome diversity.

There is debate as to the ploidy of the trypanosomes. The results of isoenzyme and RFLP analysis of genetic crosses between trypanosome clones suggest that the trypanosomes are generally diploid. However, there is evidence to suggest that some hybrids may be triploid and that changes in chromosome size may occur during genetic exchange (Kooy et al. 1989, Gibson, Garside and Bailey 1992).

One of the most interesting aspects of the trypanosomes, a major factor in their ability to produce disease and thwart the immune response, is their ability to vary the antigenic nature of their surface coat. It has been demonstrated using molecular techniques that the trypanosomes contain within their genome over 1000 different genes coding for different variant surface glycoproteins (VSG). In addition, it would appear that new variant antigen types (VAT) are constantly being created by mutations, additions, deletions and recombination during trypanosome growth.

Each trypanosome expresses only a single VSG on its surface at any given time, and the exposed epitopes of each VSG within the coat appear immunologically unique. The African trypanosomes have a large repertoire of VSG genes. It is this large number of genes and the trypanosomes' ability to switch their expression on and off, allowing them to change their surface coat, that permits the trypanosomes to escape the host's immune response. In mammals new peaks in parasitaemia appear to occur every 5–10 days (Fig. 14.4).

The kinetoplast contains a significant percentage of the cell's DNA. This DNA exists in 2 forms. There are a small number of large circular strands of DNA, called **maxicircles**. The maxicircles contain the genetic information for the synthesis of the structural and enzymic proteins of the mitochondrion. The second type consists of a large number of small interwoven **minicircles** of DNA. This DNA codes for small guide RNA (gRNA) molecules which are important in editing the maxicircles' messenger RNA (mRNA). By adding or deleting uridine molecules from mRNA the gRNAs correct the gene transcripts, making them into functional mRNA. For example, the cytochrome oxidase subunit III gene appears to differ extensively in nucleotide sequence from that in other organisms, but after RNA editing the final mRNA transcript is substantially homolgous with mRNAs of other species. The study of RNA editing is an active area of research which has been reviewed extensively (Feagin, Jasmer and Stuart 1987, Feagin, Abraham and Stuart 1988, Simpson 1990, Blum et al. 1991, Goringer et al. 1994).

The African trypanosomes have become favourite organisms for study by molecular biologists. During the past decade a variety of genes coding for housekeeping enzymes (glycolytic enzymes) (Sommer and Wang 1994); structural proteins (actin) (Seebeck et al. 1988); mitochondrial–kinetoplast enzymes and cytochromes (Simpson 1990); and major surface glycoproteins from both the procyclic and blood stages have been sequenced and characterized structurally (Blum et al. 1993, Pays, Vanhamme and Berberof 1994). In addition, a variety of molecular probes have been developed which can be used for examining trypanosomes of various isolates for both taxonomic and epidemiological purposes (Masiga et al. 1992, Myler 1993). Particular attention has been directed to cloning and sequencing of the genes coding for the VSG (the variant antigens in the surface coat, see section 2.1) and the genes involved in the regulation of VSG expression (Pays et al. 1994).

It may be concluded, based on the study of the trypanosomes in a single infected host, that considerable genetic change occurs there. The infection in a host is characterized by rapid parasite growth rates, large parasite numbers and a changing host environment during infection. This is analogous to the situation of the HIV agent in AIDS patients (Nowak et al. 1991). The rapid evolution of these organisms, like that of the HIV agent, makes their control difficult and, perhaps less significantly, complicates classification.

4 CLINICAL MANIFESTATIONS

T. b. rhodesiense and *T. b. gambiense* are similar with respect to their mechanisms of pathogenesis and the pathology they produce. However, there are differences in the clinical manifestations of the diseases they cause and in their epidemiology (Table 14.2). The major difference between them is that the disease produced by *T. b. gambiense* (also called **West African trypanosomiasis**) is chronic in nature lasting up to 4 years, whereas the disease produced by *T. b. rhodesiense* is more acute, rarely lasting more than 9 months before death occurs.

As noted earlier (see section 2.1), one of the key aspects of African trypanosomiasis is the phenomenon of antigenic variation in which waves of parasitaemia occur in the blood of infected animals (Fig. 14.4). The clinical aspects of trypanosomiasis and the chronic nature of the disease can be attributed to these waves of parasitaemia.

4.1 Phases of the disease

African trypanosomiasis in humans can be separated into 3 phases (Table 14.3).

PHASE 1

The first phase occurs just after the inoculation of the metacyclic trypomastigotes, which occurs when the fly bites. A chancre develops at the site of the bite, and the trypanosomes remain at this site for a short time. There is inflammation of the subdermal tissue at the site, with oedema, erythema, tenderness and heat. The chancre is more readily observed in white people than in black people and is most frequently found in individuals infected with *T. b. rhodesiense*.

PHASE 2

During the second phase the trypanosomes spread throughout the entire body. They move through the blood and lymphatic vessels and multiply rapidly. Clinical symptoms during this stage appear to be asso-

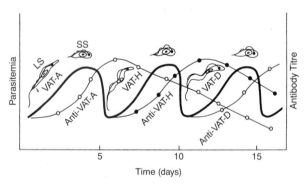

Fig. 14.4 Waves of parasitaemia and their relationship to the humoral response in a mammalian host infected with the African trypanosomes. The first wave of parasitaemia consists of a trypanosome population in which the major variant antigen type is VAT-A. The occurrence of this wave of parasitaemia is followed by an antibody response (anti-VAT-A) whose peak titre is observed shortly after this wave of parasitaemia is cleared. A minor VAT (VAT-H) present on some trypanosomes from the preceding population gives rise to the next wave of parasitaemia. This population is later cleared by host anti-VAT-H. The rise and fall of trypanosome populations continues throughout the life of the infected host. In experimentally infected rodents or rabbits a peak in parasitaemia is observed every 5–7 days. Infected rabbits may live for as long as 6 months, during which time they may experience as many as 30 waves of parasitaemia. (From Seed and Hall 1992, with permission of Academic Press.)

Table 14.2 A comparison of the biology of the subspecies of African trypanosomes: *T. (T.) b. gambiense* and *T. (T.) b. rhodesiense*[a]

Characteristic	T. (T.) b. gambiense	T. (T.) b. rhodesiense
Disease	Chronic	Acute
	Low parasitemia	High parasitemia
	Incubation period: months to years	Incubation period: days to weeks
Main tsetse vector	*G. palpalis* group	*G. morsitans* group
	G. palpalis	*G. morsitans*
	G. fuscipes	*G. pallidipas*
	G. tachinoides	*G. swynnertoni*
Transmission	Human reservoir	Animal reservoir
	↑↓ (primary)	↑↓ (primary)
	Riverine tsetse	Savanna and woodland tsetse
	↑↓ (secondary)	↑↓ (secondary)
	Animal reservoir	Human reservoir
Reservoir hosts	Possibly: kob, hartebeest, domestic pigs, dogs	Bushbuck, other antelope, hartebeest, hyena, lion, domestic cattle, possible warthog and giraffe
Geographical range	West Africa, western and north central Africa	East Africa and north central Africa

[a]Reviewed in Seed and Hall (1992).

Table 14.3 Some common clinical symptoms of African trypanosomiasis of humans

Stage of infection	Symptoms[a]
Fly bite: chancre	Localized tenderness and erythema at site of fly bite
Early parasitaemic stage	Headache, joint pain, fever, lymphadenopathy, weight erythema, itching, anemia, dizziness
Later stages: symptoms associated with particular organ systems	
Oedema:	Peripheral ascites, lung oedema, pericardial effusion
Nervous system:	Waking EEG changes and sleep–wake cycles[b,c], insomnia/somnolence, mental disorders, slurred speech, paralysis, brisk reflexes, epileptiform fits
Cardiac system:	ECG changes, congestive heart failure
Endocrine system:	Amenorrhea and impotence with hypogonadism[d], altered thyroid function[e], adrenocortical function[f], and changes in the circadian rhythms of plasma cortisol and prolactin[g]
Other:	Puffy facial appearance, diarrhoea, anorexia, splenomegaly

[a]For further details, see Seed and Hall (1992).
[b]Buguet et al. (1993).
[c]Hamon et al. (1993).
[d]Soudan et al. (1993).
[e]Reincke et al. (1993).
[f]Reincke et al. (1994).
[g]Radomski et al. (1995).

ciated with the waves of parasitaemia (Fig. 14.4). The high parasitaemias are accompanied by fever, headache, joint pain and malaise (Molyneux, DeRaadt and Seed 1984). These clinical symptoms may decrease in intensity as the disease becomes chronic. Splenomegaly and lymphadenopathy are major features of this stage of the infection. Histopathological examination of the lesions shows vasculitis with oedema and perivascular infiltration of leukocytes.

PHASE 3

Humans infected with the African trypanosomes, if untreated, eventually develop central nervous system (CNS) disorders. They may develop a wide array of behavioural changes ranging from aggressiveness to sleep-like states. The final stage involves complete somnolence (**sleeping sickness**). The common clinical symptoms of third phase infection result from damage to the heart, nervous system and other organs.

5 PATHOLOGY AND IMMUNOLOGY

Trypanosomiasis is, as noted previously, characterized by periodic waves of parasitaemia which continue during all stages of the disease. Each rise in parasitaemia is paralleled by an increase in antibody to one of the variant surface coat proteins (VSG; see section 2.1).

The variant specific antibody is involved in the removal or clearance of a major portion of the trypanosome population from the blood and other body fluids, a process which ends each wave of parasitaemia. Although this specific antibody clears a large majority of the trypanosomes present during a given wave of parasitaemia, there pre-exists within that population a minor population of trypanosomes with a different surface coat (or VSG). This minor population then gives rise to the next wave of parasitaemia. New surface coat variants appear at frequencies of 1 in 10^6 cells in syringe-passaged populations and an estimated 1 in 100 cells in fly-passaged field isolates. Antibody therefore acts as a selecting agent removing the major VSG population and allowing for other variant antigen types (VAT) that exist in the population to develop.

Although there is a strong host immune response to each of the variant antigens as they are produced, and over 99% of the trypanosomes are removed during each wave of parasitaemia, many mammalian species are not able to effect a cure. This is because the trypanosomes are able to escape the host's immune response by always producing a new parasite population with an antigenically different surface coat to replace the population removed by the host.

The first response in a given parasitaemic wave is with an antibody of IgM class. This is the antibody which clears the blood of most of the parasites present. It has been suggested that the antitrypanosome IgG antibody which is released just before or shortly after the trypanosomes in the blood are cleared by the IgM anti-trypanosome antibody is important in clearing the tissue fluids of trypanosomes because it is smaller than IgM and more readily diffuses into the tissue. It has been shown experimentally that the IgM immune response is primarily a B cell response of a type which in mice does not require T cell help.

The development of a macroglobulinaemia and a strong polyclonal B cell response are among the defining characteristics of this disease. Both anti-host and anti-trypanosome antibodies are present in the sera of infected patients and contribute to the macroglobulinaemia.

After the disease has persisted for some time the lymph nodes and spleen become enlarged and the heart is also often enlarged. The brain is oedematous and both protein and leukocyte concentrations in the cerebrospinal fluid (CSF) become elevated (Haller et al. 1986, Molyneux, DeRaadt and Seed 1984). The liver may be enlarged but the kidneys appear normal on both gross and microscopic examination.

There are inflammatory lesions in the heart and brain with perivascular infiltration by lymphocytes, plasma cells and monocytes. As the pathology progresses, oedema and haemorrhage due to changes in the vascular beds of the heart and brain develop. In the CNS there is demyelination and neuronal damage which may extend into the white matter. The perivascular cuffing and inflammatory cell infiltration extend deep into the choroid plexus. As the disease progresses chronic meningoencephalitis occurs. Changes in electroencephalograms and diurnal sleep patterns have been detected in chronically infected humans (Bentivoglio et al. 1994, Buguet et al. 1993, Hamon et al. 1993). In chronically ill patients there may be chronic inflammation of muscle and nerve fibres. These changes lead to oedema and fibrosis in patients with advanced disease; in such patients pathology visible by microscopic examination has also been seen in the lungs, spleen and liver. In the blood there is a reduction in the numbers of erythrocytes and platelets, and a reduction in haemoglobulin content. As noted above the CSF contains large numbers of white cells and contains high levels of IgM and other proteins, especially during the late stages of the disease.

Experimental data from studies of infected laboratory animals suggest that the encephalopathy observed in patients with advanced trypanosomiasis has an immunological basis (Jennings et al. 1989). It can be observed, for example, that many aspects of the pathology of African trypanosomiasis are similar to those present in animals undergoing a progressive Arthustype reaction. For example, high immunoglobulin levels, and large quantities of immune complexes are present in the blood and the CNS of experimentally infected animals and infected humans. In addition, high kinin levels with changes in prothrombin activity as well as changes in the levels of fibrin, fibrinogen and complement have been reported to occur in patients as well as in experimental animals suffering from trypanosomiasis (reviewed in Seed and Hall 1992). These last changes are not only consistent with those occurring during an Arthus reaction, but also with those induced by the activation of the coagulation system as occurs in patients with the disseminated intravascular coagulation often present in patients with the Rhodesian form of this disease. All of these changes, and others including the changes reported to occur in cytokine levels of patients, are suggestive of an immunologically mediated pathology.

The results of recent studies on patients with advanced trypanosomiasis being treated with melarsoprol are consistent with the suggestion that the reactive arsenical encephalopathy which occurs in 3–5% of the patients has an immunological basis also (Adams et al. 1986, Haller et al. 1986). The supposed immunological basis of the encephalopathy in patients with trypanosomiasis is the rationale for the use of anti-inflammatory corticosteroids in the treatment of these patients (Jennings et al. 1989).

Domestic animals infected with the African trypanosomes have high levels of the IgM in their plasma and both high levels of IgM and large numbers of morular cells in their brain tissue, but they do not develop a somnolent state.

Although immunoglobulin levels are increased in humans with trypanosomiasis and their immunological system is very active it has been found that infected humans respond as if they were immunosuppressed to secondary infections. Such immunosuppression in patients with trypanosomiasis is well documented (Greenwood, Whittle and Molyneux 1973). The actual mechanisms involved in this immunosuppression are unknown but there are a number of reasonable suggestions based on data from animal studies. These include the effects of altered cytokine levels, of suppression by T cells, by macrophages, by host prostoglandins and by toxic trypanosome products including both large molecular weight compounds, such as endotoxin-like molecules, and small molecular weight compounds, such as trypanosome catabolites. The system may also be working at capacity or driven to exhaustion in its effort to respond to the masses of antigen released by the parasites in the course of each parasitaemic wave.

In addition to the microscopic pathology and the immunopathology which the infection induces, there are extensive changes in host physiology in persons with trypanosomiasis. For example, the reproductive capacity of infected individuals is low. Low estradiol levels are reported to occur in 65% of infected females and low testosterone levels in 50% of infected males (Ikede, Elhassan and Akpavie 1988, Boersma et al. 1989, Soudan et al. 1993). Abnormalities in thyroid hormones have also been observed (Reincke et al. 1993). These observations suggest that all organ systems and physiological functions are affected by the infection. A summary of some of the physiological changes which occur in people with African trypanosomiasis is shown in Table 14.3.

African trypanosomiasis is a complex disease and it is therefore likely that a number of mechanisms contribute to production of the pathology observed in patients suffering from trypanosomiasis (Alafiatayo et al. 1993, Greenwood and Whittle 1980, Pentreath 1991, Seed and Hall 1992).

6 DIAGNOSIS

A primary consideration for diagnosis of African trypanosomiasis should be a history of travel or residence of the patient in an area of Africa where the disease occurs. This said, diagnosis of African trypanosomiasis depends upon the microscopic demonstration of trypanosomes in the blood, in lymph node aspirates or in cerebrospinal fluid. The very elevated macroglobulinaemia which occurs in patients has been considered diagnostic of African trypanosomiasis but it is only suggestive as other diseases such as leishmaniasis also cause a macroglobulinaemia.

Unfortunately, the clinical features of the disease are not sufficiently unique to be diagnostic, except possibly during the late sleeping sickness stage; the number of parasites in the blood and other body fluids is often very low, making detection difficult. Multiple sampling and concentration techniques are often required to find the parasites. In *T. b. gambiense* infected people in particular the parasitaemias can be extremely low, and therefore infection with this trypanosome is particularly difficult to diagnose (DeRaadt and Seed 1977). It should be noted that there have been attempts to develop a list of symptoms (enlarged lymph nodes, CNS associated signs, etc.)

that are common to sleeping sickness patients, which could be used by rural health personnel to make a tentative diagnosis of a *T. b. rhodesiense* infection (Boatin et al. 1986).

Examination of stained thin or thick blood films for trypanosomes is still a good diagnostic technique, and repeated daily examination can increase the probability of detection of the parasite. The use of concentration methods such as miniature anion exchange columns (Lanham and Godfrey 1970, Lumsden et al. 1979 1981), or haematocrit tube centrifugation (Woo 1971, WHO 1986, Woo and Hauck 1987, Levine, Wardlaw and Patton 1989) coupled with microscopic examination can increase the sensitivity of methods for detection of trypanosomes several fold. A modification of the haematocrit tube centrifugation test is the acridine orange quantitative buffy coat (QBC) technique (Bailey and Smith 1992). This test is simple, quick and sensitive. Since it detects trypanosomes microscopically it does not produce false positives. The concentration techniques have been modified for use in field surveys, but they are still difficult to use in field settings because of the need for a centrifuge and electrical power (WHO 1986).

If trypanosomes cannot be detected in the blood of a suspected trypanosomiasis patient, the microscopic examination of a wet preparation from an enlarged cervical lymph node may confirm the diagnosis. Once the trypanosomes are detected in the blood and lymph fluids, the CSF must also be examined in order to determine the stage of the disease. Distinguishing between the acute blood stage of the infection and the later chronic neurological stage is important in determining the appropriate chemotherapeutic regime. Centrifuged sediments of the CSF should be examined for trypanosomes. The fluid should also be examined to determine if there are elevated white cell counts and increases in protein concentration (DeRaadt and Seed 1977). Both cerebrospinal fluid and blood from patients should be examined periodically after completion of chemotherapy in order to ensure that the patient is cured.

The use of in vitro cultivation of trypanosomes or the inoculation of suspected samples into experimental animals is not currently practical for routine diagnosis, although both procedures are used extensively for research purposes. A kit for in vitro isolation of trypanosomes (KIVI) from sleeping sickness patients in the field has been developed (Aerts et al. 1992, Truc et al. 1992). This test is of value in isolating trypanosomes from infected individuals; however, because KIVI requires days for the cultures to produce detectable numbers of trypanosomes, it will probably have limited diagnostic value. Its main importance will be as a standard for evaluating other quicker diagnostic tests.

Immunodiagnostic tests can be especially useful for mass field surveys and for other epidemiological investigations as well as for the detection of latent infections. A number of serological tests have been developed and many are currently being tested in the field. Immunofluorescence, complement fixation, and card agglutination (CATT) tests have all been utilized in epidemiological studies. Several of these procedures are available in the form of commercial kits for field use. These tests are based upon the detection of antibody in the sera of infected individuals and utilize antigens from blood stage trypanosomes. For example, the CATT test employs a fixed, stained suspension of intact trypanosomes containing a mixture of various antigenic types. The various types selected are based upon the frequency with which they appear in the human population in a broad geographical area. This test is easy to perform, inexpensive, and convenient for field work. However like many indirect diagnostic tests, it is not perfect. For example, it is not equally effective in all geographical areas, nor is it equally effective for detection of the 2 forms of human trypanosomiasis. This test is also reported to give positive reactions with antibodies to species of trypanosomes infecting animals but not humans (Penchenier et al. 1991). Serological tests are also being evaluated that use the surface coat protein from the procyclic trypanosomes as antigen (Ngaira et al. 1992).

Tests that use monoclonal antibodies to detect trypanosome antigens in serum are now being developed (Komba et al. 1992, Nantulya, Doua and Molisho 1992). Antigen detection tests would be valuable since they are based on detection of trypanosome antigens in the blood and therefore active infection. Tests that detect antibody cannot distinguish between a past and a present infection, but those that detect antigen can.

The antigens produced by modern biotechnology have not yet been used for diagnostic purposes. Although molecular probes have been used successfully in epidemiological studies, hybridization and PCR technologies are not currently used for routine diagnosis because tests based on them are still too slow and cumbersome.

In a recent comparison of the CATT, the haematocrit centrifuge tube assay, the minianion exchange column technique, the QBC, the KIVI, and the thick blood film (TBF) procedures, the TBF was found to be as sensitive as any of the other procedures. It also has the advantage of being the simplest and cheapest of all the diagnostic methods. It is rapid and simple, requiring only the staining and examination of the slides (Truc et al. 1994).

7 EPIDEMIOLOGY AND CONTROL

African trypanosomiasis is restricted to Central Africa because of the ecology of the insect vector (*Glossina*, tsetse flies). The tsetse are limited by the Sahara Desert to the north and the cool, dry areas of Southern Africa to the south. The tsetse habitat is approximately the size of the USA, and it is estimated that 50 million people are at risk. It has been reported that there are more than 20 000 new cases per year. Countries such as Angola, Zaire, Sudan, Uganda, Cameroon and the Congo have the highest reported incidences of sleeping sickness. Sleeping sickness now occurs in

36 countries south of the Sahara and there are approximately 200 known disease foci (Kuzoe 1991, 1993). Because trypanosomiasis is also a disease of animals, African humans suffer additionally from a lack of meat, milk, manure and draft animals. It is estimated that Africans could raise over 120×10^6 cattle if trypanosomiasis was eliminated, but only 20×10^6 are currently maintained. Because cattle and domestic animals are preferentially raised in areas with low tsetse densities, or in areas in which the natural ecology has been modified to restrict the survival of the vector, there has been a tendency for overgrazing such areas. The heavy use of tsetse-free areas which are often not well suited ecologically for long-term livestock production has led to land degradation. Because trypanosomiasis is fatal when untreated, because the control of trypanosomiasis is costly and difficult, and because trypanosomiasis causes the loss of essential dietary proteins and work animals, it has had a significant negative impact on the economic and social development of the endemic areas (Duggan 1970, Ford 1971, Molyneux and Ashford 1983, Williams et al. 1993).

7.1 Epidemiology

The epidemiology of infection caused by *T. b. gambiense* differs from that of infection caused by *T. b. rhodesiense* in many aspects. These include the species of tsetse involved, the type of tsetse habitat, and the number and type of reservoir hosts (Table 14.2). *T. b. gambiense* is transmitted by flies of the *Glossina palpalis* group, which live primarily in the vegetation along river banks and in moist forests. Tsetse of this group feed frequently on humans in areas where contact is common, such as at river crossings and water holes. There are animals which serve as reservoir hosts of *T. b. gambiense* but people with chronic infection who have relatively mild symptoms provide the major contribution to the persistence of the Gambian type of infection (Jordan 1986, Molyneux and Ashford 1983). *T. b. rhodesiense* is transmitted by tsetse of the *G. morsitans* group. These flies inhabit low woodlands and thickets on lake shores and much of the savanna of central and east Africa. This group of flies feeds primarily on non-human hosts, and humans are only a secondary food source (Seed and Hall 1992). Fishermen, game wardens and others who enter areas with high tsetse numbers are particularly at risk (Wyatt, Boatin and Wurada 1985). In addition, epidemics of the Rhodesian infection occur when there is an increase in tsetse numbers in close association with villages, a development causing an increase in fly–human contact. The areas in which the west African infection occurs overlap the areas of infection caused by *T. b. rhodesiense* in countries such as Zaire and Uganda.

7.2 Control

In the past control of trypanosomiasis was partly based on the removal of reservoir hosts from areas near human settlements. This involved the fencing out and killing of game animals. Other early attempts at control of trypanosomiasis involved the destruction of tsetse habitats. Both the elimination of reservoir hosts and the destruction of tsetse habitats are now considered ecologically unsound. Africans have begun to realize the value of their game animals as tourist attractions also, and therefore as important sources of revenue.

The epidemiology of human African trypanosomiasis is shaped by many factors (Table 14.4). They include the type and density of the vector, the type and density of the reservoir host population and the density of the human population. The densities of the fly population and of the host population are dependent on environmental conditions such as temperature, humidity, water availability and other factors of the habitat. It is a general truth that any condition that increases the contact between tsetse, the reservoir hosts and humans, including growth of population, will increase the risk of human infection. The chronic nature of the infection in both the vector and mammalian host makes continued surveillance, and treatment of the human population and vector control, necessities if low prevalence rates are to be maintained in the human population.

All species of *Glossina* are blood feeders and as adults are totally dependent on this food source. The different species of *Glossina* have different host preferences, and both sexes take bloodmeals. In addition, tsetse are larviparous and a female produces only 8–12 larvae during her limited life span of 3–5 months. The larvae are deposited on the ground and immediately burrow into patches of moist soil or sand such as occur in shaded areas under fallen logs, rocks or bushes. The need for frequent bloodmeals and the reproduction dynamics of tsetse are important factors in shaping the epidemiology of trypanosomiasis (Molyneux and Ashford 1983).

The environmental requirements of the flies and their low reproductive rates make then vulnerable to control by a variety of techniques. The techniques used are based on our knowledge of tsetse behaviour and other aspects of epidemiology of trypanosomiasis. Control programmes using insecticide application and traps in particular are coming into wide use. Traps and insecticides such as the chlorinated hydrocarbons and synthetic pyrethroids, when properly used, cause limited environmental damage (Molyneux and Ashford 1983, Jordan 1986). Depending on the environmental conditions, application may be by spraying with individually carried sprayers or from aircraft. The latter technique is used when broad coverage is needed. Technical factors that are considered important for achieving good results in spraying programmes include appropriate formulation of the spray to obtain proper droplet size and the proper selection of insecticide. Either a residual or a non-residual insecticide may be selected, depending on the retention time desired. Selection of appropriate sites for spraying is also important. Many of the requirements for successful use of insecticides for control of tsetse are reviewed by Jordan (1986) and Molyneux and Ashford (1983). Although control by insecticide application is effective, it is also expensive and repeated application is required if results are to last.

The use of fly traps and screens impregnated with insecticides is more economical than environmental spraying and has been demonstrated to lower tsetse numbers dramatically in limited areas (Molyneux and Ashford 1983, Jordan 1986, Vale 1993). The biconical trap (Fig. 14.5a) has been shown in West Africa to be effective in reducing tsetse numbers. Detailed knowledge of fly behaviour in the area where control is attempted is required for proper design and placement of traps and screens.

Table 14.4 Some factors involved in the epidemiology of African trypanosomiasis of humans[a]

Fly	Mammal	Environmental	Parasite
Fly numbers	Host numbers	Temperature	Parasite numbers
Sex	Host species	Humidity	Genetics:
Age at infection	Habitat	Water sources	Growth rates, virulence drug resistance, human serum resistance, subspecies, strain
Symbiotic infections: viral, bacterial	Attractiveness to fly	Vegetation	
Fly behaviour: Habitat selection, host preference	Genetics	Wind direction and current	
Physiological status	Immune response		
Genetic factors:	Non-specific factors		
Species, subspecies	Race		
Stage of infection in fly	Trypanocidal factors		
	Degree of immunosuppression		
	Intercurrent infections		

[a]From Molyneux, DeRaadt and Seed (1984), Jordan (1986), Seed and Hall (1992), Vale (1993).

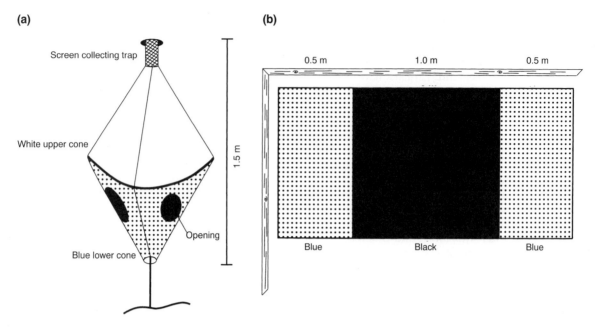

Fig. 14.5 Biconical tsetse trap (a), and insecticide impregnated screen or target (b).

There are chemicals to which tsetse are known to be attracted. These include carbon doxide and volatile compounds in the breath and urine of cattle (Vale and Hall 1985a,b; Vale et al. 1988). Some of these compounds have been identified: they include acetone, 1-octenol-3-ol, and the phenolic compounds 4-methylphenol and 3-n-propylphenol. The baiting of traps with these synthetic compounds and with carbon dioxide has been shown to increase the numbers of flies caught. There are also substances from humans that are repellent to some tsetse (Vale 1993), and these must not be permitted to contaminate traps. In addition, colour and design of traps or screens are important factors in attracting and inducing the landing of flies. In the Congo Republic a modified biconical trap is used for the control of tsetse in areas where trypanosomiasis occurs (Lancien 1981). The traps are relatively inexpensive and can be constructed and maintained by the villagers themselves if the necessary materials are provided (Okoth 1986).

In Zambia disposable screens impregnated with insecticide have replaced traps (Fig. 14.5b). The screens are 2×1 m and have a central black area of 1×1 m surrounded by 2 0.5×1 m rectangular blue areas. The screens are supported by wooden frames which can be stuck into the ground. The insecticide used, Deltamethrin, persists on the screens for months (Vale 1993). The screens are inexpensive, require no maintenance and can be utilized with or without the use of chemoattractive odours (Vale 1993). These screens are extremely effective in killing tsetse and in some areas are believed to have reduced or even eradicated tsetse populations. Similar screens have been used to control *G. pallidipes* in Kenya (Opiyo, Njogu and Omuse 1990). The use of traps and screens in the control of tsetse has been extensively discussed by Jordan (1986), Laveissiere, Vale and Gouteux (1990), and Vale (1993). They hold great promise for future control of tsetse populations and therefore African trypanosomiasis in an environmentally friendly way.

An approach related to the use of screens and traps in tsetse control has been the use of cattle dipped in insecticide. This technique has been shown to lower tsetse numbers (Fox et al. 1993). This procedure is relatively inexpensive and has the additional advantage that it also reduces the populations of ticks and other biting insects.

There have been attempts to control tsetse by the release of sterile flies. There have also been attempts to find tsetse pathogens, and to identify pheromones for use in programmes to reduce fly populations (Molyneux and Ashford 1983, Langley, Felton and Doichi 1988). An approach using biotechnology to develop a transmissible vector which would cause male sterility has been proposed, but control based on such a technique has not reached a stage of development sufficiently advanced to even permit testing. Some of the procedures being attempted are expensive and almost certainly will not be applicable in the field.

The lack of economic resources is a major factor limiting effective control of trypanosomiasis. In many of the endemic countries the per capita gross national product is less than $ 500 US, and there may be an expenditure of less than $10 US per individual for total health care. The cost of surveillance alone is estimated at approximately $1 US per individual at risk, and the cost of treatment at $35 US per patient in the early stage, and $135 US per individual treated in the late stage of the disease. In addition there are costs for vector surveillance and control (Kuzoe 1991, WHO 1986). It is obvious that the necessary resources for control of sleeping sickness are very limited in most areas of Africa, and any change in government priorities, e.g. to control political unrest, will decrease the amount of money available for long-term control activities. Civil unrest also disrupts the flow of external aid required to supplement local funds for control activities.

8 CHEMOTHERAPY

Because all forms of African trypanosomiasis are vector-borne diseases, their control requires vector control. Because the west African form of the disease is chronic and humans are the main reservoir, surveillance of the human population by mobile field teams and prompt detection of infected individuals and their treatment in health centres is vital to reduce the incidence of infection. East African trypanosomiasis is a zoonotic disease and treatment of infected humans therefore has less effect on incidence of infection in humans. Surveillance and early detection of both forms of the disease are important because the treatment protocol is shorter for patients in the early stages of the disease and drug-induced morbidity and mortality are lower than in patients in the late stages of the disease. Cure rates are also higher when infected individuals are treated early in the disease rather than during the late secondary stages. Control of both forms of sleeping sickness therefore works best if early detection and treatment are used together.

Suramin is used to treat patients with primary stage infections that do not involve the CNS. This drug is effective against both the Gambian and Rhodesian form of the disease, but because it does not cross the blood–brain barrier it is not effective against the secondary CNS stages. Suramin is a polysulfonated naphthylamine derivative of trypan red and was first found to have trypanolytic activity by Ehrlich. It is relatively toxic and may cause optic atrophy, blindness, nephrotoxicity and adrenal insufficiency in some patients (Pepin and Milord 1994). Its exact mode of action is not known, although it inhibits a wide variety of trypanosome enzymes including glycolytic enzymes and the mitochondrial glycerol phosphate oxidase enzymes.

Pentamidine isethionate and other aromatic diamidines were first examined for trypanocidal activity in the 1930s. Like suramin, the dicationic pentamidine isethionate does not cross the blood–brain barrier, and is therefore used in patients with CNS involvement only to clear the blood of trypanosomes prior to treatment with melarsoprol. Pentamidine isethionate may produce nephrotoxicity, hepatotoxicity and pancreatic toxicity in some patients (Sands, Kron and Brown 1985, WHO 1986, Goa and Campoli-Richards 1987, Kapusnik and Mills 1988, Pepin and Milord 1994). The exact mode of action of this drug is unknown, but the strongly basic dicationic molecule binds to many cellular components including a variety of trypanosome enzymes causing their inhibition. It also binds to DNA, preferentially to adenosine–thymidine rich regions in the minor groove. It has recently been shown that pentamidine isethionate is actively metabolized by the mammalian cytochrome P450 drug metabolizing system (Berger et al. 1990).

In contrast to suramin and pentamidine isethionate, Melarsoprol does cross the blood–brain barrier and is used to treat patients in the late secondary CNS stages of trypanosomiasis. Melarsoprol until very recently has been the only drug available for treatment in this stage

of the disease. It is an organic arsenical, first developed by Friedheim (1949). As with pentamidine isethionate and suramin, its exact mechanism of action is unknown, although it has been shown to inhibit a variety of trypanosome enzymes and functions in vitro. It is toxic, and in 1–10% of treated patients there is encephalopathy with mortality rates of 1–5%. Other adverse side effects include fever, headache, joint pain, gastrointestinal disturbances, renal damage and hypertension (Pepin and Milord 1994, WHO 1986). As noted above (see section 5, p. 273) the encephalopathy may have an immunological basis (Jennings et al. 1989). It has been possible to reduce the development of meningoencephalitis and perivascular cuffing in infected mice by treatment with the immunosuppressive drug azathioprine (Jennings et al. 1989).

Suramin, pentamidine isethionate and melarsoprol are still the primary drugs used to treat patients with African trypanosomiasis. The only new drug which has been developed is difluoromethylornithine (DFMO, eflornithine, Ornidyl), an inhibitor of ornithine decarboxylase which is the first enzyme in the polyamine biosynthetic pathway (Bacchi and McCann 1987). Currently it is the only drug other than melarsoprol available for treatment of late-stage trypanosomiasis (Schechter et al. 1987). DFMO is a specific irreversible inhibitor of ornithine decarboxylase. In the trypanosomes, exposure to DFMO leads to rapid depletion of putrescine and to low spermidine levels. It induces transformation of the LS to the SS form, and therefore causes an inhibition of trypanosome growth. DFMO is relatively non-toxic but adverse reactions can include anaemia, thrombocytopenia, and gastrointestinal disturbances, all of which are reversible. It is an extremely valuable chemotherapeutic agent for the treatment of late-stage patients who do not respond to melarsoprol. *T. b. gambiense* seems to be more susceptible to DFMO than is *T. b. rhodesiense*, although the reason for this difference is not clear (Bacchi et al. 1990).

Because DFMO is a specific inhibitor of ornithine decarboxylase with no other known inhibitory activity, rapid selection for drug-resistant trypanosomes has been possible in experimental studies. Resistance has also been observed in trypanosomes isolated from humans treated with DFMO. Considerable research is being conducted in an effort to find other compounds which inhibit the polyamine pathway. Treatments using combinations of drugs are also being investigated in an effort to decrease the probability of selecting for drug resistance.

The current treatment regime recommended by the WHO for reducing parasitaemia in patients with *T. b. gambiense* infection is the use of pentamidine isethionate or, where there is resistance to this drug, with suramin. This is done in patients in both early (or primary) and late (or secondary) stages of the disease. In the patients in the late stages of the disease who have CNS involvement, this treatment is followed by treating with multiple injections of melarsoprol. The treatment of patients in the early stages of a *T. b. rhode-*

Table 14.5 The protocol used in the Côte d'Ivoire for the treatment of *T. b. gambiense* in infected patients

Time (days)	Drug used	Dose (mg/kg)	Route
1 and 2	Pentamidine isethionate	4.0	IM
4	Melarsoprol	1.2	IV
5	Melarsoprol	2.4	IV
6	Melarsoprol	3.6	IV
17	Melarsoprol	1.2	IV
18	Melarsoprol	2.4	IV
19	Melarsoprol	3.6	IV
20	Melarsoprol	3.6	IV
30	Melarsoprol	1.2	IV
31	Melarsoprol	2.4	IV
32	Melarsoprol	3.6	IV
33	Melarsoprol	3.6	IV

[a]Abstracted from WHO (1986). For full details on treatment regimens for *T. b. gambiense* and *T. b. rhodesiense* infections, see Annex 5, pp. 118–21.

siense infection is with suramin. In patients with the late stages of a *T. b. rhodesiense* infection, suramin is used to clear the blood and lymph and then multiple injections of Melarsoprol are given (WHO 1986). The details of the treatment regimes are outlined in Table 14.5 (WHO 1986).

Currently the number of drugs available for the treatment of African trypanosomiasis is limited and all except DFMO are quite toxic to humans. Researchers are currently searching for better analogues of existing drugs, investigating the use of drugs in combinations, and trying to develop compounds that inhibit biochemical pathways unique to trypanosomes. Although there are new leads in this field, further research is critically required.

9 VACCINATION

Because of the phenomenon of antigenic variation (see section 3.3), no vaccine is available, and it is not anticipated that one will be developed in the near future.

10 CONCLUSION

Control of trypanosomiasis is possible, but it requires continuous surveillance of the human population and the treatment of all infected individuals. It also requires control of tsetse flies through the use of traps and insecticide impregnated screens and the judicious application of insecticides to the environment. It is possible that in the future insecticides will be required only in limited circumstances. The application of any control measure is currently limited in many areas of Africa owing to political instability as well as the lack of the resources to initiate and maintain them adequately (Williams et al. 1993).

REFERENCES

Abaru DE, 1985, Sleeping sickness in Busoga, Uganda 1876–1983, *Trop Med Parasitol*, **36:** 72–76.

Adams JH, Haller L et al., 1986, Human African trypanosomiasis (*T. b. gambiense*): A study of 16 fatal cases of sleeping sickness with some observations on acute reactive arsenical encephalopathy, *Neuropathol Appl Neurobiol*, **12:** 81–94.

Aerts D, Truc P et al., 1992, A kit for *in vitro* isolation of trypanosomes in the field: first trial with sleeping sickness patients in the Congo Repulic, *Trans R Soc Trop Med Hyg*, **86:** 394–5.

Alafiatayo RA, Crawley B et al., 1993, Endotoxins and pathogenesis of *Trypanosoma brucei brucei* infection in mice, *Parasitology*, **107:** 49–53.

Bacchi CJ, McCann PP, 1987, Parasitic protozoa and polyamines, *Inhibition of Polyamine Metabolism*, eds McCann PP, Pegg AE, Sjoerdsma A, Academic Press, New York, 317–44.

Bacchi CJ, Nathan HC et al., 1990, Differential susceptibility to DL-alpha-difluoromethylornithine in clinical isolates of *Trypanosoma brucei rhodesiense*, *Antimicrob Agents Chemother*, **34:** 1183–8.

Bailey JW, Smith DW, 1992, The use of acridine orange QBC technique in the diagnosis of African trypanosomiasis, *Trans R Soc Trop Med Hyg*, **86:** 630.

Baltz T, Baltz D et al., 1985, Cultivation in a semi-defined medium of animal infective forms of *Trypanosoma brucei, T. equiperdum, T. evansi, T. rhodesiense* and *T. gambiense, EMBO J*, **4:** 1273–7.

Bentivoglio M, Grassi-Zucconi G et al., 1994, *Trypanosoma brucei* and the nervous system, *Trends Neurosci*, **17:** 325–9.

Berger BJ, Lombardy RJ et al., 1990, Metabolic *N*-hydroxylation of pendamidine *in vitro*, *Antibicrob Agents Chemother*, **34:** 1678–85.

Blum B, Sturm NR et al., 1991, Chimeric gRNA-mRNA modecules with oligo (U) tails covalently linked at sites of RNA edit-

ing suggest that U addition occurs by transesterification, *Cell*, **65:** 543–50.

Blum ML, Down JA et al., 1993, A structural motif in the variant surface glycoproteins of *Trypanosoma brucei, Nature* (London), **362:** 603–9.

Boatin BA, Wyatt GB et al., 1986, Use of symptoms and signs for diagnosis of *Trypanosoma brucei rhodesiense* trypanosomiasis by rural health personnel, *Bull WHO*, **64:** 389–95.

Boersma A, Noireau F et al., 1989, Gondadotropic axis and *Trypanosoma brucei gambiense* infection, *Ann Soc Belge Med Trop*, **69:** 127–35.

Bowman IBR, Flynn IW, 1976, Oxidative metabolism of trypanosomes, *Biology of the Kinetoplastida*, vol 1, eds Lumsden WHR, Evans DA, Academic Press, New York, 435–76.

Brun R, Jenni L, 1985, Cultivation of African and South American trypanosomes of medical or veterinary importance, *Br Med Bull*, **41:** 122–9.

Buquet A, Bert J et al., 1993, Sleep–wake cycle in human African trypanosomiasis, *J Clin Neurophysiol*, **10:** 190–196.

Cronin CN, Nolan DP, Voorheis HP, 1989, The enzymes of the classical pentose phosphate pathway display differential activities in procyclic and bloodstream forms of *Trypanosoma brucei, FEBS Lett*, **244:** 26–30.

DeRaadt P, Seed JR, 1977, Trypanosomes causing disease in man in Africa, *Parasitic Protozoa*, vol. 1, ed Kreier JP, Academic Press, New York, 176–237.

Duggan AJ, 1970, An historical perspective, *The African Trypanosomiases*, ed Mulligan HW, Wiley-Interscience, New York.

Duszenko M, Ferguson MAJ et al., 1985, Cysteine eliminates the feeder cell requirements for cultivation of *Trypanosoma brucei* blood-stream forms *in vitro*, *J Exp Med*, **162:** 1256–63.

Enyaru JCK, Allingham R et al., 1993, The isolation and genetic heterogeneity of *Trypanosoma brucei gambiense* from the North-West Uganda, *Acta Trop*, **54:** 31–9.

Fairlamb, AH, 1989, Novel biochemical pathways in parasitic protozoa, *Parasitology*, **99**: S93–S112.

Fairlamb AH, Cerami H, 1992, Metabolism and functions of trypanothione in the kinetoplastida, *Annu Rev Microbiol*, **46**: 695–729.

Fairlamb AH, Opperdoes FR, 1986, Carbohydrate metabolism of African trypanosomes, with special reference to the glycosome, *Carbohydrate Metabolism in Cultured Cells*, ed. Morgan MJ, Plenum Press, New York, 183–224.

Feagin JE, Jasmer DP, Stuart K, 1987, Developmentally regulated addition of nucleotides within apocytochrome b transcripts in *Trypanosoma brucei*, *Cell*, **49**: 337–45.

Feagin JE, Abraham JM, Stuart K, 1988, Extensive editing of the cytochrome c oxidase III transcript in *Trypanosoma brucei*, *Cell*, **53**: 413–22.

Ford J, 1971, *The Role of the Trypanosomiases in African Ecology: A Study of the Tsetse Fly Problem*, Clarendon Press, Oxford.

Fox RGR, Monbando SD et al., 1993, Effect on herd health and productivity of controlling tsetse and trypanosomiasis by applying Deltamethrin to cattle, *Trop Anim Health Production*, **25**: 203–14.

Freidheim EAH, 1949, Mel B in the treatment of human trypanosomiasis, *Am J Trop Med*, **29**: 173–80.

Gibson W, Garside L, 1991, Genetic exchange in *Trypanosoma brucei brucei*: variable chromosomal location of house keeping genes in different trypanosome stocks, *Mol Biochem Parasitol*, **45**: 77–90.

Gibson WG, Garside L, Bailey M, 1992, Trisomy and chromosome size changes in hybrid trypanosomes from a genetic cross between *Trypanosoma brucei rhodesiense* and *T. b. brucei*, *Mol Biochem Parasitol*, **52**: 189–200.

Gibson W, Whittington H, 1993, Genetic exchange in *Trypanosoma brucei*: Selection of hybrid trypanosomes by introduction of genes conferring drug resistance, *Mol Biochem Parasitol*, **60**: 19–26.

Goa KL, Campoli-Richards DM, 1987, Pentamidine isethionate. A review of its antiprotozoal activity, pharmacokinetic properties and therapeutic use in *Pneumocystis carinii* pneumonia, *Drugs*, **33**: 242–58.

Goringer HU, Koslowsky DJ et al., 1994, The formation of mitochondrial ribonucleoprotein complexes involving guide RNA molecules in *Trypanosoma brucei*, *Proc Natl Acad Sci USA*, **91**: 1776–80.

Gray MA, Hirumi H, Gardines PR, 1987, Salivarian trypanosomes: Insect forms, In Vitro *Methods for Parasite Cultivation*, eds Taylor AER, Baker JR, Academic Press, New York, 118–52.

Greenwood BM, Whittle HC, 1980, The pathogenesis of sleeping sickness, *Trans R Soc Trop Med Hyg*, **74**: 716–25.

Greenwood BM, Whittle HC, Molyneux DH, 1973, Immunosuppression in Gambian trypanosomiasis, *Trans R Soc Trop Med Hyg*, **67**: 846–50.

Gutteridge WE, Coombs GH, 1977, *Biochemistry of Parasitic Protozoa*, University Park Press, Baltimore, 89–107.

Hajduk SL, Hager KM, Esko JD, 1994, Human high density lipoprotein killing of African trypanosomes, *Annu Rev Microbiol*, **48**: 139–62.

Haller L, Adams H et al., 1986, Clinical and pathological aspects of human African trypanosomiasis (*T. b. gambiense*) with particular reference to reactive arsenical encephalopathy, *Am J Trop Med Hyg*, **35**: 94–9.

Hamm B, Schindler A et al., 1990, Differentiation of *Trypanosoma brucei* bloodstream trypomastigotes from long slender to short stumpy-like forms in axenic cultrue, *Mol Biochem Parasitol*, **40**: 13–22.

Hammond DJ, Gutteridge WE, 1984, Purine and pyrimidine metabolism in the trypanosomatidae, *Mol Biochem Parasitol*, **13**: 242–61.

Hamon JF, Camara P et al., 1993, Waking electroencephalograms in blood lymph and encephalitic stages of Gambian trypanosomiasis, *Ann Trop Med Parasitol*, **87**: 149–55.

Hannaert V, Michels PAM, 1994, Structure, function, and biogenesis of glycosomes in Kinetoplastida, *J Bioenergetics Biomembranes*, **26**: 205–12.

Hecker H, Betschart B et al., 1995, Functional morphology of trypanosome chromatin, *Parasitol Today*, **11**: 79–83.

Hide G, Welburn, SC et al., 1994, Epidemiological relationships of *Trypanosoma brucei* stocks from South East Uganda: Evidence for different population structures in human infective and non-human infective isolates, *Parasitology*, **109**: 95–111.

Ikede BO, Elhassan E, Akpavie SO, 1988, Reproductive disorders in African trypanosomiasis: A review, *Acta Trop*, **45**: 5–10.

Jenni L, Molyneux DH et al., 1980, Feeding behavior of tsetse flies infected with salivarian trypanosomes, *Nature* (London), **283**: 383–5.

Jennings RW, McNeil PE et al., 1989, Trypanosomiasis and encephalitis: possible aetiology and treatment, *Trans R Soc Trop Med Hyg*, **83**: 578–618.

Jordan AM, 1986, *Trypanosomiasis Control and African Rural Development*, Longman, New York.

Kaminsky R, Beaudoin E, Cunningham I, 1988, Cultivation of the life cycle stage of *Trypanosoma brucei* spp., *Acta Trop*, **45**: 33–43.

Kaminsky R, Zweygarth E, 1989, Effect of *in vitro* cultivation on the stability of resistance of *Trypanosoma brucei brucei* to diminazene, isometamidium, quinapryamine, and Mel B, *J Parasitol*, **75**: 42–5.

Kapusnik JE, Mills J, 1988, Pentamidine, *The Antimicrobial Agent Annual*, vol. 3, eds Peterson PK, Verhoef J, Elsevier, New York, 299–311.

Komba E, Odiit M et al., 1992, Multicenter evaluation of an antigen-detection ELISA for the diagnosis of *Trypanosoma brucei rhodesiense* sleeping sickness, *Bull WHO*, **70**: 57–61.

Kooy RF, Hirumi H et al., 1989, Evidence for diploidy in metacyclic forms of African trypanosomes, *Proc Natl Acad Sci USA*, **86**: 5469–72.

Kuzoe FAS, 1991, Perspectives in research on and control of African trypanosomiasis, *Ann Trop Med Parasitol*, **85**: 33–41.

Kuzoe FAS, 1993, *African trypanosomiasis 6*, Tropical Disease Research Progress 1991–92. Eleventh Programme Report of the UNDP/World Bank/WHO Special Programme for Research and Training in Tropical Diseases, World Health Organization, Geneva, 57–66.

Lancien J, 1981, Descriptions du piège monoconique utilisé pour l'élimination des glossines en République de Congo, *Cah ORSTROM sér Entomol Med Parasitol*, **19**: 235–8.

Langley PA, Felton T, Doichi H, 1988, Juvenile hormone mimics as effective sterilants for the tsetse fly *Glossina morsitans morsitans*, *Med Vet Entomol*, **2**: 29–35.

Lanham SM, Godfrey DG, 1970, Isolation of salivarian trypanosomes from man and other mammals using DEAE cellulose, *Exp Parasitol*, **28**: 521–34.

Laveissiere C, Vale GA, Gouteux JP, 1990, *Appropriate Technology in Vector Control*, ed Curtis CF, CRC, Boca Raton, FL, 47–74.

Levine RA, Wardlaw SC, Patton CL, 1989, Detection of haematoparasites using quantitative buffy coat analysis tubes, *Parasitol Today*, **5**: 132–4.

Lumsden WHR, Kimber CD et al., 1979, *Trypanosoma brucei*: Miniature anion-exchange centrifugation technique for detecting low parasitemias: Adaptation for field use, *Trans R Soc Trop Med Hyg*, **73**: 312–17.

Lumsden WHR, Kimber CD et al., 1981, Field diagnosis of sleeping sickness in the Ivory Coast. I. Comparison of the miniature anion-exchange/centrifugation technique with other protozoological methods, *Trans R Soc Trop Med Hyg*, **75**: 242–50.

Lyons M, 1992, *The Colonial Disease: A Social History of Sleeping Sickness in Northern Zaire, 1900–1940*, Cambridge University Press, Cambridge.

Masiga DK, Smyth AJ et al., 1992, Sensitive detection of trypanosomes in tsetse flies by DNA amplification, *Int J Parasitol*, **22**: 909–18.

Maudlin I, Ellis D, 1985, Extrachromasomal inheritance of susceptibility to trypanosome infection in tsetse flies. I. Selection of susceptible and refractory lines of *Glossina morsitans morsitans*, *Ann Trop Med Parasitol*, **79**: 317–24.

Mellors A, Samad A, 1989, The acquisition of lipids by African trypanosomes, *Parasitol Today*, **5**: 239–44.

Molyneux DM, Ashford, RW, 1983, *The Biology of* Trypanosoma *and* Leishmania, *Parasites of Man and Domestic Animals*, Taylor and Francis, London.

Molyneux DM, DeRaadt P, Seed JR, 1984, African human trypanosomiasis, epidemiological, experimental, and clinical aspects, *Recent Advances in Tropical Medicine*, eds Labno J, Gilles HM, Churchill Livingstone, New York, 39–62.

Molyneux DM, Jefferies D, 1986, Feeding behavior of pathogen-infected vectors, *Parasitology*, **92**: 721–36.

Myler PJ, 1993, Molcular variation in trypanosomes, *Acta Trop*, **53**: 205–25.

Nantulya VM, Doua F, Molisho S, 1992, Diagnosis of *Trypanosoma brucei gambiense* sleeping sickness using an antigen detection enzyme-linked immunosorbent assay, *Trans R Soc Trop Med Hyg*, **86**: 42–5.

Ngaira JM, Olaho-Mukani W, Omuse JK, et al., 1992, Evaluation of procyclic agglutination trypanosomiasis test (PATT) for the immunodiagnosis of *Trypanosoma brucei rhodesiense* sleeping sickness in Kenya, *Trop Med Parasitol*, **43**: 29–32.

Nowak MA, Anderson RM et al., 1991, Antigenic diversity thresholds and the development of AIDS, *Science*, **254**: 963–9.

Okoth JO, 1986, Community participation in tsetse control, *Parasitol Today*, **2**: 88.

Opiyo EA, Njogu AR, Omuse JK, 1990, Use of impregnated targets for control of *Gloassina pallidipes* in Kenya, *Insect Sci Applic*, **11**: 417–425.

Opperdoes FR, 1987, Compartmentation of carbohydrate metabolism in trypanosomes, *Annu Rev Microbiol*, **41**: 127–51.

Opperdoes FR, Wierenga RK et al., 1990, Unique properties of glycosomal enzymes, *Parasites: Molecular Biology, Drug and Vaccine Design*, eds Agabian N, Cerami A, Wiley–Liss, New York, 233–46.

Otieno LH, Darji N et al., 1983, Some observations of factors associated with the development of *Trypanosoma brucei brucei* infections in *Gloassina morsitans morsitans*, *Acta Trop*, **40**: 113–20.

Paindavoine P, Zampetti-Bosseler F et al., 1989, Different allele frequencies in *Trypanosoma brucei brucei* and *Trypanosoma brucei gambiense* populations, *Mol Biochem Parasitol*, **36**: 61–72.

Pays E, Vanhamme L, Berberof M, 1994, Genetic control for the expression of surface antigens in African trypanosomes, *Annu Rev Microbiol*, **48**: 28–52.

Pegg AE, McCann PP, 1988, Polyamine metabolism and function in mammalian cells and protozoans, *ISI Atlas of Science: Biochemistry*, 11–18.

Penchenier L, Jannin J et al., 1991, Le problème de l'interpretation du CATT dans le depistage de la trypanosomiase humaine à *Trypanosoma brucei gambiense*, *Ann Soc Belge Med Trop*, **71**: 221–8.

Pentreath VW, 1991, The search for primary events causing the pathology in African sleeping sickness, *Trans R Soc Trop Med Hyg*, **85**: 145–7.

Pepin J, Milord F, 1994, The treatment of human African trypanosomiasis, *Adv Parasitol*, **33**: 2–47.

Radomski, MW, Buquet A et al., 1995, Twenty-four-hour plasma cortisol and prolactin in human African trypanosomiasis patients and healthy African controls, *Trans R Soc Trop Med Hyg*, **52**: 281–6.

Reincke M, Heppner C et al., 1994, Impairment of adrenocortical function associated with increased plasma tumor necrosis factor-alpha and interleukin-6 concentrations in African trypanosomiasis, *Neuroimmunomodulation*, **1**: 14–22.

Reincke M, Allolio B et al., 1993, Thyroid dysfunction in African

trypanosomiasis: A possible role for inflammatory cytokines, *Clin Endocrinol*, **39**: 455–61.

Sands M, Kron MA, Brown RB, 1985, Pentamidine: A review, *Rev Infect Dis*, **7**: 625–34.

Schechter PJ, Barlow JLR, Sjoerdsma A, 1987, *Inhibition of Polyamine Metabolism*, eds McCann PP, Pegg AE, Sjoerdsma A, Academic Press, New York, 345–64.

Seebeck T, Schneider A et al., 1988, The cytoskeleton of *Trypanosoma brucei* – the beauty of simplicity, *Protoplasm*, **145**: 188–94.

Seed JR, Hall JE, 1992, Trypanosomes causing disease in men in Africa, *Parasitic Protozoa*, vol 2, eds Kreier JP, Baker JR, Academic Press, New York, 85–155.

Simpson L, 1990, RNA editing – a novel genetic phenomenon?, *Science*, **250**: 512–13.

Sommer JM, Wang CC, 1994, Targeting proteins to the glycosomes of African trypanosomes, *Annu Rev Microbiol*, **48**: 105–38.

Soudan B, Boersma A et al., 1993, Hypogonadism induced by African trypanosomes in humans and animals, *Comp Biochem Physiol*, **104A**: 757–63.

Stevens JR, Godfrey DG, 1992, Numerical taxonomy of *Trypanozoon* based on polymorphisms in a reduced range of enzymes, *Parasitology*, **104**: 75–86.

Stephens JWW, Fantham HB, 1910, On the peculiar morphology of a trypanosome from a case of sleeping sickness and the possibility of its being a new species (*T. rhodesiense*), *Proc R Soc London B*, **83**: 28.

Truc P, Aerts D et al., 1992, Direct isolation *in vitro* of *Trypanosoma brucei* from man and other animals and its potential value for the diagnosis of Gambian trypanosomiasis, *Trans R Soc Trop Med Hyg*, **86**: 627–9.

Truc P, Bailey JW, Doua F et al., 1994, A comparison of parasitological methods for the diagnosis of Gambian trypanosomiasis in an area of low endemicity in Cote d'Ivoire, *Trans R Soc Trop Med Hyg*, **88**: 419–21.

Vale GA, 1993, Development of baits for tsetse flies (Diptera: Glossinidae) in Zimbabwe, *J Med Entomol*, **30**: 831–42.

Vale GA, Hall DR, 1985a, The role of 1-octen-3-ol, acetone, and carbon dioxide in the attraction of tsetse flies, *Gloassina* spp. (Diptera: Glossinidae) to ox odour, *Bull Entomol Res*, **75**: 209–17.

Vale GA, Hall DR, 1985b, The role of 1-octen-3-ol, acetone, and carbon dioxide to improve baits for tsetse flies, *Gloassina* spp. (Diptera: Glossinidae), *Bull Entomol Res*, **75**: 219–31.

Vale GA, Hall DR, Gough AJE, 1988, The olfactory responses of tsetse flies, *Glossina* spp (Diptera: Glossinidae), to phenols and urine in the field, *Bull Entomol Res*, **78**: 293–300.

Vickerman K, 1989, Trypanosome sociology and antigenic variation, *Parasitology*, **99**: S37–S47.

Vickerman K, Barry JE, 1982, African trypanosomiasis, *Immunology of Parasitic Infection*, 2nd edn, eds Cohen S, Warren KS, Blackwell Scientific Publications, Oxford, 204–60.

Vickerman K, Tetley L et al., 1988, Biology of African trypanosomes in the tsetse fly, *Biol Cell*, **64**: 109–19.

Williams B, Dransfield R et al., 1993, Where are we now? Trypanosomiasis, *Health Policy Planning*, **8**: 85–93.

Woo PTK, 1971, Evaluation of the hematocrit centrifuge and other techniques for the field diagnosis of human trypanosomiasis and filariasis, *Acta Trop*, **28**: 298–303.

Woo PTK, Hauck L, 1987, The haematocrit centrifuge smear technique for the detection of mammalian *Plasmodium*, *Trans R Soc Trop Med Hyg*, **81**: 727–8.

WHO, 1986, *Epidemiology and Control of African Trypanosomiasis*, WHO Technical Report Series No. 739, World Health Organization, Geneva.

Wyatt GB, Boatin BA, Wurapa FK, 1985, Risk factors associated with the acquisition of sleeping sickness in north-east Zambia: a case-control study, *Ann Trop Med Parasitol*, **79**: 385–92.

Chapter 15

NEW WORLD TRYPANOSOMIASIS

M A Miles

1 HISTORICAL INTRODUCTION

In 1907 the Brazilian scientist Carlos Chagas left the city of Rio de Janeiro to work as a malaria control officer at Lassance in the state of Minas Gerais. Chagas noted that poor houses in the area were infested by a large blood-sucking insect, the triatomine bug (Hemiptera, Reduviidae) (Fig. 15.1). He was aware that blood-sucking insects transmitted human diseases such as malaria and immediately suspected that triatomine bugs might also carry infectious agents. He examined bug faeces and found a flagellated protozoan parasite. At the Manguinhos Institute in Rio de Janeiro, marmosets exposed to infected bugs developed blood parasitaemias of a new trypanosome, which Chagas named *Trypanosoma cruzi* after his mentor Oswaldo Cruz.

Back in Lassance *T. cruzi* was found in the blood of sick children living in bug-infested houses (Fig. 15.2). Chagas and his distinguished colleagues, from what is now the Instituto Oswaldo Cruz, went on to describe clinical aspects of the disease, the life cycle, experimental animal models, and to discover natural mammalian hosts such as the armadillo. These discoveries were remarkable, not least because *T. cruzi* was found first in its insect vector. Chagas' early work was initially controversial, and it was not until some years later that the public health importance of Chagas disease became apparent when scientists in other Latin American countries reported its widespread distribution. The true route of transmission, through contamination with infected bug faeces, was conclusively demonstrated in 1912 by Emile Brumpt. The history of the discovery and early investigations of Chagas disease is described by Miles (1996).

Chagas disease, for those who survive the acute

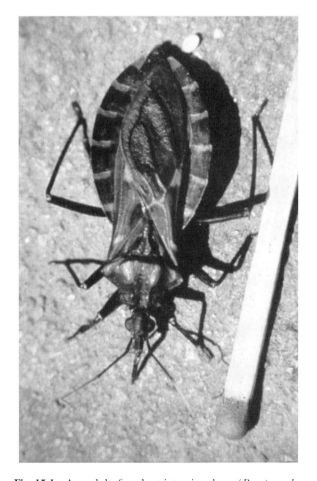

Fig. 15.1 An adult female triatomine bug (*Panstrongylus megistus*) (by courtesy of TV Barrett).

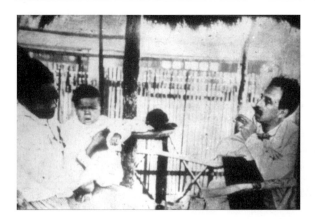

Fig. 15.2 Carlos Chagas with one of the first discovered infant cases of *Trypanosoma cruzi* infection.

phase of infection, primarily affects the heart and alimentary tract. Its pathogenesis remains enigmatic, in that many infected people remain healthy for life and the precise reasons for a poor prognosis are not fully understood. There has been an intense expansion of interest in *T. cruzi*, driven largely by a desire to understand the disease process, how the organism survives for life in the infected mammalian host and the unique features of trypanosome molecular biology. *T. cruzi* is also now known to be an opportunistic infection: in addition to being transmissible by blood and organ donors, it also relapses in immunocompromised individuals. South American trypanosomiasis is predominantly a disease of poverty. As such it is amenable to control by public health interventions to manage the insect vectors, supplemented by measures to eliminate transmission by blood transfusion.

T. cruzi is one of many trypanosome species in the New World, but only one other species is known to infect humans. Like *T. cruzi*, *Trypanosoma rangeli* was first found in triatomine bugs and later in children, but it is not considered to be pathogenic and its medical importance lies in the need to distinguish *T. cruzi* and *T. rangeli* infections during diagnosis by isolation of the parasite. Unlike *T. cruzi*, *T. rangeli* is transmitted by the bite of the vector, through infection of the triatomine bug salivary glands.

Hoare's classic monograph (1972) still contains the best introductions in the English language to the New World human trypanosomiases.

2 CLASSIFICATION

T. cruzi is a kinetoplastid protozoan parasite in the family Trypanosomatidae, which includes the disease agents of both the leishmaniases and the trypanosomiases. The taxonomic position of *T. cruzi* is summarized in Table 15.1. The genus *Trypanosoma* includes 2 species responsible for major public health problems in South America and Africa (*T. cruzi* and *Trypanosoma brucei*, respectively) and others that are not pathogenic or seldom infect humans (*T. rangeli*, *Trypanosoma vivax*, *T. lewisi*-like). *T. cruzi* falls into the section Ster-

coraria (as distinct from the section Salivaria of *T. brucei*; see Chapter 14). The stercorarian trypanosomes, with the notable exception of *T. rangeli*, are transmitted from the vector by contamination of the insect's faeces. Reproduction in the mammalian host is typically discontinuous, that is it is confined to particular life cycle stages or tissue sites. *T. cruzi* is the type species of the subgenus *Schizotrypanum* which is an assemblage of morphologically similar species comprising *T. cruzi* or *T. cruzi*-like organisms in the Americas, and a number of cosmopolitan bat trypanosomes. Trypanosome species of the subgenus *Schizotrypanum* multiply intracellularly in the mammalian host. In the blood the trypanosomes are relatively small and a proportion of them are often C-shaped, with a large kinetoplast close to a short, pointed posterior end.

As described below, chemical taxonomic methods, especially phenotypic comparisons by isoenzyme electrophoresis, and more recently comparative DNA analyses, have demonstrated that there is a remarkable diversity within the *T. cruzi* species.

3 STRUCTURE AND LIFE CYCLE

T. cruzi is a eukaryote with a nucleus, and with chromosomes that do not condense during cell division and can only be resolved by electrophoretic methods devised to separate large molecules of DNA. Extranuclear DNA is present in the form of a discrete, visible organelle, the **kinetoplast,** containing minicircle and maxicircle DNA, and associated with a large single-branched cristate mitochondrion. The kinetoplast lies adjacent to a basal body and flagellar pocket from which a **flagellum** emerges (except in the amastigote stage of the life cycle), which has 9 peripheral pairs of microtubules, a central doublet and a parallel paraxial rod. The flagellum runs alongside the main body of the organism, in a posterior to anterior direction, and adheres to it to form an undulating membrane, leading to an anterior free flagellum. Interior organelles include an endoplasmic reticulum and a Golgi apparatus and a specialized glycolytic organelle (the **glycosome**). The organism is bound by a complex network of subpellicular microtubules. Hoare (1972) gives ranges of dimensions for proven *T. cruzi* trypanosomes from humans as: length 11.7–30.4 μm; free flagellum 2.0–11.2 μm; breadth 0.7–5.9 μm. Further details of structure can be found in elegant electron microscopical studies of *T. brucei*, with which *T. cruzi* shares many features, and recent supplementary studies of *T. cruzi* (Tetley and Vickerman 1991).

There are 3 principal stages in the *T. cruzi* life cycle. The **amastigote** stage multiplies within non-phagocytic and phagocytic cells by binary fission. The **epimastigotes**, which have a kinetoplast adjacent to the nucleus and an undulating membrane that runs along approximately the anterior half of the organism, divide by binary fission in the hindgut of the triatomine bug vector. **Trypomastigotes**, with the kinetoplast at the posterior end, do not divide and are the forms found circulating in the blood of the mammalian host.

Table 15.1   Classification of *Trypanosoma cruzi*

Phylum	Euglenozoa	
Order	Kinetoplastida	
Family	Trypanosomatidae	
Genus	*Trypanosoma*	
Section	Stercoraria	Trypomastigotes with free flagellum; kinetoplast large, not terminal; posterior pointed; discontinuous reproduction in mammal; contaminative transmission (except *T. rangeli*); non-pathogenic (except *T. cruzi*).
Subgenus	*Schizotrypanum*	Trypomastigotes small and typically C-shaped with large kinetoplast near short, pointed posterior end; reproduction in mammal intracellularly as amastigote. Assemblage of morphologically indistinguishable species parasitic in diverse mammals, most restricted to New World
Species	*Trypanosoma cruzi*	

Trypomastigotes are also the infective (metacyclic) stage that occurs in the rectum of the vector and in bug faeces deposited during feeding. There are therefore some similarities between the life cycle stages of *T. cruzi* and those of both *Leishmania* and *T. brucei* in that *Leishmania* also has amastigotes that divide intracellularly (see Chapters 12 and 13) and *T. brucei* has circulating trypanosomes but, in contrast to *T. cruzi*, the latter divide in the blood by binary fission (see Chapter 14).

The life cycle is summarized in Fig. 15.3. Metacyclic trypomastigotes deposited on the mammalian host in bug faeces have the capacity to penetrate abraded skin or the wound made by the bite of the bug. They can also cross the oral and nasal mucosae, or the conjunctiva if bug faeces get into the eye. These metacyclic forms are slender, highly motile organisms, which often rapidly traverse the field of view when seen by light microscopy. Once inside the mammalian host they can penetrate phagocytic or non-phagocytic cells to form a local cutaneous or ocular lesion (see section 5.1). Within the cell, the vacuole containing the *T. cruzi* trypomastigote fuses with lysosomes to form a phagolysosome, from which the organism then escapes to lie free in the cytosol. The trypomastigote transforms to an amastigote which divides by binary fission forming a **pseudocyst,** or false cyst, so called because it has no true cyst wall but is simply bounded by the membrane of the host cell. About 5 days later within the pseudocyst there may be up to 500 amastigotes transforming to small motile C-shaped trypomastigotes (Fig. 15.4). The trypomastigotes are released into the surrounding tissue, to either infect other cells and repeat the intracellular cycle or to circulate in the blood (Fig. 15.5). When the pseudocyst ruptures not all the amastigote forms may have transformed to trypomastigotes. Amastigotes released when the cell bursts are thought to be destroyed locally but are occasionally found circulating in the blood of mice with fulminating experimental infections.

Two types of transformation from amastigote to trypomastigote have been described within the pseudocyst. The first, **fusiform transformation**, involves elongation of the body and migration of the kineto-

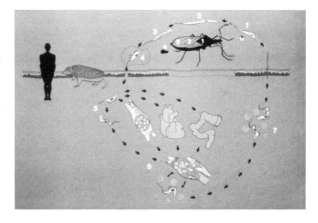

Fig. 15.3   A summary of the life cycle of *Trypanosoma cruzi* (see text) By courtesy of Meddia.

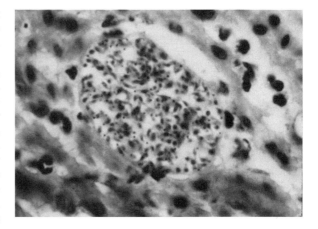

Fig. 15.4   Pseudocyst of *Trypanosoma cruzi* in umbilical cord (by courtesy of Dr Hipolito de Almeida).

plast. The second, **orbicular cycle transformation** is by unrolling of sphaeromastigotes (flagellated amastigote forms with a flagellum that encircles the body without producing an undulating membrane) that have a central vacuole: this orbicular transformation may, however, be an artefact of dry fixation and staining of tissue smears (Hoare 1972).

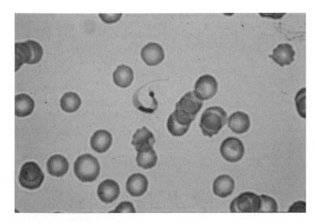

Fig. 15.5 *Trypanosoma cruzi*: C-shaped trypomastigote in circulating blood (see text).

The released trypomastigotes do not all have the same morphology and behaviour. There are 2 types; slender highly motile trypomastigotes, reminiscent of the infective metacyclic forms found in bug faeces, and smaller, broader less motile forms. The slender forms tend to traverse the field rapidly when seen microscopically, whereas the broader forms, although motile, remain for a longer time in the same field of view. The slender motile form has an elongated nucleus, a subterminal kinetoplast and a short free flagellum, whereas the broad form has an oval nucleus, almost terminal kinetoplast and a long free flagellum. The slender forms are generally only seen in the blood of experimental animals, such as mice, during the initial acute phase of infection. It has been proposed, although not proven, that the slender forms are pre-adapted to penetrating cells and renewing the intracellular cycle, whereas the shorter, broader forms may persist in the blood to be taken up by the vector with the blood-meal. Unlike *T. brucei*, however, both slender and broad forms are thought to have active mitochondria (in *T. brucei* dividing slender forms depend on glycolysis and the mitochondria are only fully active in the stumpy forms, to prepare them for life in the tsetse fly).

Except in experimental models with *T. cruzi* strains that are highly virulent to mice, the number of circulating trypomastigotes in the blood is generally quite low (less than 1 per field at × 400 magnification in a fresh blood film) and the blood parasitaemia rapidly becomes sub-patent to microscopy. Low levels of circulating organisms, which may remain for the life of the host, can then only be detected by more sensitive methods.

The development of *T. cruzi* in the triatomine bug is confined to the alimentary tract. Bugs acquire infection by feeding on an infected mammalian host (or rarely by cannibalizing other recently fed bugs) and there is no transovarial transmission from adult female to egg. Once infected, triatomine bugs retain infection throughout the moulting cycles. The development of *T. cruzi* in the vector, dependent on the stage of the insect, in general takes around 10–15 days. Trypomastigotes in the blood-meal transform to amastigotes and

sphaeromastigotes in the foregut, and multiply by binary fission. In the midgut, division is by binary fission in the epimastigote stage. In the rectum, epimastigotes attach to the epithelium and transformation to metacyclic trypomastigotes begins. More detailed descriptions of the life cycle stages can be found in Hoare (1972) and Brack (1968).

Contamination with infected bug faeces during or just after the blood-meal is not the only route of transmission. Blood transfusion transmission is commonplace where blood is not screened for presence of *T. cruzi* antibodies or not pretreated with gentian violet (WHO 1991) (see section 12). All blood donors who have resided in endemic areas and been exposed to triatomine bugs should be screened for antibodies, as should all organ donors or organ recipients with relevant histories. Antibody testing of blood donors is mandatory in some countries. It has been shown experimentally that transmission may also occur by the oral route, by consumption either of triatomine bugs or of food contaminated with bug faeces, and possibly by eating uncooked blood and tissues from infected reservoir hosts. Oral transmission may be important in sustaining prevalence rates in insectivorous mammals, particularly those that live in burrows infested with bugs, and several small outbreaks of simultaneous acute cases within families are almost certainly due to oral transmission of *T. cruzi* (see below). Congenital transmission also occurs in a small proportion of children born to seropositive mothers (WHO 1991). Sexual transmission is thought to be extremely rare, as is transmission through the milk from mother to suckling infant. Accidental transmission in the laboratory is not uncommon, usually through inoculation or ingestion. There are no other important insect vectors, although *T. cruzi* may survive in cimicid bugs and produce metacyclic trypomastigotes in the hindgut, and they are thought to have given rise to infections in primate colonies, possibly by the oral route. Persistent *T. cruzi* infections may also occur experimentally in ticks (*Ornithodorus moubata*) (Hoare 1972).

All stages of the life cycle of *T. cruzi* are reproducible in culture. Thus epimastigotes are easily grown on blood agar overlays. A wide range of mammalian cell lines can be infected to produce mature pseudocysts with motile trypomastigotes, which are seen as 'boiling cells' by phase microscopy. Emergent trypomastigotes re-enter cells in vitro such that several intracellular cycles can occur on a single cell monolayer maintained for 20 days or more (Miles 1993).

The life cycle of *T. rangeli* in the arthropod vector is quite distinct from that of *T. cruzi* in that, in bugs belonging to the genus *Rhodnius*, the haemolymph is often invaded, usually more than 40 days after the infective blood-meal. Salivary gland infections become established in a proportion of bugs that have haemolymph infections. *T. rangeli* is pathogenic to its insect vector and infected bugs may die or not moult successfully. The development of *T. rangeli* in the lumen of the bug gut and in the haemolymph is indistinguishable. Multiplication occurs in the mammalian host but blood parasitaemias are scanty. *T. rangeli* is capable of infecting an histiocytic cell line (U937) in vitro and surviving as non-dividing amastigote-like forms, but it is not clear whether such intracellular stages contribute to survival in the mammalian host (Osorio et al. 1995). The insect vector stages can be grown in vitro. The importance of *T. rangeli* as a human infective agent is secondary, in that it has to be distinguished from *T. cruzi* during diagnostic procedures (see section 8).

4 BIOCHEMISTRY, MOLECULAR BIOLOGY AND GENETICS

4.1 Biochemistry

Drug development is often quoted as the incentive for studying the biochemistry of infectious disease agents such as *T. cruzi*. Thus, the absence of some metabolic pathways may make *T. cruzi* vulnerable to drug action that is circumvented by normal mammalian metabolism and therefore not toxic to humans. Alternatively, unique features of trypanosome metabolism may expose the organism to drugs that have no equivalent target in humans. An example of absence of a metabolic pathway is the inactive mitochondrion in the blood stage form of *T. brucei*, mentioned above (and see Chapter 14), although this is not the case for *T. cruzi*. Examples of prominent differences between the biochemistry of trypanosomatids and mammals have been found in purine salvage pathways, trypanothione biosynthesis and catabolism, sterol synthesis and glycosomal metabolism. In addition, several unusual features of the molecular biology of trypanosomes have excited great interest among molecular biologists and encouraged their use as model organisms. These include the presence of the kinetoplast and radical editing of mitochondrial mRNA, discontinuous transcription and *trans*-splicing, polycistronic transcription and antigenic variation with epigenetic mechanisms of controlling gene expression.

T. cruzi utilizes sugars, especially glucose, through active transport into the cell, nevertheless it is not dependent on glucose and can survive by catabolism of amino acids and proteins: there are apparently no major reserve polysaccharides. Glucose catabolism, incomplete even in the presence of oxygen, produces succinic acids and acetic acid; anaerobic catabolism leads mainly to succinate and L-alanine. Enzymes of the glycolytic pathway, all of which have been reported, mostly occur in a specialized organelle, the glycosome, related to the peroxisome, which assists fatty acid metabolism in eukaryotes. The pentose phosphate pathway of glucose catabolism is also present. Amastigote, epimastigote and trypomastigote stages have almost all enzymes of the tricarboxylic acid cycle (Cazzulo 1994).

Glycosomes lack catalase and oxidases, which regulate hydrogen peroxide in peroxisomes, but contain enzymes for conversion of glucose and glycerol to phosphoglycerate, as well as enzymes for β-oxidation of fatty acids and for ether-lipid biosynthesis; other activities include pyrimidine biosynthesis, purine salvage and carbon dioxide fixation. Enzymes found in the glycosome of *T. cruzi* include hexokin-ase, phosphoglucose isomerase, phosphofructokinase, aldolase, triosephosphate isomerase, glyceraldehyde 3-phosphate dehydrogenase, glycerol 3-phosphate dehydrogenase, glycerol kinase, malate dehydrogenase, adenylate kinase and phosphoenolpyruvate carboxykinase: some of these enzymes are also present in the cytosol. Transport of enzymes into the glycosome does not involve larger cytosolic precursors and cleavage of signal sequences. It was once thought that 'hot spots' of positively charged amino acids on the enzymes acted as importation signals, but molecular modelling has shown that these are not conserved. Peptide recognition signals probably govern importation, as is the case for peroxisomes; some of these recognition signals occur in insertions or C-terminal extensions (Kendall et al. 1990).

Glutathione (GSH) is the low molecular weight thiol largely responsible for protection against free radicals and reactive oxygen in most aerobic organisms. In trypanosomatids glutathione is replaced by trypanothione, a glutathione dimer conjugated to spermidine. In *T. cruzi* glutathione reductase (GR) is replaced by trypanothione reductase (TR), which reduces trypanothione disulphide (T[S]$_2$) to dihydrotrypanothione (T[SH]$_2$) with NADPH as cofactor. Substrate utilization of TR is distinct from that of GR but catalytic mechanism is conserved.

The 2 negatively charged carboxyl groups on the glycyl termini of the GR substrate glutathione disulphide (GSSG) are replaced by internal amide groups in trypanothione disulphide (T[S]$_2$) and an amino group carrying a positive charge on the spermidine. Also the 2 glutathione chains in GSSG can rotate freely about the disulphide bridge whereas the T[S$_2$] is more rigid due to the linkage by spermidine. There are distinct distributions of hydrophobic and charged residues in GR and TR adjacent to the glycyl regions of the substrate. The R$_{37}$ and R$_{347}$ amino acids of GR, which are thought to bind the carboxyl groups of GSSG, are replaced by tryptophan and alanine (Taylor et al. 1994).

Studies of trypanothione metabolism in *T. cruzi* have been an interesting model for the development of rational chemotherapy: glutathionylspermidine synthetase and trypanothione synthetase enzymes of trypanothione biosynthesis are possible drug targets.

Parasitic protozoa such as *T. cruzi* rely on the salvage of free purines or re-use of purines from nucleic acids or nucleotides, whereas mammals can synthesize purines *de novo*. The hypoxanthine analogue allopurinol has been used as an inhibitor of purine salvage. The value of allopurinol as a therapeutic drug for *T. cruzi* infections is still in doubt although some reports say that allopurinol and alloprinol riboside are as effective for treatment as benznidazole and nifurtimox (see section 10).

There has been much research interest in proteinases of *T. cruzi* with the idea that they may be important for invasion of mammalian host cells, and targets for chemotherapy. Cysteine proteinases are the most prominent of the 4 main groups (aspartic, cysteine, metallo- and serine) in *T. cruzi* although metalloproteinases and serine proteinase are also present (Coombs and North 1991). There may be several other roles for *T. cruzi* proteinases, such as protection against antibody attack, or adaptation to breakdown of the blood-meal in the insect vector. Proteinase activities can be demonstrated by using electrophoresis in gels with gelatin or fluorogenic peptides as substrates. A 60 kDa cysteine proteinase named cruzipain resembles cathepsin and papain, and is also known as the GP57/51 antigen, which is recognized by sera from patients infected with *T. cruzi*. The enzyme produces a C-terminal extension domain by self-proteolysis (Stoka et al. 1995).

Glycosyl-phosphatidylinositols (GPI) and GPI-related glycolipids are abundant in trypanosomatids. They serve to anchor surface glycoproteins and, although *T. cruzi* does not have the variant surface glycoprotein (VSG) coat characteristic of the African trypanosomes (see Chapter 14), several glycoproteins are bound to the surface of *T. cruzi* by GPI anchors, including the Ssp-4 antigen of amastigotes and the 90 kDa antigen of trypomastigotes. Ferguson and his collaborators have devoted much effort to determining the GPI biosynthetic pathway in African trypanosomes, not only for the intrinsic biochemical interest but also because this pathway might present a target for trypanosome-specific chemotherapy (Güther and Ferguson 1995).

Another unique biochemical feature that is present in protozoa (also in fungi and plants) but not in vertebrates is the presence of sterol methyl transferase (SMT) which transfers a methyl group from *S*-adenosyl methionine to the sterol side chain. This has led to promising new inhibitors of sterol biosynthesis in *T. cruzi* (Urbina et al. 1995).

4.2   Molecular biology

There is a plethora of recent advances in understanding the basic molecular biology of trypanosomes, fuelled by an international interest in their unusual features and their role as models for other studies. Two molecular processes that have received detailed attention are discontinuous transcription, or *trans*-splicing, and RNA editing of transcripts from the maxicircle mitochondrial genome.

Studies of antigenic variation in African trypanosomes revealed that each primary mRNA transcript was processed by addition of 39 nucleotide spliced leader sequence transcribed from a separate chromosomal location – the **mini-exon genes**. The spliced leader is added by *trans*-splicing via Y shaped intermediates that consist of the 3′ leader precursor linked to the 5′ portion of the main transcript. *Trans*-splicing is assisted by small nuclear RNAs (sn RNAs) complexed to proteins, as is intron splicing in higher eukaryotes. Many trypanosome genes are polycistronic, with transcripts of several genes in tandem on an initial primary transcript. The mini-exon derived RNA (medRNA) is thought to be functionally equivalent to the U1-snRNA present in other eurkaryotes. Mature mRNAs of *T. cruzi* are polyadenylated. Pyrimidine (C,T)-rich regions of downstream splice acceptor sites apparently participate in the control of polyadenylation of upstream portions of the primary transcript. This may have a role in gene regulation (Matthews, Tschudi and Ullu 1994).

For many years the function of trypanosome kinetoplast minicircles was obscure. It was finally discovered that some mitochondrial maxicircle genes are condensed and that guide RNAs (gRNAs) transcribed from minicircles carry information for editing maxicircle transcripts, by the insertion (and deletion) of uridines. Editing is in the 3′ → 5′ direction and is thought to occur by 2 *trans*-esterifications involving chimaeras between the guide RNAs and mRNAs. An alternative model for RNA editing suggests that sequence-specific cleavage is followed by the addition of uridines and by ligation. It is not clear why such a complex RNA editing process is required by organisms such as *T. cruzi*, but it may be linked to developmental regulation during move-ment between host, vector and life cycle stages (Avila and Simpson 1995).

Other recent research on the molecular biology of *T. cruzi* has concerned the cloning of genes encoding products involved in cell invasion or in gene expression during transformation to the infective form (metacyclogenesis), the structural and functional analysis of genes encoding antigens recognized by the host immune response, and cloning portions of the genome identified by probing with heterologous sequences from other organisms.

T. cruzi carries a surface *trans*-sialidase which transfers sialic acid from host components to mucin-like glycoproteins on the surface of the parasite. In this way *trans*-sialidase is thought to influence adhesion and penetration of host cells and may also have a role in trypomastigote escape from the phagolysosome into the cytoplasm of the host cell (Burleigh and Andrews 1995, Salazar, Mondragon and Kelly 1996). There is a family of putative mucin genes in *T. cruzi* which share a signal peptide on the N-terminus and what is thought to be a sequence for GPI anchoring on the C-terminus (Di Noia, Sanchez and Frasch 1995). Mucins isolated from non-infective epimastigote and infective metacyclic trypomastigotes differ in lipid structure (Serrano et al. 1995). Metacyclogenesis may be induced in the triatomine bug gut by products of haemoglobin digestion: synthetic peptides corresponding to amino acids 30–49 and 35–73 of αD-globin have stimulated differentiation of epimastigotes into metacyclic trypomastigotes (Garcia et al. 1995). There is a large heterogeneous *trans*-sialidase multi-gene family in *T. cruzi* which, among other members, includes genes for *T. cruzi* neuraminidase (TCNA), shared acute phase antigen (SAPA), and the GP85 surface glycoproteins. The gene family has been classified into 4 groups. It has been proposed that changes in expression of such multigene families may provide a mechanism by which *T. cruzi* evades the host immune response, analogous to but distinct from antigenic variation in African trypanosomes (Ruef et al. 1994). *T. cruzi* genes cloned and sequenced include those for heat-shock proteins, histones, tubulin and several enzyme genes such as glyceraldehyde 3-phosphate dehydrogenase, dihydrofolate reductase-thymidylate synthase and hypoxanthine-guanine phosphoribosyltransferase.

A major technological breakthrough in research on the molecular biology of *T. cruzi* has been the development of genetic transformation systems. New plasmid and cosmid shuttle vectors allow *T. cruzi* DNA to be propagated in bacteria and reintroduced into *T. cruzi*, either episomally, or integrated into the nuclear genome by homologous recombination. In this way *T. cruzi* genes can be deleted or overexpressed so that gene structure and function can be analysed. Functional complementation of deletion mutants allows portions of the genome encoding a particular function to be identified. Structural analysis of tandem arrays or multigene families and of gene linkage are facilitated by the use of cosmid vectors carrying up to 45 kb of contiguous *T. cruzi* DNA (Kelly, Das and Tomás 1994). The wide interest in *T. cruzi* molecular biology, and availability for cosmid cloning vectors to produce representative gene libraries, has led to the establishment of a WHO-sponsored international project to map the entire *T. cruzi* genome. Automated DNA sequencing is likely to lead to exponential growth in gene sequence data available for *T. cruzi*.

4.3 Genetic diversity

Early experimental work on *T. cruzi*, its wide range of mammalian hosts and the large number of triatomine bug vector species suggested that *T. cruzi* might be genetically diverse. *T. cruzi* strains were reported to differ in their virulence and histotropism in experimental animals, in their infectivity to triatomine bug species, in their susceptibility to drug treatment, and antigenically. In addition, outcome of chronic Chagas disease appeared to show marked regional variation (Miles 1979).

In the 1970s isoenzyme electrophoresis began to be applied to study the genetic diversity and population genetics of trypanosomatids (Fig. 15.6). Isoenzyme profiles of *T. cruzi* isolates from domestic and silvatic transmission cycles in a single endemic locality (Sao Felipe, Brazil) showed that domestic and silvatic strains were very different phenotypically and, by implication, genotypically. Thus more enzyme characters separated these *T. cruzi* strains than distinguished species of *Leishmania*. *T. cruzi* isolates were subsequently characterized from many Latin American countries. Analysis of isoenzyme profiles confirmed the extensive diversity within the species, and indicated that there were 3 main strain groups, which were named principal zymodemes Z1, Z2 and Z3 (Miles 1983). Z1 appeared to be associated with marsupials, especially the genus *Didelphis* and Z3 with the armadillo, *Dasypus novemcinctus*. Host associations for Z2 were less obvious but may be linked to guinea pigs in the silvatic cycle in Bolivia, from which *Triatoma infestans* is thought to have spread to the 6 southern cone countries of South America (Argentina, Bolivia, Brazil, Chile, Paraguay, Uruguay) and to southern Peru. The zymodeme concept contributed to the description of *T. cruzi* transmission cycles as (1) non-overlapping or discontinuous, such as in Sao Felipe where distinct *T. cruzi* strains (Z2, Z1) were transmitted by domestic bugs (*Panstrongylus megistus*) and silvatic bugs (*Triatoma tibiamaculata*), as (2) overlapping or continuous, such as in Venezuela where the same principal zymodeme (Z1) was transmitted by a single bug species (*Rhodnius prolixus*) common to domestic and silvatic transmission cycles, or as (3) enzootic as in the Amazon basin and the USA, where triatomine bugs do not colonize houses and silvatic *T. cruzi* strains rarely caused human infection (Miles 1979).

One reason for such interest in the heterogeneity of *T. cruzi* is to assess whether different strains are responsible for the diverse clinical outcomes of Chagas disease. The high prevalence of *T. cruzi* Z1 in the north of South America, where megaoesophagus and megacolon (see section 5) are rare, and the abundance of Z2 in central and eastern Brazil, where megasyndromes are common, suggested that some *T. cruzi* strains were more likely to cause chronic Chagas dis-

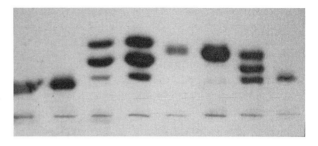

Fig. 15.6 Isoenzyme profiles of *Trypanosoma cruzi* isolates by starch-gel electrophoresis.

ease. Both Z1 and Z2 have, however, been isolated from symptomatic acute phase infections and both can recrudesce after unsuccessful treatment (Luquetti et al. 1986). Although only Z2 was isolated by the same authors from symptomatic chronic Chagas disease there is no proof that Z1 was not (also) present earlier in the infection and responsible, at least in part, for the poor prognosis. Mixed zymodeme infections have been reported from both mammalian hosts and triatomine bugs.

Identification of *T. cruzi* strains by isoenzyme profiles led to selection of biological clones representing different epidemiologies in Latin America for use as reference strains (Table 15.2) in experimental studies (together with some traditional uncloned laboratory strains) and encouraged detailed characterization by other methods, particularly by Dvorak and his collaborators (Dvorak 1984). It was found that clones of different principal *T. cruzi* zymodemes differed radically in DNA content, in kinetoplast DNA minicircle fragment patterns (schizodemes), in elemental composition of iron, zinc and potassium, in oxidative metabolism, in antigenic profiles, in extracellular and intracellular growth rates in vitro, in virulence and tropism in experimental animals, and in response to experimental chemotherapy (Nozaki and Dvorak 1993). There is broad agreement between the zymodeme and schizodeme groupings and a correlation with abundance of a particular surface antigen (Carreno et al. 1987, Chapman, Snary and Miles 1984).

Contemporary studies of allozyme frequencies in African trypanosomes suggested the presence of genetic exchange in what hitherto had been assumed to be an asexual organism. Although the genetic mechanisms are not fully understood, experimental crosses with drug resistance markers have shown that *T. brucei* undergoes recombination in the tsetse fly vector, probably in the salivary glands. Similar experiments, but without drug resistance markers, have so far failed to generate crosses between *T. cruzi* principal zymodemes, or indeed between any *T. cruzi* strains. If genetic exchange does occur in *T. cruzi* it seems most likely that it will be found, as with African trypanosomes, among undisturbed silvatic cycles of transmission. Allozyme frequencies of phosphoglucomutase (PGM) for silvatic isolates of *T. cruzi* from the Amazon basin suggest recombination in *T. cruzi* and this is supported by random amplification of polymorphic DNA (RAPD) which shows sharing of fragments between putative hybrid *T. cruzi* strains and one or other of the putative parents (Carrasco et al. 1996). Further evidence of genetic

Table 15.2 *Trypanosoma cruzi* WHO reference strains

M/HOM/PE/00/Peru
M/HOM/BR/00/12 SF
M/HOM/CO/00/Colombia
M/HOM/BR/00/Y strain
M/HOM/BR/00/CL strain
M/HOM/CH/00/Tulahuen
M/HOM/AR/74/CA-I
M/HOM/AR/74/CA-I/72*
M/HOM/AR/00/CA-I/78*
M/HOM/AR/00/Miranda 83*
M/HOM/AR/00/Miranda 88*
M/HOM/BR/82/Dm 28c*
M/HOM/BR/78?/Sylvio-X10-CL1*
M/HOM/BR/Sylvio/X-10-CL4*
M/HOM/BR/77/Esmeraldo CL3*
M/HOM/BR/68/CAN III CL1*
M/HOM/BR/68/CAN III CL2*
M/HOM/BO/80/CNT/92: 80 CL1*
I/INF/B0/80/SC43 CL1*
I/INF/PY/81/P63 CL*

*Derived from clonal populations.

recombination has come from restriction fragment length polymorphisms (RFLP) studies with gene probes for 3 *T. cruzi* enzyme genes, and suggests that homozygote and heterozygote loci for these genes occur sympatrically among clinical isolates (Bogliolo, Lauria-Pires and Gibson 1996). Genetic transformation with drug resistant markers should soon determine the potential of *T. cruzi* for genetic recombination and allow its epidemiological importance to be assessed.

Tibayrenc and colleagues have subdivided the Z1, Z2, Z3 groups into many zymodemes, performed extensive further studies on their distribution in South America and elaborated a 'clonal hypothesis' which proposes that distinct *T. cruzi* clones are propagated asexually and largely disseminated separately (Tibayrenc et al. 1993). The polymerase chain reaction (PCR) has been used to isolate kinetoplast DNA probes specific to widespread 'major clones' of *T. cruzi*. Most allozyme frequencies and measures of linkage disequilibrium support clonal propagation, and accord with single or small number of bugs invading houses and introducing a restricted number of populations of *T. cruzi*.

A link between *T. cruzi* genotypes and clinical outcome of infection remains unproven, and few attempts have yet been made to examine the role of genotypic and phenotypic diversity of the human host in influencing clinical prognosis. Multiple markers can now be used to compare genetic susceptibilities to chronic Chagas disease, although this may have little direct impact on Chagas disease control (see sections 7 and 12). Preliminary work has suggested a difference in HLA-DR antigen distributions between asymptomatic patients and patients with chronic chagasic cardiomyopathy (Goldberg et al. 1995).

5 CLINICAL ASPECTS

Shortly after his pioneering discoveries Carlos Chagas was once described as a man who searched for diseases that did not exist. Initial acute phase Chagas disease is not frequently noted and is easily confused with other clinical conditions: if present, acute symptoms usually subside within 2 months of their appearance. Patients in certain geographical regions, may suffer megaoesophagus and/or megacolon, usually with associated heart disease, but the elecrocardiographic (ECG) abnormalities and myocardiopathy of chronic Chagas disease may also be mistaken for other forms of heart problem. At least one third of the 18 million or so people thought to be infected with *T. cruzi* and surviving the initial stage of infection appear to be clinically compromised.

5.1 Clinical manifestations

The initial phase of *T. cruzi* infection may lack specific signs and symptoms. In some cases there is a lesion at the portal of entry of the organism, giving rise, in the case of entry through the skin, to a cutaneous chagoma. If metacyclic trypomastigotes cross the conjunctiva the resultant painless, inflamed, periopthalmic, unilateral oedema and conjunctivitis is known as **Romana's sign** (Fig. 15.7). There may be local infiltration of lymphocytes and monocytes and regional lymphadenopathy adjacent to these lesions. Rarely, multiple chagomas have been described during acute infections in infants. Acute infections are more common and more severe in children. Around 10% of children die during the acute stage. General clinical changes at this stage may include fever, hepatosplenomegaly, generalized lymphadenopathy, facial or generalized oedema, rash, vomiting, diarrhoea and anorexia. Early ECG changes may be sinus tachycardia, increased P–R interval, T-wave changes and low QRS voltage, and death may be due to acute myocarditis. Meningoencephalitis is infrequent, mainly found in infants and carries a very poor prognosis. In patients suffering recrudescent *T. cruzi* infection associated with AIDS the organism commonly crosses the blood–brain barrier, and causes fatal meningoencephalitis (WHO 1991).

Incubation period may be as short as 2 weeks, or several months if infection is acquired by blood transfusion. Prolonged incubation period in recipients given contaminated blood is thought to be due to the poor capacity of circulating broad blood forms to invade cells. Splenomegaly and general lymphadenopathy are frequent in such cases.

In a small proportion of seropositive mothers *T. cruzi* crosses the placenta, giving rise to abortion or premature birth. Hepatosplenomegaly is common in congenital infections and there may be fever, oedema, metastatic chagomas and neurological signs such as convulsions, tremors and weak reflexes, and apnoea. Signs of cardiac involvement are rare; ECG is usually unchanged but can show low voltage complexes, decreased T-wave height, and increased atrioventricu-

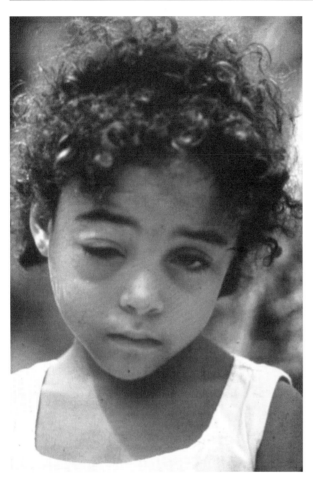

Fig. 15.7 Romana's sign.

lar (AV) conduction time. Premature birth associated with congenital Chagas disease carries a poor prognosis: symptoms are generally less severe if birth is not premature (WHO 1991).

Patients surviving the acute infection enter the indeterminate phase, in which there are no symptoms or signs of Chagas disease. Around 30% of these patients, however, develop chronic disease in which cardiac changes are most common, with arrhythmias, palpitations, chest pain, oedema, dizziness, syncope and dyspnea. The most frequent ECG abnormalities are right bundle branch block (RBB) and left anterior hemiblock (LAH) but there may also be AV conduction abnormalities, sometimes complete AV block. Many different arrhythmias may occur including sinus bradycardia, sinoatrial block, ventricular tachycardia, primary T-wave changes and abnormal Q-waves. Enlargement of the heart may be seen by chest radiography. Complications include embolism. Death is often sudden (WHO 1991).

The regions of the alimentary tract most often affected in the digestive form of chronic Chagas disease are the oesophagus and colon, with loss of peristalsis, regurgitation and dysphagia, or severe constipation, faecaloma, and with progressive dilatation of these organs.

Further details of clinical aspects of chagasic heart disease, megaoesophagus and megacolon can be found in a PAHO Expert Committee Report (PAHO 1994).

6 Immunology

In view of the intense interest in the immune response to *T. cruzi* infection it is surprising how little is understood about either the protective mechanisms or the autoimmune involvement in the pathogenesis of Chagas disease. Individuals surviving acute infection are able to mount an immune response that suppresses parasitaemia but is unable to eradicate infection. In the absence of specific treatment, infection is normally maintained for life. *T. cruzi* specific antibodies may be detectable within the first 2 weeks, and seropositivity usually remains throughout life in untreated patients. All immunoglobulin subclasses are elevated. IgM titres rise early, with increased concentrations, followed by rising IgG titres. Unlike African trypanosomiasis, in which antigenic variation stimulates a sustained increase in IgM, in Chagas disease IgM levels fall as the acute infection subsides. As anticipated for an organism dividing intracellularly, the suppressive immune response also involves cell mediated immunity (Dutra et al. 1996).

Numerous studies have been performed on the immune response to *T. cruzi* infection in mice, recently aided by transgenic mouse technology which allows the course of infection to be observed in knockout mice that are deficient in particular components of the immune response. *T. cruzi* infections in CD4⁻ and CD8⁻ knockout mice indicate that both CD4⁺ and CD8⁺ cells contribute to survival (Rottenberg et al. 1993). Hypergammaglobulinaemia (IgG2a, IgM, IgE) persists in mice until 13 weeks post infection and then IgG2a and IgM levels fall. Although mouse strains vary considerably in their antibody response and resistance to *T. cruzi*, IgG1, IgG2a, IgG2b and IgM titres are sustained throughout infection, possibly with a more dominant IgG2b isotope response in a resistant strain of mouse (Rowland, Mikhail and McCormick 1992). During the acute phase of infection in mice production of the cytokine interleukin-2 (IL-2) is severely suppressed, possibly by repression of transcription of the IL-2 gene (Soong and Tarleton 1994). Killing in macrophages is dependent on production of interferon-γ, synergistic with TNF-α, triggering macrophage activation and nitric oxide production (Munoz Fernandez, Fernandez and Fresno 1992, Silva and Vespa 1995). Nevertheless, studies in mice suggest that *T. cruzi* infection does not necessarily lead to a dominance of Th1 patterns of cytokine production (Zhang and Tarleton 1996). Infection of β₂-microglobulin deficient mice and depletion of CD8⁺T cells prior to infection indicate, however, that these cells have a role in resistance to infection, and possibly by induction of a T-helper 1 response (Tarleton et al. 1992, Hontebeyrie-Joskowicz 1994).

It is not clear how *T. cruzi* survives for life in the infected mammalian host. Immunohistochemical staining suggests that *T. cruzi* antigen can be detected in chronic, chagasic cardiomyopathy, indicating that residual pseudocysts are present. *T. cruzi* amastigotes could be found at autopsy in the hearts of 84 of 556 patients with diffuse, chronic, chagasic myocarditis

(Brener 1994). Nests of *T. cruzi* have also been found in the smooth muscle cells of the central vein of the adrenal gland at autopsy in around 50% of patients with chronic Chagas disease (Teixeira et al. 1995). Several methods have been proposed by which *T. cruzi* escapes action of antibody, including binding of the third component of complement by a specific trypomastigote surface glycoprotein to inhibit activation of the alternative complement pathway and binding of human C4b to restrict the classical pathway (Norris and Schrimpf 1994). The histopathological picture in chronic Chagas disease suggests autoimmune involvement: antibodies to host epitopes on specific proteins such as myosin and ribosomal P proteins have been reported (see p. 293).

7 PATHOLOGY

The pathology at the portal of entry is similar whether the chagoma is cutaneous or a Romana's sign, with infiltration of predominantly lymphocytes and monocytes. In the heart no inflammatory response is said to be directed towards unruptured pseudocysts but rupture is followed by infiltration of lymphocytes, monocytes and/or polymorphonuclear cells. The degree of parasitism is highly variable in clinical cases, and in experimental infections in mice – in the latter it is dependent on strain of infective organism and strain of mouse. In congenital Chagas disease amastigotes may be very widespread but are most common in cardiac and skeletal muscle or reticuloendothelial cells. If there is meningoencephalitis parasites can be found in perivascular spaces or in glial and neuronal cells with an histopathology typical of acute meningoencephalitis (WHO 1991).

In patients surviving the acute infection the inflammatory response in the heart subsides. Two principal forms of pathology have been described in chronic Chagas disease. In the first, or **neurogenic** form, the heart remains free from any progressive myocarditis, but focal lesions are found in the conducting system of the heart and there is a loss of ganglion cells, particularly from the parasympathetic nervous system. Experimental studies in dogs, in which focal cardiac lesions have been reconstructed from histology of tissue sections taken at autopsy, show a good correlation between ECG abnormalities and histopathology. Longitudinal studies of ECG abnormalities in patients with chronic chagasic heart disease followed up by postmortem histology show a similar correlation between ECG abnormalities and lesions of the conducting system. The right bundle branch is found to be most frequently affected, consistent with the frequency of right bundle branch block (RBBB) in chronic Chagas disease. The left conducting system is considered to be less vulnerable to focal lesions because of its more diffuse or bifascicular course. In a proportion of patients the inflammatory response appears to be reactivated resulting in a renewed, **myogenic** form of chronic Chagas disease and a progressive myocarditis with more diffuse lesions, a slower decline in cardiac function and less sudden death. Lymphocytes and macrophages infiltrate the heart and myocardial fibres are replaced by interstitial fibrosis (Brener and Andrade 1979).

At the gross level the heart may be enlarged (megacardia) with focal thinning of the myocardium, which may be particularly frequent and pronounced at the apex of the left ventricle, in the form of an apical aneurysm (Fig. 15.8). The presence of apical aneurysm is considered to be a pathognomonic sign of chronic chagasic heart disease. Of the intestinal sequelae chagasic megaoesophagus (Fig. 15.9) is generally more common than chagasic megacolon (Fig. 15.10), both may occur in the same individual and each is frequently associated with chagasic cardiopathy. A moderate or severe inflammatory response may be seen in the smooth muscle of the oesophagus or colon and in the myenteric or Auerbach plexus during acute infection; in chronic Chagas disease the inflammatory response in these organs is usually mild.

Qualitative observations of neurological damage in Chagas disease were recorded as early as the 1930s. Köberle and his colleagues made painstaking quantitative studies of the number of ganglion cells present in normal and chagasic sections of heart, oesophagus and colon, and demonstrated widespread and significant ganglion cell loss, especially from the parasympathetic autonomic system (Köberle 1974). Neuron loss was found in many different organs but was most fre-

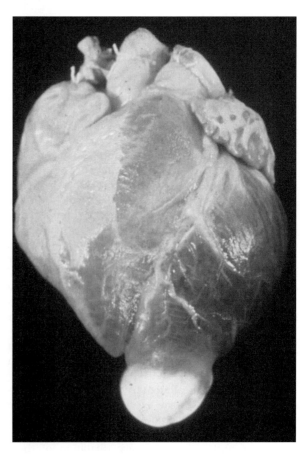

Fig. 15.8 Apical aneurysm of the left ventricle (by courtesy of Dr J. S. de Oliveira).

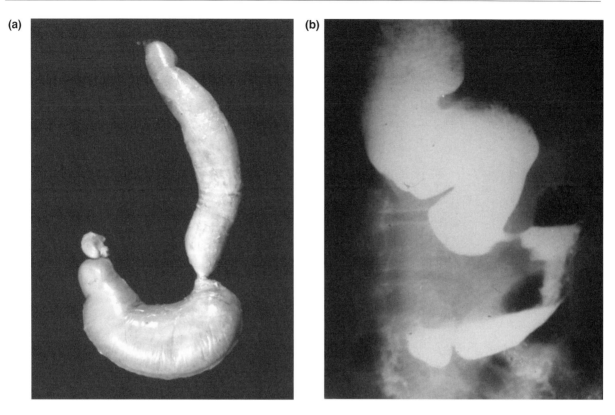

(a)

(b)

Fig. 15.9 Megaoesophagus: (a) postmortem; (b) on radiograph (by courtesy of Dr J. S. de Oliveira).

quent in the heart and alimentary tract. The variable onset of ECG abnormalities, megaoesophagus and megacolon was understandable in terms of age related neuron loss exacerbating the neurological damage attributable to *T. cruzi* infection. In addition it was proposed that different hollow organs varied in the degree to which they could tolerate neuron loss; beyond these organ-specific thresholds, functional abnormalities and dilatation would begin to appear. Several authors have confirmed neuron cell loss in chronic Chagas disease (Lázzari 1994) and experimental studies in animals have shown that this neurological damage can occur early in the acute infection. Thus, the extent of *T. cruzi* infection in the acute phase and concomitant neurological damage may govern long-term prognosis, at least as far as the neurogenic form of chronic Chagas disease is concerned. Although some nerve cells may be parasitized, it is generally considered that ganglion cells are not destroyed as a direct result of parasitism. Early ganglion cell destruction led Koberle to the conclusion that a neurotoxin was produced by *T. cruzi*. Subsequent studies in experimental animals, however, have showed adsorption of *T. cruzi* antigens to uninfected tissue following pseudocyst rupture, with the implication that a T-cell mediated immune response could give rise to focal destruction of uninfected cells. Some of the physiopathological signs of chronic Chagas disease are compatible with dominance of the sympathetic system, predictable if the parasympathetic system is more exposed to damage from *T. cruzi* infection. Indeed, Oliveira demonstrated that the pathognomonic sign of apical aneurysm could be induced in rats, in the absence of *T. cruzi* infection, by inoculation of catecholamines (Oliveira 1969, Lázzari 1994). A sympathetic dominance is also apparently associated with sudden heart failure.

The trigger that leads some patients to the renewed

inflammatory response and progressive decline of chronic myogenic Chagas disease is not clear, but the histopathological picture is highly suggestive of an autoimmune process. Release of sequestered antigens by destruction of normal cells to which *T. cruzi* antigens are adsorbed could lead to an autoimmune pathology with an unpredictable onset. Much research has been done in an attempt to elucidate the autoimmune pathogenesis of chronic Chagas disease. It seems clear that autoantibodies appear in experimental animals later than significant neuron destruction. Monoclonal antibodies to rat ganglia cross-react with *T. cruzi*; conversely some monoclonal antibodies raised to *T. cruzi* cross-react with mammalian tissues. Numerous tissue cross-reactive antibodies have also been reported from patients with chronic Chagas disease. A possible candidate for a cross-reactive epitope between *T. cruzi* and normal host components is the C-terminus of the *T. cruzi* ribosomal P protein (Kaplan et al. 1993, Ferrari, Levin et al. 1995). IgG fractions of chagasic sera contain antibodies to a motif shared by the C-terminal region of the P0 ribosomal protein, the β_1-adrenoreceptor and the M_2 muscarinic receptor, yet are absent from control sera, and antibodies affinity-purified from chagasic sera modulated receptor function in neonatal rat tissue (Ferrari, Wallukat et al. 1995). It is not clear, however, that such antibodies are markers of morbidity or a key component precipitating autoimmune pathogenesis. Putative cross-reactive epitopes have been described from mammalian proteins such as myosin: recognition of *T. cruzi* B-13 protein antigen and a corresponding epitope in

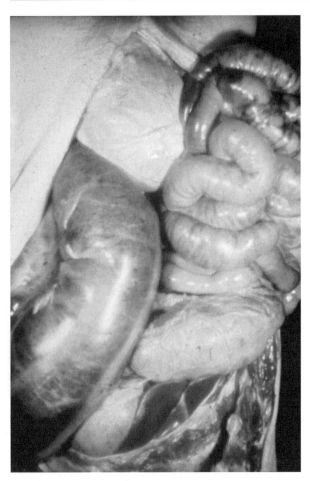

Fig. 15.10 Megacolon (by courtesy of Dr J. S. de Oliveira).

8 DIAGNOSIS

In some acute *T. cruzi* infections trypanosomes may be found transiently in the peripheral blood by direct microscopy of unstained, wet blood films. More scanty parasitaemias can be detected by microscopy of Giemsa stained thick blood films or by microscopy after concentration of trypomastigotes from blood. Concentration methods include (1) haematocrit centrifugation (with caution to avoid tube breakage and exposure to infection) followed by searching for trypomastigotes in or immediately above the buffy coat layer; (2) allowing the blood to coagulate and searching for trypomastigotes in centrifuged serum (Strout's method), or (3) lysis of red cells with 0.85% ammonium chloride and centrifugation to sediment trypomastigotes.

In the indeterminate and chronic phases of the infection *T. cruzi* is present in such low numbers in the peripheral blood that parasitaemia is not patent to microscopy even after the above concentration methods. Xenodiagnosis, in which colony-bred uninfected triatomine bugs are fed on a suspect host and dissected about 20–25 days later to detect epimastigotes, or blood culture, are employed for parasitological diagnosis of chronic infections. Xenodiagnosis is generally favoured for routine use in Latin America because, unlike blood culture, it does not require stringent aseptic precautions. Colonies of triatomine bugs are usually maintained by feeding on chicken blood, as birds are not susceptible to *T. cruzi* infection. If *T. infestans* is used, colonies must be examined periodically for presence of the monogenetic kinetoplastid *Blastocrithidia triatomae* as this may be confused with *T. cruzi* when bugs are dissected. Triatomine nymphs can survive for several months without feeding and xenodiagnosis may thus be used in rural locations, as long as the bugs are protected from high temperatures. It is advisable to use a local species of domestic vector; *R. prolixus* and *T. infestans* are favoured, *R. prolixus* feeds most avidly but may give rise to hypersensitivity skin reactions in individuals sensitized to bug bites. Precautions must be taken in dissecting infected bugs to avoid exposure to infection. Sterile diluents for bug faeces should be used so that results are not confused by motile contaminants, such as ciliates. Under ideal conditions blood culture on to a blood agar base with physiological saline overlay can be as sensitive as xenodiagnosis; cultures are inoculated 'through the cap' to minimize contamination (Miles 1993).

In central and northern South America *T. cruzi* must be distinguished from non-pathogenic *T. rangeli*, although in practice *T. rangeli* is almost never seen in human blood. *T. rangeli* and *T. cruzi* can both multiply in bugs used for xenodiagnosis. Long epimastigote forms with a small kinetoplast and pointed posterior end indicate the presence of *T. rangeli*, but such forms are not always present. In a proportion of infected bugs *T. rangeli* infections will progress to haemolymph and salivary gland infections (Hoare 1972).

Detection of parasite DNA is theoretically an attractive alternative to demonstration of the whole organism. PCR protocols have been developed that can show the presence of *T. cruzi* infection in the chronic phase. Although extremely sensitive after DNA extraction of blood samples, the PCR approach is not yet

human myosin heavy chain is said to be associated with chronic chagasic cardiopathy (Cunha Neto et al. 1995). Several attempts have been made to implicate cell mediated autoimmune pathology by studies in vitro, or by adoptive transfer of immunopathology with cells from infected donors to naive recipients: granulomata around the sciatic nerve have been induced experimentally by cell transfer and newborn syngeneic grafts were rejected by *T. cruzi* infected mice but not by control mice (Ribeiro dos Santos et al. 1992).

Thus the pathogenesis of Chagas disease remains far from understood. A tenuous unifying hypothesis emerges from these diverse considerations: in the acute phase neuron loss is precipitated by destruction of normal cells that have adsorbed *T. cruzi* antigens, which, dependent on the degree and extent of damage, is followed by a benign or catastrophic neurogenic clinical outcome; a cell-mediated autoimmune myogenic relapse occurs in an unfortunate minority of patients. Evidence for autoimmunity in chronic Chagas cardiomyopathy is reviewed by Kalil and Cunha-Neto (1996).

A comprehensive review in English of Chagas disease and the nervous system has recently been produced by a group of eminent Latin American pathologists (PAHO 1994).

simple enough for routine diagnosis. In the long term, if adaptable to a low cost, rapid assay PCR might be applicable to screening of transfusion blood or monitoring the success of chemotherapy (Britto et al. 1995a; Britto et al. 1995b).

In principle, serology detects exposure to infection rather than an active infection. In *T. cruzi* infection, however, both the infection and seropositivity are generally maintained for life unless specific anti-parasite chemotherapy has been given. Only rarely have untreated individuals become seronegative (and presumably lost their infections). A sensitive and specific complement fixation text (CFT) was developed in 1913 and is still in use, despite its complexity. Favoured serological tests are the indirect fluorescent antibody test (IFAT), the enzyme linked immunosorbent assay (ELISA) and the indirect haemagglutination test (IHAT). Care is required with the IFAT to exclude non-specific antibody binding (usually by selecting a high cut-off serum dilution between positive and negative sera, such as 1 in 80 or above). The ELISA requires careful standardization of conjugate batches, duplicate test wells, and positive and negative serum controls should be run on every plate. The IHAT is commercially available and convenient but said to be somewhat less sensitive than IFAT or ELISA. Serum or blood spots collected on filter paper can be used as the source of antibodies but serum provides a more accurate estimate of antibody titre. Cross-reactions may occur with other infectious diseases, notably visceral leishmaniasis and cutaneous leishmaniasis, which may be sympatric with Chagas disease. The advent of recombinant DNA technology has led to the testing of a series of *T. cruzi*-specific proteins selected from expression libraries, of which the CRA antigen has given sensitivity equal to that of crude *T. cruzi* antigens in one multicentre trial (Moncayo and Luquetti 1990, Krieger et al. 1992). Such recombinant antigens have yet to be incorporated, however, in a specific *T. cruzi* assay applicable throughout the Americas. Detection of IgM antibodies (with IgM specific conjugates) in newborn infants suspected of Chagas disease provides a means of helping to distinguish congenital infection from *trans*-placental transfer of IgG from mother to child.

In all cases, and especially in travellers returning from Latin America, clinical background should be explored thoroughly for a history of exposure to triatomine bites, of blood transfusion or of other sources of infection. Parasitological diagnosis is usually performed only if serology is positive. *T. cruzi* is only isolated from about 50% of seropositive individuals by xenodiagnosis, with 20 or more triatomine bugs, or by blood culture. Some clinical signs, such as RBBB, may be pathognomonic or highly indicative if associated with a supportive history. Hirschsprung's megacolon is seldom confused with chagasic megacolon because the former is rare in adults; when necessary electromanometry or radiography can help with the differential diagnosis (Miles 1994)

9 EPIDEMIOLOGY AND CONTROL

Chagas disease is essentially a public health problem that is sustained by poor housing and poverty. The later nymphal stages and adult triatomine bugs are quite large (adults of some species may be more than 4 cm long) and, although they are reclusive insects, bug infestation is a considerable nuisance to householders. Heavy bug infestations would not be tolerated if there were lesser economic and health burdens in the affected communities. It follows that economic development, access to insecticides, improved housing, and health education should interrupt vector-borne transmission of *T. cruzi*, and this has proven to be the case in several successful control campaigns (Wanderley 1993). This is, however, of little comfort for the 16 or 18 million people who are already infected with *T. cruzi*.

A single (unsatisfactory) drug is now available for the specific treatment of Chagas disease (see section 10.1); access to it may be life-saving in the initial stage of infection. Yet acute cases are seldom seen and recognized, and it is uncertain that the continued presence of the organism in the chronic stage affects the long-term prognosis, which may be dictated largely by the severity of early infection. Treatment of chronic cases thus relies on alleviation of symptoms either by drugs or by installation of pacemakers, or by elegant surgical procedures that have been pioneered in Brazil. One experimental drug looks promising (Urbina 1995) and, although new drugs are highly desirable, their epidemiological impact depends on ability to eradicate infection from the reservoir of humans already carrying *T. cruzi*: this demands drugs that are inexpensive and without side effects.

The prospects for vaccination against *T. cruzi* are remote, even though immunization has been shown to protect animals against fatal, acute phase infections, and will remain remote until autoimmune involvement in pathogenesis is fully understood and can be excluded as a complication of the antigen administration. Thus, little research is directed towards vaccine development, and it is difficult to justify in the face of successful campaigns to eliminate domestic triatomine bugs.

Elimination of domestic bug populations is an attainable goal, although eradication of *T. cruzi* is beyond reach as it is a widespread zoonosis, with numerous silvatic reservoir and vector species. The distribution of human Chagas disease is somewhat enigmatic, and changing as both the spread of domestic vectors and destruction of forest vector habitats may lead to the emergence of new endemic areas. Much remains to be learned about the complexities of the epidemiology of Chagas disease in the context of parasite, vectors and reservoir hosts.

9.1 Epidemiology (including reservoir hosts)

The blood-sucking insect vectors of Chagas disease are a subfamily (Triatominae) of the Reduviidae in the order Hemiptera. Five tribes, 14 genera and 118 species of triatomine have been described based on morphological characteristics (Lent and Wygodzinsky 1979, Schofield 1994). Thirteen species occur in the Old World, and the remaining 105 are confined to the Americas. Eight of the 13 Old World species are related to *Triatoma rubrofasciata*, which occurs worldwide in ports with its host the rat (*Rattus rattus*), to which it transmits *Trypanosoma conorhini*; the remaining 5 Old World species are grouped into the unusual Indian genus *Linshcostius*.

Most New World triatomine species have silvatic ecotopes, such as palm trees, burrows, hollow trees, rock crevices or caves, where they feed from mammals, birds or reptiles, and many of the New World species have been reported as infected with *T. cruzi*. Five species, of 3 genera, have adapted to colonize domestic habitats and are responsible for abundant and widespread household infestations; they are: *Triatoma infestans*, *Rhodnius prolixus*, *Panstrongylus megistus*, *Triatoma brasiliensis* and *Triatoma dimidiata*.

T. infestans is the main vector in the southern cone countries of South America (Argentina, Bolivia, Brazil, Chile, Paraguay, Uruguay) and in southern Peru; it is thought to have spread from the Cochabamba region of Bolivia, where it occurs in rocky silvatic ecotopes with guinea pigs: outside Bolivia *T. infestans* is said to be restricted to domestic and peridomestic habitats. *R. prolixus* is the most important vector in northern countries of South America and in central America, with *T. dimidiata* a significant secondary vector. *P. megistus* occurs along the eastern seaboard of Brazil, which was formerly covered by a continuous zone of Atlantic forest, and in central-eastern Brazil. *T. brasiliensis* is the vector in the arid northeastern region of Brazil. *Triatoma sordida*, although extremely widespread in central and eastern South America and often described as an important domestic vector, is usually associated with chickens. Many other species are reported from houses but usually as small, infrequent colonies, or as adult bugs flying into houses attracted to light.

Triatomines are considered to be obligatory blood feeders; most species take mammalian or bird blood but some feed on reptiles. At least one genus (*Eratyrus*) is known to take blood also from large invertebrates that co-inhabit its natural hollow tree ecotope (Miles, de Souza and Povoa 1981a). Each nymphal stage must take at least one blood meal before moulting to the next. Bug pheromones in faeces may lead to aggregation of vectors at feeding sites, such as roosting chickens. As there is no transovarial transmission of *T. cruzi* older bugs are more likely to have fed from an infected host and are therefore more likely to be infected.

Adults of all species are winged, with the exception of the Chilean *Triatoma spinolai*, which has wingless females and either winged or wingless males. Nevertheless, adult triatomines are not frequent flyers; they are almost never observed to fly in laboratory colonies unless artificially induced to do so, but may be seen flying in infested houses at dusk, particularly after heavy rain. Flight is known to be an important method of dispersion since adult bugs of some species commonly fly into houses. Adhesive eggs aid passive dispersion of *Rhodnius*, and nymphal stages can move from host to host by walking. The few natural predators and parasites of triatomines include wasps (*Telonomus, Gryon*) that develop in triatomine bug eggs, spiders, lizards, chickens, rodents and various other insectivores, parasitic nematodes and fungi. Immunological analysis of insect food sources can be used both to determine sources of blood in bugs and to identify their natural predators by detecting ingested bug proteins. When alarmed some triatomines produce the distinctive smell of isobutyric acid, and make sounds by stridulation, in which the proboscis is rubbed in a ridged ventral groove. *Rhodnius* has climbing organs and can scale very smooth surfaces, possibly due to the need to climb smooth trunked palms and palm frond stems in its natural arboreal habitats. The distribution of domestic vector species within houses may reflect silvatic habitat preferences: thus *R. prolixus* heavily infests roofs made of palm fronds and palm crowns are the principal habitat of the genus; *P. megistus* is most frequently found in compressed mud and wooden framed walls, and its most frequent natural habitats are hollow trees or burrows among tree roots; *T. infestans* can be found in quite good quality housing living in the walls or among tiles at the edges of roofs.

More than 150 species of 24 families of mammals have been reported as infected with *T. cruzi*, and all mammal species are considered to be susceptible. Although birds and reptiles are insusceptible to *T. cruzi* infection, domestic chickens are extremely important epidemiologically because they sustain heavy triatomine bug infestations either at roosting sites inside houses, or in neighbouring chicken houses, which may be overlooked during spraying campaigns. Important domestic hosts, apart from humans, are dogs, guinea pigs, cats, rats, mice and any other mammals sleeping inside houses and closely associated with humans. Dogs are particularly important because of high prevalence rates of infection and as they are often abundant in endemic areas. Cats, although less frequently studied, also have high prevalence rates and possibly acquire infection via the oral route, by eating either triatomine bugs or house mice that have fed upon them. Although smaller hosts, rodents may be abundant and provide an important source of infective blood meals. Pigs, goats, cattle and equines usually have indirect contact with houses and very low prevalence rates of infection, although their enclosures may be infested with bugs.

The most ubiquitous silvatic reservoir host of *T. cruzi* is the opossum, *Didelphis*, which occurs throughout much of the range of *T. cruzi* in the Americas. Multiple nesting or resting sites of *Didelphis* encompass many types of triatomine habitat. High *T. cruzi* prevalence rates may be in part due to the fact that opossums will eat triatomines and might also transmit infection via anal gland secretions, in which infective metacyclic forms typical of the vector stage of the *T. cruzi* life cycle can occur. *Didelphis* also provides an important potential link between silvatic and domestic habitats as it occasionally nests around or inside houses. Edentates (armadillos and anteaters), especially the armadillo *Dasypus novemcinctus*, are commonly infected with *T. cruzi* but less important epidemiologically as they have little direct contact with human households, except through hunting of armadillos and their consumption for food. Nevertheless, *P. geniculatus*, the silvatic triatomine bug frequently found in armadillo burrows, is one species that is attracted to light and often flies into houses. Rodents are thought to have an important epidemiological role as in times of food scarcity or drought; they might introduce triatomines and *T. cruzi* strains into new peridomestic nesting sites. Similarly, bats may roost in domestic habitats, encouraging triatomine infestation and bringing in *T. cruzi* strains. Like armadillos the numerous carnivore and primate species that may harbour *T. cruzi* have tenuous links with domestic transmission cycles.

Silvatic cycles of *T. cruzi* transmission, extend approximately from southern Argentina and Chile (latitude 46° S) to northern California (latitude 42° N). Human infection is, however, much less widespread, from 44° 45′ S in Argentina to the southern states of the USA. Prevalence estimates for human infection are based on rates of seropositivity (Miles 1982). National surveillance by serology indicates that Brazil has the largest number of infected individuals with about 5 million, in accordance with its land mass and population. Bolivia is reported to have the highest prevalence, with seropositivity rates of greater than 70% in some localities, and heavy *T. infestans* infestation of rural communities that are difficult to access. The World Health Organization has provided an outline of geographical distribution of *T. cruzi* infection within the affected countries (WHO 1991). As described above, endemic areas can be classed as having either separate domestic and silvatic transmission cycles, with separate vector species (e.g. eastern Brazil) or overlapping domestic and silvatic transmission cycles (e.g. Venezuela). Enzootic regions have rare human infections with sympatric (e.g. USA) and sometimes abundant (e.g. Amazon basin) silvatic transmission cycles (Miles, de Souza and Povoa 1981a). Locally acquired Chagas disease is rare in the USA, partly because of higher living standards and better housing. Although bugs are occasionally found inside houses, in nesting sites of animals such as opossums, they infrequently attack humans, and transmission of *T. cruzi* is less likely as the local bug species tend to defecate after feeding. Occasionally adult bugs are light attracted into camp sites. Silvatic bugs are widespread in the USA and *T. cruzi* infections common in opossums, racoons and wood rats (*Neotoma*).

Less than 100 autochthonous human *T. cruzi* infections have been reported from the vast forested Amazon basin, even though there are extensive roadside and riverine communities with houses ideally suited to colonization by triatomine bugs and *T. cruzi* infections abound among species of forest mammals. Tracing of trapped mammals to their nesting sites with a spool-and-line mammal tracking device (Miles, de Souza and Povoa 1981b) has helped to describe the ecotopes of silvatic triatomines, and show that the 13 known species of the central Amazon basin do not readily adapt to household infestation (Miles, de Souza and Povoa 1981a). *R. brethesi*, which infests the piacaba palm (*Leopoldinia piacaba*), is reported to attack forest workers harvesting the palm fronds and sleeping nearby, some of whom acquire infection. *P. geniculatus*, normally associated with high humidity within armadillo burrows and difficult to adapt to laboratory colonies, has recently been reported infesting domestic pigsties in Pará state, Brazil and attacking

the inhabitants of adjoining houses (SAS Valente, personal communication). The destruction of natural habitats around houses in the Amazon may well encourage triatomine infestation, especially as wood and palm fronds are often used in house construction, inevitably bringing some silvatic vectors into houses (Coura et al. 1994).

Non-vectorial transmission of *T. cruzi* that is epidemiologically important includes transmission by blood transfusion, congenital transmission, and oral transmission. Where prevalence is high, seropositivity rates among blood donors may reach 20% (endemic localities in Brazil and Argentina) or even higher in Bolivia (60%) (WHO 1991). In large cities where there are many migrants from rural areas and many blood transfusions, a significant proportion of recipients will become infected in the absence of serological surveillance of donors or treatment of transfusion blood to destroy *T. cruzi*; there may be thousands of blood-borne infections each year. Control of blood-borne transmission is thus an essential part of campaigns directed primarily at the elimination of domestic triatomine bugs (see section 12). In endemic areas where prevalence is high, many pregnant women will carry *T. cruzi*. Estimates vary widely but a low percentage (<5%) of infants born to seropositive mothers may acquire congenital infection (WHO 1991). Determination of rates of transplacental acquisition of infection are complicated by passive transfer of maternal IgG antibodies to *T. cruzi*, which may cause infants to be seropositive for several months after birth even in the absence of infection. There is convincing evidence of oral transmission and a high proportion of the few human cases in the Amazon basin are thought to have been acquired by this route (SAS Valente, personal communication). The most likely sources in such outbreaks are contamination of food with triatomine bugs, or with vector-like forms from opossum anal gland secretions, or through consumption of the uncooked meat or blood of an infected reservoir host. An increasing problem is the transfer of *T. cruzi* to organ recipients from infected donors, who must therefore be routinely screened for seropositivity. If already infected with *T. cruzi*, recipients risk a recrudescent acute phase infection in response to immunosuppression. Similarly, HIV positive patients who develop AIDS may reactivate *T. cruzi* infection and develop meningoencephalitis. *T. cruzi* infections in the immunocompromised will become epidemiologically more important as human migration to South American cities continues and urban HIV transmission spreads to rural areas that have endemic Chagas disease (Gorgolas and Miles 1994, Rocha et al. 1994).

10 TREATMENT

10.1 Chemotherapy

Two drugs have been used for specific chemotherapy of *T. cruzi* infection, nifurtimox and benznidazole (WHO 1991). Nifurtimox, a synthetic nitrofuran given by mouth and absorbed through the gastrointestinal tract, is no longer readily available. Dose rates employed were 8–10 mg/kg orally in 3 divided daily doses, for 90 days, using tablets of 30, 20 or 250 mg. Higher doses of 15–20 mg/kg in 4 divided daily doses for the same period were recommended for infected children. Successful treatment thus required either hospitalization or careful monitoring to ensure compliance. Side effects could include anorexia, nausea, vomiting, gastric pain, insomnia, headache, vertigo, excitability, myalgia, arthralgia, convulsions and peripheral polyneuritis, and could lead to interruption of treatment. Nifurtimox is thought to act against *T. cruzi* by increasing oxidative stress through the production of free oxygen radicals. Benznidazole is a nitroimidazol which is also absorbed from the alimentary tract. Doses are 5–7 mg/kg orally in 2 divided doses for adults, for 60 days with 100 mg tablets, and 10 mg/kg similarly for children. Adverse affects may include rashes, fever, nausea, peripheral polyneuritis, leucopenia, and rarely agranulocytosis. Benznidazole is thought to act by interaction of drug metabolites with DNA but not via oxidative stress.

Cure rates with both nifurtimox and benznidazole are not total and vary regionally. Suppression of parasitaemia during acute infection may be life-saving and treatment is therefore recommended during the acute phase. The chronic phase is seldom treated as the influence of persistent infection on long-term prognosis is unknown, and there is a significant failure rate, such that up to half of patients may remain infected after treatment. Treatment is essential for immunocompromised patients, especially if meningoencephalitis is present, in which case double or even higher dose rates may be recommended. In congenital cases either drug has been used, nifurtimox at 8–25 mg/kg daily for 30 days and benznidazole at 5–10 mg/kg daily for 30–60 days (WHO 1991). Indicators of elimination of the parasite are negative xenodiagnosis together with, in acute cases, serological reversion within a year.

Allopurinol has been suggested as a low cost, nontoxic alternative for treatment of *T. cruzi* infection, but its efficacy is in doubt. Allopurinol, a structural analogue of hypoxanthine that is metabolized via the purine salvage pathway, prevents formation of ATP, and also interferes with protein synthesis by its incorporation into RNA. Experimental drugs thought to act against the enzyme sterol methyl transferase are under development, have shown promising activities in treatment of animal infection and may proceed to clinical trial (Urbina 1995).

Additional chemotherapy is an important part of supportive treatment in both acute and chronic Chagas disease (WHO 1991). Severe acute infections may require treatment for fever, vomiting, diarrhoea and convulsions; if heart failure is present sodium intake is restricted; diuretics and digitalis may be recommended; anticonvulsants, sedatives and intravenous mannitol may assist management of acute meningoencephalitis. Chronic chagasic heart disease may require treatment of heart failure through reduced activity, limitation of sodium, diuretics, vasodilation (angiotensin converting enzyme inhibitors) and maintenance of normal serum potassium; digitalis is only advisable as a last resort for treatment because it may aggravate arrhythmias by inducing premature ventricular beats or impeding AV conduction. A pacemaker may be required to manage bradycardia that does not respond well to atropine, or atrial fibrillation with a slow ventricular response in which vagolytic drugs are not effective, or complete AV block.

Life expectancy of patients with ventricular arrhythmias may be prolonged by treatment to prevent ventricular tachycardia or ventricular fibrillation: lidocaine, mexiletine, propafenone, flecainide, β-adrenoreceptor antagonists and amiodarone are effective for treatment of ventricular extrasystoles; amiodarone is the most effective drug to treat arrhythmias, but in all cases drug treatment of arrhythmias may have an aggravating effect and patient management may be a complex combination of the use of drugs and a pacemaker. Lidocaine may be used intravenously in emergencies prior to drug administration orally. Surgical resection of arrhythmic endocardial regions may be considered, and surgical resection of ventricular aneurysms has been suggested but not extensively used. Expert reports (WHO 1991) and physicians who have specialized in management of Chagas disease should be consulted before case management can be embarked upon with confidence.

10.2 Surgical treatment

Elegant surgical procedures have been developed in Brazil to treat severe chagasic megacolon and megaoesophagus. Laxatives, colonic lavage or manual evacuation may be used to relieve symptoms of megacolon, with laparotomy if the faecaloma cannot be reached. Sigmoid volvulus can be relieved by decompressing intubation or surgery. Sigmoidostomy close to the rectosigmoid junction may simplify subsequent surgery to correct megacolon as it allows more of the colon to be retained.

Surgical treatment of megacolon is often based on the operation of Duhamel. The modified Duhamel–Haddad procedure consists of resection of the sigmoid loop, closing of the rectal stump and insertion of the descending colon through the rear wall of the rectum. The Haddad improvements introduced a 2-stage operation, the first in which the lowered colon is exteriorized through the retrorectal stump as a perineal colostomy and, the second, with peridural anaesthesia, in which the stump of the colon is sectioned into anterior and posterior halves, the anterior wall of the colon and posterior wall of the rectum held together in an inverted V, and then cut and sutured together to make a wide join between the colon and rectal stump (Fig. 15.11). A series of 624 Duhamel–Haddad operations between 1966 and 1981 had an overall associated mortality of 6.6% (Moreira et al. 1985).

Megaoesophagus can be treated by dilatation of the cardiac sphincter or the Heller–Vasconcelos surgical procedure

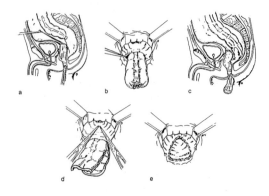

Fig. 15.11 The modified Duhamel–Haddad procedure for surgical correction of megacolon.

in which a portion of the muscle is removed from the junction of the oesophagus and stomach without disturbing the muscular control of the wall of the stomach. More severe megaoesophagus may require partial removal of the distal oesophagus and replacement with alternative portion of the alimentary tract such as jejunum. These and other surgical procedures are described in detail in the Brazilian literature (Raia 1983).

11 VACCINATION

Administration of crude *T. cruzi* lysates to experimental animals has been known for many years to suppress parasitaemia, to prevent mortality from a subsequent challenge infection, and yet not to prevent reinfection. 'Attenuated' *T. cruzi* strains have been used as experimental vaccines in human trials with small numbers of individuals, but organisms were not necessarily entirely non-infective, and are not known to have conferred resistance to infection (or superinfection). Various semi-purified or purified antigen preparations have similarly been shown in experimental models to confer protection against mortality upon challenge but not to provide a sterile immunity (Taibi et al. 1993). An autoimmune response may have a role in the pathogenesis of Chagas disease, and this does not encourage research on candidate vaccines. Without a full understanding of the autoimmune involvement in pathogenesis it is difficult to envisage clinical trials of vaccines: subjects could not be given a live challenge, and would have to be followed for many years for the appearance of vaccine induced pathology in the absence of infection. These aspects of Chagas disease suggest that resources would be most cost-effectively directed to further improvement of vector control campaigns rather than vaccine development. Immunotherapeutic modulation of progressive autoimmune damage in chronic Chagas disease has been proposed: if the intricacies of immune responses in the pathogenesis of Chagas disease can be convincingly unravelled, this may become possible for a small number of privileged patients.

12 INTEGRATED CONTROL

In 1948 successful trials of the organochlorine insecticide BHC for control of domestic triatomine bug infestation by Emmanuel Dias and Jose Pellegrino in Minas Gerais, Brazil, prompted their telegram to the Brazilian Ministry of Health suggesting that the end to vector-borne *T. cruzi* transmission was in sight (Miles 1996). The fundamental value of insecticides for control of triatomine bugs has never since been in doubt. Nevertheless, much research has been devoted to developing new methods of eliminating domestic triatomines, including the use of parasitic wasps, nematodes and fungi; sophisticated traps for catching bugs; and juvenile hormones for preventing development of nymphal instars into adults. These alternative weapons have failed to have significant impact on vector popu-

lations. The combination of insecticide spraying, health education/community participation and housing improvement has been the basis of successful national control programmes, a superb example of which is the elimination of domestic *T. infestans* populations from São Paulo State in Brazil (Wanderley 1993). João Carlos Pinto Dias, the son of Emmanuel Dias, has led the elaboration of a systematic approach to triatomine bug control (Dias 1987).

1 In the **preparatory phase**, all houses in the endemic area are mapped and sampled manually with flashlight and forceps for evidence of triatomine infestation: sampling may be assisted by spraying irritant pyrethroids on to suspect wall areas to dislodge bugs hiding in crevices. This mapping and sampling phase allows for the cost of insecticides, personnel, transport and equipment to be calculated, and for detailed planning of operations.

2 In the **attack phase**, all houses and outbuildings are sprayed irrespective of whether they are known to be infested with bugs. Failure to spray all infested domestic and peridomestic habitats may lead to rapid local re-emergence of bug populations. Spraying is repeated during the next 3 months if live bugs can still be found in houses that were infested.

3 In the **vigilance phase**, houses are sampled periodically through a surveillance system established with the local community and supported by health education. Thus, householders can report any residual infestation to a local volunteer who mobilizes an immediate insecticide spraying response. Simple surveillance kits consist of a sheet of paper pinned to walls suspected of infestation, and a plastic bag. Periodic examination of the paper may reveal either bug faeces or bugs concealed between the paper and wall; the plastic bag is used by householders to collect any live bugs, with care to avoid contamination with bug faeces. The vigilance phase is also supported by continuing contact with public health personnel. Although triatomines can sometimes be found in quite good quality housing, for example in tiled roofs (*T. infestans*) or in beds that are not regularly dismantled and cleaned, poor housing is most vulnerable to bug infestation. Encouraging and supporting the community to improve local housing, for example by plastering cracked walls, can contribute to the success of a control campaign. In houses infested by *R. prolixus* it is advisable to replace roofs of palm fronds by alternative materials.

Early spraying campaigns used chlorinated hydrocarbons but their short residual activity (30–180 days) required repeated applications. Carbonates and organophosphates have also been used but the former are expensive and the latter are not well received by communities because of their strong smell. Synthetic pyrethroids have been adopted for triatomine control since 1980 as they have a long residual activity and low toxicity, and several formulations are now available (Schofield 1994). Insecticide resistance (to dieldrin) is known only from small areas of Venezuela and has not interfered with control campaigns.

In 1991 an initiative was launched to use established triatomine control methods in a cooperative international campaign, referred to as the 'southern cone programme', and designed to eliminate domestic *T. infestans* populations from the Argentina, Bolivia, Brazil, Chile, Paraguay and Uruguay, with spraying of infested regions that spanned national frontiers intended to prevent re-infestation (Miles 1992). The strategy for this coordinated international programme incorporated World Bank recommendations on the need for clear lines of responsibility, regional integration and pragmatic local autonomy. The southern cone programme has attracted new financial support and stimulated a vigorous and sustained effort. The overall cost of the programme is estimated to be a fraction of that of dealing with the burden of new cases of Chagas disease. An international review of the programme (Schofield, personal communication 1996) indicates a huge reduction in the geographical area infested by *T. infestans* and a determination to deal with those regions still affected. Although the Amazon Basin is free of domestic bug populations, it is under threat from migration of species such as *T. infestans* and *R. prolixus* and from adaptation of local forest species to houses. A network of collaborating centres has recently been established to train local health workers in the recognition of triatomine bugs and acute cases of Chagas disease, and to plan responses to the appearance of domestic bug populations. In the past, lack of funds and poor continuity frequently interrupted control campaigns, in part because resources were diverted to resurgent malaria or outbreaks of dengue. It is essential that campaigns against different arthropod vectors are integrated, at both local and regional levels.

T. cruzi is one of several disease agents, including HIV infection, hepatitis, syphilis and malaria, that can be transmitted by contaminated transfusion blood. Screening of donors is an essential component of control campaigns and in several South American countries serological testing is mandatory. Effective serological tests include the IFAT, which can be used to distinguish maternal transfer of IgG from IgM due to congenital infections, the ELISA, the IHAT and the CFT, although the latter is now seldom used. A single standardized test may be adequate, but simultaneous use of 2 tests is often recommended, and some cross reactions with diseases such as visceral leishmaniasis are inevitable. It has been shown that CFT, IFAT, IHAT and ELISA can give comparable results. The IFAT has been employed in large scale surveys in Brazil; ELISA has distinct advantages for survey work as it is highly sensitive, relatively low cost, and does not require microscopy. In some countries, such as Chile, cross-reactions with leishmaniasis are not a problem as visceral and cutaneous leishmaniasis are not endemic. Rigorous internal and external quality control of assay performance are required with repetition of a proportion of tests in a central laboratory and in collaborating external laboratories. Sample collection and record systems must be highly efficient and integrated with spraying operations, health education and community participation aspects of control. The importance of screening blood for HIV infection in major urban areas is likely to improve access to screening for *T. cruzi* infection. Where seropositive rates are very high positive transfusion blood may be treated with 125 mg of crystal violet per 500 ml and the blood stored at 4°C for 24 hours to destroy trypomastigotes. Side effects are blue coloration of mucosae and skin in recipients of blood treated with gentian violet.

Serology is a vital and highly effective method of monitoring the success of control programmes. In its simplest form success is demonstrable by zero serological incidence in children born after the initiation of intervention measures. Thus, for a 10 year campaign, 5 years and 10 years after the beginning of vector control no vector-borne infections should occur in children aged 0–5 and 0–10 respectively. Pre-school children and school children obtaining basic/primary and junior schooling (e.g. ages 1–12 years) provide the ideal populations for serological surveillance. Baseline serological data are useful but not essential to planning serological surveillance of control: if interventions are effective no significant increase in prevalence of seropositivity should occur for any age group after the campaign begins.

Ideally all children in populations possibly exposed to vector-borne transmission should be tested, as serology is a sensitive independent aid for the detection of residual triatomine infestation. Thus one seropositive case, if congenital transmission and blood transfusion transmission are excluded, may lead to the identification of a single house that has escaped elimination of bugs. In countries such as Chile which have a relatively small population, good infrastructure, preschool rural health clinics, regional hospitals, demographic data that includes individual identification codes, and clearly defined areas of disease transmission, it is feasible to monitor the entire population exposed to transmission. In other countries, such as Brazil, with a very large population in endemic areas, it may not be possible or appropriate to survey the entire population of preschool and school children. There are 2 obvious alternatives for selection of sub-populations, the first, on a random sample basis, and the second, where effort is concentrated on highly endemic localities. The second alternative is preferred as only in areas with relatively high seroprevalence will a detectable number of the very young acquire infection. Baseline serological data are available for Bolivia, Brazil, Peru, Argentina, Paraguay and Uruguay to allow such sentinel sites of high endemicity to be selected. It might also be appropriate to survey localities at the margins of endemic areas where explosive outbreaks of disease transmission might occur in previously unexposed populations.

Social and economic development in Latin America should, in time, eliminate vector-borne and blood-borne transmission of *T. cruzi* as a major public health problem. *T. cruzi* will, however, remain as a widely distributed enzootic infection, with the threat of re-emergence and spread to new areas of human settlement. The burden of management of chronic disease will be a problem for several decades. Further research on immunological evasion and molecular pathogenesis might improve prognosis for those already infected, and a low cost, non-toxic drug may help eliminate *T. cruzi* from the human reservoir of infection. It is debatable whether other aspects of advanced research will have a significant direct impact on the control of Chagas disease but they will lead to a fuller understanding of the fascinating epidemiology and biology of trypanosomatid infections.

REFERENCES

Avila HA, Simpson L, 1995, Organization and complexity of minicircle-encoded guide RNAs in *Trypanosoma cruzi*, *RNA*, **1:** 939–47.

Bogliolo AR, Lauria-Pires L, Gibson WC, 1996, Polymorphisms in *Trypanosoma cruzi*: evidence of genetic recombination, *Acta Tropica*, **61:** 31–40.

Brack C, 1968, Elektronenmikroskopische untersuchungen zum leben szyklus von *Trypanosoma cruzi*. Unter besonderer Berücksichtigung der entwicklungsformen im ueberträger *Rhodnius prolixus*, *Acta Tropica*, **25:** 289–356.

Brener Z, 1994, The pathogenesis of Chagas' disease: an overview of current theories, *Chagas' Disease and the Nervous System*, Scientific Publication No. 547, PAHO, Washington, DC.

Brener Z, Andrade Z, 1979, Trypanosoma cruzi e Doença de Chagas, Guanabara Koogan S.A., Rio de Janeiro - RJ.

Britto C, Cardoso MA et al., 1995a, *Trypanosoma cruzi*: parasite detection and strain discrimination in chronic chagasic patients from northeastern Brazil using PCR amplification of kinetoplast DNA and nonradioactive hybridization, *Exp Parasitol*, **81:** 462–71.

Britto C, Cardoso MA et al., 1995b, Polymerase chain reaction detection of *Trypanosoma cruzi* in human blood samples as a tool for diagnosis and treatment evaluation, *Parasitology*, **110:** 241–7.

Burleigh BA, Andrews NW, 1995, The mechanisms of *Trypanosoma cruzi* invasion of mammalian cells, *Annu Rev Microbiol*, **49:** 175–200.

Carrasco HJ, Frame IA et al., 1996, Genetic exchange as a possible source of genomic diversity in sylvatic populations of *Trypanosoma cruzi*, *Am J Trop Med Hyg*, **54:** 418–424.

Carreno H, Rojas C et al., 1987, Schizodeme analyses of *Trypanosoma cruzi* zymodemes from Chile, *Exp Parasitol*, **64:** 252–260.

Cazzulo JJ, 1994, Intermediate metabolism in *Trypanosoma cruzi*, *J Bioenerg Biomembr*, **26:** 157–65.

Chapman MD, Snary D, Miles MA, 1984, Quantitative differences in the expression of a 72,000 molecular weight cell surface glycoprotein (GP72) in *T. cruzi* zymodemes, *J Immunol*, **132:** 3149–3153.

Coombs G, North M, eds, 1991, *Biochemical Protozoology*, Taylor and Francis, London.

Coura JR, Junqueira AC et al., 1994, Chagas' disease in the Brazilian Amazon. I – A short review, *Rev Inst Med Trop São Paulo*, **36:** 363–8.

Cunha Neto E, Duranti M et al., 1995, Autoimmunity in Chagas disease cardiopathy: biological relevance of a cardiac myosin-specific epitope crossreactive to an immunodominant *Trypanosoma cruzi* antigen, *Proc Natl Acad Sci USA*, **92:** 3541–5.

Dias JCP, 1987, Control of Chagas disease in Brazil, *Parasitol Today*, **3:** 336–341.

Di Noia JM, Sanchez DO, Frasch AC, 1995, The protozoan *Trypanosoma cruzi* has a family of genes resembling the mucin genes of mammalian cells, *J Biol Chem*, **270:** 24146–9.

Dutra WO, Martins Filho OA et al., 1996, Chagasic patients lack CD28 expression on many of their circulating T lymphocytes, *Scand J Immunol*, **43:** 88–93.

Dvorak JA, 1984, The natural heterogeneity of *Trypanosoma cruzi*: biological and medical implications, *J Cell Biochem*, **24:** 357–371.

Ferrari I, Levin MJ et al., 1995, Molecular mimicry between the immunodominant ribosomal protein PO of *Trypanosoma cruzi* and a functional epitope on the human beta 1-adrenergic receptor, *J Exp Med*, **182:** 59–65.

Ferrari I, Wallukat G et al., 1995, Molecular mimicry between functional epitopes on the human cardiovascular β_1-adrenergic and the M_2-muscarinic receptors and the ribosomal PO protein of *Trypanosoma cruzi*, *Mem Inst Oswaldo Cruz*, **90:** 155.

Garcia ES, Gonzalez MS et al., 1995, Induction of *Trypanosoma cruzi* metacyclogenesis in the gut of the hematophagous insect vector, *Rhodnius prolixus*, by hemoglobin and peptides carrying alpha D-globin sequences, *Exp Parasitol*, **81:** 255–61.

Goldberg AC, Cunha-Neto E et al., 1995, HLA and chronic Chagas' disease cardiomyopathy, *Mem Inst Oswaldo Cruz*, **90:** 118.

Gorgolas M de, Miles MA, 1994, Visceral leishmaniasis and AIDS, *Nature (London)*, **372:** 734.

Güther MLS, Ferguson MAJ, 1995, The role of inositol acylation and inositol deacylation in GPI biosynthesis in *Trypanosoma brucei*, *EMBO J*, **14:** 3080–93.

Hoare CA, 1972, *The Trypanosomes of Mammals*, Blackwell, Oxford.

Hontebeyrie-Joskowicz M, 1994, Humoral and cellular immunity to *Trypanosoma cruzi* infection and disease, *Chagas' Disease and the Nervous System*, Scientific Publication No. 547, PAHO, Washington, DC.

Kalil J, Cunha-Neto E, 1996, Autoimmunity in Chagas disease cardiomyopathy: fulfilling the criteria at last, *Parasitol Today*, **12:** 396–9.

Kaplan D, Vazquez M et al., 1993, The chronic presence of the parasite, and anti-P autoimmunity in Chagas disease: the *Trypanosoma cruzi* ribosomal P proteins, and their recognition by the host immune system, *Biol Res*, **26:** 273–7.

Kelly JM, Das, P, Tomás AM, 1994, An approach to functional complementation by introduction of large DNA fragments into *Trypanosoma cruzi* and *Leishmania donovani* using a cosmid shuttle vector, *Mol Biochem Parasitol*, **65:** 51–62.

Kendall G, Wilderspin AF et al., 1990, *Trypanosoma cruzi* glycosomal glyceraldehyde-3-phosphate dehydrogenase does not conform to the 'hotspot' topogenic signal model, *EMBO J*, **9:** 2751–8.

Köberle F, 1974, Pathogenesis of Chagas' disease, *Trypanosomiasis and Leishmaniasis with Special Reference to Chagas' disease*, Ciba Foundation Symposium 20 (new series), Associated Scientific Publishers, Amsterdam.

Krieger MA, Almeida E et al., 1992, Use of recombinant antigens for the accurate immunodiagnosis of Chagas' disease, *Am J Trop Med Hyg*, **46:** 427–34.

Lázzari JO, 1994, Autonomic nervous system alterations in Chagas' disease: review of the literature, *Chagas' Disease and the Nervous System*, Scientific Publication No. 547, PAHO, Washington, DC.

Lent H, Wygodzinsky P, 1979, Revision of the Triatominae (Hemiptera, Reduviidae), and their significance as vectors of Chagas' disease, *Bull Am Mus Nat Hist*, **163:** 123–520.

Luquetti AO, Miles MA et al., 1986, *Trypanosoma cruzi*: zymodemes associated with acute and chronic Chagas' disease in central Brazil, *Trans R Soc Trop Med Hyg*, **80:** 462–70.

Matthews KR, Tschudi C, Ullu E, 1994, A common pyrimidine-rich motif governs *trans*-splicing and polyadenylation of tubulin polycistronic pre-mRNA in trypanosomes, *Genes Dev*, **8:** 491–501.

Miles MA, 1979, Transmission cycles and the heterogeneity of *Trypanosoma cruzi*, *Biology of the Kinetoplastida*,, vol. 2, eds Lumsden WHR, Evans DA, Academic Press, 117–196.

Miles MA, 1982, *Trypanosoma cruzi*: epidemiology, *Perspectives in Trypanosomiasis Research*, Proceedings of the 21st Trypanosomiasis Seminar: London, 24 September 1981. ed Baker JR, Research Studies Press, 1–15.

Miles MA, 1983, The epidemiology of South American trypanosomiasis: biochemical and immunological approaches and their relevance to control, *Trans R Soc Trop Med Hyg*, **77:** 5–23.

Miles MA, 1992, Disease control has no frontiers, *Parasitol Today*, **8:** 221–2.

Miles MA, 1993, Culturing and biological cloning of *Trypanosoma cruzi*, *Protocols in Molecular Parasitology*, ed Hyde JE, Humana Press, 15–28.

Miles MA, 1994, Chagas' disease and chagasic megacolon, *Consti-*

pation, eds Kamm MA, Lennard-Jones JE, Wrightson Biomedical Publishing, Petersfield, UK and Bristol PA, USA, 205–10.

Miles MA, 1996, New World trypanosomiasis, *The Wellcome Trust Illustrated History of Tropical Diseases*, ed Cox FEG, Wellcome Trust, London, 192–205.

Miles MA, Souza AA de, Povoa M, 1981a, Chagas' disease in the Amazon basin. III. Ecotopes of ten triatomine bug species (Hemiptera: Reduviidae) from the vicinity of Belém, Pará, Brazil, *J Med Entomol*, **18:** 266–78.

Miles MA, Souza AA de, Povoa M, 1981b, Mammal tracking and nest location in Brazilian forest with an improved spool-and-line device, *J Zool*, **195:** 331–47.

Moncayo A, Luquetti AO, 1990, Multicentre double blind study for evaluation of *Trypanosoma cruzi* defined antigens as diagnostic reagents, *Mem Inst Oswaldo Cruz*, **85:** 489–95.

Moreira H, Rezende JM de et al., 1985, Chagasic megacolon, *Colo-Proctology*, **7:** 260–7.

Munoz Fernandez MA, Fernandez MA, Fresno M, 1992, Synergism between tumor necrosis factor-alpha and interferon-gamma on macrophage activation for the killing of intracellular *Trypanosoma cruzi* through a nitric oxide-dependent mechanism, *Eur J Immunol*, **22:** 301–7.

Norris KA, Schrimpf JE, 1994, Biochemical analysis of the membrane and soluble forms of the complement regulatory protein of *Trypanosoma cruzi*, *Infect Immun*, **62:** 236–43.

Nozaki T, Dvorak JA, 1993, Intraspecific diversity in the response of *Trypanosoma cruzi* to environmental stress, *J Parasitol*, **79:** 451–4.

Oliveira JSM, 1969, Cardiopatia chagásica experimental, *Rev Goiana Med*, **15:** 77–133.

Osorio Y, Travi BL et al., 1995, Infectivity of *Trypanosoma rangeli* in a promonocytic mammalian cell line, *J Parasitol*, **81:** 687–93.

PAHO, 1994, *Chagas' Disease and the Nervous System*, Scientific Publication No. 547, PAHO, Washington DC.

Raia AA, 1983, *Manifestações Digestivas da Moléstia de Chagas*, Sarvier, São Paulo, Brasil.

Ribeiro dos Santos R, Rossi MA et al., 1992, Anti-CD4 abrogates rejection and reestablishes long-term tolerance to syngeneic newborn hearts grafted in mice chronically infected with *Trypanosoma cruzi*, *J Exp Med*, **175:** 29–39.

Rocha A, Meneses AC de et al., 1994, Pathology of patients with Chagas' disease and acquired immunodeficiency syndrome, *Am J Trop Med Hyg*, **50:** 261–8.

Rottenberg ME, Bakhiet M et al., 1993, Differential susceptibilities of mice genomically deleted of CD4 and CD8 to infections with *Trypanosoma cruzi* or *Trypanosoma brucei*, *Infect Immun*, **61:** 5129–33.

Rowland EC, Mikhail KS, McCormick TS, 1992, Isotype determination of anti-*Trypanosma cruzi* antibody in murine Chagas' disease, *J Parasitol*, **78:** 557–61.

Ruef BJ, Dawson BD et al., 1994, Expression and evolution of members of the *Trypanosoma cruzi* trypomastigote surface antigen multigene family, *Mol Biochem Parasitol*, **63:** 109–20.

Salazar NA, Mondragon A, Kelly JM, 1996, Mucin-like glycoprotein genes are closely linked to members of the transsialidase super-family at multiple sites in the *Trypanosoma cruzi* genome, *Mol Biochem Parasitol*, **78:** 127–36.

Schofield CJ, 1994, *Triatominae. Biology and Control*, Eurocommunica Publications, UK.

Serrano AA, Schenkman S et al., 1995, The lipid structure of the glycosylphosphatidylinositol-anchored mucin-like sialic acid acceptors of *Trypanosoma cruzi* changes during parasite differentiation from epimastigotes to infective metacyclic trypomastigote forms, *J Biol Chem*, **270:** 27244–53.

Silva JS, Vespa GN et al., 1995, Tumor necrosis factor alpha mediates resistance to *Trypanosoma cruzi* infection in mice by inducing nitric oxide production in infected gamma interferon-activated macrophages, *Infect Immun*, **63:** 4862–7.

Soong L, Tarleton RL, 1994, *Trypanosoma cruzi* infection suppresses nuclear factors that bind to specific sites on the interleukin-2 enhancer, *Eur J Immunol*, **24:** 16–23.

Stoka V, Nycander M et al., 1995, Inhibition of cruzipain, the major cysteine proteinase of the protozoan parasite, *Trypanosoma cruzi*, by proteinase inhibitors of the cystatin superfamily, *FEBS Lett*, **370:** 101–4.

Taibi A, Plumas Marty B et al., 1993, *Trypanosoma cruzi*: immunity-induced in mice and rats by trypomastigote excretory-secretory antigens and identification of a peptide sequence containing a T cell epitope with protective activity, *J Immunol*, **151:** 2676–89.

Tarleton RL, Koller B et al., 1992, Susceptibility of β2-microglobulin-deficient mice to *Trypanosoma cruzi*, *Nature (London)*, **356:** 338–341.

Taylor MC, Kelly JM et al, 1994, The structure, organization, and expression of the *Leishmania donovani* gene encoding trypanothione reductase, *Mol Biochem Parasitol*, **64:** 293–301.

Teixeira V de P, Magalhaes E de P et al., 1995, Cardiac weight in patients with chronic Chagas disease with *Trypanosoma cruzi* nests in the central vein of the adrenal glands, *Arq Bras Cardiol*, **64:** 315–17.

Tetley L, Vickerman K, 1991, The glycosomes of trypanosomes: number and distribution as revealed by electron spectroscopic imaging and 3-D reconstruction, *J Microsc*, **162:** 83–90.

Tibayrenc M, Neubauer K et al., 1993, Genetic characterization of six parasitic protozoa: parity between random-primer DNA typing and multilocus enzyme electrophoresis, *Proc Natl Acad Sci USA*, **90:** 1335–9.

Urbina JA, 1995, Current perspectives in the treatment of Chagas disease using sterol biosynthesis inhibitors, *Mem Inst Oswaldo Cruz*, **90:** 41.

Urbina JA, Vivas J et al., 1995, Modification of the sterol composition of *Trypanosoma (Schizotrypanum) cruzi* epimastigotes by delta 24 (25)-sterol methyl transferase inhibitors and their combinations with ketoconazole, *Mol Biochem Parasitol*, **73:** 199–210.

Wanderley DM, 1993, Control of *Triatoma infestans* in the State of Sao Paulo, *Rev Soc Bras Med Trop*, **26, Suppl 3:** 17–25.

WHO, 1991, *Control of Chagas Disease*, Technical Report Series 811, World Health Organization, Geneva.

Zhang L, Tarleton RL, 1996, Characterization of cytokine production in murine *Trypanosoma cruzi* infection by *in situ* immunocytochemistry: lack of association between susceptibility and type 2 cytokine production, *Eur J Immunol*, **26:** 102–9.

Chapter 16

Toxoplasmosis

J P Dubey

1 INTRODUCTION AND HISTORY

Infection with *Toxoplasma gondii* is one of the most common parasitic infections of humans and other warm-blooded animals. It is found worldwide from Alaska to Australasia and nearly one-third of humanity has been exposed to this parasite. In most adults it does not cause serious illness but it can cause blindness and mental retardation in congenitally infected children and devastating disease in those with depressed immunity. In animals it is a common cause of abortion in goats and sheep.

T. gondii, which was discovered by Nicolle and Manceaux (1908, 1909) in Tunisia in a rodent, *Ctenodactylus gundi*, and independently in a laboratory rabbit by Splendore (1908) in São Paulo, Brazil, was recognized as a human pathogen when Wolf, Cowen and Paige (1939) reported a confirmed case of congenital toxoplasmosis in a child (see Table 16.1). The complete life cycle of *Toxoplasma gondii* was not determined until 1970 (Frenkel, Dubey and Miller 1970, Dubey, Miller and Frenkel 1970a, b). The complete life cycle clearly shows that this protozoan is a coccidian.

2 CLASSIFICATION

T. gondii is a coccidian parasite of cats with other warm-blooded animals as intermediate hosts. Coccidiosis is among the most important of parasitic infections of animals. Traditionally, all coccidia of veterinary importance were classified in the family Eimeriidae and were further classified based on the structure of the oocyst. Coccidia having oocysts with 4 sporocysts

each with 2 sporozoites (total 8 sporozoites) are classified as Eimeria, and coccidia having oocysts containing 2 sporocysts each with 4 sporozoites were classified historically as Isospora. After the discovery of the life cycle of *T. gondii*, several other genera (*Sarcocystis, Besnoitia, Hammondia* and *Frenkelia*) were also found to have isosporan oocysts with 2 sporocysts and 8 sporozoites. *T. gondii* and related genera are classified in the phylum Apicomplexa Levine, 1970, class Coccidea Leuckart, 1879, order Eimeriida Léger, 1911 (see also Chapter 228). Opinions differ regarding the placement of *T. gondii* into families and subfamilies: various authorities have placed it in one or the other of the families Eimeriidae Michin, 1903, Sarcocystidae Poche, 1913, or Toxoplasmatidae Biocca, 1956.

3 STRUCTURE AND LIFE CYCLE

The name *Toxoplasma* (*toxon* = bow, *plasma* = form) is derived from the crescent shape of the tachyzoite stage. There are 3 infectious stages of *T. gondii*: the tachyzoites (in groups), the bradyzoites (in tissue cysts), and the sporozoites (in oocysts) (Frenkel 1973).

The tachyzoite is often crescent-shaped and is approximately 2×6 μm in smears and globular to oval in sections (Fig. 16.1). Its anterior (conoidal) end is pointed and its posterior end is round. It has a pellicle (outer covering), a polar ring, a conoid, rhoptries, micronemes, mitochondria, subpellicular microtubules, endoplasmic reticulum, a Golgi apparatus, ribosomes, rough surfaced endoplasmic reticulum, a micropore and a well defined nucleus (Fig. 16.2). The nucleus is usually situated toward the posterior end or in the central area of the cell.

Table 16.1   History of *Toxoplasma gondii* and toxoplasmosis[a]

Contributors and year	Contribution
Nicolle and Manceau (1908)	Discovered in gundi
Splendore (1908)	Discovered in rabbit
Mello (1910)	Disease described in a domestic animal (dog)
Janků (1923)	Identified in human eye at necropsy
Wolf and Cowen (1937)	Congenital transmission documented
Pinkerton and Weinman (1940)	Fatal disease described in adult humans
Sabin (1942)	Disease characterized in man
Sabin and Feldman (1948)	Dye test described
Siim (1952)	Glandular toxoplasmosis described in man
Weinman and Chandler (1954)	Suggested carnivorous transmission
Hartley and Marshall (1957)	Abortions in sheep recognized
Beverley (1959)	Repeated congenital transmission observed in mice
Jacobs et al. (1960a)	Tissue cysts characterized biologically
Hutchison (1965)	Faecal transmission recognized, nematode eggs suspected
Hutchison et al. (1969, 1970, 1971); Frenkel et al. (1970); Dubey et al. (1970a,b); Sheffield and Melton (1970); Overdulve (1970)	Coccidian phase described
Frenkel et al. (1970); Miller et al. (1972)	Definitive and intermediate hosts defined
Dubey and Frenkel (1972)	Five *T. gondii* types described from feline intestinal epithelium
Wallace (1969); Munday (1972)	Confirmation of the epidemiological role of cats from studies on remote islands

[a]From Dubey (1993), where a complete bibliography may be found.

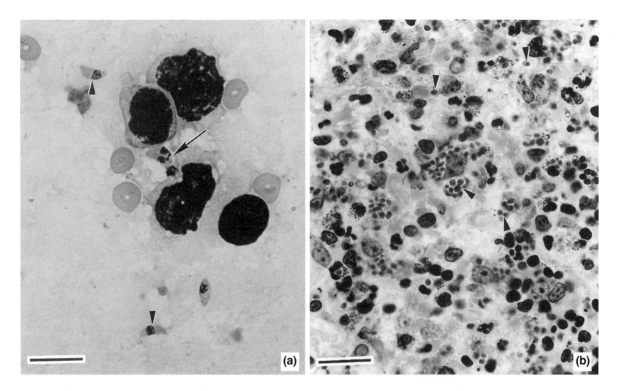

Fig. 16.1   Tachyzoites of *T. gondii*: (a) Impression smear. Note individual crescentic (arrowheads) and dividing (arrow) tachyzoites. Giemsa. Bar = 10 μm. (b) Histological section of mesenteric lymph node. Note numerous oval to round tachyzoites (arrowheads). Haematoxylin and eosin. Bar = 20 μm.

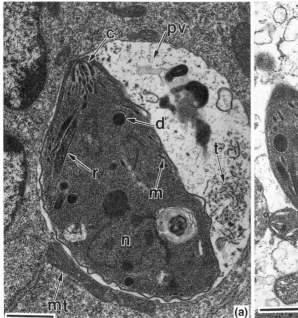
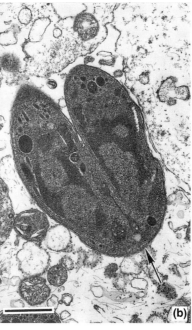

Fig. 16.2 Transmission electron micrographs of *T. gondii* tachyzoites in cell culture: (a) Tachyzoite in a parasitophorous vacuole (pv) in the cytoplasm of a host cell. Note conoid (c), rhoptries (r), micronemes (m), nucleus (n), dense granules (d), and intravacuolar tubules (t). The host cell mitochondria (mt) are closely associated with the pv. Bar = 2.1 μm. (b) Dividing tachyzoites with separated apical ends and the undivided posterior end (arrow). Bar = 1.18 μm.

The pellicle consists of 3 membranes. The inner membrane complex is discontinuous at 3 points: the anterior end (polar ring), the lateral edge (micropore), and toward the posterior end. The polar ring is an osmiophilic thickening of the inner membrane at the anterior end of the tachyzoite. The polar ring encircles a cylindrical, truncated cone (the conoid) which consists of 6–8 fibrillar elements wound like a compressed spring. There are 22 subpellicular microtubules originating from the anterior end and running longitudinally almost the entire length of the cell. Terminating within the conoid are 4–10 club-shaped organelles called rhoptries (Dubey 1977, 1993). The rhoptries are glandlike structures, often labyrinthine, with an anterior narrow neck up to 2.5 μm long. Their saclike posterior end terminates anterior to the nucleus. Micronemes (also called toxonemes) are convoluted tubelike structures which occur at the anterior end of the parasite.

The functions of the conoid, rhoptries, and micronemes are not fully known. The conoid is probably associated with the penetration of the tachyzoite through the membrane of the host cell. It can rotate, tilt, extend, and retract as the parasite searches for a host cell. *T. gondii* can move by gliding, undulating and rotating. Rhoptries have a secretory function associated with host cell penetration, secreting their contents through the conoid to the exterior. The microtubules probably provide the cytoskeleton.

The tachyzoite enters the host cell by active penetration of the host cell membrane. After entering the host cell the tachyzoite assumes an oval shape and becomes surrounded by a parasitophorous vacuole (PV) which it has been suggested is derived from both the parasite and the host. Numerous intravacuolar tubules connect the parasitophorous vacuolar membrane to the parasite pellicle (Fig. 16.2).

The tachyzoite multiplies asexually within the host cell by repeated endodyogeny (*endon* = inside, *dyo* = 2, *genesis* = birth), a specialized form of reproduction in which 2 progenies form within the parent parasite, consuming it (Fig. 16.2). Tachyzoites continue to divide by endodyogeny until the host cell is filled with parasites.

After a few divisions, *T. gondii* encysts to form tissue cysts. Tissue cysts grow and remain intracellular (Fig. 16.3) as the bradyzoites (encysted zoites) divide by endodyogeny. Tissue cysts vary in size (Fig. 16.3). Young tissue cysts may be as small as 5 μm and contain only 2 bradyzoites, although older ones may contain hundreds of organisms (Figs 16.3a, b). Tissue cysts in histological sections of brain are often circular and rarely reach a diameter of 60 μm whereas intramuscular cysts are elongated and may reach 100 μm; tissue cysts in unstained live squash preparations vary in size depending on the pressure applied to squash the tissue and the medium of suspension (Fig. 16.3b). Although tissue cysts may develop in visceral organs, including lungs, liver and kidneys, they are more prevalent in the neural and muscular tissues, such as the brain, eye and skeletal and cardiac muscle. Intact tissue cysts probably do not cause any harm and can persist for the life of the host.

The tissue cyst wall is elastic, thin (< 0.5 μm) and argyrophilic, and may enclose hundreds of crescent-shaped slender bradyzoites approximately 7 × 1.5 μm in size (Fig. 16.3). Structurally, bradyzoites differ only slightly from tachyzoites. They have a nucleus situated toward the posterior end whereas the nucleus in tachyzoites is more centrally located. The contents of rhoptries in bradyzoites in older tissue cysts are electron dense (Fig. 16.4) (Ferguson and Hutchison 1987, Dubey 1993). Bradyzoites contain several amylopectin granules which stain red with periodic acid–Schiff (PAS) reagent; such material is either in discrete particles or absent from tachyzoites. Bradyzoites are more slender than tachyzoites and less susceptible to destruction by gastric juice.

Factors influencing tissue cyst formation are not well known. Tissue cysts are more numerous in animals in the chronic stage of infection after the host has acquired immunity than during the acute stage of infection. However, tissue

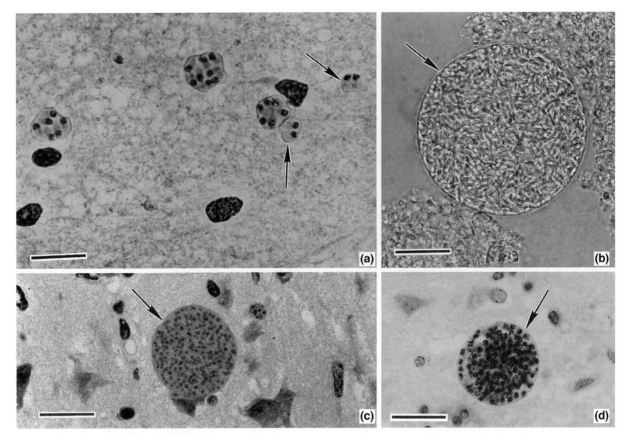

Fig. 16.3 Tissue cysts of *T. gondii* in brain: (a) Impression smear. Five young tissue cysts with silver positive cyst walls. Two tissue cysts (arrows) each have 2 bradyzoites with terminal nuclei. Silver stain. Bar = 10 μm. (b) Impression smear, unstained. This tissue cyst was freed by grinding a piece of brain in a mortar with a pestle. Note thin, elastic cyst wall (arrow) enclosing hundreds of bradyzoites. Bar = 20 μm. (c) Histological section. Note only nuclei of bradyzoites are visible. Haematoxylin and eosin. Bar = 20 μm. (d) Histological section. Note bradyzoites have PAS-positive red granules that appear black in this micrograph. The tissue cyst wall (arrow) is PAS-negative. Periodic acid–Schiff–haematoxylin. Bar = 20 μm.

cysts have been found in mice infected for only 3 days and in cells in culture systems devoid of known immune factors. It is possible, therefore, that development of functional immunity and the formation of tissue cysts are coincidental.

Cats shed oocysts (Fig. 16.5) after ingesting any of the 3 infectious stages of *T. gondii*, i.e. tachyzoites, bradyzoites or sporozoites (Frenkel, Dubey and Miller 1970, Dubey, Miller and Frenkel 1970a). Prepatent periods (time to the shedding of oocysts after initial infection) and frequency of oocyst shedding vary according to the stage ingested. Prepatent periods are 3–10 days after ingesting tissue cysts and 18 days or more after ingesting tachyzoites or oocysts (Dubey and Frenkel 1976, Freyre et al. 1989, Dubey 1996). Less than 50% of cats shed oocysts after ingesting tachyzoites or oocysts, whereas nearly all cats shed oocysts after ingesting tissue cysts.

After the ingestion of tissue cysts by cats, the cyst wall is dissolved by the proteolytic enzymes in the stomach and small intestine. The released bradyzoites penetrate the epithelial cells of the small intestine and initiate development of numerous asexual generations of *T. gondii* (Dubey and Frenkel 1972). Five morphologically distinct types (A–E) of *T. gondii* develop in intestinal epithelial cells before gameto-

gony begins. Types A–E divide asexually by endodyogeny, endopolygeny or schizogony (division into more than 2 organisms). The origin of gamonts has not been determined; probably the merozoites released from meronts of types D and E initiate gamete formation. Gamonts occur throughout the small intestine but most commonly in the ileum (Fig. 16.6). Gamonts and schizonts are located in surface epithelial cells, usually above the host cell nucleus (Fig. 16.7), where they form 3–15 days after infection. The female gamete is subspherical and contains a single centrally located nucleus (Fig. 16.7). Mature male gamonts are ovoid to ellipsoidal in shape (Fig. 16.6). When microgametogenesis takes place, the nucleus of the male gamont divides to produce 10–21 nuclei which move toward the periphery of the parasite entering protuberances formed in the pellicle of the mother parasite. One or 2 residual bodies are left in the microgamont after division into microgametes. Each microgamete has 2 flagella (Fig. 16.6) and swims to and penetrates a mature macrogamete. After penetration, oocyst wall formation begins around the fertilized gamete, and, when mature, oocysts are discharged into the intestinal lumen by the rupture of intestinal epithelial cells.

Unsporulated oocysts are subspherical to spherical, 10 × 12 μm in diameter (Fig. 16.8). The oocyst wall contains 2 colourless layers. The sporont almost fills the oocyst, and sporulation occurs outside the cat

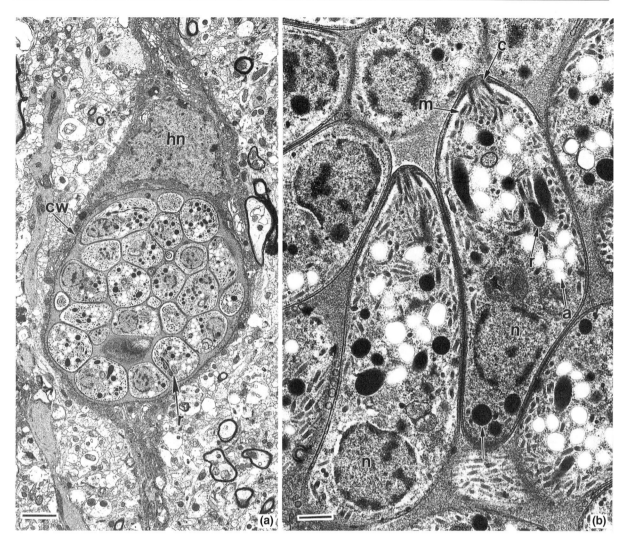

Fig. 16.4 Transmission electron micrographs of tissue cysts of *T. gondii* in brain. (a) A young intracellular cyst with well developed cyst wall (cw) is visible. The bradyzoites are plump (dividing or preparing to divide) and the contents of the rhoptries (r) in one *T. gondii* have a honeycomb structure (arrow). Bar = 4.4 μm. (b) Two longitudinally cut bradyzoites from a large cyst. Note electron-dense contents of rhoptries (r), and the terminal nuclei (n), a conoid (c), numerous micronemes (m), and amylopectin granules (a) that appear as empty spaces here. Bar = 0.77 μm.

within 1–5 days depending upon aeration and temperature. Sporulated oocysts are subspherical to ellipsoidal and each sporulated oocyst contains 2 ellipsoidal sporocysts. These lack a Stieda body (Fig. 16.8). Sporocysts measure 6 × 8 μm. There are 4 sutures with liplike thickenings in the sporocyst wall (Fig. 16.8) which open during excystation of the sporozoites. A sporocyst residuum is present, but no oocyst residuum. Each sporocyst contains 4 sporozoites, 2 × 6–8 μm in size with a subterminal to central nucleus and a few PAS-positive granules in the cytoplasm (Dubey, Miller and Frenkel 1970a). They have most of the organelles found in other coccidia except a crystalloid body and refractile globules (Fig. 16.8).

As the enteroepithelial cycle progresses, bradyzoites penetrate the lamina propria of the feline intestine and multiply as tachyzoites. Within a few hours after infection of cats, *T. gondii* may disseminate to extraintestinal tissues. *T. gondii* persists in intestinal and extra-intestinal tissues of cats for at least several months, if not for the life of the cat.

4 CULTIVATION, BIOCHEMISTRY, MOLECULAR BIOLOGY AND GENETICS

T. gondii has not been grown in cell-free media but can be cultivated in laboratory animals, chick embryos and cell cultures. Mice, hamsters, guinea pigs and rabbits are all susceptible but mice are generally used as hosts because they are more susceptible than the others and are not naturally infected when raised in the laboratory on commercial dry food free of cat faeces.

Tachyzoites of some strains of *T. gondii* grow in the peritoneal cavity of mice, sometimes producing ascites, and also grow in most other tissues after intra-

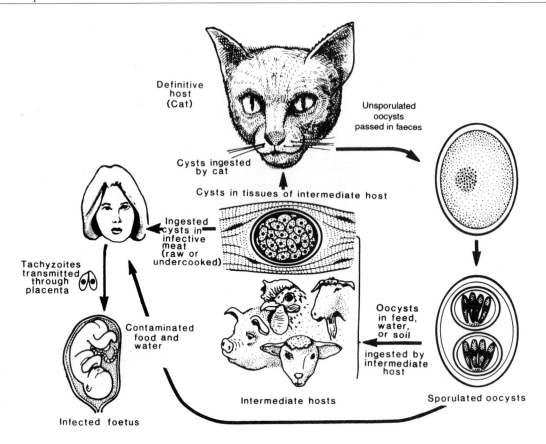

Fig. 16.5 Life cycle of *T. gondii.*

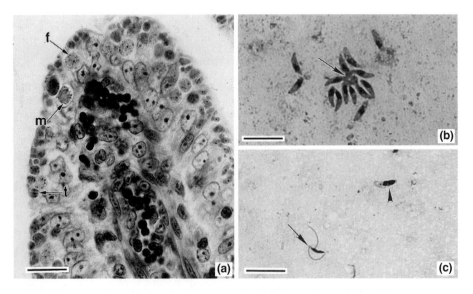

Fig. 16.6 Enteroepithelial stages of *T. gondii*, 6 days after feeding tissue cysts to a cat: (a) Histological section of a villus in small intestine. Note heavy infection of epithelial cells with *T. gondii* types (t), male gamonts (m), and numerous uninucleate female gamonts (f). Cells in the lamina propria are not infected. Haematoxylin and eosin. Bar = 15 μm. (b) Impression smear. Note a ruptured type E schizont with a residual body (arrow). Giemsa. Bar = 10 μm. (c) Impression smear. A biflagellate microgamete (arrow) and a free merozoite (arrowhead). Giemsa. Bar = 10 μm.

peritoneal inoculation with any of the 3 infectious stages, i.e. tachyzoites, bradyzoites and oocysts of *T. gondii*. Tissue cysts are prominent in the mouse brain about 8 weeks after infection. Virulent strains usually produce illness in mice and sometimes kill them

within 1–2 weeks. Most strains of *T. gondii* do not kill mice.

T. gondii tachyzoites will multiply in many cell lines in cell cultures and although most strains can develop tissue cysts in cell cultures, the yield is lower than that

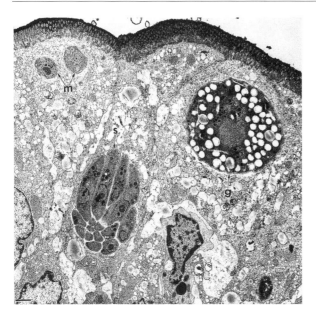

Fig. 16.7 Electron micrograph of coccidian stages of *T. gondii* in epithelial cells of ileum of a cat 6 days after ingesting tissue cysts. Note 2 merozoites (m) and a female gamont (g) located just below the microvillus border, and a schizont above the host cell nucleus. Bar = 2.5 μm.

produced in mice. The cysts can develop within 3 days of inoculation of tachyzoites in cell culture. 'Virulent' mouse strains rapidly destroy the cells whereas 'avirulent' strains grow slowly, causing minimal cell damage. The mean generation time of tachyzoites of the virulent RH strain is 5 h. Feline enteroepithelial stages of *T. gondii* have not yet been cultivated in vitro. Oocysts can be obtained by feeding tissue cysts from infected mice to *T. gondii*-free cats.

The *T. gondii* nucleus is haploid except for the zygote, in the intestine of the cat (Pfefferkorn 1990). Sporozoites result from a miotic division followed by mitotic divisions and genetic segregation seems to follow classical Mendelian laws. The total haploid genome contains approximately 8×10^7 bp. There is also a 36 kb circular mitochondrial DNA that has been partly sequenced. Nine chromosomes have been identified by pulsed field gel electrophoresis. The karyotype has been studied using probes which attach to genes of low copy number (Sibley et al. 1992). Several virulent *T. gondii* strains have been characterized genetically and comprise a single clonal linage. The α- and β-tubulin genes have been described, and both contain introns. Only the B1 gene has been found to be repeated tandemly, but other sequences, some repeated many times, have been identified. The *T. gondii* DNA has been characterized and a genetic system of nomenclature for *T. gondii* has been proposed (Sibley, Pfefferkorn and Boothroyd 1991, Sibley et al. 1992). DNA from other sources can be introduced into the *T. gondii* genome (Soldati and Boothroyd 1993).

T. gondii rRNA has the usual large and small subunit. Sequence analysis of the small rRNA suggests that *T. gondii* is closely related phylogenetically to *Sarcocystis* but distinct from *Plasmodium*. Although there are stage-specific proteins, all infective stages of *T. gondii* also share common proteins. Most of the proteins that have been characterized are from tachyzoites (Johnson 1989). *T. gondii* tachyzoites have 4 major surface proteins (22, 30, 35, and 43 kDa) of which p30 is the dominant protein and comprises 5% of the total tachyzoite protein (McLeod, Mack, and Brown 1991).

5 CLINICAL MANIFESTATIONS

T. gondii infection is widespread among humans and its prevalence varies widely from place to place. In the USA and the UK it is estimated that about 16–40% of people are infected whereas in Central and South America and continental Europe infection is esti-

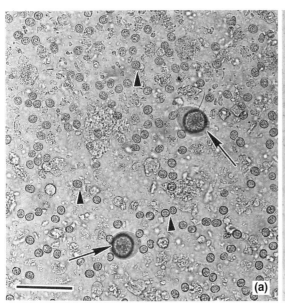

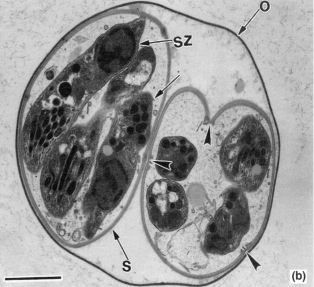

Fig. 16.8 Oocysts of *T. gondii*: (a) Unsporulated oocysts (arrowheads) and oocysts of another common feline coccidium, *Isospora felis* (arrows) in a faecal float preparation. Unstained. Bar = 50 μm. (b) Transmission electron micrograph of a sporulated oocyst. Note thin walled oocyst (o) enclosing the 2 sporocysts (s) each with 4 sporozoites (sz). Each sporocyst has 4 lip-like thickenings (arrows). Bar = 2.8 μm. (Courtesy of Dr D. S. Lindsay.)

Table 16.2   The relation of clinical toxoplasmosis in children to the time of infection in the mother[a]

Trimester infected	Children with toxoplasmosis (%)			
	Serious	**Mild**	**Subclinical**	**Total**
First	40	50	10	10
Second	17.7	45	37	62
Third	2.7	28.7	68.5	108
Undetermined	16.6	20.6	56.6	30

[a]From Couvreur et al. (1984).

mated to be 50–80% (Dubey and Beattie 1988). Most infections in humans are asymptomatic but at times the parasite can produce devastating disease. Infection may be congenitally or postnatally acquired.

5.1   Congenital infection

Congenital infection occurs only when a woman becomes infected during pregnancy and the severity of the disease may depend upon the stage of pregnancy when she becomes infected (Table 16.2) (Desmonts and Couvreur 1974, Daffos et al. 1988). Although the mother rarely has symptoms of infection she does have a temporary parasitaemia. Focal lesions develop in the placenta and the fetus may become infected. In the foetus there is generalized infection at first but later it clears from the visceral tissues and may localize in the central nervous system. A wide spectrum of clinical disease occurs in congenitally infected children (Remington, McLeod and Desmonts 1995). Mild disease may consist of slightly diminished vision only whereas severely diseased children may have the full tetrad of signs: retinochoroiditis, hydrocephalus (Fig. 16.9), convulsions, and intracerebral calcification (Fig. 16.10). Of these, hydrocephalus is the least common but most dramatic lesion of toxoplasmosis. This lesion is unique to congenitally acquired toxoplasmosis in humans and has not been reported in other animals.

By far the most common sequel of congenital toxoplasmosis is ocular disease (Guerina et al. 1994, McAu-

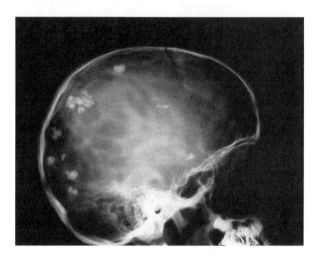

Fig. 16.10   Intracerebral calcification discovered fortuitously in a 10 year old girl, on a dental panoramic radiograph asked for by a dentist. The girl had unilateral retinochoroiditis and an IQ of 80. (Courtesy of Dr J. Couvreur).

ley et al. 1994). Except for the occasional involvement of an entire eye, in virtually in all other cases the disease is confined to the posterior chamber. Parasites proliferate in the retina leading to inflammation in the choroid, so the disease is correctly designated as retinochoroiditis. In humans the characteristic lesions of ocular toxoplasmosis in the acute or subacute stage of inflammation appear as yellowish white, cotton-like patches in the fundus (O'Connor 1975, Dutton 1989). The lesions may be single or multiple and may involve one or both eyes. During the acute stage, inflammatory exudate may cloud the vitreous fluid and may be so dense as to preclude visualization of the fundus by the examiner using an ophthalmoscope. As the inflammation subsides, the vitreous clears and the diseased retina and choroid can be seen through the ophthalmoscope. Retinal lesions may be single or multifocal small gray areas of active retinitis with minimal oedema and reaction in the vitreous humor. The punctate lesions are usually harmless unless they are located in a macular area (Fig. 16.11). Although severe infections may be detected at birth, milder infections may go undetected until they flare up in adulthood.

The socioeconomic impact of toxoplasmosis in human suffering and the cost of care of sick children, especially those with mental retardation and blindness, are enormous (Roberts and Frenkel 1990,

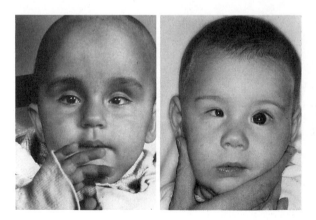

Fig. 16.9   Congenital toxoplasmosis in children. Hydrocephalus with bulging forehead (left) and microophthalmia of the left eye (right). (Courtesy of Dr J. Couvreur).

Roberts, Murrell and Marks 1994). The testing of all pregnant women for *T. gondii* infection is compulsory in France and Austria, and the cost benefits of such mass screening are being debated in many countries (Remington, McLeod and Desmonts 1995).

5.2 Postnatally acquired infection

Postnatally acquired infection may be localized or generalized. Oocyst-transmitted infections may be more severe than tissue cyst-induced infections. Lymphadenitis is the most frequently observed clinical form of toxoplasmosis in humans (Table 16.3). Although any nodes may be involved, the most frequently involved are the deep cervical nodes which, when infected, are tender, discrete but not painful; the infections resolve spontaneously in weeks or months. Lymphadenopathy may be associated with fever, malaise, fatigue, muscle pain and sore throat and headache (McCabe et al. 1987). Although the condition may be benign, its diagnosis is vital in pregnant women because of the risk to the fetus. In tissues from infected nodes examined histologically, reticular cell hyperplasia is usually present whereas necrosis and fibrosis are absent. The node architecture is preserved and usually only a few parasites are present. Diagnosis based on symptoms and histological examination can be confirmed by injection of a homogenate of the lymph node into mice, by immunohistochemical staining of the lymph tissue tagged with *T. gondii* antiserum, or by use of the polymerase chain reaction (PCR) to detect *T. gondii* DNA in tissues.

Encephalitis is the most important manifestation of toxoplasmosis in immunosuppressed patients as it causes the most severe damage to the patient. Infection may occur in any organ. Patients may have headache, disorientation, drowsiness, hemiparesis, reflex changes and convulsions, and many become comatose. Diagnosis is aided by serological examination. However, in immunosuppressed patients both inflammatory signs and antibody production may be suppressed, thus making the diagnosis very difficult. Encephalitis caused by *T. gondii* is now frequently recognized in patients treated with immunosuppressive agents.

Toxoplasmosis ranks high in the list of diseases which lead to death of patients with AIDS; approximately 10% of AIDS patients in the USA and up to 30% in Europe are estimated to die from toxoplasmosis (Luft and Remington 1992, Luft et al. 1993, Rabaud et al. 1994) Although in AIDS patients any organ may be involved, including the testis, dermis and spinal cord, infection of the brain is most frequently reported. Most AIDS patients suffering from toxoplasmosis have bilateral, severe and persistent headache which responds poorly to analgesics. As the disease progresses, the headache may give way to a condition characterized by confusion, lethargy, ataxia and coma. The predominant lesion in the brain is necrosis, especially of the thalamus.

6 IMMUNOLOGY

In those hosts which develop disease the host may die of acute toxoplasmosis but much more often recovers with the acquisition of immunity (Frenkel 1973a). In the recovering individual inflammation usually develops where there was initial necrosis. By about the third week after infection, and as recovery develops, *T. gondii* tachyzoites begin to disappear from the visceral tissues and the parasites localize as tissue cysts in neural and muscular tissues. The tachyzoites may persist longer in the spinal cord and brain than in visceral tissues because immunity there is less effective than in visceral organs; they can persist in the placenta for months after the initial infection of the mother.

T. gondii can multiply in virtually any cell of the body but how it is destroyed in immune cells is not completely known. All extracellular forms of the parasite are directly affected by antibody but intracellular forms are not. It is believed that cellular factors including lymphocytes and lymphokines are more important than humoral ones in immune mediated destruction of *T. gondii* (Frenkel 1973a). Interferon-γ is considered by some to be the main factor in cell-mediated immunity to *T. gondii* (Gazzinelli, Denkers, and Sher 1993). Under experimental conditions, infection with avirulent strains protects the host from damage but does not prevent infection with more virulent strains. In most instances, immunity following a natural *T. gondii* infection persists for the life of the host.

Immunity does not eradicate the infection. *T. gondii* tissue cysts persist for several years after acute infection, and their fate is not fully known. Whether bradyzoites can form new tissue cysts directly without transforming into tachyzoites is not known. However, the finding of new tissue cysts adjacent to old ones suggests that it might happen. It has been proposed that tissue cysts may sometimes rupture during the life of the host and the released bradyzoites may be destroyed by the host's immune responses, possibly causing local necrosis accompanied by inflammation.

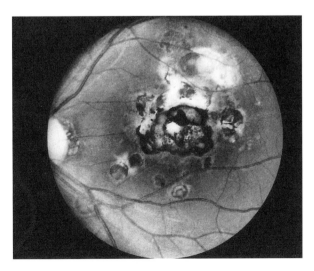

Fig. 16.11 Congenital toxoplasmosis. Retinochoroiditis in the macula of the left eye. (Courtesy of Dr R. Belfort Jr).

Table 16.3 Frequency of symptoms in people with postnatally acquired toxoplasmosis

Symptoms	Patients with symptoms (%)	
	Atlanta outbreak[a] (35 patients)	Panama outbreak[b] (35 patients)
Fever	94	90
Lymphadenopathy	88	77
Headache	88	77
Myalgia	63	68
Stiff neck	57	55
Anorexia	57	NR
Sore throat	46	NR
Artharlgia	26	29
Rash	23	0
Confusion	20	NR
Earache	17	NR
Nausea	17	36
Eye pain	14	26
Abdominal pain	11	55

[a]From Teutsch et al. (1979).
[b]From Benenson et al. (1982).
NR, not reported.

Hypersensitivity plays a major role in such reactions, which afterwards usually subside with no local renewed multiplication of *T. gondii* in the tissue. However, occasionally there may be formation of new tissue cysts.

In immunosuppressed patients, such as those given large doses of immunosuppressive agents in preparation for organ transplants and in those with AIDS, rupture of a tissue cyst may result in transformation of bradyzoites into tachyzoites and renewed multiplication. The immunosuppressed host may die from toxoplasmosis unless treated. It is not known how corticosteroids cause relapse but it is unlikely that they directly cause rupture of the tissue cysts.

Pathogenicity of *T. gondii* is determined by the virulence of the strain and the susceptibility of the host species. Strains of *T. gondii* may vary in their pathogenicity in a given host; for example, certain strains of mice are more susceptible than others and the severity of infection in individual mice within the same strain may also vary. However, mice of any age are susceptible to clinical *T. gondii* infection, whereas adult rats do not become ill although young rats can die of toxoplasmosis. Adult dogs, like adult rats, are resistant, whereas puppies are fully susceptible to clinical toxoplasmosis. Cattle and horses are among the hosts more resistant to clinical toxoplasmosis and certain marsupials and New World monkeys are the most susceptible. Nothing is known concerning genetic-related susceptibility to clinical toxoplasmosis in higher mammals, including humans.

7 PATHOLOGY

Humans acquire *T. gondii* mostly by ingestion of tissue cysts in infected meat or by ingestion of oocysts in food or water contaminated with cat faeces. The bradyzoites from the tissue cysts or sporozoites from the oocyst penetrate the intestinal epithelial cells where they multiply (Fig. 16.12) and spread first to the mesenteric lymph nodes and then to distant ones by invasion of the lymph and blood. Focal areas of necrosis may develop in many organs. The clinical picture is determined by the extent of injury, especially to vital organs such as the eye, heart and adrenals. Necrosis is caused by the intracellular growth of tachyzoites (Fig. 16.13). *T. gondii* does not produce a toxin.

Necrotic foci are the prominent lesions of toxoplasmosis, varying from microscopic (e.g. in the eye) to macroscopic. Macroscopic areas of necrosis cause encephalitis in AIDS patients. Inflammation usually follows the necrosis and is characterized by infiltration of mononuclear cells. By the time the tissue cysts are forming the inflammation has begun to subside. However, small inflammatory foci (e.g. glial nodules) may persist for months or even years after the primary infection (Fig. 16.13). The hydrocephalus of infected infants is due to a ventriculitis with a blockage of the aqueduct of Sylvius.

8 DIAGNOSIS

Diagnosis is made by biological, serological or histological methods or by some combination of these. Clinical signs are non-specific and insufficiently characteristic for a definite diagnosis because toxoplasmosis mimics several other infectious diseases.

Numerous serological procedures are available for the detection of humoral antibodies, including the Sabin–Feldman dye test, indirect haemagglutination assays, indirect fluorescent antibody assays (IFA), direct agglutination tests, latex agglutination tests,

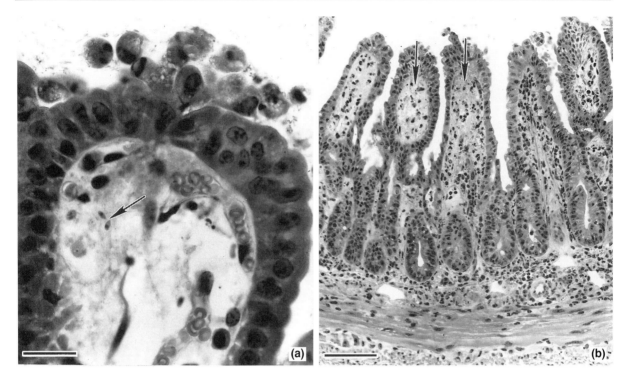

Fig. 16.12 Histological section of small intestine 6 days after feeding *T. gondii* oocysts to a mouse. Haematoxylin and eosin: (a) Intestinal villus showing oedema and necrosis of the lamina propria cells associated with tachyzoites (arrow), and extrusion of intestinal cells in the lumen. Bar = 20 μm. (b) Necrosis of lamina propria (arrows). The surface epithelium is not affected. Bar = 100 μm.

enzyme-linked immunoabsorbent assays (ELISA), and the immunoabsorbent agglutination assay test (IAAT). The IFA, IAAT and ELISA have been modified to detect IgM antibodies which appear sooner after infection than IgG and disappear faster than IgG after recovery.

The finding of antibodies to *T. gondii* in one serum sample merely establishes that the host has been infected at some time in the past, so it is best to collect 2 samples from the same individual, the second 2–4 weeks after the first. A 16-fold increase in antibody titre in the second sample indicates an acute infection. A high antibody titre sometimes persists for months after infection. A rise in antibody titre may not be associated with clinical symptoms, for as indicated earlier, most infections in humans are asymptomatic and the fact that titres persist after clinical recovery complicates the interpretation of the results of serological tests. *T. gondii* can be isolated from patients by inoculation into laboratory animals and tissue cultures of secretions, excretions, body fluids, tissues taken by biopsy and tissues with macroscopic lesions taken post-mortem. Using such specimens it is possible not only to attempt isolation of *T. gondii*, but also to search for *T. gondii* microscopically or for toxoplasmal DNA using of the PCR (Grover et al. 1990).

As just noted, diagnosis can be made by finding *T. gondii* in host tissue removed by biopsy or at necropsy. A rapid diagnosis may be made by microscopic examination of impression smears of lesions. After drying for 10–30 minutes, the smears are fixed in methyl alcohol and stained with a Romanowsky stain, Giemsa

being very satisfactory. Well preserved *T. gondii* are crescent-shaped (Fig. 16.1a). In sections, the tachyzoites usually appear round to oval (Fig. 16.1b). Electron microscopy can aid diagnosis. *T. gondii* tachyzoites are always located in vacuoles; they have few (usually 4) rhoptries and often have a honeycomb structure (Fig. 16.3a). Tissue cysts are usually spherical and lack septa, and the cyst wall stains with silver stains. The bradyzoites are strongly PAS positive. The immunohistochemical staining of parasites with fluorescent or other types of labelled *T. gondii* antiserum can aid in diagnosis (Fig. 16.13).

9 EPIDEMIOLOGY AND CONTROL

9.1 Prevalence of infection

T. gondii infection in humans is widespread and occurs throughout the world. Approximately 500 million humans have antibody to *T. gondii* (Kean 1972). Infection rates in humans and other animals differ from one geographical area of a country to another. The causes of these variations are not yet known. Environmental conditions, cultural habits of the people, and animal fauna are some of the factors that may determine the level of infection, which is more prevalent in hot and humid areas than in dry and cold climates. Only a small proportion (less than 1%) of people acquire infection congenitally.

Immunocompetent mothers of congenitally infected children have not been known to give birth to

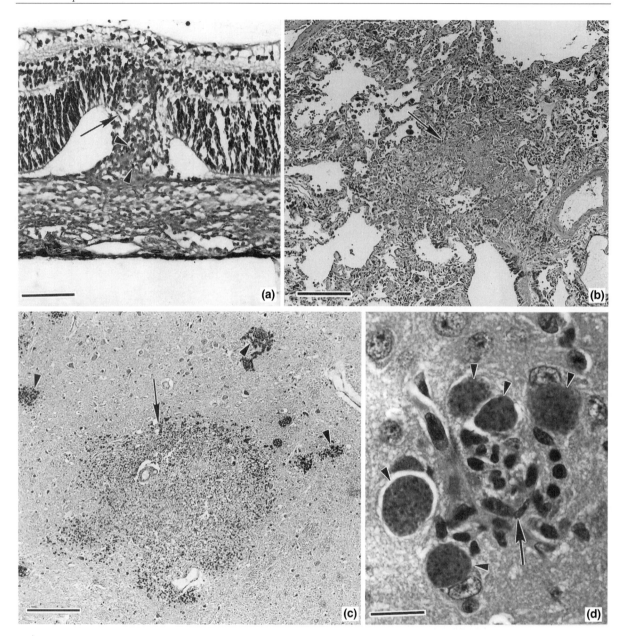

Fig. 16.13 Lesions of toxoplasmosis: (a) Focus of retinal detachment (arrow) and inflammation associated with tachyzoites (arrowheads). Haematoxylin and eosin. Bar = 80 μm. (b) Necrosis in the lung. Haematoxylin and eosin. Bar = 100 μm. (c) A large focus of necrosis (arrow) and several satellite small foci (arrowheads). Enormous numbers of *T. gondii* (all black dots) are present in the brain of an AIDS patient. Immunohistochemical stain with anti-*T. gondii* antibody. Bar = 100 μm. (d) Five tissue cysts (arrowheads) around a glial nodule (arrow) in the brain. Haematoxylin and eosin. Bar = 20 μm.

infected children in subsequent pregnancies but repeated congenital infection can occur in mice, rats, guinea pigs and hamsters (Dubey and Beattie 1988). Several litters born to an infected mouse or hamster may be infected even if there is no reinfection from outside sources. A congenitally infected mouse has been shown to be able to produce 10 generations of congenitally infected mice. In sheep, like humans, congenital infection occurs only when the ewe acquires infection during pregnancy.

9.2 Epidemiology

As noted earlier, toxoplasmosis may be acquired by ingestion of oocysts or by ingestion of tissue inhabiting stages of the parasite. The contamination of the environment by oocysts is widespread as oocysts are shed by cats, not only domestic cats but also other members of the Felidae. The domestic cat is probably the major source of contamination as oocyst formation is greatest in this extremely common animal.

Widespread natural infection of the environment is possible since a cat can excrete millions of oocysts after ingesting one infected mouse and these oocysts survive for long periods under most ordinary environmental conditions, for example in moist soil, for months and even years. Oocysts in soil do not always stay there because invertebrates such as flies, cockroaches, dung beetles and earthworms can spread them mechanically and may even carry them on to food.

Although only a few cats may be shedding *T. gondii* oocysts at any given time (as few as 1%) the enormous numbers shed and their resistance to destruction assure widespread contamination. Under experimental conditions, infected cats can shed oocysts after reinoculation with tissue cysts (Dubey 1995) and if this occurs in nature it would greatly facilitate oocyst spread. Congenital infection can also occur in cats, and congenitally infected kittens can excrete oocysts (Dubey and Carpenter 1993), providing another source of contamination. Infection rates in cats are determined by the rate of infection in local avian and rodent populations because cats are thought to become infected by eating these animals. The more oocysts in the environment the more likely prey animals are to become infected and this in turn would increase the infection rate in cats.

Infection in humans is probably most often the result of ingestion of tissue cysts contained in raw or undercooked meat as *T. gondii* is common in many animals used for food, including sheep, pigs, and rabbits. Infection in cattle is less prevalent than is infection in sheep or pigs. Tissue cysts can survive in food animals for years (Dubey and Beattie 1988).

Cultural habits may also affect the acquisition of *T. gondii* infection; for example, in France the prevalence of antibodies to *T. gondii* in humans is very high. Whereas 84% of pregnant women in Paris have antibodies to *T. gondii*, comparable figures elsewhere are 32% in New York City and 22% in London (Dubey and Beattie 1988). The high incidence of *T. gondii* infection in humans in France appears to be related in part to the French habit of eating some of their meat raw. In contrast, the high prevalence of the infection in Central and South America is in probably due to high levels of contamination of the environment by oocysts (Teutsch et al. 1979). It should be noted, however, that the relative frequency of acquisition of toxoplasmosis from eating raw meat and that due to ingestion of food contaminated by oocysts from cat faeces is very difficult to determine and statements on the subject are at best controversial.

In addition to infection as a result of ingestion of oocysts and by eating infected raw meat, transmission of toxoplasmosis can be by sexual means, by ingestion of milk or saliva and by eating eggs. The stages most likely to be involved in these transmissions are tachyzoites, which are not environmentally resistant and are killed by water.

There is little, if any, danger of *T. gondii* infection by drinking cow's milk which, in any case, is generally pasteurized or even boiled, but infection has followed drinking unboiled goat's milk. Raw hens' eggs, although an important source of *Salmonella* infection, are extremely unlikely to harbour *T. gondii*. Transmission by sexual activity including kissing is probably rare and epidemiogically unimportant.

Transmission can also occur through blood transfusions and organ transplants, transplantation being the more important; this is a recent development. In people undergoing transplantation toxoplasmosis may arise either (1) from implantation of an organ or bone marrow from an infected donor into a non-immune immunocompromised recipient or (2) from induction of disease in an immunocompromised latently infected recipient. The tissue cysts in the transplanted tissue or in the latently infected person are probably the source of the infection. In both cases the cytotoxic and immunosuppressive therapy given to the recipient is the cause of the induction of the active infection and the disease (Wreghitt et al. 1989, Slavin et al. 1994).

10 CHEMOTHERAPY

Sulphadiazine and pyrimethamine are widely used for therapy of toxoplasmosis (Guerina et al. 1994, Georgiev 1994). These drugs act synergistically by blocking the metabolic pathway involving *p*-aminobenzoic acid and the folic–folinic acid cycle respectively. The drugs are usually well tolerated; sometimes thrombocytopaenia or leukopaenia may develop, but these effects can be overcome by administering folinic acid and yeast without interfering with treatment because the vertebrate host can transport presynthesized folinic acid into its cells whereas *Toxoplasma* cannot. Although these drugs have a beneficial action when given in the acute stage of the disease when there is active multiplication of the parasite, they will not usually eradicate infection. These drugs appear to have little effect on subclinical infections, but the growth of tissue cysts in mice has been restrained with sulphonamides. Sulpha compounds are excreted within a few hours of administration, so treatment has to be administered in daily divided doses (4 doses of 500 mg each) usually for several weeks or months (WHO 1995). A loading dose (75 mg) of pyrimethamine during the first 3 days has been recommended because it is absorbed slowly and binds to tissues. From the 4th day, the dose of pyrimethamine is reduced to 25 mg, and 2–10 mg of folinic acid and 5–10 g of baker's yeast are added.

Certain other drugs, diaminodiphenylsulfone (SDDS), atovaquone, spiramycin, chlorinated lincomycin analogues, piritrexim and roxithromycin are effective in treatment of experimentally induced *T. gondii* infection in animals or cell cultures (Georgiev 1994). Spiramycin produces high tissue concentrations, particularly in the placenta, but does not cross the placental barrier, and has been used in humans without harmful effects, although it is a less effective antitoxoplasmicidal drug than sulphadiazine and pyrimethamine. Clindamycin is reported to be effective against *T. gondii* but may cause ulcerative colitis. Among all of the drugs tested atovaquone is the most cysticidal. Search for newer cysticidal drugs is continuing.

11 VACCINATION

The objectives of use of vaccines against toxoplasmosis include reducing fetal damage, reducing the number of tissue cysts in animals and preventing the formation of oocysts in cats (Araujo 1994, Dubey 1994). None of these objectives can be realized by the use of any currently available single vaccine. At present there are no effective subunit or killed vaccines for immunization against *T. gondii* but research is under way in many laboratories (Araujo 1994).

Prevention of oocyst shedding by cats is the key to controlling the spread of *T. gondii* and the oral ingestion of live bradyzoites is necessary to induce immunity to oocyst shedding, as the administration of any stage of *T. gondii* parenterally does not induce an immunity capable of inhibiting oocyst shedding (Frenkel and Smith 1982). A recently developed vaccine for use in cats contains live bradyzoites from a mutant strain (T-263) of *T. gondii*. After oral administration of T-263 bradyzoites, the cycle of development of *T. gondii* is arrested at the sexual stage because only gamonts of a single sex develop; thus oocysts are not produced (Frenkel et al. 1991). In one trial, 84% of cats vaccinated with T-263 bradyzoites failed to shed oocysts following challenge (Frenkel et al. 1991). The duration of immunity in cats induced by the vaccine has not yet been determined. This vaccine is not available commercially.

The objectives of vaccination of farm animals are to reduce the incidence of abortions in sheep and goats resulting from transplacental infection of fetuses, and to reduce the risk of human exposure resulting from ingestion of infected meat (with the subsequent risk of fetal infection). For these purposes vaccines made of non-persistent strains of *T. gondii* are under study. One vaccine that contains a strain (S48) of tachyzoites that does not persist in the tissues of sheep is available in Europe and New Zealand where it is used to reduce fetal losses attributable to toxoplasmosis (Wilkins, O'Connell and Te Punga 1988, Buxton 1993). Ewes vaccinated with the S48 strain vaccine retain immunity for at least 18 months (Buxton 1993). Another strain of *T. gondii* (RH) does not persist in tissues of swine but does induce immunity (Dubey et al. 1994). A mutant (ts-4) of the RH strain is being studied as a vaccine for immunizing hosts other than cats. It grows better at 33°C than it does at 37°C (body temperature). The ts-4 stain is non-pathogenic even to suckling pigs (Lindsay, Blagburn and Dubey 1993). These strains of *T. gondii* (S48, RH, ts-4) do not induce oocyst shedding in cats.

12 PREVENTION AND CONTROL

To prevent infection of humans by *T. gondii*, the hands of people handling meat should be washed thoroughly with soap and water before they go to other tasks. All cutting boards, sink tops, knives and other materials coming in contact with uncooked meat should also be washed with soap and water. Washing is effective because the stages of *T. gondii* in meat are killed by contact with soap and water.

Parasites in meat can be killed by exposure to extreme cold or heat; tissue cysts are killed by heating the meat throughout to 67°C (Dubey et al. 1990) or by cooling it to −13°C (Kotula et al. 1991). Tissue cysts are also killed by exposure to 0.5 Gy of γ-irradiation (Dubey and Thayer 1994). All meat should be cooked to 67°C before consumption, and tasting meat while cooking or while seasoning should be avoided. Pregnant women, especially, should avoid contact with cats, soil and raw meat. Pet cats should be fed only dry, canned or cooked food and the cat litter box should be emptied every day, preferably not by a pregnant woman. Gloves should be worn while gardening and vegetables should be washed thoroughly before eating because of possible contamination with cat faeces. Expectant mothers should be aware of the dangers of toxoplasmosis (Foulon, Naessens, and Derde 1994).

13 INFECTION IN ANIMALS OTHER THAN HUMANS

T. gondii is capable of causing severe disease in animals other than humans (Dubey and Beattie 1988) and is responsible for great losses to the livestock industry. In sheep and goats it may cause embryonic death and resorption, fetal death and mummification, abortion, stillbirth and neonatal death. Disease is more severe in goats than in sheep. Outbreaks of toxoplasmosis in pigs have been reported from several countries, especially Japan, and mortality is more common in young pigs than in adult pigs. Pneumonia, myocarditis, encephalitis and placental necrosis occur in infected pigs. Cattle and horses are more resistant to clinical toxoplasmosis than are other species of livestock. In cats and dogs the disease is most severe in young animals. Common clinical manifestations of canine toxoplasmosis are respiratory distress, ataxia and diarrhoea. In most infected dogs pneumonia is caused by a combination of *T. gondii* and distemper virus as the virus is immunosuppressive. Respiratory distress is a common clinical sign in felines with toxoplasmosis. Sporadic and widespread outbreaks of toxoplasmosis occur in rabbits, mink, birds and other domesticated and wild animals. Toxoplasmosis is severe in many species of Australian marsupials and in New World monkeys (Dubey and Beattie 1988).

REFERENCES

Araujo FG, 1994, Immunization against *Toxoplasma gondii*, *Parasitol Today*, **10:** 358–60.

Benenson MW, Takafuji ET et al., 1982, Oocyst transmitted toxoplasmosis associated with ingestion of contaminated water, *N Engl J Med*, **307:** 666–9.

Buxton D, 1993, Toxoplasmosis: the first commercial vaccine, *Parasitol Today*, **9:** 335–7.

Couvreur J, Desmonts G et al., 1984, Etude d'une série homogène de 210 cas de toxoplasmose congénitale chez des nourrissons âgés de 0 a 11 mois et dépistés de façon prospective, *Ann Pediatr (Paris)*, **31:** 815–9.

Daffos F, Forestier F et al., 1988, Prenatal management of 746 pregnancies at risk for congenital toxoplasmosis, *N Engl J Med*, **318:** 271–5.

Desmonts G, Couvreur J, 1974, Congenital toxoplasmosis. A propective study of 378 pregnancies, *N Engl J Med*, **290:** 1110–16.

Dubey JP, 1977, *Toxoplasma, Hammondia, Besnoitia, Sarcocystis,* and other tissue cyst-forming coccidia of man and animals, *Parasitic Protozoa*, 1st edn, vol. III, ed. Kreier JP, Academic Press, New York, 101–237.

Dubey JP, 1993, *Toxoplasma, Neospora, Sarcocystis,* and other tissue cyst-forming coccidia of humans and animals, *Parasitic Protozoa*, 2nd edn, vol. 6, ed. Kreier JP, Academic Press, New York, 1–158.

Dubey JP, 1994, Toxoplasmosis, *J Am Vet Med Assoc*, **205:** 1593–8.

Dubey JP, 1995, Duration of immunity to shedding of *Toxoplasma gondii* oocysts by cats, *J Parasitol*, **81:** 410–15.

Dubey JP, 1996, Infectivity and pathogenicity of *Toxoplasma gondii* oocysts for cats, *J Parasitol*, **82:** 957–61.

Dubey JP, Baker DG et al., 1994, Persistence of immunity to toxoplasmosis in pigs vaccinated with a nonpersistent strain of *Toxoplasma gondii*, *Am J Vet Res*, **55:** 982–7.

Dubey JP, Beattie CP, 1988, *Toxoplasmosis of Animals and Man*, CRC Press, Boca Raton.

Dubey JP, Carpenter JL, 1993, Neonatal toxoplasmosis in littermate cats, *J Am Vet Med Assoc*, **203:** 1546–9.

Dubey JP, Frenkel JK, 1972, Cyst-induced toxoplasmosis in cats, *J Protozool*, **19:** 155–77.

Dubey JP, Frenkel JK, 1976, Feline toxoplasmosis from acutely infected mice and the development of *Toxoplasma* cyst, *J Protozool*, **23:** 537–46.

Dubey JP, Thayer DW, 1994, Killing of different strains of *Toxoplasma gondii* tissue cysts by irradiation under defined conditions, *J Parasitol*, **80:** 764–7.

Dubey JP, Kotula AW et al., 1990, Effect of high temperature on infectivity of *Toxoplasma gondii* tissue cysts in pork, *J Parasitol*, **76:** 201–4.

Dubey JP, Miller NL, Frenkel JK, 1970a, Characterization of the new fecal form of *Toxoplasma gondii*, *J Parasitol*, **56:** 447–56.

Dubey JP, Miller NL, Frenkel JK, 1970b, The *Toxoplasma gondii* oocyst from cat feces, *J Exp Med*, **132:** 636–62.

Dutton GN, 1989, Toxoplasmic retinochoroiditis – A historical review and current concepts, *Ann Acad Med*, **18:** 214–21.

Ferguson DJP, Hutchison WM, 1987, An ultrastructural study of the early development and tissue cyst formation of *Toxoplasma gondii* in the brains of mice, *Z Parasitenkd*, **73:** 483–91.

Foulon W, Naessens A, Derde MP, 1994, Evaluation of the possibilities for preventing congenital toxoplasmosis, *Am J Perinatol*, **11:** 57–62.

Frenkel JK, 1973, *Toxoplasma* in and around us, *BioScience*, **23:** 343–52.

Frenkel JK, 1973a, Toxoplasmosis: parasite life cycle, pathology and immunology, *The Coccidia*. Eimeria, Isospora, Toxoplasma *and Related Genera*, eds. Hammond DM, Long PL,, University Park Press, Baltimore, MD, 343–410.

Frenkel JK, Dubey JP, Miller NL, 1970, *Toxoplasma gondii* in cats: fecal stages identified as coccidian oocysts, *Science*, **167:** 893–6.

Frenkel JK, Pfefferkorn ER et al., 1991, Prospective vaccine pre-pared from a new mutant of *Toxoplasma gondii* for use in cats, *Am J Vet Res*, **52:** 759–63.

Frenkel JK, Smith DD, 1982, Immunization of cats against shedding of *Toxoplasma* oocysts, *J Parasitol*, **68:** 744–8.

Freyre A, Dubey JP et al., 1989, Oocyst-induced *Toxoplasma gondii* infections in cats, *J Parasitol*, **75:** 750–5.

Gazzinelli RT, Denkers EY, Sher A, 1993, Host resistance to *Toxoplasma gondii*: model for studying the selective induction of cell-mediated immunity by intracellular parasites, *Infect Agent Dis*, **2:** 139–49.

Grover CM, Thulliez P et al., 1990, Rapid prenatal-diagnosis of congenital *Toxoplasma* infection by using polymerase chain-reaction and amniotic-fluid, *J Clin Microbiol*, **28:** 2297–301.

Guerina NG, Hsu HW et al., 1994, Neonatal serologic screening and early treatment for congenital *Toxoplasma gondii* infection, *N Engl J Med*, **330:** 1858–63.

Johnson AM, 1989, Toxoplasma vaccines: biology, pathology, immunology, and treatment, *Veterinary Protozoan and Hemoparasite Vaccines*, ed. Wright IG, CRC Press, Boca Raton, FL, 177–202.

Kean BH, 1972, Clinical toxoplasmosis – 50 years, *Trans R Soc Trop Med Hyg*, **66:** 549–71.

Kotula AW, Dubey JP et al., 1991, Effect of freezing on infectivity of *Toxoplasma gondii* tissue cysts in pork, *J Food Protection*, **54:** 687–90.

Lindsay DS, Blagburn BL, Dubey JP, 1993, Safety and results of challenge of weaned pigs given a temperature-sensitive mutant of *Toxoplasma gondii*, *J Parasitol*, **79:** 71–6.

Luft BJ, Hafner R et al., 1993, Toxoplasmic encephalitis in patients with the acquired immunodeficiency syndrome, *N Engl J Med*, **329:** 995–1000.

Luft BJ, Remington JS, 1992, Toxoplasmic encephalitis in AIDS, *Clin Infect Dis*, **15:** 211–22.

McAuley J, Boyer KM et al., 1994, Early and longitudinal evaluations of treated infants and children and untreated historical patients with congenital toxoplasmosis – the Chicago collaborative treatment trial, *Clin Infect Dis*, **18:** 38–72.

McCabe RE, Brooks RG et al., 1987, Clinical spectrum in 107 cases of toxoplasmic lymphadenopathy, *Rev Infect Dis*, **9:** 754–74.

McLeod R, Mack D, Brown C, 1991, *Toxoplasma-gondii* – new advances in cellular and molecular-biology, *Exp Parasitol*, **72:** 109–21.

Nicolle C, Manceaux L, 1908, Sur une infection à corps de Leishman (ou organismes voisins) du gondi, *C R Acad Sci Paris*, **147:** 763–6.

Nicolle C, Manceaux L, 1909, Sur un protozoaire nouveau du gondi, *C R Acad Sci Paris*, **148:** 369–72.

O'Connor GR, 1975, Ocular toxoplasmosis, *Jpn J Opthalmol*, **19:** 1–24.

Pfefferkorn ER, 1990, *Cell Biology of* Toxoplasma gondii, Freedman, New York, 26–50.

Rabaud C, May T et al., 1994, Extracerebral toxoplasmosis in patients infected with HIV. A French National Survey, *Medicine*, **73:** 306–14.

Remington JS, McLeod R, Desmonts G, 1995, Toxoplasmosis, *Infectious Diseases of the Fetus and Newborn Infant*, 4th edn, eds Remington JS, Klein JO, Saunders, Philadelphia, 140–267.

Roberts T, Frenkel JK, 1990, Estimating income losses and other preventable costs caused by congenital toxoplasmosis in people in the United States, *J Am Vet Med Assoc*, **196:** 249–56.

Roberts T, Murrell KD, Marks S, 1994, Economic losses caused by foodborne parasitic diseases, *Parasitol Today*, **10:** 419–23.

Sibley LD, LeBlanc AJ et al., 1992, Generation of a restriction fragment length polymorphism linkage map for *Toxoplasma gondii*, *Genetics*, **132:** 1003–15.

Sibley LD, Pfefferkorn ER, Boothroyd JC, 1991, Proposal for a uniform genetic nomenclature in *Toxoplasma gondii*, *Parasitol Today*, **7:** 327–8.

Slavin MA, Meyers JD et al., 1994, *Toxoplasma gondii* infection in marrow transplant recipients: A 20 year experience, *Bone Marrow Transplant*, **13:** 549–57.

Soldati D, Boothroyd JC, 1993, Transient transfection and expression in the obligate intracellular parasite *Toxoplasma gondii*, *Science*, **260:** 349–352.

Splendore A, 1908, Un nuovo protozoa parassita de' conigli. incontrato nelle lesioni anatomiche d'une malattia che ricorda in molti punti il Kala-azar dell'uomo. Nota preliminare pel, *Rev Soc Scient Sao Paulo*, **3:** 109–12.

St. Georgiev V, 1994, Management of toxoplasmosis, *Drugs*, **48:** 179–88.

Teutsch SM, Juranek DD et al., 1979, Epidemic toxoplasmosis associated with infected cats, *N Engl J Med*, **300:** 695–9.

WHO, 1995, *Drugs used in Parasitic Diseases*, 2nd edn, World Health Organization, Geneva.

Wilkins MF, O'Connell E, Te Punga WA, 1988, Toxoplasmosis in sheep III. Further evaluation of the ability of a live *Toxoplasmosis gondii* vaccine to prevent lamb losses and reduce congenital infection following experimental oral challenge, *NZ Vet J*, **36:** 86–9.

Wolf A, Cowen D, 1937, Granulomatous encephalomyelitis due to an encephalitozoon (encephalitozic encephalomyelitis): a new protozoan disease of man, *Bull Neurol Inst NY*, **6:** 306–35.

Wolf A, Cowen D, Paige B, 1939, Human toxoplasmosis: occurrence in infants as an encephalomyelitis verification by transmission to animals, *Science*, **89:** 226–7.

Wreghitt TG, Hakim M et al., 1989, Toxoplasmosis in heart and lung transplant recipients, *J Clin Pathol*, **42:** 194–9.

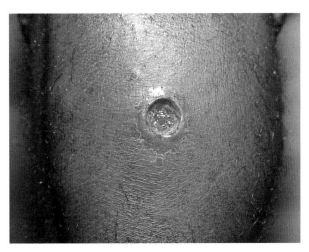

Plate 13.2 Simple skin lesion of the arm, due to *Leishmania (Viannia) braziliensis.* Pará, Brazil.

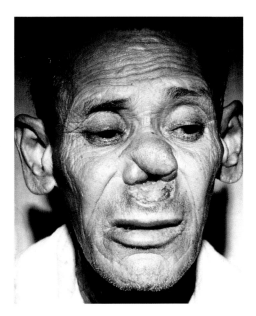

Plate 13.3 Mucocutaneous leishmaniasis, due to *L. (V.) braziliensis.* Pará, Brazil.

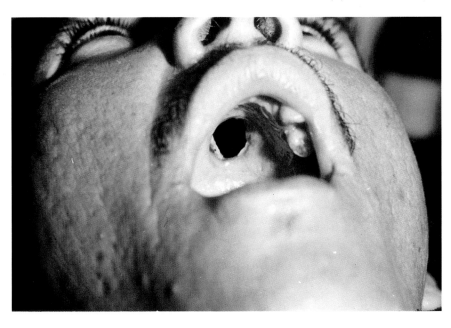

Plate 13.4 Destruction of the palate, due to *L. (V.) braziliensis.* Pará, Brazil.

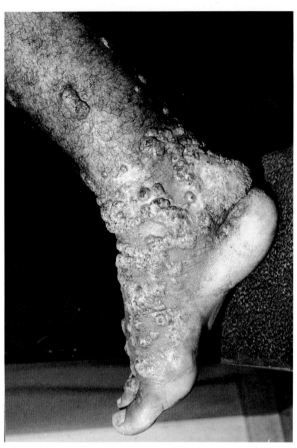

Plate 13.12 Strange multiple nodules on the foot due to *L. (V.)shawi*, clinically resembling mycotic disease.

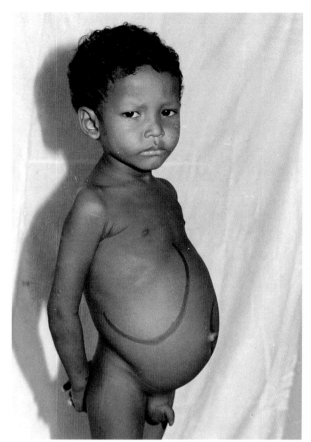

Plate 13.13 American visceral leishmaniasis (AVL), due to *L. (L.) chagasi*, in a boy from Marajó Island, Pará, Brazil. Note the greatly distended abdomen resulting from hepatosplenomegaly.

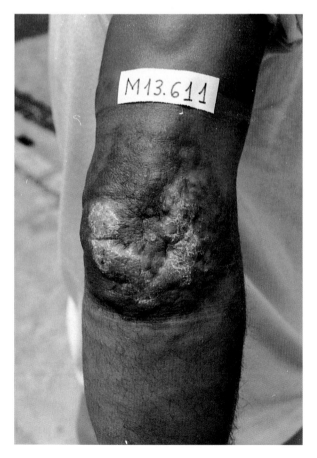

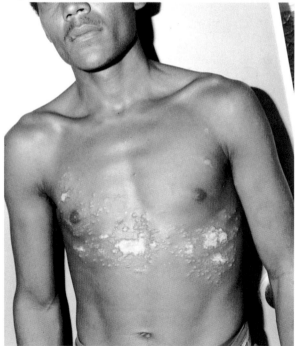

Pates 13.4 – 13.5 A variety of skin lesions due to different neotropical *Leishmania* species (also see Fig. 13.9 and Plate 13.2). Plate 13.14. Infection with *L. (L.) amazonensis*, on the elbow. Plate 13.15. A large number of small, papular satellite lesions surrounding the larger, primary lesions in a case of "pian-bois" due to *L. (V.) guyanensis*.

Chapter 17

SARCOCYSTIS, ISOSPORA AND CYCLOSPORA

J P Dubey

SARCOCYSTIS

1 HISTORY AND CLASSIFICATION

The *Sarcocystis* parasite was first found in the skeletal muscle of a house mouse (*Mus musculus*) in Switzerland in 1843 (Table 17.1). Before 1972, many of these parasites were given names based on the finding of their cysts in the muscles of a variety of hosts. The true nature of these intramuscular cysts remained unknown until the discovery of the life cycle of *Sarcocystis* in 1972 (Table 17.1).

Sarcocystis species are coccidian parasites and are classified as indicated in Table 17.2.

Table 17.2 Classification of *Sarcocystis*

Phylum	Apicomplexa Levine, 1979
Class	Coccidea Leuckart, 1879
Order	Eimeriida Léger 1911
Family	Sarcocystidae Poche, 1913
Genus	*Sarcocystis* Lankester, 1882

Table 17.1 Historical landmarks concerning *Sarcocystis*[a]

Year	Findings	Reference
1843	Sarcocysts found in muscles of a mouse	Miesher (1843)
1882	Genus *Sarcocystis* introduced	Lankaster (1882)
1943	*Sarcocystis* not transmitted from sheep to sheep, role of carnivores suspected but not proven	Scott (1943)
1972	Sexual phase cultured in vitro	Fayer (1972)
1972	Two-host life cycle found	Rommel and Heydorn (1972), Rommel et al. (1972)
1973	Vascular phase recognized and pathogenicity demonstrated	Fayer and Johnson (1975)
1975	Multiple *Sarcocystis* species within a given host recognized	Heydorn et al. (1975b)
1975	Chemotherapy demonstrated	Fayer and Johnson (1973)
1976	Abortion due to sarcocytosis recognized	Fayer et al. (1979b)
1981	Protective immunity demonstrated	Dubey (1980a)
1986	Vascular phase cultured in vitro	Speer and Dubey (1986)

[a]Reprinted with permission from Dubey, Speer, and Fayer (1989), where a complete bibliography can be found.

2 STRUCTURE AND LIFE CYCLE

Sarcocysts (Greek *sarkos* = flesh, *kystis* = bladder), the terminal asexual stage of development of these parasites, are found primarily in the striated muscles of mammals, birds, marsupials and poikilothermic animals (Fig. 17.1).

Sarcocystis has an obligatory prey–predator (2-host) life cycle (Fig. 17.2). Asexual stages develop only in the intermediate host, which in nature is often a prey animal, and sexual stages develop only in the definitive host, which is carnivorous. There are different intermediate and definitive hosts for each species of *Sarcocystis*; for example, there are 3 named species of *Sarcocystis* in cattle: *S. cruzi*, *S. hirsuta* and *S. hominis* (Dubey, Speer and Fayer 1989), the definitive hosts for these species being Canidae, Felidae and primates, respectively. Species of *Sarcocystis* are generally more specific for their intermediate hosts than for their definitive hosts; for *S. cruzi* for example, ox and bison are the only intermediate hosts whereas dogs, wolves, coyotes, raccoons, jackals and foxes can act as definitive hosts. In the following description of life cycle and structure *S. cruzi* will serve as the example because its complete life cycle is known.

The intermediate host becomes infected by ingesting sporocysts in food or water. Sporozoites excyst from sporocysts in the small intestine and first generation schizonts are formed in endothelial cells of arteries 7–15 days after inoculation. Second generation schizonts occur 19–46 days after inoculation, predominantly in capillaries virtually throughout the body (Fig. 17.3a). Merozoites are found in mononuclear blood cells 24–46 days after inoculation.

The schizonts divide by endopolygeny (*endon* = inside, *poly* = many, *genesis* = birth). The nucleus becomes lobulated and divides into several nuclei. Merozoites form at the periphery of the schizont. Both first and second generation schizonts are located within the host cytoplasm and are not surrounded by a parasitophorous vacuole. *Sarcocystis* merozoites have the same organelles as do *Toxoplasma gondii* tachyzoites except that there are no rhoptries (Dubey, Speer and Fayer 1989).

Merozoites liberated from the terminal vascular generation of the developing parasite initiate sarcocyst formation. These merozoites penetrate appropriate host cells. The intracellular merozoite which is surrounded by a parasitophorous vacuole (PV) becomes round to ovoid (metrocyte) and undergoes repeated division producing many merozoites which are released and penetrate other cells (Fig. 17.3b). After what appear to be several such cycles of reproduction some of the metrocytes, through the process of endodyogeny, produce banana-shaped zoites called bradyzoites (also called cystozoites) containing prominent amylopectin granules that stain bright red when treated with the periodic acid–Schiff (PAS) reagent. Some mature sarcocysts may contain some peripherally arranged metrocytes in addition to zoites (Fig. 17.1b). Eventually the sarcocyst is filled with bradyzoites, the stage infective for the predator definitive host. Sarcocysts generally become infectious about 75 days after infection, but in this there is considerable variation among species of *Sarcocystis*. Immature sarcocysts containing only metrocytes and schizonts are not infectious for the definitive host.

The definitive host becomes infected by ingesting

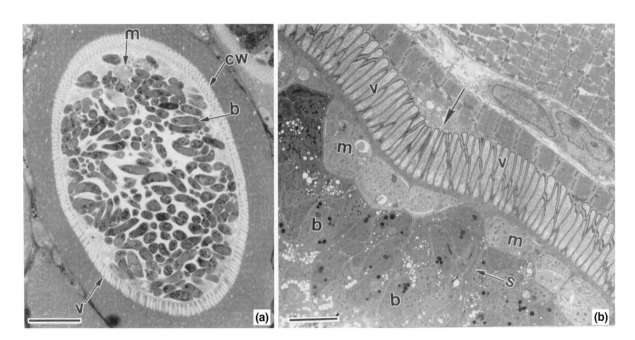

Fig. 17.1 Intramuscular *Sarcocystis hominis* sarcocysts. (a) Histological section of a mature sarcocyst. Note finger-like villar protrusions (v) on the cyst wall (cw) enclosing numerous bradyzoites (b) and a few metrocytes (m). Toluidine blue. Bar = 20 μm. (b) Transmission electron micrograph. Note villar projections (v) on the cyst wall, metrocytes (m), bradyzoites (b) and septa (s). Arrow points to border of the parasite and host cell cytoplasm. Bar = 4.3 μm.

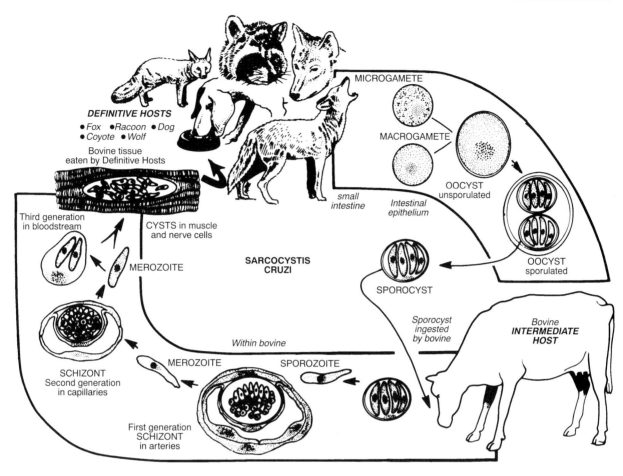

Fig. 17.2 Life cycle of *Sarcocystis cruzi* (from Dubey et al. 1989, with permission).

tissues containing mature sarcocysts. Bradyzoites liberated from the sarcocyst by digestion in the stomach and intestine penetrate the mucosa of the small intestine and transform into male (micro) and female (macro) gamonts. Within 6 h of ingesting infected tissue, gamonts are found within a PV in goblet cells near the tips of the villi (Fig. 17.3c). Macrogamonts are 10–20 μm in diameter and contain a single nucleus whereas microgamonts are 7 × 5 μm and contain 3–11 slender gametes (Fig. 17.3d). The microgametes, which are about 4 × 0.5 μm, have a compact nucleus, and 2 flagella. After fertilization of a macrogamete by a microgamete a wall develops around the zygote and an oocyst is formed. The entire process of gametogony and fertilization can be completed within 24 h. Gamonts and oocysts may be found at the same time in a host (Fig. 17.3).

Oocysts of *Sarcocystis* species sporulate in the lamina propria (Fig. 17.3e). Sporulated oocysts are generally colourless, thin-walled (< 1 μm) and contain 2 elongate sporocysts. There is neither an oocyst residuum nor a micropyle. Each sporocyst contains 4 elongated sporozoites and a granular sporocyst residuum which may be compact or dispersed. There is no Stieda body. Each sporozoite has a central to terminal nucleus, several cytoplasmic granules and a crystalloid body, but there is no refractile body. The thin oocyst wall often ruptures, releasing the sporocysts into the intes-

tinal lumen from which they are passed in the faeces. The prepatent and patent periods vary, but for most *Sarcocystis* species oocysts are first shed in faeces 7–14 days after ingesting sarcocysts.

The number of generations of schizogony and the type of host cell in which schizogony may occur vary with each species of *Sarcocystis*, but trends are apparent. For example, all species of *Sarcocystis* of large domestic animals (sheep, goats, cattle, pigs and horses) form first and second generation schizonts in the vascular endothelium whereas only a single precystic generation of schizogony has been found in *Sarcocystis* species of small mammals (mice and deer mice) and this is generally in hepatocytes (Dubey, Speer and Fayer 1989).

Sarcocysts, which are always located within a PV in the host cell cytoplasm, consist of a cyst wall that surrounds the metrocyte or the bradyzoites. The structure and thickness of the cyst wall differs among species of *Sarcocystis* and within each species as the sarcocyst matures (Tadras and Laarman 1978). Histologically, the sarcocyst wall may be smooth, striated or hirsute, or may possess complex branched protrusions. These protrusions are of taxonomic importance (Fig. 17.1). Internally, groups of zoites may be segregated into compartments by septa that originate from the sarcocyst wall or they may not be compartmentalized.

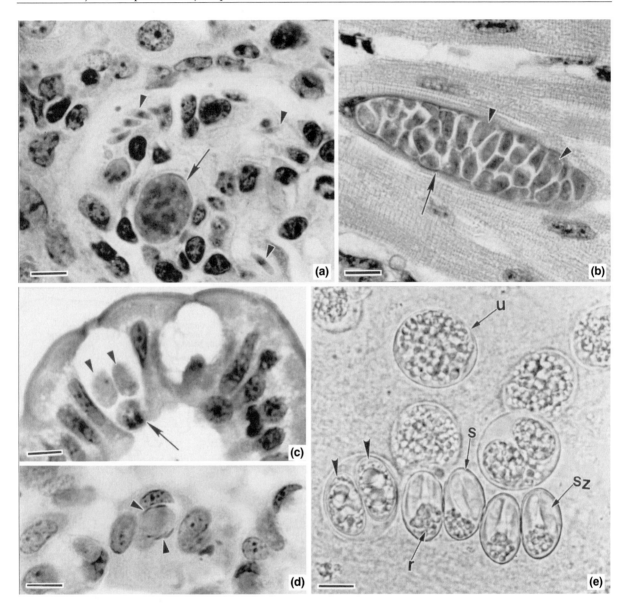

Fig. 17.3 Asexual and sexual stages of *S. cruzi*. (a) Second generation schizont (arrow) and released merozoites (arrowheads) in renal glomerulus of a calf. Haematoxylin and eosin. Bar = 10 μm. (b) Intramuscular immature sarcocyst (arrow) containing metrocytes (arrowheads). Haematoxylin and eosin. Bar = 10 μm. (c) Two female gamonts (arrowheads) and a male gamont (arrow) in a goblet cell, 6 h after infection of a coyote. Iron haematoxylin. Bar = 10 μm. (d) Mature microgamont with 5 microgametes (arrowheads) in an epithelial cell 6 h after infection of a coyote. Iron haematoxylin. Bar = 10 μm. (e) Sporogony of *S. cruzi* in the intestinal lamina propria of a coyote. Note unsporulated oocyst (u), partially sporulated oocysts with immature sporocysts (arrowheads), an oocyst with 2 sporocysts (s), and 2 fully sporulated oocysts containing sporozoites (sz) and residual body (r). Unstained. Bar = 10 μm (from Dubey et al. 1989, with permission).

Not all species of *Sarcocystis* are pathogenic (Dubey, Speer and Fayer 1989). Generally species using canids as definitive hosts are more pathogenic than those using felids. For example, of the 3 species in cattle, *S. cruzi* for which the dog is the definitive host is the most pathogenic whereas *S. hirsuta* and *S. hominis*, which undergo sexual development in cats and primates respectively, are only mildly pathogenic (Table 17.3). Pathogenicity is manifested in the intermediate host. *Sarcocystis* generally does not cause illness in definitive hosts.

3 CLINICAL IMPORTANCE OF SARCOCYSTOSIS

3.1 Sarcocystosis in humans

Humans serve as the definitive host for *S. hominis* and *S. suihominis* and also serve as accidental intermediate hosts for several unidentified species of *Sarcocystis*. Symptoms vary with the species of *Sarcocystis* causing the infection.

Table 17.3 *Sarcocystis* species in livestock

Intermediate host	*Sarcocystis* species	Reference	Sarcocysts Maximum length (mm)	Wall (mm)	Pathogenicity[a]	Definitive hosts
Cattle (*Bos taurus*)	*S. cruzi*	(Hasselmann, 1926) Wenyon, 1926	<1	7	++	Dog, coyote, red fox, raccoon, wolf
	S. hirsuta	Moulé, 1888	7	10	±	Cat
	S. hominis	(Railliet and Lucet, 1891) Dubey, 1976	7	10	±|	Man, other primates
Sheep (*Ovis aries*)	*S. tenella*	(Railliet, 1886) Moulé, 1886	0.7	14	++	Dog, coyote, red fox
	S. arieticanis	Heydorn, 1985	0.9	7	+	Dog
	S. gigantea	(Railliet, 1886) Ashford, 1977	10	21	−	Cat
	S. medusiformis	Collins, Atkinson, and Charleston, 1979	8	20	−	Cat
Goat (*Capra hircus*)	*S. capracanis*	Fisher, 1979	1	14	++	Dog, coyote, red fox
	S. hircicanis	Heydorn and Unterhozner, 1983	2.5	7	++	Dog
	S. moule	Nevu-Nemaire, 1912	7.5	7	?	Cat
Pigs (*Sus scrofa*)	*S. miescheriana*	(Künn, 1865) Labbé, 1899	1.5	10(?)	+	Dog, raccoon, wolf, red fox, jackal
	S. porcifelis	Dubey, 1976	?	?	?	Cat
	S. suihominis	(Tadros and Laarman, 1976) Heydorn, 1977	1.5	10	+	Humans, primates
Horses (*Equus caballus*)	*S. fayeri*	Dubey, Streitel, Stromberg, and Toussant, 1977	1.0	11	±	Dog
	S. equicanis	Rommel and Geisel, 1975	0.35	?	?	Dog
	S. bertrami	Doflein, 1901	12	?	?	Dog
Water buffalo (*Bubalus bubalis*)	*S. levinei*	Dissanike and Kan, 1978	1.1	7(?)	+	Dog
	S. fusiformis	(Railliet, 1897) Bernard and Bauche, 1912	3	21	−	Cat
Camel (*Camelus* spp.)	*S. cameli*	Mason, 1910	0.38	?	?	Dog
	S. sp	Mason, 1910	?	?	?	?
Chickens (*Gallus gallus*)	*S. horvathi*	Ratz, 1908	0.98	?	?	?
	S. sp	Wenzel, Erber, Boch and Schellner, 1982	?	?	?	Dog, cat
Ducks (*Anas* spp.)	*S. rileyi*	(Stiles, 1893), Michin, 1903	12	23	?	Skunk

Reprinted with permission from Dubey, Speer, and Fayer (1989), where a complete bibliography can be found.
[a] ++, very pathogenic; +, pathogenic; ±, mildly pathogenic; −, non-pathogenic; ∓, questionable pathogenicity; ?, unknown or unclassified.

3.2 Intestinal sarcocystosis

Sarcocystis hominis (Railliet and Lucet, 1891) Dubey, 1976

Infection with *S. hominis* is acquired by ingesting uncooked beef containing sarcocysts. *S. hominis* is only mildly pathogenic. A volunteer who ate raw beef from an experimentally infected calf developed nausea, stomachache and diarrhoea 3–6 h after ingesting the beef; these symptoms lasted 24–36 h and *S. hominis* sporocysts were excreted between 14–18 days after ingestion of the beef, during which time the volunteer had diarrhoea and stomachache (Heydorn 1977). Somewhat similar but milder symptoms were experienced by other volunteers who ate uncooked naturally infected beef (Rommel and Heydorn 1972, Aryeetey and Piekarski 1976, Hiepe et al. 1979).

Sarcocystis suihominis (Tadros and Laarman, 1976) Heydorn, 1977

This species, acquired by eating undercooked pork, is more pathogenic than *S. hominis*. Human volunteers developed hypersensitivity-like symptoms; nausea, vomiting, stomachache, diarrhoea and dyspnoea within 24 h of ingestion of uncooked pork from naturally or experimentally infected pigs. Sporocysts were shed 11–13 days after ingesting the infected pork (Rommel and Heydorn 1972, Piekarski et al. 1978, Hiepe et al. 1979, Kimmig, Piekarski and Heydorn 1979).

Natural prevalence of intestinal sarcocystosis of humans

Before the discovery of the life cycle of *Sarcocystis* and recognition of cattle and pigs as sources of human infection, *Sarcocystis* sporocysts in human faeces were referred to as *Isospora hominis*. Because of structural similarities between *S. hominis* and *S. suihominis* sporocysts, it is not possible to distinguish between them by microscopic examination. Intestinal sarcocystosis is more common in Europe than in other continents. *Sarcocystis* sporocysts were seen in 2% of 3500 faecal samples in France (Deluol et al. 1980), 1.6% of 1518 samples in Germany (Flentje, Jungman and Hiepe 1975, Janitschke 1975) and 10.4% of 125 faecal samples from 7–18 year old children in Poland (Plotkowiak 1976). Enteritis was associated with shedding of *Sarcocystis* sporocysts in 6 cases in Thailand and 2 cases reported from the People's Republic of China (reviewed in Dubey, Speer and Fayer 1989).

3.3 Muscular sarcocystosis

Sarcocysts have been found in striated muscles of humans, mostly as incidental findings. Judging from the published reports, sarcocysts in humans are rare (Beaver, Gadgil and Morera 1979); most reported cases are from Asia. Of the 40 histologically diagnosed reports that Beaver, Gadgil and Morera (1979) reviewed and 6 additional cases since 1982 reviewed by Dubey, Speer and Fayer (1989) 15 were from south-east Asia, 11 from India, 5 from Central and South America, 4 from Europe, 4 from Africa, 3 from the USA, 1 from China; the source of 2 was undetermined. Of the 46 confirmed cases, sarcocysts were found in skeletal muscles of 35 and in the heart of 11. The clinical significance of sarcocysts and the life cycles of sarcocysts of humans are unknown.

4 Epidemiology and control

Sarcocystis infection is common in many species of animals worldwide (Dubey, Speer and Fayer 1989). A variety of conditions permit such high prevalence: a host may harbour any of several species of *Sarcocystis;* many definitive hosts are involved in transmission; large numbers of sporocysts may be shed; *Sarcocystis* oocysts and sporocysts develop in the lamina propria, and are discharged over a period of many months; and, as oocysts and sporocysts are resistant to freezing, they can overwinter on the pasture; *Sarcocystis* sporocysts and oocysts remain viable for many months in the environment; they may be spread by invertebrate transport hosts; there is little or no immunity to reshedding of sporocysts, and therefore, each meal of infected meat can initiate a new round of sporocyst production; and the fact that *Sarcocystis* oocysts, unlike those of many other species of coccidia, are passed in faeces in the infective form frees them from dependence on weather conditions for maturation and infectivity.

Poor hygiene during handling of meat between slaughter and cooking can be a source of *Sarcocystis* infection. In one survey in India, *S. suihominis* oocysts were found in faeces of 14 of 20 3–12 year old children (Banerjee, Bhatia and Pandit 1994) indicating that meat was consumed raw at least by some because *S. suihominis* can be transmitted to humans only by the consumption of raw pork. In another study, 3–5-year-old children from a slum area were found to consume meat scraps virtually raw, and many pigs from that area harboured *S. suihominis* sarcocysts (Solanki, Shrivastava and Shah 1991). In European countries where the frequency of consumption of raw or undercooked meat is relatively high, humans are likely to have intestinal sarcocystosis. In one survey 60.7% of pigs had *S. suihominis* sarcocysts in their muscles (Boch, Mannewitz and Erber 1978).

5 Chemotherapy and control of sarcocystosis

There is no treatment for *Sarcocystis* infection of humans. On the basis of results in experimental animals, it is probable that sulfonamides and pyrimethamine may be helpful in treating sarcocystosis (Rommel, Schwerdfeger and Blenaska 1981).

There is no vaccine to protect livestock or humans against sarcocystosis. Shedding of *Sarcocystis* oocysts and sporocysts in faeces of the definitive hosts is the key factor in the spread of *Sarcocystis* infection; to interrupt this cycle, carnivores should be excluded from animal houses and from feed, water and bedding for livestock. Uncooked meat or offal should never be fed to carnivores. As freezing can drastically reduce or eliminate infectious sarcocysts, meat should be frozen if not cooked. Exposure to heat at 55°C for 20 minutes kills sarcocysts so only limited cooking or heating is required to kill sporocysts (Fayer 1975). Dead livestock should be buried or incinerated. Dead animals should never be left in the field for vultures and carnivores to eat.

6 DIAGNOSIS

The antemortem diagnosis of muscular sarcocystosis can only be made by histological examination of muscle collected by biopsy. The finding of immature sarcocysts with metrocytes suggests recently acquired infection and the finding of mature sarcocysts indicates only past infection.

The diagnosis of intestinal sarcocystosis is easily made by faecal examination. As has been mentioned, sporocysts or oocysts of sarcocystis are shed fully sporulated in faeces whereas those of *Isospora belli* are often shed unsporulated (Fig. 17.4). It is not possible to distinguish one species of *Sarcocystis* from another by the examination of sporocysts.

ISOSPORA BELLI

Isospora belli Wenyon, 1923 is uncommon in humans. Most of cases occur in the tropics and are now seen most frequently in immunocompromised patients, particularly those with AIDS (Dubey 1977, Hallak et al. 1982, DeHovitz et al. 1986, Restrepo, Macher and Radany 1987, Greenberg et al. 1988, Dubey 1993, Michiels et al. 1994).

7 STRUCTURE AND LIFE CYCLE

Unsporulated *I. belli* oocysts are elongate and ellipsoidal, measuring 20–33 × 10–19 μm (Fig. 17.4a). Sporulated oocysts contain 2 ellipsoidal sporocysts without a Stieda body. Each sporocyst is 9–14 × 7–12 μm and contains 4 crescent-shaped sporozoites and a residual body. No oocyst residuum is present. Sporulation occurs within 5 days, both within the host and in

the external environment (Brandborg, Goldberg and Breidenbach 1970, Trier et al. 1974). Both unsporulated and sporulated oocysts may thus be shed in faeces.

Infection occurs by the ingestion of food contaminated by oocysts. Merogony and gametogony occur in the upper small-intestinal epithelial cells, from the level of the crypts to the tips of the villi. Occasionally single zoites and meronts occur in the lamina propria. The number of generations of merogony is unknown. In 3 AIDS patients, zoites or groups of zoites were reported to occur in mesenteric and tracheobronchial lymph nodes (Restrepo, Macher and Radany 1987), gallbladder (Benator et al. 1994) and mesenteric and mediastinal lymph nodes, liver and spleen (Michiels et al. 1994). The zoites, surrounded by a capsule (cyst wall), had a prominent refractile or crystalloid body, indicating that the encysted organisms were sporozoites. Organisms surrounded by a cyst wall were found only in extraintestinal organs. In the patient described by Michiels et al. (1994) there were numerous encysted zoites, indicating repeated autoinfection because sporozoites do not multiply in the body (Fig. 17.5).

Most information about the life cycle of *I. belli* is based on the study of biopsy material obtained from infected patients (Brandborg, Goldberg and Breidenbach 1970, Trier et al. 1974). Intestinal stages can be found in the absence of oocysts in the faeces. It may be that oocysts sporulate and excyst in the duodenum thereby causing continued merogony and gametogony. If this type of life cycle occurs it might explain the chronic nature of the disease.

8 PATHOGENICITY

Isospora belli can cause severe clinical symptoms with an acute onset particularly in AIDS patients. Symptoms include fever, malaise, cholecystitis, persistent diarrhoea, weight loss, steatorrhoea and even death (Brandborg, Goldberg and Breidenbach 1970, Syrkis et al. 1975, Liebman et al. 1980, Butler and Deboer 1981, Guisantes, Rull and Rubio 1982, Peters et al. 1987, Restrepo, Macher and Radany 1987, Benator et al. 1994).

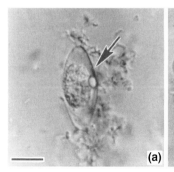 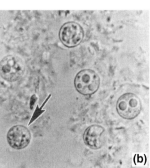 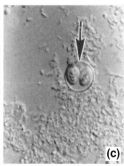

(a) **(b)** **(c)**

Fig. 17.4 Coccidian oocysts in human faeces. (a) Unsporulated *I. belli* oocyst (arrow). (b) Unsporulated (arrow) *C. cayetanesis* oocyst. (c) Sporulated (arrow) *C. cayetanesis* oocyst with 2 sporocysts. Bar = 10 μm. (Courtesy of Drs Y. Ortega and C. Sterling).

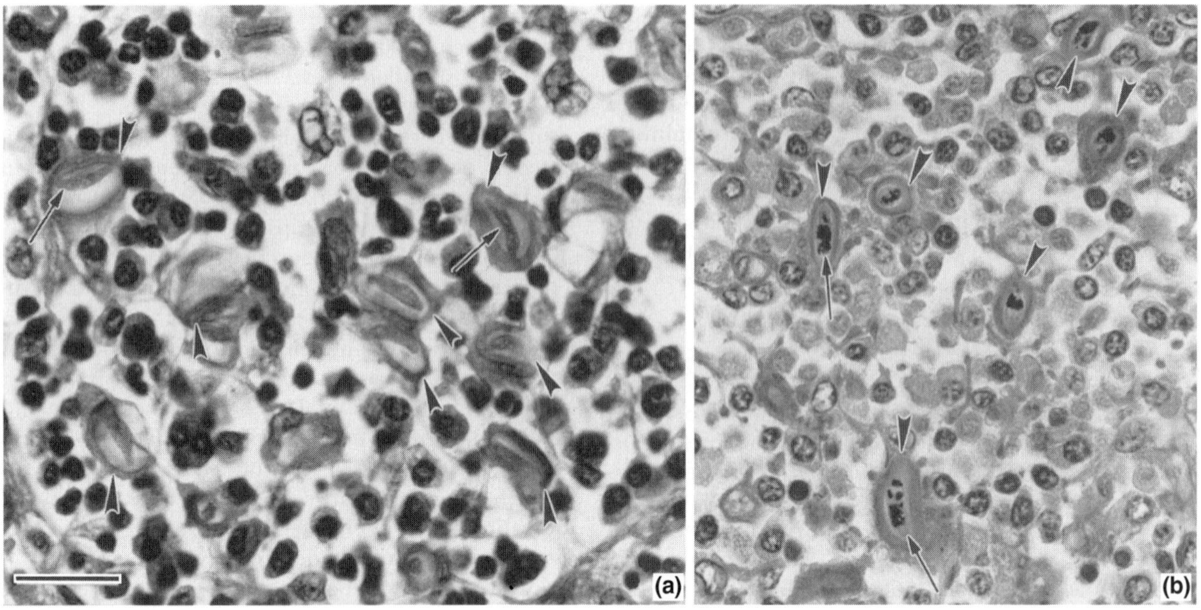

Fig. 17.5 *Isospora belli*-like single sporozoites in spleen of an AIDS patient. (a) Numerous encysted zoites (arrowheads). The cyst wall is thick and encloses one sporozoite (arrowheads). Haematoxylin and eosin. Bar = 20 μm. (b) Tissue cysts with thick PAS-negative cyst wall (arrowheads) enclosing single PAS-positive sporozoites (arrows). Periodic acid–Schiff haematoxylin. Bar = 20 μm. (Courtesy of Michiels et al. 1994.)

9 DIAGNOSIS

Diagnosis can be established by finding characteristic bell-shaped oocysts in the faeces (Fig. 17.4a) or coccidian stages in intestinal biopsy material. Affected intestinal portions have a flat mucosa similar to that which occurs in sprue. The stools during infection are fatty and at times very watery.

10 TREATMENT

Sulfonamides are considered effective against coccidiosis (St. Georgiev 1993). Trier et al. (1974) successfully treated a patient with pyrimethamine and sulfadiazine in doses similar to those used for treating toxoplasmosis (75 mg pyrimethamine and 4 g of sulfadiazine in divided doses).

CYCLOSPORA CAYETANENSIS

In 1986, unidentified 8 × 10 μm coccidian-like oocysts were first reported in faeces of humans with diarrhoea by Soave et al. (1986). Ortega, Gilman and Sterling (1994) identified the parasite and named it *Cyclospora cayetanensis*.

11 STRUCTURE AND LIFE CYCLE

Cyclospora cayetanensis oocysts are approximately 8 μm

in diameter and they contain 2 ovoid 4 × 6 μm sporocysts (Fig. 17.4b,c). Each sporocyst has 2 sporozoites. Thus there are a total of 4 sporozoites in a sporulated oocyst. Unsporulated oocysts are excreted in faeces (Fig. 17.4b). Sporulation occurs outside the body. Other stages in the life cycle are not known.

12 CLINICAL MANIFESTATIONS

C. cayetanensis infected patients of all ages both immunocompetent and immunosuppressed may have diarrhoea, fever, fatigue and abdominal cramps. Infection has been reported from several countries including the USA, Peru, Nepal and the UK (Long et al. 1991, Bendall et al. 1993, Connor et al. 1993, Ortega et al. 1993, Rijpstra and Laarman 1993, Adal 1994, Hoge et al. 1995, Soave and Johnson 1995).

13 DIAGNOSIS

Diagnosis can be made by faecal examination. *Cyclospora* oocysts are approximately 8 μm in diameter, remarkably uniform in shape and size, and contain a sporont (inner mass) that occupies most of the oocyst. They are acid-fast and may be difficult to distinguish from *Cryptosporidium muris* oocysts. Unlike cryptosporidial oocysts, *C. cayetanensis* oocysts have a much thicker oocyst wall and their contents are more granular than are those of cryptosporidial oocysts.

14 TREATMENT

No treatment is known.

REFERENCES

Adal KA, 1994, From Wisconsin to Nepal: *Cryptosporidium, Cyclospora,* and microsporidia, *Curr Opin Infect Dis,* **7:** 609–15.

Aryeetey ME, Piekarski G, 1976, Serologische *Sarcocystis*-Studien an Menschen und Ratten, *Z Parasitenkd,* **50:** 109–24.

Banerjee PS, Bhatia BB, Pandit BA, 1994, Sarcocystis *suihominis* infection in human beings in India, *J Vet Parasitol,* **8:** 57–8.

Beaver PC, Gadgil RK, Morera P, 1979, *Sarcocystis* in man: A review and report of five cases, *Am J Trop Med Hyg,* **28:** 819–44.

Benator DA, French AL et al., 1994, *Isospora belli* infection associated with acalculous cholecystitis in a patient with AIDS, *Ann Intern Med,* **121:** 663–4.

Bendall RP, Lucas S et al., 1993, Diarrhoea associated with cyanobacterium-like bodies: a new coccidian enteritis of man, *Lancet,* **341:** 590–2.

Boch J, Mannewitz U, Erber M, 1978, Sarkosporidien bei Schlachtschweinen in Süddeutschland, *Berl Münch Tierärztl Wochenschr,* **91:** 106–11.

Brandborg LL, Goldberg SB, Breidenbach WC, 1970, Human coccidiosis-A possible cause of malabsorption. The life cycle in small-bowel mucosal biopsies as a diagnostic feature, *N Engl J Med,* **283:** 1306–13.

Butler T, de Boer WGRM, 1981, *Isospora belli* infection in Australia, *Pathology,* **13:** 593–5.

Connor BA, Shlim DR et al., 1993, Pathologic changes in the small bowel in nine patients with diarrhea associated with a coccidia-like body, *Ann Intern Med,* **119:** 377–82.

DeHovitz JA, Pape JW et al., 1986, Clinical manifestations and therapy of *Isospora belli* infection in patients with the acquired immunodeficiency syndrome, *N Engl J Med,* **315:** 87–90.

Deluol AM, Mechali D et al., 1980, Incidence et aspects cliniques des coccidioses intestinales dans une consultation de médecine tropicale, *Bull Soc Pathol Exot,* **73:** 259–66.

Dubey JP, 1977, *Toxoplasma, Hammondia, Besnoitia, Sarcocystis,* and other tissue cyst-forming coccidia of man and animals, *Parasitic Protozoa,* 1st edn, vo. III, ed. Kreier JP, Academic Press, New York, 101–237.

Dubey JP, 1993, *Toxoplasma, Neospora, Sarcocystis,* and other tissue cyst-forming coccidia of humans and animals, *Parasitic Protozoa,* 2nd edn, vol. 6, ed. Kreier JP, Academic Press, New York, 1–158.

Dubey JP, Speer CA, Fayer R, 1989, *Sarcocystosis of Animals and Man,* CRC Press, Boca Raton, FL.

Fayer R, 1975, Effects of refrigeration, cooking, and freezing on *Sarcocystis* in beef from retail food stores, *Proc Helminthol Soc Wash,* **42:** 138–40.

Flentje B, Jungman R, Hiepe T, 1975, Vorkommen von *Isospora-hominis*-Sporozysten beim Menschen, *Dt Gesundh -Wesen,* **30:** 523–5.

Greenberg SJ, Davey MP et al., 1988, *Isospora belli* enteric infection in patients with human T-cell leukemia virus type I-associated adult T-cell leukemia, *Am J Med,* **85:** 435–8.

Guisantes JA, Rull S, Rubio MF, 1982, Human coccidiosis by *Isospora belli* and malabsorption, *Rev Ibér Parasitol,* **42:** 223–30.

Hallak A, Yust I et al., 1982, Malabsorption syndrome, coccidiosis, combined immune deficiency, and fulminant lymphoproliferative disease, *Arch Intern Med,* **142:** 196–7.

Heydorn AO, 1977, Sarkosporidieninfiziertes Fleisch als mögliche Krankheitsursache für den Menschen, *Arch Lebensmittelhygiene,* **28:** 27–31.

Hiepe F, Hiepe T et al., 1979, Experimentelle Infektion des Menschen und von Tieraffen (*Cercopithecus callitrichus*) mit Sarkosporidien-Zysten von Rind und Schwein, *Arch Exp Vet Med,* **33:** 819–30.

Hoge C, Shlim R et al., 1995, Placebo-controlled trial of co-trimoxazole for cyclospora infections among travellers and foreign residents in Nepal, *Lancet,* **345:** 691–93.

Janitschke K, 1975, Neue Erkenntnisse über die Kokzidien-Infektionen des Menschen. II. *Isospora*-Infektion, *Bundesgesundheitsblatt,* **18:** 419–22.

Kimmig P, Piekarski G, Heydorn AO, 1979, Zur Sarkosporidiose (*Sarcocystis suihominis*) des Menschen (II), *Immun Infekt,* **7:** 170–7.

Liebman WM, Thaler MM et al., 1980, Intractable diarrhea of infancy due to intestinal coccidiosis, *Gastroenterology,* **78:** 579–84.

Long EG, White EH et al., 1991, Morphologic and staining characteristics of a *Cyanobacterium*-like organism associated with diarrhea, *J Infect Dis,* **164:** 199–202.

Michiels JF, Hofman P et al., 1994, Intestinal and extraintestinal *Isospora belli* infection in an Aids patient. A second case report, *Pathol Res Pract,* **190:** 1089–93.

Ortega YR, Gilman RH, Sterling CR, 1994, A new coccidian parasite (Apicomplexa: Eimeriidae) from humans, *J Parasitol,* **80:** 625–9.

Ortega YR, Sterling CR et al., 1993, *Cyclospora* species: a new protozoan pathogen of humans, *N Engl J Med,* **328:** 1308–12.

Peters CS, Kathpalia SB et al., 1987, *Isospora belli* and *Cryptosporidium* sp. from a patient not suspected of having acquired immunodeficiency syndrome, *Diagn Microbiol Infect Dis,* **8:** 197–9.

Piekarski G, Heydorn AO et al., 1978, Klinische, parasitologische und serologische Untersuchungen zur Sarkosporidiose (*Sarcocystis suihominis*) des Menschen, *Immun Infekt,* **6:** 153–9.

Plotkowiak J, 1976, Wyniki dalszych badan nad wystepowaniem i epidemiologia inwazji *Isospora hominis* (Railliet I Lucet, 1891), *Wiadomosci Parazytol,* **22:** 137–47.

Restrepo C, Macher AM, Radany EH, 1987, Disseminated extraintestinal isosporiasis in a patient with acquired immune deficiency syndrome, *Am J Clin Pathol,* **87:** 536–42.

Rijpstra AC, Laarman JJ, 1993, Repeated findings of unidentified small *Isospora*-like coccidia in faecal specimens from travellers returning to the Netherlands, *Trop Geogr Med,* **45:** 280–2.

Rommel M, Heydorn AO, 1972, Beitrage zum Lebenszyklus der Sarkosporidien. III. *Isospora hominis* (Railliet und Lucet, 1891) Wenyon, 1923, eine Dauerform der Sarkosporidien des Rindes und des Schweins, *Berl Münch Tierärztl Wochenschr,* **85:** 143–5.

Rommel M, Schwerdfeger A, Blewaska S, 1981, The *Sarcocystis muris*-infection as a model for research on the chemotherapy of acute sarcocystosis of domestic animals, *Zentralbl Bakteriol Hyg I Abt Orig A,* **250:** 268–76.

Soave R, Dubey JP et al., 1986, A new intestinal pathogen?, *Clin Res,* **34:** 533A.

Soave R, Johnson WD, 1995, Cyclospora: conquest of an emerging pathogen, *Lancet,* **345:** 667–8.

Solanki PK, Shrivastava HOP, Shah HL, 1991, Prevalence of *Sarcocystis* in naturally infected pigs in Madhya-Pradesh with an epidemiological explanation for the higher prevalence of *Sarcocystis suihominis,* *Indian J Anim Sci,* **61:** 820–1.

St. Georgiev V, 1993, Opportunistic infections: treatment and developmental therapeutics of cryptosporidiosis and isosporiasis, *Drug Develop Res,* **28:** 445–59.

Syrkis I, Fried M et al., 1975, A case of severe human coccidiosis in Israel, *Israel J Med Sci,* **11:** 373–7.

Tadros W, Laarman JJ, 1978, A comparative study of the light and electron microscopic structure of the walls of the muscle cysts of several species of sarcocystid eimeriid coccidia, *Proc Konink Nederl Akad Wetensch,* **81:** 469–91.

Trier JS, Moxey PC et al., 1974, Chronic intestinal coccidiosis in man: intestinal morphology and response to treatment, *Gastroenterology,* **66:** 923–35.

CRYPTOSPORIDIOSIS

W L Current

1 HISTORICAL INTRODUCTION

Organisms of the genus *Cryptosporidium* are small coccidian parasites that infect the microvillous region of epithelial cells lining the digestive and respiratory organs of vertebrates (Angus 1983, Fayer and Ungar 1986, Current and Garcia 1991, O'Donoghue 1995). Clarke (1895) may have been the first to observe a species of *Cryptosporidium* which he described as 'swarm spores lying upon the gastric epithelium of mice'. These small organisms were probably the motile merozoites of *C. muris*, the type species named and described approximately 12 years later by the American parasitologist EE Tyzzer (1907). This small coccidian, infecting the gastric epithelium of laboratory mice, was placed in a new genus (*Cryptosporidium* = hidden sporocysts) because, unlike the previously known coccidia, the oocyst of this parasite did not have sporocysts surrounding the sporozoites. Approximately 17 years later, Tyzzer (1929) described and illustrated the developmental stages of a species of *Cryptosporidium* in the caecal epithelium of chickens.

During the 50 years following Tyzzer's original reports, *Cryptosporidium* spp. received little attention from the biomedical research community because they were not regarded as economically or medically important. Studies conducted from 1961 to 1986 that relied primarily on structural features of oocysts resulted in the naming of approximately 19 additional species of *Cryptosporidium* from fishes, reptiles, birds, and mammals (Levine 1984, Fayer and Ungar 1986, Current and Garcia 1991). Only a few of these named species, including the 2 originally described by Tyzzer, are now considered valid (see section 2, Classification).

The 1955 report of Slavin was the first to associate cryptosporidiosis with morbidity and mortality. He described a severe diarrhoea and some deaths in 10–14 day-old turkey poults and attributed the illness to a new species, *C. meleagridis* (Slavin 1955). Interest in *Cryptosporidium* by the veterinary medical profession was stimulated in 1971 when *C. parvum* was first reported to be associated with bovine diarrhoea (Panciera, Thomassen and Gardner 1971). Since then, numerous case reports from many different animals are now present in the literature and one species, *C. parvum*, is recognized as an important cause of neonatal diarrhoea in calves and lambs (Current and Garcia 1991). Another species, *C. baileyi*, causes respiratory disease in poultry (Current, Upton and Haynes 1986, Blagburn et al. 1987).

The first cases of human cryptosporidiosis were reported in 1976 (Meisel et al. 1976, Nime et al. 1976) and subsequent reports were rare until it was recognized that *C. parvum* may produce a short-term diarrhoeal illness in immunocompetent persons and a prolonged, life-threatening, cholera-like illness in immune deficient patients, especially those with the acquired immune deficiency syndrome (AIDS) (Current et al. 1983, Fayer and Ungar 1986, Crawford and Vermund 1988, Current and Garcia 1991). Additional details of the historical events outlined above can be found in review papers (Angus et al. 1983, Fayer and Ungar 1986, Crawford and Vermund 1988, Dubey, Speer and Fayer 1990, Current and Garcia 1991, O'Donoghue 1995, McDonald 1996, Fayer 1997).

2 CLASSIFICATION

Cryptosporidium is classified in the phylum Apicomplexa (Sporozoa), the same group as species of *Plasmo-dium*, causing malaria in humans, but in a different order. More closely related to *Cryptosporidium* spp. are the other true coccidia (order Eimeriida), *Cyclospora cayetanensis*, *Isospora belli*, *Sarcocystis* spp. and *Toxo-plasma gondii*, which infect humans and *Eimeria* spp. which infect other mammals and birds. Most species of *Cryptosporidium* named in the biomedical literature following Tyzzer's creation of the genus were done so with the assumption that these coccidia were as host specific as the closely related (taxonomically) species of *Eimeria* infecting mammals and birds. However, cross-transmission studies conducted in the early 1980s demonstrated little or no host specificity for 'species' of *Cryptosporidium* isolated from mammals (see O'Donoghue 1995). Lack of host specificity exhibited by mammalian isolates prompted Tzipori et al. (1980) to consider *Cryptosporidium* as a single species genus. A more realistic approach was presented by Levine (1984) who consolidated the 21 named parasites into 4 species; one each for those infecting fishes (*C. nasorum*), reptiles (*C. crotali*), birds (*C. meleagridis*), and mammals (*C. muris*). This consolidation was not entirely correct. *C. crotali* is now considered to be a species of *Sarcocystis*. At least 2 valid species, *C. baileyi* and *C. meleagridis*, infect birds (Current, Upton and Haynes 1986) and also at least 2 valid species infect mammals (*C. parvum* infecting the small intestine and *C. muris* infecting the stomach). On the basis of oocyst morphology, *C. parvum*, not *C. muris*, is associated with all well-documented cases of cryptosporidiosis in mammals (Upton and Current 1985). Thus, the species with oocysts measuring 4–5 μm that produces clinical illness in humans and other mammals should be referred to as *C. parvum*, or *Cryptosporidium* sp. if there is not enough morphologic, life-cycle, and/or host specificity data to relate it to Tyzzer's original description.

3 STRUCTURE AND LIFE CYCLE

Studies of different isolates (calf and human) of *C. parvum* in suckling mice (Current and Reese 1986) revealed that the life cycle of this parasite (Figs 18.1, 18.2) is similar to that of other true coccidia (e.g., *Eimeria* and *Isospora* spp.) infecting mammals in that it can be divided into 6 major developmental events: **excystation**, the release of infective sporozoites; **mero-gony** (schizogony), the asexual multiplication within host cells; **gametogony**, the formation of micro- and macrogametes; **fertilization**, the union of micro- and macro-gametes; oocyst **wall formation,** to produce an environmentally resistant stage that transmits infection from one host to another; and **sporogony**, the formation of infective sporozoites within the oocyst wall. The life cycle of human and calf isolates of *C. parvum* differs somewhat from that of other monoxenous (one host in life cycle) coccidia such as *Eimeria* and *Isospora* spp., parasites usually presented as the 'typical coccidia'. Each intracellular stage of *C. parvum* resides within a parasitophorous vacuole confined to

the microvillous region of the host cell, whereas comparable stages of *Eimeria* or *Isospora* spp. occupy parasitophorous vacuoles deep (perinuclear) within the host cells. Oocysts of *C. parvum* undergo sporogony while they are within the host cells and are infective when released in the faeces, whereas oocysts of *Eimeria* or *Isospora* spp. do not sporulate until they are passed from the host and exposed for 1–14 days to oxygen and temperatures below 37°C. Studies using experimentally infected mice have also shown that approximately 20% of the oocysts of *C. parvum* within host enterocytes do not form a thick, 2-layered, environmentally resistant oocyst wall. The 4 sporozoites of this autoinfective stage are surrounded only by a single unit membrane. Soon after being released from a host cell, the membrane surrounding the 4 sporozoites ruptures and these invasive forms penetrate into the microvillous region of other enterocytes and reinitiate the life cycle (Current and Reese 1986). Approximately 80% of the oocysts of *C. parvum* in enterocytes of suckling mice are similar to those of *Eimeria* and *Isospora* spp. in that they develop thick, environmentally resistant oocyst walls and are passed in the faeces. Thick-walled oocysts are the life cycle forms that transmit the infection from one host to another. Autoinfective, thin-walled oocysts and type I meronts (schizonts) that can recycle are believed to be the life cycle forms of *C. parvum* responsible for the development of severe infections in hosts exposed to only a small number of thick-walled oocysts, and for persistent, life-threatening disease in immune-deficient persons who are not exposed repeatedly to these environmentally resistant stages. Light microscopic and ultrastructural features of some of the developmental stages of *Crypto-sporidium* in enterocytes of the experimentally infected host are shown in Figs 18.2–18.4. Additional details of the ultrastructure of *Cryptosporidium* spp. can be found in several publications (Goebel and Brandler 1982, Reduker, Speer and Blixt 1985, Upton and Current 1985, Current and Reese 1986).

4 BIOCHEMISTRY, MOLECULAR BIOLOGY AND GENETICS

Although *C. parvum* is a well-known cause of gastrointestinal illness in humans and domesticated animals, surprisingly little is known about the biochemistry, molecular biology, and genetics of this obligate intracellular protozoan. The life cycles of *Cryptosporidium* spp. are similar to those of other coccidia; however, what little is known about their basic biochemistry suggests major differences. Also, studies of small-subunit ribosomal RNAs suggest that *Cryptosporidium* spp. are more closely related to *Plasmodium* spp. (the causative agents of malaria) than to the true coccidia *Eimeria*, *Isospora*, *Toxoplasma*, and *Sarcocystis* (Johnson et al. 1990). Many anticoccidial agents active against *Eimeria*, *Isospora* and/or *Toxoplasma* have little or no effect on *Cryptosporidium* (Blagburn and Soave 1997). Mitochondria present in other coccidia have not been seen in *C. parvum* (Current and Reese 1986). *Cryptospo-*

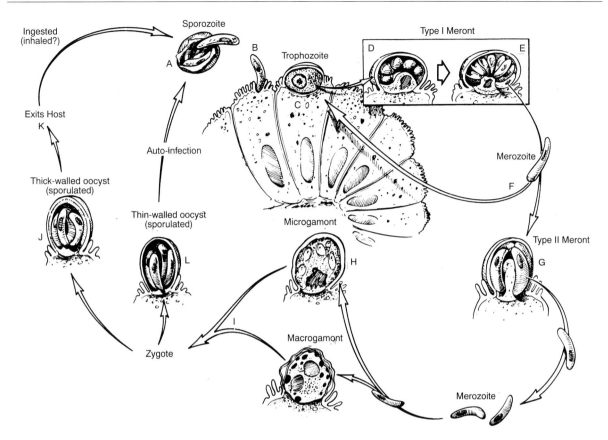

Fig. 18.1. The proposed life cycle of *C. parvum* as it occurs in the mucosal epithelium of an infected mammalian host. Living developmental stages of *C. parvum* corresponding to those labelled (A–L) here are shown in Fig. 18.2. After excysting from oocysts in the lumen of the intestine (A), sporozoites (B) penetrate into host cells, and develop into trophozoites (= uninucleate meronts) (C) within parasitophorous vacuoles confined to the microvillous region of the mucosal epithelium. Trophozoites (uninucleate meronts) (C) undergo asexual divisions (merogony = schizogony) (D) to form merozoites (E). After being released from type I meronts, the invasive merozoites enter adjacent host cells to form additional type I meronts (recycling of type I meronts) (F) or to form type II meronts (G). Type II meronts do not recycle but enter host cells to form the sexual stages, microgamonts (H) and macrogamonts. Most (c. 80%) of the zygotes (I) formed after fertilization of the microgamont by the microgametes (released from microgamont) develop into environmentally resistant, thick-walled oocysts (J) that undergo sporogony to form sporulated oocysts (K) containing 4 sporozoites. Sporulated oocysts released in faeces are the environmentally resistant life cycle forms that transmit the infection from one host to another. A smaller percentage of zygotes (c. 20%) do not form a thick, 2-layered oocyst wall, but have only a unit membrane surrounding the 4 sporozoites. These thin-walled oocysts (L) represent autoinfective life cycle forms that can maintain the parasite in the host without repeated oral exposure to the thick-walled oocysts present in the environment. (Drawing by Kip Carter, University of Georgia. Reprinted with permission from Current and Blagburn 1990.)

ridium spp. have genes with few or no introns and their genome is approximately 12–15% that of other coccidia (Tilley and Upton 1997).

4.1 Biochemistry

Coccidia, including *Cryptosporidium*, are generally not amenable to biochemical studies because the life cycle stages residing within cells of the vertebrate host are difficult to purify and continuous in vitro cultivation has not been achieved (Current 1990). Most studies have focused on the exogenous stages of the life cycle, oocysts and sporozoites, whose gene expression and intermediary metabolism are not necessarily representative of the other life cycle forms. Oocysts and sporozoites can, however, be purified in relatively large numbers (Current 1990) and have been used to elucidate the structure and function of surface antigens

and to investigate metabolic pathways of *C. parvum*. A brief account of metabolic enzymes and lipids identified in oocysts and sporozoites is followed by a summary of what we know about 2 structures specific to the coccidia – oocyst walls and the apical complex. To date biochemical investigations of *Cryptosporidium* have provided very limited data on which to base the finding of effective therapeutic agents. A brief discussion of proteins and glycoprotein antigens in the oocyst wall and in sporozoites is presented in section 6 (Immunology).

METABOLISM

Sequence data from genomic DNA of *C. parvum* suggests that this parasite has functional thymidylate synthase (Gooze et al. 1991). Folic acid has been shown to enhance in vitro development of *C. parvum* (Upton, Tilley and Brillhart 1995). These data, along

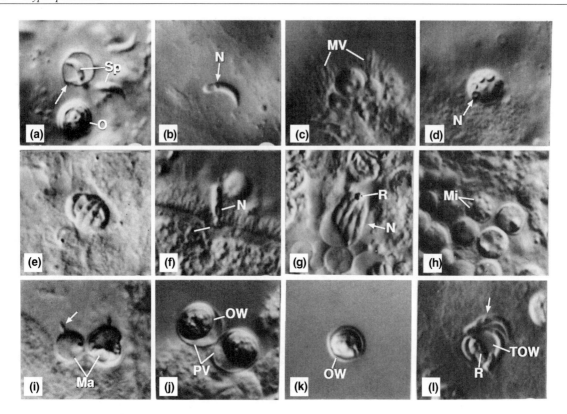

Fig. 18.2. Nomarski interference-contrast photomicrographs of developmental stages of *C. parvum* in mucosal scrapings obtained from the small intestines of experimentally infected, suckling mice: a, sporozoites (Sp) free and excysting from an oocyst (O). b, free sporozoite showing the posterior location of the nucleus (N). c, trophozoite (uninucleate meront) surrounded by hypertrophied microvilli (MV). d, Immature type I meront with peripherally located nuclei (N), 6 of which are in focus. e, Mature type I meront containing 6 or 8 merozoites. f, Merozoite penetrating into microvillous region of host enterocyte. Note the anterior location of the nucleus (N). g, Mature type II meront (schizont) showing the 4 merozoites. The residuum (R) and position of nuclei (arrows) of the 4 merozoites are shown. h. Microgamont with microgametes (Mi) budding from the surface of the residuum. i, Two macrogamonts (Ma) each with an attached microgamont (arrow points to one that is in focus). j, Two oocysts with thick walls (OW), both within parasitophorous vacuoles (PV). k, Intact thick-walled oocysts that will pass unaltered in the faeces. l, An autoinfective, thin-walled oocyst that has ruptured under coverslip pressure releasing the 4 sporozoites from the thin oocyst wall or membrane (TOW). Note the granular oocyst residuum (R) and the posterior location of the sporozoite nuclei (arrow). (Adapted from Current and Reese 1986; reprinted with permission.)

with studies showing that several sulphonamides inhibit parasite replication (Rehg 1991), suggest that *C. parvum* can incorporate exogenous folate as well as synthesizing its own folic acid.

Studies employing starch-gel zymography of isozyme extracts of oocysts of *C. parvum*, *C. muris*, and *C. baileyi* demonstrated high activity of glucose-6-phosphate isomerase and phosphoglucomutase, and weak activity of malate dehydrogenase, carboxylesterase and lactate dehydrogenase (Ogunkolade et al. 1993). No enzymatic activity has been detected for alanine aminotransferase, aspartate aminotransferase or proline iminopeptidase, suggesting but not proving lack of these enzymes.

Two enzymes of the mannitol cycle, mannitol-1-phosphate dehydrogenase and mannitol-1-phosphatase have been reported in *C. parvum* oocysts (Schmatz 1989). The mannitol cycle is common in plants, fungi and coccidia, but appears to be absent in animals and most animal-like protozoa.

Although nucleic acid metabolism has not yet been studied in *Cryptosporidium* spp., it appears that *C. parvum* is similar to *Eimeria* spp. in that it is incapable of synthesizing purines and must rely on salvage pathways requiring exogenous purines such as hypoxanthine and guanine. An anticoccidial drug, arprinocid, known to block uptake of hypoxanthine and guanine by *Eimeria* spp., is also known to inhibit growth and development of *C. parvum* in vivo (Rehg and Hancock 1990). Pyrimidines can be synthesized de novo or they can be salvaged by coccidia because they possess the enzyme uracyl phosphoribosyl transferase which converts uracil into uridylic acid. Preliminary studies suggest that *C. parvum* also possesses this enzyme since it is capable of incorporating free uracil into nucleic acids (Upton et al. 1991).

LIPIDS AND GLYCOLIPIDS

Only the basic lipid composition of sporulated oocysts of *C. parvum* has been documented (Mitschler, Welti and Upton 1994). Approximately 1.2×10^{-9} µg phospholipid per oocyst is comprised of phosphatidylcho-

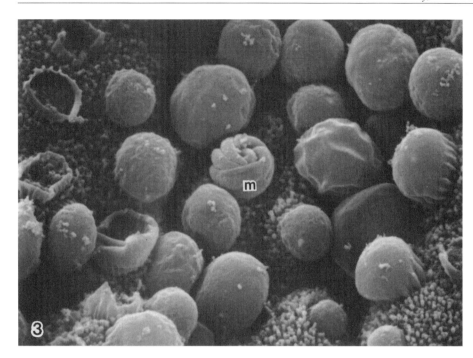

Fig. 18.3. Scanning electron micrograph showing numerous developmental stages of *Cryptosporidium* in the microvillous region of the intestinal mucosa. Each parasite is contained within a parasitophorous vacuole that bulges out from the microvillous region of the enterocyte. Some merozoites of a mature type I meront (m) are exposed as a result of a portion of the parasitophorous vacuole membrane being removed during processing. Note the craters in the mucosal surface formed by empty vacuoles that remain after the parasites are released.

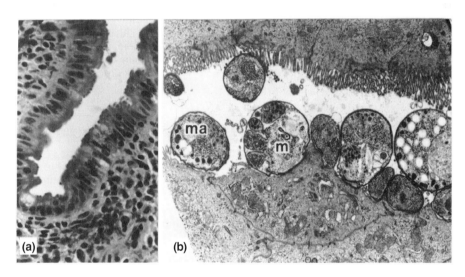

Fig. 18.4. Light photomicrograph (a) of a histological section (stained with haematoxylin and eosin) of small-bowel biopsy obtained from an immunocompromised patient with persistent cryptosporidiosis. Note the numerous developmental stages *of C. parvum* within the brush border of the enterocytes. Transmission electron micrograph (b) of developmental stages of *C. parvum* within parasitophorous vacuoles bulging from the microvillous region of ileal enterocytes of an experimentally infected mouse. Macrogametes (one labelled ma) contain the characteristic amylopectin granules near the centre and wall-forming bodies near the periphery. Several uninucleate meronts (trophozoites) and one meront (m) with budding merozoites can be seen.

line (66%), sphingomyelin (24.5%), phosphatidyle-thanolamine (7.3%), phosphatidylinositol/phos-phatidylserine (1.8%) and cardiolipin (0.9%). Major fatty acids detected were palmitic, stearic, oleic and linoleic, with smaller amounts of myristate and palmitoleate. The only sterol detected was cholesterol.

OOCYST WALL AND APICAL COMPLEX

Two structural components that are unique to protozoans in the phylum Apicomplexa, including *Cryptosporidium*, are the oocyst wall and the apical complex. Although little is known biochemically about these components, they represent potential targets for chemical and/or immunological intervention. The oocyst wall provides a highly selective barrier between the sporozoites and the environment. Preventing formation of the oocyst wall or disruption of formed oocyst walls by chemical disinfectants would circumvent survival of infective forms outside the host. The apical complex is composed of specialized organelles at the anterior of invasive forms, sporozoites and merozoites. Functional disruption of components of the apical complex, such as the rhoptries and micronemes, would block host cell invasion by *Cryptosporidium*.

The oocyst wall of *Cryptosporidium* protects the sporozoites from dehydration and harmful compounds in the environment. Because of its relatively inert nature, little is known about its structure and composition. The oocyst wall of *Cryptosporidium* is composed of 2 distinct layers which are interrupted by a protein-plugged suture through which the sporozoites escape during excystation (Current and Reese 1986). The oocyst wall of *Cryptosporidium* is similar to that of *Eimeria tenella* in that they are both rich in disulphide bonds; however, the wall of *Cryptosporidium* does not contain the fatty alcohols characteristic of *E. tenella* (Tilley and Upton 1997). More than 21 distinct bands, ranging from 14 to 200 kDa, have been identified by SDS–PAGE. The outer oocyst wall is richly glycosylated and contains several glycoproteins (250 and 40 kDa) that are highly immunogenic (Tilley and Upton 1997). The inner oocyst wall of *Cryptosporidium* contains 3 strongly immunogenic proteins of 28, 45–50 and 190 kDa (Tilley and Upton 1997).

It is believed that highly glycosylated components of the micronemes and rhoptries are released at the anterior end of sporozoites and merozoites, that these glycoproteins become associated with parasite and host cell membranes, and that they aid in host cell invasion. Many of these rhoptry and microneme glycoproteins are highly immunogenic and may represent targets for immunologic intervention (Tilley and Upton 1997)

4.2 Molecular biology and genetics

The types of molecular biology and genetics studies conducted with *Cryptosporidium* are somewhat limited because the only life cycle stage that can be purified in large numbers is the oocyst, and continuous in vitro cultivation of the parasite has not been achieved (Current 1990).

Various molecular characterization techniques have been used to determine differences among isolates of *C. parvum* and among different *Cryptosporidium* species. Polyacrylamide gel electrophoresis, one- or 2 dimensional, with or without surface iodination, has been used to demonstrate some minor differences among calf and human isolates of *C. parvum* and more marked differences between *C. parvum* and other species (Mead et al. 1990, Tilley et al. 1990). Immunoblot studies using rabbit antiserum (Nina et al. 1992) and monoclonal antibodies (Nichols, McLaughlin and Samuel 1991) have demonstrated differences between human and calf isolates of *C. parvum*. Several electrophoresis systems have been used to evaluate chromosomes obtained from sporozoites within purified oocysts of *C. parvum* (Mead et al. 1988b, Petersen 1993). Analysis by field inversion gel electrophoresis revealed 5 distinct chromosomes from 1400 to 3300 kb, whereas orthogonal field alteration gel electrophoresis clearly resolved 5 chromosomes all less than 1600 kb. Intensity of staining of some of the bands suggest that there may be 7–9 chromosomes. Differences in isolates of *C. parvum* obtained from different geographic locations have also been detected using restriction length polymorphism analysis (Ortega et al. 1991). In combination, these studies have detected significant molecular variation between different species of *Cryptosporidium* and some more subtle differences

among isolates of *C. parvum*. How these differences relate to differences in virulence, immunogenicity, host specificity, zoonotic potential and susceptibility to therapeutic agents remains to be determined.

At the time of writing there are 50 *Cryptosporidium* genes or genomic DNA fragments registered in GenBank (http://ncbi.nlm.nih.gov/cgi-bin/genbank?Cryptosporidium). Ribosomal RNA genes (18S and 5S) have been used in taxonomic investigations of *Cryptosporidium* spp. (e.g. Johnson et al. 1990), studies that have demonstrated that *C. parvum* may be more closely related to species of *Plasmodium* than to the true coccidia. Several genomic PCR fragments are listed that may prove to be useful for identification of *Cryptosporidium* in biological and environmental samples. A number of genes have been cloned from sporozoite genomic DNA of *C. parvum*, including ones encoding β-tubulin, actin, a heat shock protein (Hsp70), an elongation factor-2, an acetyl-coenzyme A synthase, a bifunctional dihydrofolate reductase-thymidylate synthase, a protein disulphide isomerase precursor, several antigenic oocyst wall proteins, and several sporozoite surface protein (glycoprotein) antigens. Cloning and characterization of *Cryptosporidium* genes is being actively pursued in a number of laboratories focusing on aspects of basic biology and taxonomy, detection and diagnosis, identification of molecular targets for therapeutic intervention, and identification of antigens useful for immunologic intervention. These efforts should, in the near future, result in many exciting advances in our understanding of the biology of *Cryptosporidium*.

5 CLINICAL ASPECTS

The most common clinical feature of cryptosporidiosis in immunocompetent and immunocompromised persons is diarrhoea, the symptom that most often leads to diagnosis. Characteristically, the diarrhoea is profuse and watery; it may contain mucus but rarely blood and leukocytes, and it is often associated with weight loss. Other less common clinical features include abdominal pain, nausea and vomiting, and low-grade fever (<39°C). Occasionally, nonspecific symptoms such as myalgia, weakness, malaise, headache and anorexia occur. Severity of these symptoms may wax and wane in individuals and this often parallels the intensity of oocyst shedding. Both the duration of symptoms and the outcome typically vary according to the immune status of the host. AIDS patients usually experience a prolonged, life-threatening illness, whereas most immunocompetent persons experience a short-term illness with complete, spontaneous recovery. However, the clinical presentation of gastrointestinal cryptosporidiosis does not always fit into one of these 2 divergent categories. Persons with the clinical and laboratory features of AIDS have been reported to clear infections after several months of diarrhoea, and individuals reported to be immunocompetent have had infections lasting more than a month (Current and Garcia 1991). Asymptomatic infections have been reported in both immunocompetent and immunodeficient persons (Current and Garcia 1991).

5.1 Clinical manifestations

IMMUNOCOMPETENT PERSONS

Most of the 18 cases of cryptosporidiosis in immunocompetent humans reported prior to 1983 and the numerous cases reported since then (cf. Current and Garcia 1991, O'Donoghue 1995) describe a self-limited, cholera-like or flu-like gastrointestinal illness. The most common symptoms reported are profuse, watery diarrhoea (cholera-like), and abdominal cramping, nausea and vomiting, low-grade fever and headache (flu-like). After reviewing the symptoms documented for 586 persons in 36 large-scale surveys, Fayer and Ungar (1986) reported that diarrhoea was the most commonly listed clinical feature (92%), followed by nausea and vomiting (51%), abdominal pain (45%) and low-grade fever (36%). In most well-nourished persons, diarrhoeal illness due to *C. parvum* infections lasts 3–12 days. Occasionally, these patients may require fluid replacement therapy, and occasionally the diarrhoeal illness may last for more than 2 weeks. In poorly nourished children with cryptosporidiosis, oral and parenteral rehydration therapy are often required because of excessive fluid loss, especially when infections last more than 3 weeks.

Failure to thrive has been reported in infants either as a result of or as a factor contributing to persistent cryptosporidiosis (Isaacs et al. 1985, Lahdevirta et al. 1987, Thomson, Benson and Wright 1987). Malnutrition may contribute to increased length of diarrhoeal illness and hospitalization, and perhaps to fatality associated with intestinal cryptosporidiosis (Bogarts et al. 1984, Sallon et al. 1986, Keren et al. 1987, MacFarline and Horner-Bryce 1987, Neira et al. 1989). For example, one study (Sallon et al. 1986) from a hospital in Jerusalem revealed that children with diarrhoea and *Cryptosporidium*-positive stools were significantly more malnourished than children with diarrhoea and no *Cryptosporidium* oocysts in their stools. Also, children with severe malnutrition and with *Cryptosporidium* oocysts in their stools had a significantly longer duration of diarrhoea than similarly malnourished children without cryptosporidiosis. Diarrhoeal illness is a major cause of morbidity and mortality, especially in young children living in developing countries. Based on the prevalence data from stool and serological surveys (see pp. 341–342) and based on reports associating cryptosporidiosis and malnutrition, it is likely that *Cryptosporidium* plays an important role in the overall health status of these children. It is also possible that *Cryptosporidium* may play a role in respiratory disease that often accompanies diarrhoeal illness in malnourished children (Current and Garcia 1991, O'Donoghue 1995).

IMMUNODEFICIENT PERSONS

Typically, the duration of diarrhoeal illness and ultimate outcome of intestinal cryptosporidiosis depend on the immune status of the patient. In the most severely immunocompromised host, such as persons with AIDS, diarrhoeal illness due to *Cryptosporidium* infection of the gastrointestinal tract becomes progressively worse with time and may be a major factor leading to death. It is believed that the infection usually begins with organisms colonizing the ileum or jejunum and develops into a life-threatening condition when a large portion of the gastrointestinal mucosa is covered with parasites (Boothe, Slavin and Dourmashkin 1980). Fluid loss in patients with AIDS and cryptosporidiosis is often excessive; 3–6 l of diarrhoeic stool per day is common, and as much as 17 l of watery stool per day has been reported (Centers for Disease Control 1982). Numerous case reports of intestinal cryptosporidiosis in AIDS patients can be found in the literature (see Current and Garcia 1991, O'Donoghue 1995).

In patients with other immune deficiencies, length and severity of illness may depend on the ability to reverse the immunosuppression. Patients included here are those on immunosuppressive chemotherapy, especially for cancer and transplantation (Collier, Miller and Meyers 1984, Kibbler et al. 1987); malnourished individuals, particularly children (Bogarts et al. 1984, Mata et al. 1984, Keren et al. 1987, Thomson, Benson, and Wright 1987, Sallon et al. 1988) and persons with concurrent viral infections such as measles, chickenpox or cytomegalovirus (Bogarts et al. 1984, Isaacs et al. 1985).

In the immune deficient patient, *C. parvum* infections are not always confined to the gastrointestinal tract, and additional clinical symptoms have been associated with these extraintestinal infections. These symptoms include a variety of respiratory problems, cholecystitis, hepatitis and pancreatitis.

Numerous case reports of *Cryptosporidium* infection of the respiratory tract have been published (see Current and Garcia 1991, O'Donoghue 1995) The symptoms associated with these infections include cough, shortness of breath, wheezing, croup, and hoarseness. Diarrhoea has not been reported in all of these patients. Oocysts have been identified in sputum samples, tracheal aspirates, bronchoalveolar lavage fluid, brush biopsy specimens and alveolar exudate obtained from lung biopsy. Most patients with severe immune deficiencies and *Cryptosporidium* in their respiratory tract do not recover.

Gallbladder disease, primarily acalculous cholecystitis and, less frequently, sclerosing cholangitis, has been has been reported in HIV-infected patients (Current and Garcia 1991). Symptoms most often reported include fever, right upper quadrant nonradiating pain, nausea, vomiting and simultaneous diarrhoea. Jaundice may also occur, and alkaline phosphatase and bilirubin have been elevated whenever measured. The gallbladder and common bile duct are usually enlarged and have thick walls and in cases of common bile duct stenosis the associated extrahepatic ducts are usually dilated. Diagnosis has generally been made by histological examination of the gallbladder epithelium or by the demonstration of oocysts in bile. Oocysts are not always found in the faeces, especially in cases of common bile duct stenosis that result in little or no release of bile into the intestine.

6 IMMUNOLOGY

6.1 Host resistance and acquired immunity

Our limited understanding of host resistance to *Crypto-sporidium* infections can be discussed within the context of data suggesting that age resistance occurs in some host species but not in others, and that acquired immunity is the usual outcome of a primary infection. Age at the time of exposure appears to have different effects, depending on host species, on the susceptibility and/or the course of infection following exposure to oocysts of *Cryptosporidium*. Available data relating to age resistance and/or acquired immunity are somewhat confusing and can best be discussed within the context of 2 different host species – mice and humans. More comprehensive reviews of host resistance and acquired immunity in different host species have been published (Current and Bick 1989, Current and Garcia 1991, O'Donoghue 1995).

MICE

The most widely used laboratory animal model for cryptosporidiosis is the suckling mouse. Suckling mice rather than adults are used routinely because of an apparent age-related resistance that occurs in most laboratory rodents. Early experience with *C. parvum* demonstrated that virtually all conventional (as opposed to germ-free or immune-deficient strains) suckling rodents – mice, rats, cotton rats, hamsters, and guinea pigs – develop heavy intestinal infections after oral inoculation of 10^3 or more oocysts of human or calf isolates (Current et al. 1983, Current and Reese 1986). However, previously unexposed rodents more than 3–4 weeks old are difficult to infect; the parasite often cannot be found even after inoculation of more than 2×10^6 oocysts, and if found they are observed in very small numbers within the intestinal mucosa. Several studies have been conducted in an attempt to address the most obvious causes of this marked difference in susceptibility between neonate and adult mice, i.e. differences in gut physiology and microflora or differences in immune status.

Our understanding of differences in the gut microflora and physiology of adult and neonate laboratory rodents which affect the ability of *C. parvum* to colonize and establish infections is limited. Harp et al. (1988) used 2 strains of adult and infant mice in an attempt to determine the effect of the adult gut microflora on establishment of *C. parvum* infections. In one experiment, using adult mice of the same strain (CD1), 7 of 9 antibiotic-treated, germ-free mice developed light to moderate infections following oral inoculation of *C. parvum* oocysts, whereas only 4 of 12 antibiotic treated, conventional mice developed light infections. Since bacteria could not be cultured from the intestines of mice in either group, the authors argue that the increased susceptibility of the germ-free mice was not due to the absence of flora that may block intestinal colonization of *C. parvum* by competing for receptor sites on host cells, producing anti-cryptosporidial agents, or stimulating gut motility. However, the authors did suggest that antigenic stimulation provided by the adult gut flora in the conventional mice could be responsible for activating components of the immune system mediating resistance against *C. parvum*. In their second experiment, none of 15 antibiotic treated or 14 non-treated adult BALB/c mice developed infections following oocyst

challenge; however, all 7 infant mice developed heavy infections. Although results of the second experiment were consistent with the authors' hypothesis that activation of the immune system by previous association with adult intestinal flora contributes to *C. parvum* resistance, additional studies are needed to confirm or refute this concept.

Our early attempts to establish infections in adult mice by the use of immunosuppressive chemotherapy were disappointing. Adult Swiss-Webster mice administered cyclophosphamide did not develop more consistent nor heavier infections than did nonimmunosuppressed mice following oral inoculation of *C. parvum* oocysts; only light infections lasting a few days could be demonstrated (by oocyst shedding and/or by microscopic examination of the intestinal mucosa) in about half of the mice in each group (Reese et al. 1982). Sherwood et al. (1982) also reported that cyclophosphamide administration did not alter the susceptibility of adult mice to *C. parvum*. Such results are difficult to interpret because immune parameters were not monitored in these mice before, during or after inoculation with the parasite. It is possible that because of insufficient T-lymphocyte depletion the overall immune status of the mice in both studies was not significantly altered. Additional studies are needed to more clearly define the effect of immunosuppressive chemotherapy on the development and intensity of *C. parvum* infection in adult mice.

Several studies have focused on the use of T-cell deficient nude (nu/nu) mice as potential laboratory models for cryptosporidiosis. One study compared oocyst-induced *C. parvum* infections in infant and adult nu/nu mice (Heine, Moon and Woodmansee 1984). Heavy intestinal infections in all infants and light infections in about half of the adults were observed when animals were monitored for approximately 2 weeks following oral inoculation of *C. parvum* oocysts into athymic nude mice and their immunocompetent, heterozygous (nu/+) littermates. When the course of experimentally induced infections in 6-day-old nu/nu mice and their nu/+, immunocompetent littermates was monitored over a longer period of time, the T-cell deficient nude mice developed diarrhoea and shed oocysts in their faeces until they died or until the experiment was terminated at 56 days; however, the heterozygous littermates did not develop diarrhoea and stopped shedding oocysts 21–30 days after inoculation. These studies suggested that host immune status at the time of parasite inoculation may not be the predominant factor determining susceptibility to *C. parvum* infection in the mouse gut; however, functional T-lymphocytes are important for the clearance of *C. parvum* from the mammalian intestine.

More recent studies suggest that this may be an oversimplistic view of the many complex events that may affect parasite colonization and subsequent development in the gut. Ungar et al. (1990) reported that severe intestinal and hepatobiliary infections with *C. parvum* were produced in adult BALB/c nu/nu mice; however, clinical signs of cryptosporidiosis and large numbers of oocysts in the faeces did not appear until 3 weeks after inoculation. Thus, it appears that adult BALB/c nu/nu mice are susceptible to *C. parvum* infection but that it takes at least 3 weeks for large numbers of parasites to develop within enterocytes of the exposed mucosal site. In contrast, heavy infections develop in neonates (immunocompetent or nu/nu) within 3–5 days after inoculation. The authors also reported that similar persistent infections could be established in immunocompetent mice if they were depleted of CD4 cells by treatment with specific monoclonal antibodies and inoculated with *C. parvum* as neonates.

From the data reviewed above, it appears that oral inoculation of *C. parvum* into adult laboratory mice may result in the establishment of a small number of parasites within the intestinal mucosa. If the inoculated mice are immunocompetent, the infection is cleared, often before the parasite population becomes large enough to detect the infection. If, however, the inoculated mice are rendered immunodeficient by depletion of T-helper lymphocytes, the small number of parasites colonizing the intestine of some mice can increase over the subsequent 3–4 weeks and become sufficiently large to produce disease.

HUMANS

In humans, age and immune status at the time of primary exposure to *C. parvum* does not appear to be the primary factor influencing susceptibility to infection – symptomatic intestinal and respiratory cryptosporidiosis has been reported in both immunocompetent and immunodeficient children and adults (Current and Garcia 1991, O'Donoghue 1995). However, host immune status does have a marked impact on the length and severity of human cryptosporidiosis. Immunocompetent persons usually develop a short-term (less than 2 weeks), self-limited, diarrhoeal illness following oral exposure to *C. parvum* oocysts, whereas most immunocompromised persons initially develop a similar illness that becomes progressively worse with time, resulting in a prolonged, life-threatening, cholera-like illness. Such prolonged, life-threatening infections have been reported in patients undergoing immunosuppressive chemotherapy with drugs that affect both T- and B-lymphocyte function (Current and Garcia 1991, O'Donoghue 1995), in at least one person with hypogammaglobulinaemia with reported normal T-lymphocyte function, and in patients with AIDS (Current and Garcia 1991, O'Donoghue 1995). These observations suggest that the marked difference in outcome between the immune-deficient and the immunocompetent person exposed to *C. parvum* can probably be best explained by the development of an acquired immune response of sufficient magnitude to clear the parasite from the intestinal mucosa. This concept is also supported by reports of persons who rapidly cleared *C. parvum* infections when their immune function was restored following discontinuation of immunosuppressive chemotherapy (Miller et al. 1983).

6.2 Antigens

From the discussions above, it is apparent that host immune status is a major determinant of the severity of cryptosporidiosis following exposure to oocysts and that acquired immunity is probably responsible for the clearance of an infection and for resistance to subsequent challenge. Each of these features has led to a search for antigens that may be important for the induction and/or expression of acquired immunity.

POTENTIAL SPOROZOITE AND OOCYST ANTIGENS

The development of techniques to purify oocysts of *Cryptosporidium* and to separate sporozoites from intact oocysts and oocyst walls (Current 1990) has allowed researchers to obtain hyperimmune sera from rabbits and other laboratory animals and hyperimmune colostrum from cows, and to employ electrophoresis and immunoblotting for general molecular weight determinations of potential antigens of these life cycle forms (Current and Bick 1990, O'Donoghue 1995). These studies have identified more than 50 bands in immunoblots of sporozoites and/or oocysts. Tilley and Upton (1990) used sodium dodecyl sulphate polyacrylamide gel electrophoresis (SDS–PAGE), immunoblotting, lectin binding and iodine-125 surface labelling to characterize the proteins and glycoproteins of purified sporozoites and oocysts of *C. parvum*, the mammalian pathogen, and *C. baileyi*, a species that infects poultry. Silver-stained profiles of freeze-thawed oocysts revealed more than 50 bands while profiles of sporozoites exhibited more than 40 bands. Surface iodination of sporozoites revealed approximately 20 surface proteins, the most heavily labelled ones forming bands corresponding to 18–20, 37–39, 48, 73–76 and 102–105 kDa. Following electrophoresis and western blotting, 4 of 12 different iodine-125 labelled lectin probes collectively bound to at least 19 bands indicating that numerous sporozoite proteins of *C. parvum* are glycosylated.

Subsequent studies employing monoclonal antibodies have localized and characterized a number of the above oocyst wall and sporozoite surface antigens, as well as microneme and rhoptry components that are highly glycosylated and immunogenic. An in depth discussion of these specific antigens is beyond the scope of this chapter, but can be found in recent reviews (O'Donoghue 1995, Tilley and Upton 1997). The functional significance of these various antigens and how different antibody preparations interact with the parasite to circumvent the infection process are the subjects of ongoing research.

ANTIGENS RECOGNIZED BY HUMANS

Several studies have demonstrated that only a few of the proteins and glycoproteins identified as potential antigens in oocyst walls and sporozoites of *C. parvum* are recognized strongly by sera obtained from humans (Ungar and Nash 1986, Mead, Arrowood, and Sterling 1988) following their recovery from intestinal cryptosporidiosis.

Ungar and Nash (1986) reported that 37 of 40 sera from persons with cryptosporidiosis (24 AIDS and 16 non-AIDS patients) recognized, by western blot analysis, a 23 kDa *C. parvum* sporozoite antigen that was separated by 5–15% SDS–PAGE using reducing conditions (5% mercaptoethanol). They also reported that 58 of 63 sera from IgM- or IgG-positive individuals, as determined by an ELISA assay, recognized the same antigen. In some of the sera, up to 3 additional bands between 125 kDa and 175 kDa were also recognized strongly and a larger number of additional bands reacted weakly. These authors proposed that the 23 kDa antigen may be useful in serodiagnosis since sera from most infected persons, including AIDS patients, react strongly to this particular band. Mead, Arrowood and Sterling (1988) reported that sera obtained from persons at various times (10 days to 1 year) after infection with *Cryptosporidium* reacted strongly with a 20 kDa antigen separated on 10–20% gradient or 10% standard SDS–PAGE using reducing (mercaptoethanol) conditions. By using a specific monoclonal antibody (C6B6) and IFA and by biotinylation of the parasite, the authors provided evidence that the 20 kDa antigen was on the surface of *C. parvum* sporozoites. They concluded that the 20 kDa sporozoite surface antigen was probably the same as the 23 kDa antigen reported by Ungar and Nash (1986), that the differences in reported molecular weights were due to differing gradient gel applications, and that the serum recognition of this antigen probably correlates with recent exposure to *C. parvum*. However, caution is advised when comparing western blots. Results of studies by Tilley and colleagues (Tilley et al. 1990a,b; Tilley and Upton 1990) compared to those of the above studies, suggest that at least 2 *C. parvum* sporozoite surface proteins are being confused. A 23 kDa molecule is weakly labelled by iodination, highly immunogenic and may have several epitopes that cross-react with some higher molecular size species. An 18–20 kDa protein, often referred to as P20, is intensely labelled by iodination and appears to be less immunogenic than P23. Galactose or galactosamine residues have been detected on P20, but P23 does not appear to be glycosylated (Ungar and Nash 1986). Effects of preparation techniques on the degree of glycosylation or perhaps strain differences may explain the variation in size of P20 reported by different investigators.

7 PATHOLOGY

Intestinal infections of *C. parvum* are relatively unremarkable from the standpoint of histopathology. Microscopically, the endogenous life cycle forms are observed in the epithelium, usually without obvious damage to host cells except that cells may be low columnar or cuboidal and microvilli may be absent at the site of parasite attachment (Figs 18.3, 18.4). Intestinal lesions include mild to severe villous atrophy, blunting and fusion of villi and inflammatory changes marked by mild to moderate infiltration of plasma cells, neutrophils, macrophages and lymphocytes into the subepithelial lamina propria (Meisel et al. 1976, Stemmerman and Frenkel 1980).

At present, the pathophysiological mechanisms of *Cryptosporidium*-induced diarrhoea are poorly defined. Studies in germ-free calves monoinfected with *C. parvum* suggest that malabsorption and impaired digestion in the small bowel coupled with malabsorption in the large intestine are major factors responsible for diarrhoea in calves with cryptosporidiosis (Heine et al. 1984). Similar malabsorption, attributed to parasite-induced villous damage, has also been reported in a neonatal pig model (Argenzio et al. 1990). This malabsorption and impaired digestion may result in an overgrowth of intestinal microflora, a change in osmotic pressure across the gut wall, and an influx of fluid into the lumen of the intestine. Malabsorption and impaired digestion have also been reported in humans infected with *C. parvum*.

The secretory (often described as cholera-like) diarrhoea common to most immune-deficient patients with cryptosporidiosis suggests a toxin-mediated hypersecretion into the gut; however, the author is not aware of reports establishing that *C. parvum* possesses enterotoxin. Several studies (Garza, Fedorak, and Soave 1986, Guarino et al. 1994) reporting changes in electrical potential of rabbit and human ileum following exposure to *C. parvum* extracts suggest, but do not establish, the presence of enterotoxins.

8 DIAGNOSIS

Prior to 1980, human cryptosporidiosis was diagnosed histologically by finding the small spherical life cycle stages of *C. parvum* in the microvillous region of the intestinal mucosa obtained by biopsy or in tissue obtained at necropsy. In haematoxylin and eosin-stained sections, developmental stages of the parasite appear as small, spherical, basophilic bodies (2–5 μm depending on stage of life cycle) within the microvillous region of the intestinal mucosa (Fig. 18.4a). Transmission electron microscopy can be used to confirm diagnosis and reveals distinct life cycle forms, each within a parasitophorous vacuole confined to the microvillous region of the host cell (Fig. 18.4b). Such invasive, expensive and time-consuming procedures are no longer required for diagnosis since a variety of techniques have been developed to identify *C. parvum* oocysts in faeces, sputum and bile; specimens that represent a sampling of the entire intestinal, respiratory or biliary tract. These specimens can be evaluated by a variety of diagnostic procedures to identify the environmentally resistant *Cryptosporidium* oocysts (Current and Garcia 1991, O'Donoghue 1995). For the diagnosis of cryptosporidiosis, stool and other body fluid specimens should be submitted as fresh material or in 10% formalin or sodium acetate–acetic acid–formalin (SAF) preservatives. Fixed specimens are recommended because of biohazard considerations. Potassium dichromate solution (2–3% w/v in water) is used routinely as a storage medium to preserve oocyst viability; it is not a fixative. Fresh or preserved stool specimens can then be examined by several concentration or staining procedures which aid in the visualization of *Cryptosporidium* oocysts.

8.1 Stool specimen collection and concentration techniques

The number of oocysts shed in stools may fluctuate, therefore, it has been recommended that a minimum of 3 specimens be collected, the same recommendation as for routine ova and parasite examination. Multiple samples are particularly important when dealing with formed stool specimens which usually contain fewer oocysts than do diarrhoeic specimens.

Stool concentration techniques that are useful for identification of *C. parvum* oocysts include flotation of oocysts in Sheather's sugar solution, in zinc sulphate (specific gravity 1.18 or 1.2) or in saturated sodium chloride (specific gravity 1.27). Stool concentration techniques using sedimentation include formalin–ether and formalin–ethyl acetate. It is important to consider that most sedimentation techniques used in the clinical microbiology laboratory were designed for the diagnosis of helminth eggs and protozoan cysts (e.g. *Giardia lamblia* and *Entamoeba* spp.) that are larger than *Cryptosporidium* spp. Therefore, after the short centrifugation times at low g-force ($300 \times g$ for 2 min) many of the oocysts may remain in the supernatant. If one is looking for *C. parvum* oocysts in stool or other body fluid samples, it is advisable to centrifuge at >500 × g for at least 10 min.

8.2 Staining of oocysts

Most recommended stains for *Cryptosporidium* oocysts cannot be performed on stools preserved in polyvinyl alcohol (PVA) fixative. The routine stains (trichrome, iron haematoxylin) used for stool diagnosis of other parasites are not acceptable for the identification of *Cryptosporidium* spp. oocysts (Garcia and Current 1989). Several widely used techniques for demonstrating *Cryptosporidium* spp. oocysts in faecal specimens from humans and animals include modified acid-fast staining, negative staining (Fig. 18.5c), and Sheather's sugar flotation (Figs. 18.5a,b) (Garcia and Current 1989, Current and Garcia 1991). Although the last 2 procedures are useful in the research laboratory, acid-fast staining is usually the method of choice for the clinical microbiology laboratory. In any of the acid-fast methods, there may be some variability in stain uptake, related to the stain itself or the age of the oocysts after prolonged storage (Garcia and Current 1989). Less common staining methods, such as auramine–rhodamine and acridine orange, are cited in a recent review (O'Donoghue 1995).

Considerable experience with the concentration and staining methods is often required to obtain an accurate diagnosis. For this reason, immunofluorescent antibody (IFA) procedures employing *Cryptosporidium*-specific polyclonal or monoclonal antibodies have been developed and may provide the most sensitive method available for the diagnosis of cryptosporidiosis (Arrowood and Sterling 1989).

8.3 Serodiagnosis

The use of serodiagnostic techniques for monitoring exposure to *Cryptosporidium* has thus far been limited to a few laboratories. Antibodies specific to *Cryptosporidium* have been detected by IFA assays using endogenous stages of *Cryptosporidium* in tissue sections as antigens (Campbell and Current 1983) or intact oocysts as antigens (D'Antonio et al. 1985, Casemore 1987, Current and Snyder 1988). These IFA procedures have been used to demonstrate seroconversion in persons who recovered from confirmed infections (Campbell and Current 1983, Casemore 1987) and for the presumptive diagnosis of cryptosporidiosis in 2 clusters of cases (D'Antonio et al. 1985, Koch et al. 1985). Specific anti-*Cryptosporidium* IgG, IgM or both have also been detected, by enzyme linked immunosorbent assays (ELISA) using crude oocyst preparations as antigens (Ungar et al. 1986, Current and Snyder 1988) and ELISA procedures have been used in seroepidemiological studies (see below). Detection of specific antibodies to *Cryptosporidium* should not be regarded as indicative of active infection, but rather as providing evidence of prior exposure.

9 EPIDEMIOLOGY AND CONTROL

Infections with *Cryptosporidium* have been recorded in over 170 different host species originating from more than 50 countries from tropical to temperate zones throughout the world (O'Donoghue 1995). Infections are presumably acquired by ingestion (or inhalation) of infective oocysts that are passed in the faeces of an infected host. Human-to-human transmission is com-

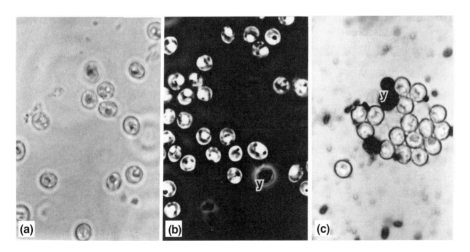

Fig. 18.5. Oocysts of *C. parvum* as seen with brightfield microscopy (a) or phase-contrast microscopy (b) following concentration by Sheather's sugar flotation. With some brightfield optics, oocysts often appear light pink. With phase contrast microscopy, oocysts appear as bright birefringent spherical bodies against a dark background. Oocysts also contain 1–4 dark granules. Yeast cells (y) are not bright and birefringent (b). Oocysts of *C. parvum* as seen with brightfield microscopy following negative-staining with carbol-fuchsin (c). Faecal debris and yeast cells (y) stain darkly, whereas the stain surrounds but does not penetrate the wall of the oocyst. Because the negative-stained preparation is covered with immersion oil, and because the interior of the oocyst wall contains water, oocysts appear bright and birefringent.

mon and has been recorded among household members, sexual partners, hospital patients and staff, and children attending day care centres. Zoonotic transmission from farm and companion animals is also well documented. Contaminated water and food are known sources of infections among international travellers and large waterborne outbreaks of cryptosporidiosis have been reported in North America and Europe. Epidemiological studies employing stool examination and serodiagnosis procedures make it clear that *Cryptosporidium* is an important, widespread cause of diarrhoeal illness in humans and some domesticated animals. Understanding the epidemiology and transmission of *Cryptosporidium* is important in the prevention and control of cryptosporidiosis because, at the time of this writing, no consistently effective therapy has been identified.

9.1 Epidemiology

TRANSMISSION BY ENVIRONMENTALLY RESISTANT OOCYSTS

Studies of experimental infections in laboratory and farm animals clearly demonstrate that *C. parvum* is transmitted by environmentally resistant oocysts that are fully sporulated and infective at the time they are passed in faeces (Current et al. 1983). As long as the thick, 2-layered wall remains intact, *Cryptosporidium* spp. oocysts are very resistant to most common disinfectants and can survive for months if kept cold and moist. One study (Sundermann, Linsday and Blagburn 1987), designed to evaluate the efficacy of commercial disinfectants, demonstrated that exposure to ammonia (50% or higher), and formalin (10% or higher) for 30 min can kill *Cryptosporidium* oocysts. When these disinfectants and others used routinely in hospitals and clinical laboratories were evaluated at the lower concentrations recommended by the manufacturers, none were effective against *Cryptosporidium* oocysts. Freeze-drying and exposure (30 min) to temperatures above +60°C and below −20°C have also been reported to kill *Cryptosporidium* oocysts (Anderson 1985). Most *C. parvum* oocysts stored at 4°C in 2.5% (weight/volume) aqueous potassium dichromate solution remain viable for 3–4 months, and some may remain infective for cell cultures and suckling mice for more than a year (Current 1990).

The recent documentation of waterborne transmission of *C. parvum* and the demonstration of oocysts in potable water samples (see p. 341) is of concern to the water industry and has prompted studies to evaluate disinfectants commonly used for water treatment. The earliest data suggesting that routine chlorination of drinking water has little or no effect on oocyst viability stemmed from procedures used routinely in several laboratories to sterilize *Cryptosporidium* oocysts prior to obtaining viable sporozoites by in vitro excystation. This procedure involves incubating oocysts in 10–50% commercial bleach (0.5–2.5% sodium hypochlorite) for 10–15 minutes in an ice bath. Sceptics argued that these data are difficult to interpret because of the low incubation temperatures, the short

incubation times and possible organic (faecal) contamination that can cause a high disinfection demand. The argument for high disinfection demand is not valid because oocysts tested in our laboratory and elsewhere were highly purified. More recent studies employing disinfectants commonly used to treat water have been performed using purified oocysts (a demand-free situation), and different incubation times and temperatures. In one carefully controlled study, oocyst viability, as determined by prevention of excystation or infectivity, was abolished following exposure to 80 ppm chlorine at 25°C, pH 7.0 for 2 h. Using these data the Ct (concentration × time required for killing) value for *C. parvum* oocysts was 9600, compared to a Ct of <15 for *Giardia* cysts (Korich et al. 1990). In this same study, ozone (another popular method for water treatment) was shown to eliminate infectivity of *C. parvum* oocysts when kept at a concentration of 1 ppm for 10 min. Results from this study also indicate that *C. parvum* oocysts are 30 times more resistant to ozone and 14 times more resistant to chlorine dioxide than are *Giardia* cysts exposed under the same conditions (Korich et al. 1990). In studies using infection in neonatal mice as a more reliable assessment of inactivation, 99% inactivation of *C. parvum* oocysts was accomplished by an integrated ozone residual of 0.5 mg l^{-1} for about 5 min in laboratory water at 22°C (Finch and Belosevic 1994). Therefore, disinfection with high levels of ozone may be of benefit in water treatment plants that do not remove *C. parvum* oocysts by filtration.

SOURCES OF HUMAN INFECTION

Data from several laboratories during the early 1980s demonstrated that calves are a source of human infection and that companion animals such as rodents, puppies and kittens may also serve as reservoir hosts (Current and Garcia 1991, O'Donoghue 1995). These findings and the realization that *C. parvum* readily crosses host species barriers led to the concept that most human infections are a result of zoonotic transmission. This view is probably correct for persons living and working in environments where exposure to faecal contamination (especially waterborne) from potential reservoir hosts is likely. However, zoonotic transmission cannot explain the large number of infections reported from persons living and working in urban areas where exposure to animal faeces is minimal. Present evidence indicates that person-to-person transmission of cryptosporidiosis is common (cf. O'Donoghue 1995). Numerous outbreaks of cryptosporidiosis among children in day-care centres have been reported, hospital-acquired infections have been investigated and a number of waterborne outbreaks have been documented, and this protozoan is now recognized as a cause of travellers' diarrhoea (Current and Garcia 1991, O'Donoghue 1995).

The highly transmissible nature of *C. parvum* infection appears to be well documented. In 1983, an accidental laboratory infection demonstrated that a human isolate of *C.*

parvum could be transmitted easily from one person to another (Blagburn and Current 1983). In the setting of an urban community in Brazil, *C. parvum* infections among household members were monitored for 6 weeks following identification of one household member who had cryptosporidiosis (Newman et al. 1994). Using the stringent criteria of at least one *Cryptosporidium*-positive stool sample or seroconversion, 51% of 31 households had at least one secondary case of cryptosporidiosis, and 19% of family contacts had documented *C. parvum* infection. This rate of transmission is similar to that documented for other highly transmissible enteric pathogens such as *Shigella* and rotavirus. In a more recent study of the infectivity of *C. parvum* in healthy volunteers, infections were detected in subjects receiving from 30 to >1000 oocysts and the median infective dose calculated by linear regression was 132 oocysts (Dupont et al. 1995). The highly transmissible nature of *C. parvum* demonstrated by the above studies underscores the risk for acquiring cryptosporidial diarrhoea when travelling in highly endemic areas or when a population is suddenly exposed to a contaminated water supply.

WATERBORNE TRANSMISSION

The first documented waterborne outbreak of cryptosporidiosis occurred in San Antonio, Texas and was linked to sewage leakage into well water (D'Antonio et al. 1986). Water from this well was chlorinated but not filtered. During the summer of 1986, drinking water from a common reservoir was considered to be the only epidemiological source link to an outbreak of cryptosporidiosis in Sheffield, England (Rush, Chapman and Ineson 1987). Similar consumption of untreated surface water appeared to be the predominant risk factor associated with cryptosporidiosis among 78 laboratory-confirmed cases of cryptosporidiosis in New Mexico during the summer of 1986 (Gallaher et al. 1989). In January and February 1987, cryptosporidiosis was associated with an estimated 13 000 cases of gastroenteritis among residents of Caroll County, Georgia, USA (Hayes et al. 1989). *Cryptosporidium* oocysts were identified in the stools of 39% of the persons examined during the outbreak and a randomized telephone survey suggested attack rates of 54% within the city of Carollton and 40% overall for the county. The only significant risk factor associated with illness was exposure to the public water supply which was filtered and chlorinated and, according to records kept during the outbreak, the treatment facility was operating within established EPA guidelines. In 1988 and 1989, 2 additional *Cryptosporidium*-related waterborne outbreaks were reported in Ayshire, Scotland and Swindon, Oxfordshire, England (Smith et al. 1988a,b). A large community outbreak in Milwaukee during March and April 1993 was investigated in which approximately one half of the people consuming water from the southern water treatment plant had diarrhoeal illness (MacKenzie et al. 1994). Among these patients, there was more than a 100-fold increase in identification of *C. parvum* oocysts, but not in other enteric pathogens. It is estimated that 403 000 people had watery diarrhoea attributed to this outbreak. It appears that oocysts in water from Lake Michigan passed through the city's southern water treatment plant. At the time of the outbreak, there was a marked increase in turbidity of treated water at the southern treatment plant and oocysts were identified in water from ice made in southern Milwaukee during these weeks.

Application of techniques to recover *Cryptosporidium* from water samples in conjunction with immunofluorescent detection methods has resulted in the demonstration of *Cryptosporidium* oocysts in surface and drinking waters, and sewage effluent samples obtained from many different geographic regions of the USA and from several other countries (Current and Garcia 1991, O'Donoghue 1995). Wastewater in the form of raw sewage and runoff from dairies and grazing lands has been identified as a likely source of oocysts that contaminate drinking and recreational water. The importance of agricultural sources of oocyst contamination should not be taken lightly since infected calves and lambs can pass up to 10^{10} oocysts per day for up to 14 days (Blewett 1989). Thus, large numbers of oocysts can enter the surface water system following a hard rain on a pasture containing infected animals.

9.2 Prevalence

STOOL DIAGNOSIS

Human infections with *Cryptosporidium* (*C. parvum*) have been reported on 6 continents. Most prevalence data contained in published surveys result from standard stool examination techniques to detect *C. parvum* oocysts. A review (Fayer and Ungar 1986) of 36 large-scale surveys of selected populations, such as children and adults seeking medical attention for diarrhoea and other gastrointestinal symptoms, demonstrates that *Cryptosporidium* is associated with diarrhoeal illness in most areas of the world and that the prevalence of cryptosporidiosis is highest in poorly developed regions. For example, prevalence rates reported in surveys from Europe (1–2%) and North America (0.6–4.3%) are lower than those reported in surveys from Asia, Australia, Africa and Central and South America (3–20%). In most of the surveys reviewed by Fayer and Ungar (1986), *Cryptosporidium* was the most common parasite found and, in several, this protozoan was considered to be the most significant of all known enteropathogens causing diarrhoeal illness. Other findings common to many of the surveys were that children usually had a significantly higher prevalence than did adults, prevalence was highest in children less than 2 years of age and infections were often seasonal, with a higher prevalence during warmer, wetter months. Another interesting finding from the standpoint of infection control was that a small number of oocysts may be present in faeces for up to 2 weeks following resolution of diarrhoea.

Several, additional reviews (Navin 1985, Crawford and Vermund 1988, Current and Garcia 1991, O'Donoghue 1995) of the published reports of cryptosporidiosis in persons residing in industrialized and developing countries support the overall conclusions presented above, and provide a more global view of the prevalence of human infection. Crawford and Vermund (1988) compared the worldwide occurrence of *Cryptosporidium* infection compiled by Navin (1985) from studies prior to 1985 with that obtained from studies published from 1985 to 1988. Data compiled from the pre- and post- 1985 studies were similar. Studies prior to 1985 suggested that the overall prevalence of *Cryptosporidium* infection in individuals with diarrhoea was 2.5% (195 of 7779) for persons living in industrialized countries and 7.2% (82 of 1135) for persons residing in developing countries (Navin 1985). The more recent studies summarized by Crawford and Vermund suggested the infection rate for individuals with diarrhoeal illness was 2.4% (285 of 11 716) for individuals in industrialized countries and 8.5% (532 of 6295) for individuals in developing countries.

A summary of more than 100 geographically based surveys (published between 1983 and 1990) for the presence of *Cryptosporidium* oocysts in stool specimens, from at least 40 countries, was presented by Current and Garcia (1991). Data from all of these surveys, excluding documented outbreaks, indicate that in the more industrialized countries of North America and Europe, the prevalence rate is 1–3%. In contrast, mean prevalence rates are higher in underdeveloped continents, ranging from approximately 5% in Asia to approximately 10% in Africa. The higher prevalence in underdeveloped countries may be due to the lack of clean water and sanitary facilities, crowded housing conditions, and large numbers of potential reservoir hosts (domestic mammals) near homes. In general it appears that cryptosporidiosis is more common in crowded urban areas in developing countries than in less crowded rural areas. The reverse appears to be true in more developed countries.

Estimates provided by Walsh and Warren (1979) suggest that in Asia, Africa and Latin America alone there are as many as 5 billion episodes of diarrhoea and 5– 10 million diarrhoea-associated deaths annually. If the estimates of Walsh and Warren are accurate and if the *Cryptosporidium* prevalence data summarized above are correct, then one may predict 250–500 million *Cryptosporidium* infections annually in persons living in Asia, Africa and Latin America.

Seroprevalence

Limited serological surveys also support the concept that *Cryptosporidium* infection is more common in developing countries compared to the more industrialized regions of North America and Europe. Seroprevalence rates in Europe and North America are usually 25–35% (Casemore 1987, O'Donoghue 1995). In contrast, approximately 64% of 389 children and adults in Lima, Peru and of 84 children in Maracaibo and Caracas, Venezuela had serologic evidence of previous infection, i.e. their sera contained antibodies (IgG and/or IgM) specific for *Cryptosporidium* (Ungar et al. 1988). In a more recent study of the household epidemiology of *Cryptosporidium* in an urban slum in northeast Brazil, 94.6% of 202 persons examined had evidence of antibodies (either IgG or IgM) to *Cryptosporidium*. At the beginning of a longitudinal serologic survey (Ungar et al. 1989) of 56 United States Peace Corps volunteers in Africa, 15 (26.8%) were seropositive. During the next year an additional 8 (14% of the 56) seroconverted. A similar rate of seroconversion occurred during the second year. These data suggest that *Cryptosporidium* infections may be more common in most regions than faecal oocyst surveys have indicated. They also point out the increased risk of infection when previously unexposed persons travel or work in areas of high prevalence.

Prevalence in HIV-infected persons

Data based on physician reporting of diagnosed cases of cryptosporidiosis to the Centers for Disease Control (CDC) have resulted in an estimated prevalence of 2–5% for late-stage HIV-infected patients in the US (Navin and Hardy 1987). Studies designed to determine if *Cryptosporidium* is associated with diarrhoeal illness in AIDS patients reveal that the prevalences reported by the CDC are an underestimation (Current and Garcia 1991). In patients with AIDS and diarrhoea, 15% of those evaluated at the National Institutes of Health in Bethesda, Maryland and 16% of those evaluated at the Johns Hopkins Hospital in Baltimore, Maryland were infected with *Cryptosporidium*, the most common pathogen in the latter study (Laughon et al. 1988, Smith et al. 1988b). In one hospital in Great Britain, 11% of AIDS patients had cryptosporidiosis (Conolly et al. 1988). In a study from France, 21.2% of 132 AIDS patients had cryptosporidiosis (Rene et al. 1989).

Since cryptosporidiosis is more prevalent among immunocompetent persons in developing countries compared to those in industrialized countries, one may predict that a similar difference exists in the AIDS population. One study reported that 27 of 29 AIDS patients from Haiti had chronic diarrhoea and that 41% (11/27) had *Cryptosporidium*-positive stools (Malebranche et al. 1983). In one report from Kinshasa, Zaire, 85% (109/128) of the patients presenting with diarrhoea of over one month duration were HIV seropositive and 22% of 106 of these patients that were studied were stool positive for *Cryptosporidium* (Loening et al. 1989). One study from a hospital in Brazil reported that 12% of the AIDS patients with diarrhoea had *Cryptosporidium*-positive stools (Dias et al. 1988). Another report from Mexico indicated that 16.7% of children with AIDS had cryptosporidiosis (Avila-Figueroa et al. 1989) The overall prevalence of intestinal and extraintestinal cryptosporidiosis in AIDS patients residing in industrialized and developing countries remains unclear; however, it is considerably higher than the 2–5% reported by the Centers for Disease Control.

10 Chemotherapy

Because immunocompromised persons often develop a prolonged life-threatening infection following exposure to *Cryptosporidium*, an effective therapy is desperately needed to treat this patient population. Despite numerous years of investigations using animal and in vitro models to evaluate chemotherapeutic agents (Blagburn and Soave 1997) and the administration of a vast array of chemotherapeutic, immuno-modulatory and pallative agents to AIDS patients (Soave 1990), we still lack a consistently effective, approved therapy for human cryptosporidiosis. A formidable list of approximately 100 ineffective compounds has been generated as a result of largely anecdotal attempts to control this life-threatening disease in immunocompromised patients (Soave 1990). Over the past decade, controlled treatment trials have been conducted but have not succeeded in identifying efficacious agents to threat this infection. A compilation of the agents evaluated for anticryptosporidial activity in animal models and humans has been published (Soave 1990, Blagburn and Soave 1997). Below is a brief discussion of some chemotherapeutic agents that have been evaluated in humans during the past decade.

MACROLIDES

Spiramycin, a macrolide with broad-spectrum antibacterial activity, has been used for many years in Europe for treatment of infections by *Toxoplasma gondii*, a coccidian closely related to *Cryptosporidium*. In the mid- to late-1980s there were approximately 5 anecdotal reports of both success and failure of spiramycin for the treatment of human cryptosporidiosis (Soave 1990). More recently conducted controlled trials also gave divergent results. The most comprehensive study was a randomized, double-blind, placebo-controlled study involving the treatment of 73 patients with AIDS and cryptosporidial diarrhoea. Approximately 3 g spiramycin 3 times daily for 3 weeks was no better than placebo (Blagburn and Soave 1997). A subsequent trial using intravenous spiramycin to circumvent absorption problems demonstrated a favourable response in 5 of 31 AIDS patients; however, administration of intravenous spiramycin was associated with adverse side effects, including paraesthesias, taste perversion, nausea and vomiting (Blagburn and Soave et al. 1997). Thus, available data suggest that spiramycin is of little benefit for the treatment of human cryptosporidiosis.

Experience with a newer macrolide, azithromycin, includes anecdotal data, a placebo-controlled study and open-label protocols. Data from these studies reviewed by Blagburn and Soave (1997) suggest that azithromycin is, at best, only marginally effective in the treatment of human cryptosporidiosis. At the time of writing, little is known about the potential effectiveness of other macrolides, including clarithromycin, roxithromycin and dirithromycin, for the treatment of human cryptosporidiosis.

BENZENEACETONITRILE DERIVATIVES

Interest in diclazuril and a better absorbed analogue, letrazuril, for the treatment of cryptosporidiosis stems from the activity of this class of compounds against related coccidia in the genus *Eimeria*. Diclazuril or letrazuril administered to AIDS patients in a randomized, double-blind, placebo-controlled, escalating

dose trial were no more efficacious than placebo (Soave et al. 1990, Blagburn and Soave 1997).

MISCELLANEOUS AGENTS

Paromomycin is a poorly absorbed aminoglycoside related to neomycin and kanamycin. There have been numerous anecdotal reports of dramatic responses of AIDS patients to this agent; however, many patients continue to shed oocysts and others relapse while on therapy. These results suggest that paromomycin is static rather than cidal for *Cryptosporidium* and that it produces only a short-term positive effect. Two placebo-controlled trials of paromomycin involving small numbers of patients showed a decrease in bowel movement frequency and some reduction in oocyst shedding. However, preliminary analysis of an NIAID-sponsored, placebo-controlled trial of 35 AIDS patients suggests that paromomycin treatment is no better than placebo.

Nitazoxanide, a nitrothiazole benzamide compound with wide spectrum activity against protozoan, helminth and bacterial pathogens, appears to have some efficacy against human cryptosporidiosis. Preliminary studies from Mexico and Mali suggests efficacy for human cryptosporidiosis in AIDS patients. Additional studies of this compound are under way in the US.

In the absence of a proven, consistent, effective treatment for cryptosporidiosis, supportive therapy can be helpful. Oral and parenteral rehydration therapy is often required by both immunodeficient and immunocompetent persons, especially young children, with severe cryptosporidial diarrhoea. Parenteral nutrition may also help sustain the nutritional status of some patients with persistent cryptosporidiosis. Antidiarrhoeal compounds may also be of some value in controlling fluid loss. Subcutaneous administration of a somatostatin analogue, octerotide, may also be of value in reducing the number of daily bowel movements and the stool volume from AIDS patients who have cryptosporidial diarrhoea (Cook et al. 1988).

A large number of drugs have also been evaluated for anticryptosporidial activity using an in vitro test system (Woods, Nesterenko and Upton 1966) or laboratory rodent models (Blagburn and Soave 1997), and some show promise. Some of the most effective compounds against cryptosporidiosis in laboratory rodents include maduramycin, lasalocid, several aromatic amadines, azithromycin, erythromycin, spiramycin, arprinocid, halofuginone sinefungin, sulphisoxazole, diclazuril, mefloquine and pentamidine (see Blagburn and Soave 1997 for complete list). Lack of efficacy in human cryptosporidiosis has already been demonstrated for some of these compounds (see above); however, others await proper evaluation in placebo-controlled trials.

11 IMMUNOLOGICAL INTERVENTION

Since immune status of the host appears to be a major factor determining the severity and duration of infection following oral exposure to *C. parvum* oocysts (Current and Bick 1989) and since a consistently effective, approved therapy for human cryptosporidiosis has not been identified, immunological intervention may be one approach to the control of cryptosporidiosis (Current and Garcia 1991, O'Donoghue 1995). Discontinuation of immunosuppressive chemotherapy, allowing restoration of immune function, has resulted in complete resolution of intestinal cryptosporidiosis in several patients (Miller et al. 1983, Stein et al. 1985). Although *Cryptosporidium*-specific IgA, IgM and IgG responses are detectable in the sera by ELISA and IFA procedures (Current and Bick 1989), the role that these antibodies play in protective immunity is questionable. Because the parasite appears to be confined to the mucosal surface and because numerous studies have failed to demonstrate a protective role for serum antibodies against closely related species of coccidia (Rose 1982), it is more probable that secretory antibodies coupled with cell-mediated immune mechanisms are responsible for the clearance of parasites from the infected mucosa and for rendering the immunocompetent host resistant to reinfection. The role of secretory antibodies as mediators of protective immunity to *Cryptosporidium* infections merits further investigation. The presence of *Cryptosporidium*-specific secretory antibodies has been reported in stools of Philippine children (Laxer and Alcantara 1990). Antibody neutralization-sensitive epitopes on the surface of *C. parvum* sporozoites have been demonstrated and several laboratories are investigating the potential immunotherapeutic utility of hyperimmune bovine colostrum (see below).

Mata and Bolanos (1984) reported that breast-fed infants in Costa Rica had a significantly lower incidence of cryptosporidiosis than did age-matched babies in the same study populations who were fed artificial diets, and they proposed that lactogenic immunity may play an important role in controlling *C. parvum* infections. Similar studies in Ecuador, Guatemala, Haiti and Liberia also revealed that breast-fed infants rarely had cryptosporidiosis (Fayer and Ungar 1986). These studies did not provide data that makes it possible to determine whether biologically active factors in milk or whether reduced exposure to contaminated food and water were responsible for the lower prevalence of cryptosporidiosis in breast-fed children.

The concept of passive lacteal immunity was subsequently tested in several studies to determine if antibodies in milk or colostrum can prevent or abrogate intestinal infections with *C. parvum*. Colostrum or milk from dairy cows that are exposed naturally to the parasite does not appear to protect calves or humans from *C. parvum* infection; however, colostrum from hyperimmunized cows may provide some protection. The fact that most calves will experience cryptosporidiosis while they are nursing from cows, most of which have colostrum antibodies to *C. parvum*, also supports the concept that natural exposure to the parasite may not result in significant lactogenic immunity. Oral administration of colostrum from a nonimmunized, naturally exposed dairy cow which contained antibodies to *C. parvum* did not alter the course of infection in an AIDS patient with cryptosporidiosis (Saxon and Weinstein 1987) A similar lack of lactogenic immunity was also reported in infant mice whose dams were immunized by oral inoculation of *C. parvum* oocysts (Arrowood and Sterling 1989).

In contrast to the above reports, several studies indicate that colostrum obtained from cows hyperimmunized with oocyst/sporozoite antigens of *C. parvum* may protect mice, calves and humans from cryptosporidiosis. Fayer et al. (1989a) demonstrated that hyperimmune bovine colostrum, obtained from cows immunized with purified *C. parvum* oocysts, neutralized sporozoites and protected mice from oocyst challenge, and that the same preparation provided prophylactic protection against cryptosporidiosis in calves (Fayer et al. 1989b). More recently, investigators reported that an immunoglobulin concentrate derived from bovine colostrum was effective in the treatment of cryptosporidiosis in a small trial of AIDS patients (Greenberg and Cello 1996). When given the immunoglobulin concentrate orally, patients with AIDS and confirmed *C. parvum* infection experienced a significant decrease in mean stool weight. Placebo-controlled trials with larger numbers of patients and with more rigorous monitoring of infections are needed to get a better assessment of this potential therapy.

REFERENCES

Anderson BC, 1985, Moist heat inactivation of *Cryptosporidium* sp., *Am J Public Health*, **75**: 1433–4.

Angus KW, 1983, Cryptosporidiosis in man, domestic animals and birds: a review, *J R Soc Med*, **76**: 62–70.

Argenzio RA, Liacos JA et al., 1990, Villous atrophy, crypt hyperplasia, cellular infiltration and impaired glucose-Na absorption in enteric cryptosporidiosis of pigs, *Gastroenterology*, **98**: 1129–40.

Arrowood MJ, Mead JR et al., 1989, Effects of immune colostrum and orally administered antisporozoite monoclonal antibodies on the outcome of *Cryptosporidium parvum* infections in neonatal mice, *Infect Immun*, **57**: 2283–8.

Arrowood MJ, Sterling CR, 1989, Comparison of conventional staining methods and monoclonal antibody–based methods for *Cryptosporidium* oocyst detection, *J Clin Microbiol*, **27**: 1490–5.

Avila-Figueroa C, Soria-Rodriguez C et al., 1989, Clinical manifestations of infection by human immunodeficiency virus in children, *Bol Med Hosp Infant Mexico*, **46**: 448–54.

Blagburn BL, Current WL, 1983, Accidental infection of a researcher with human *Cryptosporidium*, *J Infect Dis*, **148**: 772–3.

Blagburn BL, Lindsay DS et al., 1987, Experimental cryptosporidiosis in broiler chickens, *Poultry Sci*, **66**: 442–9.

Blagburn BL, Soave R, 1997, Prophylaxis and chemotherapy: Human and animal, *Cryptosporidium and Cryptosporidiosis*, ed Fayer R, CRC Press, Boca Raton, FL, 113–30.

Blewett DA, 1989, Quantitative techniques in *Cryptosporidium* research, *Proc. 1st International Workshop on Cryptosporidiosis*, eds Angus KW, Blewett DA, Moredun Research Institute, Edinburgh, Scotland, 85–96.

Bogaerts J, Lepage P et al., 1984, *Cryptosporidium* spp., a frequent cause of diarrhea in Central Africa, *J Clin Microbiol*, **20**: 874–6.

Boothe CC, Slavin G et al., 1980, Immunodeficiency and crypto-sporidiosis demonstration at the Royal College of Physicians of London, *Br Med J*, **281**: 1123–7.

Brady E, Margolis ML et al., 1984, Pulmonary cryptosporidiosis in acquired immune deficiency syndrome, *J Am Med Assoc*, **252**: 89–90.

Campbell PN, Current WL, 1983, Demonstration of serum anti-bodies to *Cryptosporidium* sp. in normal and immunodeficient humans with confirmed infections, *J Clin Microbiol*, **18**: 165–9.

Casemore DP, 1987, The antibody response to *Cryptosporidium*: development of a serological test and its use in a study of immunologically normal persons, *J Infect*, **14**: 125–34.

Centers for Disease Control, 1982, Cryptosporidiosis: an assess-ment of chemotherapy of males with acquired immune deficiency syndrome (AIDS), *Morbid Mortal Weekly Rep*, **31**: 589–92.

Clarke JJ, 1895, A study of coccidia met with in mice, *J Microsc Soc*, **37**: 277–302.

Collier AC, Miller RA et al., 1984, Cryptosporidiosis after marrow transplantation: person-to-person transmission and treatment with spiramycin, *Ann Intern Med*, **101**: 205–6.

Connolly GM, Dryden MS et al., 1988, Cryptosporidial diarrhoea in AIDS and its treatment, *Gut*, **29**: 593–7.

Cook DJ, Kelton JG et al., 1988, Somatostatin treatment for cryp-tosporidial diarrhea in a patient with AIDS, *Ann Intern Med*, **108**: 708–9.

Crawford FG, Vermund SH, 1988, Human cryptosporidiosis, *CRC Crit Rev Microbiol*, **16**: 113–59.

Current WL, 1990, Techniques and laboratory maintenance of *Cryptosporidium*, *Cryptosporidiosis In Man and Animals*, eds Dubey JP, Fayer R, Speer CA, CRC Press, Boca Raton, FL, 31–49.

Current WL, Bick PW, 1989, Immunobiology of *Cryptosporidium* spp, *Pathol Immunopathol Res*, **8**: 141–60.

Current WL, Blagburn BL, 1990, *Cryptosporidium* infections in man and domesticated animals, *Coccidiosis of Man and Domestic Animals*, ed Long PL, CRC Press, Boca Raton, FL, 155–85.

Current WL, Garcia LS, 1991, Cryptosporidiosis, *Clin Microbiol Rev*, **4**: 325–58.

Current WL, Reese NC, 1986, A comparison of endogenous development of three isolates of *Cryptosporidium* in suckling mice, *J Protozool*, **33**: 98–108.

Current WL, Reese NC et al., 1983, Human cryptosporidiosis in immunocompetent and immunodeficient persons: studies of an outbreak and experimental transmission, *N Engl J Med*, **308**: 1252–7.

Current WL, Snyder DB, 1988, Development and serologic evalu-ation of acquired immunity to *Cryptosporidium baileyi* by broiler chickens, *Poultry Sci*, **67**: 720–9.

Current WL, Upton SJ, Haynes TB, 1986, The life cycle of *Crypto-sporidium baileyi* n. sp. (Apicomplexa, Cryptosporidiidae) infecting chickens, *J Protozool*, **33**: 289–96.

D'Antonio RG, Win RE et al., 1986, A waterborne outbreak of cryptosporidiosis in normal hosts, *Ann Intern Med*, **103**: 886–8.

Dias RMDS, Mangini ACS et al., 1988, Cryptosporidiosis among patients with acquired immunodeficiency syndrome (AIDS) in the county of Sao Paulo, Brazil, *Rev Inst Med Trop São Paulo*, **30**: 310–2.

Dubey JP, Fayer R, Speer CA (eds), 1990, *Cryptosporidiosis In Man and Animals*, CRC Press, Boca Raton, FL.

Dupont HL, Chappell CL et al., 1995, The infectivity of *Cryptospo-ridium parvum* in healthy volunteers, *N Engl J Med*, **332**: 855–9.

Fayer R (ed), 1997, Cryptospordium *and Cryptosporidiosis*, CRC Press, Boca Raton, FL.

Fayer R, Andrews C et al., 1989a, Efficacy of hyperimmune bov-ine colostrum for prophylaxis of cryptosporidiosis in neonatal calves, *J Parasitol*, **75**: 393–7.

Fayer R, Perryman LE et al., 1989b, Hyperimmune bovine col-ostrum neutralizes *Cryptosporidium* sporozoites and protects mice against oocyst challenge, *J Parasitol*, **75**: 151–3.

Fayer R, Ungar PLB, 1986, *Cryptosporidium* spp. and cryptospori-diosis, *Microbiol Rev*, **50**: 458–83.

Finch GR, Belosevic M, 1994, *Ozone disinfection of* Giardia *and* Cryptosporidium, AWWA Research Foundation, Denver, 1–56.

Gallaher MM, Herndon JL et al., 1989, Cryptosporidiosis and surface water, *Am J Publ Health*, **79**: 39–42.

Garcia LS, Current WL, 1989, Cryptosporidiosis: clinical features and diagnosis, *CRC Clin Rev Lab Sci*, **27**: 439–60.

Garza DH, Fedorak RN, Soave R, 1986, Enterotoxin-like activity in cultured cryptosporidia: role in diarrhea, *Gastroenterology*, **90**: 1424.

Goebel E, Brandler U, 1982, Ultrastructure of microgametogen-esis, microgametes, and gametogony of *Cryptosporidium* sp. in the small intestine of mice, *Protistologica*, **18**: 331–4.

Gooz L, Kim K et al., 1991, Amplification of a *Cryptosporidium parvum* gene fragment encoding thymidylate synthase, *J Proto-zool*, **38**: S56–8.

Greenberg PD, Cello JP, 1996, Treatment of severe diarrhea caused by *Cryptosporidium parvum* with oral bovine immuno-globulin concentrate in patients with AIDS, *J Acquired Immune Defic Syndr Human Retrovirol*, **13**: 348–54.

Guarino A, Canani RB et al., 1994, Enterotoxic effect of stool supernatant of *Cryptosporidium*-infected calves on human jejunum, *Gasteroenterology*, **106**: 28–32.

Harp JA, Wannemuehler MW et al., 1988, Susceptibility of germ-free or antibiotic treated adult mice to *Cryptosporidium par-vum*, *Infect Immun*, **56**: 2006–10.

Hayes EB, Matte TD et al., 1989, Large community outbreak of cryptosporidiosis due to contamination of a filtered public water supply, *N Engl J Med*, **320**: 1372–6.

Heine J, Moon HW, Woodmansee DB, 1984, Persistent crypto-sporidiosis infection in congenitally athymic (nude) mice, *Infect Immun*, **43**: 856–9.

Heine J, Pohlenz JFL et al., 1984, Enteric lesions and diarrhea in gnotobiotic calves monoinfected with *Cryptosporidium* spe-cies, *J Infect Dis*, **150**: 768–75.

Isaacs D, Hunt GH et al., 1985, Cryptosporidiosis in immuno-competent children, *J Clin Pathol*, **38**: 76–81.

Johnson AM, Fielke R et al., 1990, Phylogenetic relationships of *Cryptosporidium* determined by ribosomal RNA sequence com-parison, *Int J Parasitol*, **20**: 141–7.

Keren G, Barzilai A et al., 1987, Life–threatening cryptospori-diosis in immunocompetent infants, *Eur J Pediatr*, **146**: 187–9.

Kibbler CC, Smith A et al., 1987, Pulmonary cryptosporidiosis occurring in a bone marrow transplant patient, *Scand J Infect Dis*, **19**: 581–4.

Koch KJ, Phillips DJ et al., 1985, Cryptosporidiosis in hospital personnel: evidence for person–to–person transmission, *Ann Intern Med*, **102**: 593–6.

Korich DG, Mead JR et al., 1990, Effects of ozone, chlorine diox-ide, chlorine and monochloroamine in *Cryptosporidium* oocyst viability, *Appl Environ Microbiol*, **56**: 1423–8.

Lahdevirta J, Jokipii AMM et al., 1987, Perinatal infection with *Cryptosporidium* and failure to thrive, *Lancet*, **i**: 48–9.

Laughon BE, Druckman DA et al., 1988, Prevalence of enteric pathogens in homosexual men with and without acquired immunodeficiency syndrome, *Gastroenterology*, **94**: 984–93.

Laxer MA, Alcantara AK, 1990, Immune response to cryptospori-diosis in Philippine children, *Am J Trop Med Hyg*, **42**: 131–9.

Levine ND, 1984, Taxonomy and review of the coccidian genus *Cryptosporidium* (Protozoa, Apicomplexa), *J Protozool*, **31**: 94–8.

Loening WE, Coovadia YM et al., 1989, Aetiological factors of infantile diarrhoea: A community-based study, *Ann Trop Pae-diatr*, **9**: 248–55.

MacFarlane DE, Horner-Bryce J, 1987, Cryptosporidiosis in well nourished and malnourished children, *Acta Paediatr Scand*, **76**: 474–7.

Mackinzee WR, Hoxie NJ et al., 1994, A massive outbreak in Milwaukee of *Cryptosporidium* infection transmitted through the public water supply, *N Engl J Med*, **331**: 161–7.

Malebranche R, Arnoux E et al., 1983, Acquired immunodeficiency syndrome with severe gastrointestinal manifestations in Haiti, *Lancet*, **ii**: 873–8.

Mata L, Bolanos H, 1984, Cryptosporidiosis in children from some highland Costa Rican rural and urban areas, *Am J Trop Med Hyg*, **33**: 24–9.

McDonald V, 1996, Cryptosporidiosis, *The Wellcome Illustrated History of Tropical Diseases*, ed Cox FEG, Wellcome Trust, London, 256–63.

Mead JR, Arrowood M J et al., 1988a, Antigens of *Cryptosporidium* sporozoites recognized by immune sera of infected animals and humans, *J Parasitol*, **74**: 135–43.

Mead JR, Arrowood M J et al., 1988b, Field inversion gel electrophoretic separation of *Cryptosporidium* spp. chromosome-sized DNA, *J Parasitol*, **74**: 366–9.

Mead JR, Humphreys RC et al., 1990, Identification of isolate-specific sporozoite proteins of Cryptosporidium parvum by two-dimensional gel electrophoresis, *Infect Immun*, **58**: 2071–5.

Meisel JL, Perera DR et al., 1976, Overwhelming watery diarrhea associated with *Cryptosporidium* in an immunosuppressed patient, *Gastroenterology*, **70**: 1156–60.

Miller RA, Holmberg RE, Jr, et al., 1983, Life-threatening diarrhea caused by *Cryptosporidium* in a child undergoing therapy for acute lymphocytic leukemia, *J Pediatr*, **103**: 256–9.

Mitschler RR, Welti R, Upton SJ, 1994, A comparative study of lipid compositions of *Cryptosporidium parvum* (Apicomplexa) and Madin Darby bovine kidney cells, *J Euk Biol*, **41**: 8–12.

Navin TR, Hardy AM, 1987, Cryptosporidiosis in patients with AIDS, *J Infect Dis*, **155**: 150.

Neira, P, Tardio MT et al., 1989, Cryptosporidiosis in the V region of Chile III Study of malnourished patients, 1985–1987, *Bol Chil Parasitol*, **44**: 34–6.

Newman, RD, Zu SX, et al., 1994, Household epidemiology of *Cryptosporidium parvum* infection in an urban community in northeast Brazil, *Ann Intern Med*, **120**: 500–5.

Nichols GL, McLaughlin J, Samuel D, 1991, A technique for typing *Cryptosporidium* isolates, *J Protozool*, **38**: S237–40.

Nime FA, Burek JD et al., 1976, Acute enterocolitis in a human being infected with the protozoan *Cryptosporidium*, *Gastroenterology*, **70**: 592–8.

Nina JMS, McDonald V et al., 1992, Comparative study of the antigenic composition of oocyst isolates of *Cryptosporidium parvum* from different hosts, *Parasite Immunol*, **14**: 227–32.

O'Donoghue PJ, 1995, *Cryptosporidium* and cryptosporidiosis in man and animals, *Int J Parasitol*, **25**: 139–95.

Ogunkolade BW, Robinson HA et al., 1993, Isozyme variation within the genus *Cryptosporidium*, *Parasitol Res*, **79**: 385–92.

Ortega YR, Sheehy RR et al., 1991, Restriction fragment length polymorphism analysis of *Cryptosporidium* isolates of bovine and human origin, *J Parasitol*, **38**: S40–41.

Panciera RJ, Thomassen RW, Gardner FM, 1971, Cryptosporidial infection in a calf, *Vet Pathol*, **8**: 479–84.

Petersen C, 1993, Cellular biology of *Cryptosporidium parvum*, *Parasitol Today*, **9**: 87–91.

Reducker DW, Speer CA , Blixt JA, 1985, Ultrastructure of *Cryptosporidium* oocysts and excysting sporozoites as revealed by high resolution scanning electron microscopy, *J Protozool*, **32**: 708–11.

Reese NC, Current WL et al., 1982, Cryptosporidiosis of man and calf: a case report and results of experimental infections in mice and rats, *Am J Trop Med Hyg*, **31**: 226–9.

Rehg JE, 1991, Anticryptosporidial activity associated with specific sulfonamides in immunosuppressed rats, *J Parasitol*, **77**: 238–40.

Rehg JE, Hancock ML, Woodmansee DB, 1988, Anticryptosporidial activity of sulfamethoxine, *Antimicrob Agents Chemother*, **32**: 1907–8.

Rene E, Marche C et al., 1989, Intestinal infections in patients with acquired immunodeficiency syndrome A prospective study in 132 patients, *Dig Dis Sci*, **34**: 773–80.

Rose ME, 1982, Host immune responses, *The Biology of the Coccidia*, ed Long PL, University Park Press, Baltimore, MD, 329–71.

Rush BA, Chapman PA, Ineson RW, 1987, *Cryptosporidium* and drinking water, *Lancet*, **ii**: 632–3.

Sallon S, Deckelbaum RJ et al., 1988, *Cryptosporidium*, malnutrition, and chronic diarrhea in children, *Am J Dis Child*, **142**: 312–15.

Saxon A, Weinstein W, 1987, Oral administration of bovine colostrum anti-cryptosporidia antibody fails to alter the course of human cryptosporidiosis, *J Parasitol*, **73**: 413–15.

Schmatz DM, 1989, The mannitol cycle – A new metabolic pathway in the Coccidia, *Parasitol Today*, **5**: 205–10.

Sherwood, DK, Angus KW et al., 1982, Experimental cryptosporidiosis in laboratory mice, *Infect Immun*, **38**: 471–5.

Slavin D, 1955, *Cryptosporidium meleagridis* (sp. nov.), *J Comp Pathol*, **65**: 262–6.

Smith HV, Girwood RWA et al., 1988a, Waterborne outbreak of cryptosporidiosis, *Lancet*, **ii**: 1484.

Smith PD, Lane HC et al., 1988b, Intestinal infections in patients with the acquired immunodeficiency syndrome (AIDS); etiology and response to therapy, *Ann Intern Med*, **108**: 328–33.

Soave R, 1990, Treatment strategies for cryptosporidiosis, *Ann N Y Acad Sci*, **616**: 442–8.

Soave R, Dieterich D et al., 1990, Oral diclazuril for cryptosporidiosis, *6th Ann Conf for AIDS*, **Abstr th B, 519**.

Stemmermann GN, Frenkel RI, 1980, Cryptosporidiosis: report of a fatal case complicated by disseminated toxoplasmosis, *Am J Med*, **69**: 637–42.

Stine KC, Harris JA et al., 1985, Spontaneous remission of cryptosporidiosis in a child with acute lymphocytic leukemia, *Clin Pediatr*, **24**: 722–4.

Sundermann CA, Lindsay DS, Blagburn BL, 1987, Evaluation of disinfectants for ability to kill avian *Cryptosporidium* oocysts, *Compan Anim Pract*, **2**: 36–9.

Thomson MA, Benson JWT, Wright PA, 1987, Two year study of *Cryptosporidium* infection, *Arch Dis Child*, **62**: 559–53.

Tilley M, Fayer R et al., 1990b, *Cryptosporidium parvum* (Apicomplexa: Cryptosporidiidae) oocysts and sporozoite antigens recognized by bovine colostral antibodies, *Infect Immun*, **58**: 2966–71.

Tilley M, Upton SJ, 1990, Electrophoretic characterization of *Cryptosporidium parvum* (KSU–1 isolate) (Apicomplexa: Cryptosporidiidae), *Can J Zool*, **68**: 1513–19.

Tilley M, Upton SJ, 1997, Biochemistry of *Cryptosporidium*, *Cryptosporidium and Cryptosporidiosis*, ed Fayer R, CRC Press, Boca Raton, FL, 165–81.

Tilley M, Upton SJ et al., 1990a, Identification of outer oocyst wall proteins of three *Cryptosporidium* (Apicomplexa; Cryptosporidiidae) species by ^{125}I surface labeling, *Infect Immun*, **58**: 252–3.

Tyzzer EE, 1907, A sporozoan found in the peptic glands of the common mouse, *Proc Soc Exp Biol Med*, **5**: 12–3.

Tyzzer EE, 1910, An extracellular coccidium, *Cryptosporidium muris* (gen. et sp. nov.) of the gastric glands of the common mouse, *J Med Res*, **23**: 487–516.

Tyzzer EE, 1912, *Cryptosporidium parvum* (sp. nov.) a coccidium found in the small intestine of the common mouse, *Arch Protistenkd*, **26**: 394–412.

Tzipori S, 1983, Cryptosporidiosis in animals and humans, *Microbiol Rev*, **47**: 84–96.

Tzipori S, Angus KW et al., 1980, *Cryptosporidium*: evidence for a single-species genus, *Infect Immun*, **30**: 884–6.

Ungar BLP, Burris JA et al., 1990, New mouse models for chronic *Cryptosporidium* infection in immunodeficient hosts, *Infect Immun*, **58**: 961–9.

Ungar BLP, Gilman RH et al., 1988, Seroepidemiology of *Cryptosporidium* infection in two Latin American populations, *J Infect Dis*, **157**: 551–6.

Ungar BLP, Mulligan M, Nutman TR, 1989, Serologic evidence

of *Cryptosporidium* infection in US volunteers before and during Peace Corps service in Africa, *Arch Intern Med*, **149**: 894–7.

Ungar BLP, Nash TE, 1986, Quantification of specific antibody responses to *Cryptosporidium* antigens by laser densitometry, *Infect Immun*, **53**: 124–8.

Ungar BLP, Soave R et al., 1986, Enzyme immunoassay detection of immunoglobulin M and G antibodies to *Cryptosporidium* in immunocompetent and immunocompromised persons, *J Infect Dis*, **153**: 570–8.

Upton SJ, Current WL, 1985, The species of *Cryptosporidium* (Apicomplexa, Cryptosporiidae) infecting mammals, *J Parasitol*, **71**: 625–9.

Upton SJ, Tilley M, Brillhart DB, 1995, Effects of select medium supplements on in vitro development of *Cryptosporidium parvum* in HCT–8 cells, *J Clin Microbiol*, **33**: 371–5.

Upton SJ, Tilley M et al., 1991, Incorporation of exogenous uracil by *Cryptosporidium parvum* in vitro, *J Clin Microbiol*, **29**: 1062–5.

Walsh, JA, Warren KS, 1979, Selective primary care. An interim strategy for disease control in developing countries, *N Engl J Med*, **301**: 967–74.

Woods KM, Nesterenko MV, Upton SJ, 1996, Efficacy of 101 antimicrobials and other agents on the development of *Cryptosporidium* in vitro, *Ann Trop Med Parasitol*, **90**: 603–15.

Chapter 19

BABESIOSIS OF HUMANS

S R Telford III and A Spielman

1 Historical introduction	7 Pathology
2 Classification	8 Diagnosis
3 Structure and life cycle	9 Epidemiology and control
4 Biochemistry, molecular biology and genetics	10 Chemotherapy
5 Clinical aspects of babesiosis	11 Vaccination
6 Immunology	12 Integrated control

1 HISTORICAL INTRODUCTION

Babesiosis, caused by certain tick-borne intraerythrocytic sporozoans, has affected human affairs since antiquity. The 'grievous murrain' described in Exodus IX was probably redwater fever of cattle, caused by *Babesia bovis*. Babesiosis occupies a prominent place in the history of biomedical sciences. Smith and Kilborne's landmark 1893 discovery of the role of ticks in the transmission of *B. bigemina*, the Texas cattle fever pathogen, stands as the first proof that haematophagous arthropods can transmit pathogens of vertebrates.

With the exception of the trypanosomes, *Babesia* are the most ubiquitous of the mammalian haemoprotozoa, occurring wherever certain ticks proliferate. Numerous types of mammals serve as hosts for these pathogens, certain of which, particularly *Babesia microti*, have taken a prominent place among the 'emerging infections' of humans. Babesiosis, therefore, spans human history and continues to demand our attention.

Babesia are small sporozoans that cycle between ixodid ticks and vertebrates. They undergo sexual reproduction after ingestion by ticks and replicate one to several times before reaching maturity in the vector's salivary glands. The tick, which is the definitive host, then deposits the infectious sporozoite stage of the *Babesia* within the vertebrate host's dermis. The mode of development at the site of deposition and subsequent path of dissemination remain largely unknown. Ultimately, the parasites appear as characteristic pear-shaped trophozoites (**piroplasms**) in infected erythrocytes where they multiply, appearing as simple rings, paired or single piroplasms or the pathognomonic tetrads. The parasite's 'accordion-like' intraerythrocytic gametocyte stage is only identifiable by electron microscopy or staining with DNA-specific stains. Although certain basic elements of the babesial life cycle appear to be well established, much remains to be learned about the biology of this diverse group of parasites.

2 CLASSIFICATION

The *Babesia* are Protista classified within the phylum Apicomplexa, order Piroplasmidora and family Babesiidae. Those that parasitize mammals are considered to be monophyletic, although apparent biological differences might suggest 2 main lineages, 'large' and 'small' types of *Babesia*. *Babesia* are divided informally between those with intraerythrocytic forms that are 1.0–2.5 μm in diameter and those of 2.5–5.0 μm. No pre- or exoerythrocytic forms have been described for most *Babesia*, implying that the sporozoites directly invade erythrocytes. Indeed, the absence of a pre-erythrocytic cycle has served as the main feature that distinguishes the Babesiidae from the Theileriidae (Riek 1968), *Theileria* being characterized by a lymphocytic pre-erythrocytic stage whereas *Babesia* lack such a stage in their life cycles. Direct evidence for penetration of erythrocytes by babesial sporozoites, however, is lacking. The lymphocytic exoerythrocytic forms that have been shown to occur in the life cycle of one small *Babesia*, *B. equi* (Schein et al. 1981, Mehlhorn and Schein 1987) may also occur in the life cycle of *B. microti* (Mehlhorn and Schein 1984). The existence of lymphocytic stages in the life cycle of some of the small *Babesia* raises a question about the validity of the generally accepted separation of *Babesia*, particularly the small types, from *Theileria*.

Although none of the small *Babesia* so far studied passes from generation to generation within the vector tick (**transovarial transmission**) (Walter and Weber 1981, Mehlhorn and Schein 1987, Telford, unpublished results 1988), all of the large ones appear to do so. The small *Babesia* share this exclusively intragenerational pattern of development with *Theileria*. The absence of transovarial transmission gives additional support to the suggestion that the small *Babesia* should be classified with *Theileria*. Whether all of the small *Babesia* produce pre-erythrocytic stages and whether all lack the capacity for inherited infection in the tick host remain to be determined.

Recent molecular analyses also support the long-standing inference of a phylogenetic distinction between the small and large *Babesia*. The sequences of their small subunit (ssu) ribosomal RNA genes (rDNA) indicate that all the small *Babesia* studied form a monophyletic group, or clade, with *Theileria* (Ellis et al. 1992, Thomford et al. 1994, Allsopp et al. 1994). When life cycles of additional species are determined and their DNA is studied by sequencing or similar molecular methods, and if the results are similar to those already obtained, then a formal reclassification of the small *Babesia* would seem to be in order.

At least 99 *Babesia* species infecting mammals have been described (Levine 1988), 78 of which infect non-ruminants. The vectors and other details of the life cycles of most of these species, except for those of veterinary or public health importance, remain largely undescribed. Virtually all piroplasm species were described on the basis of their microscopical appearance in Giemsa-stained blood smears, and the morphology of the blood forms and the occurrence of binary or tetrad forms as well as the host range and endemicity of the infections have formed the basis on which the species were named. Differences in the morphology of the piroplasms of a given species in different kinds of hosts, however, renders the inferred distinctions based on the morphology of the blood forms dubious. Indeed, we anticipate that the increasing use of molecular systematics will cause the combining of many of these species.

3 STRUCTURE AND LIFE CYCLE

The *Babesia* belong to a group of protists (the Apicomplexa) that are characterized by having a variety of apical complex organelles, including rhoptries and micronemes. Mature babesial sporozoites have been described as pear shaped with the anterior end the broad end (Kakoma and Mehlhorn 1994). They have one anterior rhoptry and several micronemes but lack conoids, polar rings or subpellicular microtubules. Sporozoites appear to contain free ribosomes, a smooth endoplasmic reticulum, mitochondria-like structures and coiled organelles.

Recently invaded erythrocytes contain merozoites that initially lie within a parasitophorous vacuole (Rudzinska 1981) but this invaginated host-derived membrane soon disintegrates, leaving the maturing trophozoite free in the cytoplasm. Perhaps this unique freedom from a constricting parasitophorous vacuole contributes to the frequently noted pleomorphism of the intraerythrocytic stage, which often is contorted or amoeboid.

As the asexually reproducing intraerythrocytic trophozoites of *B. microti* mature, new organelles appear, including polar rings, micronemes, larger rhoptries, subpellicular microtubules and double membrane segments (Rudzinska et al. 1979). Interestingly, no cytostome is apparent; their method for deriving nourishment from a host cell remains undescribed.

Following the ingestion of parasitized erythrocytes by feeding *Ixodes dammini* tick larvae (the main vector for *B. microti* in the northern USA), gametocytes emerge and undergo a process of development into gametes ('*Strahlenkörper*') which then fuse within the tick gut (Rudzinska et al. 1983). The existence of the ray-like *Strahlenkörper* that Koch associated with sexuality was confirmed by a demonstration of the fusion of the ray bodies emerging from neighbouring erythrocytes (Rudzinska et al. 1983). The zygotes resulting from this fusion mature and become ookinetes 14–18 h after the feeding larval tick becomes replete. The ookinetes subsequently penetrate into the haemolymph and elongate to form the kinetes which penetrate fat body cells and nephrocytes. A series of divisions within the fat body cells and nephrocytes then results in the production of secondary ookinetes which in some *Babesia* may invade the ovaries (Karakashian et al. 1986). This secondary cycle of division and invasion of the ovaries is characteristic of the large *Babesia* and may facilitate transovarial transmission. Primary ookinetes enter the salivary glands directly, where they have been observed as early as 13 days after the larva became replete.

The salivary acini become hypertrophied when ookinetes invade the salivary glands. The ookinetes in the salivary acini become sporoblasts which then remain dormant until the larval tick becomes a nymph and the nymphal tick attaches to a host. In the case of *B. microti*, this state of dormancy in its *I. dammini* vector extends naturally through the winter, a period of 9–10 months (Piesman et al. 1987). After the infected nymphal tick attaches, nuclear division occurs, resulting in the formation of about 10 000 sporozoites from each sporoblast. Many thousands of sporozoites appear to be deposited in the dermis around the tick's mouthparts during the final hours of attachment (Mehlhorn and Schein 1987). Some 10 000–25 000 syringe-injected *B. microti* sporozoites are required to infect white-footed mice and hamsters (Piesman and Spielman 1982), but the anti-inflammatory pharmacological activity of tick saliva (Ribeiro 1987) greatly facilitates infection, suggesting that ticks may transmit the infectious agents far more effectively than does a needle.

The events that follow inoculation of babesial sporozoites by the feeding vector tick are poorly understood. In the absence of evidence to the contrary, early reviews of the biology of *Babesia* by Mehlhorn and Schein (1987), Mahoney (1977), and Young and Morzaria (1986) have generally inferred that in *Babesia* no pre-erythrocytic cycle occurs. But in *B. equi*, an agent of equine babesiosis, sporozoites appear to enter lymphocytes directly, both in vitro and in vivo, where they undergo a cycle of merogony before the resulting merozoites emerge to infect erythrocytes (Schein et al. 1981). The exoerythrocytic cycle of this

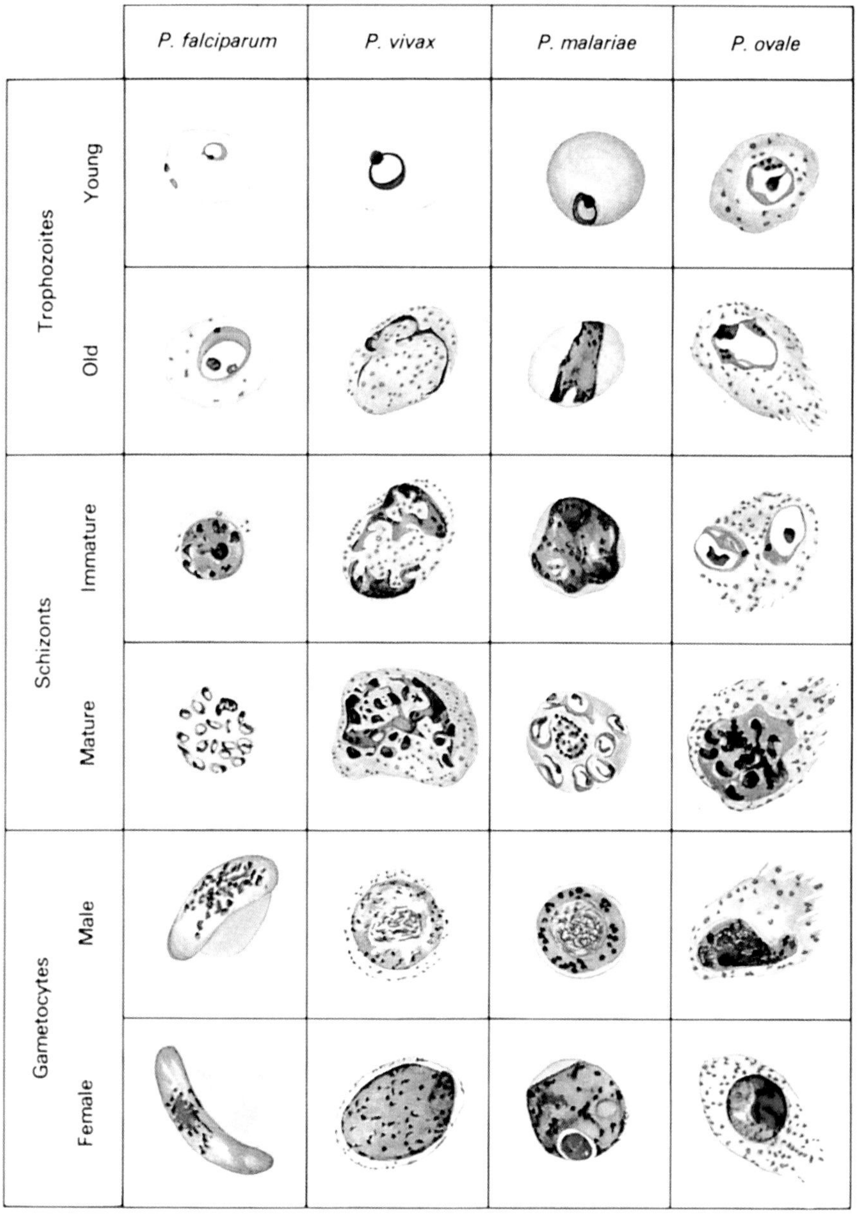

		P. falciparum	P. vivax	P. malariae	P. ovale
Trophozoites	Young				
	Old				
Schizonts	Immature				
	Mature				
Gametocytes	Male				
	Female				

Plate 20.13 Morphological characteristics of human malaria parasites.

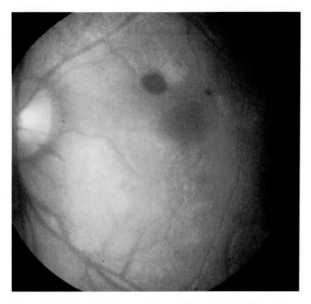

Plate 20.14 Retinal haemorrhage. (Copyright D Warrell).

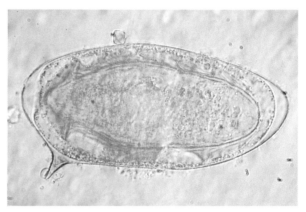

Plate 25.4 *Schistosoma mansoni* ovum.

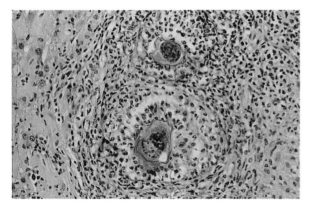

Plate 25.12 Granuloma formation around newly deposited eggs of *Schistosoma japonicum.*

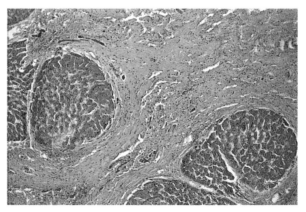

Plate 25.15 Liver cirrhosis due to *Schistosoma japonicum* infection. A case found in Yamanashi Prefecture, Japan.

small *Babesia* was only recently discovered, unlike the exoerythrocytic stages of *Theileria* which were discovered decades ago and called lymphocytic 'blue bodies' by Robert Koch.

The intraerythrocytic parasites replicate when a nucleus and other organelles migrate to a location under particular double membrane areas of the parent. These areas then develop and pinch off from the parental piroplasm in a process of budding (Rudzinska 1984). *Babesia* do not undergo synchronous budding (schizogony) as do the plasmodia, but rather one, 2 or rarely 3 bud off at one time.

In addition to the asexually reproducing trophozoites and their merozoite progeny, there are also non-reproducing 'accordion-like' gametocytes. These latter forms fail to develop the double membrane segments that become the anlage for merozoite formation and do not acquire a rhoptry; rather they just appear to grow larger, folding or coiling themselves within the confines of the erythrocyte (Mehlhorn and Schein 1987, Rudzinska et al. 1979). These 'accordion-like' forms emerge from erythrocytes within the gut of the tick and differentiate into gametes, pairs of which may fuse in a process of syngamy. Unlike the gametocytes of the plasmodia, *Babesia* gametocytes cannot be distinguished from asexual forms by light microscopy; electron microscopy must be used to make the distinction.

4 BIOCHEMISTRY, MOLECULAR BIOLOGY AND GENETICS

The biochemistry, molecular biology and genetics of the zoonotic *Babesia* have been inadequately explored. Such work as has been reported has generally had as its goal the discovery of diagnostic antigens, the elucidation of diagnostically useful DNA sequences, or the identification of variation among strains of species. Isoenzymes, for example, were examined in an attempt to distinguish various populations of *B. microti* (Momen, Chance and Peters 1979). High resolution polyacrylamide gel electrophoresis (Moss et al. 1986) was used to study the degree of polymorphism in the glucose phosphate isomerase locus in low- and high-passage Gray strain *B. microti* (the index strain for human infection) and showed that the Gray strain is heterogeneous, at least in terms of polymorphism at the locus. These preliminary results suggest that study of cloned isolates may be required to detect differences between populations.

Babesia microti infection may only slightly alter the physiology of hamster erythrocytes (Roth et al. 1981). Reduced glutathione levels double, but 2,3-diphosphoglycerate levels remain unchanged. Hamsters in which reticulocytosis is chemically induced experience similar changes, however, suggesting that the observed biochemical changes relate to anaemia and not necessarily to the presence of parasites.

The existence of sexuality in piroplasms, initially determined by observation of fusing gametes within the tick with the aid of electron microscopy (Rudzinska et al. 1983), was confirmed by fluorescence microscopy of *Babesia* stained with the DNA-specific bisbenzimide Hoechst 33258. These studies revealed the ploidy of the various life cycle stages of the cattle piroplasm *B. divergens* (Mackenstadt et al. 1990). Merozoites are haploid, 2 haploid merozoites are formed during budding within an erythrocyte, zygotes within the tick gut are diploid, kinetes are polyploid, and the polyploid sporoblasts divide to give rise to the uninuclear (haploid) infective sporozoites. Meiosis, however, has not been described.

A putative virulence-associated gene, *Bm13*, was cloned from a mung bean nuclease DNA expression library prepared from *B. microti* DNA (Tetzlaff, McMurray and Rice-Ficht 1990). Mung bean nuclease, under certain conditions, appears to cleave A–T rich DNA at sites flanking intact genes (McCutchan et al. 1984). Using hyperimmune serum from mice infected by the ATCC 30221 strain of *B. microti*, which kills murine hosts, a clone coding a 54 kDa immunodominant antigen was selected. This sequence did not hybridize with DNA prepared from the less virulent Peabody strain of *B. microti*. Further experiments characterizing the protein which is coded for by the gene and describing the protein's role in pathogenesis have not yet been published.

5 CLINICAL ASPECTS OF BABESIOSIS

The first convincingly demonstrated case of human babesial infection was reported in 1957 in a splenectomized resident of what was then Yugoslavia. The man died after an acute illness marked by anaemia, fever, haemoglobinuria and renal failure (Skrabalo and Deanovic 1957). Intraerythrocytic parasites were detected and tentatively identified as *B. bovis*, a piroplasm of cattle. In 1969, an elderly resident of Nantucket Island (USA) with no predisposing immune-compromising factors became infected with a rodent piroplasm, *B. microti* (Western 1970). Since then, infection by *B. microti* has been documented in hundreds of residents of the northeastern and upper Midwestern USA. *B. gibsoni* is a parasite of dogs, and a *B. gibsoni*-like parasite, WA-1, is now known to infect humans throughout a broad area along the Pacific coast of the USA. Human babesiosis has also been convincingly documented in Taiwan and South Africa. The public health significance of zoonotic babesiosis, then, may be greater than previously estimated.

Babesiosis is a malaria-like infection and its pathology, like that of malaria, is caused mainly by the asexually dividing intraerythrocytic forms. Non-synchronous fevers, chills, myalgia, sweats and prostration may be observed in patients with acute disease. In such patients a fulminating parasitaemia may lead to anaemia, haemoglobinuria, renal failure, disseminated intravascular coagulation and acute respiratory distress syndrome. Human infection, although occasionally severe, is usually subclinical.

5.1 Clinical manifestations

Symptoms of babesiosis caused by *B. microti* may commence 1–4 weeks after a human is bitten by an infected tick. In persons who develop clinical disease, a gradual onset of malaise, anorexia and fatigue ensues, with subsequent development (within a week) of fever as high as 40°C, drenching sweats and myalgia (Ruebush et al. 1977). Nausea, vomiting, headache, shaking chills, emotional lability and depression, haemoglobinuria and hyperaesthesia have also been reported in such patients (Golightly, Hirschhorn and Weller 1989). Pulmonary oedema may be a frequent complication in symptomatic persons (Gordon et al. 1984, Boustani et al. 1994). Splenomegaly may occur, but other findings on physical examination are unremarkable. Anaemia, thrombocytopaenia and low or generally normal WBC counts may be observed; parasitaemias range from 1% to 20% in spleen-intact patients and reach 85% in asplenic patients (Sun et al. 1983). Lactic dehydrogenase, bilirubin and transaminases may be elevated (Ruebush et al. 1977). The ambiguity of the symptoms of human babesiosis renders clinical diagnosis difficult, particularly in sites where the agents of Lyme disease and human granulocytic ehrlichiosis are co-transmitted (Telford et al. 1995). The presence of fever, malaise, headache, splenomegaly, anaemia, emotional lability and, particularly, profound fatigue provide clues useful to the physician.

As noted before, babesial infection in humans is usually subclinical or very mild. A large asymptomatic to symptomatic ratio is evident from serosurveys. For example, 8% of residents of Block Island, Rhode Island (USA) have been infected without clinically diagnosed illness (Krause et al. 1994). Even though most infections are subclinical in areas with a high level of infection, moderate to severe disease may be common. Nantucket Island reported 21 cases in 1994, which translates to 280 cases per 100 000 population, placing the community burden of this disease in a category with that of gonorrhea (Wilson 1991). The case fatality rate was estimated at 5% in a retrospective study of 136 New York cases (Meldrum et al. 1992). In certain sites, in years of particularly high transmission, babesiosis may constitute a public health burden.

Several factors appear to determine the severity of infection. There appears to be a relationship between the severity of illness and the age of the patient. The average age of 7 spleen-intact New York patients with clinically apparent disease was 63 years (Benach and Habicht 1981) as was that of 5 similar patients from Nantucket (Ruebush et al. 1977). Similarly, HIV infection appears to promote the severe manifestations of babesial infection (Ong, Stavropoulos and Inada 1990, Benezra et al. 1987, Machtinger et al. 1993). Although *B. microti* is enzootic in much of coastal New England, virtually all cases are diagnosed on Nantucket Island, eastern Long Island or in southeastern Connecticut. Parasite strain variation (as yet uncharacterized) may influence the course of infection, as well as the geographical distribution of cases.

Babesial infections acquired in Europe are due to the cattle piroplasm *B. divergens* and tend to be more severe than those in North America. Virtually all European patients had been splenectomized and the disease followed a severe course with the rapid multiplication of parasites (Gorenflot et al. 1990). Infection is usually fulminant; more than half of the 19 recorded patients died. Acute illness appears suddenly and is characterized by haemoglobinuria, which generally serves as the presenting symptom. Jaundice rapidly ensues and is accompanied by persistent non-periodic high fever (40–41°C), shaking chills, intense sweats, headaches and myalgia as well as lumbar and abdominal pain. Vomiting and diarrhoea may be present. In severe cases, renal failure ensues rapidly (in 16 of the recorded 19 cases) and is induced by intravascular haemolysis. In fatal cases, the patient loses consciousness and dies in coma.

Although only a few cases of babesiosis due to the *B. gibsoni*-like WA-1 *Babesia* have been described, the course of the infection would appear to be similar to that caused by *B. microti*. The index case (Quick et al. 1993) was a 41 year old spleen-intact man from a rural area in south central Washington (USA) with no history of travel. He was hospitalized with a 1 week history of fever, rigors, anorexia, cough and headache, which progressed to severe rigors and vomiting. Dark-coloured urine was noted, but a urine dipstick assay was only weakly positive for occult blood. Intraerythrocytic parasites were observed, including characteristic tetrad forms. The patient was treated with clindamycin and quinine and recovered uneventfully. An isolate was made by inoculating hamsters with the patient's blood, but unlike *B. microti*, this agent killed these and other rodents within 10 days of infection (unpublished results 1992). Serum reacted weakly with *B. microti* antigen but more intensely with that of *B. gibsoni*. Subsequent molecular analysis confirmed that WA-1 was more closely related to *B. gibsoni* than to other *Babesia* (Thomford et al. 1994).

Since the index case, 4 similar infections, 1 of which was fatal, have occurred in splenectomized residents of northern California (Persing et al. 1995). Seroprevalence studies using WA-1 as an antigen suggest that about 5% of residents of certain sites in northern California may have been exposed to this agent.

6 IMMUNOLOGY

The relatively greater severity of human babesiosis in patients lacking a spleen indicates that this organ plays an important role in limiting parasitaemia. In particular, early in the infection, parasitized and otherwise altered erythrocytes may be trapped and phagocytosed in the spleen. Absence of the spleen, however, does not necessarily imply that parasitaemia may not be eventually limited.

Treatment of splenectomized and intact hamsters with antilymphocyte serum (ALS) demonstrated the importance of cellular immunity because all ALS recipients died upon challenge with *B. microti*, whereas only 20% of splenectomized animals died (Wolf 1974). Persistent intense parasitaemias in athymic (nude) mice, in contrast to those of their hetero-zygous (thymus-intact) littermates, suggests the critical role of T cells in regulating the level of parasitaemia (Clark and Allison 1974). Indeed, the severe babesial disease that has been reported to occur in HIV posi-tive patients would seem to affirm the critical role of T cells in regulating this infection (Machtinger et al. 1993).

Experiments using inbred mice and murine-adapted *B. microti* have explored the possibility of a genetic basis for susceptibility, defined as the inability of mice of a given strain to regulate and eventually clear parasitaemia. Parasitaemia was lower in intact BALB/c mice than in intact mice of 4 other strains inoculated with *B. microti* but was highest in BALB/c mice when they were splenectomized (Ruebush and Hanson 1980). Intact C3H mice were most susceptible to infection. Susceptibility does not appear to be related to H-2 (major histocompatibility complex) haplotype, however, because mice of identical haplotypes develop different maximum parasitaemias. The degree of protection of mice against *B. microti* induced by *Propionibacterium acnes* inocu-lation does not correlate with H-2 haplotype (Wood and Clark 1982). On the other hand, the ability to express this induced protection trait is heritable. Some as yet undefined genetic component, then, appears to influence susceptibility to *B. microti* infection.

Various non-specific factors seem to modify susceptibility to piroplasm infection. The presence of eperythrozoa, for example, may antagonize infection (Peters 1965). Injection of various reagents and coinfection with diverse organisms may non-specifically protect mice against *B. microti* (Clark 1979). The prepatent period is increased and peak parasitae-mia reduced in mice on a severely restricted protein diet (Tetzlaff, Carlomagno and McMurray 1988). Finally, although old mice experience later and lower peak parasitae-mias than do younger animals, they fail to clear infection (Habicht et al. 1983). The factors that control susceptibility are complex.

In patients with *B. microti* babesiosis, some antibody responses are generally evident when they are first diagnosed. Seventeen patients with positive blood smears had a median IFAT (indirect fluorescent anti-body test) IgG titre of 1:1024 (negative, 1:64) with a range of 1:128–1:4096 in their serum at the time of diagnosis (Telford unpublished). The presence of antibody in their serum when they first became ill indicates that the prepatent period may be prolonged. Titre level is not related to parasitaemia, however, sug-gesting that antibody alone does not modulate infec-tion.

In one comprehensive study of immunoresponsive-ness in humans with *B. microti* babesiosis, lymphocyte responses to non-specific mitogens were markedly sup-pressed in acutely ill patients (Benach et al. 1982). The numbers of T cells bearing the IgG Fc receptor were high, as was the relative proportion of B lympho-cytes. Diminished levels of complement factors C3 and C4 in the serum of patients with acute babesiosis sug-gest activation of the classical complement pathway. In addition, the patient's blood contained a high level of circulating immune complexes. These data indicate

that *B. microti* infection profoundly alters the cellular immune status of patients.

Reinfection of those who have recovered from babesiosis has not been reported but it would not be easy to prove reinfection because of the difficulty of excluding recrudescence of an earlier infection. The concomitant immunity (or premunition) that charac-terizes babesiosis in cattle may also occur in humans. Using primers designed from species specific sequences of the small subunit ribosomal DNA (Persing et al. 1992), the PCR assay may facilitate a determination of the prevalence of chronic babesiosis in humans. Detection of non-clinical carriers is important because transfusion-acquired cases are not uncommon (Jacoby et al. 1980, Marcus et al. 1982, Smith et al. 1986).

7 PATHOLOGY

The development of the pathophysiology of babesial infection is directly related to the development of the parasitaemia. Studies on hamsters and labouratory mice infected by syringe with *B. microti* of human ori-gin have provided a wealth of information on host–parasite interactions. Intravascular and extravascular haemolysis develops as the parasitaemia rises, resulting in profound anaemia; the haematocrit may fall to 20% (Lykins et al. 1975). During this acute phase of disease, there is extramedullary haemato-poiesis and hyperplasia of the splenic red pulp, giving rise to the virtually pathognomonic gross splenomeg-aly that accompanies babesiosis in wild rodents (Fay and Rausch 1969). In addition, livers of infected ham-sters contain hypertrophied Kupffer cells, many with ingested parasitized erythrocytes but little haemo-globin breakdown products (Cullen and Levine 1987). The proximal convoluted tubules of the kidneys con-tain abundant haemosiderin, an observation consist-ent with occurrence of marked intravascular haemoly-sis (Cullen and Levine 1987).

8 DIAGNOSIS

Diagnosis of babesiosis in human hosts depends mainly on a demonstration of the organism in erythro-cytes. Examination of conventional Giemsa-stained thin blood films remains the most generally useful diagnostic procedure. Although the presence of tetrad forms ('Maltese cross') is said to be diagnostic, such elements are rarely encountered. Similarly, the absence of parasite haemozoin (malarial pigment) is often considered to be diagnostic for the piroplasms but early ring stages of malaria parasites also lack pig-ment. Diagnosis of *B. microti* (Fig. 19.1) is made by a combination of criteria, including the presence of an intense parasitaemia (1–50%), erythrocytes infected by multiple parasites, basket-shaped merozoites which are often extracellular and which often have a light coloured cytoplasm. The small *Babesia* are difficult to recognize with confidence in a thick film. Parasitaem-ias may sometimes also be exceedingly sparse, and persons with infections with low parasitimias may escape diagnosis when a thin blood film is examined. Inoculation into hamsters of a sample of patient's blood facilitates diagnosis by amplifying the parasitaemia but the blood of the hamster should be examined microscopically at weekly intervals for at least 6 weeks before the test is declared negative. Demonstration of the characteristic organisms in the hamster blood proves infection.

Serological testing is useful, particularly in diagnosing chronic *B. microti* infection. The IFAT, using antigen derived from infected hamster red cells (Chisholm et al. 1978), is sensitive and specific and is currently the serological method of choice. A serological reaction at a titre above the cutoff point of 1:64 for IgG is generally considered to be diagnostic (Krause et al. 1994). Examination of paired acute and convalescent serum samples is most useful for a diagnosis of *B. microti* infection. Detection of parasite-specific IgM may indicate that the patient has an acute infection even in the absence of a readily demonstrable parasitaemia.

In persons with *B. divergens* babesiosis, specific antibodies do not become detectable until at least 1 week after the onset of illness. Because this infection develops rapidly, serological procedures are not practical for the diagnosis of the infection in its acute form, but serological conversion serves as an aid in making a retrospective diagnosis in survivors. Of course, the high parasitaemias usually present in patients with this infection in its acute form are easily detected by examination of blood smears. Paired pyriform and accole parasites are frequently observed in

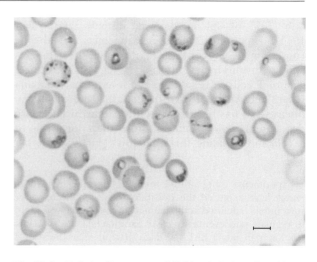

Fig. 19.2 *Babesia divergens*, gerbil blood. Pairs of pyriform organisms occur frequently and their presence helps to distinguish *B. divergens* from the other *Babesia* infecting humans. Ring-shaped organisms may also occur, as may tetrad ('Maltese cross') forms. Bar = 4.8 μm.

erythrocytes from patients with acute *B. divergens* infection (Fig. 19.2).

Infection with *Babesia* of the WA-1 strain may be readily detected by IFAT and this organism may also be detected by in vitro cultivation (Thomford et al. 1994). Its ease of cultivation facilitates production of a standardized antigen. For unknown reasons, a higher titre in the IFAT (>1:160) is required for diagnosis of WA-1 infection than for diagnosis of infection with *B. microti*. Tetrad forms are more frequently seen in blood smears from patients and rodents with WA-1 infection (Fig. 19.3) than in those with *B. microti* infections, but otherwise infection with this agent is difficult to distinguish from that with *B. microti*.

The PCR should supplant the hamster inoculation test

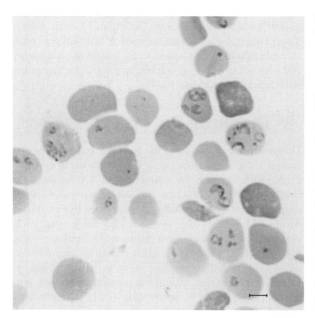

Fig. 19.1 *Babesia microti*, hamster blood. Note the varied morphology of the parasites, ranging from that of merozoites to that of mature trophiozoites. The occurrence of multiple infection of single erythrocytes is a characteristic which helps to distinguish these ring-shaped parasites from *Plasmodium falciparum*. Bar = 4 μm.

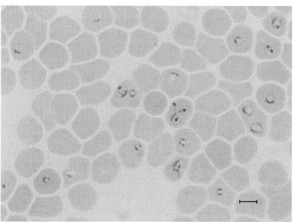

Fig. 19.3 *Babesia* sp. (WA-1), hamster blood. Although its morphology is very similar to that of *B. microti*, WA-1 may more frequently occur as tetrads than does *B. microti*; multiple infection of erythrocytes occurs less frequently in blood infected with WA-1 than in blood infected with *B. microti*. Bar = 5 μm.

when laboratory proficiency certification mechanisms for use of this procedure are instituted. In experienced hands, the PCR test detects *Babesia* DNA accurately and usually within a single working day. Hamster inoculation, long thought to be the gold standard for confirmatory diagnosis, has its problems. For example, it requires at least a week and often more than a month for incubation before results are obtained. Blood samples for hamster inoculation must also be taken prior to initiating treatment. An additional problem with use of hamster inoculation for diagnosis is that in many instances infection is transient in hamsters and may be missed if monitoring of blood smears is done only weekly. Finally, an infection due to a *Babesia* other than *B. microti*, *B. divergens* or WA-1, might be missed entirely if it lacks the ability to infect hamsters. These problems are avoided if diagnosis is made with the aid of a genus-specific DNA amplification assay.

9 EPIDEMIOLOGY AND CONTROL

The acquisition of babesiosis due to *B. divergens* or *B. microti* depends on contact with the minute subadult stages of certain *Ixodes* ticks. The vector of WA-1, however, has not yet been described. Environmental disturbance, increasing recreational use of the wilderness and suburbanization promote contact between people, ticks and the pathogens that they maintain (Spielman 1988).

Three epidemiological patterns are apparent in human babesiosis. The first (pattern I) involves splenectomized or otherwise immunologically compromised people, a *Babesia* of cattle (usually *B. divergens*) and the tick *I. ricinus*. In contrast to this 'European' pattern of infection, the risk of acquiring human babesiosis in the northeastern and northern Midwestern USA does not appear to depend on splenectomy. This second epidemiological pattern (pattern II) involves infection by the rodent piroplasm *B. microti* and being bitten by *I. dammini* ticks. A third epidemiological pattern (pattern III) is emerging in the western USA due to infection by WA-1 or similar *Babesia*. Although similar to pattern I in that splenectomy appears to be the major determinant of risk, pattern III infections are not associated with cattle. The vector is unknown.

A fourth pattern of infection is becoming evident as a result of the increasing prevalence of HIV infection in many parts of the world, which may diminish the ratio of non-apparent to apparent cases for a variety of opportunistic pathogens. Babesiosis is particularly severe in individuals with HIV and some case reports of babesiosis in AIDS patients already exist in the literature (Machtinger et al. 1993). The diversity of *Babesia* species and the ubiquity of ticks suggest a high potential for the emergence of *Babesia* as zoonotic agents. Tropical areas would seem to be at particular risk, although most babesial infections of humans to date have been observed in temperate regions of Europe and the USA. It is at least possible that some 'chloroquine-resistant' malaria parasites may eventually be identified as *Babesia* (Young and Morzaria 1986). Whether this is the case will be determined by careful microscopy, complemented by the use of molecular diagnostic techniques by people

aware of the possibility of babesial infection in humans.

9.1 Epidemiology and ecology

The ecology of *B. microti* is the best understood of the 3 known zoonotic piroplasms. The enzootic cycle of *B. microti* clearly depends upon the interaction of subadult *I. dammini* and their main host, the white-footed mouse (*Peromyscus leucopus*). Deer (*Odocoileus virginianus*) serve as the host upon which adult ticks commonly feed, but deer are not reservoirs for *B. microti* (Piesman et al. 1979). Adult ticks feed during the autumn, overwinter, feed and engorge again and lay eggs during the spring (Yuval and Spielman 1990). The eggs hatch synchronously in late July, with larvae feeding on mice mainly during August and September, when they acquire babesial infection; the prevalence of *Babesia* infection in the mice appears to be about 60% (Etkind et al. 1980).

Fed larvae overwinter and moult to the nymphal stage during the spring. Thus, non-infected mice resulting from reproduction during May and June are inoculated by nymphs infected as larvae during the preceding fall. About 40% of nymphal ticks on Nantucket Island (USA) may contain babesial sporozoites in their salivary glands during June. People become exposed mainly during June (Piesman et al. 1987) when they visit zoonotic sites for recreation or inhabit summer homes located in such sites. The population of Nantucket Island increases from about 7000 winter residents to over 35 000 summer residents after Memorial Day (at the end of May). The small size of nymphal *I. dammini* makes its detection and prompt removal difficult. Failure to remove a feeding tick promptly determines risk because the probability that the tick will transfer the *Babesia* to the host on which it feeds is directly proportional to the duration of feeding by the tick (Piesman et al. 1986).

The life cycle of the tick is completed when nymphs that have fed on a host moult to the adult stage in the fall. Thus, *I. dammini* ticks develop from egg to egg over a span of at least 2 years (Yuval and Spielman 1990), permitting cohorts of nymphal ticks to overlap, thereby buffering the tick population against years of host scarcity.

The epizootiology of *B. divergens* and the role of its presumed vector, *I. ricinus*, in the spread of infection is poorly understood. In Ireland, a high incidence in cattle is associated with elevated air temperature, which is when there is much tick activity. As in the case of *I. dammini*, nymphs may become active in the spring before the larvae hatch, but incrimination of the vector stage responsible for transmitting infection is confounded by the presence of adult ticks concurrently with nymphs (Gray 1980). Most cases of babesiosis due to *B. divergens* in humans have occurred in farmers or others who are frequently in contact with cattle (Clarke, Rogers and Egan 1989). Interestingly, although *B. microti* is enzootic in many European sites, human babesiosis due to this parasite has not been observed there, possibly because a uniquely mouse-specific tick, *I. trianguliceps*, maintains *B. microti* in Europe, although the aggressively human-biting *I. ricinus* may densely infest the same sites. Perhaps European strains of *B. microti* are not pathogenic to humans.

Neither the vector nor the reservoir of the WA-1 *Babesia* are known. Although closely related to *B. gibsoni*, the WA-1 agent does not infect dogs (PA Conrad personal communication 1993) but will parasitize and kill most rodents. Three ticks are prevalent in sites where cases of WA-1 babesiosis have occurred: *I. pacificus*, *Dermacentor variabilis*, and *Ornithodoros coriaceus*. We have not been able to infect the deer tick, *I. dammini*, in our laboratory (SR Telford unpublished results 1994), a result suggesting that *I. pacificus* may not serve as the vector of this *Babesia*.

Residents of few countries outside the USA and Europe appear to have experienced clinical babesiosis. One case has been observed in China (Li and Meng 1984) and 2 in South Africa (Bush et al. 1990). The species of *Babesia* involved in these cases has not been determined. One fatal case due to infection by *B. caucasica* has been observed in the former Soviet Union (Rabinovich et al. 1978). Unidentified *Babesia* were isolated by hamster inoculation from asymptomatic residents of Mexico (Osorno et al. 1976). A serosurvey conducted in Venezuela revealed that there was a low prevalence of antibody against *B. bovis* in the Venezuelan population (Montenegro-James, James and Lopez 1990). In Asia, serosurveys using *B. microti* antigen indicated exposure of a few residents of Taiwan (Hsu and Cross 1977) and recently 3 cases of human babesiosis, caused by an agent that infected hamsters and whose 16s rDNA sequence closely resembles *B. microti*, were observed (CM Shih, unpublished results). Asymptomatic *Babesia* infections have been observed in Africa. A survey conducted in Nigeria indicated that 54% of 173 men from the northwestern border may have been infected (Leeflang et al. 1976) and a serological survey in Mozambique suggested that *B. bovis* may infect residents there (Rodriguez et al. 1984).

Two human infections have been ascribed to *Entopolypoides* (Wolf et al. 1978). Organisms in this genus, however, are now generally considered to be *Babesia*, perhaps *B. microti* (Levine 1988). The status of this parasite should be considered to be uncertain pending study by electron microscopy or by other definitive methods of analysis.

10 CHEMOTHERAPY

Because of its use for malaria, orally administered chloroquine was used in the treatment of the first few Americans in whom *Babesia* infections were observed. Symptomatic improvement was described, but parasitaemia tended to continue (Ruebush et al. 1977). Indeed, administration of chloroquine, sulphadiazine or pyrimethamine fails to reduce parasitaemia in hamsters (Miller, Neva and Gill 1978). Although pentamidine appears to have been useful in several patients who were treated with this drug, such therapy fails to eliminate the parasitaemia completely (Francioli et al. 1981). The treatment of choice for babesiosis in

humans caused by *B. microti* is quinine and clindamycin, administered in combination (Dammin et al. 1983). Quinine should be administered orally in a regimen of 650 mg, 3 times daily and clindamycin intravenously at 1200 mg, 2 times a day. Alternatively, clindamycin can be administered in an oral regimen of 600 mg, 3 times a day. The treatment should be continued for at least 7 days (Anonymous 1986) or until the parasitaemia is eliminated, whichever comes first. This treatment generally is effective, except in those who are immunosuppressed (Smith et al. 1986) or infected by HIV (Benezra et al. 1987, Ong et al. 1990). In fulminating cases, exchange transfusion is life-saving (Jacoby et al. 1980, Cahill et al. 1981, Sun et al. 1983).

Any person with babesiosis acquired in Europe should be treated on an emergency basis. In addition to supportive treatment, such patients should receive prompt specific therapy designed to reduce parasitaemia and to prevent the extensive haemolysis and consequent renal failure that may follow. Massive exchange transfusion (2–3 blood volumes) should be followed by administration of 600 mg clindamycin intravenously, 3–4 times daily, together with quinine (600 mg base) administered orally 3 times a day (Gorenflot et al. 1990, Gorenflot et al. 1987, Unoo et al. 1992). Indeed, because of the rapidly increasing parasitaemia characteristic of the disease, exchange transfusion should be instituted upon the first signs of disease due to *B. divergens* infection. The time element becomes crucial because the request for medical attention generally follows the onset of haemoglobinuria, a manifestation of the disease that signals a fulminating parasitaemia. Unless blood exchange is promptly undertaken prognosis is poor, as the rapidly increasing intravascular haemolysis leads to renal failure.

Babesiosis due to WA-1 appears to respond to quinine and clindamycin, although too few cases have been reported to gauge the efficacy of this treatment regimen.

11 VACCINATION

Strong immunity in cattle against bovine babesiosis has been induced by injection of attenuated parasites (Callow 1971) or exoantigen preparations (Smith and Ristic 1981). Less successful vaccines have been prepared from recombinant antigens. Crude parasite lysates serve to immunize hamsters against infection by *B. microti* (Benach et al. 1984). Culture-derived parasites, crude culture supernatants and purified exoantigen preparations will protect gerbils and cattle against *B. divergens* (Gorenflot et al. 1992). These reports suggest that vaccination might serve as an effective means of prevention of babesiosis in humans. Other than for those individuals who are splenectomized or otherwise immunocompromised or living in certain high risk areas, however, the value of an anti-babesial vaccine for prevention of babesiosis in humans is doubtful.

12 INTEGRATED CONTROL

The accepted public health strategies to protect human populations against zoonotic babesial infection depend upon reducing the density of ticks. The spraying of acaricidal emulsions (Stafford 1991) has been used to reduce the abundance of ticks on vegetation. Less environmentally intrusive methods of application of acaricides, one particularly based on fibre-formulated permethrin may be more acceptable (Mather, Ribeiro and Spielman 1987). These methods interrupt transmission of *B. microti* infection by depositing acaricide in the nests and on the coats of rodent reservoir hosts. Tick infestations may also be reduced locally by destroying the animals (i.e. deer) that serve as host to the adult stage of the tick (Wilson et al. 1988). An effort to reduce the abundance of the hosts of subadult ticks might be counterproductive because the absence of these hosts might increase the density of ticks seeking alternative hosts (Spielman, Etkind and Piesman 1981). Acaricides applied to the coats of cattle could reduce the possible transmission of cattle babesiosis to humans.

Repellents are useful for personal protection, particularly permethrin-based formulations applied to clothing (Schreck et al. 1986). Even volatile compounds such as diethyltoluamide (DEET) may provide a certain measure of protection. Personal protection, based on daily examination of the body surface of a person who has visited a site where transmission is intense, is the most effective means of reducing the risk of contracting babesiosis. All ticks found should be promptly disposed of to prevent their attachment. Ticks already attached should be removed by means of forceps to take advantage of the initial 50–60 h 'grace period' during which attached ticks rarely transmit infection.

ACKNOWLEDGEMENTS

Our work is supported by grants from the National Institutes of Health (AI 19693 and AI 37993), Smith Kline Beecham Pharmaceuticals, the Chace Fund, the Gibson Island Corporation, and David Arnold.

REFERENCES

Allsopp MT, Cavalier-Smith T et al., 1994, Phylogeny and evolution of the piroplasms, *Parasitology*, **108**: 147–52.

Anonymous, 1986, Drugs for parasitic infections, *Medical Letter Drugs Therapeutics*, **28**: 9–16.

Benach JL, Habicht GS, 1981, Clinical characteristics of human babesiosis, *J Infect Dis*, **144**: 48.

Benach JL, Habicht GS, Hamburger MI, 1982, Immunoresponsiveness in acute babesiosis in humans, *J Infect Dis*, **146**: 369–80.

Benach JL, Habicht GS et al., 1982, Glucan as an adjuvant for a murine *Babesia microti* immunisation trial, *Infect Immun*, **35**: 947–51.

Benezra D, Brown AE et al., 1987, Babesiosis and infection with human immunodeficiency virus (HIV), *Ann Intern Med*, **107**: 944.

Boustani MR, Lepore TJ et al., 1994, Acute respiratory failure in patients treated for babesiosis, *Am J Resp Crit Care Med*, **149**: 1689–91.

Bush JB, Isaacson M et al., 1990, Human babesiosis: a preliminary report of 2 suspect cases in southern Africa, *S Afr J Med*, **78**: 699.

Cahill KM, Benach JL et al., 1981, Red cell exchange: Treatment of babesiosis in a splenectomized patient, *Transfusion*, **21**: 193–8.

Callow LL, 1971, The control of babesiosis with a highly effective attenuated vaccine, *Proc World Vet Congress*, **1**: 357–60.

Chisholm ES, Ruebush TK II et al., 1978, *Babesia microti* infection in man: evaluation of an indirect immunofluorescent antibody test, *Am J Trop Med Hyg*, **27**: 14–19.

Clark IA, 1979, Protection of mice against *Babesia microti* with cord factor, COAM, zymosan, glucan, *Salmonella* and *Listeria*, *Parasite Immunol*, **1**: 179–96.

Clark IA, Allison AC, 1974, *Babesia microti* and *Plasmodium berghei yoelii* infections in nude mice, *Nature* (London), **252**: 328–9.

Clarke CS, Rogers ET, Egan EL, 1989, Babesiosis: under-reporting or case-clustering?, *Postgrad Med J*, **65**: 591–93.

Cullen JM, Levine JF, 1987, Pathology of experimental *Babesia microti* infection in the Syrian hamster, *Lab Anim Sci*, **37**: 640–3.

Dammin GJ, Spielman A et al., 1983, Clindamycin and quinine treatment for *Babesia microti* infections, *Morbid Mortality Reports*, **32**: 65–6.

Ellis J, Hefford C et al., 1992, Ribosomal DNA sequence comparison of *Babesia* and *Theileria*, *Mol Biochem Parasitol*, **54**: 87–96.

Etkind P, Piesman J et al., 1980, Methods for detecting *Babesia microti* infection in wild rodents, *J Parasitol*, **66**: 107–10.

Fay FG, Rausch RL, 1969, Parasitic organisms in the blood of arvicoline rodents in Alaska, *J Parasitol*, **55**: 1258–65.

Francioli PB, Keithly JS et al., 1981, Response of babesiosis to pentamidine therapy, *Ann Intern Med*, **94**: 326–30.

Golightly LM, Hirschhorn LR, Weller, PF, 1989, Fever and headache in a splenectomized woman, *Rev Infect Dis*, **11**: 629–37.

Gordon S, Cordon RA et al., 1984, Adult respiratory distress syndrome in babesiosis, *Chest*, **86**: 633–4.

Gorenflot A, Precigout E et al., 1987, Mem Inst Oswaldo Cruz, **87 (suppl 3)**: 279–81.

Gorenflot A, Brasseur P et al., 1990, Deux cas de babesiose humaine grave traités avec succes, *Presse Med*, **19**: 335.

Gray JS, 1980, Studies on the activity of *Ixodes ricinus* in relation to the epidemiology of babesiosis in County Meath, Ireland, *Br Vet J*, **136**: 427–36.

Habicht GS, Benach JL et al., 1983, The effect of age on the infection and immunoresponsiveness of mice to *Babesia microti*, *Mech Aging Dev*, **23**: 357–69.

Hsu NHM, Cross JH, 1977, Serologic survey for human babesiosis on Taiwan, *J Formosan Med Assoc*, **76**: 950–4.

Jacoby GA, Hunt JV et al., 1980, Treatment of transfusion-transmitted babesiosis by exchange transfusion, *N Engl J Med*, **303**: 1098–100.

Kakoma I, Mehlhorn H, *Babesia* of domestic animals, *Parasitic Protozoa*, 2nd edn, ed. Kreier JP, Academic Press, San Diego, 141–216.

Karakashian SJ, Rudzinska MA et al., 1986, Primary and secondary ookinetes of *Babesia microti* in the larval and nymphal stages of the tick, *Ixodes dammini*, *Can J Zool*, **64**: 328–39.

Krause PJ, Telford SR III et al., 1994, Diagnosis of babesiosis: evaluation of a serologic test for the detection of *Babesia microti* antibody, *J Infect Dis*, **169**: 923–6.

Leeflang P, Oomen JMV et al., 1976, The presence of *Babesia* antibody in Nigerians, *Int J Parasitol*, **6**: 159–61.

Levine ND, 1988, *The Protozoan Phylum Apicomplexa*, vol. II, CRC Press, Boca Raton, FL, 151.

Li JF, Meng DB, 1984, The discovery of human babesiosis in China, *Chin J Vet Med*, **10**: 19–20.

Lykins JD, Ristic M et al., 1975, *Babesia microti*: pathogenesis of parasite of human origin in the hamster, *Exp Parasitol*, **37**: 388–97.

Machtinger L, Telford SR III et al., 1993, Treatment of babesiosis by red blood cell exchange in an HIV positive splenectomised patient, *J Clin Apheresis*, **8**: 78–81.

Mackenstedt U, Gauer M et al., 1990, Sexual cycle of *Babesia divergens* confirmed by DNA measurements, *Parasitol Res*, **76**: 199–206.

Mahoney DF, 1977, Babesiosis of domestic animals, *Parasitic Protozoa*, vol. IV, ed. Kreier JP, Academic Press, New York, 1–52.

Marcus LC, Valigorsky JM et al., 1982, A case report of transfusion induced babesiosis, *JAMA*, **248**: 465–7.

Mather TN, Ribeiro JMC, Spielman A, 1987, Lyme disease and babesiosis: acaricide focused on potentially infected ticks, *Am J Trop Med Hyg*, **36**: 609–14.

McCutchan TF Hansen JL et al., 1984, Mung bean nuclease cleaves *Plasmodium* genomic DNA at sites before and after genes, *Science*, **225**: 625–8.

Mehlhorn H, Schein E, 1987, The piroplasms: life, cycle and sexual stages, *Adv Parasitol*, **23**: 37–103.

Meldrum SC, Birkhead GS et al., 1992, Human babesiosis in New York state: an epidemiological description of 136 cases, *Clin Infect Dis*, **15**: 1019–23.

Miller LH, Neva FA, Gill F, 1978, Failure of chloroquine in human babesiosis (*Babesia microti*): case report and chemotherapeutic trials in hamsters, *Ann Intern Med*, **88**: 200–2.

Momen H, Chance ML, Peters W, 1979, Biochemistry of intra-erythrocytic parasites III Biochemical taxonomy of rodent *Babesia*, *Ann Trop Med Parasitol*, **73**: 203–12.

Montenegro-James S, James MA, Lopez R, 1990, Seroprevalence of human babesiosis in Venezuela, *Annual Meeting, American Society of Tropical Medicine and Hygiene*, New Orleans, LA.

Moss DM, Healy, GR Dickerson, JW et al., 1986, Isoenzyme analysis of *Babesia microti* infections in humans, *J Protozool*, **33**: 213–15.

Ong KR, Stavropoulos C, Inada Y, 1990, Babesiosis, asplenia, and AIDS, *Lancet*, **336**: 112.

Osorno BM, Vega C, Ristic M et al., 1976, Isolation of *Babesia* spp. from asymptomatic human beings, *Vet Parasitol*, **2**: 111–20.

Persing DH, Herwaldt BL, Glaser C et al., 1995, Infection with a *Babesia*-like organism in northern California, *N Engl J Med*, **332**: 298–303.

Persing DH, Mathiesen D et al., 1992, Detection of *Babesia microti* by polymerase chain reaction, *J Clin Microbiol*, **30**: 2097–103.

Peters W, 1965, Competitive relationship between *Eperythrozoon coccoides* and *Plasmodium berghei* in the mouse, *Exp Parasitol*, **16**: 158–66.

Piesman J, Spielman A, 1982, *Babesia microti*: infectivity of parasites from ticks from hamsters and white-footed mice, *Exp Parasitol*, **53**: 242–48.

Piesman J, Mather TN et al., 1987, Seasonal variation of transmission risk of Lyme disease and human babesiosis, *Am J Epidemiol*, **126**: 1187–9.

Piesman J, Mather TN et al., 1986, Duration of tick attachment and *Borrelia burgdorferi* transmission, *J Clin Microbiol*, **25**: 557–58.

Piesman J, Spielman A et al., 1979, Role of deer in the epizootiology of *Babesia microti* in Massachusetts, USA, *J Med Entomol*, **15**: 537–40.

Quick RE, Herwaldt BL et al., 1993, Babesiosis in Washington state: a new species of *Babesia*?, *Ann Intern Med*, **119**: 284–90.

Rabinovich SA, Voronina ZK et al., 1978, First detection of human babesiosis in the USSR and brief analysis of cases described in the literature, *Med Parazitol*, **47**: 97–107.

Ribeiro JMC, 1987, Role of saliva in blood-feeding by arthropods, *Annu Rev Entomol*, **32**: 463–78.

Riek RF, 1968, Babesiosis, *Infectious Blood Diseases of Man and Animals*, vol. 2, eds Weinman D, Ristic M, Academic Press, New York, 220–68.

Rodriguez ON, Dias M, Rodriguez P, 1984, Reporte de la infeccion por *Babesia bovis* (Babes) en la poblacion humana de la Republica popular de Mozambique, *Rev Cubana Cien Vet*, **15**: 41–50.

Roth EF Jr, Tanowitz H et al., 1981, *Babesia microti*: biochemistry and function of hamster erythrocytes infected from a human source, *Exp Parasitol*, **51**: 116–23.

Rudzinska MA, 1981, Morphological aspects of host-cell-parasite relationships in babesiosis, *Babesiosis*, eds Ristic M, Kreier JP, Academic Press, New York, 87–141.

Rudzinska MA, Spielman A et al., 1979, Intraerythrocytic 'gametocytes' of *Babesia microti* and their maturation in ticks, *Can J Zool*, **57**: 424–34.

Rudzinska MA, Spielman A et al., 1983, Sexuality in piroplasms as revealed by electron microscopy in *Babesia microti*, *Proc Natl Acad Sci USA*, **80**: 2966–70.

Ruebush MJ, Hanson WL, 1979, Susceptibility of five strains of mice to *Babesia microti* of human origin, *J Parasitol*, **65**: 430–3.

Ruebush MJ, Hanson WL, 1980, Thymus dependence of resistance to infection with *Babesia microti* of human origin in mice, *Am J Trop Med Hyg*, **29**: 507–15.

Ruebush TK, Cassaday PB et al., 1977, Human babesiosis on Nantucket Island: clinical features, *Ann Intern Med*, **86**: 6–9.

Schein E, Reihbein G et al., 1981, *Babesi equi* (Laveran 1901) 1 Development in horses and in lymphocyte culture, *Z Parasitenk*, **34**: 68–94.

Schreck CE, Snoddy EL, Spielman A, 1986, Pressurized sprays of permethrin or deet on military clothing for personal protection against *Ixodes dammini* (Acari: Ixodidae), *J Med Entomol*, **23**: 396–9.

Skrabalo Z, Deanovic Z, 1957, Piroplasmosis in man. Report on a case, *Doc Med Geogr Trop*, **9**: 11–16.

Smith RP, Evans AT et al., 1986, Tranfusion-acquired babesiosis and failure of antibiotic treatment, *JAMA*, **256**: 2726–7.

Smith T, Kilbourne FL, 1893, *Investigation into the Nature, Causation, and Prevention of Texas or Southern Cattle Fever*, Bureau of Animal Industries Bulletin No. 1, US Department of Agriculture, Washington, DC.

Smith RD, Ristic M, 1981, Immunization against babesiosis with culture derived antigens, *Babesiosis*, eds Ristic M, Kreier JP, Academic Press, New York, 485–507.

Spielman A, 1988, Lyme disease and human babesiosis: evidence incriminating vector and reservoir hosts, *The Biology of Parasitism*, Englund PT, Sher A eds, AR Liss, New York, 147–65.

Spielman A, Etkind P, Piesman J, 1981, Reservoir hosts of human babesiosis on Nantucket Island, *Am J Trop Med Hyg*, **30**: 560–5.

Stafford KC, 1991, Effectiveness of carbaryl applications for the control of *Ixodes dammini* (Acari:Ixodidae) nymphs in an endemic residential area, *J Med Entomol*, **28**: 32–6.

Sun T, Tenenbaum MJ et al., 1983, Morphologic and clinical observations in human infection with *Babesia microti*, *J Infect Dis*, **148**: 239–48.

Telford SR III, Lepore TJ et al., 1995, Human granulocytic ehrlichiosis in Massachusetts, *Ann Intern Med*, **123**: 277–9.

Tetzlaff CL, Carlomagno MA, McMurray DN, 1988, Reduced dietary protein content suppresses infection with *Babesia microti*, *Med Microbiol Immunol*, **177**: 305–15.

Tetzlaff CL, McMurray DN, Rice-Ficht AC, 1990, Isolation and characterisation of a gene associated with a virulent strain of *Babesia microti*, *Mol Biochem Parasitol*, **40**: 183–92.

Thomford JW, Conrad PA et al., 1994, Cultivation and characterisation of a newly recognised human pathogenic protozoan, *J Infect Dis*, **169**: 1050–6.

Uhnoo I, Cars O et al., 1992, First documented case of human babesiosis in Sweden, *Scan J Infect Dis*, **24**: 541–7.

Walter G, Weber G, 1981, Untersuchung zur Ubertragung (transstadial, transovarial) von *Babesia microti* in Stamm 'Hannover I', in *Ixodes ricinus*, *Tropenmed Parasitol*, **32**: 228–30.

Western KA, Benson GD, Gleason NN, 1970, Babesiosis in a Massachusetts resident, *N Engl J Med*, **283:** 854–6.

Wilson ME, 1991, *A World Guide to Infections*, Oxford University Press, New York.

Wilson ML, Telford SR III et al., 1988, Reduced abundance of immature *Ixodes dammini* (Acari: Ixodidae) following elimination of deer, *J Med Ent*, **25:** 224–8.

Winger CM, Canning EU, Culverhouse JD, 1987, A monoclonal antibody to *Babesia divergens* which inhibits merozoite invasion, *Parasitology*, **94:** 17–27.

Wolf RE, 1974, Effects of antilymphocyte serum and splenectomy on resistance to *Babesia microti* infection in hamsters, *Clin Immunol Immunopathol*, **2:** 381–94.

Wolf RE, Gleason NN et al., 1978, Intraerythrocytic parasitosis in humans with *Entopolypoides* species (Family Babesiidae), *Ann Intern Med*, **88:** 769–73.

Wood PR, Clark IA, 1982, Genetic control of *Propionibacterium acnes*-induced protection of mice against *Babesia microti*, *Infect Immun*, **35:** 52–7.

Young AS, Morzaria SP, 1986, Biology of *Babesia*, *Parasitol Today*, **2:** 211–19.

Yuval B, Spielman A, 1990, Duration and regulation of the developmental cycle of *Ixodes dammini* (Acari:Ixodidae), *J Med Entomol*, **27:** 196–201.

Chapter 20

MALARIA

M Hommel and H M Gilles

1 INTRODUCTION

Malaria is the most important of all the tropical diseases in terms of morbidity and mortality. World wide, some 2 billion individuals are at risk; 100 million develop overt clinical disease and 1.5–2.7 million die every year. Nearly 85% of the cases and 90% of carriers (many asymptomatic) are found in tropical Africa, where in some countries 20–30% of deaths in childhood are attributed to the disease (Greenwood et al. 1987, Defo 1995).

Drug and insecticide resistance have aggravated the complexity of the malaria problem world wide. Thus, among the countries where falciparum malaria persists, only those of Central America have not recorded the resistance of *Plasmodium falciparum* to chloroquine. In contrast, in the Mekong region in south east Asia, multidrug resistance to chloroquine, sulphadoxine-pyrimethamine and even mefloquine now occurs and the sensitivity to quinine is also diminishing (WHO 1994a).

Maps showing the global distribution of malaria and the countries from which *P. falciparum* resistance to chloroquine and other antimalarial drugs has been reported are given in Figs 20.1 and 20.2. It should be emphasized that degrees of resistance vary within individual countries; for example, in Cambodia multidrug resistance occurs in one part of the country, whereas in another part of the country *P. falciparum* parasites are still sensitive to chloroquine.

2 CLASSIFICATION

Malaria parasites belong to the genus *Plasmodium* which includes over 125 species infecting reptiles, birds and mammals. *Plasmodium* is the only genus in the family Plasmodiidae, the class Haematozoea, the phylum Apicomplexa (see Volume 5, Chapter 7). The characteristic feature of the Apicomplexa is the presence, at specific stages of the life-cycle, of an apical complex consisting of a number of specialized organelles, which may include a conoid, polar rings, rhoptries and micronemes.

The genus *Plasmodium* is subdivided into 10 subgenera. Human and primate malaria parasites are all included in the subgenera *P. (Plasmodium)* and *P. (Laverania)*, whereas all other species infecting mammals are members of the heterogeneous sub-genus *P. (Vinckeia)*. Four species of malaria parasites normally infecting humans are: *P. (Laverania) falciparum*, *P. (Plasmodium) malariae*, *P. (P.) vivax* and *P.(P.) ovale*. The taxonomic status of these 4 species within the genus and their relationships with other important species of malaria parasites are illustrated in Fig. 20.3.

Morphological characteristics and features of the life-cycle, the major criteria used in Garnham's classification (1966), include the shape of the trophozoite, the gametocyte and the oöcyst, the number of nuclei in the erythrocytic and exoerythrocytic schizonts, the aspect and distribution of the pigment and the nature of the damage induced by the parasite in the host cell (e.g. 'Maurer's clefts' or 'Schüffner's dots'). The main biological criteria include the host range, the type of host cell infected, the duration of the different stages in the life-cycle, the presence or absence of relapse (with or without recrudescences), the nature of the vector and the geographical distribution. While none of these criteria are ideal taxonomic markers, they have in most cases been considered broadly adequate to differentiate and classify species. The analysis of sequence homologies of the circumsporozoite (CS)

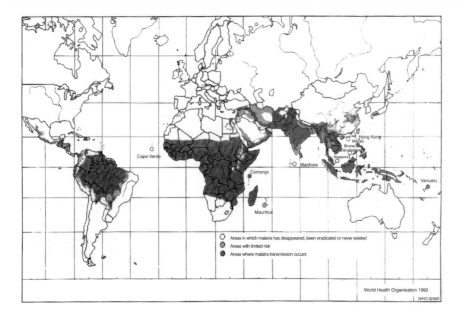

Fig. 20.1 Global distribution of malaria in 1995 (Courtesy of WHO, from Weekly Epidemiological Record, 1992, 22, 162).

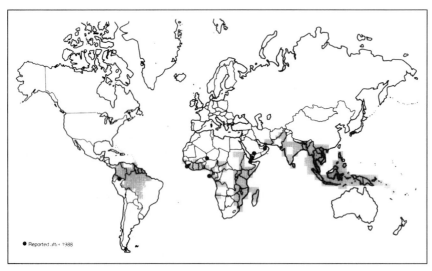

Fig. 20.2 Distribution of chloroquine resistance (Courtesy of WHO, from Weekly Epidemiological Record, 1992, 22, 162).

gene in different species (McCutchan et al. 1984) and the comparison of different small subunit ribosomal RNA genes (Waters 1994) have provided new information, such as the fact that murine plasmodia have segregated from other mammalian parasites and that *P. falciparum* is more closely related to avian than to mammalian plasmodia.

The nomenclature for referring to parasite populations is confusing and terms such as isolate, strain and line are often used interchangeably in the malaria literature. A useful nomenclature was proposed by a WHO working group on trypanosomes in 1978, and this may be applied to malaria with a few modifications (as discussed by Cox 1988):

1 Isolate (or primary isolate): a population of parasites isolated from a naturally infected host.
2 Stock: a population of parasites derived by serial passage (in animals or in culture) from a primary isolate.
3 Strain: a population of parasites derived from a primary isolate and possessing defined characteristics (i.e. a strain is a well defined stock).
4 Line: a population of parasites derived from a named

strain, but having characteristics that are different from the parental strain or other lines of the same strain (e.g. more virulent, different drug sensitivity pattern, etc.).
5 Stabilate: a population of parasites preserved by cryopreservation on a single occasion (this may refer to a primary isolate or a line).
6 Clone: a population of parasites derived from a single individual asexual parasite.

Although some of these terms may imply a degree of stability in the characteristics of the population, this should be regarded as relative stability only, because the parasite has considerable genomic fluidity and is capable of variation in the expression of certain genes at a rate of 2% in every asexual cycle (Roberts et al. 1992). A primary isolate is rarely a homogenous entity and on occasions when clones have been derived from parasite stocks (i.e. primary isolates established in culture), many clones with different characteristics have been isolated (Thaithong et al. 1984). Some strains of malaria parasites have such characteristic individual features that they have given a 'subspecies' status.

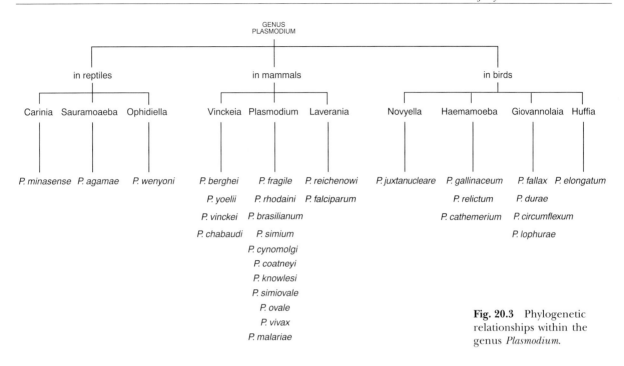

Fig. 20.3 Phylogenetic relationships within the genus *Plasmodium*.

3 LIFE-CYCLE AND STRUCTURE

3.1 Life-cycle

Human malaria parasites undergo a complex cycle of development, including stages in a female *Anopheles* mosquito. The infection starts with the bite of an infected mosquito, when the sporozoite is introduced into the skin together with mosquito saliva. The sporozoite rapidly makes its way to the liver, where it invades a hepatocyte. Within the hepatocyte, the parasite undergoes a period of differentiation and multiplication to produce the extra-erythrocytic schizont, containing a few thousand merozoites. The merozoite, when released from the hepatocyte, enters the bloodstream and invades an erythrocyte to start a characteristic periodic phase of differentiation and asexual multiplication leading to the erythrocytic schizont. This contains a small number of merozoites, which in turn invade new erythrocytes. At some stage, a proportion of merozoites undergo sexual differentiation and gametocytogenesis. The male and female gametocytes produced remain dormant in the bloodstream waiting to be picked up in the blood meal of a new biting mosquito. In the acidic, low-temperature environment of the insect midgut, gametocytes released from the erythrocytes transform into gametes, which fertilize to form first a zygote, then an oökinete. The motile oökinete crosses the epithelial wall of the midgut before transforming into an oöcyst, which divides by schizogony to produce thousands of sporozoites. These undergo a final differentiation into their infective forms while migrating to the salivary glands of the insect, where they stay until the next bite, thus completing the cycle. Figure 20.4 illustrates the life-cycle of *P. falciparum*.

3.2 Structure

The various stages of malarial parasites exhibit dramatically different morphological features, which reflect both their very different function and the various microenvironments inhabited. Only the sporozoite, merozoite and oökinete (which are designed for the invasion of, respectively, the hepatocyte, erythrocyte or midgut epithelial cell of the mosquito) possess a surface coat and the specialized apical end characteristic of Apicomplexa. The surface coat is responsible for host cell recognition and adherence, and the invasion organelles allow the parasite to actively enter the target cell. In contrast, other stages of the life-cycle, which are designed for growth and development within the host cell, lack these invasion organelles, but possess structures involved in respiration, intake of food or digestion of nutrients (e.g. mitochondrion, cytostome, food vacuoles and pigment). The sexual stages of the parasite undergo a complex differentiation in order to become equipped for the fertilization process that takes place within the mosquito midgut; the zygote (oökinete) is the only part of the life-cycle in which the organism is diploid and where meiosis is observed.

The nucleus of plasmodia is variable, depending on the stage in the life-cycle. Individual chromosomes cannot be seen by electron microscopy, but 14 chromosomal units have been identified using either pulse field gradient electrophoresis (PFGE) (Kemp et al. 1987) or the counting of centromeres by tridimensional microscopy of mitotic spindles (Prensier and Slomniany 1986). Cellular division is by schizogony, a form of mitotic division in which multiple nuclear divisions take place before the segmentation of the cytoplasm occurs.

Plasmodium spp. possess a single mitochondrion (Fry

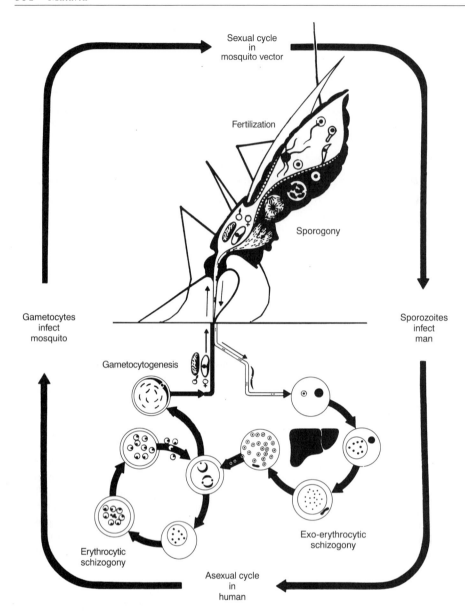

Fig. 20.4 Life cycle of
Plasmodium falciparum.

1991), which seems to play a very different function during
the vertebrate stage (when it is almost acristate, particularly
in mammalian plasmodia) and the invertebrate stage (when
it is always fully cristate). A switch of enzymatic activity takes
place as the parasite differentiates from one stage to the
other. Mitochondria are self-replicating and each stage of
the life-cycle carries at least one, albeit rudimentary in
some cases.

Malarial parasites are unable to ingest particulate food and
are entirely dependent upon the intake of soluble cellular
macromolecules. Early trophozoites feed by micropinocytosis, pinching off small portions of the erythrocyte cytoplasm and producing small digestive vesicles. Later trophozoites are equipped with a cytostome (i.e. primitive 'mouth')
which becomes functional when micropinocytosis ceases. For
most growing stages, the cytostome represents the major
route for food intake.

Within the food vacuole, the digestion of haemoglobin
leaves an insoluble waste product consisting of haematin and
ferriprotoporphyrin coupled to partially degraded globin
and plasmodial proteins; this forms malaria pigment or
haemozoin. When the mature schizont finally breaks up, lib-

erating merozoites, the pigment is left behind in the
'residual body'; these bodies will eventually accumulate and
remain within the cells of the reticuloendothelial system for
many years.

The plasma membrane, the interface between the parasite
and its host, provides both an effective protection against
host defence mechanisms (e.g. proteolytic enzymes, cytokines or antibodies) and the means for a selective permeability and macromolecular exchanges. In the extracellular stages (merozoites, gametes, oökinetes or sporozoites),
the cell membrane is specifically designed for survival in a
hostile environment and for the recognition of and binding
to host cells. In contrast, the intracellular stages have lost
the membrane components involved in protection, mobility
or cell recognition in order to allow for more effective
uptake and excretion of macromolecules, crucial for parasite
growth and development. The parasitophorous vacuole
membrane, which separates the intracellular parasite from
the host cell cytoplasm is involved in the complex molecular
trafficking events required for macromolecular exchange
between the parasite and its host. The host cell membrane
itself may be altered during parasite development to serve
the metabolic needs of the growing parasite.

The merozoite, oökinete and sporozoite stages of the parasite have organelles at their apical end, characteristic of the phylum Apicomplexa, represented by a short, truncated cone-shaped projection of the cell membrane, which extends and retracts with parasite movement. It is assumed that this differentiation of the apical end is specifically designed for boring into host tissues and for host cell recognition and invasion. A duct open at the centre of the tip of the apical end represents the final effluent of a network of ductules linking the secretory organelles; these are all electron-dense by transmission electron microscopy and may include 2 club-shaped rhoptries and a series of round micronemes and dense granules. During cell invasion, the contents of the various secretory organelles are released and are believed to play a crucial role in destabilizing the host cell membrane and in the formation of the parasitophorous vacuole.

EXOERYTHROCYTIC STAGE

The sporozoite enters the bloodstream and is rapidly carried to the liver. The sporozoite enters a hepatocyte and undergoes drastic changes in morphology, losing the apical complex and the surface coat and transforming into a round or oval trophozoite. Development takes place within a parasitophorous vacuole in the hepatocyte. The nucleus divides many times and the cytoplasmic mass grows substantially; the number of nuclear divisions and the duration of schizogony varies considerably from one species to another, as does the ultimate size of the exoerythrocytic schizont (which reaches a diameter of 60 μm in *P. falciparum*, and contains more than 30 000 nuclei) (Fig. 20.5).

After completion of nuclear divisions, the cytoplasmic segments and individual merozoites are formed. The duration of exoerythrocytic schizogony is characteristic for each species; for instance, minimum maturation time is 5.5 days in *P. falciparum* and 15 days in *P. malariae*.

In mammalian plasmodia, it is now generally accepted that merozoites arising from exoerythrocytic schizogony can invade only red cells (i.e. they cannot invade hepatocytes or start a secondary exoerythrocytic schizogony).

ERYTHROCYTIC STAGE

After invading the erythrocyte, the parasite loses its specific invasion organelles and dedifferentiates into a round trophozoite located within a parasitophorous vacuole in the red cell cytoplasm. The young trophozoite (termed the 'ring' stage, because of its morphology on stained blood films) grows substantially before undergoing several nuclear divisions; the number of nuclear divisions and the duration of schizogony both vary from one species to another. The timing of the different stages of the erythrocytic schizogony of *P. falciparum* is illustrated in Fig. 20.6.

The length of the intraerythrocytic development is variable: 48 h for *P. falciparum*, *P. vivax* and *P. ovale*, and 72 h for *P. malariae*. At the end of schizogonic development, new merozoites are formed that have a very short extracellular viability (probably less than 30 min) and can only invade erythrocytes.

The development of the parasite within the erythrocyte produces a series of alterations of the host cell, including the presence in the cytoplasm of the red cell of vacuoles or clefts and morphological changes of the erythrocyte membrane (e.g. 'knobs' or 'caveolae'). Some of these alterations are visible in stained parasites and represent useful taxonomic features (e.g. Maurer's clefts in *P. falciparum* or Schüffner's dots in *P. vivax*) (Fig. 20.7).

The metabolism of the malaria parasite is largely dependent on the digestion of red cell haemoglobin, which is transformed into malaria pigment. Pigment is absent in the ring stage and becomes detectable only in the late trophozoite and the schizont. The aspect and distribution of the pigment in the parasite may vary from species to species and represents another useful distinguishing feature.

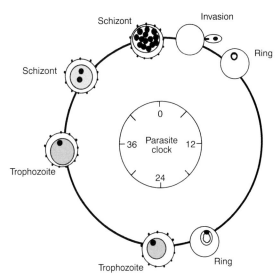

Fig. 20.6 Timing of the intra-erythrocytic cycle of *Plasmodium falciparum*. The fact that the ring stage parasite takes almost 24 hours to develop and that all the later stages express knobs on the erythrocyte surface (•) and are sequestered in capillaries, is crucial to the understanding of pathophysiological events.

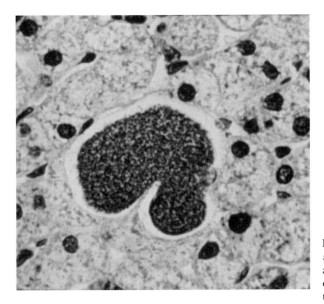

Fig. 20.5 Liver pre-erythrocytic schizont.

Diagram of ultrastructure of malaria-infected red blood cells

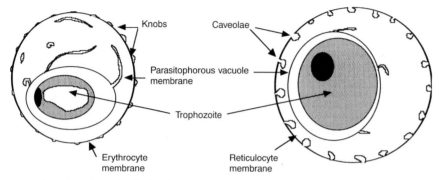

Diagram of infected cells as visualized on Romanovsky-stained thin blood films

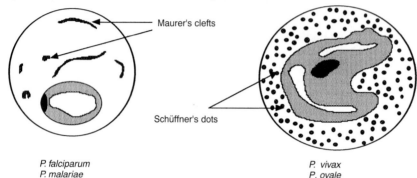

P. falciparum
P. malariae

P. vivax
P. ovale

Fig. 20.7 Diagram describing the differences between Maurer's clefts and Schüffner's dots. The ultrastructure shows the objects identified as Schüffner's dots on a Romanowsky-stained thin film are caveolae on the surface of infected reticulocytes, while Maurer's clefts correspond to expansions of the parasitophorous vacuole membrane and vesicles derived from this membrane.

GAMETOCYTES, GAMETES AND FERTILIZATION

Some merozoites develop into a male or a female gametocyte but the factors that induce sexual differentiation, rather than schizogonic development, are essentially unknown. Mature gametocytes of *P. vivax*, *P. ovale* and *P. malariae*, like most mammalian species, are round but the gametocytes of *P. falciparum* (like the malarial parasites of birds and reptiles) are elongated or crescent-shaped (Fig. 20.8).

Although the longevity of mature gametocytes may exceed several weeks, their half-life in the bloodstream may be only 2 or 3 days, while waiting in an arrested state of development to be taken up by a mosquito.

When taken up by a suitable mosquito vector, the gametocytes transform into gametes, stimulated by the drop in temperature and the biochemical features of the new environment, including a rise in pH and the presence of a vector-specific 'mosquito exflagellation factor' (Carter and Graves 1988). The maturation of the female gametocyte into a macrogamete takes place without major morphological changes. In the extracellular male gamete, the nucleus divides 3 times and each of the 8 nuclei formed combines with cytoplasm to form 8 thread-like microgametes ('exflagellation'). Microgametes are very motile, highly differentiated stages, which move actively towards the macrogametes. The invasion of the macrogamete by the microgamete starts the process of fertilization and the sexual stage of the parasite's life-cycle.

SPOROGONY

Immediately after fertilization, the zygote is formed and elongates to become an oökinete. The slowly motile oökinete crosses the peritrophic membrane of the midgut (probably by means of a chitinase), then passes through the single cell layer of the midgut epithelium and establishes itself beneath the basal lamina, forming an oöcyst.

Surrounded by a smooth, thin cyst wall, the oöcyst grows to reach a diameter of 40–50 μm after 4–21 days, the speed of maturation being largely dependent on environmental temperature. Each infected mosquito may carry a few hundred oöcysts (as many as 1600 have been found in laboratory infected mosquitoes) (Fig. 20.9), but normally the number of oöcysts per mosquito is much smaller (<100). The size of the mature oöcyst and the distribution of pigment are characteristic for each species and may be used as taxonomic markers.

At the end of the maturation period, sporozoites are formed, the number of which varies from species to species (e.g. c. 10 000–20 000 in *P. falciparum*). The immature sporozoites emerge through the oöcyst wall into the haemolymph and migrate to the salivary glands of the mosquito. Infected salivary glands contain 10 000–200 000 sporozoites. At the time of the mosquito bite, each drop of saliva carries with it a small number of sporozoites which are injected into the skin of a host. An infective bite from a single mosquito will characteristically represent between 5 and a few hundred sporozoites (Rosenberg et al. 1990) sufficient to induce an infection in the host. The completion of the sporogony takes between 7 days and 8 weeks, depending on the parasite species, the nature of the vector and, more importantly, the environmental conditions (particularly temperature and relative humidity).

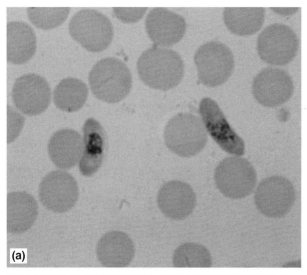

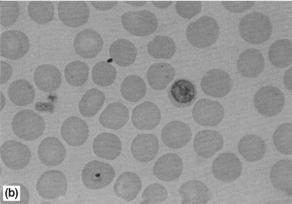

Fig. 20.8 Gametocytes of (a) *P. falciparum* and (b) *P. vivax*.

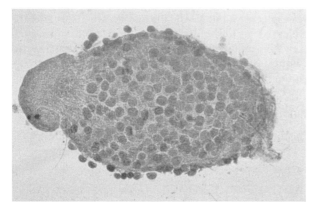

Fig. 20.9 Oocysts in the mosquito.

3.3 Relationship between the life-cycle and manifestations of malaria

RECRUDESCENCE AND RELAPSE

Some sporozoites develop immediately after entering the hepatocyte and a few days later, when the exoerythrocytic schizont is mature, produce merozoites that infect red blood cells. This first wave of parasitaemia is responsible for the primary attack of malaria

and may, in the absence of specific antimalarial treatment, last from a few weeks to a few months in a non-immune individual (ranging from 2–3 weeks in some *P. falciparum* infections to 4–6 months in *P. malariae* infections). Further waves of parasitaemia may follow a few weeks, months or years after the primary attack. In the absence of reinfection, there are 3 possible causes for such secondary attacks:

1 A secondary exoerythrocytic schizogony. This is known to take place in *Plasmodium* spp. of birds and reptiles, but not in species infecting mammals.
2 The presence of dormant parasites or 'hypnozoites'. This is a situation in which some of the sporozoites do not immediately start to grow and divide, but remain in a dormant stage for weeks or months (Krotoski et al. 1980). The duration of latency is variable from one hypnozoite to another and the factors that eventually trigger growth are not known; this explains how a single infection can be responsible for a series of waves of parasitaemia or 'relapses'. *P. vivax* and *P. ovale* are the only 2 human malaria parasites that produce hypnozoites and, thus, relapses. Different strains of parasites have their own characteristic pattern of relapse. Lengthy pre-patencies or delayed relapses seem to be a feature of parasites endemic in temperate rather than tropical areas (Brumpt 1949).
3 Parasites that do not form hypnozoites (*P. malariae* or *P. falciparum*) may, nevertheless, produce secondary waves of parasitaemia called 'recrudescences', either by long-term survival of erythrocytic stages (e.g., within a 'sequestration' site) or the continuation, at a low or undetectable level, of erythrocytic schizogony in the peripheral bloodstream. The basis for this latent survival of parasites has not, so far, been elucidated. In the case of *P. malariae*, recurrences have been described as long as 60 years after the primary attack (Brumpt 1949). Drug resistance creates a situation in which the initial peak of parasitaemia is only partially controlled and a recrudescence of resistant parasites occurs shortly after. Figure 20.10 illustrates the differences between reinfection, recrudescence and relapse.

The main practical difference between relapse and recrudescence is that, whereas latent erythrocytic stages are susceptible to standard chemotherapy, hypnozoites (being cells of low metabolic activity) require a specific treatment (e.g. with primaquine). A true relapse is, therefore, always exoerythrocytic in nature and may be defined as the 'reappearance of parasitaemia in a sporozoite-induced infection following adequate blood schizonticidal therapy' (Cogswell 1992). This also means that a blood-induced infection (e.g. by blood transfusion) cannot relapse.

Hypnozoites are uninucleate forms within hepatocytes, but they are very difficult to identify on routinely stained pathology specimens, which is probably why this stage of the life-cycle was elucidated only in 1980 by Krostoski and colleagues.

POSSIBLE OUTCOME OF MALARIA INFECTIONS

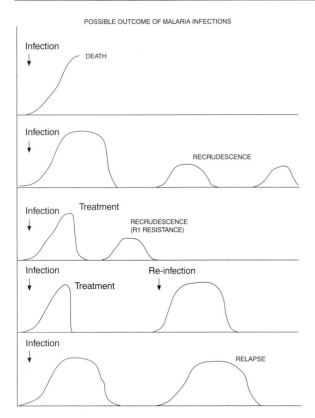

Fig. 20.10 Relapse, recrudescence, reinfection and drug resistance. Potential outcomes of an infection, including death, complete recovery and secondary infection, are illustrated in this figure.

Synchronicity

One of the striking features of the erythrocytic cycle of mammalian malarial parasites is the fact that the parasites tend to grow in synchrony. The consequence is that parasites examined on a patient's blood film are frequently all at the same developmental stage and that clinical symptoms (e.g. fever paroxysms) often tend to occur at regular intervals of time (e.g. 48 h in tertian malaria or 72 h in quartan malaria). This synchronous life-cycle of the parasite is determined, at least in part, by host factors. In *P. falciparum*, a parasite in which synchronicity is particularly striking, it has been suggested that it is the paroxysms of fever themselves that sharpen the level of synchronicity (Kwiatkowski and Greenwood 1989), in consequence of which the periodicity of fever becomes more regular as the malaria infection progresses. The host's circadian rhythm is also a determining factor in controlling the timing of parasite development; this very accurate 'biological clock' of the parasite is believed to represent an adaptation designed to facilitate the transmission of the parasite by night biting mosquitoes (Hawking 1975).

Sequestration

The overall distribution of both asexual forms and gametocytes in the blood is not always random and there are circumstances in which parasites may be removed from the peripheral bloodstream and be retained or 'sequestered' in various host tissues.

In *P. falciparum*, only the early trophozoites ('rings') are present in the peripheral circulation and later developmental stages are sequestered within the capillaries of various organs. This sequestration is caused by the adherence of infected erythrocytes to capillary endothelial cells by means of a specific interaction between a parasite-derived molecule present at the surface of the malaria infected red cell and specific host cell receptors (Hommel 1990). Adherent malaria infected red cells can be found in various tissues, including the heart, the liver and the brain (Fig. 20.11).

It is believed that the packing of cerebral capillaries with these adherent, highly metabolically active cells is responsible for local metabolic defects (including hypoglycaemia and hypoxia), which may in turn lead to coma and 'cerebral malaria', the most severe complication of the disease (Warrell 1987). Sequestration has important consequences for the diagnosis of falciparum malaria, because it means that parasites may not be found on a blood film at a time when the clinical picture is most suggestive.

During pregnancy, infected erythrocytes are preferentially retained in the placenta. This is believed to be a mechanical phenomenon, resulting from sluggish blood flow of the placenta, rather than because of any interaction between infected erythrocytes and specific receptors on the surface of syncytiotrophoblasts (Galbraith et al. 1980).

A radically different form of sequestration is responsible for the removal of immature gametocytes of *P. falciparum* from the peripheral circulation. As early as the first 24 h of gametocytogenesis, the immature gametocytes are retained within the bone marrow and the spleen (Smalley, Abdalla and Brown 1980) and are released into the peripheral circulation only after reaching maturity, 8–10 days later. In contrast to the sequestration of immature gametocytes, which is unique to *P. falciparum*, mature gametocytes of all species may be submitted to intermittent sequestration, controlled by the diurnal rhythm of the host; it is conceivable that this sequestration may take place in the capillaries of the upper layer of the skin, which

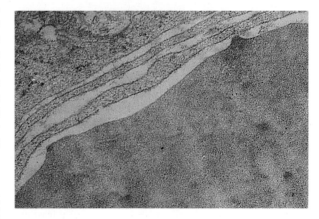

Fig. 20.11 Cytoadherence of *P. falciparum*.

are more accessible to the feeding mosquito. This would explain why the number of gametocytes in the blood meal may be far greater than that present in the peripheral circulation of the host (Carter and Graves 1988).

INTERACTION OF PARASITE AND HOST CELL

Invasion of the erythrocyte

In order to invade the erythrocyte, the merozoite has to recognize, and attach to, its surface components. Several groups of molecules have been described on the surface of human erythrocytes with a function in merozoite attachment. The nature of the erythrocyte receptor involved varies from one merozoite to another, because each species of parasite has specific host cell preferences (Hadley and Miller 1988, Bannister and Dluzewski 1990). In *P. falciparum*, a parasite that can invade erythrocytes of all ages, the receptor varies from one group of isolates to another (Perkins and Holt 1988) and optional receptors include sialic acid (Facer 1983), glycophorins (Pasvol, Wainscoat and Weatherall 1982) and band 3 (Okoye and Bennett 1985). In *P. vivax*, a parasite that is restricted to reticulocytes, attachment to 2 additional receptors is required: one is reticulocyte-specific, the other is associated with a glycoprotein serologically defined by the Duffy (FyFy) blood group determinant (Wertheimer and Barnwell 1989). The red cell receptor preferences of *P. ovale* and *P. malariae* are presumed to be different from those of *P. falciparum* and *P. vivax*. *P. ovale* can infect Duffy negative red cells, which is compatible with the fact that the species is found in West Africa (where the Duffy negative phenotype is highly prevalent), whereas *P. malariae* is said to have a predilection for senescent red cells.

Invasion of the hepatocyte

After a sporozoite has entered the bloodstream, it rapidly 'homes in' towards liver sinusoids and establishes itself within a hepatocyte. In view of the technical difficulties inherent in the study of this biological event, many questions remain unanswered; for instance the following points are not clear:

1 Whether there is a specific liver-homing mechanism.
2 Whether sporozoites enter the hepatocyte directly (e.g. into the space of Disse through gaps in the endothelial lining) or whether they first cross a Kupffer cell.
3 Which parasite and host cell receptors and ligands are involved in hepatocyte invasion (Verhave and Meis 1984).

The membrane of the sporozoite is believed to be entirely covered by the CS protein, which is likely to be responsible for the initial attachment to the hepatocyte surface.

Invasion of mosquito gut epithelial cells

The oökinete, which is equipped with the characteristic apical complex of invasive stages, is believed to recognize and attach to a specific receptor on the midgut epithelial cell, and then to invade the cell (Garnham, Bird and Baker 1962). After crossing the cell, it is thought to exit either into the intercellular space or directly into the basal region, where it will attach to the basal lamina and differentiate into an oöcyst.

Alterations of host cells

After infection by the malarial parasite, the host cell undergoes a variety of structural changes, which may substantially alter its function, appearance or antigenicity. The nature of the alterations induced vary from one species to another. These host cell alterations have been studied most comprehensively in the erythrocytic stage of the parasite (Hommel and Semoff 1988), but it is conceivable that they may also exist in the other intracellular stages.

The alterations identified so far in the membranes of malaria infected erythrocytes include the following: a visible change of shape and reduced deformability; the presence of electron-dense protrusions or 'knobs' (in *P. falciparum* and *P. malariae*) (Fig. 20.12); the presence of small depressions, or 'caveolae', at the surface of the erythrocyte, connected by a network of small vesicles and clefts (in *P. vivax* or *P. ovale*) (Aikawa 1988); the expression of new sugar moieties, particularly galactose (David, Hommel and Oligino 1981); the cytoadherence to endothelial cells or rosetting with normal erythrocytes (Wahlgren, Carlson and Udomsangpetch 1987); the presence of new metabolic channels (Ginsburg et al. 1985); the evidence of new parasite-specific antigens associated with the red cell membrane (Hommel, David and Oligino 1983); and the reorganization of normal erythrocyte components (e.g. disruption of spectrin or conformational changes of band 3) (Yuthavong et al. 1979, Winograd and Sherman 1989).

3.4 Characteristics of human malaria parasites

The main features of human malaria parasites, as observed on Romanowsky-stained thin blood films, are shown in Fig. 20.13.

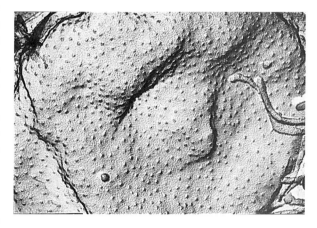

Fig. 20.12 Knobs on *P. falciparum*-infected erythrocytes.

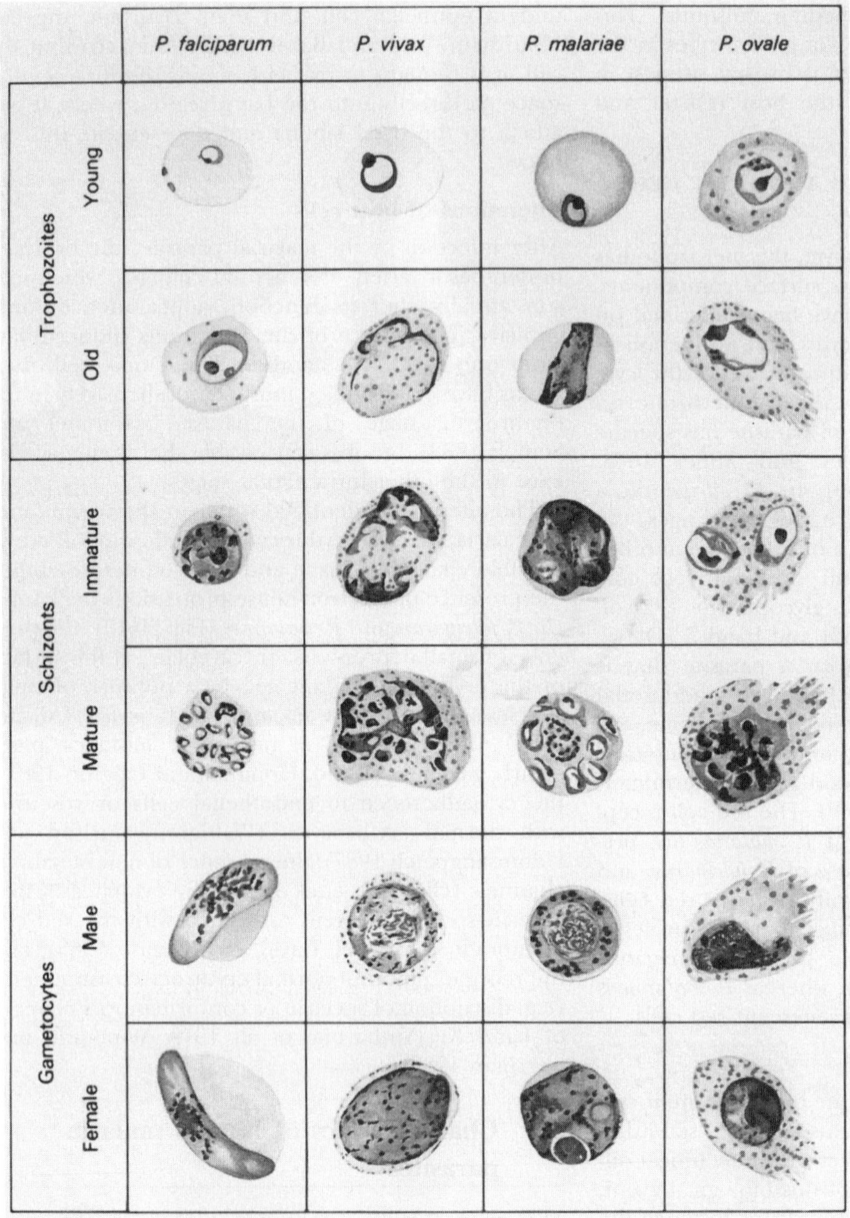

		P. falciparum	P. vivax	P. malariae	P. ovale
Trophozoites	Young				
	Old				
Schizonts	Immature				
	Mature				
Gametocytes	Male				
	Female				

Fig. 20.13 Morphological characteristics of human malaria parasites. See also Plate 20.13.

PLASMODIUM (LAVERANIA) FALCIPARUM

Of all the human malaria parasites, *P. falciparum* is the most highly pathogenic and is responsible for 'malignant tertian malaria', a form of the disease which runs an acute course in non-immune patients and which frequently is fatal if untreated. This parasite is the major cause of malaria in tropical Africa and is also responsible for the great regional epidemics that sometimes occur in north west India or Sri Lanka; it is generally confined to tropical or subtropical areas because its development in the mosquito is greatly retarded when the temperature falls below 20°C. The most characteristic biological features of *P. falciparum* are as follows:

1   It infects mature and young erythrocytes.
2   The surface of erythrocytes infected with late-stage trophozoites or schizonts is altered in such a way as to make them stick to endothelial cells in various tissues (this cytoadherence is responsible for the sequestration of the parasite).
3   The pre-erythrocytic cycle starts immediately after injection of sporozoites by the mosquito, without the production of hypnozoites (i.e. there are no relapses).
4   Schizogony is particularly prolific in all stages (pre-erythrocytic schizogony produces up to 30 000 merozoites, erythrocytic schizogony produces 16–18 merozoites and sporogony produces up to 20 000 sporozoites) and this may be the cause of its success as a species and its virulence.
5   Infection in the peripheral blood is characterized by the predominant presence of ring forms and gametocytes, whereas late trophozoites and schizonts are seen only exceptionally; the level of parasitaemia may be high and multiple infection in a single erythrocyte is common.

6 The gametocytes are characteristically crescent-shaped and, unlike the gametocytes of other species, are very slow to reach maturity (up to 10 days) and early forms of gametocytes are sequestered.

PLASMODIUM VIVAX

P. vivax occurs throughout most of the temperate zones as well as large areas of the tropics (but is mainly absent from tropical West Africa). It causes 'benign tertian' malaria, the pattern of which varies with different parasite strains. As a species, *P. vivax* is particularly polymorphic and the subspecies status proposed for some strains may be justified on morphological grounds (e.g. *P. vivax multinucleatum*, found in China, seems to have a characteristic oöcyst), on biological grounds (e.g. *P. vivax hibernans*, found in Russia, whose sporozoites produce only hypnozoites), or on molecular grounds (e.g. a series of *P. vivax* isolates with substantial differences in their genetic make-up have been identified, including a *P. vivax*-like parasite indistinguishable from the simian parasite *P. simiovale* found in humans in Papua New Guinea, Brazil and Madagascar) (Qari et al. 1993).

The distinctive biological features of *P. vivax* are:

1 A restriction of erythrocyte invasion to reticulocytes bearing Duffy blood group determinants, a feature that explains why red blood cells infected with trophozoites of *P. vivax* are sometimes described as 'larger' than normal.

2 The presence of caveolar structures on the surface of the infected erythrocyte membrane, that communicate with underlying cytoplasmic vesicles; these structures readily take up the Romanowsky stain and appear, to the microscopist, as a reddish cytoplasmic stippling or 'Schüffner's dots'.

3 After invading the hepatocyte some, or all, of the sporozoites may transform into hypnozoites, then remain latent for months or years and be responsible for subsequent relapses.

PLASMODIUM OVALE

P. ovale is a species truly distinct from *P. vivax*, not only with respect to minor morphological differences (e.g. oval shape of infected red cell with ragged or fimbriated margin, smaller number of merozoites in schizont, aspect of gametocytes), but also presenting antigenic and molecular differences. Nevertheless, most of the biological and clinical features are identical. The major biological difference is that *P. ovale* can infect Duffy negative reticulocytes, whereas *P. vivax* cannot.

PLASMODIUM MALARIAE

P. malariae differs from the other 3 human malaria parasites in its slow development and in its longer asexual cycle. Development is slow in both the vector and the human host, because of less efficient schizogony (pre-erythrocytic schizonts have 6000 merozoites, erythrocytic schizonts have 6–12 merozoites). The asexual cycle is 72 h instead of 48 h, and this feature has given the clinical form of *P. malariae* its name,

quartan malaria, because fever paroxysms occur every fourth day according to the Roman custom of regarding day 0 as day 1. The biological characteristics of the parasite are:

1 An apparent erythrocytic preference for old erythrocytes, explaining why infected cells are often described as 'smaller' by microscopists (this feature is poorly documented because of the absence of an in vitro culture system).

2 The presence of 'knobs' at the surface of infected erythrocytes; similar to *P. falciparum*, but these cells do not exhibit any cytoadherence (and therefore no sequestration). The surfaces of infected cells do not exhibit any caveolar vesicle complexes and, consequently, Schüffner's dots are absent.

3 Sporozoites of *P. malariae* do not transform into hypnozoites and, hence, there are no relapses. However, *P. malariae* can survive for a considerable time in the peripheral blood (10 years or more) at a very low level of parasitaemia, occasionally producing detectable peaks with a recrudescence of clinical symptoms.

4 BIOCHEMISTRY, MOLECULAR BIOLOGY AND GENETICS

4.1 Metabolic pathways

Much of what is known about the metabolism of malaria parasites has been derived from studies of blood stages, either isolated from their vertebrate host or produced in culture. Our knowledge of the biochemical pathways and metabolic requirements of malarial parasites is still limited and probably often inaccurate (e.g. owing to contamination by host material or the damaging effect of methods used to separate the parasites from their host cells) (Homewood and Neame 1980). With the exception of the invasive forms of the parasite, which are short lived and presumed to be in a state of low metabolic activity, all developmental stages are intracellular. One of the major issues of parasite metabolism is access to nutrients from the host cell cytoplasm and extracellular environment.

ACCESS TO NUTRIENTS

The passage of nutrients from the extracellular space to the parasite involves transfer through the host cell membrane, the parasitophorous membrane and the parasite's own membrane; it is difficult to identify the respective barrier functions of these 3 separate membranes and, in most studies, the transfer measured represents the overall result. Transfer across membranes may be achieved by a variety of mechanisms, including diffusion along a gradient of substrate and carrier-mediated transport. Because of rapid parasite growth and replication, the normal transport mechanisms of the red cell are not sufficient to cope with the increased demand (e.g. an infected red cell uses almost 100 times more glucose than a normal red cell) (Roth et al. 1982). Increased traffic across the membrane is achieved not only by an increase in the transmembrane gradient of substrate (created by increased consumption of nutrients by the growing parasite) but also by new permeation pathways introduced by the parasite into the host cells (Sherman 1988, Cabantchik 1990). The need for such new pathways is probably greater for parasites restricted to adult erythrocytes, because these cells are relatively impermeable to many of the nutrients needed for parasite growth (e.g. L-glutamine) (Elford 1986) and the presence of such pathways may represent a target for new antimalarials (e.g. the derivatives of the Chinese antimalarial qinghaosu are potent inhibitors of the L-glutamine influx).

Most nutrients required by the parasite originate from the extracellular space (e.g. host plasma); these include glucose, purines and pyrimidines, amino acids, anions, cations, iron, zinc, vitamins, fatty acids and phospholipids. Some of these nutrients may also be obtained from the host cytoplasm either by transport across the membranes or by uptake through the cytostome, e.g. the uptake of haemoglobin and its breakdown to form malarial pigment. The uptake of antimalarial drugs follows the same pathways as the transport of nutrients and, to some extent, these pathways may also function in the opposite direction for the disposal of waste products such as lactate.

Carbohydrate metabolism

The intraerythrocytic malaria parasites lack reserves of glycogen and other polysaccharides and are, consequently, dependent on glucose as their primary source of energy. Glucose utilization by the parasite is relatively inefficient, because oxidization stops at the lactate stage; this also means that a large amount of lactate is generated, which reduces the internal pH and which has to be efficiently disposed of. All the malarial enzymes of the glycolytic pathway have been identified and found to be isoenzymes that differ from host enzymes (Roth 1990). Although the hexose monophosphate shunt pathway is operative and represents an essential source of NADPH, the activity of the parasite-encoded glucose-6-phosphate-dehydrogenase (G6PD) is only about 5% of that of the host cell enzyme (Ling and Wilson 1988). This suggests that the host enzyme normally initiates the pathway and that the parasite enzyme may be upregulated only when the parasite is in a G6PD-deficient red cell; this would explain why the in vitro growth of *P. falciparum* in G6PD-deficient cells is initially impaired but may be overcome after a few cycles of growth.

There is still considerable doubt concerning the presence or absence of a functional citric acid cycle in malaria parasites and the only citric acid cycle enzyme identified with any certainty in blood stage plasmodia is malate dehydrogenase (Sherman 1979). All malaria parasites seem to be capable of fixing CO_2, producing α-ketoglutarate and oxaloacetate as first intermediates; it has been suggested that a branched pathway from the oxaloacetate thus produced may be preferred by malaria parasites to the Krebs cycle for the production of aspartate, glutamate, malate and citrate (Scheibel 1988).

Protein and polyamine synthesis

The molecular mechanisms involved in plasmodial protein synthesis are typically eukaryotic. The parasite obtains most of the amino acids it needs either from the digestion of red cell proteins (particularly haemoglobin) or from the free amino acid pool in the plasma; some are biosynthesized by the parasite itself (e.g. glutamic acid from glucose). The minimal amino acid requirements of the parasite are not yet known. Haemoglobin is broken down within the parasite food vacuoles, into haem (the major component of haemozoin, the malarial pigment) and globin, which is further hydrolysed to free amino acids by a series of parasite proteases (including serine, aspartic and cysteine proteases) (Schrevel et al. 1990); up to 75% of the haemoglobin of an infected cell may be degraded by the parasite. Protein synthesis does not occur at a constant rate during the life-cycle and maximum activity occurs during schizogony.

Three steps are critical in the biosynthesis of polyamines: the decarboxylation of ornithine to putrescine via ornithine decarboxylase (ODC), the formation of S-adenosylmethionine (AdoMet) from L-methionine and ATP, and the decarboxylation of AdoMet which provides the aminopropyl groups required for the synthesis of spermidine and spermine (Assaraf et al. 1984). All 3 steps represent potential targets for chemotherapy.

Nucleic acid metabolism

The amount of DNA in a malaria parasite is approximately 10^{-13} g and there is about 2–5 times more RNA than DNA (Gutteridge and Trigg 1970). DNA synthesis occurs mostly in the late trophozoite and the early part of schizogony (29–44 h in the *P. falciparum* cycle). The nuclear DNA base composition of malaria parasites is characteristically adenine and thymidine (A + T) rich. Because of its rapid schizogonic development (e.g. a merozoite may generate 8–20 new merozoites in 48 h), the parasite needs to possess an effective method of nucleic acid synthesis and this implies access to nucleic acid precursors. The mature human erythrocyte has no requirements for pyrimidine and, lacking the capacity for purine synthesis *de novo*, relies on the salvage of preformed purines (mostly for its ATP synthesis). Nucleosides are transported into erythrocytes by means of a specific transport protein in the membrane and adenosine, hypoxanthine and guanine can thus be salvaged from the plasma. In infected erythrocytes, the influx of purines into the red cell is increased and there is evidence to suggest that the erythrocyte's ATP is broken down to AMP and hypoxanthine; although hypoxanthine seems to be the major purine incorporated into the parasite, the parasite does have a range of purine salvage pathway enzymes (Reyes et al. 1982).

Malaria parasites must synthesize pyrimidines *de novo*, because the erythrocyte cannot supply them; the small amount of uridine and thymidine taken up by the erythrocyte does not seem to be incorporated by the parasite. The parasite has all the enzymes required for the synthesis of UMP from glutamine, ATP and CO_2 (Gero and O'Sullivan 1990); some of these enzymes are functionally different from the corresponding host enzymes.

The synthesis of pyrimidines is intimately linked to folate metabolism. All 3 enzymes of the folate cycle have been studied in malaria parasites, particularly dihydrofolate reductase (DHFR) and thymidylate synthetase (TS), 2 enzymes which in parasites are part of a single bifunctional protein (DHFR-TS) (Snewin et al. 1989). It seems that the parasite relies more on the *de novo* folate pathway than folate salvage, which explains the synergy of the antimalarial activity of sulpha drugs (which inhibit *de novo* synthesis) and pyrimethamine (this inhibits the parasite DHFR, which is considerably more sensitive to the drug than the host enzyme). The synthesis of pyrimidines also involves the vitamin *para*-amino benzoic acid (PABA) and several authors have shown that the growth of plasmodia in experimental hosts is affected by the absence of PABA in the diet (Ferone 1977).

Lipid metabolism

The growth of the parasite within the host erythrocyte requires a substantial increase of its total membranes; lipids generally constitute about 50% of the membrane mass. The lipid content of infected erythrocytes is higher than in normal ones (Homewood and Neame 1980) and the relative distribution of various lipids reflects the separate contributions that are made to erythrocyte membrane, parasitophorous vacuole membrane, external parasite membrane and parasite organelles membranes.

During the erythrocytic cycle of the parasite, there is a 500–700% increase in phospholipid levels and the 4 major types of phospholipids are found in infected cells (Vial et al. 1990). Although infected cells can incorporate some intact phospholipids from the plasma (probably by means of a specific phospholipid transfer molecule), it is thought that *de novo* synthesis and conversion from one phospholipid species to another represent the 2 major sources of new phospholipids.

As there seems to be no fatty acid synthesis in infected cells, nor the capacity for retailoring available molecules (by elongation or desaturation processes) (Holz 1977), the host plasma must represent the main source of fatty acids. Infected cells incorporate considerable amounts of palmitic, stearic, oleic, arachidonic and linoleic acids. Parasites have a high acyl-CoA synthetase activity (20 times more active than in normal erythrocytes), which produces fatty acyl-CoA, the usual fatty acid donor molecule in biosynthesis pathways. Choline enters the infected cell by means of a transport-mediated process, similar to that of normal erythrocytes.

ION METABOLISM

The uptake of extracellular calcium (Ca^{2+}) is essential for the growth of malaria parasites. The in vitro growth of *P. falciparum* trophozoites and merozoite invasion is inhibited after depletion of Ca^{2+} by EGTA. This is consistent with the presence of calmodulin, one of the Ca^{2+}-binding proteins, both in the parasite cytoplasm and in apical organelles (Scheibel et al. 1987). The Ca^{2+} content of infected cells increases as the parasite matures, due to an increased permeability of infected cells to external Ca^{2+} (Tanabe 1990). Because malaria infected cells actively incorporate extracellular Ca^{2+}, it is not surprising that blockers of Ca^{2+} channels (e.g. verapamil) or antagonists of calmodulin (e.g. diltiazem or calmidazolium) may arrest parasite development.

Malaria parasites, like most eukaryotic cells, are capable of maintaining a high level of K^+ and a low level of Na^+ in their cytoplasm by means of a Na^+, K^+-ATPase and at the expense of the host cell ionic environment. It is interesting that the ATPase has been identified in the parasitophorous vacuole membrane (not in the parasite membrane) and this implies that the parasite is living in a low Na^+, high K^+ extracellular environment. This unusual feature is consistent with the observation that it is necessary to use a low Na^+, high K^+ medium to grow trophozoites extracellularly in vitro (Trager and Williams 1992).

The requirement for iron in a number of metabolic pathways, including the synthesis of DNA, explains why the parasite may be inhibited by relatively low amounts of desferrioxamine (Raventos-Suarez, Pollack and Nagel 1982). Although haemoglobin is degraded within its food vacuoles, most of the haem released is transformed into crystalline haemozoin and is not a usable source of free iron. It has been suggested that extracellular iron may be taken up by the parasite either by the binding of ferrotransferrin (from serum transferrin) to a parasite transferrin receptor in the infected erythrocyte membrane (Rodriguez and Jungery 1986) or by means of a transferrin-independent mechanism (Sanchez-Lopez and Haldar 1992). The role of iron in the viability of malaria parasites is a matter of controversy, because iron deficiency protects mice against *P. chabaudi*, whereas people with iron deficiency are still susceptible to malaria, but may have an increased parasitaemia if given iron supplementation (Murray et al. 1978).

OXYGEN UPTAKE AND REDOX STATUS

Low oxygen levels have a beneficial effect on the in vitro growth of *P. falciparum* and increased oxygen uptake is observed in infected erythrocytes in the presence of glucose, suggesting that malaria parasites are essentially microaerophilic (Scheibel, Ashton and Trager 1979). For many years, there was little tangible evidence of the existence of respiration or the presence of an electron transport chain in the parasite. The isolation of purified mitochondria from *P. falciparum* has allowed an unambiguous measurement of the cytochrome content of these organelles and confirmed the existence of a classic respiratory chain including the presence of cytochromes (Fry 1991).

The status of reduction-oxidation ('redox') reactions of the infected red cell is complex because it involves a combination of the oxidative stress exerted by the parasite on the host cell, the ability of the host cell to mount antioxidant defences to prevent oxidative damage, oxidative stress exerted by the host on the parasite (which may include the effect of immune responses and antimalarial drugs) and, finally, the ability of the parasite to mount its own antioxidant defences (Hunt and Stocker 1990). The generation of reactive oxygen intermediates (ROIs) is the major factor of oxidative stress both in the parasite and in the host cell. Parasites are susceptible to various ROIs, and hydrogen peroxide, *t*-butyl-hydroperoxide, xanthine-xanthine oxidase and alloxan all have antiparasitic activity (Clark, Cowden and Chaudhri 1989). A number of antimalarial drugs (e.g. primaquine and qinghaosu) also seem to act by means of oxidation. The reduced growth of parasites in erythrocytes with certain genetic abnormalities (sickle cell disease, α- and β-thalassaemia, persistence of haemoglobin E) may be explained either by a reduced ability to mount antioxidant defences or by an increased level of oxidative stress. Among the antioxidant mechanisms used both by the red cell and the parasite, detoxification by the glutathione cycle (by means of glutathione reductase and NADPH) plays a crucial role (Fritsch et al. 1987). Vitamins C and E are found in increased amounts in infected cells and are thought to have a protective role, particularly in preventing the peroxidation of membrane lipids and in preventing the formation of methaemoglobin. Both host cell and parasite superoxide dismutases (SODs) have been identified in *P. falciparum*-infected cells, the parasite SOD being cyanide insensitive (Fairfield et al. 1988).

4.2 Molecular biology and genetics

The genome of malaria parasites is complex, presenting a high degree of diversity, not only from species to species, but also from one isolate to another. Diversity is generated either by cross-fertilization during meiosis or by genomic reorganization during mitosis. The genome is haploid throughout most of the life-cycle, apart from a short time after zygote formation; it consists of 14 chromosomes of various sizes.

GENOME STRUCTURE

Measured sizes of the haploid genomes of malaria parasites range between 20 and 40 Mb, values comparable to the genome of yeast but 3–4 times greater than that of *E. coli*. The base composition of the genome of all malaria parasites is always A + T rich (from 70 to 83% A + T, depending on the species) (Weber 1988). Codon usage by malaria parasites is not random and for some genes (e.g. the repeat region of the CS protein) the usage of synonymous codons may be highly biased. Over 150 different malaria genes have already been identified, partially sequenced and mapped on chromosomes; so far low-resolution physical maps of 9 of the 14 chromosomes have been published (Triglia, Wellems and Kemp 1992) and the Malaria Genome Project has completed the physical map of 6 of 14 chromosomes.

Analysis of chromosomes by PFGE has shown that *P. falciparum* chromosomes not only differ from each other in size (from 0.6 to 3 Mb), but also that individual chromosomes may vary considerably from one isolate to another (Corcoran et al. 1986); chromosome size can change during the sexual part of the life-cycle, and also during mitosis.

The extreme diversity of the genomic make-up of malaria isolates has also been demonstrated by the use of Southern blot fingerprinting which measures restriction fragment length polymorphisms (RFLPs) with various DNA probes (e.g. rep20). This has revealed a different fingerprint pattern for almost every single isolate from a given geographical area (Langsley et al. 1988, Hughes, Hommel and Crampton 1989). The genetic polymorphism of parasite isolates may be used as a molecular epidemiological tool. The sequencing of malaria genes (mostly in the context of a search for a malaria vaccine) has shown that many genes present a high frequency of tandem repeats, but also that a number of malarial antigens may have regions of sequence homology. Repeat regions are often assumed to have a functional significance (e.g. as receptor binding sites or as a decoy against the host immune response) and this has been particularly well studied for the CS gene, which presents a comparable repeat region in the genes of all malaria species, whereas the repeated sequence itself and the number of repeats are substantially different from one species to another. The tandem repeats generally evolve more rapidly than the non-repeated flanking regions and the number of repeats may vary between different alleles of the same gene; there is considerable allelic polymorphism for all the malarial genes studied so far.

Apart from nuclear DNA, malaria parasites have 2 other extrachromosomal forms of DNA; a 6 kb element that is related to the mitochondrial DNA of other species and a 35 kb circular element that seems to be related to the chloroplast element found in algae (Gardner et al. 1993). A complete map of the latter is now available and includes small subunit RNA genes and genes for RNA proteins.

Malaria genetics

Genetic recombination in malaria parasites occurs in the mosquito where fertilization of gametes, zygote formation and meiosis take place For recombination to occur, the parasites picked up by the mosquito must consist of more than one population of parasites of the same species (cross-fertilization between gametes of 2 different species is believed not to be possible).

During recombination, each member of a pair of chromosomes segregates randomly into the haploid progeny and crossing-over events take place between homologous chromosomes; this results in complex changes between the parental and the various progeny lines, in which the number of recombinant parasites generated by a given cross is usually much higher than would be predicted (Walliker et al. 1987). The subtelomeric regions of chromosomes represent 'hotspots' of recombination, being subject to the greatest degree of variability and genetic rearrangements. In view of the fact that malarial infections observed in humans are rarely clonal, but more often a mixture of 3–9 different parasite clones, it is surprising that the level of recombination actually observed in mosquitoes is lower than expected (1.5–2 on average); this may be explained by the fact that different populations are present at the same time and the different populations are rarely synchronized with regard to gametocytogenesis, thus making homozygote crosses more likely than heterozygote crosses.

5 Clinical aspects

5.1 Introduction

Malaria is the most important parasitic disease in terms of morbidity and mortality on a global scale. Almost all of the 2 million deaths attributed to it yearly are due to falciparum malaria. In Africa, it is responsible for the death of 1 out of 20 children, before the age of 5 years. Malaria can mimic many diseases and there are no absolute diagnostic clinical features. The classic periodicity of febrile paroxysms every 48 h for *P. falciparum*, *P. vivax* and *P. ovale* (days 1 and 3) or every 72 h for *P. malariae* (days 1 and 4) are usually absent at the beginning of the disease. Periodicity develops only as a result of a delay in treatment when a sufficient number of schizonts rupture at the same time and the infection becomes synchronized.

5.2 Clinical manifestations

Falciparum malaria ('malignant tertian malaria')

In non-immune people, falciparum malaria is a medical emergency, as there are few conditions in tropical medicine that can change so dramatically from a relatively benign illness to a catastrophic and fatal one (Gilles and Phillips 1988, Molyneux and Fox 1993, Warrell 1993).

The incubation period is generally 9–14 days, but it can be as short as 7 days. The symptoms are non-specific with headache and pains in the back and limbs, simulating influenza; anorexia; nausea; and a feeling of chill rather than a distinct cold phase (as in vivax malaria). Fever is very common but not invariable; it is continuous or remittent, not tertian. The physical findings include prostration, a tinge of jaundice often misdiagnosed as viral hepatitis, *Herpes simplex* of the lips and tender hepatosplenomegaly. An ophthalmoscopic examination should always be carried out, because in many parts of the world the presence of retinal haemorrhages in adults is associated with imminent coma.

Complications of severe falciparum malaria

Cerebral malaria is the most common presentation of severe malaria in adults. They have usually been ill for 4–5 days with fever, slowly lapsing into coma, with or without convulsions. The usual neurological picture is of a symmetrical upper motor neuron lesion with increased muscle tone, brisk, tender reflexes, ankle clonus and extensor plantar responses. The abdominal reflexes are absent. A number of bizarre neurological signs can occur; dysconjugate gaze is common. A whole variety of other neurological signs have been described (Warrell 1993). Retinal haemorrhages occur in about 15% of adults and carry a bad prognosis (Fig. 20.14). Even when good standards of care can be provided, the mortality is about 15–20%.

Malarial anaemia is common in young children (see section 5.2, p. 376), in pregnant women (see section 5.2, p. 377) and in adults with severe malaria in whom it correlates with parasitaemia.

Biochemical evidence of renal dysfunction progressing to oliguria, anuria and acute renal failure is present in about 10% of cases.

Hypoglycaemia is common in patients with hyperparasitaemia or as a result of treatment with quinine. The classic symptoms of hypoglycaemia may not be present, the only sign being a deterioration in the level of consciousness.

Pulmonary oedema is the most dreaded complication of malaria, with a mortality of over 50%. It is sometimes precipitated by excessive parenteral fluid therapy and, as such, may be avoidable. The earliest signs are an increase in respiratory rate, dyspnoea and crepitations. In most patients, however, it is not iatrogenically produced and the picture is similar to that of the adult respiratory distress syndrome (ARDS) (Charoenpan et al. 1990).

Malarial haemoglobinuria is now usually associated with hyperparasitaemia resulting in severe intravascu-

lar haemolysis. Some patients are mistakenly labelled as such when in fact the haemoglobinuria is due to G6PD deficiency, triggered by a variety of drugs including the oxidant antimalarial primaquine (Gilles and Ikeme 1960). The known complications of severe falciparum malaria are given in Table 20.1.

VIVAX AND OVALE MALARIA ('BENIGN TERTIAN MALARIA')

The incubation period of vivax malaria is usually 12–17 days but with some strains it can be as long as 250–637 days; that of ovale malaria is usually 16–18 days but it may also be longer. The clinical manifestations are similar.

After 2–3 days of non-specific symptoms similar to those described for falciparum malaria, the classic febrile paroxysm occurs. The cold stage, which lasts for 15–60 min, is characterized by violent rigors, a high core temperature, a cold, dry skin due to intense peripheral vasoconstriction and a rapid, low-volume pulse. The hot stage follows, the patient becoming unbearably hot. The temperature rises to 40–41°C accompanied by a severe throbbing headache, palpitations, prostration, confusion and delirium. The skin is flushed, the pulse rapid and full. The patient looks ill, may be anaemic and mildly jaundiced, and the liver and spleen are enlarged and tender. The hot stage lasts 2–6 h. It is followed by the sweating stage characterized by drenching sweats, defervescence and exhausted sleep. Unless treated, the febrile paroxysms recur every other day. Thrombocytopenia is common and the only serious (often fatal) complication is splenic rupture. Untreated or inadequately treated cases relapse after a period of quiescence at intervals varying from 8 to 40 weeks or more, depending on the strain of the parasite.

MALARIAE MALARIA ('QUARTAN MALARIA')

The incubation period of quartan malaria is 18–40 days. The clinical picture is similar to that of benign tertian malaria, the febrile paroxysms occurring every 72 h. Symptomatic recrudescences, which can occur up to 52 years after the last exposure to infection, are due to persistent undetectable parasitaemia, not to hypnozoites. In several parts of the world there is strong epidemiological evidence that *P. malariae* is an

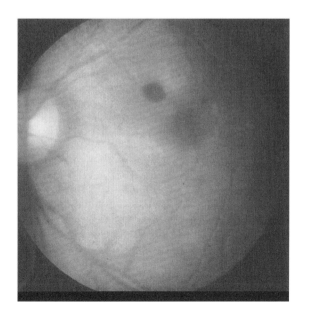

Fig. 20.14 Retinal haemorrhage. See also Plate 20.14. (Copyright D. Warrell.)

Table 20.1 Complications of severe falciparum malaria

Cerebral malaria
Anaemia
Renal failure
Hypoglycaemia
Hyperparasitaemia
Malarial haemoglobinuria
Fluid, electrolyte and acid base disturbances
Pulmonary oedema
Circulatory collapse ('algid malaria')
Bleeding and clotting disturbances
Hyperpyrexia

important cause of nephrotic syndrome especially in children under 15 years of age.

MALARIA IN CHILDREN

The manifestations of the primary attack of malaria in non-immune children are very variable, consisting of any of the following symptoms, or combinations thereof: restlessness or drowsiness, refusal to eat or suck, headache, vomiting, loose stools and cough. In the majority, the temperature is high (40°C), the child is flushed and febrile convulsions are common, lasting only a few minutes. If the child does not regain consciousness within 30 min following the convulsion, cerebral malaria must be suspected. The liver is often enlarged and tender; splenomegaly develops later. Ocular fundus findings such as papilloedema indicate a poor prognosis (Lewallen et al. 1993).

Children living in highly endemic malarious areas are equally vulnerable until the age of about 5 years, after which they achieve a relative immunity to malaria infection. Many, especially in tropical Africa, are either asymptomatic or have a mild illness, despite a parasitaemia of 10–30%. Hepatosplenomegaly occurs in 80% of these individuals.

Many of the clinical features of severe malaria (described in section 5.2, page 375) also occur in children. The commonest and most important complications are cerebral malaria, severe anaemia and metabolic acidosis. Cerebral malaria is the commonest presentation in The Gambia and in Burkina Faso (Waller et al. 1995, Modiano et al. 1995), whereas anaemia is the most frequent presentation in Kenya and in Papua New Guinea (Marsh et al. 1995, Allen et al. 1996).

Cerebral malaria

In holoendemic areas of malaria, cerebral malaria occurs in children between 6 months and 5 years old, most commonly in children aged 3–4 years. The earliest symptom is usually fever (37.5–41°C) followed by failure to eat or drink. Vomiting and cough are common; diarrhoea is unusual. The history of symptoms preceding coma may be very brief (1 or 2 days). Hypoglycaemia is a particularly common presenting feature in children under 3 years and in those with convulsions, hyperparasitaemia or profound coma (White et al. 1987, Taylor et al. 1988). In the latter, corneal and vestibular-ocular reflexes may be absent. Extreme opisthotonos is sometimes seen (Fig. 20.15) and is easily mistaken for tetanus or meningitis.

Some children are in a state of shock. CSF opening pressure is often raised, sometimes markedly so. Intracranial hypertension and neurological evidence of cerebral herniation have been documented (Newton et al. 1991). Convulsions are common before or after the onset of coma; they are significantly associated with morbidity and sequelae. Neurological sequelae which occur in about 10% of children include: hemiparesis, cerebellar ataxia, cortical blindness, severe hypotonia, mental retardation, generalized spasticity and aphasia (Molyneux et al. 1989, Newton et al. 1994).

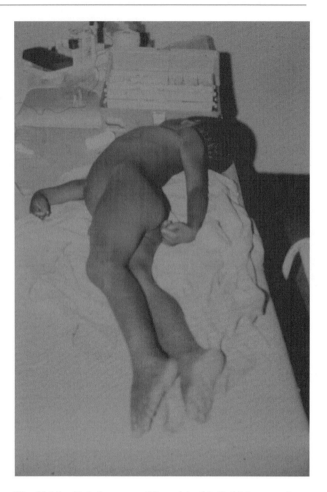

Fig. 20.15 Opisthotonos. (Copyright M. E. Molyneaux.)

Anaemia

This is particularly common in children aged between 6 months and 2 years. It is often the result of repeated untreated or partially treated episodes of uncomplicated malaria. Parasitaemia is often scanty, although numerous pigmented monocytes are seen in the peripheral blood. The anaemia is normochromic with prominent dyserythropoietic changes in the bone marrow. In older children the anaemia is acute and haemolytic and associated with hyperparasitaemia.

Children with severe anaemia may present with tachycardia, dyspnoea, respiratory distress, confusion, restlessness, coma, retinal haemorrhages, cardiac failure and pulmonary oedema.

Metabolic acidosis

Metabolic acidosis is an important feature of severe malaria. It may present separately or in combination with cerebral malaria or anaemia (Taylor and Voller 1993, Marsh et al. 1995). Deep breathing is a good clinical indicator of the presence of acidosis. Lactic acidosis is a major contributor to acidaemia (Krishna et al. 1994). Metabolic acidosis is associated with a poor prognosis.

The differences between severe malaria in adults and in children are given in Table 20.2. The reasons for these differences have yet to be fully elucidated.

Table 20.2   Differences between severe malaria in adults and in children

Sign or Symptom	Adults	Children
Cough	Uncommon	Common
Convulsions	Common	Very common
Jaundice	Common	Uncommon
Duration of antecedent illness	5–7 days	1–2 days
Pre-treatment hypoglycaemia	Uncommon	Common
Resolution of coma	2–4 days	1–2 days
CSF opening pressure	Usually normal	Often raised
Abnormality of brain stem reflexes (e.g. oculovestibular, oculocervical)	Rare	More common
Neurological sequelae	Uncommon	Occurs in about 10%
Pulmonary oedema	Common	Rare
Renal failure	Common	Rare
Bleeding, clotting disturbances	Up to 10%	Rare

MALARIA IN PREGNANCY

Non-immune pregnant women are susceptible to all the usual manifestations of malaria. Moreover, they have an increased risk of abortion, stillbirth, premature delivery and of low birth weight of their infant. Mortality from severe malaria is higher than in non-pregnant patients (Wickramasuriya 1937, Menon 1972, Bray and Anderson 1979, Brabin 1983, Looaresuwan et al. 1985, Brabin et al. 1993).

Pregnant women are particularly prone to hypoglycaemia which may occur on admission in severe disease, in otherwise uncomplicated malaria and as a complication of quinine therapy. It is commonly asymptomatic, although it may be associated with fetal bradycardia and other signs of fetal distress. In the quinine-induced hyperinsulinaemic hypoglycaemia, abnormal behaviour, sweating and sudden loss of consciousness usually occur (White et al. 1983).

Pulmonary oedema may occur in pregnant women on admission, may develop suddenly and unexpectedly several days after admission, or may develop immediately after childbirth (Fig. 20.16).

In holoendemic areas of malaria, partially immune pregnant women, especially primigravidae, are susceptible to abortion, stillbirth, premature delivery and low-birth-weight infants (Archibald 1956, Bray and

Anderson 1979, McGregor, Wilson and Billewicz 1983, Greenwood et al. 1994, Morgan 1994). Significant increases in parasite rates and densities occur, particularly in primigravidae. In the second trimester primiparae are prone to develop a severe haemolytic anaemia that bears little relation to their peripheral parasitaemia (Gilles et al. 1969, Rougemont et al. 1977, Brabin 1983, McGregor 1984, Fleming et al. 1986, Steketee et al. 1994a). The other complications of severe malaria are, however, rarely encountered.

Vertical transmission of malaria across the placenta from mother to fetus occurs and in endemic areas it is not uncommon for neonates to have cord-blood and peripheral parasitaemia that disappears within a day or 2. Congenital malaria (i.e. symptoms or signs resulting from malarial infection in the neonate) is more common in infants born to non-immune mothers and during epidemics of malaria. In malaria endemic regions, the incidence is low, despite a high prevalence of placental infection.

HYPERACTIVE MALARIAL SPLENOMEGALY (TROPICAL SPLENOMEGALY SYNDROME)

In some malaria endemic regions of the world and particularly in parts of Papua New Guinea and sub-Saharan Africa, adults develop a progressive, sometimes massive enlargement of the spleen (more than 10 cm below the costal margin). The spleen may weigh over 4 kg. The liver is often enlarged with dilated sinuses containing lymphocytes. Hypersplenism can cause a normocytic anaemia, leucopenia and thrombocytopenia. Pregnant women may suffer attacks of acute haemolysis. There is a gradual onset of early lethargy that can progress to an incapacitating weakness. Left upper quadrant pain is common. Physical examination reveals gross splenomegaly with an obvious notch in an afebrile patient, evidence of hypovolaemia and moderate anaemia.

The syndrome seems to be an abnormal immune response to recurrent malaria infections with excessive production of IgM. Raised titres of IgM and IgG malaria antibodies and sinusoidal lymphocytic infiltration of hepatic sinuses are also often found.

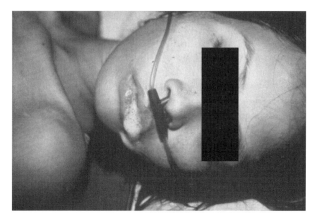

Fig. 20.16   Pulmonary oedema. (Copyright D. Warrell.)

Patients respond well both clinically and immunologically within 3 months of starting continuous antimalarial chemoprophylaxis (Fakunle 1981, Crane 1986).

6 IMMUNOLOGY

Susceptibility to malaria is restricted by a variety of genetic features of the host, generally referred to as 'natural immunity' or 'innate resistance'. When infection does occur, the host's immune system responds in a variety of ways, some of which may eventually lead to the clearance of parasites and protection against subsequent infection. In many circumstances the development of protective immunity is slow and this may be explained by both the extreme antigenic diversity of the parasite and the existence of efficient escape mechanisms.

6.1 Innate resistance

The relationship between malaria parasites and their host is a delicately balanced one, which may be affected by a variety of host and parasite features (Miller 1976). When different hosts are exposed to a given *Plasmodium*, their susceptibility may range from negligible to fatal. This is the case, for example, for *P. knowlesi* which produces a chronic but low-level infection in *Macaca fascicularis* (the natural host), a low-level and rapidly self-limiting infection in humans (accidental host) and a fulminant, fatal infection in *M. mulatta* (experimental host). The degree of susceptibility may vary with time, particularly after serial subinoculations of the parasite, and there may be 'adaptation' to an artificial host. For example, *P. knowlesi* was extensively used for malariotherapy of neurosyphilitic patients in Rumania and after a number of subinoculations the strain became so highly virulent to humans that it was unmanageable (Coatney et al. 1971).

Susceptibility to infection is primarily determined by the ability of the parasite to invade and survive in appropriate host cells (e.g. hepatocyte and erythrocyte in the mammalian host). With regard to human malaria parasites, specific receptors for hepatocyte invasion are still unknown and there is no evidence to suggest differential susceptibility or resistance in any particular human ethnic group or in association with any specific genetic characteristic of hepatocytes. The maturity of the hepatocyte is crucial, as fetal hepatocytes seem to be resistant to infection.

The susceptibility to erythrocytic infection may be determined at the level of merozoite invasion, intracellular growth or erythrocytic lysis at the time of merozoite release. *P. vivax* is restricted to reticulocytes and Duffy positive cells, whereas *P. falciparum* invasion may be substantially reduced in red cells with glycophorin abnormalities, e.g. the En(a-) or the S-s-U phenotypes (Pasvol and Wilson 1982).

Resistance to parasite entry is observed in cells with cytoskeleton abnormalities; ovalocytosis confers resistance to all malarial species whereas elliptocytosis, due to the absence of band 4.1, may hinder the entry of

P. falciparum (Nagel 1990). Intraerythrocytic development of *P. falciparum* is reduced or retarded in red cells presenting various haemoglobinopathies, including HbS, HbE, HbF, HbC, G6PD deficiency or β-thalassaemia. The reduced growth of *P. falciparum* in HbC/C cells has been attributed to an increased resistance to red cell lysis and to intracellular degenerescence, compatible with an incapacity of parasites to induce merozoite release. In some cases, reduced growth may be observed only in the initial cycle of development in abnormal cells, for instance, when *P. falciparum* is grown in G6PD deficient cells, in which the parasite can 'adapt' by switching on its own enzyme.

Resistance to infection may also be caused by the antiparasitic effect of components of the host serum. The serum of Sudanese adults living in endemic areas for malaria may cause intraerythrocytic death of *P. falciparum*; the toxic component of serum, named 'crisis forming factor', is independent of host immunity (Jensen et al. 1983). The nutritional status of the host is also crucial and children with severe forms of malnutrition, marasmus or kwashiorkor, are less likely to present with severe malaria.

Apart from innate resistance to infection, the degree of individual susceptibility to severe disease may also be variable; for instance, it has been estimated that *P. falciparum* leads to cerebral malaria in only a small percentage of cases in an endemic area (estimated at 1:200) and that only a percentage of those are fatal (Greenwood, Marsh and Snow 1991). In The Gambia, individuals heterozygous for the HLA-B53 haplotype have a significantly decreased susceptibility to severe falciparum disease (Hill et al. 1991) whereas individuals with the type-2 allele of the TNFα promoter gene are 7 times more likely to die of cerebral malaria (McGuire et al. 1994).

6.2 Immune effector mechanisms

ANTIBODIES

A rapid increase of immunoglobulin levels is observed in the course of malaria, but only a small percentage of these antibodies is directed against the parasite (5–10% of immunoglobulins produced) (Cohen and Butcher 1971); most of the characteristic hypergammaglobulinaemia observed during acute malaria may be attributed to polyclonal activation (Rosenberg 1978). The role of antibodies in protection has best been demonstrated by the passive transfer of serum from immune donors to infected recipients; the infection of neurosyphilitic patients with *P. vivax* (Sotiriades 1936) or the natural infection of Gambian children with *P. falciparum* (Cohen, McGregor and Carrington 1961) have both been completely cleared within 48 h of the transfer of immune serum. Similarly, in the new-born child of an immune mother, the passive transfer of IgG across the placenta protects the child during the early months of life (Edozien, Gilles and Udeozo 1962).

Individuals living in an area endemic for malaria have high levels of antibodies against many malarial antigens as demonstrated by the use of enzyme-linked immunosorbent assay (ELISA) or immunofluorescence antibody tests (IFAT) (Voller and O'Neill 1971, Ambroise-Thomas et al. 1976). These antibodies are generally directed against immunodominant epitopes of the parasite, but are not necessarily protective. Protective antibodies may either act directly on the parasite or parasitized cells, or act in synergy with various effector cells. Depending on the expected mode of action of the protective antibodies and the target stage in the life-cycle, various in vitro correlates for protection have been described including circumsporozoite precipitation (Spitalny, Rivera-Ortiz and Nussenzweig 1973), inhibition of merozoite reinvasion (Butcher, Mitchell and Cohen 1978), inhibition of merozoite dispersal from schizonts (Green et al. 1981), recognition of the ring-infected erythrocyte surface antigen (RESA) (Perlmann et al. 1984), recognition of the surface of infected erythrocytes (Hommel et al. 1991), inhibition or reversal of cytoadherence (Singh et al. 1988) or inhibition of rosette formation (Carlson et al. 1990). Each of these in vitro tests has a degree of correlation with protection but none is perfect; when a number of such tests were compared and related to clinical outcome in a study of Gambian children, it was shown that, although high antibody titres had a predictable age distribution, none of the individual tests had a significant correlation with protection (Marsh et al. 1989).

The activity of antibodies may be a consequence of opsonization, as suggested by the fact that the passive transfer of immune serum is more effective in intact than in splenectomized recipients (Brown and Phillips 1974). Although it has been convincingly demonstrated that immune phagocytosis is an important mechanism for the removal of dead parasites (Shear, Nussenzweig and Bianco 1979), the true role of opsonization in parasite killing and elimination remains unclear. In contrast to several other infectious diseases, the phenomenon in which some isotypes of immunoglobulins are more effective than others in mediating protection has not been reported in human malaria to date. The cytophilic nature of the antibodies may be more crucial than the isotype and there is evidence to support the view that co-operation between antibodies and macrophages is always required (which may explain the poor correlation between in vitro antibody assays and protection) (Bouharoun-Tayoun et al. 1990).

MACROPHAGES

The role of macrophages in malaria was recognized by early pathologists, who observed an increased number of macrophages in the spleen, liver and bone marrow of infected animals (Taliaferro and Cannon 1936). The increased number of macrophages in the spleen has been related to the release of T cell cytokines, which seems to trigger a major cellular influx, leading to splenomegaly (Wozencraft et al. 1984). During the parasitic 'crisis' (when parasitaemia starts to decrease under the influence of acquired immunity) there is a considerable increase in phago-

cytosis of malaria parasites, infected erythrocytes and malarial debris (particularly residual bodies and pigment). In rodent malaria, the phagocytic activity of splenic macrophages has been estimated to be 20– to 50–fold greater than that of normal macrophages (Zuckerman 1977). This increase in phagocytic activity has been linked both to a specific activation of macrophages and to humoral factors, particularly opsonizing antibodies, which act in synergy with macrophages to enhance the destruction of parasites. Despite this massive deployment of defence mechanisms against the parasite, the process is not very effective in eliminating the infection; it has been suggested that an impairment of macrophage functions occurs during malarial infection (Schwarzer et al. 1992), perhaps due to the suppressive effect of the malarial pigment ingested (Arese, Turini and Ginsburg 1991).

In addition to their phagocytic activity, macrophages and monocytes can produce a variety of toxic substances which may damage or destroy malaria parasites; the production of these toxic molecules is generally enhanced in activated macrophages. Effector functions of macrophages include the release of reactive oxygen intermediates (hydrogen peroxide and hydroxyl radicals) (Clark and Hunt 1983), the production of tumour necrosis factor (TNF) (Taverne, Bate and Playfair 1990) and the production at least 80 other cytokines and enzymes, some of which may adversely affect the parasite (e.g. polyamine oxidase which can kill *P. falciparum* in vitro) (Kumaratilake and Ferrante 1994). In addition to damaging parasites within erythrocytes (producing 'crisis forms'), the activated macrophage-derived toxic products may also damage the parasite in its exoerythrocytic cycle, either directly or by means of the production of nitrogen monoxide (nitric oxide, NO) (Green et al. 1990). The infectivity of gametocytes may also be reduced as a result of the presence of macrophage products (e.g. TNF) (Mendis et al. 1990).

T CELLS

It is well documented that T cells are crucial for malaria immunity (Weidanz and Long 1988, Ho and Webster 1989). As far as immunity to the erythrocytic stage of the parasite is concerned, the major functions of T cells seem to be to provide help for the production of antibodies and to activate macrophages. It is conceivable that during the early days of infection, the immune response is essentially of a Th-1 type, which may be sufficient to maintain the infection in check (avoiding the kind of fulminant, rapidly lethal infection that occurs in T-deficient mice) but not sufficient to eliminate parasites altogether. Later, the immune response may switch to an essentially Th-2 mode, antibody-mediated mechanisms playing a major role in the eventual elimination of parasites.

Neither cytotoxic CD4+ or CD8+ T cells (CTLs) nor antibody-dependent cellular cytotoxicity (ADCC) have been conclusively implicated in immunity to erythrocytic parasites. In contrast, the exoerythrocytic stages reside within hepatocytes, that bear the MHC Class I antigens required for CTL activity. In experimental models, CTLs from mice immunized with X-irradiated sporozoites can kill malaria parasites grown in vitro in mouse hepatocytes and seem to be involved in the destruction of exoerythrocytic parasites in the livers of immunized mice (Hoffman et al. 1989). C-reactive protein, interferon-γ, interleukin-1 (IL-1), IL-6, TNF and NO have all been incriminated in the killing of exoerythrocytic stages, probably in the form of a cascade of events triggered by T-cell recognition of sporozoite or liver stage antigens and involving both hepatocytes and Kupffer cells (Suhrbier 1991). There is now a reasonable body of evidence to implicate CTLs in protection against the exo-erythrocytic stages of malaria parasites in humans (Lalvani et al. 1994).

γδ T CELLS

The γδ T cell receptor is normally expressed in only a small percentage of peripheral lymphocytes and, although the number of γδ T cells may be increased in certain infections, the role of these cells in immunity is not well understood. A substantial increase in the number of γδ cells has been reported both in experimental mouse malaria (Langhorne, Pells and Eichmann 1993) and during the acute stage of *P. falciparum* and *P. vivax* infection in humans (Ho et al. 1994, Perera et al. 1994). In addition, the presence of high levels of activated γδ cells may contribute to the increased production of cytokines, particularly TNFα, and thus be involved in the pathophysiological events leading to the disease (Grau and Behr 1994).

ANTI-DISEASE IMMUNITY

Acquired immunity to malaria in humans is a mixture of 'anti-disease' immunity, which results in decreased clinical manifestations despite infection, and of 'anti-parasite' immunity, which results in control of the infection itself. The mechanisms of these 2 types of immunity are clearly distinct as anti-disease immunity usually occurs much earlier than anti-parasite immunity. Consequently an individual living in a highly endemic area of the world may harbour very heavy parasite loads and be clinically well (Miller 1958). Little is known of the mechanisms leading to anti-disease immunity but the most attractive hypothesis proposed to date is that host immunity interrupts a cascade of events, initially triggered by the production of a series of inflammatory cytokines (including TNFα) in response to malarial 'toxins' (Playfair et al. 1990). The lipidic nature of the immunogens involved is suggestive of T cell-independent mechanisms, which may explain why anti-disease (or 'anti-toxic') immunity is acquired only slowly and requires frequent boosting in order to be sustained. This reduced susceptibility to clinical malaria may be due to a form of non-sterile immunity described as 'premunition' by early malariologists (Sergent, Parrot and Donatien 1924), but never adequately elucidated.

6.3 Evasion of host immunity

Protective immunity against malaria parasites is slow to develop and it may be necessary for a child born in a malaria endemic zone to be exposed to successive infections for a number of years before developing any resistance; complete protection may never be achieved. This 'real-life' situation is in sharp contrast to that which is observed in experimental situations where solid, sterile immunity can be achieved. The apparent inefficiency of antimalarial immunity may be explained by the ability of the malaria parasite to evade host immunity, by the intrinsically poor immunogenicity of its antigens, by sequestration, by antigenic diversity and variation, or by an alteration of the host's immune response (Mercereau-Puijalon et al. 1991).

POOR IMMUNOGENICITY

Crucial antigens involved in protection may be poorly immunogenic either because of their intrinsic molecular structure, their analogy to host molecules, or because of immune restriction which may impair recognition. The presence of multiple repeat sequences on a number of highly immunogenic erythrocytic stage antigens (e.g. RESA, S-antigens or FIRA) has been interpreted as an evasion mechanism, as such immunodominant structures may act as a 'smoke screen' preventing the development of effective immunity to more relevant epitopes. The existence of cross-reactivity between repetitive epitopes of different malarial antigens (e.g. between RESA, FIRA, Pf11.1, Ag332 and an S-antigen) has been interpreted as a further cause of poor immunogenicity as the presence of these epitopes may interfere with the normal maturation of the immune response towards a progressively increasing percentage of high affinity antibodies (Anders 1986).

SEQUESTRATION

The ability of parasites to remain sequestered by cytoadherence to the capillary lining of certain tissues must be regarded as a selective advantage as such parasites can avoid frequent passage through the spleen and thus exposure to immune effector mechanisms. *P. falciparum* isolates are able to switch rapidly from one endothelial receptor to another (Ockenhouse et al. 1992) and this may be part of a parasite survival strategy, particularly as the change of receptor requirements may be in response to a changing environment of the host (acute malaria infection induces cytokine production which in turn upregulates certain endothelial cell surface antigens).

ALTERATION OF THE IMMUNE RESPONSE

Several reports demonstrate that malaria infection can induce a suppression of host immune responsiveness, including increased severity of *Salmonella* infections (Bennett and Hook 1959), decreased efficiency of tetanus vaccination (McGregor and Barr 1962) and the strong association between malaria and Burkitt's lymphoma (Marsh and Greenwood 1986). The paradox of malaria during pregnancy, when a previously immune woman becomes fully susceptible to severe malaria, may represent another facet of such immunosuppression (McGregor, Wilson and Billewicz 1983).

Various mechanisms of immunosuppression have been proposed, including polyclonal activation, macrophage dysfunction, abnormal antigenic presentation, disruption of lymphatic and splenic tissue architecture, activation of suppressor cells and antigenic competition. These mechanisms may affect not only the outcome of concurrent infections, but also the ability of the host to mount an effective immune response to the malaria parasite itself.

ANTIGENIC DIVERSITY

In addition to the marked species- and stage-specificity of immunity to malaria parasites, there are also marked differences between isolates of the same species. Studies of S-antigens confirm the concept that field isolates of *P. falciparum* may vary in their antigenic structure (Wilson, McGregor and Williams 1975), More specific methods of analysis (using isoenzymes, two-dimensional gel electrophoresis, monoclonal antibodies or RFLP polymorphism) have provided further evidence of considerable diversity of the phenotype and genotype of field isolates.

The extent of diversity varies from one antigen to another and several types of polymorphisms have been described. The differences between different alleles of a given gene represent a relatively restricted form of polymorphism; there are substantial differences in the primary sequence, but the number of alleles is limited for a given locus (e.g. alleles of MSP-1). In contrast, much more extensive polymorphism is generated by variation of the repeat domain (as described for molecules like S-antigens, Pf 11.1 or FIRA), where the presence of repeat degeneracies adds a further level of polymorphism (Stahl et al. 1987, Scherf et al. 1992). In addition to the diversity observed in highly polymorphic antigens, a degree of polymorphism may exist in limited domains of otherwise highly conserved molecules and this may be generated by point mutations. The antigens expressed on the surface of infected erythrocytes (e.g. PfEMP-1) seem to be particularly polymorphic (Howard 1987).

The considerable diversity between field isolates may be the major reason why a long time is required to develop immunity, as an individual living in an endemic area would need to be exposed to a vast repertoire of local strains (Day and Marsh 1991). However, before accepting that antigenic diversity is a likely explanation for the slow development of immunity, it is necessary to assume that strain-specific immunity can ultimately be transcended by a broader species-specific immunity; in the absence of such a transcending immunity, it would be difficult to understand why infections become rarer in adults, as adults continue to be exposed to new isolates. The constant fluctuation of isolates 'in circulation' in a given geographical area has best been demonstrated in a study of the distribution of S-antigens over time in villages of Papua New Guinea (Forsyth et al. 1989)

ANTIGENIC VARIATION

Malaria parasites, like many other micro-organisms, are capable of periodically changing the expression of their antigens; this provides the parasite with a powerful means for evading host immunity particularly when antigenic variation occurs in conditions in which a selective pressure is exerted. In all examples of antigenic variation, the common feature is the presence of successive peaks of infection in which each new peak is antigenically distinct from the previous one (the latter having been eliminated by host immunity) (Hommel 1985). Surface antigens, which are most exposed to immune pressure, are obviously most likely to exhibit antigenic variation.

In malaria, antigenic variation was first described in the *P. knowlesi* and rhesus monkey model (Brown and Brown 1965), but it has since been shown to exist also in *P. falciparum*, in *P. chabaudi* in mice and in *P. fragile* in monkeys. Considering that the demonstration of variation requires both the availability of a precise methodology for identifying individual parasite populations and an experimental design that actively selects for emerging variant populations, it is conceivable that the phenomenon might be more widespread. For instance, although antigenic variation has not yet been demonstrated for *P. malariae* or *P. vivax*, the long chronicity of the former and the presence of successive waves of recrudescence in the latter suggest the existence of either a fluctuating immunity or of antigenic variation.

Many studies on antigenic variation have concentrated on the molecules expressed on the surface of infected erythrocytes (e.g. PfEMP-1). In one study, a single isolate of *P. falciparum* was able to express at least 10 different variant surface antigens when subinoculated in squirrel monkeys; for reasons that remain unclear, the set of variant antigens observed was different in intact and splenectomized animals (Hommel et al. 1991). In *P. fragile* (in contrast to other malaria parasites), the expression of new variant antigens seemed to follow a predetermined sequence (Handunetti, Mendis and David 1987) suggesting that some variant populations may possess an inherently higher 'switch rate' and would therefore be more likely to be selected early. The rate of switching from one set of antigens to another is thought to be very fast. In an in vitro study of *P. falciparum*, 2% of parasites switched to a new antigen in every erythrocytic cycle (Roberts et al. 1992). Antigenic variation of *P. falciparum* has been linked to a large gene family (the *var* genes), which seem to be differentially expressed in different individual parasites (Smith et al. 1995, Su et al. 1995); it has been calculated that the genome of a given clone of malaria parasites has 50–150 different *var* genes (i.e., approximately 6% of the total genome) and that *var* genes are scattered over most of the malarial chromosomes. It has also been suggested that only one *var* gene may be expressed at a time in a given parasite.

Besides PfEMP-1, other malarial antigens may have the ability to switch to alternative gene expression, particularly when submitted to a strong selective pressure. The 140 kDa antigen expressed on the surface of merozoites of *P. knowlesi* seems to be highly conserved in all isolates tested, but when a clone of *P. knowlesi* was injected into an animal previously immunized with the 140 kDa antigen, a breakthrough population exhibited a novel merozoite surface antigen unrelated to 140 kDa (David et al. 1985).

6.4   Important malarial antigens

Knowledge of the antigenic structure of malaria parasites has been derived mainly from studies aimed at identifying protective antigens with a view to the development of an antimalarial vaccine. In addition, it has long been known, mainly from observations made in neurosyphilitic patients treated by malariotherapy (Jeffery 1966), that there is no cross-protection between different species of human parasites, or between different stages of the life-cycle of a given parasite. Table 20.3 lists the *P. falciparum* antigens that have been considered important in antimalarial immunity, because they are expressed on the surface of extracellular infective forms, on the surface of malaria infected cells or because their recognition by patients' antibodies seems to be consistent with the development of protective immunity. In many cases, these *P. falciparum* molecules are representative of a family of antigens and similar, if not always biochemically identical, antigens may be found in all malarial species. The reader may refer to other reviews for a fuller description of these molecules (Phillips 1994, Coppel 1995).

7   PATHOLOGY

Infection by malarial parasites may lead to a variety of clinical syndromes, depending on a combination of different elements, including the 'virulence' of the parasite isolate and a variety of host-related factors, such as the status of host immunity and genetic make-up. The development of asexual parasites in the blood plays the central role in disease pathophysiology and, for most malarial species, it is the rupture of the schizont which triggers off the major events leading to the characteristic symptoms of the malarial paroxysm.

7.1   Direct effects of the parasite on the host

The rupture of the mature schizont has 3 consequences: (1) the liberation of merozoites, which leads to further invasion and a sharp increase in parasitaemia; (2) the destruction of infected erythrocytes; and (3) the liberation of malarial antigens, pigment and malarial toxins.

Although erythrocyte destruction may contribute to the anaemia observed in malaria, this is only of importance in chronic infections of semi-immune individuals in whom high parasitaemias (e.g. 5–15%) are relatively well tolerated. In non-immune individuals, the malarial paroxysms occur at very low parasitaemia (less than 1%) and the effects of massive erythrocyte destruction are negligible at this stage. In contrast, it is the release of malarial antigens, pigment and toxins

which is responsible for most of the pathology. Most of these effects are indirect, occurring via a cascade of pathological events in the host (see section 7.2). Nevertheless, 2 of the parasite products released have direct pathological effects: (1) malarial pigment, which is taken up by monocytes and inhibits some of the phagocytic and immunological functions of these cells and thus contributes to the immunosuppression observed (particularly as pigment remains in the reticuloendothelial system for many years after infection) (Arese, Turini and Ginsburg 1991); (2) some malarial lipid antigens may be responsible for the induction of hypoglycaemia by acting directly on glucose uptake by adipocytes in synergy with insulin (Taylor et al. 1992).

7.2   Indirect effects of the parasite on the host

These effects are by far the most important and the production of cytokines, particularly tumour necrosis factor (TNFα), induced by the release of parasite products during schizont rupture, seems to play the central role in the pathophysiology of most of the symptoms of malaria.

TUMOUR NECROSIS FACTOR

Several lines of evidence support the hypothesis that TNFα plays a central role: the experimental injection of TNFα in humans produces symptoms and signs that closely resemble a malarial paroxysm (Clark, Cowden and Chaudri 1989); the rise in temperature during *P. vivax* paroxysms closely follows the rise in circulating levels of TNFα (Karunaweera et al. 1992); the levels of TNFα are higher in severe than in mild forms of falciparum malaria and are particularly high in fatal cases (Grau et al. 1989); the injection of anti-TNFα monoclonal antibodies into children with severe malaria abolishes some of the symptoms, particularly fever (Kwiatkowski et al. 1993); and there are many similarities between severe malaria and sepsis, and TNFα and phospholipase-A2 are substantially increased in both (Vadas et al. 1993).

The multifaceted effects of TNFα are illustrated in Fig. 20.17.

At physiological levels, TNFα may destroy intracellular parasites or reduce the infectivity of gametocytes to mosquitoes (Mendis et al. 1990). At increased levels, TNFα induces fever, depresses erythropoeisis and increases erythrophagocytosis, thus contributing to anaemia (Weatherall 1988, Means 1994) and directly causes many of the non-specific symptoms of malaria (nausea, vomiting, diarrhoea, etc.).

Although the circulating levels of other 'endogenous pyrogens', such as IL-1 and IL-6, are also increased during malaria (Kern et al. 1989), they seem to play only a modest pathophysiological role in severe malaria, probably in synergy with TNFα, as suggested by Rockett et al. (1994). IL-6 may play a role in the induction of hyper-gammaglobulinaemia and contribute to some of the complications of malaria (e.g. glomerulonephritis and increased frequency of Burkitt's lymphoma) (Grau et al. 1990).

Table 20.3 Important antigens of *Plasmodium falciparum*

Antigen	Full name and alternative	Location
Intra-erythrocytic stages		
hsp70-1	heat shock protein-1, p75	parasite cytoplasm
hsp70-2	heat shock protein-2, Pfgrp	parasite cytoplasm
aldolase	aldolase	parasite cytoplasm
ARP	asparagine-rich protein	parasite cytoplasm
CARP	clustered asparagine-rich protein	parasite cytoplasm
RESA	ring-infected erythrocyte surface antigen, Pf155	RBC internal surface, merozoite dense granule
MESA	mature erythrocyte-parasite infected surface antigen-2, PfEMP-2	RBC internal surface
HRP-1	histidine-rich protein-1, KAHRP, KP	RBC internal surface
HRP-2	histidine-rich protein-2	RBC internal surface and secreted
HRP-3	histidine-rich protein-3, SHARP	parasite cytoplasm
Ag332	Ag332	RBC internal surface
41-2	41-2	RBC internal surface
GBP	glycophorin-binding protein, Pf120,	RBC cytoplasm
FIRA	Falciparum interspersed repeat antigen	RBC cytoplasm
S-antigen	S-antigen	parasitophorous vacuole
SERA	serine-rich antigen, SERP, p113, p126, Pf140	parasitophorous vacuole
GLURP	glutamate-rich protein	parasitophorous vacuole
ABRA	acidic basic repeat antigen, p101	parasitophorous vacuole
ORA	octapeptide repeat antigen	parasitophorous vacuole
PfEMP-1	erythrocyte membrane-associated malaria protein-1	RBC external surface
Merozoite		
MSP-1	merozoite surface antigen-1, MSA-1, PMMSA, P190, gp185	merozoite surface, surface of schizont
MSP-2	merozoite surface antigen-2, MSA-2, gp56, QF122, GYMMSA	merozoite surface
MSP-3	merozoite surface antigen-3, SPAM	merozoite surface, parasitophorous vacuole
AMA-1	apical membrane antigen-1, Pf83	apical region, merozoite surface
EBA-175	erythrocyte-binding antigen, SABP	micronemes, merozoite surface
RAP-1	rhoptry-associated protein-1	rhoptries
RAP-2	rhoptry-associated protein-2, pf41	rhoptries
RhopH3	RhopH3	rhoptries
Ag512	Ag512	rhoptries
Sporozoite and pre-erythrocytic stages		
CSP-1	circumsporozoite protein, CSP	sporozoite surface, infected hepatocyte
SSP-2	sporozoite surface protein-2	sporozoite surface
LSA-1	liver-specific antigen-1	infected hepatocyte
LSA-2	liver-specific antigen-2	infected hepatocyte
LSA-3	liver-specific antigen-3	infected hepatocyte
STARP	sporozoite threonine and asparagine-rich protein	sporozoite surface, infected hepatocyte
Sexual stages		
Pfs230	Pfs230	gametocytes, surface gametes
Pfs45/48	Pfs45/48	gametocytes, surface gametes
Pfs25	Pfs25	surface öokinete
Pfs16	Pfs16	gametes and sporozoite
11.1	11.1	parasite cytoplasm

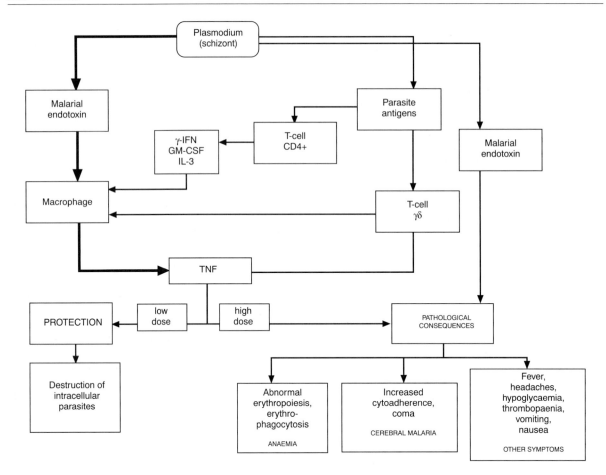

Fig. 20.17   Role of TNF in the pathophysiology of malaria.

INDUCTION OF CYTOKINE PRODUCTION

The induction of inflammatory cytokines is determined by 2 independent pathways: 1) the direct action of malarial toxins on host macrophages and Tγδ cells and 2) the immune response against malarial antigens and the production of Th1 cytokines (particularly IFN-γ), which upregulate the production of inflammatory cytokines and act in synergy with them (Clark and Rockett 1994).

The nature of malarial toxins is still controversial, e.g. whether toxicity is due to haemozoin (Sherry et al. 1995), a proteolipid (Bate and Kwiatkowski 1994) or a glycosylphosphatidylinositol (GPI) (Schofield et al. 1993). Nevertheless, most authors agree that the toxin is released at the time of schizont rupture, that it is at least partly lipidic in nature and that it is probably associated with the pigment-containing 'residual body'. Such a toxin can induce TNFα production by host cells in vitro and this production may be blocked by anti-toxic antibodies, which, notably, are not malaria-species-specific (Bate et al. 1992). Different isolates of *P. falciparum* vary considerably in their ability to induce TNFα and this may be one explanation for the observed differences in clinical responses (Allan, Rowe and Kwiatkowski 1993).

UPREGULATION OF CYTOADHERENCE RECEPTORS

One of the major features of cerebral malaria is cytoadherence of infected erythrocytes in capillaries of the brain (McPherson et al. 1985). Different isolates of *P. falciparum* are more or less cytoadherent to a variety of receptor molecules, including CD36, ICAM-1, thrombospondin, E-selectin, VCAM-1 and chondroitin sulphate (see reviews by Hommel 1993, Roberts et al. 1993). These differences in cytoadherence characteristics may represent a virulence factor and there is some evidence of a correlation between high cytoadherence or rosetting and cerebral malaria (Carlson et al. 1990, Ho et al. 1991). One of the effects of inflammatory cytokines in malaria is to upregulate the expression of certain cytoadherence receptors (e.g. ICAM-1 or VCAM-1) and to focus sequestration to certain tissues; cerebral malaria occurs when this increased cytoadherence takes place preferentially in the brain. Receptor upregulation may also require a Th1 immune response (particularly γIFN) (Grau and Behr 1994) and the development of cerebral complications may be avoided by the injection of Th2 mediators, such as IL-10 (Ho et al. 1995).

The cascade of events leading to cerebral malaria

or severe anaemia is a complex one, particularly as it is influenced both by parasite and by host factors (including host immunity and genetic 'susceptibility' factors). Fig. 20.18 shows the sequence of events leading to cerebral malaria, taking into account the 2 most relevant features of the parasite (i.e. ability to cytoadhere and ability of parasite toxins to induce inflammatory cytokines) as well as the various points in the cascade where host factors may intervene.

Further details on the pathogenesis of malaria may be found in one of the many excellent reviews of the subject (White 1992, Miller, Good and Milon 1994, Pasvol et al. 1995). Parasitization is greatest in the following organs (in descending order) : brain, heart, liver, lung kidney and blood.

The histopathological changes of falciparum malaria have been described in detail on previously (Edington 1967, Edington and Gilles 1976, Lucas 1992, Frances and Warrell 1993).

7.3 Immunopathology

The fact that the host's immune system seems to have considerable difficulties in controlling the malarial infection is probably the reason why so many aberrant responses have been described. Aberrant responses are generally caused by an over-reaction in a host whose immunologically inappropriate response has no

effect on the parasite, but which may have immuno-pathological consequences of various degrees of severity. Table 20.4 gives a list of immunopathological complications of malaria, some of which have already been briefly described (see section 6.2, page 378); detailed descriptions of these complications may be found in reviews by Marsh and Greenwood (1986) and by Ho and Sexton (1995).

8 DIAGNOSIS

The diagnosis of malaria can be conveniently subdivided into clinical, parasitological, biochemical, serological and molecular biological detection.

8.1 Clinical diagnosis

The most important factor in the clinical diagnosis of malaria is a high index of suspicion (Doherty, Grant and Bryceson 1995). A history of travel is mandatory in these days of widespread geographical movement, and should be elicited in all patients, particularly febrile ones. In this context, it is also important to remember that population movements are common within countries where malaria is not uniformly endemic.

Malaria can mimic many diseases and the differen-

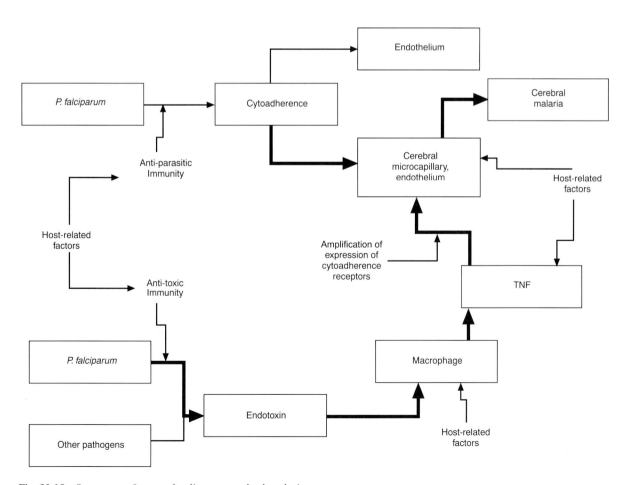

Fig. 20.18 Sequence of events leading to cerebral malaria.

Table 20.4 Immunopathology of malaria

Pathology	Possible mechanisms
Hypergammaglobulinaemia	Antigen induced cytokine production (IL-6)
	Antigenic variation
	Polyclonal activation
Immunosuppression	Antigenic competition
	Structural disruption of germinal centres
	Disruption of spleen function
	Macrophage dysfunction
	Polyclonal activation and immune "exhaustion"
Nephrotic syndrome	Immune complex deposition
	Autoimmunity
Autoimmunity	Auto-antibodies
	Anti-nuclear antibodies
Anaemia	Anti-erythrocyte antibodies
	Dyserythropoiesis (e.g. effect of TNF)
	Excessive erythrophagocytosis
Thrombocytopaenia	Excessive removal of platelets
	Coating of platelets with malaria antigen
Hyperreactive malarial splenomegaly	Genetic predisposition
	Hypergammaglobulinaemia
	Chronic increase of lymphocyte proliferation
Burkitt's Lymphoma	Co-endemicity with Epstein-Barr virus
	Polyclonal activation
	Antigen induced cytokine production

tial diagnosis is an extensive one. The golden rule is always to exclude malaria, irrespective of the clinical presentation, if a history of exposure is elicited. The commonest misdiagnoses in non-immune individuals are influenza, viral hepatitis, viral encephalitis, meningitis, psychosis and viral haemorrhagic fever.

Clinical diagnosis can be further guided by epidemiological considerations, e.g. acute febrile illness in high risk groups, such as pregnant women or children under 5 years of age in holoendemic areas. Also, association with particular locations such as forest or forest fringe areas may be strongly correlated with malaria infection and may serve as a pointer to diagnosis.

The discovery of parasitaemia provides an explanation for symptoms and signs in a non-immune patient, but this is not necessarily the case in semi-immune individuals in whom parasitaemia may be incidental. In these patients, the diagnosis is more difficult and no 'gold standard' exists. A reasonable set of guidelines is as follows: (1) a clinical illness compatible with malaria including objective evidence of fever; (2) exclusion of any other likely cause of fever following physical examination; (3) malaria parasitaemia above $10\,000\ \mu l^{-1}$; and (4) appropriate response to treatment.

8.2 Parasitological methods

Despite the wide range of serological, immunological and molecular techniques currently available, the only certain means of diagnosing all 4 species of human malaria parasite is the detection of the *Plasmodium* spp. by microscopic examination of the blood (Fig. 20.19).

Both thick and thin blood films should be prepared. The thick film method, which concentrates layers of red blood cells on a small surface by a factor of 20–30, is the most sensitive and considerably the most superior for clinical use. The thin film is useful for species identification in cases of doubt. Technical details for preparation and microscopic examination of blood films are outside the scope of this chapter and can readily be found elsewhere (Shute 1988, WHO 1988). Giemsa is the most commonly used of the Romanowsky stains and is the best for routine diagnosis because of its applicability to both thick and thin smears, its stability on storage and its constant and reproducible staining quality over a wide range of temperatures. Clear, good

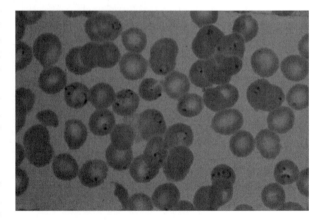

Fig. 20.19 Blood film of *P. falciparum* infected blood showing the presence of ring stage parasites.

quality glass slides are essential. In the absence of a positive blood film, a thrombocytopenia (platelet count $<150\,000\ \mu l^{-1}$) is strongly suggestive of malaria. Diagnostic characteristics of human malaria parasites, as seen in a well stained thick or thin film, are given in Table 20.5.

The main problem with microscopic diagnosis is that it is time-consuming and must be performed by skilled microscopists. Various methods have been designed to enhance the examination of blood films in order to reduce the time spent reading the slides or to enable less trained personnel to achieve equally reliable results. The staining of films with acridine orange, which can be read either on a fluorescence microscope or a microscope equipped with an interference filter system (Kawamoto 1991), allows quicker screening of films, because parasites are more readily recognized and a lower power lens may be used. The quantitative buffy coat (QBC®) method is also based on acridine-orange staining, but in this case the blood is centrifuged in a specially designed and patented micro-capillary tube fitted with a plastic float. The float spreads the buffy coat against the edge of the tube; parasites and leucocytes take up the dye, which is fluorescent when examined under ultraviolet light (Fig. 20.20).

This elegant method is easy to perform, fast and easy to read, but requires specialized equipment (a microcentrifuge and a fluorescence microscope) and the purchase of expensive QBC capillary tubes (Spielman and Perrone 1989, Petersen and Marbiah 1994). The sensitivity of QBC, when used in field conditions, is comparable to, or marginally better, than that of thick films. Both acridine orange staining

Table 20.5 Differential diagnosis of human *Plasmodium* species in stained thin blood films

	P. falciparum	*P. malariae*	*P. vivax*	*P. ovale*
Appearance of infected red blood cells (size and shape)	Both normal	Normal shape; size normal or smaller	$1\frac{1}{2}$ to 2 times larger than normal; shape normal or oval	As for *P. vivax*, but some have irregular frayed edges
Schüffner's dots (eosinophilic stippling)	None (but presence of occasional comma-like red Maurer's dots)	None	Present in all stages, except early ring form	As for *P. vivax*
Red cells with multiple parasites per cell	Common	Rare	Occasional	As for *P. vivax*
Stages present in peripheral blood	Rings and gametocytes Schizonts rarely seen	All stages	All stages	All stages
Ring form (young trophozoite)	Delicate, small ring; scanty cytoplasm; sometimes at edge of cell ("accolé" form)	Ring $\frac{1}{3}$ diameter of cell; heavy chromatin dots; vacuole sometimes "filled in"	Ring $\frac{1}{3}$ to $\frac{1}{2}$ diameter of red cell; heavy chromatin dots	As for *P. vivax*
Schizont	Rarely seen in peripheral blood; 16–18 merozoites	6–12 merozoites in rosette; coarse pigment clump in centre	12–24 merozoites in rosette filling the entire RBC; central pigment	8–12 merozoites in rosette
Gametocyte	"Crescent" shape characteristic	Round or oval; coarse pigment	Round or oval	Round or oval (smaller than *P. vivax*)
Main criteria	Only rings and crescent shaped gametocytes in blood; multiple infection; level of infection high; normal RBC shape; no Schüffner dots	All stages in blood; trophozoites compact and intensily stained; band forms suggestive; coarse pigment; normal/small RBC; no Schüffner dots	Large pale RBC; presence of Schüffner dots; round gametocytes; large amoeboid trophozoite with pale pigment	Generally like *P. vivax*, oval RBC with fimbriated edges characteristic but not always present

Fig. 20.20 Quantitative buffy coat (QBC). Blood infected with *P. falciparum* as seen in QBC capillary tubes. The large fluorescent cells are white blood cells, the small fluorescent dots in the dark area are ring-stage parasites within non-fluorescing erythrocytes. (Courtesy of Beckton-Dickinson Tropical Disease Diagnostics, USA).

techniques are inferior to Romanowsky staining for the precise identification of malaria species or their accurate enumeration. In situations in which it is necessary to identify parasite species with precision, the use of blood films stained by immunocytochemical methods using species monoclonal antibodies may be envisaged (Lindergard 1995, Perez et al. 1995).

Despite its shortcomings, microscopy has qualitative and quantitative features that are not associated with most other techniques. For example, when carefully examined by an experienced microscopist, a thin film with *P. falciparum* can provide clues regarding the degree of disease severity, which include not only the high level of parasitaemia but also the presence of more 'mature' ring-stage parasites (linked to the existence of a greater sequestered biomass of parasites) (Silamut and White 1993) or the presence of an unusually high number of circulating schizonts. In addition to the observation of the parasites themselves, the overall examination of a blood film may provide other clues. It has been reported, in a study performed in Vietnam, that the presence of visible malarial pigment in neutrophils or monocytes may be used as a criterion of poor prognosis (a fatal outcome was associated with pigment in more than 5% neutrophils) (Nguyen Hoan Phu et al. 1995). One must, however, be careful not to over-interpret such observations, as pigmented monocytes are not uncommon in asymptomatic African children.

8.3 Immunological methods

Instead of identifying the parasite itself, immunological methods provide the means for detecting either the parasite antigens or the host antibodies directed against the parasite. The detection of antigens may be an acceptable alternative to parasite detection, particularly if the assay is robust, inexpensive, easy to use in field conditions and does not require a microscope, but the detection of antibodies merely provides information on past malaria experience and is of limited use for individual diagnosis.

SEROLOGY

Serological methods have been used since the early 1960s, when indirect fluorescent antibody tests (IFAT) and indirect haemagglutination assays (IHA) were described. Because such tests detect antimalarial antibodies, they cannot distinguish between current or past infection and they are therefore of limited value as a guide to the treatment or management of the disease. At best, a negative serological assay may help to eliminate the possibility of malaria, as antibody levels become detectable a few days after the blood is invaded. Detailed description of the various methods may be found elsewhere (Voller 1988, Gilles 1993).

IFAT is the main method for routine serodiagnosis, because it is relatively easy to make antigen slides for all human malarial parasites (commercial IFAT slides for malaria are also available from various sources) (Fig. 20.21).

The disadvantages of the method are the requirement for a fluorescence microscope, the subjectivity of the reading and the fact that the method is relatively labour-intensive, which limits its application to specialized centres with a relatively small through-put of samples.

ELISA uses a soluble malarial antigen (generally prepared from asexual stages of *P. falciparum*, which can be readily grown in vitro) (Trager and Jensen 1976), coated on the wells of a microtitre plate; this enables a large number of samples to be processed at the same time and produces quantitative results, when the assay is read on a spectrophotometer (portable, battery-operated ELISA readers are available for field use). In addition to crude extracts of malarial antigens, ELISA has been applied to a variety of defined, synthetic or recombinant malarial antigens (e.g. MSP-1, RESA or CSP) (Zavala, Tam and Masuda 1986, Del Giudice et al. 1987, Riley et al. 1992); such studies have been useful for elucidating the role of target malarial antigen in immunity and protection.

A variety of other serological test formats have been explored, including radioimmunoassays, latex agglutination, indirect haemagglutination, solid-phase dipstick and membrane dot-blot, which may have specific advantages in given situations.

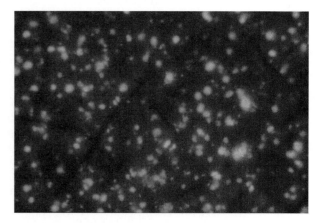

Fig. 20.21 Positive immunofluorescent antibody test with malarial antigen. (Courtesy of Dr W. Bailey, Liverpool School of Tropical Medicine).

Antigen detection

In contrast to serology, a positive antigen detection assay should detect a current infection. The ideal target antigen should not persist after parasitaemia disappears, should be abundant in the blood (or other bodily fluids, such as urine) to maximize sensitivity and should be malaria specific without cross-reactions with other micro-organisms. If the assay is intended to be useful in field conditions (e.g. to replace microscopy at the primary care level), it should also be robust, inexpensive, easy to perform and to interpret; in addition, it would be useful if the assay was to some extent quantitative, given that a qualitative assay is always more difficult to interpret. Such an assay does not yet exist, but a number of assays have been described which possess at least some of these features.

Experimental tests for detecting malarial antigens are based on either an antigen-capture or an antigen-competition format and often use ELISA or the radioimmunoassay (RIA) methodology. Once optimal reagents have been identified (i.e. monoclonal or polyclonal antibodies to specific malarial antigens), the assay may be simplified using a simple agglutination or dipstick method. The best antigen detection assays described have a maximum sensitivity of 0.01–0.001% parasitaemia and are 5–10 times inferior to good quality microscopy (Mackey et al. 1982, Fortier et al. 1987, Khusmith et al. 1987, Taylor and Voller 1993).

ParaSight™-F (Shiff, Premij and Minjas 1993) is a commercial detection test in dipstick format (Fig. 20.22), in which a monoclonal antibody captures a specific antigen of *P. falciparum* (PfHRP-2, a molecule present in the parasite throughout the erythrocytic cycle); if antigen is present, a positive result is indicated by a second anti-HRP2 antibody labelled with a coloured marker, which produces a visible line on the dipstick.

The whole test takes only 10 min and gives a sensitivity almost comparable to that of thick films. This simple, robust assay requires no additional equipment and can be taught to village health workers, as reading

of the result is a straightforward positive or negative assessment (Premij, Minjas and Shiff 1994). The high cost of the assay, and the fact that it is not quantitative in its current form, are serious limitations to its use in the very field situations for which it was designed.

The detection of parasite lactate dehydrogenase (pLDH), originally developed as a way to monitor in vitro drug susceptibility assays (Makler and Hinrichs 1993) has the potential of being useful for the detection of *Plasmodium* parasitaemia (Knobloch and Henk 1995). The principle of the assay is that pLDH has different biochemical characteristics from human LDH and may therefore be differentially measured using a simple colorimetric assay. Such assays are not species specific, can detect a parasitaemia as low as 0.1% (a level of parasitaemia just below the threshold of 10 000 parasites μl^{-1} and thus potentially useful as a marker for clinical malaria in endemic areas) and can be used as a quantitative assay above that threshold. The assay is currently being improved, by combining it with an antigen capture method using a monoclonal antibody to pLDH; this improves sensitivity 100 times (Piper et al. 1995).

8.4 Molecular methods

The application of DNA or RNA hybridization to malaria diagnosis has several advantages over traditional methods. Although the methodology is never likely to be useful at the peripheral level of health care in its present form, it may have a place as a research tool to monitor malaria control programmes, to perform quality control checks on microscopic diagnoses or to determine the distribution of important genes (e.g. genes associated with drug resistance).

The presence of parasites in the blood means that there is parasite DNA and RNA present and various methods based on the principle of nucleic acid hybridization have been developed in order to detect these molecules. In these methods, a known sequence of nucleic acid (oligonucleotide) is synthesized and labelled either with radioactive ^{32}P or a non-radioactive colorimetric reagent and this 'probe' is used to detect parasite nucleic acid, taking advantage of the fact that complementary sequences will hybridize. The simplest version of this technique is the use of DNA probes to detect parasites directly in a drop of patient's blood immobilized on a filter paper (Franzen et al. 1984); in this test format, the sensitivity and specificity of the technique depends largely upon the choice of nucleic acid sequence. In order to achieve a higher degree of sensitivity, most of the first generation DNA probes were directed towards repetitive sequences of parasite genes; the *rep20* subtelomeric repeat of *P. falciparum* was considered to be of particular interest because of its specificity for *P. falciparum*. Since the availability of amplification methods, such as the polymerase chain reaction (PCR), in which the number of copies of any target sequence may be increased many times, the sensitivity of nucleic acid probes has exponentially increased. This has made it possible to use probes against non-repetitive sequences, for example, to examine the association of *Pfmdr* genes with chloroquine resistance (Foote et al. 1989, Wellems et al. 1990) or to use species specific small subunit ribosomal RNA sequences to differen-

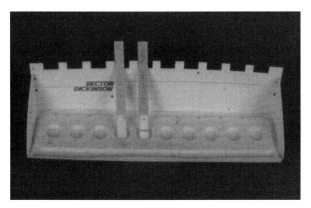

Fig. 20.22 Positive and negative malarial antigenaemia using the ParaSight F dipstick. (Courtesy of Dr W Bailey, Liverpool School of Tropical Medicine).

tiate between *P. falciparum*, *P. vivax*, *P. ovale* or *P. malariae* (Snounou et al. 1993) (Fig. 20.23).

The gain in sensitivity of PCR over the original dot DNA probes has been accompanied by an increased technical complexity, including the need for PCR equipment to perform automatically the thermal recycling used for amplification and the need to separate the amplified material by agarose gel electrophoresis. In addition, the risk of sample contamination is an intrinsic problem with any form of amplification and scrupulous care must be taken when handling samples, in order to avoid this problem. Many technical refinements of the PCR method have been described, some of which have been applied to malaria diagnosis (e.g., methods for the detection of immobilized amplified nucleic acid, or liquid phase hybridization, which provide a test format akin to ELISA methods) (Oliveira et al. 1995). Various ways have also been described to make the PCR technique more user-friendly under field conditions by reducing the manipulation of the samples and the likely contamination of specimens (e.g. by collection of blood on filter paper) (Long et al. 1995).

It has been claimed that PCR is capable of detecting parasitaemia of less than 0.00002% when used in the best possible conditions and is theoretically capable of detecting the presence of a single parasite in the sample, although this is rarely achieved, partly because the blood contains poorly defined products which may inhibit the PCR reaction. The detection of a parasitaemia of 0.00002%, which corresponds to one parasite per mm^3 or 5 parasites per 5 µl sample of blood, is a detection threshold at least 5 times lower than the detection threshold achieved by means of a thick film performed in optimal conditions (i.e. 0.0001%), (assuming that a competent microscopist has spent at least 10 min examining 100 fields of an adequately stained thick film, i.e. a 0.2 µl fraction of a 5–10 µl drop of blood). A sensitivity of 1 parasite per 20 µl of blood, as reported by Tirasophon and colleagues (1991) would, therefore, correspond to a sensitivity 100 times better than a thick film. In reality, the sensitivity of PCR is rarely as good, particularly when performed in field conditions and may be considered comparable or only marginally better than that of the microscopic examination of a thick film (Laserson et al. 1994). In contrast, the specificity of PCR is generally considered to be better than microscopy.

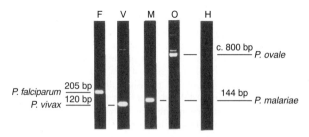

Fig. 20.23 Polymerase chain reaction (PCR) detection of human *Plasmodium* species. (Courtesy of Dr G Snounou, Imperial College School of Medicine, London). Genomic DNA samples purified from the four human malaria parasites were separately subjected to nested PCR analysis (as described by Snounou et al., 1993) and PCR products were resolved by electrophoresis on a 2% agarose gel and visualized under UV light after ethidium bromide staining. A characteristic DNA band is observed for each of the malaria species; no species PCR products are observed when oligonucleotide primers specific to one parasite species are used with DNA templates from any of the other three malaria species, or from uninfected human blood.

8.5   Appraisal of the relative value of diagnostic methods

Whatever the method used, a diagnostic test should be able to differentiate correctly between individuals who are infected and those who are not; consequently, the validity of a test is usually determined by its sensitivity (i.e. the test with the highest sensitivity has the lowest number of false negatives) and its specificity (i.e. the test with the highest specificity has the lowest number of false positives). In reality, it is generally more important to know the ability of a positive assay to predict the probability of infection, i.e. its positive predictive value.

INDIVIDUAL DIAGNOSIS

In most situations, the 'gold standard' for individual diagnosis is the microscopic examination of thick and thin films. There are, however, situations in which this may not apply.

In areas of high endemicity, clinical diagnosis alone is usually the only feasible and cost effective method for recommending the first line of treatment, i.e. chloroquine, or Fansidar or Mefloquine. In a country where the annual budget for health per individual is US $2, it is difficult to justify diagnostic assays costing US $1 or more, if the full treatment dose of Fansidar is only US $0.04 (Foster 1991); even if this first line treatment was given inappropriately in 75% of cases, this would still mean that 6 patients were treated appropriately for the cost of one diagnostic test. Unfortunately, modern diagnostic assays are all likely to cost over US $1 and the use of less costly microscopy requires a health care infrastructure and expertise which often does not exist (Payne 1988). When microscopy is not available a variety of clinical features may be used as predictive markers of disease (Genton et al. 1994).

The optimal use of methods like QBC, PCR or Para-Sight is in sophisticated laboratories in developed countries that can afford the cost of the assays and that have expertise in complex technologies but that have been unable to maintain competency in malaria microscopy. Paradoxically in these situations, because of the need for a quantitative evaluation of the level of parasitaemia as a means to monitor treatment efficacy, it may be necessary to perform a microscopic examination of blood films as a second-line test in a specialized centre.

When microscopy is used in areas of high endemicity, it is usually necessary to redefine the critical threshold for each situation, i.e. a level above which parasitaemia may have a clinical significance. A parasitaemia above 5000–10 000 parasites µl^{-1} is usually suggested as a guideline, but precise counting may not always be feasible; Coosemans and colleagues have proposed the sensible 'rule of thumb' that a 100% field positivity on a thick film may be used as a good morbidity indicator (1994).

EPIDEMIOLOGICAL SURVEILLANCE

Active or passive surveillance of malaria prevalence is an important tool for malaria control, particularly when the efficacy of control measures is being evaluated. Microscopy and, by extension, antigen detection or PCR, have serious limitations for such an evaluation, because these techniques only measure a 'point prevalence' of the infection at the time of the survey (particularly unhelpful in situations in which malaria transmission is seasonal). In contrast, seroepidemiology may help to delineate those areas where there is malaria transmission, may provide information on species-prevalence or age-related prevalence and may also chart the changes that are taking place as a result of the control intervention.

Another issue in diagnosis for epidemiological purposes is the follow-up of the distribution in a community of isolates with specific features (e.g. antigens of interest, in the context of a vaccination programme or drug resistance markers, for the definition of treatment policies). PCR, the specificity of which can be changed at will by changing the primer sequences used, is ideally suited for this purpose and is increasingly being used for isolate-specific surveys (Contamin et al. 1995).

TRANSFUSION MALARIA

The transmission of malaria by blood transfusion is a serious risk, as the diagnosis of malaria in the recipient is unexpected, and thus is often missed. Microscopic examination of donor blood is highly unsatisfactory as most donor infections are at a sub-microscopic level. Outside endemic areas, the policy of screening the donor's history for known episodes of clinical malaria or for tropical travel in the past 5 years is generally sufficient. In view of the increasing frequency of tropical travel in the general population, the policy in some countries is to reject only donors whose malaria serology is positive (generally using IFAT with homologous antigens for *P. falciparum*, *P. vivax* and *P. malariae* for maximum assay sensitivity). This screening method is not perfect, but a negative serology gives a high probability of freedom from infection. The use of PCR (which has been explored by the Blood Transfusion Centre of Ho Chi Minh City in Vietnam) is not, despite its much increased sensitivity, a complete guarantee of safe blood, because the absence of parasites in a 20 µl sample does not exclude the possibility of infection in the remaining volume of the 450 ml blood unit (Vu thi Ty Hang et al. 1995). In endemic areas, the only safe prevention of transfusion malaria is appropriate preventive antimalarial therapy of the recipient.

9 EPIDEMIOLOGY AND CONTROL

9.1 Introduction

The epidemiology of malaria can be described in at least 4 different ways, each of which is complementary: (1) the classical approach; (2) the ecological classification with 8 paradigms; (3) a clinico-epidemiological approach; (4) a conceptual diagram which merely elaborates on the above 3 aspects.

In addition to transmission by various species of anopheline mosquitoes, malaria can also be transmitted by blood transfusion, by infected needles among drug users and by organ transplantation. Mosquitoes surviving an aeroplane journey from an endemic country may infect persons in a non-endemic area ('airport malaria' or 'baggage malaria'). For all practical purposes animal reservoirs play no part in the epidemiology of human malaria.

9.2 The classical macro-epidemiology approach

Two epidemiological extremes are described; stable and unstable malaria. The salient differences are shown in Table 20.6.

In between these 2 extremes, variable degrees of transmission occur. Moreover the prevalence of malaria can vary considerably within the same country. For example, in Bangladesh holoendemic *P. falciparum* malaria occurs in one area, unstable (or epidemic prone) malaria occurs in another, whereas in the majority of the country malaria transmission is low and is predominantly due to *P. vivax*.

The four major determinants that are relevant to the dynamics of malaria transmission are (1) the parasite, (2) the vector, (3) the human host and (4) the environment.

THE PARASITE

Differences in the biology of the different species of human malaria parasites are important factors in the epidemiology of malaria. Thus, the pre-patency period is shortest in *P. falciparum* (6–25 days) and longest in *P. malariae* (18–27 days) whereas the incubation period for *P. falciparum* is 7–27, days in contrast to that for *P. malariae* which is 23–69 days. The parasite life span is usually only 1 year for *P. falciparum* whereas for *P. malariae* it is many decades. The appearance of gametocytes occurs simultaneously with the asexual parasitaemia in *P. vivax*, *P. ovale* and *P. malariae*, in contrast with *P. falciparum* in which viable gametocytes appear in the circulation only 8–15 days after blood infection. Genetic diversity in *P. falciparum* antigens is well documented and has already been discussed. The potential for multiplication and ability to relapse in the human host varies with the different species of parasite.

THE VECTOR

Many factors affect the susceptibility of anophelines (of which around 60 species can transmit malaria) to specific *Plasmodium* species. Air temperature, relative humidity and types of breeding places can affect gonotrophic maturation, the longevity of the adult mosquito and the development of the aquatic stages. The density of the vectors in relation to humans, their parous rates, the frequency of mosquitoes feeding on humans or animals (anthropophilic or zoophilic), the

Table 20.6 The epidemiological features of stable and unstable malaria

	Stable malaria	Unstable malaria
Transmission pattern	Transmission occurs throughout the year. Fairly uniform intensity. Pattern repeats annually	Seasonal transmission variable in intensity. Liable to flare up in dramatic epidemics
Immunity	Potent resistance in the community due to prevailing intense transmission	General lack of communal immunity due to low level and variable intensity of transmission
Impact	Mainly young children	All age groups
Control	Difficult	Much easier than stable malaria
Occurrence	Rural West Africa and East Africa, coastal areas of PNG	Plateau of Ethiopia, Plateau of Madagascar, Sri Lanka, North West India

duration of sporogony, the sporozoite rates, the peak biting time, the preference for biting indoors or outdoors (endophagy, exophagy) and the choice of resting place (endophily, exophily), are important determinants which affect the transmission dynamics and which are usually measured to quantify the malaria risk (Bockarie et al. 1994, Service 1993).

THE HOST

Human biological factors, human-parasite interactions and human behaviour all influence the epidemiology of malaria.

Several genetic factors prevent parasite development in the red cell and conclusive evidence of protection against *P. falciparum* malaria is now available for the inherited genes for haemoglobin S, β-thalassaemia, G6PD deficiency and ovalocytosis (Allison 1954, Edington 1967, Gilles et al. 1967, Willcox 1975, Cattani 1987, Hill 1992, Ruwenda et al. 1995).

Miller et al. (1979), demonstrated natural selection to *P. vivax* malaria in individuals in whom the Duffy blood group antigen is absent (Fy^{a-b-} phenotype). Subsequently, it was found that 2 HLA types (HLA-BW53 and a haplotype bearing the DRW13.02 antigen) confer a degree of protection against cerebral malaria and malarial anaemia in The Gambia (Hill et al. 1991). In contrast, in the same population, homozygotes for the TNF2 allele (a variant of the TNFα gene promoter region) have a relatively higher risk of death or severe neurological sequelae due to cerebral malaria (McGuire et al. 1994).

Acquired immunity is discussed in Section 6 (see section 6, p. 378). Other human variables such as pregnancy (especially in primigravidae) modify malaria prevalence and density, as well as the birth weight of infants and the incidence of anaemia (Brabin et al. 1993). Nutritional factors seem to have a paradoxical effect. Severe malaria is seldom evident at necropsy in children who die with marasmus or kwashiorkor in West Africa (Edington 1967). On the other hand correction of severe malnutrition, either on its own or in combination with iron deficiency, may cause latent *P. falciparum* malaria to flare up. Human behaviour, e.g. sleeping habits, types of housing, occupational activities and political and social factors can

all be responsible for changes in the epidemiology of malaria.

THE ENVIRONMENT

The physical environment has a direct effect on both the parasite and the vector. Thus, altitude, temperature, rainfall, the rate of flow of rivers and streams, the presence of collections of water and the availability of animals all influence human malaria transmission.

The effect of global warming could represent a risk of epidemics in the highland areas of tropical Africa, by pushing malaria transmission uphill into these populated areas (Bradley 1995). The following can all have a significant impact on malaria endemicity: increases in agricultural colonization; the construction of large economic projects such as dams, irrigation schemes and highways; mining; deforestation; and the mobilization of large migrant labour forces. The cultivation of rice and cotton cultivation is often associated with increased malaria risk; the creation of new microclimates following deforestation in urban areas of west Africa seems to have favoured the establishment of *A. arabiensis*, a savannah species, at the expense of *A. gambiae* (Coluzzi et al. 1979). Environmental factors may interact with social, political and economic pressures, e.g. movements of large numbers of refugees, smuggling, illegal logging and gem mining, and the existence of ethnic and marginalized communities. The Garki Project is probably the best example of a study in which many of the parameters of malaria epidemiology have been critically examined (Molineaux and Grammicia 1980).

9.3   The ecological classification

A pragmatic approach to the epidemiological stratification of malaria has been developed by Najera Liese and Hamer (1991), defining 8 major ecological prototypes: (1) African savannah; (2) plains and valleys outside Africa (areas of traditional agriculture); (3) forest and forest fringe; (4) desert and highland fringe; (5) coastal and marshland; (6) urban slums; (7) agricultural developments; and (8) sociopolitical disturbances. For each paradigm a description of the circumstances that are responsible for the transmission of malaria is given and the salient features of the impact of the disease are described.

9.4 A clinico-epidemiological approach

The natural history of 'stable' malaria infection has been extensively documented. The salient features are as follows: infants born from semi-immune mothers are protected for the first 3–6 months of life predominantly by passive immunity acquired from their mothers and possibly other factors such as a high concentration of foetal haemoglobin. Although parasitaemia occurs during this period, severe and complicated malaria is seldom encountered. From 6 months to 5 years or more (depending on the level of transmission and other factors, e.g. availability of antimalarial drugs, bed nets etc.) the child is susceptible to severe attacks of malaria resulting in death in a proportion of children exposed. In The Gambia it was estimated that 25% of all childhood deaths under 5 years in the late 1980s were due to malaria (Greenwood et al. 1987a). After this danger period, when the cause of death is usually either malarial anaemia or cerebral malaria, immunity is gradually acquired and clinical disease is rare except in primigravidae. This sequence of events is graphically presented in Fig. 20.24.

The timescale given was based on close observation of cohorts of children from birth to 6 years in The Gambia in the 1950s when transmission was apparently much higher than it is today. The clinical description and duration are governed by the various factors known to affect malaria transmission and will therefore be place-dependent, but the chronology is characteristic of all the stable malaria areas of Africa. In these areas daily parasitaemia is sometimes encountered. One example is a Gambian child aged 1 year 2 months in whom parasitaemia lasted for 106 continuous days, but who did not appear ill or require antimalarial treatment for many days (see Fig. 20.25). He was eventually treated when regular monitoring revealed that his haemoglobin level had dropped to 8 g. This insidious onset of malarial anaemia is not uncommon in children under 2 years old.

9.5 A conceptual diagram

A conceptual diagram of the epidemiology of malaria is given in Fig. 20.26.

Various factors are known to determine the relative sizes of the circles in various communities. For example, in 'stable' areas of malaria a substantial proportion of the population will have asymptomatic parasitaemia at any one time, whereas comparatively few will have clinical malaria and fewer still will have severe malaria; this will occur mainly in children, of whom a small proportion (estimated at 0.1%) will die. Nevertheless, this amounts to the alarming figure of 1 million children under 5 years in Africa alone. In contrast, in 'unstable' areas the largest circle will be that for uncomplicated malaria, as most of those who become infected usually develop clinical illness.

We have only just begun to determine the factors that might determine which circle an individual patient falls into. For example, some genetic factors that protect against the development of severe disease have already been identified (see section 9.1, p. 391), but many questions remain unanswered.

9.6 Imported malaria

Malaria continues to be imported into countries from which it has been eliminated. In the USA in 1991, 1170 cases of malaria were reported to the Centers for Disease Control (CDC), whereas in Australia, this figure was 939. In Europe some 8000 cases were notified to WHO but it is thought that the actual number of cases is considerably higher. For the UK, the number of cases for the years 1972–1994 are given in Figure 20.27.

P. falciparum was responsible for 11 deaths in 1992, for 7 deaths in 1993 for 11 deaths in 1994. The most dangerous risk areas were west and east Africa.

10 CHEMOTHERAPY

Although chemotherapy is mandatory in the treatment of malaria (White 1988), correct management of the patient and the complications that occur with severe malaria is also vital (Gilles and Warrell 1993, Molyneux and Fox 1993, Wilkinson et al 1994). A summary of the management of severe and complicated malaria is given in Table 20.7 (Gilles 1991).

For uncomplicated *P. falciparum* malaria, oral therapy is the administration of choice and parenteral therapy should be considered only if the patient presents with severe nausea and vomiting. For severe and complicated falciparum malaria parenteral therapy is always indicated but reversal to oral therapy should be instituted as soon as the patient's condition has improved enough for drugs to be taken by mouth.

The antimalarial drugs in common use are: chloroquine; quinine; mefloquine; halofantrine; sulphadoxine/pyrimethamine; artemether; artesunate; and primaquine. When choosing a treatment it is important to be aware of the treatment regimen recommended for the specific geographical area in question, both by the national malaria control programme and by WHO.

The treatment of uncomplicated *P. falciparum* malaria is given in Table 20.8; of severe and complicated malaria in Table 20.9; of *P. vivax* and *P. ovale* malaria in Table 20.10 and *P. malariae* in Table 20.11 (Gilles and Warrell 1993).

Although the proposed regimen for *P. malariae* is that which is usually recommended, the authors feel that a 4 day treatment would be more logical for this parasite, in view of its longer intraerythrocytic cycle (i.e. 72 h as opposed to 48 h for the other human malaria species). This approach may help to deal with the 'lesser susceptibility' of this parasite to chloroquine treatment, which has been reported but which has not been thoroughly documented.

In the greater Mekong region (i.e. the region

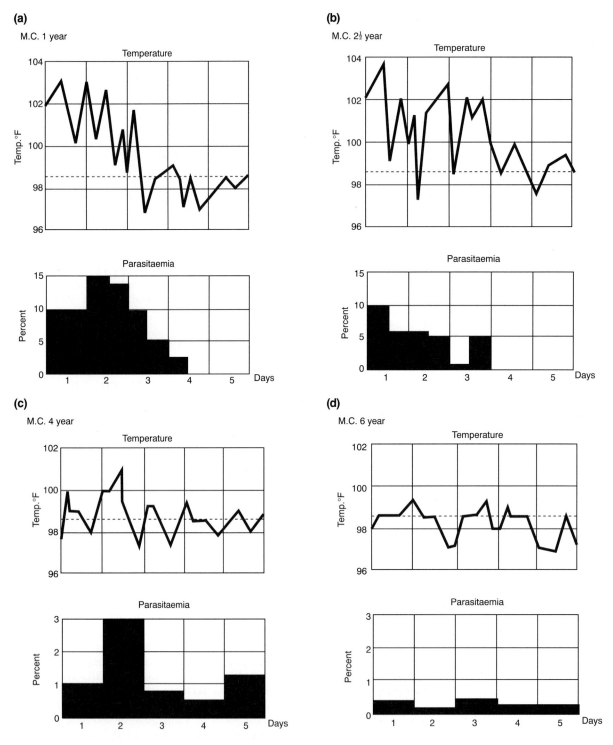

Fig. 20.24 Natural history of *Plasmodium falciparum* malaria in a 'stable' area, showing how clinical immunity develops in a child. With each subsequent phase there is first a decline in the febrile response to infection and subsequently a decline in parasitaemia. (a) Child looks ill, has high temperature and heavy parasitaemia. (b) Child does not look ill, despite high temperature and heavy parasitaemia. (c) Child does not look ill, has mild temperature despite appreciable parasitaemia. (d) Child does not look ill, has no temperature and light parasitaemia.

including Thailand, Vietnam, Laos PDR, Cambodia and Myanmar), where multidrug resistance has been recognized, the treatment of choice is with qinghaosu and its analogues (Jing-Bo Jiang et al 1982, Karbwang and Harinasuta 1992, Looareesuwan et al 1992, Hien and White 1993, Bunnag et al 1995). The recommended regimens for this area are given in Tables 20.12 and 20.13.

Longest continuous parasitaemia (F. G. D. O. B. 11.5.56)

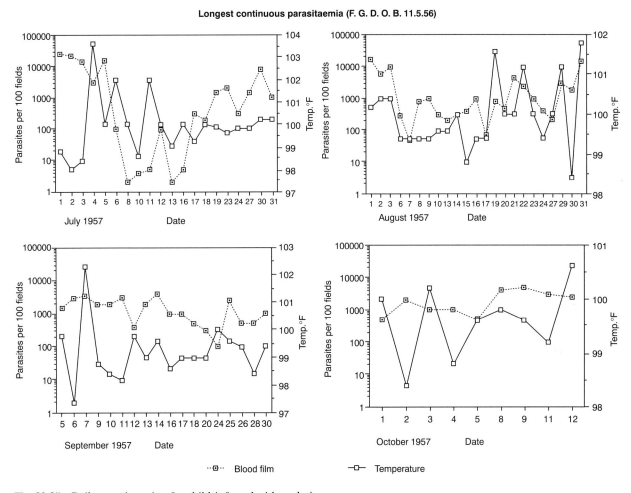

Fig. 20.25 Daily parasitaemia of a child infected with malaria.

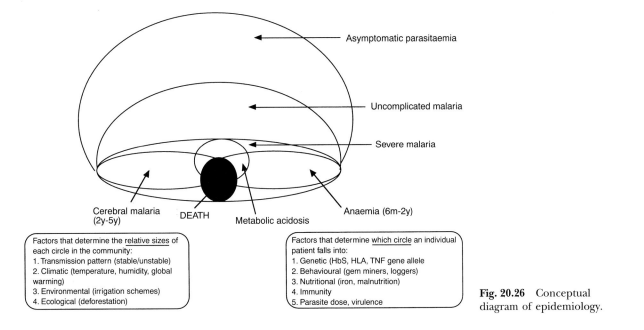

Factors that determine the relative sizes of each circle in the community:
1. Transmission pattern (stable/unstable)
2. Climatic (temperature, humidity, global warming)
3. Environmental (irrigation schemes)
4. Ecological (deforestation)

Factors that determine which circle an individual patient falls into:
1. Genetic (HbS, HLA, TNF gene allele)
2. Behavioural (gem miners, loggers)
3. Nutritional (iron, malnutrition)
4. Immunity
5. Parasite dose, virulence

Fig. 20.26 Conceptual diagram of epidemiology.

10.1 Drug resistance

Monitoring the spread of drug resistance is one of the most important functions of malaria control pro-grammes and such monitoring provides the basis for recommending therapeutic regimens appropriate for each given geographical area, but the available meth-odologies for determining parasite resistance have no

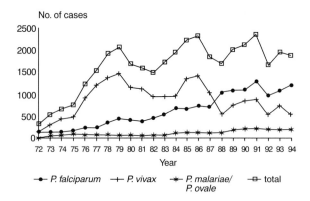

No. of cases

—●— *P. falciparum* —+— *P. vivax* —✳— *P. malariae/ P. ovale* —□— total

Fig. 20.27 Annual number of imported cases of malaria in the United Kingdom. (Based on data from the Malaria Reference Laboratory.)

place in individual patient treatment. Either in vitro or in vivo drug assays may be used to monitor resistance.

In vitro assays provide a quantitative measurement of the level of sensitivity of a given parasite isolate to a drug and are considered to be invaluable operational tools. Such assays are based on brief in vitro cultivation of *P. falciparum* from an infected individual (e.g. the microtest developed by Rieckmann et al., 1978) and the measurement of parasite growth (either as a 24-h schizont maturation assay or as a 48-h growth inhibition assay, depending on the drug tested). In vivo assays are performed in patients and measure the more complex interaction between parasite, drug and host (including the confounding effect of immunity and the effect of host metabolism on drug pharmacokinetics). Although in vivo tests are cumbersome to perform and require a long-term follow-up of treated individuals, with daily blood film examination

Table 20.7 Summary of the management of severe and complicated falciparum malaria

Manifestation/complication	Immediate management[a]
1. Coma (cerebral malaria)	Maintain airway; nurse on side; exclude other treatable causes of coma (eg hypoglycaemia, bacterial meningoencephalitis). Give prophylactic anticonvulsant (10 mg of phenobarbital sodium per kg of body weight intramuscularly). Avoid harmful adjuvant treatments such as corticosteroids, heparin and epinephrine (adrenaline)
2. Convulsions	(Prevent with intramuscular phenobarbital sodium, see above). Maintain airway; treat with diazepam given intravenously or per rectum (0.15 mg/kg to a maximum of 10 mg) or intramuscular paraldehyde injection (0.1 ml/kg from a glass syringe)
3. Severe anaemia	Transfuse fresh whole blood or packed cells
4. Acute renal failure	Exclude dehydration; maintain strict fluid balance; carry out peritoneal dialysis (or haemodialysis if available)
5. Hypoglycaemia	Measure blood glucose, give 50% glucose injection 50 ml (1 ml/kg for children) followed by 5% or 10% glucose infusion
6. Metabolic acidosis	Exclude or treat hypoglycaemia, hypovolaemia and Gram-negative septicaemia. Give oxygen. Correct arterial pH to 7.2 or above. Blood transfusion. Crystalloid infusion
7. Acute pulmonary oedema	Prevent by avoiding excessive rehydration. Prop patient up; give oxygen. If the pulmonary oedema is due to overhydration, stop intravenous fluids, give diuretic (frusemide 40 mg intravenously) and withdraw 250 ml of blood by venesection into a donor bag
8. Shock, algid malaria	Suspect Gram-negative septicaemia; take blood samples for culture. Give parenteral antimicrobials; correct haemodynamic disturbances
9. Spontaneous bleeding and coagulopathy	Transfuse fresh whole blood or clotting factors; give vitamin K injection
10. Hyperpyrexia	Use tepid sponging and fanning; give antipyretic (paracetamol 15 mg/kg of body weight)
11. Hyperparasitaemia	Give initial dose of parenteral antimalarial therapy. If parasitaemia in a severely ill patient exceeds 10%, carry out exchange or partial exchange transfusion
12. Malarial haemoglobinuria	Continue antimalarial treatment; transfuse fresh blood to maintain haematocrit above 20%; give frusemide 20 mg intravenously
13. Aspiration pneumonia	Give parenteral antimicrobials; change position of patient; give physiotherapy; give oxygen

[a]In all cases infusion or injection of an appropriate antimalarial drug should be started immediately.

Table 20.8 Antimalarial chemotherapy for uncomplicated falciparum malaria

Chloroquine-sensitive areas	Chloroquine-resistant areas or sensitivity unknown
Chloroquine Adults: 600 mg base on days 1 and 2 300 mg base on day 3 Children: 10 mg base/kg on days 1 and 2 5 mg base/kg on day 3	1. Mefloquine Adults: 15–25 mg base/kg given as 2 doses 6 hours apart Children: 25 mg base/kg given as 2 doses 6 hours apart OR 2. Halofantrine[a] Adults: 500 mg of the salt every 6 hours × 3 doses with food Children: 8 mg/kg every 6 hours × 3 doses OR 3. Quinine[b] Adults: 600 mg of the salt 3 times daily for 7 days Children: 10 mg of the salt/kg 3 times daily for 7 days OR 4. Sulphonamide-pyrimethamine[c] Sulphadoxine (500 mg per tablet) or sulfalene (500 mg) plus pyrimethamine 25 mg Adults: 3 tablets as single dose Children: <5 years ½ tablet, <9 years 1 tablet, <15 years 2 tablets

[a]Not to pregnant or lactating women, or patients with conduction defects or taking drugs known to prolong the QT interval. In non-immune repeat same treatment on day 7.
[b]In areas of quinine resistance (eg Mekong region) add tetracycline 250 mg 4 times daily or doxycycline 100 mg daily for 7 days except in children <8 years and pregnant women. For these two groups, clindamycin may be considered instead.
[c]Contraindicated if patient has shown sulfomamide hypersensitivity or is pregnant or lactating.

Table 20.9 Antimalarial chemotherapy for severe falciparum malaria (adults or children)

Chloroquine-sensitive areas	Chloroquine-resistant areas or sensitivity unknown
1. Chloroquine 25 mg base/kg diluted in isotonic fluid by continuous iv infusion over 30 hours OR 2. Chloroquine 2.5 mg base/kg every 4 hours im or sc. *Total dose:* 25 mg base/kg OR 3. Quinine (See right-hand column)	1. Quinine[a] Adults: 20 mg salt/kg (loading dose)[b] diluted in 10 ml/kg 5% dextrose saline by iv infusion over 4 hours, then 10 mg salt/kg over 4 hours, 8–12 hourly until patients can swallow[c]. The 7 day course should be completed with quinine tablets 10 mg salt/kg 3 times daily[d] OR 2. Quinine[a] 20 mg salt/kg (loading dose)[b] im (anterior thigh), then 10 mg salt/kg until patients can swallow[c]. Complete course as above.

[a]In patients requiring more than 48 hours parenteral therapy reduce the quinine dose by one half to one third (i.e. 5–7 mg salt/kg).
[b]Loading dose must not be used if patient has had quinine or mefloquine within preceding 24 hours. 1st dose should be 10 mg salt/kg in these circumstances.
[c]After parenteral quinine, *oral* quinine therapy can be continued as above. Mefloquine should not be used in severe malaria.
[d]In areas of quinine resistance add tetracycline 250 mg 4 times daily or doxycycline 100 mg daily for 7 days except for children under 8 years and pregnant women.

Table 20.10 Antimalarial chemotherapy for vivax and ovale malaria

1. Chloroquine
10 mg base/kg on days 1 and 2
5 mg base/kg on day 3
plus for radical cure
2. Primaquine[a]
0.25–033 mg[b] base/kg daily on days 4–17.

[a]Contraindicated for pregnant and lactating women.
  For G6PD-deficient patients daily doses of primaquine are also contraindicated but radical cure can be obtained using 0.75 mg/kg once weekly for 8 weeks, with minimal risk of haemolysis.
[b]For Oceania and South East Asia strains.

Table 20.11 Antimalarial chemotherapy for *P. malariae*

Chloroquine
10 mg base/kg on days 1 and 2
5 mg base/kg on day 3 and 4

for 7 days, 28 days or longer, they allow a very useful grading of resistance from sensitive (S) to one of three levels of resistance (RI, RII and RIII) (see Table 20.14 for the definition of different resistance levels).

There may be a discrepancy between in vitro and in vivo drug assays particularly when comparing the results performed in non-immune and semi-immune individuals or when comparing the results from symptomatic and asymptomatic individuals (Wernsdorfer and Payne 1988).

The mechanism of drug resistance of malaria parasites is only well understood for antifolate drugs. The four groups of drugs (sulphonamides, sulphones, pyrimethamine and proguanil) act at different points of the parasite pathway for folate production, with 2 major target enzymes: dihydropteroate synthetase (DHPS) and dihydrofolate reductase (DHFR). Resistance to antifolates is generally induced by one or more mutations on either of these genes and these mutations tend to occur in a limited number of sites on the molecules (Foote, Galatis and Cowman 1990). It is therefore feasible to use molecular techniques (e.g. PCR) as an alternative to in vitro assays to monitor the spread of such mutations in an area where antifolate drug resistance has been reported.

The mechanism of resistance to chloroquine and other quinoline type drugs is less well understood. The mode of action of chloroquine involves concentration of the drug in the food vacuole of the parasite and antimalarial activity related to inhibition of the polymerization of haem. This leads to the accumulation of free haem which is toxic to the parasite (Slater and Cerami 1992). Chloroquine resistant parasites seem to accumulate less chloroquine due either to a diminished intake of the drug (as suggested by

Table 20.12 Treatment of uncomplicated falciparum malaria in areas where *P. falciparum* is multidrug resistant

1.   Artesunate or Arthemether[a] orally 3.2 mg/kg[a] (loading dose) Day 1
then
Artesunate or Arthemether[a] orally 1.5 mg/kg daily for 6 days
OR
2.   Artesunate or Arthemether[a] orally 3.2 mg/kg[a] (loading dose) Day 1
then
Artesunate or Arthemether[a] orally 2.0 mg/kg daily for 4 days
plus
Mefloquine[b] 25 m/kg orally (in two divided dose)—15 mg/kg initially followed 12 hours later by 10 mg/kg

[a]Not to be used in 1st trimester.
[b]Not to be used in severe malaria.

Table 20.13 Treatment of severe and complicated falciparum malaria (adults) in areas where *P. falciparum* is multidrug resistant

1.   Artesunate 2.4 mg/kg intravenously[a] or intramuscularly (loading dose) followed by Artesunate 1.2 mg/kg at 12 hours and then daily for 6 days
OR
2.   Arthemether[b] 3.2 mg/kg intramuscularly (loading dose) followed by Arthemether (imi) 1.6 mg/kg daily for 6 days

[a]Artesunate intravenously is given *by injection not infusion*.
[b]Not to be used in 1st trimester—Use quinine as in Table 20.9.

Table 20.14 Definition of in vivo antimalarial drug response

Sensitive: (S)	if asexual parasites have cleared by day 6 from the beginning of treatment without subsequent recrudescence until day 28
Resistance grade I: (RI)	if the asexual parasites have cleared for at least two consecutive days, latest on day 6 from the beginning of treatment, followed by recrudescence. Two types of recrudescence may be differentiated: i) early (before day 14) and ii) late (between days 15 and 28)
Resistance grade II: (RII)	showing a marked reduction of asexual parasitaemia to less than 25% of the pretreatment count within 48 hours of the initiation of treatment, but no subsequent disappearance of parasitaemia (positive on day 6)
Resistance Grade III: (RIII)	showing only a modest reduction, no change or an increase in asexual parasitaemia, during the first 48 hours following the implementation of treatment and no subsequent clearance of asexual parasites

Ginsburg and Stein 1991) or a greater efflux of the drug, presumably linked to the presence of a molecule capable of pumping the drug out of the cell (similar to the P-glycoprotein responsible for multi-drug resistance, *mdr*, in tumour cells) (Krogstadt et al. 1987). The theory of an increased efflux is strengthened by the observation that drug resistance of *P. falciparum* may be reversed by compounds known to inhibit such pumps (e.g. verapamil or desipramine). Two P-glycoprotein-like genes have been identified in *P. falciparum*, namely *Pfmdr1* and *Pfmdr2* and amplification of gene expression occurs in association with certain mutations (Foote et al. 1989). Although several alleles of *Pfmdr* have a strong correlation with chloroquine resistance (Foote et al. 1990), this correlation is not perfect and many resistant parasite seem to have the same *Pfmdr* genes as sensitive isolates (Haruki et al. 1994). The situation is further complicated by the demonstration by Wellems, Walker and Panton (1991), using a genetic cross experiment of malaria parasites in a chimpanzee, that chloroquine resistance was associated with a single gene locus on chromosome 7, whereas there had previously been a consensus that chloroquine resistance was a multigenic event.

10.2 Chemoprophylaxis of malaria

Drug resistance of *P. falciparum* to chloroquine and other antimalarial drugs continues to increase in both intensity and geographical distribution. In the greater Mekong region multidrug resistance has been well documented. The situation is a dynamic one and advice on the current chemoprophylaxis recommendations for travellers should be sought from the various specialized centres in respective countries (Steffen et al. 1993, Bradley and Warhurst 1995, Lobel et al. 1995). To date, resistance of *P. vivax* to chloroquine has been reported only occasionally from Indonesia, Papua New Guinea and Vanuatu, and these reports do not yet justify a recommendation for alternative chemoprophylaxis in these areas.

The principles of prevention that should be borne in mind are:

1 Awareness of the malaria risk coupled with a high index of suspicion if fever occurs while in a malarious country or within 3–12 months of return, even if all recommended precautions have been taken.
2 Personal protection to diminish contact between human and vector is very important. This includes (1) sleeping in screened rooms and spraying the room with a knockdown insecticide before sleeping to kill any mosquitoes that have entered during the day; (2) using bed nets impregnated with pyrethroids; (3) using an electric mat to vaporize synthetic pyrethroids, or burning mosquito coils; (4) wearing long-sleeved clothing and trousers after sunset; and (5) application of repellents containing diethyltaluanide to exposed skin.
3 Strict compliance with the chemoprophylaxis regimens recommended (Bradley and Warhurst 1995).

Chemoprophylaxis at the community level is a contentious issue, which at present is not advised by WHO for a variety of reasons: potential dangers of drug resistance; poor compliance in areas of perennial transmission; possible delay in the development of natural immunity; cost; toxicity of drugs; regularity of supply and logistics of delivery. Nevertheless, there may be a place for community chemoprophylaxis targeted to young children and pregnant women in areas where transmission is seasonal and short and where the population is very co-operative and well educated with regard to malaria (as is the case in The Gambia) (Greenwood et al. 1991).

Chemoprophylaxis in pregnancy has long been recommended, particularly in primigravidae (Gilles et al. 1969, Fleming et al. 1986, Greenwood et al. 1989, Steketee and Wirima 1994, WHO 1994b). The advent of drug resistance, increasing evidence of poor compliance, unacceptable adverse drug reactions and economic considerations have resulted in alternative strategies being sought. For instance, in Malawi, a 2-dose regimen of sulphadoxine-pyrimethamine given at first attendance in the 2nd trimester of pregnancy and repeated at the beginning of the 3rd trimester, was found to be a cost effective intervention to reduce the incidence of low birth weight infants (Schultz et al. 1995). Further studies are required before this regimen can be generally recommended. Meanwhile, a curative treatment with chloroquine given at first attendance, followed by prophylaxis continued throughout pregnancy is recommended in areas where chloroquine resistance is still predominantly at the RI level, particularly for primigravidae and secundogravidae mothers (WHO 1994b).

11 VACCINATION

The prevention of malaria by vaccination is a conceivable goal, which may eventually have a place in malaria control. Unfortunately, no effective malaria vaccine is as yet available and, despite very intensive research since the mid 1970s, none is likely to be available at an operational level for many years. The topic of malaria vaccines is vast and complex and has been reviewed at length elsewhere (Mitchell 1989, Hommel 1991, Mendis 1991, Nardin and Nussenzweig 1993, Phillips 1994).

The aim of a vaccine is to reduce morbidity and mortality due to malaria and this may be achieved in one of 2 ways: either by interrupting infection at one of the stages of the parasite life-cycle, or by using an anti-disease vaccine to reduce the pathophysiological effects triggered by the release of malarial toxins (as proposed by Playfair et al. 1990). The interruption of the life-cycle may take place at the time of entry of the sporozoite into the host, at the level of schizogony in the hepatocyte, at the time of erythrocyte invasion and intra-erythrocytic parasite development, or by interruption of the sexual development within the mosquito. Fig. 20.28 illustrates the potential vaccine targets and indicates which possible parasite molecules may be used as a vaccine in each situation.

The methods by which host immunity will control the infection are variable, depending on the target and this will have implications for the choice of immunogen. For example, a pre-erythrocytic vaccine is likely to rely more on the production of CTLs than antibodies, whereas a transmission-blocking vaccine is likely to rely essentially on antibodies to sexual stages. It follows that new methods for immunization using DNA injection are likely to be particularly useful for pre-erythrocytic stages (as they are good for producing CTLs) and perhaps less useful for transmission-blocking vaccines.

A number of vaccine candidates have been tested in human volunteers with variable success: the best results were obtained with X-irradiated sporozoites (Clyde et al. 1973), whereas synthetic and recombinant antigens have so far given disappointing results. This is illustrated by the following examples: one out of 34 volunteers were protected in a trial using a recombinant CS epitope (Ballou et al. 1987); 0 out of 20 volunteers vaccinated with a recombinant CS co-expressed in yeast with hepatitis B surface antigen were protected (Gordon et al. 1995); a 31% efficacy was reported for the synthetic 'SPf66' vaccine when tested in Tanzania (Alonso et al. 1994), but only a 3% efficacy for the same molecule when tested in The Gambia (D'Alessandro et al. 1995). Current research trends in vaccine development are geared towards 'cocktail' vaccines including a combination of multiple epitopes from different malarial antigens and from different stages of the parasite life-cycle; these may include a combination of CSP, LSA-1/3, MSP-1/2, SERA, AMA-1, Pfs48/45, Pfs25, STARP and SSP-2 (currently the most likely vaccine candidates).

The predicted impact of a malaria vaccine in controlling the disease has been discussed and analyzed with a variety of mathematical models and with various degrees of optimism (Halloran, Struchiner and Spielman 1989, Saul 1992).

12 INTEGRATED CONTROL

Between 1898 and 1940 malaria control was effected by the use of quinine (prophylactically as well as therapeutically) and mosquito larval control.

The second world war (1940–1945) revolutionized malaria control through the development of the synthetic antimalarials (atebrin, chloroquine, proguanil) for effective prophylaxis and treatment, and the first residual insecticide (DDT) which made possible the control of adult mosquitoes by house spraying. Between 1945 and 1955, house spraying with DDT, combined with chloroquine treatment of cases, eliminated malaria from several countries in Europe, giving rise to the concept of malaria eradication as opposed to malaria control. Thus in 1956, the WHO World Health Assembly recommended that WHO should implement a programme that would eliminate malaria from the world and this policy was pursued until 1975 when it was abandoned. The reasons for failure can be listed as follows: (1) eradication was an unrealistic objective, particularly for tropical Africa; (2) inflationary price increases of equipment, fuel and insecticides; (3) political instability; (4) financial and administrative shortcomings; (5) vector resistance; (6) vector-exophily; (7) parasite resistance; and (8) uncontrolled population movements.

In 1976 the WHO World Health Assembly adopted an integrated malaria control strategy, the elements of which are shown in Fig. 20.29.

Nevertheless, even this reduced goal has proven to be over-ambitious and unachievable in most of the endemic malaria countries, especially those in tropical Africa, and in 1985 the World Health Assembly recommended that malaria control should be developed as an integrated part of national primary health care systems.

The malaria control strategy now being promoted by the Ministerial Conference on Malaria (WHO 1992) recognizes 4 basic technical elements: to provide early diagnosis and prompt treatment; to plan and implement selective and sustainable preventive measures against the parasite as well as the vector; to detect early, contain or prevent epidemics; and to reassess regularly a country's malaria situation, in particular the ecological, social and economic determinants of the disease. This strategy involves a radical shift from the primary emphasis on transmission control of the parasite to the present focus on reduction of malarial disease.

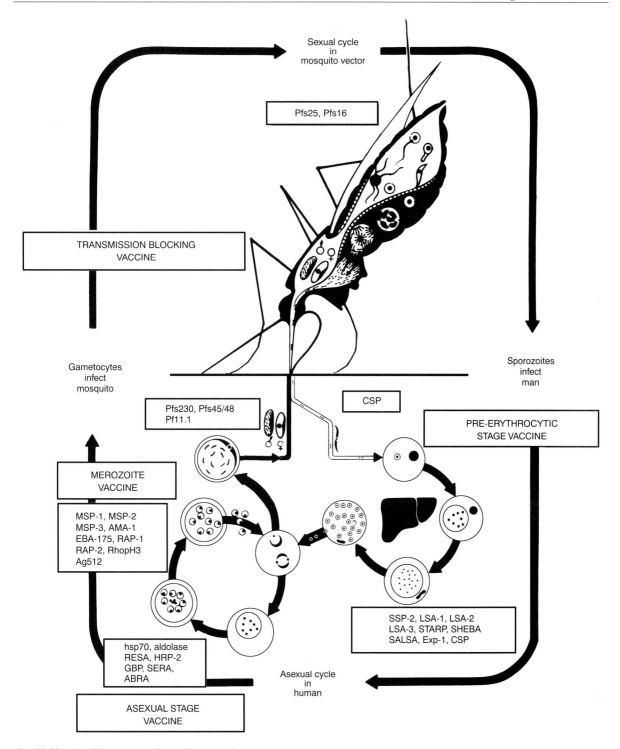

Fig. 20.28 Possible targets of a malaria vaccine.

In this context the use of impregnated bed nets is of particular interest. Pyrethroid treated bed nets have reduced malarial morbidity in certain areas, e.g. China and The Gambia. In areas of intense perennial malarial transmission there is evidence of reduction of *P. falciparum* parasitaemia, reduction in transmission and reduction in rate of reinfection. In some trials but not in others, widespread community use of insecticide treated bednets protect even non-users of nets (Greenwood and Baker 1993, Smith et al 1993, Bockarie et al 1994, Somboon et al 1995, WHO 1995). Sustained utilization of nets is clearly important and remains an unsolved challenge. (Meek 1995). The existing vector control tools can still be effective, but they must be selectively deployed, cost-effective and sustainable.

In the long term, the impact of any malaria control measure (including early diagnosis and treatment, indoor residual spraying, personal protection or environmental management) depends on the impor-

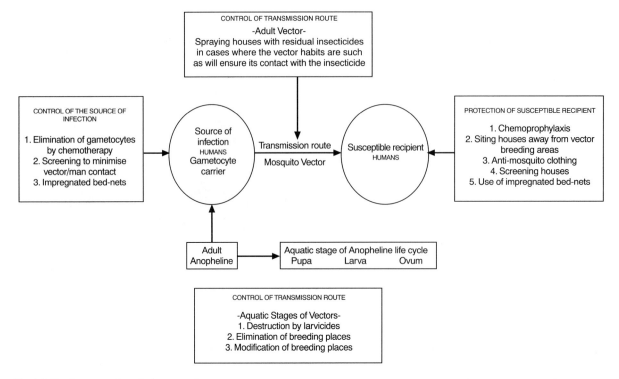

Fig. 20.29 Integrated malaria control strategy.

tance given to these measures by the community at risk and on their understanding of and involvement in their application (WHO 1995). The long neglected social, behavioural and economic aspects of malaria and its control are being increasingly recognized (Combie 1994, Manderson 1994, Ruiz and Kroeger 1994, Agyepong et al. 1995).

It would be wrong to assume that the involvement of primary health care in malaria control in endemic countries is an easy way of solving the difficulties related to administrative, social or economic obstacles. The following must all be achieved: a proper degree

of co-operation between the different levels of the health care system; inter-sectorial co-ordination; substantial political commitment; adequate human and financial resources; and the full partnership of communities. In addition to these obstacles, the appropriate choice of antimalarial in areas of increasing parasite resistance must also be made, if the relatively modest goal of reducing malaria morbidity and mortality is to be achieved (Naimoli et al. 1994, Steketee et al. 1994a, Steketee et al. 1994b)

REFERENCES

Agyepong IA, Aryce B et al., 1995, *The Malaria Manual*, GenevaTDR/SER/MSR/95.1, WHO, 17.

Aikawa M, 1988, Morphological changes in erythrocytes induced by malarial parasites, *Biol Cell*, **64**: 169–77.

Allan RJ, Rowe A, Kwiatkowski D, 1993, *Plasmodium falciparum* varies in its ability to induce tumor necrosis factor, *Infect Immun*, **61**: 4772–6.

Allen SJ, O'Donnell A et al., 1996, Severe malaria in children from Madang, Papua New Guinea, *Q J Med*, **89**: 779–88.

Allison AC, 1954, Protection afforded by the sickle cell trail against subtertian malarial infection, *Br Med J*, **1**: 290–4.

Alonso P, Smith T et al., 1994, Randomised trial of efficacy of Spf66 vaccine against *Plasmodium falciparum* in children in Southern Tanzania, *Lancet*, **344**: 1175–81.

Ambroise-Thomas P, Wernsdorfer WH et al., 1976, Etude séro-épidémiologique longitudinale sur le paludisme en Tunisie, *Bull W H O*, **54**: 355–67.

Anders RF, 1986, Multiple cross-reactivities among antigens of *Plasmodium falciparum* impair the development of protective immunity against malaria, *Parasite Immunol*, **8**: 529–39.

Archibald HM, 1956, The influence of malarial infection of the placenta on the incidence of prematurity, *Bull W H O*, **15**: 842–5.

Arese P, Turini F, Ginsburg H, 1991, Erythrophagocytosis in malaria: host defence or menace to the macrophage, *Parasitol Today*, **7**: 25–8.

Assaraf YG, Golenser J et al., 1984, Polyamine levels and the activity of their biosynthetic enzymes in human erythrocytes infected with the malarial parasite, *Plasmodium falciparum*, *Biochem J*, **222**: 815–19.

Ballou WR, Hoffman SL et al., 1987, Safety and efficacy of a recombinant DNA *Plasmodium falciparum* sporozoite vaccine, *Lancet*, **1**: 1277–81.

Bannister LH, Dluzewski AR, 1990, The ultrastructure of red cell invasion in malaria infection: a review, *Blood Cells*, **16**: 257–92.

Bate CAW, Kwiatkowski D, 1994, A monoclonal antibody that recognizes phosphatidylinositol inhibits induction of tumor necrosis factor alpha by different strains of *Plasmodium falciparum*, *Infect Immun*, **62**: 5261–6.

Bate CAW, Taverne J et al., 1992, Serological relationship of tumour necrosis factor-inducing exoantigens of *Plasmodium falciparum* and *P. vivax*, *Infect Immun*, **60**: 1241–3.

Bennett IL, Hook EW, 1959, Infectious diseases (some aspects of salmonellosis), *Annu Rev Med*, **16**: 1–19.

Bockarie MJ, Service MW et al., 1994, Malaria in a rural area of Sierra Leone. III Vector ecology and disease transmission, *Ann Trop Med Parasitol*, **88**: 251–62.

Bouharoun-Tayoun H, Attanah P et al., 1990, Antibodies which protect man against *Plasmodium falciparum* blood stages do not on their own inhibit parasite growth and invasion in vitro but act in cooperation with monocytes, *J Exp Med*, **172:** 1633–41.

Brabin BJ, 1983, An analysis of malaria in pregnancy in Africa, *Bull W H O*, **61:** 1005–16.

Brabin BJ, Maxwell S et al., 1993, A study of the consequences of malarial infection in pregnant women and their infants, *Parassitologia*, **35, Suppl.:** 9–11.

Bradley DJ, 1995, The Epidemiology of Malaria in the Tropics and in Travellers, *Baillière's Clinical Infectious Diseases – Malaria*, ed Pasvol G, Baillière Tindall, London, 211–26.

Bradley DJ, Warhurst DC, 1995, Malaria prophylaxis: Guidelines for travellers from Britain, *Br Med J*, **310:** 709–14.

Bray RS, Anderson MJ, 1979, Falciparum malaria in pregnancy, *Trans R Soc Trop Med Hyg*, **73:** 427–31.

Brown KN, Brown IN, 1965, Immunity to malaria: antigenic variation in chronic infections of *Plasmodium knowlesi*, *Nature (London)*, **208:** 1286–90.

Brown KN, Phillips RS, 1974, Immunity to *Plasmodium berghei* in rats: passive serum transfer and role of the spleen, *Infect Immun*, **10:** 1213–18.

Brumpt E, 1949, The human parasites of the genus *Plasmodium*, *Malariology*, vol.1, ed Boyd MF, WB Saunders, Philadelphia, 65–121.

Bunnag D, Kanda T et al., 1995, Artemether-mefloquine combination in multidrug-resistant falciparum malaria, *Trans R Soc Trop Med Hyg*, **89:** 213–15.

Butcher GA, Mitchell GH, Cohen S, 1978, Antibody mediated mechanisms of immunity to malaria induced by vaccination with *P. knowlesi* merozoites, *Immunology*, **34:** 77–86.

Cabantchik ZI, 1990, Properties of permeation pathways induced in the human red cell membrane by malaria parasites, *Blood Cells*, **16:** 421–32.

Carlson J, Helmby H et al., 1990, Human cerebral malaria: association with erythrocyte rosetting and lack of anti-rosette antibodies, *Lancet*, **336:** 1457–60.

Carter R, Graves PM, 1988, Gametocytes, *Malaria. Principles and Practice of Malariology*, vol 1, eds Wernsdorfer WH and McGregor I, Churchill Livingstone, Edinburgh, 253–305.

Cattani, JA, 1987, Hereditary ovalocytosis and reduced susceptibility to malaria in Papua New Guinea, *Trans R Soc Trop Med Hyg*, **81:** 705–9.

Charoenpan P, Indraprasit S et al., 1990, Pulmonary oedema in severe malaria. Haemodynamic study and clinicopathological correlation, *Chest*, **97:** 1190–7.

Clark IA, Hunt NH, 1983, Evidence for reactive oxygen intermediates causing hemolysis and parasite death in malaria, *Infect Immun*, **39:** 1–6.

Clark IA, Rockett KA, 1994, T cells and malarial pathology, *Res Immunol*, **145:** 437–41.

Clark IA, Chaudri G, Cowden WB, 1989, Role of tumour necrosis factor in the illness and pathology of malaria, *Trans R Soc Trop Med Hyg*, **83:** 436–40.

Clark IA, Cowden WB, Chaudhri G, 1989, Possible roles for oxidants, through tumor necrosis factor, in malarial anemia, *Malaria and the Red Cell*, vol 2, eds Eaton JW, Meshnick SR, Brewer GJ, Alan R.Liss Inc., New York, 73–82.

Clyde DF, Most H et al., 1973, Immunization of man against sporozoite-induced falciparum malaria, *Am J Med Sci*, **266:** 169–77.

Coatney GR, 1971, The simian malarias: zoonoses, anthropozoonoses or both?, *Am J Trop Med Hyg*, **20:** 795–803.

Coatney GR, Collins W et al., 1971, *The Primate Malarias*, US Dept Health Educ and Welfare.

Cogswell FB, 1992, The hypnozoite and relapse in primate malaria, *Clin Microbiol Rev*, **5:** 26–35.

Cohen S, Butcher GA, 1971, Serum antibody in acquired malarial immunity, *Trans R Soc Trop Med Hyg*, **65:** 125–8.

Cohen S, McGregor IA, Carrington S, 1961, Gamma globulin and acquired immunity to human malaria, *Nature (London)*, **192:** 733–7.

Collins WE, 1988, Major animal models in malaria research: simian, *Malaria. Principles and Practice of Malariology*, vol 2, eds Wernsdorfer WH and McGregor I, Churchill Livingstone, Edinburgh, 1473–501.

Coluzzi M, Sabatini A et al., 1979, Chromosomal differentiation and adaptation to human environments in the *A. gambiae* complex, *Trans R Soc Trop Med Hyg*, **73:** 483–97.

Combie SC, 1994, Treatment seeking for malaria. TDR/SER/RP/94.1, Reference Paper No. 2. TDR Geneva, 29.

Contamin H, Fandeur T et al., 1995, PCR typing of field isolates of *Plasmodium falciparum*, *J Clin Microbiol*, **33:** 944–51.

Coosemans M, Van der Stuyft P, Delacollette C, 1994, A hundred per cent of fields positive in a thick film: a useful indicator of relative changes in morbidity in areas with seasonal malaria, *Ann Trop Med Parasitol*, **88:** 581–6.

Coppel RL, 1995, The contribution of molecular biology to our understanding of malaria, *Baillière's Clinical Infectious Diseases – Malaria*, ed Pasvol G, Baillière Tindall, London, 351–69.

Corcoran LM, Forsyth KP et al., 1986, Chromosome size polymorphisms in *Plasmodium falciparum* can involve deletions and are frequent in natural parasite populations, *Cell*, **44:** 87–95.

Cox FEG, 1988, Major animal models in malaria research: rodent, *Malaria. Principles and Practice of Malariology*, vol 2, eds Wernsdorfer WH and McGregor I, Churchill Livingstone, Edinburgh, 1503–43.

Crane GC, 1986, Hyperreactive malarious splenomegaly (Tropical splenomegaly syndrome), *Parasitol Today*, **2:** 4–9.

D'Alessandro U, Leach A et al., 1995, Efficacy trial of malaria vaccine Spf66 in Gambian infants, *Lancet*, **346:** 462–7.

David PH, Hommel M, Oligino LD, 1981, Interactions of *Plasmodium falciparum*-infected erythrocytes with ligand coated agarose beads, *Mol Biochem Parasitol*, **4:** 195–204.

David PH, Hudson DE et al., 1985, Immunisation of monkeys with 140 kDa merozoite surface protein of *Plasmodium knowlesi*: appearance of alternate forms of this protein, *J Immunol*, **134:** 4146–52.

Day KP, Marsh K, 1991, Naturally acquired immunity to *Plasmodium falciparum*, *Parasitol Today*, **7:** 68–71.

Defo BK, 1995, Epidemiology and control of infant and early childhood malaria: A competing risks analysis, *Int J Epidemiol*, **24:** 204–17.

Del Giudice G, Biro S et al., 1987, Antibodies to the repetitive epitope of *Plasmodium falciparum* circumsporozoite protein in a rural Tanzanian community. A longitudinal study of 132 children, *Am J Trop Med Hyg*, **36:** 203–12.

Doherty JF, Grant AD, Bryceson ADM, 1995, Fever as the presenting complaint of travellers returning from the tropics, *Q J Med*, **88:** 277–81.

Edington GH, 1967, Pathology of malaria in West Africa, *Br Med J*, **1:** 715–18.

Edington GH, Gilles HM, 1976, Malaria, *Pathology in the Tropics*, 2nd edn, Edward Arnold, London, 10–33.

Edozien JC, Gilles HM, Udeozo IO, 1962, Adult and cord blood gammaglobulins and immunity to malaria in Nigerians, *Lancet*, **2:** 951–5.

Elford BC, 1986, L-Glutamine influx in malaria-infected erythrocytes: a target for antimalarials?, *Parasitol Today*, **2:** 309–11.

Facer CA, 1983, Erythrocyte sialoglycoproteins and *Plasmodium falciparum* isolates, *Trans R Soc Trop Med Hyg*, **77:** 524–30.

Fairfield AS, Abosch A et al., 1988, Oxidant defense enzymes of *Plasmodium falciparum*, *Mol Biochem Parasitol*, **30:** 77–82.

Fakunle YM, 1981, Tropical splenomegaly. Part 1. Tropical Africa, *Clin Haematol*, **10:** 963–75.

Ferone R, 1977, Folate metabolism in malaria, *Bull W H O*, **55:** 291–8.

Fleming AF, Ghatoura GB et al., 1986, The prevention of anaemia in pregnancy in primigravidae in the guinea savanna of Nigeria, *Ann Trop Med Parasitol*, **80:** 211–33.

Foote SJ, Galatis, Cowman AF, 1990, Amino acids in the dihydrofolate reductase-thymidylate synthase gene of *Plasmodium falciparum* involved in cycloguanil resistance differ from those involved in pyrimethamine resistance, *Proc Natl Acad Sci USA*, **87:** 3014–17.

Foote SJ, Kemp DJ, 1989, Chromosomes of malaria parasites, *Trends Genet*, **5:** 337–42.

Foote SJ, Thompson JK et al., 1989, Amplification of the multidrug-resistance gene in some chloroquine resistant isolates of *Plasmodium falciparum*, *Cell*, **57:** 921–30.

Foote SJ, Kyle DE et al., 1990, Several alleles of multidrug-resistance gene are closely linked to chloroquine resistance in *Plasmodium falciparum*, *Nature (London)*, **345:** 255–8.

Forsyth KP, Anders RF et al., 1989, Small area variation in prevalence of an S-antigen serotype of *Plasmodium falciparum* in villages of Madang, Papua New Guinea, *Am J Trop Med Hyg.*, **40:** 344–50.

Fortier B, Delplace JF et al., 1987, Enzyme immunoassay for detection of antigen in acute *Plasmodium falciparum* malaria, *Eur J Clin Microbiol Infect Dis*, **6:** 596–8.

Foster SO, 1991, Pricing, distribution and use of antimalarial drugs, *Bull W H O*, **69:** 349–63.

Francis N, Warrell DA, 1993, Pathology and pathophysiology of human malaria, *Bruce-Chwatt's Essential Malariology*, 3rd edn, eds Gilles HM, Warrell DA, Edward Arnold, London, 50–9.

Franzen L, Shabo B et al., 1984, Analysis of clinical specimens by hybridization with a probe containing repetitive DNA for *Plasmodium falciparum* malaria, *Lancet*, **1:** 525–7.

Fritsch B, Dieckmann A et al., 1987, Glutathione and peroxide metabolism in malaria-parasitized erythrocytes, *Parasitol Res*, **73:** 515–17.

Fry M, 1991, Mitochondria of *Plasmodium*, *Biochemical Protozoology*, eds Coombs GH, North MJ, Taylor and Francis, London, 154–67.

Galbraith RM, Fox H et al., 1980, The human materno-foetal relationship in malaria. II. Histological, ultrastructural and immunopathological studies of placenta, *Trans R Soc Trop Med Hyg*, **74:** 61–72.

Gardner MJ, Feagin JE et al., 1993, Sequence and organization of large subunit rRNA genes from the extrachromosomal 35 kb circular DNA of the malaria parasite *Plasmodium falciparum*, *Nucleic Acids Res*, **21:** 1067–71.

Garnham PCC, 1966, *Malaria Parasites and Other* Haemosporidia, 1st edn, Blackwell Scientific, Oxford.

Garnham PCC, Bird RG, Baker JR, 1962, Electron microscope studies of motile stages of malaria parasites. III. The oökinetes of *Haemamoeba* and *Plasmodium*, *Trans R Soc Trop Med Hyg*, **56:** 116–20.

Genton B, Smith T et al., 1994, Malaria – How useful are clinical criteria for improving the diagnosis in a highly endemic area?, *Trans R Soc Trop Med Hyg*, **88:** 537–41.

Gero AM, O'Sullivan WJ, 1990, Purines and pyrimidines in malarial parasites, *Blood Cells*, **16:** 467–84.

Gilles HM, 1991, *Management of Severe and Complicated Malaria. A Practical Handbook*, WHO, Geneva.

Gilles HM, 1993, Diagnostic methods in malaria, *Bruce-Chwatt's Essential Malariology*, 3rd edn, eds Gilles HM, Warrell DA, Edward Arnold, London, 78–95.

Gilles HM, Hendrickse RG et al., 1967, Glucose-6-phosphate dehydrogenase deficiency, sickling and malaria in African children in South Western Nigeria, *Lancet*, **1:** 138–40.

Gilles HM, Ikeme AC, 1960, Haemoglobinuria among adult Nigerians due to glucose phosphate dehydrogenase deficiency with drug sensitivity, *Lancet*, **2:** 889–91.

Gilles HM, Phillips RE, 1988, Malaria, *Medicine International – Infections*, eds Gilles HM, Warrell DA, 2220–5.

Gilles HM, Warrell DA, 1993, *Bruce-Chwatt's Essential Malariology*, 3rd edn, Edward Arnold, London.

Gilles HM, Lawson JB et al., 1969, Malaria, anaemia and pregnancy, *Ann Trop Med Parasitol*, **63:** 245–63.

Ginsburg H, Stein WD, 1991, Kinetic modelling of chloroquine uptake by malaria-infected erythrocytes. Assessment of the factors that may determine drug resistance, *Biochem Pharmacol*, **41:** 1463–70.

Ginsburg H, Krugliak M et al., 1985, New permeability pathways induced in membranes of *Plasmodium falciparum*-infected erythrocytes, *Mol Biochem Parasitol*, **8:** 177–90.

Gordon DM, McGovern TW et al., 1995, Safety, immunogenicity, and efficacy of a recombinantly produced *Plasmodium falciparum* circumsporozoite protein-hepatitis B surface antigen subunit vaccine, *J Infect Dis*, **171:** 1576–85.

Grau GE, Behr C, 1994, T cells and malaria: is Th1 cell activation a prerequisite for pathology?, *Res Immunol*, **145:** 441–54.

Grau GE, Taylor TE et al., 1989, Tumour necrosis factor and disease severity in children with falciparum malaria, *N Engl J Med*, **320:** 1586–91.

Grau GE, Frei K et al., 1990, Interleukin-6 production in experimental cerebral malaria. Modulation by anti-cytokine antibodies and possible role in hyper gammaglobulinemia, *J Exp Med*, **172:** 1505–8.

Green SJ, Mellouk S et al., 1990, Cellular mechanisms of non-specific immunity to intracellular infection: cytokine-induced synthesis of toxic nitrogen oxides from L-Arginine by macrophages and hepatocytes, *Immunol Lett*, **25:** 15–20.

Green TJ, Morhardt M et al., 1981, Serum inhibition of merozoite dispersal from *Plasmodium falciparum* schizonts; indicator of immune status, *Infect Immun*, **31:** 1203–8.

Greenwood AM, Greenwood BM et al., 1987, A prospective study of the outcome of pregnancy in a rural area of the Gambia, *Bull W H O*, **65:** 635–43.

Greenwood AM, Menendez C et al., 1994, The distribution of birthweight in Gambian women who received malaria chemoprophylaxis during their first pregnancy and in control women, *Trans R Soc Trop Med Hyg*, **88:** 311–12.

Greenwood BM, Baker JR, 1993, A malaria control trial using insecticide-treated bed nets and targeted chemoprophylaxis in a rural area of the Gambia, West Africa, *Trans R Soc Trop Med Hyg*, **87, Suppl. 2:** 60.

Greenwood BM, Marsh K, Snow R, 1991, Why do some African children develop severe malaria?, *Parasitol Today*, **7:** 277–81.

Greenwood BM, Bradley AH et al., 1987, Mortality and morbidity from malaria among children in a rural area of The Gambia, West Africa, *Trans R Soc Trop Med Hyg*, **81:** 478–86.

Greenwood BM, Greenwood AM et al., 1989, The effects of malaria chemoprophylaxis given by traditional birth attendants on the course and outcome of pregnancy, *Trans R Soc Trop Med Hyg*, **83:** 589–94.

Gutteridge WE, Trigg PI, 1970, Incorporation of radioactive precursors into DNA and RNA of *Plasmodium knowlesi* in vitro, *J Protozool*, **17:** 89–96.

Hadley TJ, Miller LH, 1988, Invasion of erythrocytes by malaria parasites; erythrocyte ligands and parasite receptors, *Prog Allerg*, **41:** 49–71.

Haldar K, Henderson CL, Cross GAM, 1986, Identification of the parasite transferrin receptor of *Plasmodium falciparum*-infected erythrocytes and its acylation via 1,2-diacyl-sn-glycerol, *Proc Natl Acad Sci USA*, **83:** 8565–9.

Halloran ME, Struchiner CJ, Spielman A, 1989, Modelling malaria vaccines. II. Population effects of stage-specific malaria vaccines dependent on natural boosting, *Math Bioscience*, **94:** 115–49.

Handunetti SM, Mendis KN, David PH, 1987, Antigenic variation of cloned *Plasmodium fragile* in its natural host *Macaca sinica*. Sequential appearance of successive variant antigenic types, *J Exp Med*, **165:** 1269–83.

Haruki K, Bray PG et al., 1994, Chloroquine resistance in *Plasmodium falciparum*: further evidence for a lack of association with mutations of the Pfmdr1 gene, *Trans R Soc Trop Med Hyg*, **88:** 694.

Hawking F, 1975, Circadian and other rhythms of parasites, *Adv Parasitol*, **13**: 123–82.

Hien TT, White NJ, 1993, Qinghaosu, *Lancet*, **341**: 603–8.

Hill AVS, 1992, Malaria resistance genes: a natural selection, *Trans R Soc Trop Med Hyg*, **86**: 225–6.

Hill AVS, Allsopp CEM et al., 1991, Common West African HLA antigens are associated with protection from malaria, *Nature (London)*, **352**: 595–60.

Ho M, Webster HK, 1989, Immunology of human malaria. A cellular perspective, *Parasite Immunol*, **11**: 105–16.

Ho M, Sexton MM, 1995, Clinical immunology of malaria, *Baillière's Clinical Infectious Diseases – Malaria*, ed Pasvol G, Baillère Tindall, London, 227–47.

Ho M, Singh B et al., 1991, Clinical correlates of in vitro *Plasmodium falciparum* cytoadherence, *Infect Immun*, **59**: 873–8.

Ho M, Tongstawe P et al., 1994, Polyclonal expansion of peripheral γδ T cells in human *Plasmodium falciparum* malaria, *Infect Immun*, **62**: 855–62.

Ho M, Sexton MM et al., 1995, Interleukin-10 inhibits tumor necrosis factor production but not antigen-specific lymphoproliferation in acute *Plasmodium falciparum* malaria, *J Infect Dis*, **172**: 838–44.

Hoffman SL, Isenbarger D et al., 1989, Sporozoite vaccine induces genetically restricted T cell elimination of malaria from hepatocytes, *Science*, **244**: 1078–81.

Holz GG, 1977, Lipids and the malaria parasite, *Bull W H O*, **55**: 237–48.

Homewood CA, Neame KD, 1980, Biochemistry of malarial parasites, *Malaria*, vol 1, ed Kreier JP, Academic Press, New York, 345–405.

Hommel M, 1985, Antigenic variation in malaria parasites, *Immunol Today*, **6**: 28–33.

Hommel M, 1990, Cytoadherence of malaria-infected erythrocytes, *Blood Cells*, **16**: 605–19.

Hommel M, 1991, Steps towards a malaria vaccine, *Res Immunol*, **142**: 611–38.

Hommel M, 1993, Amplification of cytoadherence in cerebral malaria: towards a more rational explanation of disease pathophysiology, *Ann Trop Med Parasitol*, **87**: 627–35.

Hommel M, David PH, Oligino LD, 1983, Surface alterations of erythrocytes in *Plasmodium falciparum* malaria, *J Exp Med*, **157**: 1137–48.

Hommel M, Semoff S, 1988, Expression and function of erythrocyte-associated surface antigens in malaria, *Biol Cell*, **64**: 183–204.

Hommel M, Hughes M, Bond PM et al., 1991, Antibody and DNA probes used to analyse variant populations of the Indochina-1 strain of *Plasmodium falciparum*, *Infect Immun*, **59**: 3975–81.

Howard RJ, 1987, Antigenic variation and antigenic diversity in malaria, *Contrib Microbiol Immunol*, **8**: 176–218.

Hughes MA, Hommel M, Crampton JM, 1989, The use of biotin-labelled oligomers for the detection and identification of *Plasmodium falciparum*, *Parasitology*, **100**: 382–7.

Hunt NH, Stocker R, 1990, Oxidative stress and redox status of malaria-infected erythrocytes, *Blood Cells*, **16**: 499–526.

Jeffery GM, 1966, Epidemiological significance of repeated infections with homologous and heterologous strains and species of *Plasmodium*, *Bull W H O*, **35**: 873–82.

Jensen JB, Boland MT et al., 1983, Association between human serum induced crisis forms in cultured *Plasmodium falciparum* and clinical immunity to malaria in Sudan, *Infect Immun*, **41**: 1302–11.

Jing-Bo-Jiang, Xing-Bo-Go et al., 1982, Antimalarial activity of mefloquine and qinghaosu, *Lancet*, **323**: 285–288.

Karbwang J, Harinasuta T, 1992, *Chemotherapy of Malaria in Southeast Asia*, Ruantasan, Bangkok.

Karunaweera ND, Grau GE et al., 1992, Dynamics of fever and serum levels of tumour necrosis factor are closely associated during clinical paroxysms in *Plasmodium vivax* malaria, *Proc Natl Acad Sci USA*, **89**: 3200–3.

Kawamoto F, 1991, Rapid detection of *Plasmodium* by a new thick smear method using transmission fluorescence microscopy: direct staining with acridine orange, *J Protozool Res*, **1**: 27–34.

Kemp DJ, Thompson JK et al., 1987, Molecular karyotype of *Plasmodium falciparum*: conserved linkage groups and expendable histidine-rich protein genes, *Proc Natl Acad Sci USA*, **84**: 7672–6.

Kern P, Hemmer CJ et al., 1989, Elevated tumour necrosis factor alpha and interleukin-6 serum levels as markers for complicated *Plasmodium falciparum* malaria, *Am J Med*, **57**: 139–43.

Khusmith S, Tharavanij S et al., 1987, Two-site immunoradiometric assay for detection of *Plasmodium falciparum* antigen in blood using monoclonal and polyclonal antibodies, *J Clin Microbiol*, **25**: 1467–71.

Knobloch J, Henk M, 1995, Screening for malaria by determination of parasite-specific lactate dehydrogenase, *Trans R Soc Trop Med Hyg*, **89**: 269–70.

Krishna S, Weller DW et al., 1994, Lactic acidosis and hypoglycaemia in children with severe malaria: pathophysiological and prognostic significance, *Trans R Soc Trop Med Hyg*, **88**: 67–73.

Krogstadt DJ, Gluzman IY et al., 1987, Efflux of chloroquine from *Plasmodium falciparum*: mechanism of chloroquine resistance, *Science*, **235**: 1283–5.

Krotoski WA, Krotoski DM et al., 1980, Relapses in primate malaria: discovery of two populations of exoerythrocytic stages. Preliminary note, *Br Med J*, **1**: 153–4.

Kumaratilake LM, Ferrante A, 1994, T-cell cytokines in malaria: their role in the regulation of neutrophil- and macrophage-mediated killing of *Plasmodium falciparum* asexual blood forms, *Res Immunol*, **145**: 423–9.

Kwiatkowski D, Greenwood BM, 1989, Why is malaria fever periodic? A hypothesis, *Parasitol Today*, **5**: 264–8.

Kwiatkowski D, Molyneux M et al., 1993, Anti-TNF therapy inhibits fever in cerebral malaria, *Q J Med*, **86**: 91–8.

Lalvani A, Aidoo M et al., 1994, An HLA-based approach to the design of a CTL-inducing vaccine against *Plasmodium falciparum*, *Res Immunol*, **145**: 461–8.

Langhorne J, Pells S, Eichmann K, 1993, Phenotypic characterization of splenic T cells from mice infected with *Plasmodium chabaudi chabaudi*, *Scand J Immunol*, **38**: 521–8.

Langsley G, Patarapotikul J et al., 1988, *Plasmodium vivax*: karyotype polymorphism of field isolates, *Exp Parasitol*, **67**: 301–6.

Laserson KF, Petralanda I et al., 1994, Use of polymerase chain reaction to directly detect malaria parasites in blood samples from the Venezuelan Amazon, *Am J Trop Med Hyg*, **50**: 169–80.

Lewallen S, Taylor TE et al., 1993, Ocular fundus filings in Malawian children with cerebral malaria, *Ophthalmologie*, **100**: 857–61.

Lindergard G, 1995, Tools for the evaluation of *Plasmodium malariae* endemicity, MSc Dissertation, University of Liverpool.

Ling IT, Wilson RJM, 1988, Glucose-6-phosphate dehydrogenase activity of the malarial parasite *Plasmodium falciparum*, *Mol Biochem Parasitol*, **31**: 47–56.

Lobel HO, Miani M et al., 1995, Long-term malaria prophylaxis with weekly mefloquine, *Lancet*, **341**: 848–51.

Long GW, Fries L et al., 1995, Polymerase chain reaction amplification from *Plasmodium falciparum* on dried blood spots, *Am J Trop Med Hyg*, **52**: 344–6.

Looaresuwan S, Phillips RE et al., 1985, Quinine and severe falciparum malaria in late pregnancy, *Lancet*, **2**: 4–8.

Looaresuwan S, Viravan C et al., 1992, Randomised trial of artesunate and mefloquine alone and in sequence for acute uncomplicated falciparum malaria, *Lancet*, **339**: 82–4.

Lucas S, 1992, Malaria, *Muir's Textbook of Pathology*, 13th edn, Edward Arnold, London.

Mackey LJ, McGregor IA et al., 1982, Diagnosis of *Plasmodium falciparum* infection in man: detection of parasite antigens by ELISA, *Bull W H O*, **60**: 69–75.

McCutchan TF, Dame JB et al., 1984, Evolutionary relatedness of *Plasmodium* species as determined by the structure of DNA, *Science*, **225**: 808–11.

McGregor IA, 1984, Epidemiology, malaria and pregnancy, *Am J Trop Med Hyg*, **33**: 517–25.

McGregor IA, Barr M, 1962, Antibody response to tetanus toxoid inoculation in malarious and non-malarious Gambian children, *Trans R Soc Trop Med Hyg*, **56**: 364–7.

McGregor IA, Wilson ME, Billewicz WZ, 1983, Malaria infection of the placenta in The Gambia. Its incidence and relationship to stillbirth and placental weight, *Trans R Soc Trop Med Hyg*, **77**: 232–44.

McGuire W, Hill AVS et al., 1994, Variation in the TNF-alpha promoter region associated with susceptibility to cerebral malaria, *Nature (London)*, **371**: 508–10.

MacPherson G, Warrell MJ et al., 1985, Human cerebral malaria: a quantitative ultrastructural analysis of parasitized erythrocytes, *Am J Pathol*, **119**: 385–401.

Makler MT, Hinrichs DJ, 1993, Measurement of the lactate dehydrogenase activity of *Plasmodium falciparum* as an assessment of parasitaemia, *Am J Trop Med Hyg*, **48**: 205–10.

Manderson L, 1994, Community participation and malaria control in Southeast Asia: Defining the principles of involvement, *Southeast Asian J Trop Med Public Health*, **23**: 9–17.

Marsh K, Greenwood BM, 1986, The immunopathology of malaria, *Malaria, Clinics in Tropical Medicine and Communicable Diseases, vol.1*, WB Saunders Company, London, 91–125.

Marsh K, Otoo L et al., 1989, Antibodies to blood stage antigens of *Plasmodium falciparum* in rural Gambians and their relation to protection against infection, *Trans R Soc Trop Med Hyg*, **83**: 293–303.

Marsh K, Forster D et al., 1995, Indicators of life-threatening malaria in African children, *N Engl J Med*, **332**: 1399–404.

Means RT, 1994, Pathogenesis of the anemia of chronic diseases: a cytokine-mediated anemia, *Stem Cells*, **13**: 32–7.

Meek SR, 1995, Vector control in some countries of South East Asia: Comparing the vectors and the strategies, *Ann Trop Med Parasitol*, **89**: 135–47.

Mendis KN, 1991, Malaria vaccine research – a game of chess, *Waiting for the Vaccine*, ed Targett GAT, John Wiley & Sons, Chichester, 183–97.

Mendis KN, Naotunne TD et al., 1990, Anti-parasite effects of cytokines in malaria, *Immunol Lett*, **25**: 217–20.

Menon R, 1972, Pregnancy and malaria, *Med J Malaysia*, **27**: 115–19.

Mercereau-Puijalon O, Fandeur T et al., 1991, Parasite features impeding malaria immunity: antigenic diversity, antigenic variation and poor immunogenicity, *Res Immunol*, **142**: 690–7.

Miller LH, 1976, Innate resistance in malaria, *Exp Parasitol*, **40**: 132–46.

Miller LH, Good MF, Milon G, 1994, Malaria pathogenesis, *Science*, **264**: 1878–83.

Miller LH, Mason SJ et al., 1979, The resistance factor to *Plasmodium vivax* in blacks. The Duffy blood group genotype, *N Engl J Med*, **295**: 302–4.

Miller MF, 1958, Observations on the natural history of malaria in semi-resistant West Africans, *Trans R Soc Trop Med Hyg*, **52**: 152–68.

Mitchell GH, 1989, An update on candidate malaria vaccines, *Parasitology*, **98**, **Suppl.**: S29–S47.

Modiano D, Sawadogo A, Pagnoni F, 1995, Indicators of life-threatening malaria, *N Engl J Med*, **333**: 1011.

Molineaux L, Grammiccia G, 1980, *The Garki Project*, World Health Organisation, Geneva.

Molyneux ME, Fox R, 1993, Diagnosis and treatment of malaria in Britain, *Br Med J*, **306**: 1175–80.

Molyneux ME, Taylor TE et al., 1989, Clinical features and prognostic indicators in paediatric cerebral malaria: a study of 131 comatose Malawian children, *Q J Med*, **71**: 441–59.

Morgan HG, 1994, Placental malaria and low birthweight neonates in urban Sierra Leone, *Ann Trop Med Parasitol*, **88**: 575–80.

Murray MJ, Murray AB et al., 1978, The adverse effect of iron repletion on the course of certain infections, *Br Med J*, **2**: 1113–5.

Nagel RL, 1990, Innate resistance to malaria: the intraerythrocytic cycle, *Blood Cells*, **16**: 321–39.

Naimoli J, Nguyen-Dink et al., 1994, Controlling malaria in Francophone Africa: taking the initiative, USA ID Africa Regional Project (698-0421), 68.

Najera J, Liese B, Hamer JS, 1991, Malaria, *Disease Control Priorities in Developing Countries*, eds Jameson DT, Mosley WH, Oxford University Press, Oxford, 200–10.

Nardin EH, Nussenzweig RS, 1993, T-cell responses to pre-erythrocytic stages of malaria: role in protection and vaccine development against pre-erythrocytic stages, *Ann Rev Immunol*, **11**: 687–727.

Newton CR, Kirkham FJ et al., 1991, Intracranial pressure in African children with cerebral malaria, *Lancet*, **338**: 573–6.

Newton CR, Peshu N et al., 1994, Brain swelling and ischaemia in Kenyans with cerebral malaria, *Arch Dis Child*, **70**: 281–7.

Nguyen Hoan Phu, Day N et al., 1995, Intraleucocytic malaria pigment and prognosis in severe malaria, *Trans R Soc Trop Med Hyg*, **89**: 200–4.

Ockenhouse CF, Tegosho T et al., 1992, Endothelial cell adhesion receptors for *Plasmodium falciparum*-infected erythrocytes: roles for endothelial leukocyte adhesion molecule 1 and vascular cell adhesion molecule 1, *J Exp Med*, **176**: 1183–9.

Okoye VC, Bennett V, 1985, *Plasmodium falciparum* malaria: band 3 as a possible receptor during invasion of human erythrocytes, *Science*, **227**: 169–71.

Oliveira DA, Holloway BP et al., 1995, Polymerase chain reaction and a liquid-phase, nonisotopic hybridization for species-specific and sensitive detection of malaria infection, *Am J Trop Med Hyg*, **52**: 139–44.

Pasvol G, Wilson RJM, 1982, The interaction of malaria parasites with red blood cells, *Br Med Bull*, **38**: 133–40.

Pasvol G, Wainscoat JS, Weatherall DJ, 1982, Erythrocytes deficienct in glycophorin resist invasion by the malarial parasite *Plasmodium falciparum*, *Nature (London)*, **297**: 64–6.

Pasvol G, Clough et al., 1995, The pathogenesis of severe falciparum malaria, *Baillière's Clinical Infectious Diseases – Malaria*, ed Pasvol G, Baillère Tindall, London, 249–70.

Payne D, 1988, Use and limitations of light microscopy for diagnosing malaria at the primary health care level, *Bull WHO*, **66**: 621–6.

Perera MK, Carter R et al., 1994, Transient increase in circulating γδ T cells during *Plasmodium vivax* malarial paroxysms, *J Exp Med*, **179**: 311–5.

Perez HA, Wide A et al., 1995, *Plasmodium vivax*: detection of blood parasites using fluorochrome labelled monoclonal antibodies, *Parasite Immunol*, **17**: 305–12.

Perkins ME, 1992, Rhoptry organelles of apicomplexan parasites, *Parasitol Today*, **8**: 28–32.

Perkins ME, Holt EH, 1988, Erythrocyte receptor varies in *Plasmodium falciparum* isolates, *Mol Biochem Parasitol*, **27**: 23–34.

Perlmann H, Berzins K et al., 1984, Antibodies in malaria sera to parasite antigens in the membrane of erythrocytes infected with early asexual stages of *Plasmodium falciparum*, *J Exp Med*, **159**: 1686–1704.

Peters W, 1980, Chemotherapy of malaria, *Malaria*, vol 1, ed Kreier JP, Academic Press, New York, 145–284.

Petersen E, Marbiah NT, 1994, QBC® and thick films for malaria diagnosis under field conditions, *Trans R Soc Trop Med Hyg*, **88**: 416–7.

Phillips RS, 1994, Malaria vaccines – a problem solved or simply a promising start?, *Protozool Abstr*, **18**: 459–86.

Piper RC, Van Der Jagt DL et al., 1996, Malarial lactate dehydrogenase: target for diagnosis and drug development, *Ann Trop Med Parasitol*, **90**: 433.

Playfair JHL, Taverne J et al., 1990, The malaria vaccine: anti-parasite or anti-disease?, *Immunol Today*, **11**: 25–7.

Premij Z, Minjas JN, Shiff CJ, 1994, Laboratory diagnosis of malaria by village health-workers using the rapid manual ParaSight™-F test, *Trans R Soc Trop Med Hyg*, **88**: 418.

Prensier G, Slomniany CH, 1986, The karyotype of *Plasmodium falciparum* determined by ultrastructural serial sectioning and 3D reconstruction, *J Parasitol*, **72**: 731–6.

Qari SH, Shi YP et al., 1993, Identification of *Plasmodium vivax*-like human malaria parasites, *Lancet*, **341**: 780–3.

Raventos-Suarez C, Pollack S, Nagel RL, 1982, *Plasmodium falciparum*: inhibition of in vitro growth by desferrioxamine, *Am J Trop Med Hyg*, **31**: 919–22.

Reyes P, Rathod P et al., 1982, Enzymes of purine and pyrimidine metabolism from the human malaria parasite, *Plasmodium falciparum*, *Mol Biochem Parasitol*, **5**: 275–90.

Rieckmann KH, Campbell GH et al., 1978, Drug sensitivity of *Plasmodium falciparum*. An in vitro micro technique, *Lancet*, **1**: 22–3.

Riley EM, Allen SJ et al., 1992, Naturally acquired cellular and humoral immune responses to the major merozoite surface antigens (Pf MSP-1) of *Plasmodium falciparum* are associated with reduced malaria morbidity, *Parasite Immunol*, **14**: 321–37.

Roberts DJ, Craig AG et al., 1992, Rapid switching to multiple antigenic and adhesive phenotypes in malaria, *Nature (London)*, **357**: 689–91.

Roberts DJ, Biggs BA et al., 1993, Protection, pathogenesis and phenotypic plasticity in *Plasmodium falciparum* malaria, *Parasitol Today*, **9**: 281–6.

Rockett KA, Awburn MM et al., 1994, Tumor necrosis factor and interleukin-1 synergy in the context of malaria pathology, *Am J Trop Med Hyg*, **50**: 735–42.

Rodriguez MH, Jungery M, 1986, A protein on *Plasmodium falciparum*-infected erythrocytes functions as a transferrin receptor, *Nature (London)*, **324**: 388–91.

Rosenberg R, Wirtz RA et al., 1990, An estimation of the number of malaria sporozoites ejected by a feeding mosquito, *Trans R Soc Trop Med Hyg*, **84**: 209–12.

Rosenberg YJ, 1978, Autoimmune and polyclonal B cell responses during murine malaria, *Nature (London)*, **274**: 170–2.

Roth E, 1990, *Plasmodium falciparum* carbohydrate metabolism: a connection between host cell and parasite, *Blood Cells*, **16**: 453–60.

Roth EF, Raventos-Suarez C et al., 1982, Glutathione stability and oxidative stress in *Plasmodium falciparum* infection in vitro: response of normal and G6PD deficient cells, *Biochem Biophys Res Commun*, **109**: 355–62.

Rougemont A, Boisson ME et al., 1977, Paludisme et anémie de la grossesse en zone de savane africaine, *Bull Soc Pathol Exot Filiales*, **70**: 265–73.

Ruiz W, Kroeger A, 1994, The socioeconomic impact of malaria in Colombia and Ecuador, *Health Policy and Planning*, **9**: 144–54.

Ruwenda C, Khoo SC et al., 1995, Natural selection of hemizygotes and heterozygotes for glucose 6-phosphate dehydrogenase deficiency in Africa by resistance to severe malaria, *Nature (London)*, **376**: 246–9.

Sanchez-Lopez R, Haldar K, 1992, A transferrin-independent iron uptake activity in *Plasmodium falciparum*-infected and uninfected erythrocytes, *Mol Biochem Parasitol*, **55**: 9–20.

Saul A, 1992, Towards a malaria vaccine: riding the rollercoaster between unrealistic optimism and lethal pessimism, *Southeast Asian J Trop Med Public Health*, **23**: 656–71.

Scheibel LW, 1988, Plasmodial metabolism and related organellar function during various stages of the life-cycle: carbohydrates, *Malaria. Principles and Practice of Malariology*, vol 1, eds Wernsdorfer WH and McGregor I, Churchill Livingstone, Edinburgh, 171–217.

Scheibel LW, Ashton SH, Trager W, 1979, *Plasmodium falciparum*: microaerophilic requirements in human red cells, *Exp Parasitol*, **47**: 410–18.

Scheibel LW, Colombani PM et al., 1987, Calcium and calmodulin antagonists inhibit human malaria parasites (*Plasmodium falciparum*): implications for drug design, *Proc Natl Acad Sci USA*, **84**: 7310–14.

Scherf A, Hilbich C et al., 1992, The 11.1 gene of *Plasmodium falciparum* codes for distinct fast evolving repeats, *EMBO J*, **7**: 1129–37.

Schofield L, Vivas L et al., 1993, Neutralizing monoclonal antibodies to glycosylphosphatidylinositol, the dominant TNF-α inducing toxin of *Plasmodium falciparum*: prospects for the immunotherapy of severe malaria, *Ann Trop Med Parasitol*, **87**: 617–26.

Schrevel J, Deguercy A et al., 1990, Proteases in malaria-infected red blood cells, *Blood Cells*, **16**: 563–84.

Schultz, Steketee RW et al., 1995, Antimalarials during pregnancy: a cost effectiveness analysis, *Bull W H O*, **73**: 207–14.

Schwarzer W, Turrini F, Ulliers D, 1992, Impairment of macrophage functions after ingestion of *Plasmodium falciparum*-infected erythrocytes or isolated malarial pigment, *J Exp Med*, **176**: 1033–41.

Sergent E, Parrot L, Donatien A, 1924, Une question de terminologie: immuniser et prémunir, *Bull Soc Pathol Exot Filiales*, **17**: 37–8.

Service M, 1993, The *Anopheles* vector, *Bruce-Chwatt's Essential Malariology*, 3rd edn, eds Gilles HM, Warrell DA, Edward Arnold, London, 97–123.

Shear HL, Nussenzweig RS, Bianco C, 1979, Immune phagocytosis in murine malaria, *J Exp Med*, **149**: 1288–93.

Sherman IW, 1979, Biochemistry of malarial parasites, *Microbiol Rev*, **43**: 453–95.

Sherman IW, 1988, Mechanisms of molecular trafficking in malaria, *Parasitology*, **96**: 857–81.

Sherry BA, Alava G et al., 1995, Malaria-specific metabolite hemozoin mediates the release of several potent endogenous pyrogens (TNF, MIP-1α and MIP-1β) in vitro and alters thermoregulation in vivo, *J Inflammation*, **45**: 85–96.

Shiff CJ, Premij Z, Minjas JN, 1993, The rapid ParaSight™-F test. A new diagnostic tool for *Plasmodium falciparum* infection, *Trans R Soc Trop Med Hyg*, **87**: 29–31.

Shute GT, 1988, The microscopic diagnosis of malaria, *Malaria. Principles and Practice of malariology*, vol 1, eds Wernsdorfer WH and McGregor I, Churchill Livingstone, Edinburgh, 781–814.

Silamut K, White NJ, 1993, Relation of the stage of parasite development in the peripheral blood to prognosis in severe falciparum malaria, *Trans R Soc Trop Med Hyg*, **87**: 436–43.

Singh B, Ho M et al., 1988, *Plasmodium falciparum*: Inhibition/reversal of cytoadherence of Thai isolates to melanoma cells by local immune sera, *Clin Exp Immunol*, **72**: 145–50.

Slater AF, Cerami A, 1992, Inhibition by chloroquine of a novel haem polymerase in malaria trophozoites, *Nature (London)*, **335**: 167–9.

Smalley ME, Abdalla S, Brown J, 1980, The distribution of *Plasmodium falciparum* in the peripheral blood and bone marrow of Gambian children, *Trans R Soc Trop Med Hyg*, **75**: 103–5.

Smith JD, Chitnis CE et al., 1995, Switches in expression of *Plasmodium falciparum var* genes correlate with changes in antigenic and cytoadherent phenotypes of infected erythrocytes, *Cell*, **82**: 101–10.

Smith T, Charlwood JD et al., 1993, Absence of seasonal variation in malarial parasitaemia in an area of intense seasonal transmission, *Acta Trop*, **54**: 55–72.

Snewin VA, England SM et al., 1989, Characterization of the dihydrofolate reductase-thymidylate synthetase gene from human malaria parasites highly resistant to pyrimethamine, *Gene*, **76**: 41–52.

Snounou G, Viriyakosol S et al., 1993, Identification of the four human malaria parasite species in field samples by the polymerase chain reaction and detection of a high prevalence of mixed infections, *Mol Biochem Parasitol*, **58**: 283–92.

Somboon P, Lines J et al., 1995, Entomological evaluation of community-wide use of lambdacyhalothian-impregnated bed nets against malaria in a border area of North West Thailand, *Trans R Soc Trop Med Hyg*, **89:** 248–54.

Sotiriades D, 1936, Passive immunity in experimental and natural malaria, *J Trop Med Hyg*, **39:** 257–60.

Spielman A, Perrone JB, 1989, Rapid diagnosis of malaria, *Lancet*, **1:** 727.

Spitalny GL, Rivera-Ortiz CI, Nussenzweig RS, 1973, *Plasmodium berghei*: relationship between protective immunity and antisporozoite (CSP) antibody in mice, *Exp Parasitol*, **33:** 168–78.

Stahl HD, Crewther PE et al., 1987, Structure of the FIRA gene of *Plasmodium falciparum*, *Mol Biochem Parasitol*, **4:** 199–211.

Steffen R, Fuchs E et al., 1993, Mefloquine compared with other chemoprophylactic regimens in tourists visiting East Africa, *Lancet*, **341:** 1299–303.

Steketee RW, Wirima JJ, 1994, Malaria prevention in pregnancy: The Mangochi malaria research project, USA ID Africa Regional Project (698-0421), 125.

Steketee RW, Taylor T et al., 1994a, Addressing the challenges of malaria control in Africa, USAID Africa Regional Project (698-0421), 59.

Steketee RW, Dioine B et al., 1994b, Controlling malaria in Africa: Progress and priorities, USAID Africa Regional Project (698-0421), 118.

Su XZ, Heatwole VM et al., 1995, The large diverse gene family *var* encodes proteins involved in cytoadherence and antigenic variation of *Plasmodium falciparum*-infected erythrocytes, *Cell*, **82:** 89–100.

Suhrbier A, 1991, Immunity to the liver stage of malaria, *Parasitol Today*, **7:** 160–3.

Taliaferro WH, Cannon PR, 1936, The cellular reactions during primary infections and superinfections of *Plasmodium brasilianum* in Panamian monkeys, *J Infect Dis*, **59:** 72–125.

Tanabe K, 1990, Ion metabolism in malaria-infected erythrocytes, *Blood Cells*, **16:** 437–49.

Taverne J, Bate CA, Playfair JH, 1990, Malaria exoantigens induce TNF, are toxic and are blocked by T-independent antibody, *Immunol Lett*, **25:** 207–12.

Taylor DW, Voller A, 1993, The development and validation of a simple antigen detection ELISA for *Plasmodium falciparum* malaria, *Trans R Soc Trop Med Hyg*, **87:** 29–31.

Taylor K, Bate CAW et al., 1992, Phospholipid containing toxic malaria antigens induce hypoglycaemia, *Clin Exp Immunol*, **90:** 1–5.

Taylor TE, Borgstein A, Molyneux ME, 1993, Acid-base status in paediatric *Plasmodium falciparum* malaria, *Q J Med*, **86:** 99–109.

Taylor TE, Molyneux ME, 1988, Blood glucose levels in Malawian children before and during the administration of intravenous quinine for severe falciparum malaria, *N Engl J Med*, **319:** 1040–7.

Thaithong S, Beale GH et al., 1984, Clonal diversity in a single isolate of the malaria parasite, *Plasmodium falciparum*, *Trans R Soc Trop Med Hyg*, **78:** 242–5.

Tirasophon W, Ponglikitmonghol M et al., 1991, A novel detection of a single *Plasmodium falciparum* in infected blood, *Biochem Biophys Res Comm*, **175:** 179–84.

Trager W, Jensen JB, 1976, Human malaria parasites in continuous culture, *Science*, **193:** 125–9.

Trager W, Williams J, 1992, Extracellular (axenic) development in vitro of the erythrocytic cycle of *Plasmodium falciparum*, *Proc Natl Acad Sci USA*, **89:** 5351–5.

Triglia T, Wellems TE, Kemp DJ, 1992, Towards a high-resolution map of the *Plasmodium falciparum* genome, *Parasitol Today*, **8:** 225–9.

Vadas P, Taylor TE et al., 1993, Increased serum phospholipase A2 activity in Malawian children with falciparum malaria, *Am J Trop Med Hyg*, **49:** 455–9.

Verhave JP, Meis JFG, 1984, The biology of tissue forms and other sexual stages in mammalian plasmodia, *Experientia*, **40:** 1317–29.

Vial HJ, Ancelin ML et al., 1990, Biosynthesis and dynamics of lipids in *Plasmodium falciparum*-infected mature mammalian erythrocytes, *Blood Cells*, **16:** 531–55.

Voller A, 1988, The immunodiagnosis of malaria, *Malaria. Principles and Practice of Malariology*, Vol. 1, eds Wernsdorfer WH and McGregor I, Churchill Livingstone, Edinburgh, 815–25.

Voller A, O'Neill P, 1971, Immunofluorescence method suitable for large scale application to malaria, *Bull W H O*, **45:** 524–9.

Vu thi Ty Hang, Tran Van Be et al., 1995, Screening donor blood for malaria by polymerase chain reaction, *Trans R Soc Trop Med Hyg*, **89:** 44–7.

Wahlgren M, Carlson J, Udomsangpetch R, 1987, Why do *Plasmodium falciparum*-infected erythrocytes form spontaneous rosettes?, *Parasitol Today*, **5:** 183–5.

Waller D, Krishna S et al., 1995, Clinical features and outcome of severe malaria in Gambian children, *Clin Infect Dis*, **21:** 577–87.

Walliker D, Quakyi IA et al., 1987, Genetic analysis of the human malaria parasite *Plasmodium falciparum*, *Science*, **236:** 1661–6.

Warrell DA, 1987, Pathophysiology of severe falciparum malaria in man, *Parasitology*, **94, Suppl.:** S63–S76.

Warrell DA, 1989, Cerebral malaria, *Q J Med*, **71:** 369–71.

Warrell DA, 1993, Clinical features of malaria, *Bruce-Chwatt's Essential Malariology*, 3rd edn, eds Gilles HM, Warrell DA, Edward Arnold, London, 35–49.

Waters AP, 1994, The ribosomal RNA genes of *Plasmodium*, *Adv Parasitol*, **34:** 246–50.

Weatherall DJ, 1988, The anaemia of malaria, *Malaria: Principles and Practice of Malariology*, vol 1, eds Wernsdorfer WH and McGregor I, Churchill Livingstone, Edinburgh, 735–51.

Weber JL, 1988, Molecular biology of malaria parasites, *Exp Parasitol*, **66:** 143–70.

Weidanz WP, Long CA, 1988, The role of T-cells in immunity to malaria, *Malaria Immunology*, vol 41, eds Perlmann P, Wigzell H, Karger, Basel, 215–22.

Wellems TE, Walker JA, Panton LJ, 1991, Genetic mapping of the chloroquine-resistance locus on *Plasmodium falciparum* chromosome 7, *Proc Natl Acad Sci USA*, **88:** 3382–6.

Wellems TE, Panton LJ et al., 1990, Chloroquine resistance not linked to mdr-like genes in a *Plasmodium falciparum* cross, *Science*, **345:** 253–8.

Wernsdorfer WH, Payne D, 1988, Drug sensitivity tests in malaria parasites, *Malaria. Principles and Practice of Malariology*, vol 2, eds Wernsdorfer WH and McGregor I, Churchill Livingstone, Edinburgh, 1765–1800.

Wertheimer SP, Barnwell JW, 1989, *Plasmodium vivax* interaction with the human blood group glycoprotein: identification of a parasite receptor-like protein, *Exp Parasitol*, **69:** 340–50.

White NJ, 1988, Drug treatment and prevention of malaria, *J Pharmacol*, **34:** 1–14.

White NJ, 1992, The pathophysiology of malaria, *Adv Parasitol*, **31:** 83–173.

White NJ, Warrell DA et al., 1983, Severe hypoglycaemia and hyperinsulinaemia in falciparum malaria, *N Engl J Med*, **309:** 61–6.

White NJ, Miller KD et al., 1987, Hypoglycaemia in African children with severe malaria, *Lancet*, **1:** 708–11.

Wickramasuriya GWA, 1937, *Malaria and Ankylostomiasis in Pregnant Women*, Oxford University Press, Oxford, 5–90.

Wilkinson RJ, Brown JL et al., 1994, Severe falciparum malaria: Predicting the effect of exchange transfusion, *Q J Med*, **87:** 553–5.

Willcox, MC, 1975, Thalassaemia in Northern Liberia: a survey in the Mount Nimba area, *J Med Genet*, **12:** 55–63.

Wilson RJM, McGregor IA, Williams K, 1975, Occurrence of S-antigens in serum in *Plasmodium falciparum* infections in man, *Trans R Soc Trop Med Hyg*, **69:** 453–9.

Winograd E, Sherman IW, 1989, Characterization of a modified red cell membrane protein expressed on erythrocytes infected with the human malaria parasite *Plasmodium falciparum*: possible role as a cytoadherence mediating protein, *J Cell Biol*, **108:** 23–30.

World Health Organization, 1978, Proposals for the nomenclature of salivarian trypanosomes and for the maintenance of reference collections, *Bull W H O*, **56:** 467–80.

World Health Organization, 1988, Malaria diagnosis: memorandum from a WHO meeting, *Bull W H O*, **66:** 575–94.

World Health Organization, 1992, Global malaria control strategy (Conference on Malaria, Amsterdam, 26–27 October 1992), *Document CTD/MCM/92-3.*

World Health Organization, 1994a, World Malaria situation in 1992, *Wkly Epidemiol Rec No. 42, 309-314: No. 43, 317–321: No. 44, 325–330.*

World Health Organization, 1994b, Antimalarial drug policies. Report of an informal consultation, WHO/Mal/94.1070, Geneva 14–18 March 1994, 67.

World Health Organization, 1995, Vector Control for malaria and other mosquito-borne diseases, *WHO Technical Report Series 857*, 99.

Wozencraft AO, Dockrell HM et al., 1984, Killing of human malaria parasites by macrophage secretory products, *Infect Immun*, **43:** 664–9.

Yuthavong Y, Wilairat P et al., 1979, Alterations in membrane proteins of mouse erythrocytes infected with different species and strains of malaria parasites, *Comp Biochem Physiol*, **63B:** 83–5.

Zavala F, Tam JP, Masuda A, 1986, Synthetic peptides as antigens for the detection of humoral immunity to *Plasmodium falciparum* sporozoites, *J Immunol Methods*, **93:** 55–61.

Zuckerman A, 1977, Current status of the immunology of blood and tissue protozoa. II. Plasmodium, *Exp Parasitol*, **42:** 374–446.

MICROSPORIDIANS

A Curry

Protozoa of the phylum *Microspora* are all obligate intracellular parasites with a unique mode of entering host cells via a polar tube within a spore. Microsporidians are among the most successful and widespread groups of intracellular parasites in animals (Sprague and Vávra 1977, Canning and Lom 1986, Weidner 1991), infecting other protozoa (Ball 1969, Cali 1991), bryozoans, arthropods, fish, amphibians, reptiles, birds and mammals. Some are hyperparasites (Hussey 1971). Microsporidians are eukaryotes of ancient origin (Canning and Lom 1986, Vossbrinck et al. 1987) and about 100 genera and about 1000 species are currently recognized worldwide (Sprague, Becnel and Hazard 1992). They lack mitochondria and their ribosomes are similar to those found in prokaryotes. Relatively few microsporidian species infect homeothermic vertebrates (birds and mammals) and before the recognition of human immunodeficiency virus (HIV) infection and the acquired immunodeficiency syndrome (AIDS), only a handful of human infections were reported in the literature. However, with the spread of HIV infection and AIDS, microsporidia are becoming increasingly recognized as important causes of opportunistic disease in infected individuals. Several previously unrecognized microsporidian species, some of which may be unique to humans, have recently been described.

1 CLASSIFICATION AND TAXONOMIC CHARACTERISTICS

Much of the current taxonomy is based on light microscopy, ultrastructural features, host species and organ or tissue specificity. Important ultrastructural features include nuclear arrangement (mono- or diplokaryotic), mode of division, development of proliferative forms in direct contact with host cell cyto-

plasm or within a parasitophorous vacuole, sporogony producing spores dispersed or aggregated in a sporophorous vesicle and spore structure. Many amendments and revisions to the current classification are likely as extensive molecular studies are undertaken and this will significantly alter the currently accepted classification.

1.1 *Encephalitozoon*

See Canning and Lom (1986). Unpaired (isolated) nuclei in all stages of development. Development occurs in parasitophorous vacuoles, which contain a finely granular matrix. Meronts lie attached to the vacuolar membrane, whereas sporogony, which is generally disporoblastic, occurs within the lumen of the parasitophorous vacuole. Merogony typically by binary fission supplies abundant potential sporonts and the vacuole concomitantly expands to accommodate the growing numbers of parasites. Vacuoles contain mature and maturing spores. Spores are small with a thick endospore layer and a rugose exospore.

Three species of *Encephalitozoon* have been recognized in humans: *E. cuniculi* (type species), *E. hellem* and *E. intestinalis* (synonym for *Septata intestinalis*). Spores of *E. cuniculi* measure about 2.5–3.2 × 1.2–1.6 μm, with 4–6 coils of the polar tube (Canning and Lom 1986). Spores of *E. hellem* measure 2–2.5 × 1–1.5 μm, with 6–8 coils of the polar tube (Didier ES et al. 1991). Spores of *E. intestinalis* measure 2.2 × 1.2 μm, with 5–7 coils of the polar tube (Canning et al. 1994).

1.2 *Enterocytozoon*

See Desportes et al. (1985), Cali and Owen (1990). Unpaired nuclei in all stages of development. Merogonic and sporogonic stages lie in direct contact with the host cell cytoplasm. Proliferative stages develop into sporogonial plasmodia which produce sporoblasts by multiple fission. Membrane-bound electron-lucent clefts conspicuous in both meronts and sporonts. In the multinucleated sporogonial plasmodia, polar tube precursors form as electron-dense discs adjacent to the clefts. A unique characteristic of this genus is the complete differentiation of the polar tube within the sporogonial plasmodium, prior to fission (Wongtavatchai, Conrad and Hedrick 1995). On division into sporoblasts and maturation of these into spores, each becomes dispersed within the host cell cytoplasm.

One species has been recorded from humans, the type species *Enterocytozoon bieneusi*. Spores are very small (1.8 × about 1 μm), with 4–6 coils of the polar tube in 2 rows. Endospore layer is thin. To avoid confusion with species of *Encephalitozoon*, *Enterocytozoon bieneusi* will be referred to as *Ent. bieneusi*, as used in Canning et al. (1993).

1.3 *Trachipleistophora*

See Hollister et al. (1996). Unpaired nuclei in all stages of development. Plasma membrane of meronts is overlain by a dense surface coat which extends outwards as branched and anastomosing processes. Meronts divide by binary fission or plasmotomy. At the onset of sporogony, the surface coat separates and becomes the thick envelope of the sporophorous vesicle. Sporonts divide repeatedly by binary fission of binucleate stages to give a variable number of uninucleate sporoblasts and spores. Multinucleate sporogonial plasmodia are not formed.

One species has been recorded from humans, the type species *T. hominis*. Spores measure 5.2 × 2.4 μm, with about 11 coils of the polar tube. Endospore is thick.

1.4 *Pleistophora*

See Canning and Lom (1986). Unpaired nuclei in all stages of development. Meronts form as multinucleate plasmodia which possess a thick amorphous electron-dense surface coat external to the plasma membrane. Division into smaller segments occurs. Surface coat becomes the wall of the sporophorous vesicles (**pansporoblast membranes**). Sporogony is polysporoblastic. Division of the sporogonial plasmodium is by repeated segmentation, finally producing uninucleate sporoblasts which mature into spores. The number of spores produced within the sporophorous vesicles is large and variable (**polysporoblastic**).

A few cases of human infection have been ascribed to parasites belonging to the genus *Pleistophora* but the species have not been named nor has their full development been described. These parasites may not be true species of *Pleistophora* and some may have to be reclassified within the genus *Trachipleistophora* (Hollister et al. 1996). Spores from human infections measure 3.2–3.4 × 2.8 μm, with 11 coils of the polar tube (Ledford et al. 1985) or about 4 × 2 μm, with 9–12 coils of the polar tube (Chupp et al. 1993).

1.5 *Vittaforma*

See Silveira and Canning (1995). Nuclei in diplokaryotic arrangement throughout the life cycle. All stages individually enveloped by cisternae of the host cell rough endoplasmic reticulum. Merogony is by binary fission and sporogony is polysporoblastic, giving rise to 4–8 linearly arranged sporoblasts.

One species has been recorded from humans, the type species *Vittaforma corneae*. Spores, still enveloped by host endoplasmic reticulum, measure 3.8 × 1.2 μm, with 5–7 coils of the polar tube.

1.6 *Nosema*

See Canning and Lom (1986). Nuclei in diplokaryotic arrangement throughout the life cycle. Parasites are in direct contact with the host cell cytoplasm. Merogony is by binary fission and sporogony is disporoblastic giving rise to spores which are dispersed in host cell cytoplasm.

Three species have been recorded from humans, *N. connori* (Sprague 1974, Shadduck, Kelsoe and Helmke 1979). Spores measure 4–4.5 × 2–2.5 μm, with 10–11 coils of the polar tube, *N. corneum* (Shadduck et al. 1990) (synonym for *V. corneae*) and *N. ocularum* (Cali et al. 1991a). Spores measure 3 × 5 μm, with 9–12 coils of the polar tube.

1.7 '*Microsporidium*'

See Canning and Lom (1986). An assemblage of identifiable species for which the generic positions are uncertain because of insufficient taxonomic detail. These include *M. ceylonensis* (Ashton and Wirasinha 1973) in which the spores measure 3.5 × 1.5 μm and with about 9 coils of the polar tube and *M. africanum* (Pinnolis et al. 1981) 4.5–5 × 2.5–3 μm, with 11–13 coils of the polar tube.

2 STRUCTURE AND LIFE CYCLE

The most familar stage of microsporidia is the small highly resistant, gram-positive staining spore (Fig. 21.1). Spores contain a coiled filament (**polar filament** or **polar tube**) and an infective sporoplasm. The polar tube and its associated organelles are responsible for the unique mode of entering host cells exhibited by microsporidia. Several reviews of the ultrastructure and general biology of microsporidia have been published (Canning and Lom 1986, Cali 1991, Perkins 1991, Canning 1993).

Microsporidian spores are small, more or less ovoid, with a double-layered spore wall. The outer layer, or **exospore**, is proteinaceous and electron-dense and, according to Weidner and Halonen (1993), is partially stabilized by kera-

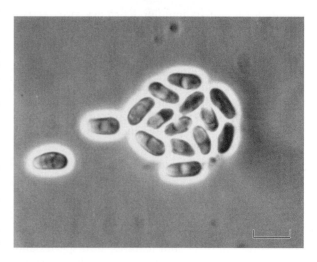

Fig. 21.1 Light micrograph of spores of *Trachipleistophora hominis* showing shape and posterior vacuole. Bar = 4 μm. (Reproduced with permission from WS Hollister and EU Canning.)

tins. The inner layer, or **endospore**, is chitinous and electron-lucent. The plasma membrane lines the inside of the spore wall. Organelles within the cytoplasm are the polar sac, polar tube, polaroplast, nucleus and posterior vacuole (Figs. 21.2, 21.3). All forms lack mitochondria, centrioles, peroxisomes and a classical Golgi apparatus (Canning 1988, Cali 1991). Ribosomes are of prokaryotic size. The polar sac (or anchoring disc), shaped like the cap of a mushroom, is continuous with the polar tube, the base of which appears like the stalk of the mushroom. A thin layer of cytoplasm separates the polar sac from the spore wall. The endospore layer immediately above the polar sac is thinned. From its insertion in the polar sac, the polar tube is initially straight (the **manubrium**) before coiling into loops around the inside of the spore wall (Fig. 21.4). This polar tube is a complex organelle with intricate anatomical relationships to the other structures of the mature spore (Jensen and Wellings 1972). The structure of the polar tube in the ungerminated spore appears to be tubular, with a filled lumen and concentric rings (Weidner 1982), and appears to be composed of a single polypeptide of low molecular weight (Weidner 1976). It is surrounded by a membrane. Around the manubrium is located the **polaroplast**, which is a component of the extrusion apparatus. Ultrastructurally, the polaroplast is composed of a stack of closely apposed membranes. By light microscopy, the polaroplast region appears transparent and is often referred to as the anterior vacuole. The nucleus is surrounded by a nuclear envelope. In some microsporidial species, nuclei are paired with apposed membranes flattened against one another in a diplokaryon arrangement. The posterior region of the spore is occupied by a membrane-bound posterior vacuole.

On entering a suitable host, the emergence of the polar tube is initiated within a fraction of a second (Weidner 1976). The extruded tube can be very long compared with the size of the spore and is a flexible structure the purpose of which is to penetrate a host cell and allow entry of the infective sporoplasm. The extrusion process appears to be initiated by swelling of the spore stimulated by a rise in pH and the presence of calcium ions (Weidner and Byrd 1982).

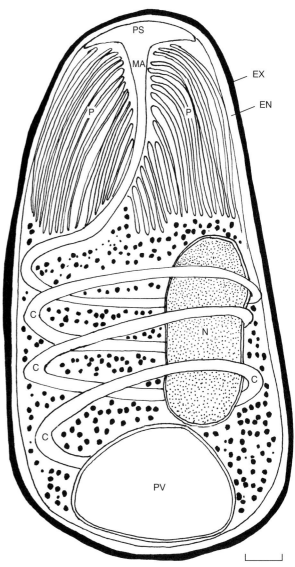

Fig. 21.3 Diagram showing general features of a microsporidian spore. C, coils of polar tube; EN, endospore; EX, exospore; MA, manubrium; N, nucleus; P, polaroplast; PS, polar sac; PV, posterior vacuole.

Swelling of the polar sac and polaroplast causes the thin anterior area of the spore wall to rupture, a prerequisite for polar tube eversion. The polar tube is proteinaceous in nature and is believed to be extruded as a solid cylinder, the interior of which flows outward at the growing tip to form a hollow cylinder (Weidner 1982). Once fully everted, the migration of the sporoplasm commences, driven by processes associated with the posterior vacuole. The multilamellar nature of the polaroplast diminishes during extrusion and provides the plasma membrane surrounding the sporoplasm as it arrives within the host cell cytoplasm (Weidner 1982). The migration of the sporoplasm through the lumen of the extruded polar tube occurs within 5–30 s (Weidner 1976) and causes some slight distension of the tube.

Discharged spores, devoid of the sporoplasm, appear empty and show that the proximal part of the polar tube is funnel-shaped, perhaps to guide the sporoplasm cytoplasm into the tube lumen. Little remains of the polaroplast membranes and the externalized polar tube has a flaccid appearance after passage of the sporoplasm cytoplasm.

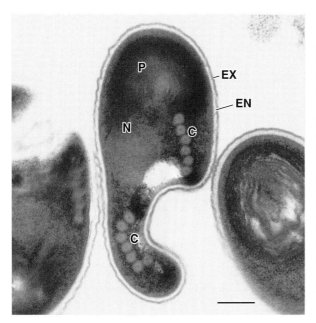

Fig. 21.2 Electron micrograph of a section through a spore of *Encephalitozoon hellem*, showing the coiled polar tube (C), electron-dense exospore (EX), electron-lucent endospore (EN), nucleus (N), polaroplast (P). Bar = 0.18 μm.

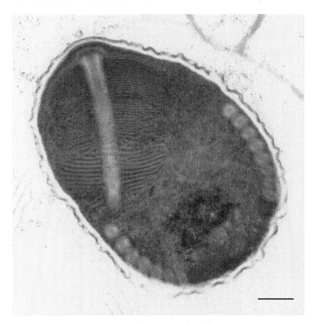

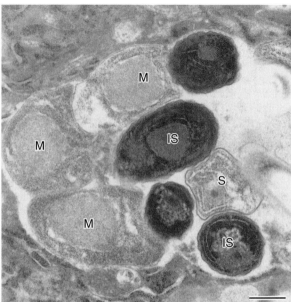

Fig. 21.4 Electron micrograph of a mature spore of *Trachipleistophora hominis*, showing manubrium, polaroplast and coiled polar tube. Bar = 0.48 μm. (Reproduced with permission from Andrew S Field.)

Fig. 21.5 *Encephalitozoon hellem* from nasal epithelium. Electron micrograph showing parasitophorous vacuole containing meronts (M), a sporont (S) and immature spores (IS). Bar = 0.37 μm.

In some species, penetration into a host cell occurs by the polar tube punching a hole in the host cell plasma membrane without loss of cytoplasm. In other species, penetration appears to induce host-cell plasma membrane expansion to cover the emerging sporoplasm, which is itself covered by a membrane thought to be derived from the polaroplast: an example is *Encephalitozoon* (Canning et al. 1992).

Inside the host cell, proliferation begins and 2 major phases are recognized, **merogony** and **sporogony**. In both these phases, the parasite nuclei divide without breakdown of the nuclear envelope. Nutrients are absorbed from the host cell to fuel parasite development (Canning and Lom 1986).

Meronts are rounded, irregular or elongated cells with little differentiation of the cytoplasm and are surrounded by a plasma membrane. In most species, the meronts are in direct contact with the host cell cytoplasm (e.g. *Ent. bieneusi*). However, meronts of *Encephalitozoon* are surrounded by a membrane derived from the host cell which ultimately forms the margin of a parasitophorous vacuole seen in the later stages of parasite development. Meronts may divide by binary fission, multiple fission of a multinucleate meront, or **plasmotomy** (fission of multinucleate parasite to form multinucleate offspring by division of the cytoplasm without relation to that of the nuclei).

Meronts develop into sporonts characterized by the presence of an electron-dense surface coat, on the outside of the plasma membrane, which will ultimately become the exospore layer of the mature spore wall (Fig. 21.5). Sporonts may divide by binary fission directly into **sporoblasts** (cells that differentiate into spores without further division) or may become multinucleate and form **sporogonial plasmodia** (Fig. 21.6). Sporogonial plasmodia undergo multiple (sequential) fission to produce sporoblasts which ultimately develop into spores. The endospore layer of the spore wall is synthesized between the dense exospore layer and the plasma membrane. Spores may be liberated by lysis of the host cell, although in some species, such as *E. hellem*, mature spores

may germinate and infect other neighbouring cells without lysis of the host cell (Canning et al. 1992) (Fig. 21.7).

Chromosomal separation during mitosis is facilitated by an intranuclear spindle. The mitotic apparatus consists of 2 centriolar plaques (electron-dense regions associated with nuclear pores) at the spindle apices, on which the spindle microtubules converge (Canning 1988). Sexual processes, as indicated by synaptonemal complexes (reported in some

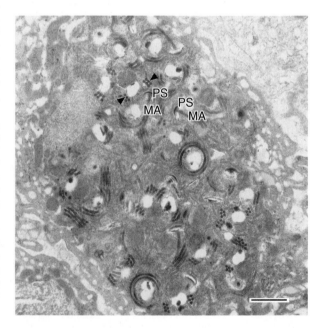

Fig. 21.6 Late sporogonial sporoplasm of *Enterocytozoon bieneusi* showing many copies of spore organelles. Multiple fission will produce sporoblasts which will mature into spores. Note manubrium (MA), polar sac (PS) and 6 coils in 2 rows of a polar tube (arrowheads). Bar = 0.64 μm.

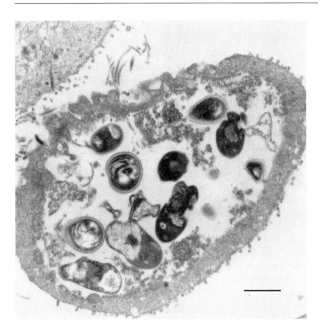

Fig. 21.7 *Encephalitozoon hellem* from conjunctival epithelium. Parasitophorous vacuole containing spores. Note that some have germinated as indicated by the presence of prophiles of polar tubes between and around the spores. Bar = 1 μm.

genera parasitizing invertebrates) are poorly understood (Canning 1988, Raikov 1995). Among the genera that infect vertebrates, meiosis is either unknown or unconfirmed.

3 CLINICAL ASPECTS

3.1 Historical aspects of human infection

The historical aspects of human microsporidial infection have been reviewed by Canning and Lom (1986). There were several reports in the 1920s and 1930s but in none of these was the microsporidial nature of the infection determined and some may have been due to other parasites such as *Toxoplasma gondii*.

In 1927, Torres (1927a,b,c) described 3 fatal cases in humans ascribed to infection by *Encephalitozoon* but, unfortunately, the type material has been lost and confirmation of the microsporidial nature of these infections cannot now be determined (Weiser 1964).

The first authenicated case of human microsporidial infection was by Matsubayashi and colleagues (1959) who described a case of microsporidial infection in a 9 year old Japanese boy suffering a severe convulsive illness and admitted to hospital unconscious and with a fever. Organisms resembling *E. cuniculi* were isolated on day 5 of the illness from the cerebrospinal fluid and on the days 13–15 spores were identified from the urine. On regaining consciousness, headache and vomiting were recurrent symptoms but the boy is reported to have made a full recovery.

A 3 year old Colombian child suffered a similar convulsive illness (Bergquist et al. 1984) and spores of *E. cuniculi* were isolated from the urine. After anticonvulsive therapy, the child made a full recovery. Ashton and Wirasinha (1973) described a case of corneal infection in an 11 year old Sri

Lankan boy. Although it was not specifically identified by the original authors, Canning and Lom (1986) transferred this organism to the collective group *Microsporidium* and named it *M. ceylonensis*. Margileth and colleagues (1973) described a case history of an overwhelming disseminated infection in a 4 month old infant with a defective lymphoid system. After an illness lasting 4 months, characterized by diarrhoea and malabsorption and concurrent infection with *Pneumocystis carinii*, the child died. Microsporidian spores were seen in both cardiac and smooth muscle, diaphragm, myocardium, kidney tubules, liver, lungs and adrenal cortex and within the walls of arteries in many organs. On the basis of the cytoplasmic and ultrastructural features of the sporoblasts, immature and mature spores, particularly the diplokarya and about 11 coils of the polar tube, the organism was tentatively classified as *Nosema connori* (Sprague 1974, Shadduck, Kelsoe and Helmke 1979, Canning and Lom 1986).

Since the recognition of HIV and AIDS in the late 1970s and early 1980s several previously rare or unknown human parasitic protozoa have been recognized in this immunocompromised group (Curry, Turner and Lucas 1991). In 1985, a new microsporidian was identified in the duodeno-jejunal enterocytes of an AIDS patient with a 5 month history of diarrhoea, weight loss, epigastric pain and fever (Desportes et al. 1985, Modigliani et al. 1985). The organism involved, *Enterocytozoon bieneusi*, has now been recognized as one of the commonest enteric infections found in AIDS patients. Since this description several more species and sites of infection have been described in patients with HIV but it is not known whether such microsporidial infections are acquired from a zoonotic source or whether they involve reactivation of a latent asymptomatic or clinically transient infection (Weber and Bryan 1994).

3.2 Serological surveys of microsporidial infection in humans

Before our recent awareness of human microsporidial infections, one of the few species known to infect homeothermic vertebrates was *E. cuniculi* (Levine 1985, Canning and Lom 1986) which has a worldwide distribution in many mammals including rodents, lagomorphs, carnivores and primates. It is a multiorgan pathogen found in the brain, kidneys, liver, spleen and other organs. In the past it caused many problems in animal houses, and serological tests are now available to test for such infections (Canning and Lom 1986). Considering its wide host range in homeothermic vertebrates, it is not surprising that encephalitozoonosis has also been reported in humans. Bergquist and colleagues (1984) reported the results of a serological survey for *E. cuniculi* in 22 serum samples from human patients with disorders of the central nervous system (all of uncertain origin); one sample gave clearly positive results. The patient was an apparently healthy Colombian boy, adopted when just over 1 year old by a Swedish family, who was admitted to hospital a year later with generalized convulsive seizures. Based on an indirect immunofluorescence technique, a serum sample taken from the boy about the time of adoption (a year before initial admission to hospital) showed a positive IgM antibody response to *E. cuniculi*. This original serum sample and those taken during his subsequent admissions to hospital also showed high titres of IgG against *E. cuniculi*. Sedimented urine, obtained during his first stay in hospital, contained gram-positive spores measuring 1.5 × 2.5 μm, which reacted with a fluorescent anti-*E. cuniculi* conjugate. Urine-derived organisms were injected intraperitoneally into 5 mice known to be free of encephalitozoonosis and, after 3 weeks, 2 became infected with parasites indistinguishable from *E. cuniculi*. Haematological testing revealed that the child had a lymphocyte abnormality. The child was given prophylactic anticonvulsive therapy and recovered.

A later serological survey for antibodies to *E. cuniculi* using ELISA and utilizing spores harvested from cell culture, demonstrated antibodies to *E. cuniculi* in some patients with psychiatric disorders and also some of those previously exposed to schistosomiasis and malaria (Hollister and Canning 1987).

A more comprehensive survey of human sera (Hollister, Canning and Willcox 1991) utilizing ELISA and also immunofluorescence, immunoperoxidase and western blots of SDS–PAGE protein profiles of *E. cuniculi* spores concluded that human *E. cuniculi* infections were common in the tropics and that reactivation of such infections could account for the occurrence of infections in AIDS patients. Hollister and colleagues (1993) in a retrospective analysis of stored serum samples from an AIDS patient, detected antibodies to *Encephalitozoon* sp. 32 months before signs of keratoconjunctivitis developed and 3 years before nasal obstruction became a problem (Hollister et al. 1993).

3.3 Ocular microsporidioses

Two types of ocular infection have been described: the first involves the conjunctival and corneal epithelium and occurs concomitantly with HIV. The microsporidian involved is a species of *Encephalitozoon*. The second type involves the corneal stroma and leads to ulceration and suppurative keratitis and occurs in immunocompetent individuals, free of HIV infection (Shadduck et al. 1990).

Corneal stromal infections

In 1981, Pinnolis and colleagues published a report of a 26 year old Botswanan woman with a perforated corneal ulcer, who became blind and underwent enucleation. Microsporidial spores were identified mainly in the cytoplasm of corneal histiocytes. The description of the parasite suggested that this was a new species of indeterminate genus and Canning and Lom (1986) named it *Microsporidium africanum*. Shadduck and colleagues (1990) reported a case of a 45 year old HIV-seronegative man with an 18 month history of central disciform keratitis, recurrent patchy infiltration of the anterior stroma and iritis. At biopsy, microsporidia were seen in the corneal stroma by light and electron microscopy. He was treated with topical steroids and broad spectrum antibiotics but ultimately required a corneal transplant. During the transplantation, part of the explanted cornea was inoc-

lated into cell cultures and an infection was established. The organism contained diplokarya, division was by binary fission and the parasite was in intimate contact with the host cell cytoplasm for all stages of the life cycle. Because of these features, it was named *Nosema corneum* and differentiated from *N. connori* (Margileth et al. 1973) by having 6 coils of the polar tube, compared with 10–11 coils in *N. connori*.

Cali and colleagues (1991a) described a case of a 39 year old man with irritation and blurred vision of his left eye. A foreign body was removed but visual problems and a corneal ulcer persisted. A biopsy revealed microsporidia in direct contact with host cell cytoplasm. The nuclei of the parasites were in a diplokaryotic arrangement. The spore size was 3 × 5 μm, with 9–12 coils of the polar tube. The organism was placed in the genus *Nosema* and named *N. ocularum* n. sp.

Silveira, Canning and Shadduck (1993) established an infection of *N. corneum* in athymic mice. Subsequently, Silveira and Canning (1995) revised the classification of this microsporidian based on the ultrastructural development of the organism in the mouse hepatocytes and concluded that it was not a species of *Nosema*, as only the diplokaryotic arrangement of the nuclei was consistent with that genus (Fig. 21.8). Sporogony was polysporoblastic and sporonts were ribbon-shaped, dividing to produce linear arrays of sporoblasts. Each parasite was also completely enveloped by endoplasmic reticulum derived from the host cell (Fig. 21.8). Based on these new taxonomically significant features, the organism was placed in a new genus, *Vittaforma* and specifically named *V. corneae*. *V. corneae* has not yet been described from AIDS patients, but experimental infection in athymic mice suggests that, if established, it could spread systemically and not be restricted to the eyes (Silveira, Canning and Shadduck 1993).

3.4 HIV disease and microsporidial infections

Current information indicates that patients with severe cellular immunodeficiency (as in HIV disease) are at the greatest risk of developing microsporidial disease (Weber and Bryan 1994). Experimental evidence in mice supports this view (Schmidt and Shadduck 1983) and that resistance to lethal disease appears to be T-cell dependent. *E. cuniculi* causes chronic but not life threatening infections in euthymic BALB mice, whereas athymic mice succumb to infection. Serum antibodies are not protective.

Predominantly ocular infections in HIV disease

In the USA in 1990 5 homosexual men with AIDS were diagnosed as having bilateral microsporidial keratoconjunctivitis (Friedberg et al. 1990, Lowder et al. 1990, Orenstein et al. 1990b, Yee et al. 1991). Clinical manifestations included conjunctivitis, foreign-body sensation, blurred vision and photophobia. Concomitant unilateral cytomegalovirus retinitis was noted in 2 patients. Ophthalmic examination revealed a diffuse punctate keratopathy. Histological sections of corneal or conjunctival scrapings contained numerous oval spores, confirmed as being microsporidial by electron microscopy. Seven further cases of ocular microsporidiosis, 5 in homosexual men, one in a male intravenous drug user and one in a woman whose previous

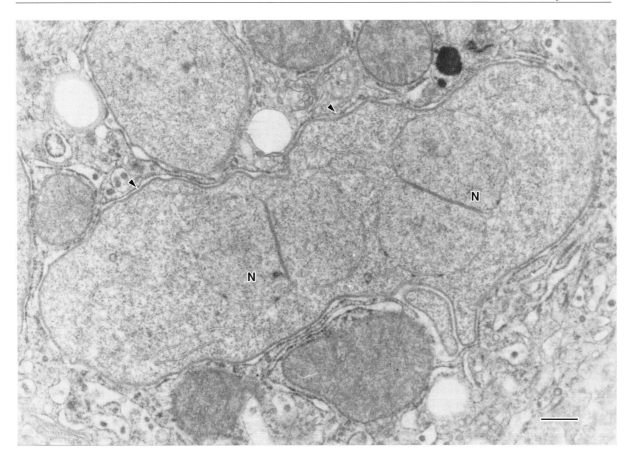

Fig. 21.8 Electron micrograph of a meronts of *Vittaforma corneae* with 2 diplokaryotic nuclei (N). Note that parasite is enveloped by host endoplasmic reticulum (arrowheads) Bar = 0.26 μm. (Reproduced from Silveira and Canning 1995, with permission of authors and publisher.)

sexual partner was an intravenous drug user, have subsequently been reported from the USA (Schwartz et al. 1993a). In the 6 patients for whom data were available, CD4$^+$ lymphocytes were profoundly decreased (mean $26 \times 10^6/l$; range 2–50). The microsporidial species involved was stated to be either *Encephalitozoon* sp. or *E. cuniculi*.

Additional cases of ocular infection from other parts of the world have followed these initial reports. Metcalfe and colleagues (1992) reported a case of keratoconjunctivitis from the UK and McCluskey et al. (1993) reported one from Australia. The Australian case was a homosexual male, with a CD4 count of 83 $\times 10^6/l$, and an *Encephalitozoon*-like species was thought likely to be the microsporidian involved.

The case reported from the UK involved a married man who had homosexual activity before marriage. In contrast to the other published cases, his symptoms of ocular infection had been noted 2 years before diagnosis of microsporidial infection, when his CD4 count was of the order of 200 $\times 10^6/l$. In this individual, both corneae were diffusely covered with fine punctate epithelial opacities and there was also some punctate staining of the interpalpetral bulbar conjunctiva of both eyes. Conjunctival scrapings established the microsporidial nature of the infection (Fig. 21.7). The taxonomic features of this parasite were consistent with a species of the genus *Encephalitozoon* and further study confirmed this

as unpaired nuclei were present at all stages, sporogony was disporoblastic and development in the host cell took place in a vacuole (Canning et al. 1992).

This patient also had nasal obstruction and discharge (Lacey et al. 1992). ENT examination showed multiple nasal polyps and CT showed extensive opacities in the maxillary antra, and ethmoid and sphenoid sinuses, as well as minor cerebral atrophy. A nasal polypectomy was performed and on both histological and electron microscopical examination, many superficial epithelial cells were found to contain microsporidial spores, identical to those found in the corneal and conjunctival scrapings. An interesting feature of the ultrastructural examination was the presence of discharged (or germinated) spores within intact parasitophorous vacuoles (Canning et al. 1992). These would have probably contributed to the chronic nature of this infection (Lacey et al. 1992) if spores discharged their sporogonial contents into adjacent epithelial cells without release from the cell in which development occurred. Cali and colleagues have also noted this premature germination (Cali et al. 1991b).

It is possible that in the UK case infection was initially caused by inoculation of spores into corneal abrasions and infection could have spread from the corneal epithelium through the lacrimal canaliculi and nasolacrimal ducts that drain secretions from the eyes into the nasal sinuses (Curry and Canning 1993). However, ocular infection may possibly be acquired by reverse passage from a respiratory source, as microsporidial infection has been identified within the tracheobronchial epithelium (Weber et al. 1992b, Schwartz et al. 1993b).

The microsporidian species involved in all these AIDS cases was originally described as *E. cuniculi*-like or as *Encepalitozoon* sp., based on morphological characteristics. Isolates from conjunctival or corneal scrapings obtained from 3 American AIDS patients, grown in cultures of Madin–Darby kidney cells (MDCK cells) by Didier ES and colleagues (1991), were all identical by SDS–PAGE analysis but were different from a well-characterized isolate of *E. cuniculi*. Identical banding patterns on western immunoblotting were obtained from each patient's serum, whereas murine antisera to *E. cuniculi* reacted to only some antigens from the tissue culture grown isolates. The differences were sufficient for Didier ES et al. (1991) to propose that the ocular isolates from the AIDS patients studied should be redesignated as a new species, *E. hellem*.

Electron microscopical studies indicate that *E. hellem* and *E. cuniculi* are indistinguishable on ultrastructural grounds (Didier PJ et al. 1991, Vossbrinck et al. 1993, Schwartz et al. 1993a, Visvesvara et al. 1994, Weber et al. 1994). Comparison by SDS–PAGE and western blotting with murine antisera raised to *E. cuniculi*, *E. hellem* and the UK nasal isolate showed significant similarities between *E. hellem* and the nasal isolate, but differences when compared with *E. cuniculi*. Minor protein differences between the nasal isolate and *E. hellem* were not considered sufficient to separate them at the species level and thus the UK isolate was also considered to be *E. hellem*. Ultrastructural studies of the UK isolate of *E. hellem* compared with *E. cuniculi* (Canning et al. 1993, Hollister et al. 1993) demonstrated that in *E. cuniculi* the surface coat of the sporont is secreted as a series of parallel strips which ultimately coalesce to form a uniform coating. By contrast, the sporont coat of *E. hellem* appears to be secreted almost simultaneously over the whole surface of the sporont. Such ultrastructural differences are potentially useful for differentiating the 2 species without recourse to in vitro culture and protein analysis.

PREDOMINANTLY ENTERIC INFECTIONS IN HIV DISEASE

Diarrhoea, malabsorption and wasting are frequently encountered in AIDS patients (Modigliani et al. 1985, Dobbins and Weinstein 1985) and many microbiological causes have been identified for these enteric symptoms; among the parasitic protozoa, both *Cryptosporidium parvum* and microsporidial infections are significant causes of morbidity.

The first reported case of enteric microsporidial infection in an AIDS patient was from France by Desportes et al. (1985). The patient was a 29 year old non-homosexual Haitian patient with AIDS, who had severe diarrhoea and *Giardia duodenalis* in stool specimens. Electron microscopic investigations of duodenal–jejunal and ileal biopsies revealed the presence of developmental stages of a microsporidian parasite in the enterocytes (Fig. 21.6). The ultrastructural details of the development of this microsporidian supported the view that the microsporidial species involved was distinctive enough to merit classification as a new species within a new genus. The name allocated was *Enterocytozoon bieneusi*. As originally described by Desportes et al. (1985), *Ent. bieneusi* appeared to contain closely paired nuclei (diplokarya) but as further cases involving the same organism were reported from the USA (Dobbins and Weinstein 1985) the occurrence of diplokarya was found to be incorrect, as nuclei were never found in a closely abutted arrangement typical of true diplokaryotic nuclei (Cali and Owen 1990).

Enterocytozoon bieneusi has now been reported from several other countries around the world including the UK (Curry et al. 1988), the Netherlands (Rijpstra et al. 1988), Africa (Lucas et al. 1989) and Australia (Field et al. 1993b) and it is now recognized that the majority of microsporidial infections found in patients infected with HIV are attributable to this species (Weber and Bryan 1994). *Ent. bieneusi* infection in the small bowel can show histological changes such as villous blunting or ballooning (Orenstein et al. 1990a, Kotler et al. 1993, Asmuth et al. 1994), although some biopsies show more or less normal villous architecture (Eeftinck Schattenkerk et al. 1991). Crypt hyperplasia may also be found (Field, Marriott and Hing 1993). Inflammation in infected tissues is often minimal (Lucas 1989, Orenstein 1991). Such a variability of changes seen in biopsies may reflect the degree of infection, with heavy infections causing the most cellular and histological changes. *Ent. bieneusi* infection is generally restricted to the enterocytes of the small bowel but infection in other sites has been reported. The biliary tract can be infected, leading to cholangitis (Beaugerie et al. 1992). Such infection may be caused by spread along the intestinal–bile duct epithelium. In addition, there are reports of *Ent. bieneusi* infection in nasal (Hollister and Canning unpublished results, quoted in Canning et al. 1993) and bronchial (Weber et al. 1992b) epithelia and the liver (Pol et al. 1993). Such non-small-intestinal sites of infection involving *Ent. bieneusi* appear to be uncommon, and the mechanism of spread is uncertain.

Association of *Enterocytozoon bieneusi* with symptoms of diarrhoea

A significant number of patients with intestinal microsporidiosis are co-infected with other potential enteric pathogens (Weber and Bryan 1994) making the pathogenic role of microsporidia difficult to assess. However, most prevalence studies of intestinal microsporidiosis in HIV positive patients have shown a strong association with diarrhoea. Greenson et al. (1991) investigated 35 patients with advanced HIV infection, of which 22 had chronic diarrhoea and 13 had no diarrhoea. Five patients (23%) with diarrhoea had *Ent. bieneusi* but no microsporidia were found in the group without diarrhoea. Weber, Bryan and colleagues (Weber et al. 1992a) investigated 134 HIV positive patients and found 4 (3%) positive for *Ent. bieneusi*, all of whom had chronic watery diarrhoea. Microsporidia were not found in any patient with acute diarrhoea or without diarrhoea. Studies from developed countries other than the USA show similar results. In London, Peacock et al. (1991) investigated 59 HIV positive patients with diarrhoea and 20 HIV positive patients with weight loss but no diarrhoea. Of these, 8 patients (13%) were found to be infected with *Ent. bieneusi*, in 5 of whom *Ent. bieneusi* was the sole pathogen found. Again, microsporidia were not found in the group without diarrhoea. In Australia, Field and colleagues (1993) investigated 180 consecutive

HIV infected patients, 109 with chronic diarrhoea and 71 without diarrhoea: 33% (36 of 109 patients) had microsporidial infection, whereas only one patient of the group without diarrhoea was positive; 33 of the total of 37 positives were infected with *Ent. bieneusi*. Eeftinck Schattenkerk et al. (1991) investigated 2 groups of HIV positive patients in the Netherlands, one group with diarrhoea and the second without; 27% (15 of 55 patients) of the group with diarrhoea had *Ent. bieneusi* infection compared with 3% (1 of 38 patients) without diarrhoea. In a further study from the Netherlands, Van Gool et al. (1993), found 16 of 143 (11%) consecutive stool samples from HIV seropositive patients with diarrhoea to contain microsporidial spores. *Ent. bieneusi* occurred in 11 and *Encephalitozoon* (probably *E. intestinalis*) in 5. Three of these were also excreting spores in their urine and spores were identified in maxillary sinus aspirate of 2 of them, suggesting disseminated infection (see 'Disseminated infections involving species of *Encephalitozoon*', p. 420).

In contrast, Rabeneck and colleagues (1993) found that the association between enteric microsporidial infection and diarrhoea was not as strong as previous studies had suggested. No significant difference in the prevalence of microsporidial infection was observed in a group of patients with chronic diarrhoea (33%; 18 of 55) and those without (25%; 13 of 51). This is the only study not to link microsporidial infection to symptoms of chronic diarrhoea in HIV disease.

Prevalence of *Enterocytozoon bieneusi* infection in Africa

In developing countries, such as those in central Africa, diarrhoea and weight loss are important indicators for the clinical diagnosis of AIDS (Kelly et al. 1994). These common manifestations are often referred to as enteropathic AIDS or 'slim disease' (Serwadda et al. 1985, Lucas et al. 1993). Lucas et al. (1989) identified a lower prevalence of microsporidial infection from Uganda and Zambia than in developed countries; 6.5% (5 of 77 patients with chronic diarrhoea and wasting) had *Ent. bieneusi* infection. This low prevalence suggested that patients were dying from other causes (particularly tuberculosis) before their CD4 count had dropped to the critical level of about $100 \times 10^6/l$, where microsporidial infection becomes significant (Canning et al. 1993).

Bretagne et al. (1993) in a survey of children of unknown HIV status from an area of Africa (Niamey, Niger) with a low occurrence of HIV, to determine the prevalence of microsporidial spores in stool samples found that in 990 samples tested, 6 of 593 (1%) with diarrhoea and 2 of 397 (0.5%) without diarrhoea contained *Ent. bieneusi* spores.

A second enteric species, *Encephalitozoon* (=*Septata*) *intestinalis*

A second enteric microsporidian parasite has been found more recently. Originally described as resembling *E. cuniculi* (Orenstein, Dieterich and Kotler 1992, Orenstein et al. 1992), it was subsequently assigned to a new genus and named *Sepata intestinalis* (Cali, Kotler and Orenstein 1993). Unlike *Ent. bieneusi*, intracellular development takes place within a lobed parasitophorous vacuole bounded by a membrane (Fig. 21.9). Within the vacuole, parasites are separated by granular septa secreted by the parasite (Cali, Kotler and Orenstein 1993). It is not confined to epithelial cells as it

is also found in macrophages in the lamina propria. This microsporidian appears to have a primary infection site in the small bowel, but can disseminate to the viscera (see below, p. 420) and has been found in epithelial enterocytes and the lamina propria of the duodenum, jejunum (Orenstein et al. 1992), ileum, colon (Field et al. 1993a), kidney (Orenstein, Dieterich and Kotler 1992, Field et al. 1993a), liver and gallbladder (Orenstein, Dieterich and Kotler 1992) and other sites, including the lower airways (Schwartz et al. 1993b).

This second enteric microsporidian species has been found in AIDS patients in the USA (Orenstein, Dieterich and Kotler 1992), UK (Blanshard et al. 1992b), Australia (Field et al. 1993a) and Africa (Kelly et al. 1994). Recent observations on the ultrastructure of the parasite from 4 Australian AIDS patients have shown that the parasitophorous vacuolar membrane is present throughout development including around isolated meronts, that the granular matrix, normally associated with the production of septa in this species, is evenly distributed in vacuoles containing only meronts (Canning et al. 1994) and that sporogony is mainly disporoblastic, although tetrasporogony cannot be excluded. It has there-

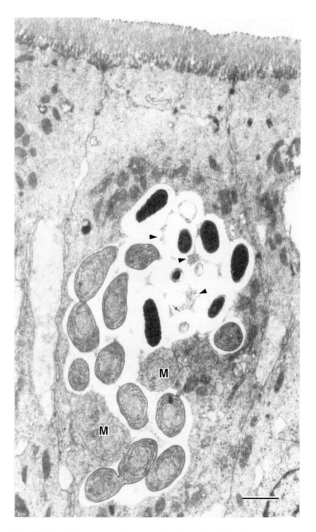

Fig. 21.9 Electron micrograph of a duodenal enterocyte with a parasitophorous vacuole containing *Encephalitozoon intestinalis*. Note meronts (M) apposed to vacuolar membrane and granular septal material between parasites (arrowheads). Bar = 0.53 μm. (Reproduced with permission, Canning et al. 1994.)

fore been suggested that the description of the genus *Septata* should be modified as these characteristics are already associated with the well established genus *Encephalitozoon*.

Nucleotide sequencing of the well conserved 16S rDNA gene suggests that *E. intestinalis* is similar to both *E. cuniculi* and *E. hellem*, but is distinct enough to be separated from these species at the generic level (Doultree et al. 1995). However, Hartskeerl et al. (1995) consider that this organism should be classified as *Encephalitozoon intestinalis*, on the basis of restriction fragment length polymorphism analysis of amplified ribosomal RNA sequences which shows about 90% identity with *E. cuniculi* and *E. hellem*. In addition, western blots reveal a significant cross-reactivity between these 3 species. Hartskeerl and colleagues concluded that *E. intestinalis* should be regarded as a species within the genus *Encephalitozoon* and this is what is accepted in this chapter.

The prevalence of *E. intestinalis* in small-intestinal biopsies appears to be significantly less than *Ent. bieneusi* infection to which there are now numerous references (Canning et al. 1993). Kelly et al. (1994) found 2 of 75 (3%) patients with HIV-related diarrhoea infected with *E. intestinalis* in an African (Zambia) study and the prevalence is similar to that found in other studies elsewhere.

Concurrent infections with *Ent. bieneusi* have been reported (Blanshard et al. 1992b, Orenstein, Dieterich and Kotler 1992, Cali et al. 1991c). Van Gool et al. (1994), in an attempt to culture *Ent. bieneusi* from stool samples from 4 AIDS patients with biopsy-proven *Ent. bieneusi* infections, established cultures but the organism was identified as *E. intestinalis*. A possible explanation for this somewhat unexpected result is that *Ent. bieneusi* and *E. intestinalis* are dimorphic forms of the same species. Despite any evidence of *E. intestinalis* infection in the original biopsies, Van Gool and colleagues (1994) dismissed this explanation and suggested that all the patients from whom stool samples were obtained had heavy infections of *Ent. bieneusi* and light infections of *E. intestinalis*. Critical re-examination of the stool samples revealed abundant *Ent. bieneusi* spores and rarely seen, larger spores, which could possibly have been *E. intestinalis*. These results suggest that *E. intestinalis* can occur as an inapparent infection and that its true prevalence may be much higher than previously thought.

Clinical features of enteric microsporidial infections in AIDS

Asmuth et al. (1994) retrospectively reviewed 20 patients who had small-intestinal microsporidiosis. Mean CD4 count was $35 \pm 29 \times 10^6/l$ and most had been lower than $100 \times 10^6/l$ for at least 16 months. Mean duration of diarrhoeal symptoms was 8.5 ± 6.9 months, with stool frequency at the time of diagnosis 5.7 ± 2 per day. Abdominal cramping was present, but fever was absent. Within this group of 20 patients 18 had their microsporidial parasites identified to species level, 14 (78%) were infected with *Ent. bieneusi* and 4 (22%) with *E. intestinalis*. Biochemical findings suggest that the enteric microsporidia have the ability to turn on secretory processes within the small intestine and to induce diarrhoea.

OTHER SITES OF INFECTION AND OTHER SPECIES

E. cuniculi has been reported from a number of AIDS cases. A case of peritonitis was reported by Zender et al. (1989) and a case of hepatitis by Terada et al. (1987). Several cases of renal infection involving spec-

ies of *Encephalitozoon* have been reported (Orenstein, Dieterich and Kotler 1992, Cali, Kotler and Orenstein 1993, Aarons et al. 1994, Dore et al. 1995). Aarons and colleagues (1994) describe a case of renal failure in an HIV-seropositive patient, caused by a species of *Encephalitozoon*, which was reversible on treatment with albendazole and correlated with the disappearance of the parasite from the urine. In another AIDS patient with disseminated *E. intestinalis* infection and with evidence of impairment of renal function, after a course of treatment with albendazole, renal function returned to normal (Dore et al. 1995).

The genus *Pleistophora* is normally associated with infections of fish (Canning and Lom 1986) but a few cases of myositis caused by *Pleistophora sp.* have been reported in humans (Chupp et al. 1993, Ledford et al. 1985: Macher et al. 1988). In the case reported by Ledford and colleagues, the patient was immunodeficient but HIV seronegative. The other reported cases were from AIDS patients. In the case described by Chupp and colleagues, the patient was a 33 year old Haitian man with AIDS with pain and weakness spreading to the posterior thighs and upper extremities and daily fevers. Electromyography findings were consistent with a diffuse, active myopathic process including denervation characteristic of inflammatory myopathy. The patient died without the cause of death being immediately known but a muscle biopsy taken before death showed, in one area, that all the fibres were atrophic and contained intracellular basophilic organisms. Electron microscopy revealed all the developmental stages of a microsporidian, which was ascribed to the genus *Pleistophora*.

A case originating from Australia (Hollister et al. 1996) was similar, but the organism was diagnosed from a muscle biopsy and was also present in corneal epithelium, urine and nasopharyngeal washings, suggesting disseminated infection. All stages were surrounded by an electron-dense surface coat. Further studies of this organism in culture and athymic mice (Fig. 21.10), indicate that the parasite differs from established species of *Pleistophora* and it has therefore been reclassified as *Trachipleistophora hominis*. This organism does not form multinucleate sporogonial plasmodia, the sporophorous vesicle enlarges during sporogony and the vesicle wall is not a multilayered structure. The AIDS patient involved was treated with albendazole and there was a complete clinical and biochemical (muscle enzymes) cure (Andrew Field, personal communication 1995).

DISSEMINATED INFECTIONS INVOLVING SPECIES OF *ENCEPHALITOZOON*

In addition to intestinal and ocular microsporidiosis, there are now several reports of multiorgan infection (Gunnarsson et al. 1995) or systemic dissemination (Orenstein, Dieterich and Kotler 1992, Cali, Kotler and Orenstein 1993, Doultree et al. 1995). In patients presenting with symptoms localized to one organ system, consideration must be given to the possibility of systemic infection, particularly if species of *Encephalitozoon* are involved (Schwartz et al. 1993b). Dore et al. (1995) suggest that a distinguishing feature of disseminated infection with *E. intestinalis* is the prevalence of

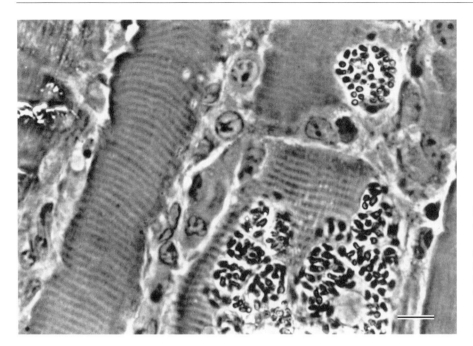

Fig. 21.10 Light micrograph of *Trachipleistophora hominis* in skeletal muscle fibres of an athymic mouse. Note that muscle fibre is packed with spores. Bar = 10 μm. (Reproduced with permission from WS Hollister and EU Canning.)

symptoms of chronic rhinosinusitis. De Groote and colleagues (1995) describe a case of disseminated *E. cuniculi* infection in which the patient had advanced renal failure. The organism was found in urine and sputum and many tests, including the polymerase chain reaction and indirect immunofluorescence, confirmed the presence of *E. cuniculi*. Once again, treatment with albendazole resulted in improvement of symptoms.

Schwartz et al. (1993b) describe a case of a patient previously diagnosed as having keratoconjunctivitis involving *E. hellem* infection, but who subsequently presented with respiratory problems and fever. A chest radiograph revealed a left lower lobe interstitial infiltrate. Bronchoscopy with biopsy and bronchoalveolar lavage revealed abundant *E. hellem* spores within epithelial cells. Sputum and urine samples also contained the same microsporidian.

Molina and colleagues (1995) describe 5 cases of disseminated infection due to *E. intestinalis*. Symptoms included chronic diarrhoea, fever, cholangitis, sinusitis and bronchitis. Albendazole cleared the stool samples of all 5 patients but the urine of only 3 patients. Other disseminated infections involving *E. intestinalis* have been reported (Orenstein, Dieterich and Kotler 1992, Cali, Kotler and Orenstein 1993).

The reports outlined above strongly suggest that AIDS patients with low CD4 counts presenting with infections involving any species of *Encephalitozoon* may have unsuspected disseminated infection. Early treatment with albendazole can result in significant improvement of symptoms in most cases. The mechanism of dissemination of microsporidia is uncertain, but infected macrophages may play a significant role in this process (Doultree et al. 1995).

3.5 *Enterocytozoon bieneusi* infection in an immunocompetent individual

Ent. bieneusi has been described in a non-HIV infected, non-immunocompromised patient with acute diarrhoea following a journey through Jordan and Egypt (Sandfort et al. 1993, Sandfort et al. 1994). With increased awareness of human microsporidial infections, this finding may lead to greater recognition of such infections within the immunocompetent population, a situation very much like that associated with *Cryptosporidium parvum* infection.

4 DIAGNOSIS

Microsporidiosis in AIDS patients is probably significantly under-reported because of diagnostic difficulties (Aldras et al. 1994). Diagnosing microsporidial infections depends on recognizing that the patient could be infected with microsporidia, particularly when the CD4 lymphocyte count drops below $100 \times 10^6/l$, thus allowing the most appropriate specimens to be taken and the laboratory to choose the most appropriate methods of testing. Laboratory diagnosis of microsporidial infections in tissues is not easily accomplished because of the intracellular nature of these parasites, their small size and poor staining properties (particularly of proliferative stages) with routinely used histological stains. In addition, the histopathologist requires experience in detecting such organisms. Equally, microbiological examination of a faecal sample must include appropriate stains for identifying microsporidial spores and the use of an appropriately configured microscope.

4.1 Small-intestinal biopsies

Enteric infection is the most common type of microsporidial infection. Until about 1990, diagnosis required both light microscopic and electron microscopic examination of small-intestinal biopsy sections (Orenstein et al. 1990a) or touch preparations of biopsies (Rijpstra et al. 1988). Microsporidia stain poorly with conventional histopathology stains and appropriate special stains should be chosen for the tissue sections, although these are not always considered. Diagnostic workers interested in microsporidial detection have tried many alternative staining methods and often advocate their own particular favourite. Stains used include haematoxylin and eosin, Giemsa, tissue Gram stain (Rabeneck et al. 1993) and periodic acid–Schiff reagent (Field, Hing et al. 1993). A tissue stain which shows great promise is Warthin–Starry (Field et al. 1993a,b, Field, Marriot and Hing 1993), which stains some sporogonic stages and spores (Fig. 21.11).

Microsporidial infections can be misdiagnosed in tissues. Furuta et al. (1991) thought that pulmonary lesions found in autopsy material from leprosy patients involved microsporidia, but after immunohistochemical staining it was concluded that these lesions were, in fact, caused by *Cryptococcus neoformans*. Resin-embedded tissue stained with toluidine blue can also be useful, but mucus granules in goblet cells also take up stain and can cause confusion. The excellent preservation and thin tissue sections (1 μm) enhance the resolution of the cellular detail compared with wax-embedded material. This intermediate step of resin embedding naturally leads to possible electron microscopic examination of ultrathin tissue sections, and electron microscopy remains the gold standard for confirmation of microsporidial infection in tissues (Weber et al. 1994, Rabeneck et al. 1993, Asmuth et al. 1994, Field, Hing et al. 1993). Demonstration of the coiled polar tube within spores is pathognomic of

microsporidial infection (Fig. 21.2) and identification to generic and sometimes species level can be made from ultrastructural features (Cali 1991). The identification of the species involved in new patients is important, as effective drug therapies can be instigated with this knowledge. Some workers regard electron microscopy as cumbersome and time-consuming (Visvesvara et al. 1994), but efficiently run, experienced units can produce confident results in a matter of days.

Immunofluorescent or immunoperoxidase antibody staining of microsporidia in tissue sections would be useful if such antibodies were commercially available. Visvesvara et al. (1994) produced both polyclonal and monoclonal antibodies to *E. hellem* that successfully differentiated this organism from other species in both clinical specimens and established cultures. Other studies (Schwartz et al. 1993a) have shown that, using the indirect fluorescent antibody test (IFAT) with species specific antibodies, it is possible to identify microsporidial infection in sections of corneal biopsies.

Because *E. cuniculi*, *E. hellem* and *E. intestinalis* can be grown in culture (Schwartz et al. 1993a, Hollister et al. 1993, Beauvais et al. 1994, Van Gool et al. 1994, Visvesvara et al. 1995, Doultree et al. 1995), purified spore preparations can be harvested for inoculation into rabbits or mice. Aldras et al. (1994) describe the production of monoclonal antibodies raised against *E. hellem* and polyclonal antibodies raised against *E. cuniculi* and *E. hellem* which used in IFAT, were able to specifically identify the presence of microsporidial spores, including those of *Ent. bieneusi*, in stool samples. Commercial availability of such antisera would be diagnostically useful, particularly if they could also be used on tissue sections and species specific antibodies would also be useful as mentioned above.

4.2 Microsporidial spores in stool samples

Simple non-invasive techniques have been developed for the detection of microsporidial spores in, for example, stool samples. The contents of the duodenum–jejunum can also be examined for microsporidial spores using the Entero-test (HDC Corporation) method, which is often used to obtain luminal contents for detection of *Giardia* (Hamour, Curry and Mandal, personal communication 1995). The staining properties of the microsporidian spore wall differentiates them from most other micro-organisms. Spore staining methods utilizing a modified Trichrome stain (chromotrope 2R stain) (Weber et al. 1992a), Giemsa (Van Gool et al. 1990) or fluorescent dyes (optical brightening agents) (Van Gool et al. 1993, Vavra et al. 1993) have been described and all these microscopical methods require adequate illumination, high magnification objectives (oil immersion) (Weber et al. 1994), examination of multiple stool samples and an adequately long examination time (minimum 10 min) (Wuhib et al. 1994) or examination of at least 100 high power fields (Bendall and Chiodini 1993) for reliable diagnosis.

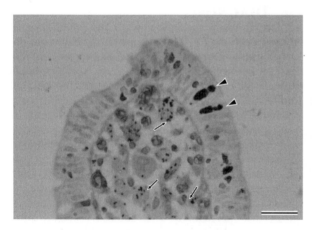

Fig. 21.11 Light micrograph of a tip of a duodenal villus showing aggregates of *Encephalitozoon*-like species in enterocytes (arrowheads) and macrophages in the lamina propria (arrows). Warthin–Starry stain. (Reproduced from Field et al. 1993b, with permission of the authors and publisher.)

Weber's method (Weber et al. 1992a) utilizing chromotrope 2R has become a routine diagnostic staining method in many laboratories, particularly in the USA. Microsporidial spores stain pink and surrounding bacteria light green in thin stool smears. A number of modifications to Weber's method have been published. In one, aniline blue is substituted for fast green and there is a reduction in the level of phosphotungstic acid (Ryan et al. 1993). In the other, processing time is reduced by raising the temperature of staining (Kokoskin et al. 1994). Both modified methods are claimed to give superior results compared to the original method (Weber et al. 1992a).

Microsporidial spores are of the same order of size as bacteria and any diagnostic staining method must allow differentiation between spores and faecal bacteria. In addition, the microscopist must be able to differentiate between microsporidial spores and those of fungi and yeasts, as well as oocysts of coccidian protozoal parasites. Of the fluorescent dyes, Uvitex 2B (Ciba-Geigy 48) and Calcofluor (Sigma), are useful for faecal screening as they both stain chitin, found in the endospore layer of microsporidial spores. They are quick to use, but require an epi-illumination, fluorescence microscope fitted with a 350–380 nm excitation filter and a light source which emits such wavelengths (e.g. a mercury vapour lamp). Spores are identified by their size, shape and staining properties (Fig. 21.12). Fungal and yeast spores also contain chitin and therefore putative positive microsporidial samples should be confirmed by another method such as Giemsa or Trichrome staining or electron microscopy (Corcoran et al. 1995). Experience is required for confident results.

Some caution may be needed in ascribing the finding of microsporidial spores in stool samples to patient symptoms. McDougall et al. (1993) report the finding of microsporidian spores in a stool sample from an AIDS patient with chronic diarrhoea, anorexia and lethargy. Further investigations suggested that the microsporidia found had been ingested as food in heavily infected muscle and were, therefore, an incidental finding. This situation is, perhaps, not uncommon. Levine (1985) has reported that oocysts of a number of animal coccidian parasites ingested in food and found in human faeces have been mistaken for parasites of humans.

Concurrent infections involving both microsporidia and *Cryptosporidium parvum* may also be common. Garcia, Shimizu and Bruckner (1994) showed that 17 of 60 (28%) mainly immunocompromised patients with diarrhoea had simultaneous *Cryptosporidium* and microsporidial infections. The

finding of one parasite should not preclude further examination by a different diagnostic method for other parasites. In addition, enteric infection with both *Ent. bieneusi* and *E. intestinalis* may not be unusual (Van Gool et al. 1994) and this may have important implications for treatment, as *E. intestinalis* appears to be fully susceptible to treatment with albendazole, whereas the response of *Ent. bieneusi* is variable.

4.3 Culture of microsporidia from clinical samples

Microsporidial spores from clinical samples such as urine (Visvesvara et al. 1991, Bocket et al. 1992, Hollister, Canning and Colbourn 1993, Visvesvara et al. 1995, Hollister et al. 1995), nasal polyps (Hollister et al. 1993), nasopharyngeal aspirates (Doultree et al. 1995), faeces (Van Gool et al. 1994) and muscle biopsies (Hollister et al. 1995) can sometimes be cultured in various cell lines. Once established in culture, enough spores can be produced from the original human sample to allow further tests, such as SDS–PAGE or the polymerase chain reaction, to be carried out, which can help to establish the species involved. *Ent. bieneusi* has yet to be cultured.

4.4 Polymerase chain reaction

Recently it has become possible to generate sequence data rapidly by direct sequencing of amplified ribosomal DNA using the polymerase chain reaction (PCR). This technique has identified sequence variation and shows considerable promise for the specific identification of microsporidian species.

Vossbrinck et al. (1993) sequenced a segment of ribosomal DNA about 1350 bp long and demonstrated that both *E. cuniculi* and *E. hellem* could be specifically identified. A comparison of the sequence data showed relatively high sequence homology, justifying the same generic status of these organisms but also confirmed that the isolates of *E. hellem* and *E. cuniculi* were not of the same species. Restriction digests of the amplified region of ribosmal DNA provides the potential for a rapid method of distinguishing between *E. hellem* and *E. cuniculi*. Visvesvara and colleagues (1994) using direct sequencing of PCR amplified small-subunit rRNA (SSU-rRNA) demonstrated similar specific differences between these 2 species. Techniques based on PCR still largely depend on cultured organisms from clinical sources, which limits their usefulness in rapid diagnosis, but amplification directly from clinical specimens should improve the speed of diagnosis (Visvesvara et al. 1994, Zhu et al. 1994).

A PCR assay of stool samples from AIDS patients known to be infected with microsporidia (identified by chromotrope 2R stain) not only detected microsporidial infection but also identified the enteric species involved (Fedorko, Nelson and Cartwright 1995). However, this assay required a laborious 4-day extraction procedure and was strongly inhibited by fresh stools, although this could be overcome with the addition of sodium hypochlorite. Cultured spores of *E. intestinalis* were added to a stool specimen positive

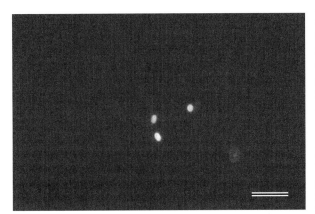

Fig. 21.12 Spores of *Enterocytozoon bieneusi* from a stool sample stained with calcofluor and examined with 350–380 nm wavelength illumination under an epi-illumination fluorescence microscope. Note ovoid shape of spores.

for *Ent. bieneusi* to simulate a dual infection. A single primer (PMP2) complementary to conserved sequences of the SSU-rRNA enabled amplification of DNA from both species. An important observation was that whereas *Ent. bieneusi* lacks a Pst1 restriction site in the amplicon, that of *E. intestinalis* cut into 2 distinct fragments, thus enabling differentiation of the 2 species. The authors suggest that PCR may become the method of choice for identification of microsporidia in clinical specimens. Laboratories able to undertake molecular studies on microsporidial samples are currently restricted to research centres.

Canning and colleagues (1993) also demonstrated differences between *Nosema corneum* (=*Vittaforma corneae*), *E. cuniculi* and *E. hellem* using a random amplified polymorphic DNA polymerase chain reaction (RAPD).

Vossbrink and colleagues (1993) suggested that sequence information appropriate for comparison with other microsporidial species should be included in future species descriptions for the specific identification and phylogenetic comparisons of microsporidia.

5 EPIDEMIOLOGY AND CONTROL

5.1 Possible animal reservoirs

Microsporidial infections have only become well recognized in humans since the advent of HIV and AIDS, and such infection may have been previously unrecognized. The open question is whether the organisms involved are solely human infections or are some episodes of zoonotic origin. Any explanation of the current situation, where microsporidial infections are becoming increasingly commonly recognized, albeit in immunocompromised individuals, must consider possible zoonotic transmission (Glaser, Angulo and Rooney 1994) but such links have not yet been established or are tenuous.

As microsporidia are ubiquitous in the wild, both in animals and in environmental situations exposed to spores excreted in urine, humans must inevitably become exposed to these parasites. Theoretically many potential animal reservoirs exist but no studies have shown definitive zoonotic transmission. Domestic animals, such as dogs, would seem to be a possible source for human infection; *E. cuniculi*, in particular, is known to occur in dogs and a wide range of other animal species commonly associated with humans. Future work is necessary to clarify the taxonomic status of individual species and isolates, within the *Encephalitozoon*-group before zoonotic links, if any, can be identified.

Another possibility is that the microsporidia found in humans are dimorphic forms of infections in other animals. Microsporidial dimorphism between certain animal hosts is well recognized but poorly understood (Canning 1988, Canning and Lom 1986). Care must be taken to exclude microsporidial species that occur in animals associated with humans or which can contaminate their food.

Many arthropods live on (such as lice and fleas) or near humans (such as cockroaches and house flies) and some have considerable medical importance (Smith 1973). Fleas do not feed exclusively on the blood of a single host and are, therefore, potential carriers and transmitters of disease-producing organisms. Infections transmitted to man in this way are well documented (Smit 1973). Microsporidia have been identified in the cat flea (*Ctenocephalides felis*), which frequently infests human dwellings (Beard, Butler and Becnel 1990). Other biting arthropods can harbour microsporidial infections, such as ticks (Weiser and Rehacek 1975) and mosquitoes (Hazard and Fukuda 1974, Becnel and Sweeney 1990). However, there is no evidence of microsporidial transmission from biting insects to humans.

Other homeothermic pests of human habitation, such as rats and mice may be involved, and could contaminate the environment with spores excreted in urine. Both brown rats (Webster and MacDonald 1995) and house mice (Chalmers et al. 1994) have recently been shown to act as potential reservoirs for *Cryptosporidium parvum*, which is commonly found in AIDS patients, sometimes with concurrent enteric microsporidia (Garcia, Shimizu and Bruckner 1994). Such small mammal hosts can also harbour *E. cuniculi* (Canning and Lom 1986). Ingestion of spores by severely immunocompromised individuals with low CD4 lymphocyte counts (below $100 \times 10^6/l$), could result in disease but although no evidence for such a transmission route is known, it remains a possibility.

Infected fish muscle is also emerging as a possible source of human infection. Species of *Pleistophora* are common fish pathogens. A number of cases of *Pleistophora* infection in humans have now been described, all involving skeletal muscle infection. Poorly cooked infected fish may have a role in these infections, and some evidence for this comes from the incidental finding of microsporidial spores in a human stool sample from an AIDS patient with diarrhoea (McDougall et al. 1993) which also contained muscle fibres (meat) infected with microsporidia; it was suggested that infected fish had been consumed and that spores had passed through the gut largely intact. However, a recent ultrastructural study on a *Pleistophora*-like organism has concluded that the species infecting humans is distinctive enough to be renamed as *Trachipleistophora hominis* (Hollister et al. 1996).

A second species of *Enterocytozoon*, *Ent. salmonensis*, has been identified in chinook salmon (*Oncorhynchus tshawytscha*) (Chilmonczyk, Cox and Hedrick 1991, Wongtavatchai, Conrad and Hedrick 1995). This parasite replicates within host cell nuclei of haemopoietic cells in the spleen, kidney and leucocytes, which makes it distinct from *Ent. bieneusi*. Given the prevalence of *Ent. bieneusi* in AIDS patients, it is highly unlikely that any causal relationship could be established with chinook salmon. Indeed, some workers consider that *Ent. bieneusi* is a natural human parasite without a zoonotic origin (Canning and Hollister 1990). Clearly, further investigation needs to be undertaken to establish if there are any links between microsporidial species found in fish and those found in humans.

The likelihood of microsporidial species from poikilothermic hosts being able to infect homeothermic humans, particularly if severely immunosuppressed (as in HIV disease) needs to be explored and demonstrated (Hollister et al. 1996). Clearly, considerable work remains to be undertaken before any zoonotic routes of transmission can be accepted. Although we must remain open minded, in the absence of compelling evidence to the contrary many of the microsporidial infections recently recognized in humans may be previously unrecognized and exclusively human microsporidial parasites.

5.2 Control

SUSCEPTIBILITY TO PHYSICAL AND CHEMICAL AGENTS

Disinfection of surfaces contaminated with microsporidia has received little attention. That spores are highly resistant has been demonstrated in the laboratory, where they have been found to be viable after storage for up to 10 years in distilled water (Sprague and Vávra 1977). Shadduck and Polley (1978) used a rabbit isolate of *E. cuniculi* grown in a rabbit choroid plexus cell line to evaluate various factors influencing the infectivity and replication of this organism. *E. cuniculi* was not affected by penicillin, streptomycin or gentamicin, nor was it affected by sonication, freezing and thawing or distilled water. Organisms survived 60 but not 120 min at 56°C. They were, however, killed after 10 min of autoclaving at 120°C, or exposure to 2% (v/v) lysol, 10% (v/v) formalin or 70% (v/v) ethyl alcohol for 10 min. Whether all microsporidian species are affected by these physical conditions to the same degree as *E. cuniculi* is not known.

Undeen and Vander Meer (1990) subjected spores of *N. algerae* to ultraviolet radiation and found that very high dosages ($3.8 \, \text{J}/\text{cm}^2$) were required to inhibit germination. Similar results had been obtained with γ-radiation (Undeen et al. 1984) and it was concluded that spore germination did not involve nuclear function. Significantly, after receiving γ-radiation above 0.5 kGy, this microsporidian was unable to infect its mosquito host, but spore germination rate remained unaffected up to 10 kGy.

In recent work on the inhibition of polar tube extrusion in purified spores derived from cell cultures infected with *E. hellem* undertaken by Leitch et al. (1993) germination was found to be pH dependent and was enhanced in the presence of calcium in the medium. Under experimental conditions, 4 agents inhibited polar tube extrusion: cytochalasin D disrupts microfilaments, demecolcine disrupts microtubules, nifedipine is a calcium channel blocker and itraconazole an antifungal agent. As a result of this work it was concluded that future clinical trials employing drug combinations may be useful in treating microsporidiosis.

6 CHEMOTHERAPY

6.1 Problems of treatment

Microsporidial infections are difficult to treat because of their intracellular habitat and the resistant nature of the spores. Enteric infections have been treated with varying degrees of success with several drugs, but carefully controlled comparative treatment trials are lacking.

6.2 Treatment of keratoconjunctivitis

Various topical antimicrobial, lubricating and anti-inflammatory agents have been used to treat eyes infected with microsporidia. Itraconazole (Yee et al. 1991) was responsible, at least in part, for the resolution of a corneal infection with *Encephalitozoon* sp. (later identified as *E. hellem* by Didier ES et al. 1991). Treatment with propamidine isethionate resolved symptoms in a UK patient infected with *Encephalitozoon* sp. (Metcalfe et al. 1992) (also later identified as *E. hellem* by Hollister et al. 1993). The symptoms returned when treatment was discontinued (Metcalfe et al. 1992) but albendazole treatment improved the nasal infection, with significant regression of sinus opacification. The patient remained free from nasal symptoms until his death from AIDS dementia complex (Lacey et al. 1992). Independently of the UK case treated with propamidine isethionate (Metcalfe et al. 1992), an Australian case was also treated with propamidine isethionate eye ointment, with similar resolution of symptoms (McCuskey et al. 1993).

Fumagillin has been known for some time to control *Nosema* infection in honey bees, where infection causes severe economic loss (Katznelson and Jamieson 1952). Shadduck (1980) observed the in vitro effects of fumagillin on *E. cuniculi* and observed that it protected non-infected cells but did not eliminate the parasite from infected ones. This anti-microsporidial agent is toxic to humans (McCowen, Callender and Lawles 1951), but has been used topically to resolve ocular infection by *E. hellem*. Fumagillin is insoluble in water, but a derivative, Fumidil B, is soluble. A Fumidil B preparation applied topically reduced the keratoconjunctivitis in 2 AIDS patients (Diesenhouse et al. 1993). No toxic side effects were observed but infection recurred when treatment was stopped, just as had been found with propamidine isethionate (Metcalfe et al. 1992). Both these topical antimicrosporidial agents appear to be inhibitory rather than parasiticidal in action. Rosberger et al. (1993) has also reported successful treatment of keratoconjunctivitis with topical fumagillin.

6.3 Treatment of enteric microsporidial infections

Octreotide produced a partial remission in one patient infected by *Ent. bieneusi* (Simon et al. 1991) and metronidazole caused some remission in most (10 of 13 patients) of a small group of HIV seropositive patients with mild microsporidial diarrhoea caused by *Ent. bieneusi* (Eeftinck Schattenkerk et al. 1991). Blanshard et al. (1992a) treated 6 AIDS patients with diarrhoea and biopsy confirmed infection with *Ent. bieneusi*, but no other identified cause of symptoms. Albendazole, a broad-spectrum antiparasitic agent with activity against protozoa, was used and was found to be well tolerated. Within 7 days of treatment, there was a marked reduction in stool frequency, volume and incontinence, with all patients either gaining weight or weight loss being arrested. Four patients relapsed within a month of cessation of treatment, 3 of whom responded to a further course of albendazole treatment. It was concluded that albendazole had a partial parasitostatic effect, rather than a parasiticidal action. Further studies by Blanshard et al. (1993) confirmed this conclusion. In biopsy material taken from patients being treated with albendazole, damage to developmental stages of *Ent. bieneusi*, causing a partial inhibition of parasite replication, was apparent. Dieterich et al. (1994) showed a similar reduction of symptoms in patients treated with albendazole, but again concluded that *Ent. bieneusi* was not eliminated.

In contrast to *Ent. bieneusi*, *E. intestinalis* appears to be more susceptible to treatment with albendazole, as demonstrated by the disappearance of the parasite from the intestine of a case of disseminated infection (Orenstein, Dieterich and Kotler 1993). Gunnarson et al. (1995) used albendazole to treat 5 patients with evidence of multiorgan infection with *E. intestinalis*. After treatment, most clinical samples were negative for microsporidia and there was a significant improvement of symptoms. Treatment of one patient was stopped, however, because of nausea and vomiting induced by albendazole.

The direct effect of albendazole on cell cultures infected with *E. cuniculi* has been examined by Colbourn et al. (1994). Many of the proliferative stages of the parasite became grossly enlarged and devoid of nuclei. As albendazole prevents the polymerization of microtubules, which are only known to occur within the intranuclear spindles of dividing nuclei in microsporidia, parasite growth continues in the absence of nuclear division.

Albendazole was administered to 5 AIDS patients (400 mg orally twice a day) with evidence of disseminated microsporidiosis caused by *E. intestinalis* (Molina et al. 1995). Symptoms included chronic diarrhoea, usually associated with fever, cholangitis, sinusitis, bronchitis, or mild bilateral conjunctivitis. Spores of *E. intestinalis* were detected in stool and urine samples and confirmed by transmission electron microscopy of duodenal biopsies. There was a rapid clinical response to therapy, with spores being cleared from faeces of all patients and from the urine of 3. However, during follow up, spores were detected in faeces and mild diarrhoea recurred in 2 patients. It was concluded that albendazole has a significant effect on *E. intestinalis* infection, but that its effects are transient.

Asmuth et al. (1994) also suggested that benefit could be derived from nutritional therapy directed at minimizing malabsorption. Low-fat diets and introduction of simple carbohydrates could also induce an improvement in symptoms.

7   CONCLUSION

Much remains to be learned about microsporidia, particularly in relation to human infection (Current and Blagburn 1991) and almost nothing is known about the epidemiology or pathogenesis of these parasites in humans. Whether there are animal sources of human infection will become clearer as epidemiological and experimental studies become better established. Molecular techniques are becoming more commonly available and should provide incontrovertible evidence of microsporidial infection and latent infection and also establish the phylogenetic and taxonomic relationships of the species involved (Zhu et al. 1994). Further developments in treatment are needed, particularly in relation to *Ent. bieneusi* infection.

REFERENCES

Aarons EJ, Woodrow D et al., 1994, Reversible renal failure caused by a microsporidian infection, *AIDS*, **8:** 1119–21.

Aldras AM, Orenstein JM et al., 1994, Detection of microsporidia by indirect immunofluorescence antibody test using polyclonal and monoclonal antibodies, *J Clin Microbiol*, **32:** 608–12.

Ashton N, Wirasinha PA, 1973, Encephalitozoonosis of the cornea, *Br J Ophthalmol*, **57:** 669–74.

Asmuth DM, DeGirolami PC et al., 1994, Clinical features of microsporidiosis in patients with AIDS, *Clin Infect Dis*, **18:** 819–25.

Ball GH, 1969, Organisms living on and in protozoa, *Research in Protozoology*., vol. 3, ed Chen TT, Pergamon Press, New York, 565–718.

Beard CB, Butler JF, Becnel JJ, 1990, *Nolleria pulicis* n. gen., n. sp. (Microsporidia: Chytridiopsidae), a microsporidian parasite of the cat flea, *Ctenocepalides felis* (Siphonaptera: Pulicidae), *J Protozool*, **37:** 90–9.

Beaugerie L, Teilhac MF et al., 1992, Cholangiopathy associated with microsporidia infection of the common bile duct mucosa in a patient with HIV infection, *Ann Intern Med*, **117:** 401–2.

Beauvais B, Sarfati C et al., 1994, In vitro model to assess effect of antimicrobial agents on *Encephalitozoon cuniculi*, *Antimicrob Agents Chemother*, **38:** 2440–8.

Becnel JJ, Sweeney AW, 1990, *Amblyospora trinus* n. sp. (Microsporida:Amblyosporidae) in the Australian mosquito *Culex halifaxi* (Diptera: Culicidae), *J Protozool*, **37:** 584–92.

Bendall RP, Chiodini PL, 1993, New diagnostic methods for parasitic infections, *Curr Opin Infect Dis*, **6:** 318–23.

Bergquist NR, Stintzing G et al., 1984, Diagnosis of encephalitozoonosis in man by serological tests, *Br Med J*, **288:** 902.

Blanshard C, Ellis DS et al., 1992a, Treatment of intestinal microsporidiosis with albendazole in patients with AIDS, *AIDS*, **6:** 311–13.

Blanshard C, Ellis DS et al., 1993, Electron microscopic changes in *Enterocytozoon bieneusi* following treatment with albendazole, *J Clin Pathol*, **46:** 898–902.

Blanshard C, Hollister WS et al., 1992b, Simultaneous infection with two types of intestinal microsporidia in a patient with AIDS, *Gut*, **33:** 418–20.

Bocket L, Marquette CH et al., 1992, Isolation and replication in human fibroblast cells (MRC-5) of a microsporidian from an AIDS patient, *Microb Pathog*, **12:** 187–91.

Bretagne S, Foulet F et al., 1993, Prevalance of microsporidial spores in stools from children in Niamey, Niger, *AIDS*, **7:** S34–S35.

Cali A, 1991, General microsporidian features and recent findings on AIDS isolates, *J Protozool*, **38:** 625–630.

Cali A, Owen RL, 1990, Intracellular development of *Enterocytozoon*, a unique microsporidian found in the intestine of AIDS patients, *J Protozool*, **37:** 145–55.

Cali A, Meisler DM et al., 1991a, Corneal microsporidioses: characterization and identification, *J Protozool*, **38:** 215S–217S.

Cali A, Meisler DM et al., 1991b, Corneal microsporidiosis in a patient with AIDS, *Am J Trop Med Hyg*, **44:** 463–8.

Cali A, Orenstein JM et al., 1991c, A comparison of two microsporidian parasites in enterocytes of AIDS patients with chronic diarrhea, *J Protozool*, **38:** 96S–98S.

Cali A, Kotler DP, Orenstein JM, 1993, *Septata intestinalis* n.g. n.sp., an intestinal microsporidian associated with chronic diarrhea and dissemination in AIDS patients, *J Euk Microbiol*, **40:** 101–12.

Canning EU, 1988, Nuclear division and chromosome cycle in microsporidia, *BioSystems*, **21:** 333–40.

Canning EU, 1993, Microsporidia, *Parasitic Protozoa*, 2nd edn, vol. 6, eds. Kreier JP, Baker JR, Academic Press, New York, 299–370.

Canning EU, Hollister WS, 1990, *Enterocytozoon bieneusi* (microspora): prevalence and pathogenicity in AIDS patients, *Trans R Soc Trop Med Hyg*, **84:** 181–6.

Canning EU, Lom J, 1986, *The Microsporidia of Vertebrates*, Academic Press, London.

Canning EU, Curry A et al., 1992, Ultrastructure of *Encephalitozoon sp.* infecting the conjunctival, corneal and nasal epithelia of a patient with AIDS, *Eur J Protistol*, **28:** 226–37.

Canning EU, Hollister WS et al., 1993, Human microsporidioses: site specificity, prevalence and species identification, *AIDS*, **7 (suppl 3):** S3–S7.

Canning EU, Field AS et al., 1994, Further observations on the ultrastructure of *Septata intestinalis* Cali, Kotler and Orenstein, 1993, *Eur J Protistol*, **30:** 414–22.

Chalmers RM, Sturdee AP et al., 1994, *Cryptosporidium muris* in wild house mice (*Mus musculus*): first report in the UK, *Eur J Protistol*, **30:** 151–5.

Chilmonczyk S, Cox WT, Hedrick RP, 1991, *Enterocytozoon salmonenis* n. sp.: an intranuclear microsporidium from salmonid fish, *J Protozool*, **38:** 264–9.

Chupp GL, Alroy J et al., 1993, Myositis due to *Pleistophora* (microsporidia) in a patient with AIDS, *Clin Infect Dis*, **16:** 15–21.

Colbourn NI, Hollister WS et al., 1994, Activity of albendazole against *Encephalitozoon cuniculi* in vitro, *Eur J Protistol*, **30:** 211–20.

Corcoran GD, Tovey DG et al., 1995, Detection and identification of gastrointestinal microsporidia using non-invasive techniques, *J Clin Pathol*, **48:** 725–7.

Current WL, Blagburn BL, 1991, *Cryptosporidium* and microsporidia: some closing comments, *J Protozool*, **38:** 244S–245S.

Curry A, Canning EU, 1993, Human microsporidiosis, *J Infect*, **27:** 229–236.

Curry A, McWilliam LJ et al., 1988, Microsporidiosis in a British AIDS patient, *J Clin Pathol*, **41:** 477–8.

Curry A, Turner AJ, Lucas S, 1991, Opportunistic protozoan infections in human immunodeficiency virus disease : review highlighting diagnostic and therapeutic aspects, *J Clin Pathol*, **44:** 182–93.

De Groote MA, Visvesvara G et al., 1995, Polymerase chain reaction and culture confirmation of disseminated *Encephalitozoon*

cuniculi in a patient with AIDS: successful therapy with albendazole, *J Infect Dis*, **171:** 1375–8.

Desportes I, Le Charpentier Y et al., 1985, Occurrence of a new microsporidian : *Enterocytozoon bieneusi* n. g., n. sp. in the enterocytes of a human patient with AIDS, *J Protozool*, **32:** 250–4.

Didier ES, Didier PJ et al., 1991, Isolation and characterization of a new microsporidian, *Encephalitozoon hellem* (n. sp.), from three AIDS patients with keratoconjunctivitis, *J Infect Dis*, **163:** 617–21.

Didier PJ, Didier ES et al., 1991, Fine structure of a new human microsporidian, *Encephalitozoon hellem*, in culture, *J Protozool*, **38:** 502–7.

Diesenhouse MC, Wilson LA et al., 1993, Treatment of microsporidial keratoconjunctivitis with topical fumagillin, *Am J Opthalmol*, **115:** 293–8.

Dieterich DT, Lew EA et al., 1994, Treatment with albendazole for intestinal diseases due to *Enterocytozoon bieneusi* in patients with AIDS, *J Infect Dis*, **169:** 178–83.

Dobbins WO, Weinstein WN, 1985, Electron microscopy of the intestine and rectum in acquired immunodeficiency syndrome, *Gastroenterology*, **88:** 738–49.

Dore GJ, Marriott DJ et al., 1995, Disseminated microsporidiosis due to *Septata intestinalis* in nine patients infected with the human immunodeficiency virus: response to therapy with albendazole, *Clin Infect Dis*, **21:** 70–6.

Doultree JC, Maerz AL et al., 1995, *In vitro* growth of the microsporidian *Septata intestinalis* from an AIDS patient with disseminated illness, *J Clin Microbiol*, **33:** 463–70.

Eeftinck Schattenkerk JKM, van Gool T et al., 1991, Clinical significance of small-intestinal microsporidiosis in HIV-1-infected individuals, *Lancet*, **337:** 895–8.

Fedorko DP, Nelson NA, Cartwright CP, 1995, Identification of microsporidia in stool specimens using PCR and restriction endonucleases, *J Clin Microbiol*, **33:** 1739–41.

Field AS, Canning EU et al., 1993a, Microsporidia in HIV-infected patients in Sydney, Australia: a report of 37 cases, a new diagnostic technique and the light microscopy and ultrastructure of a disseminated species, *AIDS*, **7 (suppl 3):** S27–S33.

Field AS, Hing MC et al., 1993b, Microsporidia in the small intestine of HIV-infected patients. A new diagnostic technique and a new species, *Med J Aust*, **158:** 390–4.

Field AS, Marriott DJ, Hing MC, 1993, The Warthin–Starry stain in the diagnosis of small intestinal microsporidiosis in HIV-infected patients, *Folia Parasitol*, **40:** 261–6.

Friedberg DN, Stenson SM et al., 1990, Microsporidial keratoconjunctivitis in acquired immunodeficiency syndrome, *Arch Ophthalmol*, **108:** 504–8.

Furuta M, Oara A et al., 1991, *Cryptococcus neoformans* can be misidentified as a microsporidian: studies of lung lesions in leprosy patients, *J Protozool*, **38:** 95S–96S.

Garcia LS, Shimizu RY, Bruckner DA, 1994, Detection of microsporidial spores in fecal specimens from patients diagnosed with cryptosporidiosis, *J Clin Microbiol*, **32:** 1739–41.

Glaser CA, Angulo FJ, Rooney JA, 1994, Animal-associated opportunistic infections among persons infected with the human immunodeficiency virus, *Clin Infect Dis*, **18:** 14–24.

Greenson JK, Belitsos PC et al., 1991, AIDS enteropathy: occult enteric infections and duodenal mucosal alterations in chronic diarrhea, *Ann Intern Med*, **114:** 366–72.

Gunnarson G, Hurlbut D et al., 1995, Multiorgan microsporidiosis: report of five cases and review, *Clin Infect Dis*, **21:** 37–44.

Hartskeerl RA, Van Gool T et al., 1995, Genetic and immunological characterization of the microsporidian *Septata intestinalis* Cali, Kotler and Orenstein, 1993 : reclassification to *Encephalitozoon intestinalis*, *Parasitology*, **110:** 277–85.

Hazard E, Fukuda T, 1974, *Stempellia milleri* sp. n. (Microsporida: Nosematidae) in the mosquito *Culex pipiens quinquefasciatus* Say, *J Protozool*, **21:** 497–504.

Hollister WS, Canning EU, 1987, An enzyme-linked immuno-sorbent assay (ELISA) for detection of antibodies to *Encephalitozoon cuniculi* and its use in determination of infections in man, *Parasitology*, **94:** 209–19.

Hollister WS, Canning EU, Colbourn NI, 1993, A species of *Encephalitozoon* isolated from an AIDS patient: criteria for species differentiation, *Folia Parasitol*, **40:** 293–5.

Hollister WS, Canning EU, Willcox A, 1991, Evidence for widespread occurrence of antibodies to *Encephalitozoon cuniculi* (Microspora) in man provided by ELISA and other serological tests, *Parasitology*, **102:** 33–43.

Hollister WS, Canning EU et al., 1993, Characterization of *Encephalitozoon hellem* (Microspora) isolated from the nasal mucosa of a patient with AIDS, *Parasitology*, **107:** 351–8.

Hollister WS, Canning EU et al., 1995, *Encephalitozoon cuniculi* isolated from the urine of an AIDS patient, which differs from canine and murine isolates, *J Euk Microbiol*, **42:** 367–72.

Hollister WS, Canning EU et al., 1996, Development and ultrastructure of *Trachipleistophora hominis* n.g., n.sp. after *in vitro* isolation from an AIDS patient and inoculation into athymic mice, *Parasitology*, **112:** 143–54.

Hussey KL, 1971, A microsporidan hyperparasite of strigeoid trematodes, *Nosema strigeoideae* sp. n, *J Protozool*, **18:** 676–9.

Jensen HM, Wellings SR, 1972, Development of the polar filament–polaroplast complex in a microsporidian parasite, *J Protozool*, **19:** 297–305.

Katznelson H, Jamieson CA, 1952, Control of nosema disease of honey bees with fumagillin, *Science*, **115:** 70–1.

Kelly P, McPhail G et al., 1994, *Septata intestinalis*: a new microsporidian in Africa, *Lancet*, **344:** 271–2.

Kokoskin E, Gyorkos TW et al., 1994, Modified technique for efficient detection of microsporidia, *J Clin Microbiol*, **32:** 1074–5.

Kotler DP, Reka S et al., 1993, Effects of enteric parasitoses and HIV infection upon small intestinal structure and function in patients with AIDS, *J Clin Gastroenterol*, **16:** 10–15.

Lacey CJN, Clarke AMT et al., 1992, Chronic microsporidian infection of the nasal mucosae, sinuses and conjunctivae in HIV disease, *Genitourin Med*, **68:** 179–81.

Ledford DK, Overman MD et al., 1985, Microsporidiosis myositis in a patient with the acquired immunodeficiency syndrome, *Ann Intern Med*, **102:** 628–30.

Leitch GJ, He Q et al., 1993, Inhibition of the spore polar filament extrusion of the microsporidium, *Encephalitozoon hellem*, isolated from an AIDS patient, *J Euk Microbiol*, **40:** 711–17.

Levine ND, 1985, *Veterinary Protozoology*, Iowa State University Press. Ames.

Lowder CY, Meisler DM et al., 1990, Microsporidia infection of the cornea in a man seropositive for human immunodeficiency virus, *Am J Ophthalmol*, **109:** 242–4.

Lucas SB, 1989, Aspects of infectious disease, *Recent Advances in Histopathology*, no. 14, eds. Anthony PP, MacSween RNM., Churchill Livingstone, Edinburgh, 281–302.

Lucas SB, Hounnou A et al., 1993, The mortality and pathology of HIV infection in a West African city, *AIDS*, **7:** 1569–79.

Lucas SB, Papadaki L et al., 1989, Diagnosis of intestinal microsporidiosis in patients with AIDS. Letters to the editor, *J Clin Pathol*, **42:** 885–90.

McCluskey PJ, Goonan PV et al., 1993, Microsporidial keratoconjunctivitis in AIDS, *Eye*, **7:** 80–83.

McCowen MC, Callender ME, Lawles JF Jr, 1951, Fumagillin (H-3), a new antibiotic with amebicidal properties, *Science*, **113:** 202–3.

McDougall RJ, Tandy MW et al., 1993, Incidental finding of a microsporidian parasite from an AIDS patient, *J Clin Microbiol*, **31:** 436–9.

Macher AM, Neafie R et al., 1988, Microsporidial myositis and the acquired immunodeficiency syndrome (AIDS): a four year follow up (letter), *Ann Intern Med*, **109:** 343.

Margileth AM, Strano AJ et al., 1973, Disseminated nosematosis in an immunologically compromised infant, *Arch Pathol*, **95:** 145–50.

Matsubayashi H, Koike T et al., 1959, A case of *Encephalitozoon*-like body infection in man, *Arch Pathol*, **67:** 181–7.

Metcalfe TW, Doran RML et al., 1992, Microsporidial keratoconjunctivitis in a patient with AIDS, *Br J Ophthalmol*, **76:** 177–8.

Modigliani R, Bories C et al., 1985, Diarrhoea and malabsorption in acquired immune deficiency syndrome: a study of four cases with special emphasis on opportunistic protozoan infestations, *Gut*, **26:** 179–87.

Molina J-M, Oksenhendler E et al., 1995, Disseminated microsporidiosis due to *Septata intestinalis* in patients with AIDS: clinical features and response to albendazole therapy, *J Infect Dis*, **171:** 245–9.

Orenstein JM, 1991, Microsporidiosis in the acquired immunodeficiency syndrome, *J Parasitol*, **77:** 843–64.

Orenstein JM, Chiang J et al., 1990a, Intestinal microsporidiosis as a cause of diarrhea in human immunodeficiency virus-infected patients: a report of 20 cases, *Hum Pathol*, **21:** 475–81.

Orenstein JM, Seedor J et al., 1990b, Microsporidian keratoconjunctivitis in patients with AIDS, *MMWR*, **39:** 188–9.

Orenstein JM, Dieterich DT, Kotler DP, 1992, Systemic dissemination by a newly recognised intestinal microsporidia species in AIDS, *AIDS*, **6:** 1143–50.

Orenstein JM, Tenner M et al., 1992, A microsporidian previously undescribed in humans infecting enterocytes and macrophages, and associated with diarrhea in an acquired immunodeficiency syndrome patient, *Hum Pathol*, **23:** 722–8.

Orenstein JM, Dieterich DT, Kotler DP, 1993, Albendazole as a treatment for disseminated microsporidiosis due to *Septata intestinalis* in AIDS patients : a report of four patients, *AIDS*, **7 (suppl 3):** S40–S42.

Peacock CS, Blanshard C et al., 1991, Histological diagnosis of intestinal microsporidiosis in patients with AIDS, *J Clin Pathol*, **44:** 558–63.

Perkins FO, 1991, 'Sporozoa': Apicomplexa, Microsporidia, Haplosporidia, Paramyxea, Myxosporidia and Actinosporidia, *Microscopic Anatomy of Invertebrates 1. Protozoa*, eds Harrison FW, Corliss JO, Wiley-Liss, New York, 288–302.

Pinnolis M, Egbert PR et al., 1981, Nosematosis of the cornea. Case report, including electron microscopic studies, *Arch Ophthalmol*, **99:** 1044–7.

Pol S, Romania CA et al., 1993, Microsporidia infection in patients with the human immunodeficiency virus and unexplained cholangitis, *N Engl J Med*, **328:** 95–9.

Rabeneck L, Gyorkey F et al., 1993, The role of *Microsporidia* in the pathogenesis of HIV-related chronic diarrhea, *Ann Int Med*, **119:** 895–9.

Raikov IB, 1995, Meiosis in protists: recent advances and persisting problems, *Eur J Protistol*, **31:** 1–7.

Rijpstra AC, Canning EU et al., 1988, Use of light microscopy to diagnose small-intestinal microsporidiosis in patients with AIDS, *J Infect Dis*, **157:** 827–31.

Rosberger DF, Serdarevic ON et al., 1993, Successful treatment of microsporidia keratoconjunctivitis with topical fumagillin in a patient with AIDS, *Cornea*, **12:** 261–5.

Ryan NJ, Sutherland G et al., 1993, A new trichrome-blue stain for detection of microsporidial species in urine, stool, nasopharyngeal specimens, *J Clin Microbiol*, **31:** 3264–9.

Sandfort J, Hannemann A et al., 1993, *Enterocytozoon bieneusi* in a patient not infected with HIV. Abstract 433, *Proceedings of the IX International Congress of Protozoology, Berlin, 25–31 July*, 111.

Sandfort J, Hannemann A et al., 1994, *Enterocytozoon bieneusi* infection in an immunocompetent patient who had acute diarrhea and who was not infected with the human immunodeficiency virus, *Clin Infect Dis*, **19:** 514–16.

Schmidt EC, Shadduck JA, 1983, Murine encephalitozoonosis model for studying the host parasite relationship of a chronic infection, *Infect Immun*, **40:** 936–42.

Schwartz DA, Visvesvara GS et al., 1993a, Pathological features and immunofluorescent antibody demonstration of ocular microsporidiosis (*Encephalitozoon hellem*) in seven patients with acquired immunodeficiency syndrome, *Am J Ophthalmol*, **115:** 285–92.

Schwartz DA, Visvesvara GS et al., 1993b, Pathology of symptomatic microsporidial (*Encephalitozoon hellem*) bronchiolitis in the acquired immunodeficiency syndrome: a new respiratory pathogen diagnosed from lung biopsy, bronchoalveolar lavage, sputum, and tissue culture, *Hum Pathol*, **24:** 937–43.

Serwadda D, Mugerwa RD et al., 1985, Slim disease: a new disease in Uganda and its association with HTLV-III infection, *Lancet*, **ii:** 849–52.

Shadduck JA, 1980, Effect of fumagillin on *in vitro* multiplication of *Encephalitozoon cuniculi*, *J Protozool*, **27:** 202–8.

Shadduck JA, Polley MB, 1978, Some factors influencing the in vitro infectivity and replication of *Encephalitozoon cuniculi*, *J Protozool*, **25:** 491–6.

Shadduck JA, Kelsoe G, Helmke J, 1979, A microsporidian contaminant of a non-human primate cell culture: ultrastructural comparison with *Nosema connori*, *J Parasitol*, **65:** 185–8.

Shadduck JA, Meccoli RA et al., 1990, Isolation of a microsporidian from a human patient, *J Infect Dis*, **162:** 773–776.

Silveira H, Canning EU, 1995, *Vittaforma corneae* n. comb. for the human microsporidium *Nosema corneum* Shadduck, Meccoli, Davis & Font, 1990. based on its ultrastructure in the liver of experimentally infected athymic mice, *J Euk Microbiol*, **42:** 158–65.

Silveira H, Canning EU, Shadduck JA, 1993, Experimental infection of athymic mice with the human microsporidian *Nosema corneum*, *Parasitology*, **107:** 489–96.

Simon D, Weiss LM et al., 1991, The light microscopic diagnosis of human microsporidiosis and variable response to octreotide, *Gastroenterology*, **100:** 271–3.

Smit FGAM, 1973, Siphonaptera (fleas), *Insects and Other Arthropods of Medical Importance*, ed Smith KGV, Trustees of the British Museum (Natural History), London, 325–71.

Smith KGV (ed), 1973, *Insects and Other Arthropods of Medical Importance*, Trustees of the British Museum (Natural History), London.

Sprague V, 1974, *Nosema connori* n.sp., microsporidian parasite of man, *Trans Amer Microsc Soc*, **93:** 400–3.

Sprague V, Vávra J, 1977, Systematics of the microsporidia, *Comparative Pathobiology*, vol 2, eds Bulla LA Jr, Cheng TC, Plenum Press, New York.

Sprague V, Becnel JJ, Hazard EI, 1992, Taxonomy of phylum microspora, *Crit Rev Microbiol*, **18:** 285–395.

Terada S, Reddy KR et al., 1987, Microsporidian hepatitis in the acquired immunodeficiency syndrome. (brief report), *Ann Intern Med*, **107:** 61–2.

Torres CM, 1927a, Sur une nouvelle maladie de l'homme, caractérisée par la présence d'un parasite intracellulaire, très proche de *Toxoplasma* et de l'*Encephalitozoon*, dans le tissu musculaire cardique, les muscles du squelette, le tissu cellulaire sous-cutane et le tissu nerveux, *C R Soc Biol Paris*, **97:** 1778–81.

Torres CM, 1927b, Morphologie d'un nouveau de l'homme, *Encephalitozoon chagasi*, n. sp. observé dans un cas de méningo-encéphalomyélite congenitale avec myosite et myocardite, *CR Soc Biol Paris*, **97:** 1787–90.

Torres CM, 1927c, Affinités de l'*Encephalitozoon chagasi*, agent étiologique d'une méningo-encéphalite-myélite congenitale avec myocardite et myosite chez l'homme, *C R Soc Biol Paris*, **97:** 1998–9.

Undeen AH, Vander Meer RK, 1990, The effect of ultraviolet radiation on the germination of *Nosema algerae* Vávra and Undeen (Microsporidia: Nosematidae) spores, *J Protozool*, **37:** 194–9.

Undeen AH, Vander Meer RK et al., 1984, The effect of gamma radiation on *Nosema algerae* (Microspora: Nosematidae) spore viability and germination, *J Protozool*, **31:** 479–82.

Van Gool T, Canning EU et al., 1994, *Septata intestinalis* fre-

quently isolated from stools of AIDS patients with a new cultivation method, *Parasitology*, **109:** 281–9.

Van Gool T, Hollister WS et al., 1990, Diagnosis of *Enterocytozoon bieneusi* microsporidiosis in AIDS patients by recovery of spores from faeces, *Lancet*, **336:** 697–8.

Van Gool T, Snijders F et al., 1993, Diagnosis of intestinal and disseminated microsporidial infections in HIV-infected individuals with a new rapid fluorescent technique, *J Clin Pathol*, **46:** 694–9.

Vavra J, Dahbiova et al., 1993, Staining of microsporidian spores by optical brighteners with remarks on the use of brighteners for the diagnosis of AIDS associated human microsporidiosis, *Folia Parastiol*, **40:** 267–72.

Visvesvara GS, Leitch GJ et al., 1991, Culture, electron microscopy, and immunoblot studies on a microsporidian parasite isolated from the urine of a patient with AIDS, *J Protozool*, **38:** 105S–111S.

Visvesvara GS, Leitch GJ et al., 1994, Polyclonal and monoclonal antibody and PCR-amplified small-subunit rRNA identification of a microsporidian, *Encephalitozoon hellem*, isolated from an AIDS patient with disseminated infection, *J Clin Microbiol*, **32:** 2760–8.

Visvesvara GS, Da Silva AJ et al., 1995, In vitro culture and serological and molecular identification of *Septata intestinalis* isolated from urine of a patient with AIDS, *J Clin Microbiol*, **33:** 930–6.

Vossbrinck CR, Maddox JV et al., 1987, Ribosomal RNA sequence suggests microsporidia are extremely ancient eukaryotes, *Nature (London)*, **326:** 411–14.

Vossbrinck CR, Baker MD et al., 1993, Ribosomal DNA sequences of *Encephalitozoon hellem* and *Encephalitozoon cuniculi*: species identification and phylogenetic construction, *J Euk Microbiol*, **40:** 354–62.

Weber R, Bryan RT, 1994, Microsporidial infections in immunodeficient and immunocompetent patients, *Clin Infect Dis*, **19:** 517–21.

Weber R, Bryan RT et al., 1992a, Improved light-microscopical detection of microsporidia spores in stool and duodenal aspirates, *N Engl J Med*, **326:** 161–6.

Weber R, Bryan RT et al., 1994, Human microsporidial infections, *Clin Microbiol Rev*, **7:** 426–461.

Weber R, Kuster H et al., 1992b, Pulmonary and intestinal microsporidiosis in a patient with the acquired immunodeficiency syndrome, *Am Rev Respir Dis*, **146:** 1603–5.

Webster JP, MacDonald DW, 1995, Cryptosporidiosis reservoir in wild brown rats (*Rattus norvegicus*) in the UK, *Epidemiol Infect*, **115:** 207–9.

Weidner E, 1976, The microsporidian invasion tube. The ultrastructure isolation and characterisation of the protein comprising the tube, *J Cell Biol*, **71:** 23–34.

Weidner E, 1982, The microsporidian spore invasion tube. III. Tube extrusion and assembly, *J Cell Biol*, **93:** 976–9.

Weidner E, 1991, Closing remarks on opportunistic microsporidians in humans, *J Protozool*, **38:** 638.

Weidner E, Byrd W, 1982, The microsporidian spore invasion tube. II. Role of calcium in the activation of invasion tube discharge, *J Cell Biol*, **93:** 970–5.

Weidner E, Halonen SK, 1993, Microsporidian spore envelope keratins phosphorylate and disassemble during spore activation, *J Euk Microbiol*, **40:** 783–8.

Weiser J, 1964, On the taxonomic position of the genus *Encephalitozoon* Levaditi, Nicolau & Schoen, 1923 (Protozoa, Microsporidia), *Parasitology*, **54:** 749–51.

Weiser J, Rehacek J, 1975, *Nosema slovaca* sp. n. : a second microsporidian of the tick *Ixodes ricinus*, *J Invert Pathol*, **26:** 411.

Wongtavatchai J, Conrad PA, Hedrick RP, 1995, In vitro characteristics of the microsporidian: *Enterocytozoon salmonis*, *J Euk Microbiol*, **42:** 401–5.

Wuhib T, Silva TMJ et al., 1994, Cryptosporidial and microsporidial infections in human immunodeficiency virus-infected patients in northeastern Brazil, *J Infect Dis*, **170**: 494–7.

Yee RW, Tio FO et al., 1991, Resolution of microsporidial epithelial keratopathy in a patient with AIDS, *Ophthalmology*, **98**: 196–201.

Zender HO, Arrigoni E et al., 1989, A case of *Encephalitozoon cuniculi* peritonitis in a patient with AIDS, *Am J Clin Pathol*, **92**: 352–6.

Zhu X, Wittner M et al., 1994, Ribosomal RNA sequences of *Enterocytozoon bieneusi*, *Septata intestinalis* and *Ameson michaelis*: phylogenetic construction and structural correspondence, *J Euk Microbiol*, **41**: 204–9.

Chapter 22

PNEUMOCYSTOSIS

H Fujioka and M Aikawa

Pneumocystosis or *Pneumocystis carinii* pneumonia (PCP) is an acute pneumonitis. In the 1960s and 1970s, *P. carinii* was found to be an important pathogen causing opportunistic pneumonia in immunosuppressed hosts, and in the 1980s *P. carinii* emerged as the most significant opportunistic pathogen in patients with acquired immunodeficiency syndrome (AIDS). *P. carinii* is an unicellular eukaryote that usually develops extracellularly in the lungs of host animals and undergoes encystment during one phase of its life cycle. There is no general agreement on the taxonomic position of this protistan parasite, which has biological characteristics that resemble those of both the fungi and the protozoa. The development of an in vitro culture system would be very useful in obtaining an understanding of the biological characteristics of *P. carinii*. However, despite intensive effort, *P. carinii* has not yet been grown in any completely satisfactory in vitro culture system.

1 CLASSIFICATION

Carlos Chagas probably recognized the organism and related lung pathology in 1909 while studying the histopathology of experimental *Trypanosoma cruzi* infections in guinea pigs. Chagas also reported that organisms similar to *P. carinii* occurred in the pneumonic lungs of a Chagas disease patient (Chagas 1911). However, until 1914, the organism was believed to be a form of *T. cruzi*. This error was corrected when Delanoe and Delanoe (1914) proved that this microorganism was distinct from *T. cruzi*, and assigned the descriptive genetic name *Pneumocystis carinii* to it.

Because it forms cysts, *P. carinii* has been variously classified as a fungus or as a protozoan (Vávra and Kucera 1970). The organism is probably not a sporozoan as the very specialized apical organelles (conoids, polar rings, rhoptries and subpellicular tubules), which are found in all members of the Sporozoa, are completely lacking in any stage of *P. carinii*. Some of the investigators who have decided that *P. carinii* is a protozoan (Balachandran, Jones and Humphrey 1990, Vossen et al. 1976), have proposed that it may belong in an independent taxonomic position (Matsumoto Matsuda and Tegoshi 1989, Yoshida 1989). Historically, all the therapeutic compounds which are effective against *P. carinii* are anti-protozoal agents, while no clinically used anti-fungal agents are effective (Burke and Good 1992). Various researchers have nevertheless decided it is a fungus (Bedrossian 1989, Dyer et al. 1992, Li and Edling 1994, Riis et al. 1990, Ruffolo, Cushion and Walzer 1989, ul Haque et al. 1987, Wakefield et al. 1992), on the basis of molecular and biochemical data. For example, the base sequences of the *P. carinii* 16S-like rRNA (Edman et al. 1988, Stringer et al. 1989), of the dihydrofolate reductase gene (Edman et al. 1989a), of the thymidilate synthase gene (Edman et al. 1989b), and of the mitochondrial DNA (Pixley et al. 1991) have been characterized. A phylogenic analysis of the 5S RNA gene of *P. carinii* has also been reported (Watanabe et al. 1989). These studies suggest that the closest phylogenetic affinities of *P. carinii* are with the fungi (see Volume 4, Chapter 35).

2 STRUCTURE AND LIFE CYCLE

The terminology for stages in the life cyle of *P. carinii*

(trophozoite, cyst, intracystic body, etc.) are drawn from terminology used for describing protozoan rather than fungal morphology. Since this is the most commonly used terminology it will be used in this chapter.

Our knowledge of the life cycle of *P. carinii*, including the mode of transmission, reservoir hosts and the nature of the transmissible form, remains incomplete. The developmental forms of *P. carinii* within mammalian lungs have been studied using specimens from humans or experimentally infected animals. Cultured organisms have also been studied. Light microscopy and electron microscopy have both been used in these studies. It appears likely that, with rare exceptions, the primary site of infection is the lungs, and it is possible that the entire life cycle of *P. carinii* may take place within the alveoli of infected lungs. *P. carinii* organisms may produce 10^8–10^9 cysts and 10^9–10^{10} nuclei per lung when the infection reaches peak intensity.

P. carinii assumes 4 basic morphological forms during its life cycle: (1) trophozoites, (2) precysts, (3) cysts and (4) intracystic bodies. The trophic forms (trophozoites) are of 2 distinct types, small spherical to oval forms and larger amoeboid types. Morphologically and ultrastructurally, the small trophic forms closely resemble the intracystic bodies within the mature cyst of *P. carinii*.

The small trophic form, unlike the large trophic form, has very few or no tubular extensions of its surface. The pellicle, 29–30 nm in thickness, consists of an electron-dense outer layer and an inner plasma membrane. The cytoplasm contains a double membrane-bound nucleus, a single mitochondrion with few cristae, endoplasmic reticulum, ribosomes and a few osmiophilic bodies. The glycogen content of the small form is less than that of the larger trophozoite. A single mitochondrion with a budding area is the main organelle of the small trophozoite (Palluault et al. 1991a). Mitochondrial processes for energy production seem to be the main physiological processes in the small trophozoite.

Large trophozoites are very irregular in shape (i.e. pleomorphic or amoeboid) having lobopodic pseudopodia as well as deep surface invaginations (Fig. 22.1). On the surface of mature large trophozoites, numerous long thin tubular expansions occur. The trophozoites form complicated infoldings and interdigitations with the type I pneumocytes (Del-Cas et al. 1991, Henshaw, Carson and Collier 1985, Itatani and Marshall 1988, Settnes and Nielsen 1991, Yoneda and Walzer 1983), forming a tight cluster of cells on the wall of the alveolar cavity (Fig. 22.2) (Itatani and Marshall 1988).

The membrane of the large trophozoites appears to be a typical unit membrane, and is covered externally by an electron-dense layer (about 15 nm thick) of extracellular material (the fuzzy coat) (Ruffolo, Cushion and Walzer 1989). The structure of the membrane of *P. carinii* has been revealed in great detail by freeze-fracture techniques (Yoneda et al. 1982, Yoshida 1989). There are more intermembranous particles (IMP) on the protoplasmic face of the split membrane than on the exoplasmic face in organisms in every stage of development. The IMP density decreases during development of the cyst from the trophozoite (Yoshida 1989). The cytoplasm of the large trophozoite appears to be less dense than that of the small trophozoite. The large trophozoite contains a single nucleus, a mitochondrion, endoplasmic reticulum, ribosomes, glycogen particles and osmiophilic round bodies (about 100 nm in diameter). Some investigators have described Golgi-like vesicles

(Palluault et al. 1990, Palluault et al. 1991a,b), but other investigators have reported that there is no Golgi apparatus in the trophozoites (Ruffolo, Cushion and Walzer 1989, Yoshida 1989). Neither microtubules nor microfilaments have been demonstrated in the non-dividing stage of the large trophozoites.

The precyst is considered to be an intermediate stage between the trophozoite and the cyst (Campbell 1972). It is oval in shape and 4–5 μm in diameter, with a large nucleus. As development proceeds, the thin double-layered pellicle of the precyst becomes thickened by the appearance of a new electron-lucent middle layer (Fig. 22.3). As development continues, the precyst becomes more spherical and the pellicle increases to 40–120 nm in thickness (Yoshikawa and Yoshida 1986). In the early stage of development of the precyst, a synaptonemal complex, indicative of a meiotic prophase, has been observed (Matsumoto and Yoshida 1984, Yoshida 1989). Following the disappearance of this complex, nuclear divisions occur. The 4 haploid nuclei are produced by a second meiosis and then 8 nuclei are produced by mitosis. During the process of nuclear division, a mitochondrion is developed. Ribosomes, glycogen granules and round bodies are also present in the cytoplasm of precysts.

The mature cyst is round and smooth (4–6 μm in diameter) and contains 8 intracystic bodies. The cyst wall is very thick (100–160 nm) and consists of an electron-dense outer layer, an electron-lucent middle layer and an inner plasmalemma (Fig. 22.4). The pellicle of the cyst has a thickened area 1–2 μm in diameter and 200–300 nm in thickness (Fig. 22.5). The function of this structure is unclear; some investigators have proposed that it is involved in excystation of the intracystic bodies. The main compartment of the electron-lucent layer of the cyst wall is β-1,3-glucan (Fig. 22.6) (Hidalgo et al. 1991, Matsumoto, Matsuda and Tegoshi 1991, Nollstadt et al. 1994), and inhibitors of β-1,3-glucan biosynthesis have been shown to effectively prevent *P. carinii* cyst development in pneumocystis of murine origin (Matsumoto, Matsuda and Tegoshi 1991, Nollstadt et al. 1994).

The intracystic body has a single nucleus, a mitochondrion, abundant endoplasmic reticulum and ribosomes. There are 3 types of intracystic bodies: a spherical form, a banana-shaped form and a pleomorphic ameboid form. After excystation, empty cysts frequently collapse into a crescent shape (Fig. 22.1).

In the initial stage of infection, small, haploid trophozoites (1.5–2 μm) without filopodia attach to the type I alveolar epithelial cells. These thin-walled stages increase in size (>10 μm): and assume a polymorphic shape. These haplophasic trophozoites transform into diplophasic trophozoites following a sexual process. The enlarged diploid trophozoites may develop in one of 2 ways.

In one way, reproducing asexual forms are produced by a process of binary fission (Richardson et al. 1989, Yoshida 1989). The mature trophozoites which develop by this process and which have a thin limiting pellicle (20–30 nm), are the precysts and transform into cysts. The precyst, as noted before, is an intermediate stage in the sexual cycle. The presence of synaptonemal complexes, which have been observed in the early precysts of *P. carinii*, indicate that this is a meiotic stage (Matsumoto and Yoshida 1986, Yoshida 1989). The precyst is ovoid. As development of this form progresses, the cyst wall becomes thicker by for-

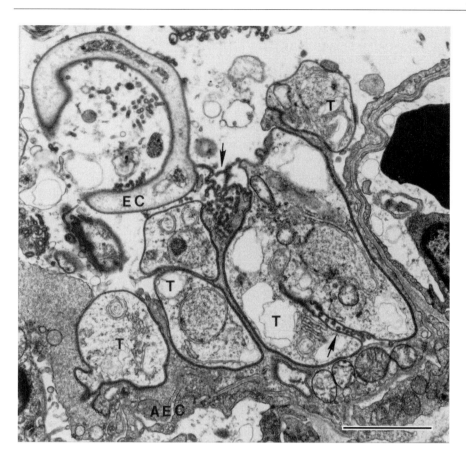

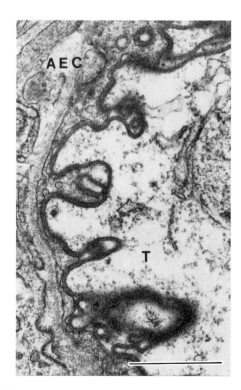

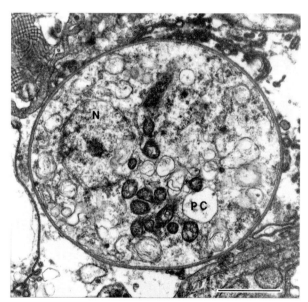

Fig. 22.1 Electron micrograph of *P. carinii* in rat lung tissue. The alveolus is occluded by cell debris and surfactant granules. Trophozoites (T) of *P. carinii* attached to type I alveolar epithelial cell (AEC). An empty cyst (EC) is collapsed into a crescent shape. Tubular expansions (arrows) can be seen around a large trophozoite but not around small trophozoites. Bar=2 μm. (*P. carinii* infected tissues were kindly provided by Dr DM Schmatz.)

Fig. 22.3 Electron micrograph of a intermediate precyst (PC) of *P. carinii* in rat lung tissue. The cell is spherical and the cell wall is thick. Nucleus (N) is located at the periphery of the cell near the plasma membrane. Bar=1 μm.

Fig. 22.2 Electron micrograph of *P. carinii* in rat lung tissue. Interdigitations form between type I epithelium cells (AEC) and trophozoite (T). Note the fingerlike projections of cytoplasm from the type I pneumocyte. Bar=1 μm.

mation of an inner electron-lucent and an outer electron-dense layer. During encystment, the diploid nucleus undergoes first and second meiotic divisions, followed by a postmeiotic mitosis to produce 8 haploid nuclei. These nuclei are incorporated in the intracystic bodies. The 8 intracystic bodies thus formed

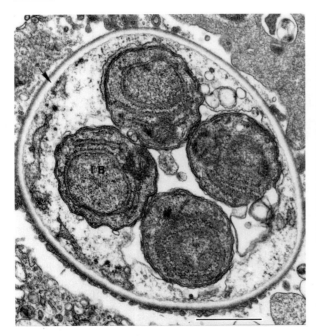

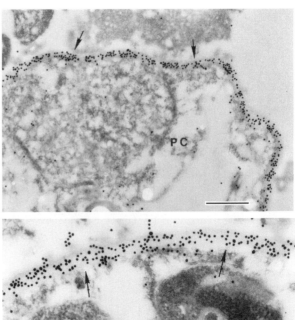

Fig. 22.4   Electron micrograph of a cyst of *P. carinii* in rat lung tissue. The cyst contains spherical intracystic bodies (IB). An electron-lucent middle layer (arrow) is shown between the electron-dense layer and the plasma membrane of the cyst. Bar=1 μm.

Fig. 22.6   Immunoelectron micrographs of a precyst (PC) and a mature cyst (C) containing intracystic bodies (IB) of *P. carinii*. Gold particles are associated with the distribution of β-1,3-glucan on the electron-lucent layer (arrows) of the precyst and cyst. Bar=0.5 μm. (Rabbit anti-β-1,3-glucan serum was kindly supplied by Dr DM Schmatz.)

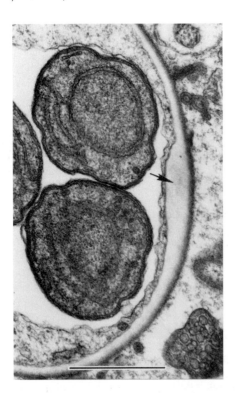

Fig. 22.5   Electron micrograph showing a thickened portion (arrow) of the cyst wall of *P. carinii*. Bar=1 μm.

diploid trophozoites may follow involves another cycle producing thin-walled cysts (Matsumoto and Yoshida 1986, Vossen et al. 1978). In a mature thin-walled cyst produced by this process pleomorphic daughter cells develop. The significance of these forms is not understand.

3   BIOCHEMISTRY, MOLECULAR GENETICS AND ANTIGENIC PROPERTIES

Although numerous attempts to cultivate *P. carinii* using a variety of media and feeder cell layer systems have been reported (Latorre, Sulzer and Norman 1977, Pifer, Wood and Hughes 1978b, Bartlett, Vervanac and Smith 1979, Smith and Bartlet 1984, Cushion, DeStefano and Walzer 1985, Tegoshi 1988, Cushion 1989, Durkin et al. 1989, Armstrong et al. 1991), a completely satisfactory in vitro system has not yet been achieved (Sloand et al. 1993). Further work is urgently needed in this area as good in vitro cultivation systems would greatly aid studies of the metabolism, biochemistry, molecular genetics, antigenic properties and mode of transmission of *P. carinii* and

remain for a time within the mature cyst. After cyst formation is complete, excystation occurs and the spherical or elongated intracystic bodies are released from the cyst (Shiota 1984).

The second path of development that the enlarged

thus facilitate the development of diagnostic and therapeutic techniques.

The haploid genome of rat-derived *P. carinii* is organized into 15–18 chromosomes containing 700– 1000 kbp of DNA (Hong et al. 1990, Lundgren et al. 1990). The chromosomes size is similar to that of fungi, and like that of fungi, *P. carinii* DNA is rich in adenine and thymine (Worley, Ivey and Graves 1989, Hong et al. 1990, Lundgren et al. 1990). *P. carinii* cysts contain 8 times more DNA than the trophozoites do (Yamada et al. 1986). This supports conclusions drawn from morphological observations based on the fact that the cyst has 8 intracystic bodies. *P. carinii* organisms from different hosts are substantially different in electrophoretic karyotype, and in DNA sequences (Liu et al. 1992, Cushion et al. 1993, Liu and Leibowitz 1993, Stringer et al. 1993). These studies indicate that organisms identified as *P. carinii* have diverse genotypes.

The total protein content per cyst has been estimated as approximately 62 pg (Gradus, Gilmore and Lerner 1988), and many enzymes, such as ATPase (Meade and Stringer 1991), glucose-6-phosphate dehydrogenase (Mazer et al. 1987) and lactic dehydrogenase (Mazer et al. 1987) have been identified in the organism by direct and indirect methods. In cysts there is very little glucose-6-phosphate dehydrogenase (Mazer et al. 1987). This enzyme in *P. carinii* has been reported to be very different from that of rat host cells (Pesanti 1989a). A highly developed mitochondrion is present in trophozoites and precysts (Palluault et al. 1991a,b), so *P. carinii* would seem to have aerobic metabolic capacities.

Cholesterol is the major sterol of *P. carinii* (Kaneshiro et al. 1989). On the basis of electron microscopic studies it has been proposed that the osmiophilic cytoplasmic bodies of *P. carinii* are the organs in which lipids are stored. It has been suggested that *P. carinii* can incorporate low molecular weight nutrient substances from the alveolar fluid of the host lungs (Itatani and Marshall 1988), and Paulsrud and Queener (1994) demonstrated the in vitro incorporation of fatty acids, leucine and methionine. Ultrastructural studies have failed to demonstrate phagocytosis or pinocytosis.

Glucose is the major sugar in *P. carinii*, with mannose, galactose and *N*-acetylglucosamine also having been demonstrated in the organism by use of a lectin binding assay (Yoshikawa, Tegoshi and Yoshida 1987, Cushion, DeStefano and Walzer 1988, Pesanti and Shanley 1988, DeStefano et al. 1989, DeStefano et al. 1992). Glycogen, α-1,4-glucan, β-1,3-glucan and chitin have also been demonstrated in the cyst wall by assays using enzymes and immunocytochemistry (Schmatz et al. 1990, Williams et al. 1991, Garner, Walker and Horst 1991, Nollstadt et al. 1994). Studies using immunoelectron microscopy have show that a high concentration of β-1,3-glucan is present in the electron-lucent layer of the *P. carinii* cyst wall, although it is not present in the intracystic bodies and trophozoites (Nollstadt et al. 1994). Moreover, the β-1,3-glucan synthesis inhibitor, L733,560, has a significant effect on cyst development. These data suggest that the synthesis of β-1,3-glucan is required for cyst wall formation (Nollstadt et al. 1994).

Pneumocystis organisms contain a large surface glycoprotein (90–120 kDa). Such glycoproteins have been found in various *Pneumocystis* isolated from animals of various species including glycoprotein A (gpA) from a *Pneumocystis* infecting ferrets (Haidaris et al. 1992), a major surface glycoprotein (MSG) from one infecting rats (Kovacs et al. 1993, Wada et al. 1993); and gpA from one infecting humans (Walzer and Linke 1987, Lundgren, Lipschik and Kovacs 1991). It has been suggested that MSG/gpA may play a major role in binding *Pneumocystis* organisms to host cells by a system mediated by fibronectin (Pottratz and Martin 1990) or a lectin (Baughman, Hull and Whitsett 1992).

4 CLINICAL ASPECTS

Epidemics of pneumocystosis had occurred in Europe before the 1940s, but this interstitial plasma cell pneumonitis was not common in humans. After the 1960s, immunosuppressive therapies using corticosteroids and cytotoxic agents came into general use in patients, and the incidence of pneumocystosis increased as many immunocompromised patients developed it. Before the acquired immunodeficiency syndrome (AIDS) epidemic, Hodgkin's disease and renal transplantation were the conditions most often associated with pneumocystosis. After the beginning of the AIDS epidemic, the number of cases of pneumocystosis increased dramatically. More than 60% of AIDS patients in the United States and Europe were estimated to develop pneumocystosis and many of them died of the disease before methods of prophylaxis for *P. carinii* infection were developed. Pneumocystosis is usually a bilateral and diffuse pneumonitis caused by pulmonary infection. The incidence of extrapulmonary *P. carinii* infections has been increasing. The lymph nodes, the spleen, the liver, and the bone marrow are the organs most commonly involved in patients with extrapulmonary infection.

4.1 Clinical manifestations

Pneumocystis carinii is widely distributed in nature with many mammal species serving as natural hosts. For the most part, the infections are latent without any clinical signs. For example, serological studies have shown that approximately 75–83% of normal individuals have acquired antibody against *P. carinii* by 4 years of age (Meuwissen et al. 1977, Pifer et al. 1978a). These data show clearly that *P.carinii* infection does not usually cause disease in individuals who have normal immune responses.

In individuals developing disease, *P. carinii* organisms are often found adhering to the alveolar epithelium in clusters. The adhering parasite cluster is a prime factor in the production of the pathophysiology of the infection and its mass may cause blockage of the alveolar capillaries with disturbances in blood oxygenation in the alveoli. The CD4 count is a very useful aid in making a prognosis for immunocompromised patients; with *P. carinii* infection, low counts indicate a poor prognosis.

There are 4 types of *P. carinii* infections: (1) asymptomatic infections (2) infections causing interstitial plasma cell pneumonitis in infants (3) infections causing sporadic pneumonitis in immunosuppressed children and adults and (4) extrapulmonary infections.

Asymptomatic infections are common but are of no clinical importance except that they may act as reservoirs of infection for susceptible individuals.

The first clinical signs of infantile interstitial plasma cell pneumonitis caused by *P. carinii* are subtle. They include poor appetite and diarrhoea. Cough, coryza and fever are usually absent early in the course of the disease. After 1–2 weeks, severe tachypnoea, dyspnoea, cyanosis, intercostal and sternal retraction and rales become obvious. Without treatment, many of the affected infants die. The histopathological appearance of lung tissue samples is typically characterized by mild chronic interstitial inflammation with proliferation of type II pneumocytes (Weber, Askin and Zenner 1977)

The clinical features of pneumocystosis in immunosuppressed children and adults are remarkably uniform, being characterized by dyspnoea, tachypnoea, fever and cough in patients both with and without HIV infection (Kovacs et al. 1984). There is usually a non-productive cough with chest tightness or pain and haemoptysis (Kovacs et al. 1984, Mascarenhas, Vasudevan and Vaidya 1991). Chest radiographs reveal fine, perihilar, diffuse 'ground-glass' infiltrates in the lungs. The infiltration progresses to form an interstitial alveolar butterfly pattern (DeLorenzo et al. 1987). In pneumocystosis patients with HIV infection, the lung inflammation is less and there are fewer neutrophils than in immunosuppressed patients without HIV infection. In the HIV-infected patients a large number of *P. carinii* organisms are present in fluids obtained by bronchoalveolar lavage (Limper et al. 1989).

Extrapulmonary *Pneumocystis carinii*-infected lesions have been detected in increasing numbers of patients (Northfelt, Clement and Safrin 1990, Cohen and Stoeckle 1991), but they are more common in AIDS patients than in other immunocompromised individuals. Extrapulmonary lesions have been observed in the lymph nodes, spleen, liver, bone marrow, adrenal glands, thyroid, heart, pancreas, eyes, ears, skin, gastrointestinal tract, and genitourinary tract (Raviglione 1990, Cohen and Stoeckle 1991).

5 IMMUNOLOGY

P. carinii is an opportunistic pathogen which causes disease in immunosuppressed hosts whose immune systems are functioning abnormally for a variety of reasons including inhibition by immunosuppressive drugs. The evidence available suggests that both the humoral and cell-mediated immune systems are important for protection from the consequences of infection and for elimination of infection.

Walzer and Rutledge (1982) concluded that normal mice carrying subclinical *P. carinii* infection develop serum antibodies to *P. carinii*, that the antibody titre is generally suppressed by steroid administration, that the infection becomes patent during steroid administration, and that the titre rises and the infection again becomes subclinical when the treatment is discontinued. They observed that the major immunoglobulin class produced is IgG and that antibody production requires an intact functioning thymus (Walzer

and Rutledge 1982).They also observed that athymic nude mice cannot produce antibodies against *P. carinii*, and that outbred nude mouse strains vary in their susceptibility to *P. carinii* infection. Several other studies also suggest that serum IgG antibody titres are developed upon recovery from *P. carinii* infection in nu/+ mice, nu/+ rats, nu/nu mice and rats, and severe combined immunodeficiency (SCID) mice (Walzer and Rutledge 1982, Furuta, Ueda and Fujiwara 1984, Furuta et al. 1985b). Similar findings have also been obtained in humans (Hofmann et al. 1988, Peglow et al. 1990, Pifer et al. 1978a), but contradictory results have been obtained in assays for IgA or IgM antibodies against *P. carinii* in infected animals (Walzer and Rutledge 1982, Furuta, Ueda and Fujiwara 1984, Furuta, Fujiwara and Yamonouchi 1985a, Walzer et al. 1987) and also in humans (Hofmann et al. 1985, Hofmann et al. 1988). AIDS patients with or without pneumocystosis have an IgA titre similar to that of the healthy controls (Hofmann et al. 1988). These results support the belief that IgM and IgA immune responses to *P. carinii* are not consistent.

Antibodies to *P. carinii* are not fully protective against pneumocystosis and are not fully effective in bringing about recovery from infection. Much evidence suggests that cell-mediated immunity is important in host defence; the T cell mediated immune system, in particular that portion controlled by the CD4[+] T cells, has been shown to be the major component in the host defence against disease caused by *P. carinii* infection (Furuta, Ueda and Fujiwara 1984, Roths and Sidman 1992). Roths and Sidman (1992), using an adoptive transfer system in SCID mice, demonstrated that CD4[+] cells are essential for resistance to disease caused by *P. carinii* infection, but that CD8[+] T cells are not, at least in the absence of antibody. They also showed that humoral immunity (in the absence of T cells) cannot fully protect. Roifman et al. (1989), however, suggested that CD8[+] T cells alone may play a role in resistance to infantile *P. carinii* pneumocystosis.

Histological evidence indicates that macrophages in the alveolar spaces are critical in control of *P. carinii* organisms. Opsonic antibody enhances the ingestion of *P. carinii* by alveolar macrophages (Masur and Jones 1978). Tumour necrosis factor (TNF)-α has been shown to be directly toxic to the pneumocystosis agent (Pesanti 1989b). Tamburrini et al. (1991) demonstrated that *P. carinii* stimulated the production of TNF-α by human macrophages. Its production by alveolar macrophages in AIDS patients with pneumocystosis increases during the course of the disease (Krishnan et al. 1990).

6 PATHOLOGY

The lungs are usually enlarged and heavy with a firm rubbery consistency. The principal finding on examination of lung sections stained with haematoxylin and eosin is the presence in the alveoli of a hyaline foamy granular eosinophilic exudate with a honeycomb form (Figs 22.7). The alveolar septa are thickened and there is typically interstitial inflammation with proliferation of type II pneumocytes.

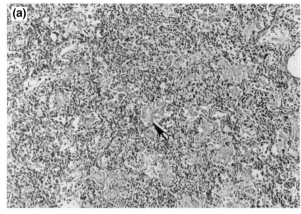

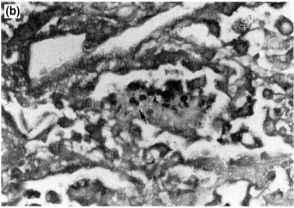

Fig. 22.7 (a) Low magnification light micrograph of a paraffin-embedded haematoxylin and eosin stained section of human lung tissue infected with *P. carinii*. This section shows the distended alveoli which are commonly observed in overt cases of *P. carinii* (arrow) infection on histopathological examination. (b) High magnification light micrograph of a silver stained section of *P. carinii* infected human lung tissue. With the silver staining techniques, in contrast to haematoxylin and eosin techniques, both the *P. carinii* organisms (arrow) and the foamy material are clearly shown. Reproduced with permission from Seed and Aikawa, 1977.

The preceding were the typical histological features found in patients before the AIDS epidemic. Pneumocystosis patients with AIDS frequently manifest atypical histological features. They may not have an alveolar exudate, and often have pulmonary cysts and cavities (Judson, Postic and Weiman 1990). The pulmonary cysts in AIDS patients with pneumocystosis are usually found in the upper lobes.

In patients with the disseminated (extrapulmonary) form of pneumocystosis, there are pathological findings throughout the body (Northfelt, Clement and Sarin 1990, Cohen and Stoeckle 1991). Such patients may develop granulomatous inflammations, lymphatic interstital infiltrates and microscarification in infected organs (Weber, Askin and Dehner 1977, Blumenfeld et al. 1988, Murphy et al. 1989, Travis et al. 1990). Extensive invasion of an organ by *P. carinii* can lead to its failure and to the patient's death (Cote et al. 1990).

7 DIAGNOSIS

The diagnosis of pneumocystosis is usually based on (1) patient history, physical examination and white cell counts (2) radiological and sonographic examination (3) histopathological examination and direct microscopic detection of *P. carinii* organisms in lung and other specimens (4) serological tests, and (5) detection of *P. carinii* specific DNA.

An evaluation of the patient's history and a physical examination are universally used for diagnosis when pneumocystosis is suspected. The patient with *P. carinii* pneumonia has an increasing dyspnoea. Severe hypoxaemia often develops in patients who exercise. Rapid breathing and a non-productive cough are also common clinical features. In general, patients with human immunodeficiency virus (HIV) infection are at high risk of developing pneumocystosis when the CD4 count is below $250/\text{mm}^3$ (Phair et al. 1990). The CD4 count is particularly useful as an aid to prognosis for HIV positive immunocompromised patients with *P. carinii* infection (Siminski et al. 1991). Low counts indicate a poor prognosis.

A chest radiograph is a most useful aid in diagnosis and prognosis, but it does not provide a conclusive diagnosis of pneumocystis infection. The typical radiographic appearance of lungs in patients with pneumocystosis is a diffuse opacity that appears early in the infection. These areas of opacity transform into irregular patches of consolidation as the infection progresses, and they may disappear during chemotherapy. Sonography and computed tomography can also be a useful aid in diagnosis of extrapulmonary infection (Lubat et al. 1990).

A positive diagnosis is made by identifying the aetiological agent in sputum (Pitchenik et al. 1986) or within specimens taken by open-lung biopy (Fitzgerald et al. 1987), by transbronchial biopsy (Broaddus et al. 1985), by bronchoscopy (Gal et al. 1987) or at necropsy. A diagnosis may also in part be based on finding the characteristic hyaline eosinophilic exudate with its honeycomb structure in the lung tissues examined (see section 6). The presence of an eosinophilic alveolar exudate has been considered to be the key sign in the diagnosis of pneumocystosis, but this may not be true for AIDS patients and even others, as recent studies have indicated that the percentage of patients lacking alveolar exudate ranges from 19% to 47% (Weber, Askin and Dehner 1977, Travis et al. 1990).

Several staining procedures are available for preparation of specimens. Gomori's methenamine silver stain is the most common silver stain employed (Mahan and Sale 1978, Shimano and Hartman 1986) and is the best and easiest method for staining *P. carinii* cysts. Toluidine blue O stain may also be used (Gosey et al. 1985). Papanicolaou (Greaves and Strigle 1985) or Wright–Giemsa stain (Domingo and Waksal 1984) is used for staining the trophozoites. Conventional light microscopy and electron microscopy are used for detection of *P. carinii* organisms. Tests based on direct and indirect immunofluorescent stains are said to be more sensitive than tests based on conventional staining methods (Kovacs et al. 1988, Cregan et al. 1990, Ng et al. 1990).

Kovacs et al. (1986) have developed many monoclonal antibodies against major cell wall and surface antigens of *P. carinii*, and these can be used in a variety of immunological diagnostic procedures. Serological examinations are of limited diagnostic use because most normal people have antibodies against *P. carinii* in their blood, presumably from subclinical infection in childhood (Peglow et al. 1990).

DNA hybridization techniques, using the polymerase chain reaction (PCR) and oligonucleotide probes, have also been developed (Wakefield et al. 1990, Becker-Hapak, Liberator and Graves 1991, Galman et al. 1991, Kitada et al. 1991, Wakefield et al. 1991) and should facilitate diagnosis of *P. carinii* infection.

8 EPIDEMIOLOGY AND CONTROL

P. carinii has been found in the lungs of humans and a variety of domestic and wild animals in most countries of the world. It is not known if infection is normally passed from one species to another. Airborne animal to animal transmission has been demonstrated (see section 8.1). Human to human transmission seems to occur both by the airborne route and by direct or close contact transmission. Endemic clusters of human *P. carinii* infection have been observed and this suggests that direct or close contact transmission is an important route of infection. As noted above (see section 5, 'Immunology'), serological surveys indicate that 19% of infants younger than 1 year of age have acquired antibody against *P. carinii* and the incidence increases to 83% by 4 years of age (Pifer et al. 1978a). This observation suggests the existence of a reservoir from which the young became infected.

The prevention of pneumocystosis and its treatment are wholly dependent on chemotherapeutic agents, and unfortunately the drugs currently available have severe side effects. An understanding of the life cycle, modes of transmission and species specificity of *P. carinii* might help us to develop programmes for control of infections caused by this organism. At present no vacccine is available.

8.1 Epidemiology (including reservoir hosts)

The many domestic and wild animals which have been found to harbour *P. carinii* include rats, mice, dogs, guinea pigs, monkeys, sheep, goats and horses (Robbins 1967), but whether the *P. carinii* in all these animals are really of the same species is not known. Poelma (1975) reported that no *P. carinii* organisms were detected in birds in zoos in Holland. *P. carinii* organisms can grow in cells of human cell lines at temperatures of 35–37°C, but replication was inhibited at 41°C (Cushion et al. 1985), suggesting that *P. carinii* has very specific temperature requirements for growth. The body temperature of birds is over 40°C, which may explain the absence of infection.

There are 3 epidemiological types of human pneumocystosis; (1) classical plasma cell pneumonia in infants (2) pneumocystosis in hosts immunocompromised as a result of immunosuppressive or cytotoxic therapies (3) pneumocystosis in AIDS patients. The first type is an endemic disease usually affecting malnourished premature infants. The second epidemically distinct form of human pneumocystosis was first recognized in the 1960s and 1970s and appeared with the development of procedures for control of cancer by means of cytotoxic agents, and of therapies which suppress or compromise the immune systems of organ transplant recipients. Children with severely compromised immune systems, especially those with impaired cell mediated responses, are at particular risk of contracting pneumocystosis, and *P. carinii* is now recognized as the major cause of pneumonia in such children. The third distinct endemic type of pneumocystosis has been recognized since the 1980s and appeared with the AIDS epidemic in almost every country of the world. Pneumocystis in AIDS patients is characterized by some unique clinical features, such as the spread of the organisms to organs other than the lungs and a high frequency of recurrence after treatment.

The source of *P. carinii* in people with clinical disease is unclear. Exogenous *P. carinii* may be the cause of infection, or possibly a latent organism in the lungs is activated in the immunosuppressed hosts. Infection may be only from other humans, or a non-human reservoir may exist. It is believed that *P. carinii* is maintained in humans primarily by direct transmission from infected individuals to uninfected ones.

Soulez et al. (1991) demonstrated that the transmission of *P. carinii* of mice occurred by an airborne route and that the young were not infected at birth. In these studies *P. carinii*-free SCID mice were bred in cages isolated by air filters from *P. carinii*-infected mice, and the isolated mice did not develop *P. carinii* infection. However, infection did occur in *P. carinii*-free mice exposed only to unfiltered air from infected mice housed in separate cages. This clearly demonstrated that the mice were not latently infected with *P. carinii* organisms, but could be infected by an airborne route. The fact that corticosteroid treatment induced infection in the healthy normal mice used as a source of infection in these experiments indicates the widespread occurence of latent infection in normal mice.

9 CHEMOTHERAPY

The key to effective treatment is early diagnosis. Without treatment, pneumocystosis is usually fatal to compromised hosts. The current therapeutic approach consists of (1) specific chemotherapy and (2) supporting therapy. The standard treatment is the administration of trimethoprim–sulfamethaxazole (TMP-SMX, co-trimoxazole) or parenteral pentamidine isethionate.

Trimethoprim and sulfamethaxazole are both inhibitors of microbial folate production, each inhibiting a different step in folate production: trimethoprim inhibits the dihydrofolate reductase, and sulfamethaxazole inhibits the dihydropteroate synthetase of *P. carinii*. The standard dose of co-trimoxazole for patients with pneumocystosis is 12–20 mg/kg of the trimethoprim component per day. The dose is administered orally or intravenously for 14–21 days. In AIDS patients, co-trimoxazole therapy has been associated with a high rate of allergic reactions, such as rash, fever, leucopenia and thrombocytopenia 8–12 days after co-trimoxazole treatment (Gordin et al. 1984).

Pentamidine isethionate is a diamidine compound to which *P. carinii* (like many protozoa) is very sensitive. It is administered either intravenously or intramuscularly, but intravenous administration is preferable because it minimizes severe adverse effects (Kovacs et al. 1984, Conte, Hollander and Golden 1987, Sattler et al. 1988). Discontinuation of therapy was required due to major toxicity in up to 47% of patients receiving the drug by the intramuscular route. Azotaemia, pancreatitis, dysglycaemia, hypocalcaemia and leucopenia are among the most severe toxic effects of the drug (Salmeron et al. 1986, Zuger et al. 1986, Sattler et al. 1988). The standard dose of pentamidine isethionate is 4 mg/kg once daily for 14–21 days. In AIDS patients, the dosage can be reduced to a level causing less toxicity (Conte, Hollander and Golden 1987, Sattler et al. 1988). In an attempt to reduce the undesirable effects that result from parenteral administration, aerosolized pentamidine (AP) has been given by inhalation in treatment of patients with acute pneumocystosis (Conte and Golden 1988).

A combination of trimethoprim and dapsone has been used for treatment of AIDS patients with mild to moderate pneumocystosis (Leoung et al. 1986). Trimethoprim–dapsone therapy caused fewer adverse effects than co-trimoxazole therapy, and many physicians now consider that trimthoprim–dapsone is the first choice for initial therapy (Medina et al. 1990).

Several other agents are now being evaluated for use against *P. carinii* and 2 of them, trimetrexate and hydroxynaphthoquinone (BW 566C80), have given promising results in trials and seem to have potent anti-*P. carinii* activities (Allegra et al. 1987a; Hughes et al. 1990, Hughes et al. 1993). Trimetrexate is an inhibitor of the dihydrofolate reductase of *P. carinii* (Allegra et al. 1987b) and BW 566C80 is known to be an inhibitor of the dihydroorotate dehydrogenase of plasmodia (Hammond, Burchell and Pudney 1985).

Great efforts are being made to discover and evaluate new anti-*P. carinii* drugs. Recently tested compounds that show some promise include (1) folate antagonists (Walzer et al. 1988, Kovacs et al. 1989), (2) various compounds of the diamidine class (Jones et al. 1990, Tidwell et al. 1990), (3) 8-aminoquinolines (Queener et al. 1992), (4) β-1,3-glucan synthesis inhibitors (Schmatz et al. 1991, Nollstadt et al. 1994) and (5) acridone alkaloid derivatives (Queener et al. 1991).

Supplemental therapies aimed at the elevation of arterial oxygen presure are helpful to AIDS patients who are receiving chemotherapy for moderate or severe pneumocystosis. The administration of corticosteroids is of significant benefit (El-Sadr and Simberkoff 1988, Bozzette et al. 1990, National Institutes of Health–University of California Expert Panel 1990). Many patients with pneumocystosis develop pulmonary dysfunction 3–5 days after treatment for *P. carinii* infection. The administration of therapy to support lung function along with specific anti-*P. carinii* agents reduces the frequency of mortality in such patients.

10 VACCINATION

Propagation of *P. carinii* can easily occur in patients suffering from malnutrition, in premature infants, in people with congenital immunodeficiency diseases, or undergoing immunosuppressive therapy and in those with AIDS. In people with any of these conditions cell mediated immunity is depressed, in particular that controlled by T cells (Gleason and Roodman 1977, Bujes et al. 1981, Rao and Gelfand 1983, Slade and Hepburn 1983). However, there are data to suggest that both the humoral and cellular immunity systems are important for protection and recovery from pneumocystosis (Harmsen and Stankiewicz 1990, Peglow et al. 1990, Shellito et al. 1990). Although the antibodies specific for *P. carinii* are produced by B cells, they require the co-operation of helper T cells (Gigliotti and Hughes 1988, Harmsen and Stankiewicz 1991), and therefore any condition that destroys T cells may also effect humoral immunity. Any immunization procedure, active or passive, that would compensate for these defects would be useful. Some examples of such treatments include the demonstration by Gigliotti and Hughes (1988) that administration of a monoclonal antibody against a major antigen of *P. carinii* reduced the numbers of *P. carinii* in rats and ferrets immunosuppressed by steroid treatment, and the demonstration by Roths and Sidman (1993) that administration of anti-*P. carinii*-hyperimmune serum reduced the numbers of *P. carinii* in SCID mice with pneumocystosis. These data suggest that a vaccine that induces antibody specific for *P. carinii* may be of some use for immunotherapy and immunoprophylaxis against pneumocystosis. No such vaccine is at present available, and if it were it would probably not help individuals whose immunological system were badly damaged, but administration of immune serum would possibly be of some help to patients with pneumocystosis.

11 INTEGRATED CONTROL

Prophylaxis against *P. carinii* infection is necessary for patients suffering from conditions such as AIDS, AIDS-related complex (ARC) diseases and acute lymphoblastic leukaemia, and in those receiving bone marrow and solid organ transplants. Prophylaxis is usually based on administration of appropriate drugs to high risk patients. Approximately 90% of heart–lung and lung allograft recipients will develope pneumocystosis in the absence of prophylaxis (Gryzan et al. 1988). Pneumocystosis can be prevented by the administration of co-trimoxazole and AP. The prophylactic dosage is 160 mg trimethoprim and 800 mg sulfame-thoxazole orally in adults, and 75 mg trimethoprim and 375 mg sulfamethaxazole intravenously in children. Although co-trimoxazole is commonly used for treatment and chemoprophylaxis to prevent pneumocystosis, up to 50% of patients so treated develop adverse reactions. Pentamidine isethionate given by inhalation (AP) is extensively used for prophylaxis. The prophylactic dose is 300 mg of pentamidine isethionate each month inhaled with the aid of a nebulizer. This treatment is used in adults and in children over 5 years of age. Although some undesirable side effects may occur in patients on AP treatment, for example moderate to severe cough, the proportion of the patients suffering undesirable affects so severe as to require termination of the AP therapy is lower than the proportion of those on co-trimoxazole treatment requiring termination because of side effects.

12 CONCLUSIONS

Chemotherapy is available for treatment and prophylaxis of patients suffering from or at risk of pneumocystosis. Better drugs, less toxic ones for example, are needed, but the ones we have are better than nothing considering the difficulties in producing any type of cure in immunodepressed patients. Control of transmission of *P. carinii* is very important. Unfortunately its mode of transmission, the transmissive form and the source of infection are not well understood. If we had accurate information on these subjects, transmission could possibly be controlled. Our lack of understanding of the life cycle of this parasite and the lack of a satisfactory culture system are obstacles to the management of *P. carinii* infections. Useful genetic information is gradually becoming available. Analysis of the *P. carinii* genome demonstrates that there are distinct differences in the genomes of *P. carinii*, depending on the host from which the parasite was isolated (Pneumocystis Workshop 1994). Analysis of the thymidylate synthase gene of *P. carinii* also revealed genomic differences among *P. carinii* isolated from different hosts (Mazars et al. 1995). These results indicate that there may be different species in different hosts. The study of characterized strains for their ability to infect a variety of hosts could help us understand the relationships between *P. carinii* in possible reservoir animals and in humans and thus aid planning of programmes to control its transmission. What is really needed, however, is application of available public health measures to reduce the proportion of immunocompromised people in the population. If this could be done, pneumocystosis would again become the rare disease it used to be.

ACKNOWLEDGEMENTS

This work was supported in part by grants from the US Agency for International Development (DPE936 600129) and the USPHS/NIH AI35827.

REFERENCES

Allegra CJ, Chabner BA et al., 1987a, Trimetrexate for the treatment of *Pneumocystis carinii* pneumonia in the patients with the acquired immunodeficiency syndrome, *N Engl J Med*, **317:** 978–85.

Allegra CJ, Kovacs JA et al., 1987b, Activity of antifolates against *Pneumocystis carinii* dihydrofolate reductase and identification of a potent new agent, *J Exp Med*, **165:** 926–31.

Armstrong MYK, Koziel H et al., 1991, Indicators of *Pneumocystis carinii* viability in short-term cell culture, *J Protozool*, **38:** 88–90S.

Balachandran I, Jones DB, Humphrey DM, 1990, A case of *Pneumocystis carinii* in pleural fluid with cytologic, histologic and ultrastructural documentation, *Acta Cytol*, **34:** 486–90.

Bartlett MS, Vervanac PA, Smith JW, 1979, Cultivation of *Pneumocystis carinii* with WI38 cell, *J Clin Microbiol*, **10:** 796–9.

Baughman RP, Hull W, Whitsett JA, 1992, *Pneumocystis carinii* alters surfactant associated protein-A concentrations found in bronchoalveolar fluid, *J Clin Res*, **40:** 412A.

Becker-Hapak M, Liberator P, Graves D, 1991, Detection of *P. carinii* by polymerase chain reaction, *J Protozool*, **38:** 1915–45.

Bedrossian CWM, 1989, Ultrastructure of *Pneumocystis carinii* : a review of internal and surface characteristics, *Semin Diagn Pathol*, **6:** 212–37.

Blumenfeld W, Basgoz N et al., 1988, Granulomatous pulmonary lesions in patients with the acquired immunodeficiency syndrome (AIDS) and *Pneumocystis carinii* infection, *Ann Intern Med*, **109:** 505–7.

Bozzette SA, Sattler FR et al., 1990, A controlled trial of early adjunctive treatment with corticosteroids for *Pneumocystis carinii* pneumonia in the acquired immunodeficiency syndrome, *N Engl J Med*, **323:** 1451–7.

Broaddus C, Dake MD et al., 1985, Bronchoalveolar lavage and transbronchial biopsy for the diagnosis of pulmonary infections in the acquired immunodeficiency syndrome, *Ann Intern Med*, **102:** 747–52.

Bujes D, Hardt C et al., 1981, Cyclosporin A mediates immunosuppression of primary cytotoxic T cell responses by impairing the release of interleukin 1 and interleukin 2, *Eur J Immunol*, **11:** 657–61.

Burke BA, Good RA, 1992, *Pneumocystis carinii* : infection and commentary by WT Hughes, *Medicine (Baltimore)*, **71:** 165–78.

Campbell WG, 1972, Ultrastructure of *Pneumocystis carinii* in human lung. Life cycle in human pneumocystosis, *Arch Pathol*, **93:** 312–24.

Chagas C, 1911, Nova entidade morbida do homen; rezumo geral de estudos etiolojicos e clinicos, *Mem Inst Oswaldo Cruz*, **3:** 219–75.

Cohen OJ, Stoeckle MY, 1991, Extrapulmonary *Pneumocystis carinii* infections in the acquired immunodeficiency syndrome, *Arch Intern Med*, **151:** 1205–14.

Conte JE, Golden JA, 1988, Concentrations of aerosolized pentamidine in bronchoalveolar lavage, systemic absorption and excretion, *Antimicrob Agents Chemother*, **32:** 1490–3.

Conte JE Jr, Hollander H, Golden JA, 1987, Inhaled or reduced-dense intravenous pentamidine for *Pneumocystis carinii* pneumonia, *Ann Intern Med*, **107:** 495–8.

Cote RJ, Rosenblum M et al., 1990, Disseminated *Pneumocystis carinii* infection causing extrapulmonary organ failure: clinical, pathologic, and immunohistochemical analysis, *Mol Pathol*, **3:** 25–30.

Cregan P, Yamamoto A et al., 1990, Comparison of four methods for rapid detection of *Pneumocystis carinii* respiratory specimens, *J Clin Microbiol*, **28:** 2432–6.

Cushion MI, 1989, In vitro studies of *Pneumocystis carinii*, *J Protozool*, **36:** 45–52.

Cushion MT, DeStefano JA, Walzer PD, 1988, *Pneumocystis carinii*: surface reactive carbohydrates detected by lectin probes, *Exp Parasitol*, **67**: 137–47.

Cushion MT, Ruffolo JJ et al., 1985, *Pneumocystis carinii* : growth variables and estimates in the A549 and WI38 VA13 human cell lines, *Exp Parasitol*, **60**: 43–54.

Cushion MT, Zhang J et al., 1993, Evidence for two genetic variants of *Pneumocystis carinii* coinfecting laboratory rats, *J Clin Microbiol*, **31**: 1217–23.

Delanoe P, Delanoe P, 1914, De la rareté de *Pneumocystis carinii* chez les cobayes de la region de Paris : absence de kystes chez d'autres animaux lapin, grenouille, 3 anguilles, *Bull Soc Pathol Exot Filiales*, **7**: 291.

Del-Cas E, Jackson H et al., 1991, Ultrastructural observation of the attachment of *Pneumocystis carinii* in vitro, *J Protozool*, **38**: 205–7S.

DeLorenzo LJ, Huang CT et al., 1987, Roentgenographic patterns of *Pneumocystis carinii* pneumonia in 104 patients with AIDS, *Chest*, **91**: 323–7.

DeStefano JA, Cushion MT et al., 1989, Lectins as probes to *Pneumocystis carinii* glycocomplexes, *J Protozool*, **36**: 65–6S.

DeStefano JA, Trinkle LS et al., 1992, Flow cytometric analysis of lectin binding to *Pneumocystis carinii* surface carbohydrates, *Parasitology*, **78**: 271–80.

Domingo J, Waksal HW, 1984, Wright's staining in rapid diagnosis of *Pneumocystis carinii*, *Am J Clin Pathol*, **81**: 511–14.

Durkin MM, Bartlett MS et al., 1989, A culture method allowing production of relatively pure *Pneumocystis carinii* trophozoites, *J Protozool*, **36**: 31–2S.

Dyer M, Volpe F et al., 1992, Cloning and sequence of a β-tubulin cDNA from *Pneumocystis carinii*: possible implications for drug therapy, *Mol Microbiol*, **68**: 991–1001.

Edman JC, Deman V et al., 1989a, Isolation and expression of the *Pneumocystis carinii* dihydrofolate reductase gene, *Proc Natl Acad Sci USA*, **86**: 8625–9.

Edman V, Edman JC et al., 1989b, Isolation and expression of the *Pneumocystis carinii* thymidylate synthase gene, *Proc Natl Acad Sci USA*, **86**: 6503–7.

Edman JC, Kovacs JA et al., 1988, Ribosomal RNA sequence shows *Pneumocystis carinii* to be member of the fungi, *Nature (London)*, **334**: 519–22.

El-Sadr W, Simberkoff MS, 1988, Survival and prognostic factors in severe *Pneumocystis carinii* pneumonia requiring mechanical ventilation, *Am Rev Respir Dis*, **137**: 1264–7.

Fitzgerald W, Bevelaqua FA et al., 1987, The role of open lung biopsy in patients with the acquired immunodeficiency syndrome, *Chest*, **91**: 659–61.

Furuta T, Ueda K, Fujiwara K, 1984, Experimental *Pneumocystis carinii* infection in nude rats, *Jpn J Exp Med*, **54**: 65–72.

Furuta T, Fujiwara K, Yamanouchi K, 1985a, Detection of antibodies to *Pneumocystis carinii* by enzyme-linked immunosorbent assay in experimentally infected mice, *J Parasitol*, **71**: 522–3.

Furuta T, Ueda K et al., 1985b, Cellular and humoral immune responses of mice subclinically infected with NK *Pneumocystis carinii*, *Infect Immun*, **47**: 544–8.

Gal AA, Klatt EC et al., 1987, The effectiveness of bronchoscopy in the diagnosis of *Pneumocystis carinii* and cytomegalovirus pulmonary infections in acquired immunodeficiency syndrome, *Arch Pathol Lab Med*, **111**: 238–41.

Galman F, Olivier JL et al., 1991, Detection of *Pneumocystis carinii* DNA by polymerase chain reaction in bronchoscopic lavage compared to direct microscopy and immunofluorescence, *J Protozool*, **38**: 1995–2005.

Garner RE, Walker AN, Horst MN, 1991, Morphologic and biochemical studies of chitin expression in *Pneumocystis carinii*, *J Protozool*, **38**: 12–4S.

Gigliotti F, Hughes WT, 1988, Passive immunoprophylaxis with specific monoclonal antibody confers partial protection against *Pneumocystis carinii* pneumonia in animal model, *J Clin Invest*, **81**: 1666–8.

Gleason WA Jr, Roodman ST, 1977, Reversible T cell depression in malnourished infants with *Pneumocystis carinii* pneumonia, *J Pediatr*, **90**: 1032–3.

Gordin FM, Simon GL et al., 1984, Adverse reactions to trimethoprimsulfamethoxazole in patients with the acquired immunodeficiency syndrome, *Ann Infect Med*, **100**: 495–9.

Gosey LL, Howard RM et al., 1985, Advantages of modified toluidine blue O stain and bronchoalveolar lavage for the diagnosis of *Pneumocystis carinii* pneumonia, *J Clin Microbiol*, **22**: 803–7.

Gradus MS, Gilmore M, Lerner M, 1988, An isolation method of DNA from *Pneumocystis carinii*: a quantitative comparison to known parasitic protozoan DNA, *Comp Biochem Physiol B*, **89**: 75–7.

Greaves TS, Strinlie SM, 1985, The recognition of *Pneumocystis carinii* in routine Papanicolaou stained smear, *Acta Cytol*, **29**: 714–21.

Gryzan S, Paradis IL et al., 1988, Unexpected high incidence of *Pneumocystis carinii* infection after heart-lung infection transplantation, *Am Rev Respir Dis*, **137**: 1268–74.

Haidaris PJ, Wright YW et al., 1992, Expression and characterization of a cDNA clone encoding an immunodominant surface glycoprotein of *Pneumocystis carinii*, *J Infect Dis*, **166**: 1113–23.

Hammond DJ, Burchell JR, Pudney MR, 1985, Inhibition of pyrimidine biosyntheses de novo in *Plasmodium falciparum* by 2-(4-*t*-butylcyclohexyl)-3-hydroxyl-1,4-naphthoquinone in vitro, *Mol Biochem Parasitol*, **14**: 97–109.

Harmsen AG, Stankiewicz M, 1990, Requirement for CD4+ cells in resistance of *Pneumocystis carinii* in mice, *J Exp Med*, **172**: 937–45.

Hamrsen AG, Stankiewicz M, 1991, T cells are not sufficient for resistance to *Pneumocystis carinii* pneumonia in mice, *J Parasitol*, **38**: 44–5.

Henshaw NG, Carson JL, Collier AM, 1985, Ultrastructural observation in *Pneumocystis carinii* attachment to rat lung, *J Infect Dis*, **151**: 181–6.

Hidalgo HA, Helmke RJ et al., 1991, Role of the zymolyase-sensitive cyst wall of *Pneumocystis carinii* in the oxidative burst of macrophages, *J Protozool*, **38**: 30–1S.

Hofmann B, Nielsen PB et al., 1988, Humoral and cellular responces to *Pneumocystis carinii*, CMV, and herpes simplex in patients with AIDS and in controls, *Scand J Infect Dis*, **20**: 389–94.

Hofmann B, Ødum N et al., 1985, Humoral responces to *Pneumocystis carinii* in patients with acquired immunodeficiency syndrome and immunocompromised homosexual man, *J Infect Dis*, **152**: 838–40.

Hong ST, Steele PE et al., 1990, *Pneumocystis carinii* karyotypes, *J Clin Microbiol*, **28**: 1785–95.

Hughes WT, Gray VI et al., 1990, Efficacy of a hydroxynaphthoquinone, 566C80, in experimental *Pneumocystis carinii* pneumonia, *Antimicrob Agents Chemother*, **34**: 225–8.

Hughes WT, Leoung G et al., 1993, Comparison of 566C80 and trimethoprimsulfamethoxazole for the treatment of *P. carinii* pneumonitis, *N Engl J Med*, **328**: 1521–7.

Itatani CA, Marshall GJ, 1988, Ultrastructural morphology and staining characteristics of *Pneumocystis carinii* in situ and from bronchoalveolar lavage, *J Parasitol*, **74**: 700–12.

Jones SK, Hall JE et al., 1990, Novel pentamidine analogs in the treatment of experimental *Pneumocystis carinii* pneumonia, *Antimicrob Agents Chemother*, **34**: 1026–30.

Judson MA, Postic B, Weiman DS, 1990, *Pneumocystis carinii* pneumonia manifested as a hilar mass and cavitary lesion: an atypical presentation in a patient receiving aerosolized pentamidine prophylaxis, *South Med J*, **83**: 1309–12.

Kaneshiro ES, Cushion MT et al., 1989, Analysis of *Pneumocystis* fatty acids, *J Protozool*, **36**: 69–72S.

Kitada K, Oka S et al., 1991, Detection of *Pneumocystis carinii* sequences by polymerase chain reaction: animal model and clinical application to noninvasive specimens, *J Clin Microbiol*, **29:** 1885–90.

Kovacs JA, Allegra CJ et al., 1989, Characterization of de novo folate synthesis in *Pneumocystis carinii* and *Toxoplasma gondii*: potential for screening therapeutic agents, *I Infect Dis*, **160:** 312–20.

Kovacs JA, Gill CV et al., 1986, Prospective evaluation of a monoclonal antibody in diagnosis of *Pneumocystis carinii* pneumonia, *Lancet*, **2:** 1–3.

Kovacs JA, Hiemenz JW et al., 1984, *Pneumocystis carinii* pneumonia: a comparison between patients with the acquired immunodeficiency syndrome and patients with other immunodeficiencies, *Ann Intern Med*, **100:** 663–71.

Kovacs, JA, Ng VL et al., 1988, Diagnosis of *Pneumocystis carinii* pneumonia: improved detection in sputum with use of monoclonal antibodies, *N Engl J Med*, **318:** 589–93.

Kovacs JA, Powell F et al., 1993, Multiple gene encode the major surface glycoprotein of *Pneumocystis carinii*, *J Biol Chem*, **268:** 6034–40.

Krishnan VL, Meager LA et al., 1990, Alveolar macrophages in AIDS patients: increased spontaneous tumor necrosis factor alpha production in *Pneumocystis carinii* pneumonia, *Clin Exp Immunol*, **80:** 156–60.

Latorre CR, Sulzer AT, Norman LG, 1977, Serial propagation of *Pneumocystis carinii* in cell line cultures, *Appl Environ Microbiol*, **33:** 1204–6.

Leoung GS, Mills J et al., 1986, Dapsonetrimethoprim for *Pneumocystis carinii* pneumonia in the acquired immunodeficiency syndrome, *Ann Intern Med*, **105:** 45–8.

Li J, Edling T, 1994, Phylogeny of *Pneumocystis carinii* based on β-tubulin sequence, *J Euk Microbiol*, **41:** 97S.

Limper AH, Offord KP et al., 1989, *Pneumocystis carinii* pneumonia. Differences in lung parasite number and inflammation in patients with and without AIDS, *Am Rev Respir Dis*, **140:** 1204–9.

Liu Y, Leibowitz MJ, 1993, Variation and in vitro splicing of group I introns in rRNA gene of *Pneumocystis carinii*, *Nucleic Acids Res*, **21:** 2415–21.

Liu Y, Rocourt M et al., 1992, Sequence and variabirity of the 5.8S and 26S rRNA gene of *Pneumocystis carinii*, *Nucleic Acids Res*, **20:** 3763–72.

Lubat E, Megibow AJ et al., 1990, Extrapulmonary *Pneumocystis carinii* infection in AIDS: CT findings, *Radiology*, **174:** 157–60.

Lundgren B, Cotton R et al., 1990, Identification of *Pneumocystis carinii* chromosomes and mapping of five genes, *Infect Immun*, **58:** 1705–10.

Lundgren B, Lipschik GY, Kovacs JA, 1991, Purification and characterization of major human *Pneumocystis carinii* surface antigen, *J Clin Invest*, **87:** 163–70.

Mahan CT, Sale GE, 1978, Rapid methenamine silver stain for *Pneumocystis* and fungi, *Arch Pathol Lab Med*, **102:** 351–2.

Mascarenhas DAN, Vasudevan VP, Vaidya KP, 1991, *Pneumocystis carinii* pneumonia. Rare cause of hemoptysis, *Chest*, **99:** 251–3.

Masur H, Jones TC, 1978, The infection in vitro of *Pneumocystis carinii* with macrophages and L-cells, *J Exp Med*, **147:** 157–70.

Matsumoto Y, Matsuda S, Tegoshi T, 1989, Yeast glucan in the cyst wall of *Pneumocystis carinii*, *J Protozool*, **36:** 21–2S.

Matsumoto Y, Yamada M, Amagai T, 1991, Yeast glucan of *Pneumocystis carinii* cyst wall: an excellent target for chemotherapy, *J Protozool*, **38:** 6–7S.

Matsumoto Y, Yoshida Y, 1984, Sporogony in *Pneumocystis carinii*: synaptonemal complexes and meiotic nuclear divisions observed in precysts, *J Protozool*, **31:** 420–8.

Matsumoto Y, Yoshida Y, 1986, Advances in *Pneumocystis* biology, *Parasitol Today*, **2:** 137–42.

Mazars E, Ödberg-Ferragut C et al., 1995, Polymorphism of the thymidylate synthase gene of *Pneumocystis carinii* from different host species, *J Euk Microbiol*, **42:** 26–32.

Mazer MA, Kovacs JA et al., 1987, Histoenzymological study of selected dehydrogenase enzymes in *Pneumocystis carinii*, *Infect Immun*, **55:** 727–30.

Meade JC, Stringer JR, 1991, PCR amplification of DNA sequences from the transcription factor IID and cation transporting ATPase genes in *Pneumocystis carinii*, *J Protozool*, **38:** 66–8S.

Medina I, Mills J et al., 1990, Oral therapy for *Pneumocystis carinii* pneumonia in the acquired immunodeficiency syndrome: a controlled trial of trimethoprimsulfamethoxazole versus trimethoprim dapsone, *N Engl J Med*, **323:** 776–82.

Meuwissen JHET, Tanker I et al., 1977, Parasitology and serologic observation of infection with *Pneumocystis carinii* in human, *J Infect Dis*, **136:** 43–8.

Murphy PM, Fox C et al., 1989, Acquired immunodeficiency syndrome may preset as serve restrictive lung disease, *Am J Med*, **86:** 237–40.

Ng VL, Virani NA et al., 1990, Rapid detection of *Pneumocystis carinii* using a direct fluorescent monoclonal antibody stain, *J Clin Microbiol*, **28:** 2228–33.

Nollstadt KH, Powles MA et al., 1994, Use of β-1,3-glucan-specific antibody to study the cyst wall of *Pneumocystis carinii* and effects of pneumocandin B 0 analog L733,560, *Antimicrob Agents Chemother*, **38:** 2258–65.

Northfelt DW, Clement MJ, Safrin S, 1990, Extrapulmonary pneumocystosis: clinical features in human immunodeficiency virus infection, *Medicine (Baltimore)*, **69:** 392–8.

Palluault F, Dei-Cas E et al., 1990, Golgi complex and lysosomes in rabbit derived *Pneumocystis carinii*, *Biol Cell*, **70:** 73–82.

Palluault F, Pietrzyk B et al., 1991a, Three-dimensional reconstruction of rabbit-derived *Pneumocystis carinii* from serial-thin sections I: Trophozoite, *J Protozool*, **38:** 402–7.

Palluault F, Pietrzyk B et al., 1991b, Three dimensional reconstruction of rabbit-derived *Pnemocystis carinii* from serial thin sections II: Intermediate precyst, *J Protozool*, **38:** 407–11.

Paulsrud JR, Queener SF, 1994, Incorporation of fatty acids and amino acids by cultured *Pneumocystis carinii*, *J Euk Microbiol*, **41:** 633–8.

Peglow SL, Smulian AG et al., 1990, Serologic responses to *Pneumocystis carinii* antigens in health and disease, *J Infect Dis*, **161:** 296–306.

Pesanti EL, 1989a, Enzymes of *Pneumocystis carinii*: electrophoretic mobility on starch gels, *J Protozool*, **36:** 2–3S.

Pesanti EL, 1989b, Interaction of *Pneumocystis carinii* with secretions of alveolar macrophages and type II epithelial cells, *J Protozool*, **36:** 47–50S.

Pesanti EL, Shanley JD, 1988, Glycoproteins of *Pneumocystis carinii*: characterization by electrophoresis and microscopy, *J Infect Dis*, **158:** 1353–9.

Phair J, Munoz A et al., 1990, The rise of *Pneumocystis carinii* pneumonia among men infected with human immunodeficiency virus type 1. Multicenter AIDS cohort study group, *N Engl J Med*, **332:** 161–5.

Pifer LL, Hughes WT et al., 1978a, *Pneumocystis carinii* infection: evidence for high prevalence in normal and immunosuppressed children, *Pediatrics*, **61:** 35–41.

Pifer LL, Woods D, Hughes WT, 1978b, Propagation of *Pneumocystis carinii* in Vero cell culture, *Infec Immun*, **20:** 66–8.

Pitchenik AE, Ganjei P et al., 1986, Sputum examination for the diagnosis of *Pneumocystis carinii* pneumonia in the acquired immunodeficiency syndrome, *Am Rev Respir Dis*, **133:** 226–9.

Pixley FJ, Wakefield AE et al., 1991, Mitochondrial sequences show fungal homology for *Pneumocystis carinii*, *Mol Microbiol*, **5:** 1347–51.

Pneumocystis Workshop, 1994, Revised nomenclature for *Pneumocystis carinii*, *J Euk Microbiol*, **41:** 121–2S.

Poelma FG, 1975, *Pneumocystis carinii* infections in zoo animals, *Z Parasitenkd*, **46:** 61–8.

Pottratz ST, Martin WJ, 1990, Role of fibronectine in *Pneumocystis carinii* attachment to cultured lung cells, *J Clin Invest*, **85:** 351–6.

Queener SF, Dean RA et al., 1992, Efficacy of intermittent dosage of 8-aminoqunolines for therapy of prophylaxis of pneumocystis pneumonia in rats, *J Infec Dis*, **165:** 764–8.

Queener SF, Fujioka H et al., 1991, In vitro activities of acridone alkaloids against *Pneumocystis carinii*, *Antimicrob Agents Chemother*, **35**: 377–9.

Rao CP, Gelfand EW, 1983, *Pneumocystis carinii* pneumonitis in patients with hypogammaglobulinemia and intact T cell immunity, *J Pediatr*, **103**: 410–12.

Raviglione MC, 1990, Extrapulmonary pneumocystosis: the first 50 cases, *Rev Infect Dis*, **12**: 1127–38.

Richardson JD, Queener SE et al., 1989, Binary fission of *Pneumocystis carinii* trophozoites grow in vitro, *J Protozool*, **36**: 27–9S.

Riis B, Rattan SIC et al., 1990, Eukaryotic protein elongation factors, *Trends Biochem Sci*, **15**: 420–4.

Robbins JB, 1967, *Pneumocystis carinii* pneumonitis. A review, *Pediatr Res*, **1**: 131–58.

Roifman CM, Hummel D et al., 1989, Depletion of CD8+ cells in human thymic medulla results in selective immune deficiency, *J Exp Med*, **170**: 2177–82.

Roths JB, Sidman CL, 1992, Both immunity and hyperresponsiveness to *Pneumocystis carinii* result from transfer of CD4+ but not CD8+ T cells into severe combined immunodeficiency mice, *J Clin Invest*, **90**: 673–8.

Roths JB, Sidman CL, 1993, Single and combined humoral and cellmediated immunotherapy of *Pneumocystis carinii* pneumonia in immunodeficient *scid* mice, *Infect Immun*, **61**: 1641–9.

Ruffolo JJ, Cushion MT, Walzer PD, 1989, Ultrastructural observation on life cycle stages of *Pneumocystis carinii*, *J Protozool*, **36**: 53–4S.

Salmeron S, Petitpretz P et al., 1986, Pentamidine and pancreatis (letter), *Ann Intern Med*, **105**: 140–1.

Sattler FR, Cowan R et al., 1988, Trimethoprim-sulfamethoxazole compared with pentamidine for treatment of *Pneumocystis carinii* pneumonia in the acquired immunodeficiency syndrome: a prospective, noncrossover study, *Ann Intern Med*, **109**: 280–7.

Schmatz DM, Powles MA et al., 1991, Treatment and prevention of *Pneumocystis carinii* pneumonia and further elucidation of the *P. carinii* life cycle with 1,3-β-glucan synthesis inhibitor L671,329, *J Protozool*, **38**: 151–3S.

Schmatz DM, Romancheck MA et al., 1990, Treatment of *Pneumocystis carinii* pneumonia with 1,3-β-glucan synthesis inhibitors, *Proc Natl Acad Aci USA*, **87**: 5950–4.

Seed TM, Aikawa M, 1977, Pneumocystis, *Parasitic Protozoa*, vol 4, ed Kreier JP, Academic Press, New York.

Settnes OP, Nielsen MJ, 1991, Host–parasite relationship in *Pneumocystis carinii* infection: Activation of the ov plasmalemmal vesicular system in type I alveolar epithelial cells, *J Protozool*, **38**: 174–6S.

Shimono LH, Hartman B, 1986, A simple and reliable rapid methenamine silver stain for *Pneumocystis carinii* and fungi, *Arch Pathol Lab Med*, **110**: 855–6.

Shellito J, Suzara VV et al., 1990, A new model of *Pneumocystis carinii* infection in mice selectively depleted of helper T lymphocytes, *J Clin Invest*, **85**: 1686–93.

Shiota T, 1984, Morphology and development of *Pneumocystis carinii* observed by phasecontrast microscopy and semiultrathin section of light-microscopy, *Jpn J Parasitol*, **33**: 443–55.

Siminski J, Kidd P et al., 1991, Reversed helper / suppressor T-lymphocyte ratio in bronchoalveolar lavage fluid from patients with breast cancer and *Pneumocystis carinii* pneumonia, *Am Rev Respir Dis*, **143**: 437–40.

Slade JD, Hepburn B, 1983, Prednisone-induced alterations of circulating human lymphocyte subsets, *J Lab Clin Med*, **101**: 479–87.

Sloand E, Laughon B et al., 1993, The challenge of *Pneumocystis carinii* culture, *J Euk Microbiol*, **40**: 188–95.

Smith JW, Bartlet MS, 1984, In vitro cultivation of *Pneumocystis carinii*, Pneumocystis carinii *pneumonia*, ed. Young L, Marcel Dekker, New York, 107–37.

Soulez B, Palluault F et al., 1991, Introduction of *Pneumocystis carinii* in a colony of SCID mice, *J Protozool*, **38**: 123–5S.

Stringer SL, Stringer JR et al., 1989, *Pneumocystis carinii*: sequence from ribosomal RNA implies a close relationship with fungi, *Exp Parasitol*, **68**: 450–61.

Stringer JR, Stringer SL et al., 1993, Molecular genetics distinction of *Pneumocystis carinii* from rats and humans, *J Euk Microbiol*, **40**: 733–41.

Tamburrini E, DeLuca A et al., 1991, *Pneumocystis carinii* stimulates in vitro production of tumor necrosis factor-α by human macrophages, *Med Microbiol Immunol (Berlin)*, **180**: 15–20.

Tegoshi T, 1988, New system of in vitro cultivation of *Pneumocystis carinii* without feeder cells, *J Kyoto Pref Univ Med*, **97**: 1473–82.

The National Institute of Health–University of California Expert Panel, 1990, Consensus statement on the use of corticosteroids as adjunctive therapy for pneumocystis pneumonia in the acquired immunodeficiency syndrome, *N Engl J Med*, **323**: 1500–4.

Tidwell RR, Jones SK et al., 1990, Development of pentamidine analogues as new agents for treatment of *Pneumocystis carinii* pneumonia, *Ann NY Acad Sci*, **616**: 421–41.

Travis WD, Pittaluga S et al., 1990, Atypical pathologic manifestations of *Pneumocystis carinii* pneumonia in the acquired immune deficiency syndrome. Review of 123 lung biopsies from 76 patients with emphasis on cysts, vascular invasion, vasculitis, and granulomas, *Am J Surg Pathol*, **14**: 615–25.

ul Haque A, Plattner SB et al., 1987, *Pneumocystis carinii*. Taxonomy as viewed by electron microscopy, *Am J Clin Pathol*, **87**: 504–10.

Vávra J, Kucera K, 1970, *Pneumocystis carinii* Delanoe, its ultrastructure and ultrastructural affinities, *J Protozool*, **17**: 463–83.

Vossen MEMH, Beckers PJA et al., 1976, Microtubules in *Pneumocystis carinii*, *Z Parasitenkd*, **49**: 291–2.

Vossen MEMH, Beckers PJA et al., 1978, Developmental biology of *Pneumocystis carinii*, an alternative view on the life cycle of the parasite, *Z Parasitenkd*, **55**: 101–18.

Wada M, Kitada K et al., 1993, cDNA sequence diversity and genomic clusters of major surface glycoprotein gene of *Pneumocystis carinii*, *J Infec Dis*, **168**: 979–85.

Wakefield AE, Guiver L, Miller RF, Hopkin JM, 1991, DNA amplification on induced sputum samples for diagnosis of *Pneumocystis carinii* pneumonia, *Lancet*, **337**: 1378–9.

Wakefield AE, Peters SE, et al., 1992, *Pneumocystis carinii* shows DNA homology with the Ustomycetous red yeast fungi, *Mol Microbiol*, **6**: 1903–11.

Wakefield AE, Pixley FJ et al., 1990, Detection of *Pneumocystis carinii* with DNA amplification, *Lancet*, **336**: 451–3.

Walzer PD, Kim CK et al., 1988, Inhibitors of folic acid synthesis in the treatment of experimental *Pneumocystis carinii* pneumonia, *Antimicrob Agents Chemother*, **32**: 96–103.

Walzer PD, Linke KJ, 1987, A comparison of the antigenic characteristics of rat and human *Pneumocystis carinii* pneumonia in the United States: epidemiologic, clinical and diagnostic features, *Ann Intern Med*, **80**: 83–93.

Walzer PD, Rutledge ME, 1982, Serum antibody responses to *Pneumocystis carinii* among different strains of normal and athymic mice, *Infect Immun*, **35**: 620–6.

Walzer PD, Stanforth D et al., 1987, *Pneumocystis carinii*: immunoblotting and immunofluorescent analyses of serum antibodies during rat infection and recovery, *Exp Parasitol*, **63**: 319–28.

Watanabe J, Hori H et al., 1989, Phylogenetic association of *Pneumocystis carinii* with the 'Rhizopod / Myxomycotoa / Zygomycota' group indicated by comparison of 5S ribosomal RNA sequences, *Mol Biochem Parasitol*, **32**: 163–8.

Weber WR, Askin FB, Dehner LP, 1977, Lung biopsy in *Pneumocystis carinii* pneumonia: a histopathologic study of typical and atypical features, *Am J Clin Pathol*, **67**: 11–9.

Williams DJ, Radding JA et al., 1991, Glucan synthesis in *Pneumocystis carinii*, *J Protozool*, **38**: 427–37.

Worley MA, Ivey MH, Graves DC, 1989, Characterization and cloning of *Pneumocystis carinii* nucleic acid, *J Protozool*, **36**: 9–11S.

Yamada M, Matsumoto Y et al., 1986, Demonstration and determination of DNA in *Pneumocystis carinii* by fluorescence microscopy with 4,6-diamidino-2-phenylinodole (DAPI), *Zentralbl Baktiol Hyg*, **262:** 240–6.

Yoneda K, Walzer PD, 1983, Attachment of *Pneumocystis carinii* to type I alveolar cells; study by freeze fracture electron microscopy, *Infect Immun*, **40:** 812–5.

Yoneda K, Walzer PD et al., 1982, *Pneumocystis carinii*: freeze-fracture study of stages of the organism, *Exp Parasitol*, **53:** 68–76.

Yoshida Y, 1989, Ultrastructural studies of *Pneumocystis carinii*, *J Protozool*, **36:** 53–60.

Yoshikawa H, Tegoshi T, Yoshida Y, 1987, Detection of surface carbohydrates on *Pneumocystis carinii* by fluorescein-conjugated lectins, *Parasitol Res*, **74:** 43–9.

Yoshikawa H, Yoshida Y, 1986, Freeze-fracture studies on *Pneumocystis carinii*. I Structural alteration of the pellicle during the development from trophozoite to cyst, *Z Parasitenkd*, **72:** 463–77.

Zuger A, Wolf BZ et al., 1986, Pentamidine-associated fatal acute pancreatitis, *JAMA*, **256:** 2383–5.

Chapter 23

BALANTIDIUM COLI

V Zaman

1 HISTORICAL INTRODUCTION

Balantidium coli is the only ciliate known to infect humans. Human infection is uncommon and only 722 cases of balantidial dysentery had been reported up to 1960 (Woody and Woody 1960). In contrast to this, infection in pigs is extremely common and it is generally believed that pigs act as the main reservoir for human infection. The subject has been reviewed by Zaman (1993).

Historically, the genus *Balantidium* was first recognized by Claparède and Lachmann (1858) who found the parasites in the rectum of frogs. Since then it has been observed in a variety of animals, and a number of species have been described (Levine 1973). Malmsten (1857), the first to describe the human form in a patient with acute dysentery, named it *Paramecium coli* in view of its close resemblance to *Paramecium*. Leukart (1861) discovered a similar organism in the large intestine of a pig. Stein (1863) pointed out that the human parasite described by Malmsten (1857) and the pig ciliate described by Leukart (1861) were morphologically identical and named them *Balantidium coli*.

2 CLASSIFICATION

The genus *Balantidium* belongs to the phylum Ciliophora, class Litostomatea, subclass Trichostomatia, order Vestibuliferida and family Balantidiidae (Lee, Hutner and Bovee 1985). McDonald (1922) proposed that pig and human species be separated as *B. suis* and *B. coli*. This separation has not been accepted (Hoare 1962, Levine 1973) and the parasites in the 2 hosts continue to be regarded as a single species by most authors.

3 STRUCTURE AND LIFE CYCLE

3.1 Structure

Balantidium coli has a trophozoite and a cyst stage. The trophozoite is actively motile and is the invasive stage; the cyst is the resistant form and the infective stage. The length of the trophozoite varies from 30 to 300 μm and the width from 30 to 100 μm. The body shape is variable but is generally ovoid and slightly flattened on one side (Figs. 23.1, 23.2). At the anterior end of the trophozoite there is a funnel-shaped depression or mouth through which food is ingested. The mouth can be considered to consist of a peristome, cytopharynx and cytosome. The food passes from the peristome to the elongated cytopharynx and then to the cytosome. The cytopharynx, not visible when the parasite is filled with food, is often small but sometimes reaches about half the length of the parasite. The peristome appears as a rigid structure with striations when observed with the aid of a scanning electron microscope (SEM) (Figs. 23.3, 23.4).

The cilia, the organs of locomotion, cover the whole parasite and are embedded in the pellicle in longitudinal rows known as **kineties**. The number of kineties varies from 36 to 106 (Krascheninnikow 1962). The ciliary movement can be easily observed with the aid of a light microscope and the structure of the cilia is readily seen by SEM (Figs. 23.3, 23.4). The peristomal cilia are larger than those on the body (the somatic cilia). The peristomal cilia are used for propelling food into the cytopharynx (Fig. 23.5). The food particles on being ingested become surrounded by a vacuolar membrane and digestion takes place inside the vacuoles. The parasite is capable of ingesting a variety of food particles, such as bacteria, starch grains,

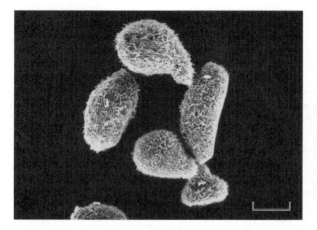

Fig. 23.1 *Balantidium coli* trophozoites, showing variability in size and shape. SEM; bar = 30 μm.

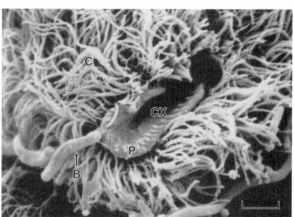

Fig. 23.4 *B. coli* trophozoite, showing peristome (P) with striations. A bacterium (b) is lying close to the peristome. CX, cytopharynx. SEM; bar = 1.5 μm.

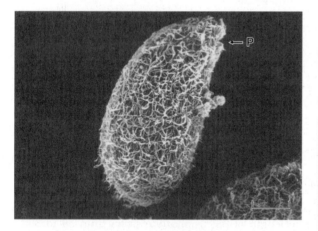

Fig. 23.2 *B. coli* trophozoite, showing peristome (P) at the anterior end. SEM; bar = 15 μm.

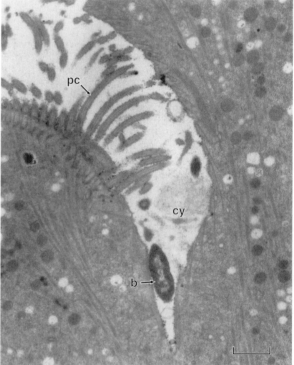

Fig. 23.5 *B. coli* trophozoite, showing peristomal cilia (PC) and cytopharynx (CY). A bacterium (b) is lying inside the cytopharynx. TEM; bar = 0.8 μm.

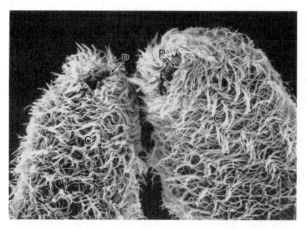

Fig. 23.3 *B. coli* trophozoites, showing peristome (P) and cilia (C) covering the body. SEM; bar = 3 μm.

red cells, fat droplets, etc. The parasite has a excretory opening at the posterior end known as the **cytopyge**, which is circular and much smaller than the peristome (Fig. 23.6).

There are 2 contractile vacuoles which may lie side by side or one above the other. They are easily visible to an observer using a light microscope with interference or phase-contrast capability (Fig. 23.7). These vacuoles are responsible for maintaining the proper osmotic pressure in the cell by drawing excess water from the cytoplasm and ejecting it to the exterior.

The trophozoite has 2 nuclei which are visible in stained preparations (Fig. 23.8). A macronucleus, which is large and situated near the middle of the body, may be spherical, curved, elongate, or kidney shaped (Fig. 23.9). It is enclosed in a nuclear membrane and can be removed intact by breaking the cell

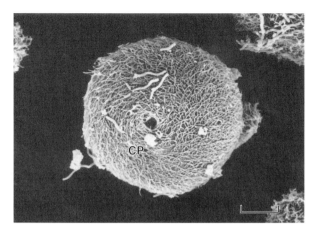

Fig. 23.6 *B. coli* trophozoite, showing the cytopyge (CP) at the posterior end. SEM; bar = 1.5 μm.

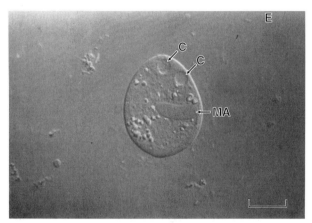

Fig. 23.7 *B. coli* trophozoite. Live organism showing macronucleus (MA) and 2 contractile vacuoles (C). Interference contrast; bar = 6 μm.

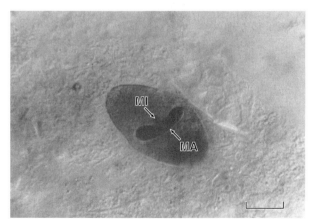

Fig. 23.8 *B. coli* trophozoite, showing macronucleus (MA) and micronucleus (MI). Trichrome stain; bar = 6 μm.

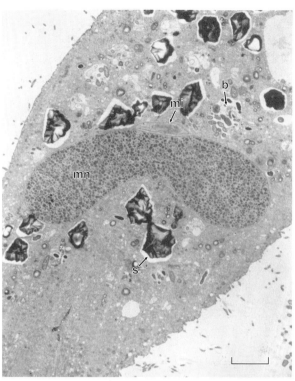

Fig. 23.9 *B. coli* trophozoite, showing the macronucleus (MN) and a small spindle-shaped micronucleus (MI). Ingested bacteria (b) and starch (S) are seen in the cytoplasm. TEM; bar = 3 μm.

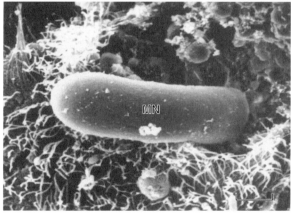

Fig. 23.10 *B. coli* trophozoite, showing the macronucleus after disruption of the cell membrane. SEM; bar = 3 μm.

membrane (Fig. 23.10). At the ultrastructural level numerous small nucleoli are visible inside the macronucleus (Fig. 23.11). The micronucleus is small and lies in close proximity to the macronucleus (Figs. 23.8, 23.9).

The cyst of *B. coli* is spherical to ovoid with a diameter of 40–60 μm (Fig. 23.12). The cyst wall is thick and transparent. In electron microscopic images it is 400–500 nm thick (Figs. 23.11, 23.13). The parasite is visible inside the cyst. In newly formed cysts it shows movement, but as the cyst matures the cilia are absorbed and the movement ceases. The cyst has a macro- and micronucleus, as does the trophozoite.

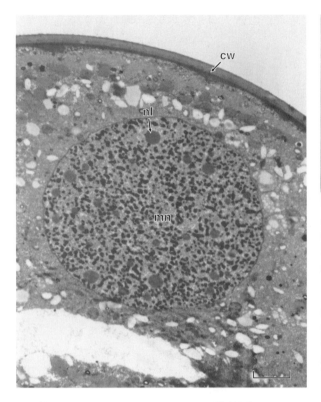

Fig. 23.11 *B. coli* cyst, showing the cyst wall (CW), macronucleus (mn) and nucleoli (nl). TEM,; bar = 1 μm.

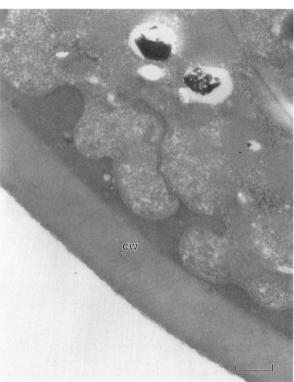

Fig. 23.13 *B. coli* cyst, showing the cyst wall (CW) at high magnification. TEM; bar = 0.2 μm.

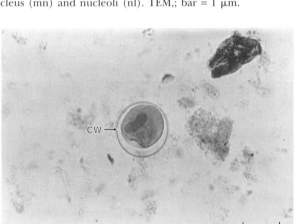

Fig. 23.12 *B. coli* cyst. The transparent cyst wall (CW) and the macronucleus are visible. Trichrome stain; bar = 15 μm.

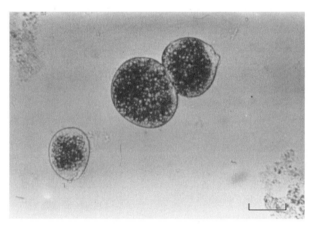

Fig. 23.14 *B. coli* undergoing binary fission. Live preparation; bar = 15 μm.

3.2 Life cycle

The parasite is transmitted by the oral–faecal route and the cyst is the infective stage. Excystation probably occurs in the small intestine and multiplication occurs in the large intestine.

Multiplication is by binary fission and the earliest indication of it is the elongation of the organism. Elongation is followed by the formation of a transverse structure through the middle of the body. The body gradually begins to constrict and finally separates into 2 parasites (Fig. 23.14). The ciliary activity continues during this process; the anterior cell develops a new excretory pore and the posterior cell a new mouth.

Sexual union (**syngamy**) is an important aspect of this parasite's life cycle and occurs by a process of conjugation, in which 2 cells come in contact with each other at their anterior ends and exchange nuclear material (Fig. 23.15). Conjugation lasts for a few moments, after which the cells detach. There is no increase in numbers as a result of conjugation.

In the infected animal the parasite may be passed in the faeces as a trophozoite or a cyst. The trophozoite does not encyst outside the body and disintegrates. The passed cyst survives and may contaminate food and water and, as a result, may then be passed to other animals or humans. Pig-to-pig transmission is very

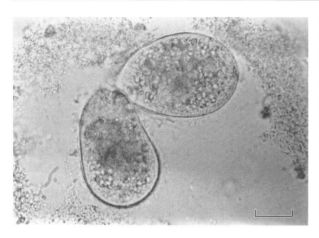

Fig. 23.15 *B. coli* under conjugation. Attachment occurs at the anterior end. Live preparation; bar = 15 μm.

common and virtually 100% infection occurs in some piggeries where hygienic conditions are poor.

4 BIOCHEMISTRY

Agosin and von Brand (1953) found that *B. coli* is capable of consuming considerable amounts of oxygen despite the fact that it normally lives in the large intestine where little if any oxygen is available. The parasite prefers anaerobic conditions and in the absence of oxygen it produces a large amount of carbon dioxide. Carbohydrates are the main source of energy. Templis and Lysenko (1957) found that *B. coli* can produce hyaluronidase, which probably helps it in its invasion of the host tissues by dissolution of the intracellular ground substance.

5 CLINICAL FORMS OF THE INFECTION

5.1 The asymptomatic carrier condition

Asymptomatic carriers have no symptoms and continue to pass cysts in their faeces. They are responsible for spreading infection, especially in insanitary institutional environments such as long-stay psychiatric units.

5.2 The chronic case

Patients with chronic disease have periods in which frequent bowel movements alternate with periods of constipation. The faeces are mucoid and rarely bloody. The organism is not easily seen in the faeces and repeated stool examination may be necessary for its detection.

5.3 The acute case

In acute disease, patients have diarrhoea and the faeces contain a lot of mucus and blood (Castro *et al.* 1983). The clinical presentation is identical to that of acute amoebic dysentery. There may be fever and other intestinal symptoms such as anorexia, nausea, epigastric pain, vomiting and intestinal colic. This may lead to severe dehydration, and sometimes to renal insufficiency. There is usually pain and tenderness in the caecal region. The symptoms may mimic those of appendicitis. In a majority of patients recovery occurs in 3–4 days even without treatment. In some patients, especially immunocompromised and malnourished ones, death may occur due to extensive destruction of the large intestine, involvement of the appendix, perforation, peritonitis, dehydration and renal failure. In patients with acute infection, extraintestinal involvement such as liver abscess formation, pleuritis and pneumonia may occur.

6 IMMUNOLOGY

It is possible to differentiate *Balantidium* from pigs (*B. coli*), guinea pigs (*B. caviae*) and spider monkeys (*B. wenrichi*) by antigenic analysis (Krascheninnikow and Jeska 1961). Using immobilization reactions Zaman (1964) could also differentiate human strains of *Balantidium* from pig strains. The epidemiological significance of these observations is not known. It is possible that only some pig strains are capable of infecting humans, thus explaining the relative infrequency of human disease.

7 PATHOLOGY

The gross pathologic appearance of the large intestine in patients with *Balantidium* infection is similar to that in patients with amoebiasis. On rare occasions the terminal ileum may also be infected. The gross changes consist of multiple ulcers with necrotic bases and undermined edges. The intervening mucosa may or may not be inflamed. On microscopic examination parasites are frequently seen in clusters in the submucosa or at the bases of crypts. They can easily be recognized because of the presence of the macronucleus which stains deeply with haematoxylin and eosin (Fig. 23.16). The cellular response is mainly lymphocytic, with some plasma cells being present. Neutrophils are few unless there is a superimposed bacterial infection. Sometimes the parasites may invade the regional lymph nodes and then they may be detected inside the lymphatic tissues.

8 DIAGNOSIS

Diagnosis is based on faecal examination, which reveals mainly trophozoites in acutely infected patients and cysts in patients with chronic infections. Diagnosis can also be made by the examination of biopsy specimens taken with the aid of a sigmoidoscope or by examination of scrapings of an ulcer. *Balantidium* can be cultured in all the media that support the growth of *Entamoeba histolytica*. However, culture is rarely attempted for diagnosis, as the parasites are more

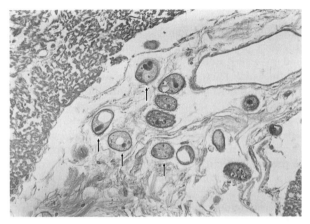

Fig. 23.16 *B. coli* in intestine. Many trophozoites (arrows) are lying in the submucosa. Haematoxylin and eosin; bar = 30 μm.

easily detected in faeces by microscopy and in tissues on histological examination.

9 EPIDEMIOLOGY

The main endemic areas are in the tropical and subtropical regions of the world including South and Central America, the Philippines, Iran, Central Asia, Papua New Guinea and some Pacific islands. In China the parasite appears to be endemic in Yunan province with infection rates of up to 4.24% in some villages (Yang et al. 1995). However, the highest prevalence (up to 20%) has been reported in the mountain districts of West Irian (Indonesia), where there is a close association between humans and pigs. McCarey (1952) has reviewed the prevalence of balantidiasis in Iran – an endemic area of unusual interest, as there

is no pig farming there because of the Moslem ban on eating pork. The transmission is from human to human and the animal host, if any, is not known.

A single outbreak of balantidiasis of epidemic proportions was reported from the Pacific island of Truk (Walzer and Healy 1982). The outbreak involved 110 persons in a short period of time. The epidemic occurred as a result of contamination of the water supply by pig faeces during a typhoon.

Balantidiasis has been frequently observed in psychiatric units in the USA and many other countries. Here the transmission occurs by human-to-human contact and is due to a lack of hygienic conditions and to coprophagy.

10 CHEMOTHERAPY

At present tetracycline and metronidazole are the drugs of choice. Tetracycline, 500 mg, 4 times a day for 10 days, is recommended although clearance generally occurs in 2–3 days. Alternatively, metronidazole, 750 mg, 3 times a day for 5–7 days, can be used with equal efficacy. No relapse of the infection after treatment and no resistance to these antibiotics have been reported. Treatment should be given to carriers in institutions to prevent the spread of infection to susceptible patients.

11 INTEGRATED CONTROL

Control consists of hygienic rearing of pigs and preventing the human–pig contact which can lead to human infections. Improved hygiene in psychiatric institutions will prevent human-to-human transmission in these settings, and treatment of humans shedding cysts will prevent human-to-human transmission.

REFERENCES

Agosin M, von Brand T, 1953, Studies on the respiratory metabolism of *Balantidium coli*, *J Infect Dis*, **93**: 101–6.

Claparède E, Lachmann J, 1858, Etudes sur les infusores et les rhizopodes, Geneva, Switzerland (cited by Wenyon, 1926).

Castro J, Vazquez-Iglesias JL, Arnal-Monreal F, 1983, Dysentery caused by *Balantidium coli* – Report of two cases, *Endoscopy*, **15**: 272–4.

Hoare CA, 1962, Reservoir hosts and natural foci of human *Entamoeba histolytica*, *Acta Trop*, **19**: 281–317.

Krascheninnikow S, 1962, Variability in number of kineties in *Balantidium coli*, *J Parasitol*, **48**: 192.

Krascheninnikow S, Jeska EL, 1961, Agar diffusion studies on the species specificity of *Balantidium coli*, *B. caviae* and *B. wenrichi*, *Immunology*, **4**: 282–8.

Lee JJ, Hutner SH, Bovee EC, 1985, *An Illustrated Guide to the Protozoa*, Society of Protozoologists, Lawrence, KA.

Leukart R, 1861, Über *Paramecium coli* Malmsten, *Arch Natureqesch*, **27**: 81 (cited by Wenyon, 1926).

Levine ND, 1973, *Protozoan Parasites of Domestic Animals and Man*, Burgess, Minneapolis, MN, 369–73.

Malmsten PH, 1857, Infusorien als intestinal-tiere beim Menschen, *Pathol Anal Physiol Klin Med*, **12**: 302 (cited by Wenyon, 1926).

McCarey AG, 1952, Balantidiasis in South Persia, *Br Med J*, **1**: 629–31.

McDonald JD, 1922, On *Balantidium coli* and *B. suis* (sp. nov.), *Univ California Publ Zool*, **20**: 243–6.

Stein F, 1863, Über *Paramecium coli* Malmst., *Amtl Ber Dtsch Naturfors Artz*, **37**: 165 (cited by Wenyon, 1926).

Templis CH, Lysenko MG, 1957, The production of hyaluronidase by *Balantidium coli*, *Exp Parasitol*, **6**: 31–6.

Walzer PD, Healy GR, 1982, Balantidiasis, *CRC Handbook Series in Zoonoses*, vol. 1, ed Jacobs L, CRC Press, Boca Raton, FL, 15–24.

Wenyon CM, 1926, *Protozoology*, Baillière, Tindall and Cox, London, 1201–10.

Woody NC, Woody HB, 1960, Balantidiasis in infancy. Review of the literature and report of a case, *J Pediatr*, **56**: 485–9.

Yang Yuezhong, Zeng Li, Li Mingkun, Zhou Jinlu, 1995, Diarrhoea in piglets and monkeys experimentally infected with *Balantidium coli* isolated from human faeces, *J Trop Med Hyg*, **98**: 69–72.

Zaman V, 1993, *Balantidium coli*, *Parasitic Protozoa*, 2nd edn, vol. 3, eds Kreier JP, Baker JR, Academic Press, New York, 43–60.

Zaman V, 1964, Studies on the immobilization reaction in the genus *Balantidium*, *Trans Roy Soc Trop Med Hyg*, **59**: 255–9.

Part III

HELMINTHS

Nature and Classification of Parasitic Helminths

D I Gibson

---

1 **General introduction**	**3** **Phylum Nematoda**
2 **Phylum Platyhelminthes**	**4** **Phylum Acanthocephala**

The parasitic worms, or helminths, which occur in humans comprise 4 major groups: 2 groups of flatworms (phylum Platyhelminthes), the **trematodes** or **digeneans** (flukes) and **cestodes** (tapeworms), the **nematodes** (or roundworms; phylum Nematoda) and the **acanthocephalans** (or thorny-headed worms; phylum Acanthocephala). Other groups have been reported as parasites of humans, for example free-living flatworms (turbellarians), hairworms (or gordiids; Phylum Nematomorpha) free-living nematodes (such as mermithids) and even earthworms (oligochaete annelids). Although these groups may be seen at the site of a toilet (in WCs, after defaecation or urination on the ground, etc.) they are very unlikely to have passed through the human digestive system.

1 GENERAL INTRODUCTION

1.1 Nomenclature

The more important levels used in the classification of parasites, in descending order of status, and the suffixes by which they can be often be recognized, are shown in Table 24.1. Those above the family level vary because they are not covered by the International Code for Zoological Nomenclature. Vernacular versions are derived from some groups by the addition of -s or -es to the root, e.g. platyhelminths, diplostomids, diplostomines. The genus and species together, e.g. *Schistosoma mansoni*, form the scientific name of an organism. Any personal name and date following this name indicate the original authority for the name.

A **direct life cycle** is one in which the final host is reinfected directly without the involvement of intermediate hosts. An **indirect life cycle** is one in which intermediate hosts or paratenic hosts harbour one or more life history stages. The **final** or **definitive host** harbours the adult (sexual adult in the case of the Digenea). **Intermediate hosts** are those in which one or more larval stages develop as a neces-

sary part of the life cycle. A **paratenic host** is one which larval stages may survive but do not normally develop; they are often not a necessary part of the life cycle.

1.2 Identification and morphometric analysis

The identification of parasitic worms is possible in certain cases using a variety of techniques, such as: (1) the identification of eggs found during coprological examination (e.g. Thienpont, Rochette and Van Parijs 1986); (2) the recognition of worm sections in histological investigations (e.g. Chitwood and Lichtenfels 1972); (3) immunodiagnosis (e.g. Lightowlers and Gottstein 1995); (4) enzyme electrophoresis (e.g. Wright and Ross 1980); and (5) molecular biological approaches (e.g. De Clercq et al. 1994); but in the majority of cases the most effective method is still morphometrics. Although this may well change in the future, helminth classification, whether it involves the intuitive approach of the specialist or the more rigorous protocols of cladistics (a method based upon the use of derived characters as indicators of evolutionary events), still relies mainly upon morphological features.

FIXATION

Morphometric analysis relies upon having material in good condition, and, in order to achieve this, it is best if specimens are fixed live. In many cases, for example when worms are voided after the administration of anthelmintics, this is not possible, and any conventional fixative, such as 10% formalin or 70–80% alcohol, may be used. Live material is best fixed in Berland's fluid (19 parts glacial acetic acid to 1 part pure formalin) or (especially in the case of cestodes) a very hot conventional fixative or boiling water. After fixation for a minute or so, the specimens are best stored in 80% alcohol. Specimens should not be fixed under the pressure (e.g. a

Table 24.1 Levels used in the classification of helminth parasites

Classification level	Example	Common suffix
Phylum	Platyhelminthes	Varies
Class	Trematoda	Commonly -a
Subclass	Digenea	-ea, -a
Order	Ascaridida	-ida, -idea, -iformes
Superfamily	Diplostomoidea	-oidea
Family	Diplostomidae	-idae
Subfamily	Diplostominae	-inae
Genus	*Schistosoma*	Varies, if used
Species	*mansoni*	Varies, but depends on its derivation and certain rules

coverslip, glass slide or other device) except in the case of large tapeworms and acanthocephlans; some pressure or prior soaking in tap water may help evert the proboscis of live acanthocephalans.

MOUNTING

Nematodes and acanthocephalans are best examined as temporary mounts between a glass slide and a coverslip in a clearing agent, such as beechwood creosote, lactophenol or glycerine: the latter is really only useful for smaller worms (<15 mm in length). Trematodes and cestodes (or fragments of the latter; usually the head and mature segments) need to be mounted on slides permanently. This requires the staining of the worms in a good carmine-based stain such as Mayer's paracarmine for 1–20 min, depending upon size, destaining in acid alcohol until the worm is a pale pink colour, dehydrating , clearing and mounting in Canada balsam or some other mountant.

HISTOLOGY

In some cases, serial histological sections of specimens are required for identification. In this procedure, orientation is usually critical, so it must be done manually. The technique was outlined in detail by Cooper (1988).

SPECIALIST HELP

Help may be obtained from specialist laboratories which are usually in museums or similar institutes and where there are helminth taxonomists. Contact should be made before sending material, and any material sent should be very well packed, well dried in the case of slidemounts and in strong plastic (not glass) containers in the case of wet material.

1.3 The helminth groups

An account of the helminth groups which might occur as parasites in humans is given below. The higher taxa dealt with tend to be those generally considered important in the systematics of the group, with most information being given at the family level. The account is presented in the form of a summary of the gross morphological features by which that group is recognized, detailed information on many organs and organ systems being omitted. This is followed by: a section listing the genera involved and some idea of the basic recognition features of the group; information on the life history, how humans become infected and any control measures relating to the life history; and information on the pathogenicity of the worm which might relate to its morphology, mode of

existence or life history. The information was gathered from a variety of sources, but Muller (1975), Coombs and Crompton (1991) and Garcia and Bruckner (1993) were useful references for non-systematic data.

2 PHYLUM PLATYHELMINTHES

The platyhelminths or flatworms are bilaterally symmetrical, dorsoventrally flattened worms with a definite head end and lacking a body cavity. They include a variety of free-living turbellarians, which occur in aquatic and terrestrial conditions (a small number are parasitic), and a number of entirely parasitic groups. These comprise 3 classes: the Monogenea (mainly ectoparasites of fishes); the Cestoidea (tapeworms; endoparasites); and the Trematoda (endoparasitic flukes; mainly digeneans). Only the latter 2 classes infect humans.

2.1 Class Cestoidea Rudolphi, 1808

Main features. Platyhelminthes. Primarily intestinal parasites of vertebrates. Usually with single generation in life cycle and sexual adult in vertebrate; rarely with asexual reproduction in intermediate host. Life cycle invariably indirect (one exception); wide variety of invertebrates and vertebrates used as intermediate hosts. Adult segmented or not; with duplication of reproductive organs along body (polyzoic) or not (monozoic); segmented forms polyzoic; unsegmented forms monozoic or polyzoic. Distinct scolex (head) present or absent. Syncytial tegument usually but not always unarmed (at light microscope level). Gut absent. (See Fig. 24.1.)

The cestodes, or tapeworms, occur as intestinal parasites of all groups of vertebrates. Their closest relatives are the monogeneans, ectoparasitic flukes mainly of fishes, from which they are likely to have been derived. There are 2 subclasses, the Cestodaria, which are monozoic forms, lacking a scolex (head) and parasitic in fishes and turtles, and the Eucestoda, the majority of which are segmented and polyzoic. Only the latter subclass parasitizes humans.

The higher classification of the cestodes is controversial and complex (see, for example, Brooks 1989). The classification used here (see Table 24.2) at ordinal and subordinal taxonomic levels follows that of Khalil, Jones and Bray (1994).

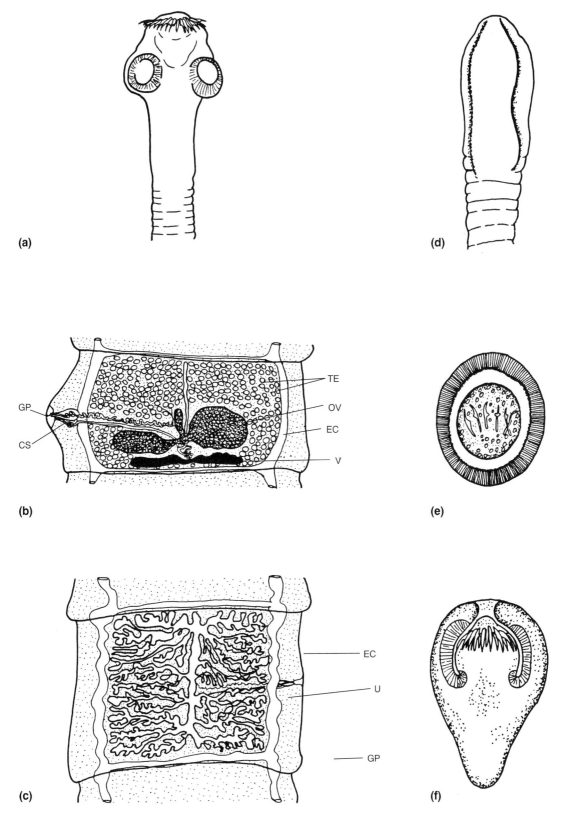

Fig. 24.1 Cestodes: (a) Scolex (head) of *Taenia* (Taeniidae) with armed rostellum and four suckers; (b) Mature segment of *Taenia*; (c). Gravid segment of *Taenia*; (d) Scolex of *Diphyllobothrium* (Diphyllobothriidae); (e) Egg of *Taenia* containing hexacanth larva; (f) Taeniid cysticercus larva (these can occur singly or, in certain genera, in large numbers within a cyst following asexual multiplication). *Abbreviations*: CS, cirrus sac; EC, excretory canal; GP, genital pore; OV, ovary; TE, testes; U, uterus; V, vitellarium. (Adapted from: (a–d), Khalil et al. 1994; (e) Abuladze 1964; (f), Fuhrmann 1931).

Table 24.2 Classification of cestodes found in humans

Order	Family
Pseudophyllidea	Diphyllobothriidae
Cyclophyllidea	Anoplocephalidae
	Davaineidae
	Dipylidiidae
	Hymenolepididae
	Mesocestoididae
	Taeniidae

SUBCLASS EUCESTODA SOUTHWELL, 1930

Main features. Cestoidea. Usually segmented; usually polyzoic, with one or more sets of reproductive organs per segment. Distinct scolex (head) normally present. Invariably parasitic in intestine of vertebrates.

The tapeworms of this subclass which infect humans are all segmented as adults (Fig. 24.1), with one or more copies of the reproductive system in each segment (proglottid) along the body (strobila). There are 2 orders involved: the Pseudophyllidea, recognizable by the fact that the scolex (head) lacks suckers and hooks, the attachment organ being a pair of bothria (dorsal and ventral longitudinal grooves on the scolex); and the Cyclophyllidea, whose scolex is armed with a ring of 4 suckers and sometimes one or more rings of apical hooks. In some cases, humans can also become infected with the larval stages of tapeworms; these normally reside in the tissues (see sections on Diphyllobothriidae, p. 456 and Taeniidae, p. 458).

Cestodes generally have a life cycle involving one or 2 intermediate hosts. Only one species (see *Hymenolepis*, p. 458) is capable of autoinfection without the use of intermediate hosts. Since adult cestodes are intestinal parasites of vertebrates, the eggs or gravid segments containing eggs pass out with the faeces. In the cyclophyllideans, if the eggs are eaten by a suitable intermediate host, which may be a terrestrial invertebrate (commonly an arthropod) or a vertebrate, they hatch to release a **hexacanth** (6-hooked) larva, called an **onchosphere**. In the case of the pseudophyllideans, the eggs hatch in water to release a ciliated, motile hexacanth, called a **coracidium**, which is eaten by an aquatic arthropod, such as a copepod. Once in the intermediate host the hexacanth usually penetrates the gut wall and develops in the body cavity into a **procercoid**. This develops further, either in the same host or in a second intermediate host, if the first host is eaten, into a resting, normally encysted, stage, which takes on a variety of names, depending upon its form, e.g. **cysticercus, cysticercoid, plerocercoid**. The final host acquires the parasite when it feeds upon the host harbouring the encysted stage. In a few instances (see Taeniidae, p. 458) some asexual multiplication of larval heads (protoscoleces) can occur when vertebrates act as an intermediate host.

The form of the attachment organ on the scolex differs markedly in different forms and can be readily used to distinguish the various orders. The form and armament of the scolex distinguishes genera, and the number and morphometrics of the hooks which comprise the armature are useful at the specific level. Other important characters relate to the shape of the segments and the arrangement and form of the reproductive system(s) within the segments, e.g. the position of the genital pore, the nature of the vitellarium, the size of the cirrus sac, the shape of the ovary and the nature of the uterus.

Since adult tapeworms are intestinal parasites which absorb nutrients though their tegument rather than browse, except perhaps at the point of attachment, the worms tend to do little physical damage to their host, apart from the possibility of bowel obstruction in the case of large infections. Their presence in humans, when apparent, is often accompanied by diarrhoea and loss of appetite. In some cases the absorption of certain nutrients is a factor (see *Diphyllobothrium*, p. 456, for selective absorption), especially in the malnourished. The presence of encysted larval tapeworms in the tissues is much more serious, notably in certain organs, such as the brain, liver and lungs, since the cysts can, in some cases, reach a large size. Control is dependent upon the life cycle of the worm, but it in most cases it can be effected by the cooking or freezing of meat (especially that of game, fish or other wild animals) and insects intended for ingestion, or the removal of insects from salad and other plant material to be eaten.

ORDER PSEUDOPHYLLIDEA CARUS, 1863

Main features. Eucestoda. Without suckers or hooks on scolex; but normally with pair of longitudinal grooves (bothria) which aid attachment. Polyzoic (segmented). First larval stage in crustaceans; second usually in fish. Adults in all vertebrate groups, especially fish.

Family Diphyllobothriidae Lühe, 1910

Main features. Pseudophyllidea. Strobila medium to large. Scolex occasionally poorly developed. Bothria usually well developed. Set of reproductive organs in each segment usually single, occasionally double or multiple. Second larval stage (plerocercoid) usually in fish, occasionally in reptiles and mammals. Adults in reptiles, birds and mammals.

Diphyllobothriids are usually parasitic in piscivorous higher vertebrates. One genus, *Diphyllobothrium* Cobbold, 1858, regularly occurs as an adult in humans, *Diplogonoporus* Lönnberg, 1892 occurs occasionally and other genera on rare occasions. These may be huge worms, reaching many metres in length. Diphyllobothriids in humans are recognizable by the absence of suckers and hooks on the scolex (head). One genus, *Spirometra* Faust, Campbell and Kellog, 1929, occurs in humans as a **plerocercoid** larva (called a **sparganum**).

Adult diphyllobothriids live in the intestine of their final host, producing huge numbers of eggs which pass out with the faeces and hatch in water to release a ciliated larva (a **coracidium**). If the coracidium is eaten by a suitable copepod, they develop in the haemocoel as a **procercoid** larva. If the infected copepod is eaten by a suitable vertebrate host, usually a fish, the larva penetrates the tissues and develops (sometimes encysting) in the body cavity, muscles or other tissues as a **plerocercoid** larva. If this host is eaten by a suitable higher vertebrate, the plerocercoid develops to an adult in the intestine. Humans become infected with adult diphyllobothriids by feeding upon raw, lightly marinated or inadequately cooked freshwater or, less frequently, marine fishes. Since these parasites are more usually parasitic in other mammals, little can be done to control the presence of larvae in fishes, but the freezing or cooking of fish and fish products kills the worms. Larval forms (*Spirometra*) are acquired by humans by drinking water containing infected copepods, by feeding upon raw or poorly cooked amphibians, reptiles or mammals and, apparently, by using flesh of reptiles or other species as a poultice for wounds, etc. Control is effected by filtering water and avoiding the consumption or contact with raw flesh which might harbour the plerocercoid larva.

The adult worms are large and absorb nutrients from the gut, notably vitamin B_{12}, absorption of which results in pernicious anaemia. Large infections can also result in obstruction of the bowel. Infections with plerocercoids (spargana) are more of a problem, as these larvae wander through the tissues before becoming encysted in a fibrous nodule reaching c.2 cm in diameter. These can be painful in subcutaneous regions, but can be much more serious if they end up in the eye, lymphatic system, brain, etc. (See Chapter 27.)

ORDER CYCLOPHYLLIDEA VAN BENEDEN IN BRAUN, 1900

Main features. Eucestoda. Scolex normally with 4 suckers. Rostellum (apical protrusion on scolex) usually present, sometimes absent; armed with hooks or not. Polyzoic (segmented). Parasitic as adults in all vertebrate groups except fish; normally in intestine.

Family Anoplocephalidae Cholodkowsky, 1902

Main features. Cyclophyllidea. Small to large worms. Scolex without rostellum. Suckers unarmed. Segments craspedote (posterior border overlaps anterior border of next segment) or not. Single or double set of reproductive organs per segment. In mammals, birds and reptiles.

Several genera have been recorded as occasional or accidental parasites of humans, including *Bertiella* Stiles and Hassall, 1902 (species normally occurring in primates), *Inermicapsifer* Janicki, 1910 and *Mathevotaenia* Akhumyan, 1946 (species normally occurring in rodents) and *Moniezia* Blanchard, 1891 (species normally parasitic in domesticated ruminants). A general, but not infallible, recognition feature of anoplocephalids is the absence of both hooks and a rostellum (muscular apical organ) on the scolex.

The eggs of anoplocephalids leave with the faeces either freely or in the form of gravid segments. If eaten by a suitable terrestrial arthropod, such as a soil mite, the egg hatches and the embryo (**onchosphere**)

develops into a **cysticercoid** larva in the haemocoel. Herbivorous vertebrates become infected when they feed upon infected arthropods or accidentally ingest them with vegetation. Humans acquire infections by accidentally ingesting mites with raw vegetation (*Bertiella* and *Moniezia*) or by eating larger insects, e.g. beetles, either as food or as medical remedies (*Mathevotaenia* and probably *Inermicapsifer*). Control measures include the careful washing of salad and other items of vegetation intended to be eaten raw and the avoidance or cooking or freezing of insects intended to be eaten.

Little is known regarding the pathogenicity of anoplocephalid infections in humans (diarrhoea has been reported), but it is likely that these unarmed worms cause little harm.

Family Davaineidae Braun, 1900

Main features. Cyclophyllidea. Body small to large. Rostellum usually present, rarely rudimentary; armed with crown of hooks usually but not always in 2 rows; crown of hooks round, oval or undulating, interrupted or not. Hooks characteristically numerous, small, hammer-shaped. Suckers normally present; armed with small spines or not. Segments normally numerous. One or 2 sets of reproductive organs per segment. Adults in birds and mammals.

Several species of *Raillietina* Furhmann, 1920, normally parasites of rodents, have been recorded as occasional parasites of humans. Davaineids are usually recognizable by the presence of a rostellum on the scolex armed with 2 rings of many minute, hammer-shaped hooks.

The adult worms release gravid segments which pass out in the faeces. Eggs eaten by suitable terrestrial insects develop in the haemocoel into a **cysticercoid** larva. The vertebrate host picks up the parasite by feeding upon the infected intermediate host. Humans are thought to acquire *Raillietina* by ingesting insects, such as ants, beetles or cockroaches, either accidentally with food or as part of the diet. Control can be effected by the careful washing of raw and cold food, keeping cold food in a meat safe or refrigerator and cooking or freezing of insects intended for ingestion.

Family Dipylidiidae Stiles, 1896

Main features. Cyclophyllidea. Body small to medium-sized. Scolex with protrusible rostellum armed with several rows of hooks. Hooks usually rose-thorn-shaped. Rostellar sac absent. Suckers unarmed. Segments numerous; mature and gravid segments longer than wide. Two sets of reproductive organs per segment. Larval stages in insects, amphibians or reptiles. Adults in carnivorous mammals.

One genus, *Dipylidium* Leuckart, 1863, occurs in humans. Dipylidiids are recognizable by the absence of a rostellar sac and the presence of 2 sets of reproductive organs in each segment.

Dipylidiid tapeworms normally occur in the intestine of carnivorous mammals. The gravid segments break off and leave with the faeces, releasing large numbers of eggs. This group of tapeworms appear to have 2 life cycle strategies. It seems likely that all use insects as intermediate hosts in which the larval cysticercoid stage develops. In some cases the mammalian host becomes infected when these insects are ingested; in other cases insectivorous amphibians or reptiles act as second intermediate or paratenic hosts. In the case of *Dipylidium*, dogs, cats, humans (usually children), etc. become infected by feeding upon fleas harbouring the cysticercoid larvae. Control relates to improvements in hygiene and the regular de-worming and de-fleaing of pets.

Although the rostellum of these worms is armed with hooks, they appear not to be very pathogenic, causing only slight indigestion and loss of appetite. Infection may only become apparent when segments are observed in stools.

Family Hymenolepididae Perrier, 1897

Main features. Cyclophyllidea. Rostellum usually present, occasionally lacking or rudimentary; unarmed or armed with single, rarely double, crown of hooks (hooks may be very small). Suckers armed or not. Segments broader than long, craspedote. Single (rarely double) set of reproductive organs in each segment. Normally 1–3 (usually 3) testes per segment. Adults in birds and mammals.

Two genera, *Hymenolepis* Weinland, 1858 and *Rodentolepis* Spasskii, 1954, occur relatively commonly in humans; both normally parasitize rodents. Although previously considered as *Hymenolepis*, species of *Rodentolepis* differ from *Hymenolepis* in that the rostellum is armed with a crown of hooks. Another genus, *Drepanidotaenia* Railliet, 1892, a parasite of anseriform birds, has also been reported in humans. Hymenolepidids are relatively small tapeworms generally recognizable by the fact that each segment has only 3 testes.

Hymenolepidids are intestinal parasites. Their eggs leave with the faeces and are ingested by arthropods, within which develops a cysticercoid larva. The vertebrate host normally becomes infected by swallowing arthropods harbouring this stage. In terrestrial forms (e.g. *Hymenolepis* and *Rodentolepis*) the usual intermediate hosts are beetles and fleas; whereas in aquatic forms (e.g. *Drepanidotaenia*) they are copepods. One species of *Rodentolepis* (*R. nana*), which occurs in humans, is unique for a tapeworm in that direct infection is possible, either by reinfection (autoinfection) of the intestinal mucosa by eggs in the gut or by swallowing eggs which have passed in the faeces. Humans also become infected with hymenolepidids by accidentally eating beetles and fleas, and, in the rare cases of *Depanidotaenia*, by drinking water containing infected copepods. Control is effected by rodent control, personal hygiene, care when handling laboratory animals, especially where these parasites are used as laboratory models, de-fleaing laboratory rodents, and filtering drinking water.

These worms cause few symptoms, although heavy infections of *R. nana* caused by autoinfection may result in enteritis. This is thought to be caused more by the waste-products of these worms than damage at the site of attachment resulting from the armed scolex. (See Chapter 27.)

Family Mesocestoididae Lühe, 1894

Main features. Cyclophyllidea. Body narrow; with numerous segments. Rostellum absent. Mature segments wider than long; gravid segments may be longer than wide. Single set of reproductive organs in each segment; with median genital pore. Larval stage (tetrathyridium) in amphibians, reptiles, birds and mammals. Adults in mammals, rarely birds.

One genus, *Mesocestoides* Lühe, 1894, has been reported from humans, the species concerned being natural parasites of carnivorous mammals, such as foxes, racoons, skunks, etc. Mesocestoidids are recognizable by the absence of a rostellum on the scolex and the median position of the genital pore on the segments.

Eggs pass out with the faeces in gravid segments. If these are eaten by a suitable arthropod, probably an insect, the onchosphere develops in the haemocoel as a procercoid larva. If the arthropod is eaten by vertebrates such as amphibians, reptiles, birds and mammals, the worms develop in the tissue as a type of plerocercoid referred to as a **tetrathyridium**. The final host acquires the parasite by feeding upon the vertebrate intermediate host. Infections in humans appear to have been caused by people feeding upon poorly cooked game, raw birds and especially raw snake livers. Control is by the proper cooking or freezing of meat of all sorts obtained from the wild.

These unarmed worms appear not to be very pathogenic, but diarrhoea, poor appetite, and some anaemia has been reported in relation to human infections.

Family Taeniidae Ludwig, 1886

Main features. Cyclophyllidea. Strobila ribbon-like, usually with many segments. Rostellum usually well developed; usually bearing 2 rows of hooks. Anterior row of hooks usually larger and alternating with second row. Single set of reproductive organs in each segment. Larval stage either cysticercus or large cystic structure producing multiple protoscoleces asexually within brood capsules. Larval stage and adult in mammals.

Taeniid tapeworms may occur in humans in both larval and adult form. Two genera frequently parasitize humans, *Taenia* Linnaeus, 1758 (now includes *Multiceps* Goeze, 1782 and *Taeniarhynchus* Weinland, 1858) and *Echinococcus* Rudolphi, 1801, the latter only in its larval form.

Taeniids normally occur as adults in the intestine of carnivorous mammals, such as canids and felids. Eggs or segments containing eggs leave with the faeces. If the eggs fall on grass or other vegetation and are eaten by herbivorous mammals, the egg hatches in the gut and releases a larva (the onchosphere) which penetrates the gut wall and enters the blood system. These larvae are transported via the circulation until they reach the body muscles, where they encyst and develop as a **cysticercus** larva which has an invaginated scolex (protoscolex). Carnivores become infected with the adult parasite when they feed upon herbivorous mammals. Similarly, humans become infected by feeding upon raw or poorly cooked meat, especially pork and beef. Humans can also harbour the larval stage (cysticercus), when the eggs passed by infected humans or carnivores are accidentally ingested. In some species this larva (a **coenurus**) produces within its body many small protoscoleces (heads), each one of which can develop into an adult worm if eaten by a suitable host; another (the **hydatid cyst** of *Echinococcus*) contains huge number of 'brood capsules' within each of which develop numerous protoscoleces. In the latter case the cysts may be huge, reaching 30 cm in diameter. A consequence of this asexual reproduction is that the adult worms are much smaller, have fewer segments and produce fewer eggs than more conventional taeniids. Control includes the proper cooking (or freezing) of meat, regular deworming of dogs, especially farm dogs, not feeding raw offal and other parts of slaughtered animals to dogs, keeping dog (and human) faeces away from farm animals and vegetable crops, and the proper washing of raw vegetation intended as food.

Adult worms in the intestine cause few symptoms, although diarrhoea, bowel discomfort, weight loss, irritation at the site of attachment in the case of species armed with hooks, and bowel obstruction have been reported. The presence of segments in the stools or crawling out of the anus may be the only evidence of infection. The presence of larval stages (cysticercosis, hydatid disease, coenurosis) in the tissues is another matter, as, depending upon size and location, the cysts can be very dangerous. These larvae may live for many years and may have to be removed surgically. Hydatid cysts can occur in many parts of the body; the commonest site is the liver and another frequent site is the lungs. Symptoms are similar to those of a slow-growing tumour. The cysticerci and coenurus larvae of *Taenia* spp. (including *Multiceps*) frequently occur in the brain in humans, sometimes in the eye or under the skin. Symptoms of brain infections are similar to those caused by any space-filling lesion, including epileptic seizures, paraplegia, etc. (See Chapters 27 and 28.)

2.2 Class Trematoda Rudolphi, 1808

Main features. Platyhelminthes. Primarily permanent parasites of tissues of molluscs; with single or multiple generation in life history; life cycle may or may not involve other additional hosts. Mollusc normally harbours asexual generations or single sexual generation. Additional host usually a vertebrate; harbours adult sexual stage, especially in gut and associated organs. Sexual adult usually with 2 organs of attachment organs (normally suckers or sucker-like structures); one generally anterior and one ventral or posterior. Syncytial tegument armed with spines or smooth. Gut or its vestige always present.

The trematodes or 'flukes' are flatworms which originally evolved as parasites of molluscs and virtually all species retain a molluscan element in the their life history. There are 2 subgroups, the Digenea and the Aspidogastrea, but only the former occurs in humans and other mammals.

There is no modern accepted classification of the Trematoda or the Digenea. Brooks, O'Grady and Glen (1985, 1989) presented a version based on a cladistic analysis, but this has been heavily criticized by, *inter alia*, Pearson (1992). The classification in Table 24.3 follows the general outline indicated by Gibson and Bray (1994).

Subclass Digenea Carus, 1863

Main features. Trematoda. With alternation of generations; normally 2 (sometimes more) asexual generations in mollusc and single sexual generation in vertebrate (occasionally invertebrate). Normally hermaphroditic, occasionally partly or entirely dioecious. Generally small elongate-oval to tubular worms, but various other forms, including round and filamentous, occur. Body smooth or armed with spines. Usually with 2 muscular suckers, sometimes one, occasionally none. Form of testes variable; one to many, often 2. Muscular sac, e.g. cirrus sac, often envelopes all or part of male terminal genitalia. Genital atrium (chamber into which male and female ducts open; opens via genital pore) present or absent. Common genital pore normally present; position variable, usually ventral on anterior body, occasionally terminal. Ovary normally single, occasionally multiple; position variable. Uterus variable in size, form and distribution. Eggs normally oval and operculate; normally tanned; occasionally with spine or filament(s). Vitellarium (yolk gland) variable in shape and distribution, exhibiting all forms between follicular and single compact mass. Parasitic as sexual adult in all vertebrate groups, occasionally in invertebrates; usually present in gut or other body cavities, occasionally in blood or other tissues, rarely ectoparasitic.

Those trematodes (i.e. digeneans) which occur in humans are readily recognized by the fact that they possess 2 suckers which act as attachment organs, they have only a single set of reproductive organs and they have a functional gut (Fig. 24.2). They are endoparasites occurring in humans mainly in the gut, liver, bile ducts, lungs or blood system.

Digeneans have a unique life cycle which, usually involves 3 generations, 2 asexual generations in a mollusc and a sexual generation in a vertebrate. The eggs leave the vertebrate, normally with the faeces, and hatch to release a ciliated larva, the **miracidium**, which penetrates a particular molluscan host; sometimes the egg is eaten by this host prior to release of the miracidium. Within the mollusc the miracidium develops into a sac-like parthenogenetic adult, the **mother sporocyst**. Within this stage develop daughter stages called **daughter sporocysts** or, if a sac-like gut is present, **rediae**. Within this second parthenogenetic generation develop a short-lived, usually tailed, larval stage, the **cercaria**, often in huge numbers (Fig. 24.2). These larvae usually escape from the mollusc and swim or crawl to the next host. Some cercariae penetrate the final vertebrate host directly, but the majority penetrate or settle upon in its food as a long-lived resting stage called the **metacercaria**. Metacercariae are normally encysted within invertebrates or other vertebrates, which act as intermediate hosts, or upon vegetation. The final vertebrate hosts become infected by feeding upon prey or vegetation harbouring metacercariae. Digeneans tend to be very specific in relation to their mollucsan host, relatively unspecific for inter-

Table 24.3 Classification of digeneans found in humans

Order	Superfamily	Family
Strigeida	Diplostomoidea	Diplostomidae
	Gymnophalloidea	Gymnophallidae
	Schistosomatoidea	Schistosomatidae
Echinostomida	Echinostomatoidea	Echinostomatidae
		Fasciolidae
	Paramphistomatoidea	Zygocotylidae
Plagiorchiida	Dicrocoelioidea	Dicrocoeliidea
	Opsithorchioidea	Heterophyidae
		Opsithorchiidae
	Plagiorchioidea	Lecithodendriidae
		Paragonimidae
		Plagiorchiidae
		Troglotrematidae

mediate hosts and exhibit various levels of specificity for their final vertebrate host.

Some digeneans differ considerably in shape and morphology, but the majority are similar in overall appearance. Features used to distinguish groups include the presence or absence of spines on the tegument, the position and number of suckers, the form and arrangement of the reproductive organs, and the shape the gut and excretory vesicle. At the specific level, details such as sucker ratio and egg size are important.

Although, like tapeworms, digeneans can take in nutrients through their body surface, they also tend to feed by browsing. In the gut this is usually not a great problem, especially in light infestations, but in other sites the damage, irritation and toxins produced can result in inflammation, tissue reactions, fibrosis, obstruction, etc. The body spines of some worms, which help it maintain its position, may also cause irritation. In view of the nature of the life cycle, obvious targets for the control of digenean infections are the molluscan host and the development of sewage systems and standards of hygiene which prevent contact between worm eggs and molluscs. Similarly, transmission to humans can be pre-empted by avoidance of contact between bare skin and water containing cercariae, where these penetrate the skin directly, or by changes in food preparation and eating habits.

SUPERFAMILY DIPLOSTOMOIDEA POIRIER, 1886

Family Diplostomidae Poirier, 1886

Main features. Diplostomoidea. Body usually divided into 2 regions; anterior region wide, foliate with ventral depression; hindbody cylindrical. Oral and ventral suckers well developed, sometimes small; latter in base of ventral concavity. Pseudosuckers often present lateral to oral sucker. Cirrus sac absent. Metacercaria in fishes or amphibians. Adults in intestine of birds and mammals.

One species of the genus, *Neodiplostomum* Railliet, 1919, which is more commonly a parasite of rats, has been recorded in the intestine of humans in Korea on several occasions. Diplostomids are recognizable by

the bipartite nature of the body and wide, ventrally concave forebody.

Eggs of diplostomids leave with the faeces. If they enter water, the miracidium is released; after penetrating an aquatic snail, it transforms into a mother sporocyst. The mother sporocyst produces daughter sporocysts which release fork-tailed cercariae. The latter leave the snail and encyst as metacercariae usually in fishes, but in the case of *Neodiplostomum* in frogs. Snakes, which acquire the parasites by feeding upon frogs, act as paratenic hosts. Humans may become infected by feeding upon raw or poorly cooked frogs or snakes. Control can be effected by the proper cooking of amphibians or reptiles used as food. Little is known about the pathogenicity of these worms in humans.

SUPERFAMILY GYMNOPHALLOIDEA ODHNER, 1905

Family Gymnophallidae Odhner, 1905

Main features. Gymnophalloidea. Body small; oval to pear-shaped; flattened. Tegument armed with small spines. Oral sucker large, often very large; may support pair of lateral papillae. Ventral sucker small; in anterior or posterior half of body (posterior for *Gymnophalloides*). Cirrus sac absent. In intestine, bursa of Fabricius or gallbladder of birds (mainly) and mammals.

Gymnophallids are usually parasites of birds. Only one genus, *Gymnophalloides* Fujita, 1925, is parasitic in humans; this is a very small worm which can occur in the intestine, or possibly the biliary system, in huge numbers in Korea. An obvious recognition feature is that the small ventral sucker occurs in the posterior quarter of the body. It is readily distinguished from paramphistomoids (see p. 463) by its smaller size, spiny tegument and smaller, non-terminal ventral sucker.

Its full life cycle is not known, but the intermediate host is presumed to be a marine oyster or clam. The asexual generations of gymnophallids usually occur in bivalves; but there is no free-living cercarial stage, as the metacercariae encyst directly inside the daughter sporocyst. Consequently, the final host acquires the

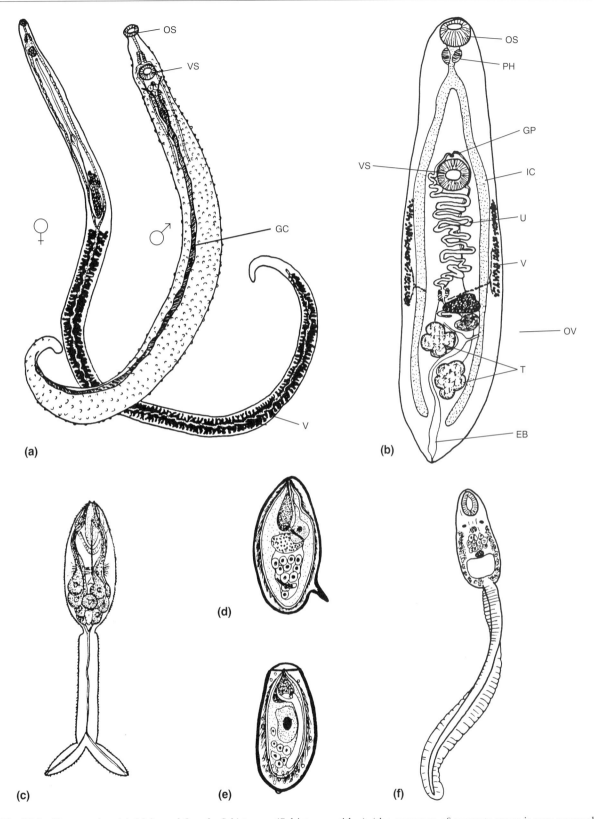

Fig. 24.2 Trematodes: (a) Male and female *Schistosoma* (Schistosomatidae) (the presence of separate sexes is very unusual for a flatworm); (b) *Opisthorchis* (Opisthorchiidae) with more conventional trematode morphology; (c) Cercaria (larva) of *Schistosoma* with bifid tail; (d) Egg of *Schistosoma* containing miracidium (ciliated larva); (e) Egg of *Opisthorchis* with lid (operculum) through which miracidium escapes; (f) Cercaria of *Opisthorchis*. *Abbreviations:* EB, excretory bladder; GC, gynae-cophoric canal within which female lies; GP, genital pore; IC, intestinal caecum; OS, oral sucker; OV, ovary; PH, pharynx; T, testes; U, uterus; V, vitellarium; VS, ventral sucker. (Adapted from: (a), Schell 1985; (b,e,f), Vogel 1934; (c,d), Cort, 1919).

parasite by feeding upon bivalve molluscs. Control can, therefore, be implemented by the avoidance of feeding upon raw bivalves or at least those which have not been treated by freezing to kill the parasite.

Little is known about this parasite, but it appears to cause gastric discomfort, indigestion and diarrhoea, and possibly, pancreatitis or cholecystitis. Presumably, when they are present in large numbers, the spined tegument of these worms can cause local irritation to the tissues.

SUPERFAMILY SCHISTOSOMATOIDEA STILES AND HASSALL, 1898

Family Schistosomatidae Stiles and Hassall, 1898

Main features. Schistosomatoidea. Dioecious. Elongate worms; females narrower and longer than males; female clasped in gynaecophoric canal (longitudinal groove) of male. Oral and ventral suckers normally present. Eggs non-operculate; with or without spine. Parasitic in blood system of birds and mammals.

Only one genus of schistosome, i.e. *Schistosoma* Weinland, 1858, occurs as an adult in humans. The fact that the sexes are separate and their presence in the blood system makes the group readily recognizable (Fig. 24.2).

Eggs leave the body with the faeces or urine. The miracidium hatches from the egg, penetrates an aquatic snail and transforms into a mother sporocyst. This gives rise to daughter sporocysts, which produce cercariae. The life cycle in this group is different from the majority of digeneans in that there is no metacercarial stage and no intermediate host between the molluscan and vertebrate hosts: the fork-tailed cercariae leave the molluscan host, swim and penetrate the skin of the final host, and enter the blood system. The mode of transmission means that avoidance of contact between the skin and water containing cercariae is important in preventing infection, as are control of the relevant species of molluscs, general sanitation and hygiene.

Since schistosomes occur in the blood system, there is no direct route for the voiding of eggs, which become lodged in small blood vessels in various parts of the body, including the liver and lungs, causing blockages, local granulomata and abscesses which form around the eggs and aid their passage into the lumen of the gut or bladder. These worms are therefore very pathogenic and cause a variety of symptoms. In addition, the fact that the cercariae penetrate the skin means that local immune responses are elicited, with a resulting skin reaction known as **cercarial dermatitis**: this reaction is caused not only by species of *Schistosoma* of humans and other mammals but also by avian schistosomes of the genera *Trichobilharzia* Skrjabin and Zakharov, 1920 and *Ornithobilharzia* Odhner,

1912 where the reaction is often more pronounced. (See Chapter 25.)

SUPERFAMILY ECHINOSTOMATOIDEA LOOSS, 1899

Family Echinostomatidae Looss, 1899

Main features. Echinostomatoidea. Body oval to elongate. Tegument armed with small spines. Head collar present; usually armed with single or double crown of spines. Suckers well developed. Encysted as metacercariae in or on molluscs, annelids, fishes, tadpoles, etc. Eggs relatively large. Adults mainly in intestine, occasionally other organs, of birds, mammals and occasionally reptiles.

Several echinostomatid genera, the most common of which is *Echinostoma* Rudolphi, 1809, occur in humans especially in parts of southeast Asia. Other genera include *Echinochasmus* Dietz, 1909, *Echinoparyphium* Dietz, 1909 and *Hypoderaeum* Dietz, 1909; these are primarily parasites of birds and mammals and infect humans only accidentally. Echinostomatids, which occur in the intestine, are readily recognized by the single or double crown of large circumoral spines; but worms must be in good condition when they are fixed, since the spines are readily lost in frozen or poorly preserved material.

The life cycle involves 2 intermediate hosts, both of which may be snails. The eggs pass out from the vertebrate host with the faeces and hatch to release the ciliated miracidium. This penetrates a snail and develops into a mother sporocyst. Within this develops a brood of rediae. When these are released into the mollusc's tissues, they produce cercariae which leave the mollusc and then encyst in or on the same snail or neighbouring snails. The metacercarial stage of echinostomatids tends to occur, therefore, in or on snails, but some species also encyst in or on annelids, fishes and tadpoles. Humans acquire this parasite by feeding on uncooked snails or, more likely, on poorly washed salad or other raw vegetation harbouring the snails. Control is, therefore, possible by avoiding the ingestion of snails, by the careful washing or cooking of vegetation intended as food, and by limiting the use of human faeces as a fertilizer. *Echinostoma* is not specific to humans and occurs in other mammals; rats and dogs are especially noted for carrying infections.

These worms attach to the wall of the intestine and cause local inflammation, presumably due in part to the large oral spines and general body spination. The oral spines are used by the worm for abrading the gut wall. Heavy infections can cause ulceration of the bowel, diarrhoea and abdominal pain.

Family Fasciolidae Railliet, 1895

Main features. Echinostomatoidea. Body large; flattened; often broad, sometimes narrow. Forebody short. Tegument normally armed with small spines. Head collar and circumoral crown of spines absent. Intestinal caeca with or without dendritic lateral branches. Testes usually deeply lobed; sometimes unlobed. In intestine and biliary system of mammals.

Two genera occur in humans, *Fasciola* Linnaeus, 1758 and *Fasciolopsis* Looss, 1899. These are large, broad, leaf-like worms, recognizable by the presence of deeply lobed gonads, the lobes being so deep that the gonads appear dendritic. *Fasciola,* the common liver fluke of sheep, occurs in the biliary system, whereas *Fasciolopisis* occurs in the intestine and is restricted to southeast Asia. The 2 genera are readily distinguished as *Fasciola* has branched intestinal caeca.

The eggs of fasciolids, whether they be in the intestine or biliary system, pass out with the faeces. The miracidia infect freshwater snails, within which the mother sporocyst develops and produces rediae. Accounts of the life history within the molluscan host vary; but, apparently, within the rediae may develop a second or even third generation of rediae and any generation of redia may produce cercariae. The latter leave the snail and encyst as metacercariae usually on vegetation. Encysted metacercariae are especially common on grass close to water and on plants such as watercress and water chestnut. The final hosts, normally herbivorores but occasionally humans, become infected by feeding upon vegetation harbouring the encysted metacercariae. Metacercariae of *Fasciola* migrate through the liver *en route* for the bile ducts, where the adults live. These parasites are very common in domesticated animals, such sheep, pigs and cattle, which form huge reservoirs of infection. Control is, therefore, facilitated by the avoidance of raw (or unpeeled) vegetables or other plant material which has been associated with water-bodies. Similarly, control can be assisted by avoidance where possible of the links between human and animal faeces and bodies of water, e.g. by the use of drinking troughs and the draining of pasture land.

Fasciolids cause inflammation at the site of attachment, which may lead to ulceration and haemorrhage, as these spine-covered worms browse on the tissues. The amount of damage caused depends on the worm burden. In the liver the presence of these worms can cause traumatic damage resulting in necrosis ('liver rot'); in the bile ducts mechanical irritation can cause hyperplasia and fibrosis. When flukes are present in large numbers, their large size can result in blockages of the bile ducts or even the intestine. (See Chapter 26.)

Superfamily Paramphistomoidea Fischoeder, 1901

Family Zygocotylidae Ward, 1917

Main features. Paramphistomoidea. Body stout, often large; pear-shaped to elongate-oval; ventrally flattened. Tegument unarmed; tegumentary papillae present or absent. Appears to have suckers at each end of body. Oral sucker absent. Pharynx resembles oral sucker; terminal at anterior extremity; opening via mouth; with one or 2 posterolateral sacs. Posterior (ventral) sucker normally occurs ventroterminally at posterior end of body; well developed, often very large. Eggs very large, numerous. In intestine of mammals and birds (mainly herbivores) .

Two genera of zygocotylid paramphistomoids occur in humans, *Gastrodiscoides* Leiper, 1913 and *Watsonius* Näsmark, 1937. These relatively large worms are read-ily recognizable by the apparent presence of a sucker at each end of the body, hence their vernacular name, 'amphistomes'. The 2 genera can be distinguished by shape; in *Gastrodiscoides* the body consists of a posterior discoid region and a narrower anterior region.

The zygocotylid life cycle commences with eggs passed out with the faeces. When the eggs reach water, they hatch and the released larva, the miracidium, penetrates aquatic gastropod molluscs. Within the mollusc the miracidium transforms into a mother sporocyst, within which develop rediae (some authors maintain that only a single mother redia derives from the mother sporocyst and this produces a second generation, **daughter rediae**.) Cercariae, which develop within the rediae, are released from the mollusc and encyst as metacercariae on the substratum, especially on vegetation and the snail host. The final host, a bird or mammal, normally becomes infected by feeding upon vegetation or snails harbouring the metacercarial stage.

The general similarity in transmission between the zygocotylids and the fasciolids means that the method of human infection and control measures linked to the worms' life cycles are essentially the same, i.e. avoiding the consumption of uncooked vegetation which has originated from or close to water bodies. There is a difference, however, in that primates rather than domesticated herbivores tend to act as reservoir hosts, although pigs, rats and other rodents may also be involved. Human faeces should be kept away from water-bodies.

Little pathogenicity is observed in light infections, but inflammation of the intestinal mucosa may occur where the large posterior sucker attaches. Heavy infestations may cause oedema of the intestinal wall and diarrhoea.

Superfamily Opisthorchioidea Looss, 1899

Family Heterophyidae Leiper, 1909

Main features. Opisthorchioidea. Body small; oval to elongate. Tegument spined. Oral and ventral suckers present. Ventral sucker occasionally small or submedian, often associated with genital atrium forming ventrogenital complex. Cirrus sac absent. Gonotyl(s) (genital sucker = muscular structure associated with genital atrium) may or may not be developed; armed or unarmed. Eggs small. Metacercariae on skin and fins and in tissues of fishes. Adults in piscivorous birds and mammals.

Two heterophyid genera occur relatively commonly in humans, *Heterophyes* Cobbold, 1886 in lands bordering the western Mediterranean and both *Heterophyes* and *Metagonimus* Katsurada, 1913 in China, Korea, Japan and neighbouring regions. Other genera, such as *Centrocestus* Looss, 1899, *Stellantchasmus* Onji and Nishio, 1915 and *Haplorchis* Looss, 1899, may also occur on rare occasions. *Heterophyes* and *Metagonimus* can be distinguished by the fact that in the latter the mouth of the ventrogenital sac is directed anteriorly, there is no muscular gonotyl (genital sucker) present and the genital pore is anterior to the ventral sucker. Heterophyids are small worms recognizable by the fact that the genital atrium is associated with the ventral sucker to form a ventrogenital complex.

Heterophyids in humans are intestinal parasites. Their eggs pass out with the faeces and hatch to release miracidia which penetrate aquatic snails. Within the snail there are two generations of rediae. Cercariae produced by the rediae leave the mollusc and encyst under the scales and in the superficial muscles of freshwater fishes. Humans and other piscivorous mammals obtain the infection by feeding upon raw, pickled or poorly cooked fish harbouring the metacercaria. Infection can be avoided by ensuring that fish intended as food are well-cooked or frozen prior to ingestion. A reduction in the likelihood of infection may also occur if the fish in the food of reservoir hosts, such as cats, dogs and pigs, is treated in the same way. Improvements in sanitation also help disrupt the life cycle.

In small numbers, these small, spined worms cause little damage to the intestine apart from local inflammation at the site of attachment; but more serious damage, including ulceration, may occur when large numbers are present. Occasionally the worms may penetrate the gut wall and eggs may end up in various parts of the body, including the heart and brain.

Family Opisthorchiidae Looss, 1899

Main features. Opisthorchioidea. Body small to medium-sized; flattened; elongate-oval to fusiform; often translucent. Tegument spined. Suckers well developed. Cirrus sac absent. Gonotyl and ventrogenital sac (see Heterophyidae) absent. Metacercariae present in tissues of freshwater fishes. Adults in piscivorous mammals and birds.

Two genera of opisthorchiids occur in humans, *Opisthorchis* Blanchard, 1895 and *Clonorchis* Looss, 1907. They can be distinguished by the fact that in *Clonorchis* the testes are tandem and have long, branched lobes which overlap the intestinal caeca. Both are parasitic in the biliary system and are most common in southeast Asia. They can be distinguished from heterophyids by their greater size, more elongate shape and the absence of a ventrogenital complex. Body spines are very small and commonly lost in preserved specimens.

Worms in the bile ducts release eggs that pass into the intestine to be voided with the faeces. If an egg finds its way to water and is ingested by a suitable aquatic gastropod snail, it hatches in the gut and releases the miracidium, which penetrates the mollusc and develops into a mother sporocyst. Within the latter stage develop rediae, which in turn give rise to cercariae. These leave the snail, swim and encyst as metacercariae under the scales or in the superficial tissues of freshwater fishes. Piscivorous mammals and birds become infected by feeding upon fishes harbouring the metacercarial stage. Control measures are similar to those outlined for heterophyids, i.e. primarily the avoidance of raw, pickled or poorly cooked fishes. Opisthorchiids are not primarily parasites of

humans, as those infecting humans also occur commonly in many piscivorous mammals, including cats, foxes, dogs, pigs, etc., which act as reservoir hosts. Avoidance of the link between both human and animal faeces and water-bodies is needed to break the life cycle.

Light infections are not pathogenic, but heavier infections of these spine-covered worms cause abdominal discomfort, diarrhoea and even acute pain. This results from inflammation of the biliary epithelium and thickening of the bile ducts as a consequence of mechanical irritation and their browsing activity. The presence of worms may cause gallstones, cirrhosis of the liver and perhaps even carcinoma of the bile ducts. (See Chapter 26.)

Superfamily Dicrocoelioidea Looss, 1899

Family Dicrocoeliidae Looss, 1899

Main features. Plagiorchiida. Body oval, lanceolate or filiform; flattened; often translucent. Tegument usually spined. Oral sucker subterminal. Ventral sucker in anterior third of body; occasionally very reduced or absent. Cirrus sac present; close to ventral sucker. Metacercaria occurs in terrestrial arthropods. In biliary system or pancreatic ducts of reptiles, birds and mammals.

Only one dicrocoeliid genus, *Dicrocoelium* Dujardin, 1845, occurs in humans and then only rarely. It normally parasitizes a wide range of mammals and even birds, but is very common in domesticated ruminants, especially sheep. Dicrocoeliids can be distinguished from other digeneans occurring in the biliary system of humans in that the testes occur close to the ventral sucker and the vitelline fields are in the post-testicular region of the hindbody.

As in the case of other parasites of the biliary system, the eggs pass out with the faeces, but, in contrast to other digeneans, occurring in humans, the snail host is a terrestrial gastropod. Inside the mollusc the miracidium transforms into a mother sporocyst within which form daughter sporocysts. The latter give rise to cercariae which end up in slime balls produced by the snail. When the slime balls are eaten by ants, the parasite encysts as a metacercaria in these insects. Herbivores, and humans, become infected with the parasite when ants are eaten accidentally with vegetation. Human infection can, therefore, be avoided by careful washing of salad material and other items of vegetation eaten raw.

Little is known regarding the pathogenicity of these worms in humans, but, since infections are likely to be light, they are presumably similar to mild infections of fasciolids or opisthorchiids.

Superfamily Plagiorchioidea Lühe, 1901

Family Lecithodendriidae Lühe, 1901

Main features. Plagiorchioidea. Body spherical to elongate. Tegument usually spined. Oral sucker well developed. Ventral sucker often small; near middle of body. Testes usually symmetrical and widely separated near middle of body. Cirrus sac usually present. Vitelline follicles in forebody, occasionally hindbody. Eggs small. Metacercariae in aquatic insects. In gut of amphibians, reptiles, birds and mammals (especially bats).

Lecithodendriids occur in a wide variety of insectivorous vertebrates and are noted parasites of bats. Only one genus, *Phaneropsolus* Looss, 1899, regularly parasitizes humans, although others, such as *Paralecithodendrium* Odhner, 1910 and *Prosthodendrium* Dollfus, 1931 have also been reported. These minute parasites are recognizable by the fact that the gonads and vitelline follicles are in the forebody or at least level with the ventral sucker.

Lecithodendriid eggs pass into water with the host's faeces. The miracidium enters the tissues of aquatic snails and transforms into a mother sporocyst. It is likely that these produce daughter sporocysts, which, in turn, produce cercariae. The cercariae leave the snail and some are eaten by or penetrate the larvae of aquatic insects, within which they encyst as cercariae. The final vertebrate host acquires the parasite by feeding upon larval or adult insects harbouring the parasite. It is not clear how people in southeast Asia (Thailand and Indonesia) become infected with lecithodendriids, but it is presumably by feeding upon larval or adult insects in regions where these are local delicacies or by accidentally ingesting insect larvae with aquatic vegetation or water. Control measures include the filtering or heating of water, the cleaning of vegetable material and the cooking or freezing of insects intended as food.

Virtually nothing is known concerning the pathogenicity of lecithodendriids in humans, but it seems likely that some local irritation occurs, similar to that caused by mild infections of other small, intestinal digeneans armed with spines, such as heterophyids.

Family Paragonimidae Dollfus, 1939

Main features. Plagiorchioidea. Body oval to fusiform. Tegument spinose. Suckers relatively small; ventral sucker near middle of body. Testes symmetrical; lobed; in hindbody. Cirrus sac absent. Genital pore closely posterior to ventral sucker. Metacercariae in tissues of crustaceans. In lungs of mammals.

Numerous species of the genus, *Paragonimus* Braun, 1899, occur in the lungs of humans in parts of Africa, South America and especially southeast Asia. They are medium-sized worms readily recognizable by their site in the lungs and the position of the genital pore posterior to the ventral sucker. They can be distinguished from the closely related troglotrematids by the absence of a cirrus sac. Paragonimids are usually parasitic in carnivores, especially felids and others likely to feed upon freshwater crabs and other large crustaceans.

The eggs pass out of the lungs with mucus, are swallowed and then voided with the faeces or voided in sputum. The hatched miracidium penetrates freshwater snails and develops into a mother sporocyst. Two generations of rediae are then produced. The second generation gives rise to cercariae, which leave the snail and encyst in the tissues (especially muscles

and gills) of crustaceans (usually crabs or crayfish); the latter may apparently also become infected by feeding directly upon infected snails. Humans acquire the parasite by eating raw or inadequately cooked crustaceans, the young flukes penetrating the gut wall and finding their way to the lungs via the abdominal cavity, diaphragm and pleural cavity. Control is effected by the cooking of crustaceans intended as food and sanitary measures which break the link between human and, where possible, carnivore faeces and water bodies.

Paragonimids are covered with small spines and presumably browse on the walls of the bronchi, so their presence in the lungs causes local inflammation, resulting in a tissue reaction, cyst formation and fibrosis. The net result is coughing, bloodstained sputum, chest pains and bronchitis, which occur when the cysts rupture. The migration of the young worms through the body tissues does not cause any serious problems; but occasionally worms reach other parts of the body where problems may arise, especially when worms reach the brain where they may cause paralysis or even death. (See Chapter 26.)

Family Plagiorchiidae Lühe, 1901

Main features. Plagiorchioidea. Body oval, pyriform, lanceolate or elongate. Tegument armed with spines. Suckers well developed. Ventral sucker normally in anterior half of body. Testes in hindbody; usually diagonal. Cirrus sac present; usually long. Genital pore anterior to ventral sucker. Ovary pretesticular. Uterus in hindbody. In intestine, occasionally biliary system, of vertebrates, especially birds and mammals.

Species of the genus *Plagiorchis* Lühe, 1899 have occasionally been recorded from the intestine of humans in parts of southeast Asia. Plagiorchiids are parasites of insectivorous vertebrates, especially mammals. Although some nominal species are known only from humans, it is not known whether they are zoonotic infections or specifically human parasites. The worms differ from other plagiorchioids found in humans in that the testes tend to be diagonal to tandem rather than symmetrical.

Plagiorchiid eggs leave with the faeces and the miracidium enters an aquatic snail and develops into a mother sporocyst. These give rise to daughter sporocysts from which cercariae emerge. These leave the snail and find their way into the larval stages of aquatic insects which act as intermediate hosts. The vertebrate host becomes infected by feeding upon larval or adult insects harbouring cercariae. Humans are thought to become infected by eating insect grubs.

Little is known regarding the pathogenicity of these worms, but infections are likely to be light and effect similar local responses to those of other small, spined digeneans parasitic in the gut, such as heterophyids.

Family Troglotrematidae Odhner, 1914

Main features. Plagiorchioidea. Body oval. Tegument spinose. Suckers well developed; often similar in size. Ventral sucker in middle or anterior half of body. Testes symmetrical. Cirrus sac present. Genital pore usually closely posterior to ventral sucker. Metacercaria in tissues of fishes or crustaceans. In intestine, body sinuses, kidney, liver, etc. of mammals.

One genus of troglotrematid, *Nanophyetus* Chapin, 1927, occasionally occurs in humans. These worms normally occur as parasites of piscivorous carnivores in North America. This group appears closely related to the paragonimids and, like the latter group, tends not to be parasitic in the alimentary system (though *Nanophyetus* is an intestinal parasite) and be recognizable by the position of the genital pore posterior to the ventral sucker.

Eggs leave with the faeces. The miracidium enters aquatic snails, within which a generation of rediae produce more rediae and cercariae. The cercariae leave the snail, become attached to fish, encysting under the scales as metacercariae (some troglotrematid cercariae encyst in crustaceans). Carnivores become infected by feeding upon fish carrying the metacercariae. Similarly, humans become infected by eating raw, smoked or poorly cooked freshwater fish. Obvious control measures involve the skinning, cooking or freezing of fish prior to consumption.

Little is known concerning the pathogenicity of these worms, but, as they have body spines and may be acquired in some numbers, some irritation and inflammation of the bowel is to be expected.

3 PHYLUM NEMATODA

Nematodes are probably the most abundant and widespread animal group, often occurring in huge numbers in environments ranging from the polar regions to hot springs. In addition to free-living marine and freshwater forms, there are free-living forms in the soil and parasitic forms in both animals and plants. Nematodes are symmetrically bilateral, unsegmented, normally dioecious worms which are usually filiform; they have a body cavity with a high hydrostatic pressure, a straight digestive tract with an anteriorly terminal mouth and posteriorly subterminal anus, no circulatory system, a simple excretory system and a body wall consisting of an outer layer of cuticle and an inner layer of longitudinal muscles (Fig. 24.3). As animal parasites they occur in virtually all groups, both invertebrate and vertebrate. The phylum is divided into 2 classes, the Adenophora and the Secernentea; both groups have evolved parasitic members, although the majority of animal parasites belong to the latter group. The differences between the groups reflect the presence and absence of small sensory structures (phasmids) on the tail and the nature of the excretory system; but there is a fundamental biological difference in the parasitic members, since in the Adenophora the first stage larva is infective to the definitive (final) host, whereas in the Secernentea it is the third stage larva.

All nematodes have 5 life history stages, 4 larval and one adult, which are separated by a moult of the cuticle. It is common for the first one or 2 moults to occur within the egg. The life cycle may be direct or indirect. Except in the case of the Adenophora, the stage infective to the final host is the third stage larva. Direct life cycles can involve the ingestion of eggs or larvae with

food or, in some cases, direct penetration of larvae through the skin. Indirect life cycles usually utilize invertebrate intermediate hosts but sometimes vertebrates (or other invertebrates) may act as intermediate or paratenic hosts. The larvae normally reside, often encysted, in the tissues of intermediate hosts. The majority of nematode parasites of vertebrates occur in the alimentary canal; those in other parts of the body often require the migration of larvae through the body to reach these sites. Some groups also have a larval migration from the gut and into the tissues and back to the gut; this represents the vestige of an indirect life cycle in its evolutionary past. Whichever mode of transmission is utilized, the chance of a particular egg or larva developing into an adult worm is very slight; this is compensated for in many cases by a huge output of eggs, which in some cases reaches as high as 200 000 per female per day.

The morphological features by which nematodes are recognized vary from group to group, but at higher taxonomic levels, the nature of the anterior regions of the alimentary canal, e.g. the oesophagus, the form of the head (presence, number of lips, teeth, etc.) and the form of the male tail are usually important. At the specific level details of the male tail, such as the arrangement of caudal papillae (sensory structures used during copulation) and the length and shape of the spicule(s) (sclerotized copulatory aids) are important. In the majority of cases, males carry more taxonomically useful information than females, the latter often being unidentifiable at the specific level in the absence of males.

The pathogenicity of nematodes in their final host varies considerably, usually being dependent upon the size of the infection. Those, such as hookworm, which are heavily armed with teeth or other sclerotized mouthparts and browse upon the gut wall can cause considerable damage. Similarly, forms which migrate around the body, both adults in the tissues and larvae (termed **larva migrans**), can cause serious problems, especially if they reach sensitive regions such as the brain, liver or eyes (see Chapter 31).

The classification of the nematodes presented in Table 24.4 is based on that of Anderson, Chabaud and Willmott (1974–83). It includes most of the forms which have been recorded from humans regularly, but accidental infections of other forms do occur infrequently.

3.1 Class Adenophorea Dougherty, 1958

Main features. Nematoda. Tail occasionally modified to form sucker. Oesophagus with normal appearance or modified, with oesophageal gland cells forming row of large gland cells (stichocytes) or reserve organ (trophosome). Oviparous or viviparous; eggs with plug at either end. Excretory system without lateral canals. Caudal papillae absent or few. Phasmids absent. First larval stage usually infective to final host.

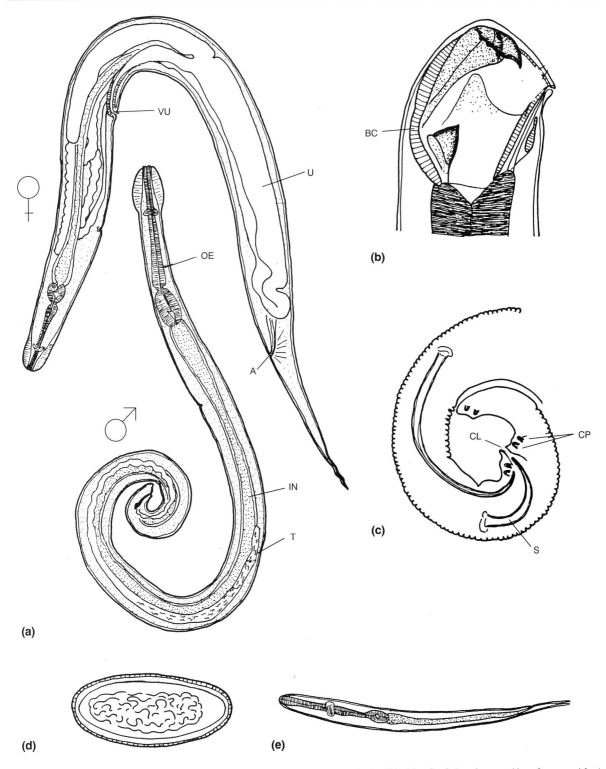

Fig. 24.3 Nematodes: (a) Male and female *Strongyloides* (Strongyloididae); (b). Head of *Ancylostoma* (Ancylostomatidae) (hookworm) with cuticularized buccal capsule armed with teeth; (c) Caudal end of male *Onchocerca* (Onchocercidae); (d) Egg of *Strongyloides*; (e) Third-stage larva of *Strongyloides*. *Abbreviations*: A, anus; BC, buccal capsule; CL, cloaca (in the male, the gut and reproductive system open through the same aperture); CP, caudal papillae; IN, intestine; OE, oesophagus; S, spicule; T, testis; U, uterus; VU, vulva. (Adapted from: (a,d,e), Hugot and Tourte-Schaefer 1985; (b), Yorke and Maplestone 1926; (c), Caballero 1944).

Table 24.4   Classification of nematodes found in humans

Class	Superfamily	Family
Adenophorea	Trichinelloidea	Trichinellidae
		Trichuridae
Secernentea	Ancylostomatoidea	Ancylostomatidae
	Ascaridoidea	Anisakidae
		Ascarididae
	Dracunculoidea	Dracunculidae
	Filarioidea	Onchocercidae
	Gnathostomatoidea	Gnathostomatidae
	Metastrongyloidea	Angiostrongylidae
	Oxyuroidea	Oxyuridae
	Physalopteroidea	Physalopteridae
	Rhabditoidea	Rhabditidae
		Strongyloididae
	Spiruroidea	Gongylonematidae
	Strongyloidea	Chabertiidae
		Syngamidae
	Thelazioidea	Thelaziidae
	Trichostrongyloidea	Trichostrongylidae

SUPERFAMILY TRICHINELLOIDEA WARD, 1907

Family Trichinellidae Ward, 1907

Main features. Trichinelloidea. Modified oesophagus with one row of stichocytes (large oesophageal gland cells). Intestine unmodified. Anus present. Vulva of female close to middle of oesophagus. Viviparous. Spicule in male absent. Larval stage in muscles of mammals. Adults usually in intestine of carnivorous mammals.

One genus, *Trichinella* Railliet, 1895, occurs in humans both as an adult in the intestine (usually gut wall) and as a larval stage in the tissues (usually muscles). The adult worms are very small, thread-like and recognizable by the row of large gland cells (stichocytes) surrounding the oesophagus and the absence of spicules in the male.

Adult worms occur in the intestine and intestinal mucosa. Females are viviparous and release first stage larvae into the intestinal mucosa. These larvae migrate via the blood and lymphatic system to muscles where they encyst in a coiled form. Transmission to another host occurs when the host is eaten by a carnivore or omnivore; here the larvae moult 4 times in the gut prior to reaching the adult stage. The same animal may serve, therefore, as both intermediate and definitive host. Humans usually become infected by feeding upon raw or inadequately cooked meat, especially pork, but also wild carnivores, such as bears. Control is effected by the cooking or freezing of meat, preventing pigs eating raw meat and offal, and getting rid of rats (which may harbour the infection) on pig farms.

The effects of *Trichinella* infection range from diarrhoea and nausea during the intestinal phase to eosinophilia, general weakness due to muscle damage, and difficulties in breathing and myocarditis caused by larvae in the muscles. Heavy infection can result in death, especially in cases where the heart or brain is involved. (See Chapter 31.)

Family Trichuridae Ransom, 1911

Main features. Trichinelloidea. Modified oesophagus with one to 3 rows of stichocytes. Intestine unmodified. Vulva of female close to posterior end of oesophagus. Oviparous; eggs with plug at each end. Single spicule and spicule sheath usually present. In alimentary canal, tissues and various organs of vertebrates.

Several trichurid genera are known to infect humans, including *Trichuris* Roederer, 1761, *Aonchotheca* Lopez-Neyra, 1947, *Calodium* Dujardin, 1845 and *Eucoleus* Dujardin, 1845; the latter 3 genera are still commonly referred to as *Capillaria* Zeder, 1800, when the latter is used in its wide sense (see Moravec, 1982, for generic differences). *Trichuris* is a common parasite of humans, whereas the capillariines are normally parasites of wild animals which occasionally infect humans. Like trichinellids, these worms have a row of stichocytes around the oesophagus, but they can be distinguished by the presence of thick-shelled eggs with terminal plugs in the females and a spicule in the male.

Trichurids inhabit the intestine, intestinal mucosa, liver, lungs and other tissues of vertebrates, depending upon the species involved. Eggs pass out with the faeces, or remain in the body until the host dies or is eaten by a predator or scavenger and are voided with its faeces. Again, depending upon the species involved, the life cycle may be direct (*Trichuris, Aonchotheca, Eucoleus*), in which case the definitive host becomes infected by feeding upon eggs, or indirect (e.g. *Calodium*) and involve an intermediate host which has swallowed the eggs. Humans become infected by ingesting eggs in soil (especially children) or on vegetation, or, in the case of *Calodium*, by ingesting raw fish harbouring the larva. Control is effected by modern sewage disposal and improvements in personal hygiene, the proper cooking of fish (*Calodium)* and the control of rats and other rodents which act as reservoirs (*Aonchotheca*).

Symptoms of infection vary according to the species, but in the case of *Aonchotheca* in the liver they resemble hepatitis as eggs are deposited in the liver parenchyma. Intestinal forms may cause diarrhoea, dysentery and weight loss as the worms penetrate the mucosa, but the severity depends upon the size of the infection. In extreme cases rectal prolapse, muscle wasting and death can occur. (See Chapters 29, 30.)

3.2   Class Secernentea Dougherty, 1958

Main features. Nematoda. Oesophagus without stichocytes or reserve organ (trophosome). Oviparous or viviparous; eggs without plug at either end. Excretory system with lateral canals. Caudal papillae numerous. Phasmids present. Third larval stage infective to final host.

SUPERFAMILY ANCYLOSTOMATOIDEA LOOSS, 1905

Family Ancylostomatidae Looss, 1905

Main features. Ancylostomatoidea. Buccal cavity large; cuticularized; subglobular. Mouth not surrounded by lips or comblike leaf-crown(s); armed with teeth or cutting plates, or unarmed. Oesophagus claviform; not divided into 2 regions. Male with caudal bursa normally supported by rays. In alimentary canal of mammals.

Two genera of ancylostomatids ('**hookworms**'), *Ancylostoma* Dubini, 1843 and *Necator* Stiles, 1903, occur in humans mainly in the tropics. These are intestinal parasites recognizable by their large globular, cuticularized buccal cavity, mouth armed with teeth or cutting plates and dorsally curved anterior extremity. Other genera may occur as accidental parasites on rare occasions.

The life cycle is direct. Eggs laid by female worms in the intestine are voided with the faeces and hatch in the soil. The larva feeds upon bacteria in the soil and moults twice. The third stage larvae penetrate the skin of a suitable mammalian host and then migrate via the blood system to the lungs; here they pass from the blood system into the alveoli, ascend the bronchi and trachea and are then swallowed. Once in the intestine they moult twice and mature. Humans become infected via their bare feet, the skin of which is penetrated by the larvae. Human infection is also possible from larvae swallowed with salad or other raw vegetation. Control is effected by sewage management, the wearing of shoes and the careful washing of salad material.

The penetration of the skin by larvae can cause an itching and the migrating larvae can result in coughing and bronchitis. The heavy armature of the mouth parts of adults, as they feed upon the tissues and blood of the host, damages the intestinal wall, resulting in blood loss, abdominal pain, general weakness and sometimes even death. (See Chapter 29.)

SUPERFAMILY ASCARIDOIDEA BAIRD, 1853

Family Ascarididae Baird, 1853

Main features. Ascaridoidea. Head with 3 well-defined lips. Lips sometimes separated by interlabia; unadorned by spines or cuticular embellishments posteriorly; single row of denticles on anterior margin present or absent. Buccal cavity absent or weakly developed. Oesophagus cylindrical; occasionally divided into 2 regions (when posterior glandular ventriculus is present); without posterior muscular bulb. Excretory system symmetrical, 2-sided, tubular; excretory pore at level of nerve ring. In all vertebrate groups; mainly, but not always, terrestrial forms.

Three genera of ascaridid nematode, *Ascaris* Linnaeus, 1758, *Toxocara* Stiles, 1905 and *Toxascaris* Leiper, 1907, regularly occur as parasites of humans, although only *Ascaris* is a true human parasite, the other 2 being common parasites of dogs or cats. Other genera occurring in wild animals, such as *Baylisascaris* Sprent, 1968 and *Lagochilascaris* Leiper, 1909, have also been recorded from humans on rare occasions. Only *Ascaris* normally occurs in humans as an adult; the others are present in the tissues in larval form only. Ascaridids are related to anisakids, and like that group have 3 distinct lips; they differ in that (with the exception of the subfamily Heterocheilinae) their life cycle is linked to terrestrial rather than aquatic conditions.

Ascaridids occur in all vertebrate groups and have a variety of life cycles. Most involve invertebrate or vertebrate intermediate hosts, or both; but those occurring in humans normally have a direct life cycle. Nevertheless, even in these forms the vestige of an indirect life cycle is apparent in the form of a larval migration through the tissues of the host prior to maturation in the intestine. In these cases eggs pass out with the faeces and the first 2 larval moults occur within the egg. If the eggs are eaten by a suitable host, the third stage larvae hatch in the gut, penetrate the gut wall and are transported by the blood to the lungs. After a short period in the lungs where they moult twice, they escape into the alveoli, pass up the bronchi and trachea with mucus and are swallowed. Once they reach the intestine they mature. There are variations: in some genera developing in mammals, migrating larvae in the blood can result in transplacental or transmammary infections of young; and occasionally insects and rodents may act as intermediate hosts. Humans, especially children, become infected by accidentally ingesting soil or food contaminated with eggs. Control is effected by careful sewage management, avoiding the use of human faeces as manure, improvements in personal hygiene, keeping children away from the faeces of domesticated animals, especially dogs, the regular de-worming of pets and the careful washing of salad material, fruit, etc.

Despite the fact that *Ascaris* is a large worm, its presence in the intestine does not cause many symptoms unless the worm burden is high. Light infections can cause nausea and other bowel disorders; heavy infections can result in bowel obstruction or peritonitis and even death. The migration of the larval stage of *Ascaris* and especially the other ascaridids mentioned above can be more serious. Larvae passing through the lungs cause some pneumonitis, but larva migrans which lodge in other tissues, such as the liver, spleen, kidneys, placenta and especially the eye and CNS (e.g. *Toxocara*) can represent a danger, producing inflammation and granulomata in these sensitive areas. (See Chapters 29, 31.)

Family Anisakidae Railliet and Henry, 1912

Main features. Ascaridoidea. Head with 3 well-defined lips. Lips sometimes separated by interlabia; unadorned by spines or cuticular embellishments posteriorly; single row of denticles on anterior margin present or absent. Buccal cavity absent or weakly developed. Oesophagus with posterior ventriculus. Gut caeca present or absent. Excretory system asymmetrical, entirely or mainly one-sided, tubular or ribbon-like; excretory pore at level of nerve ring or ventral interlabium. Larval stages in fishes or invertebrates or both. In piscivorous vertebrates.

Anisakids capable of accidentally infecting humans are normally parasites of the stomach of marine mammals. The group occurs in all vertebrate groups, but those parasitic as adults in other hosts, such as fishes, are not capable of infecting humans. There are 2 main genera involved, *Anisakis* Dujardin, 1845 and *Pseudoterranova* Mozgovoi, 1950; the former is the more widely reported. Since humans do not provide a suitable environment for the development of these parasites, they do not reach maturity and usually attempt to penetrate the gut wall in order to re-encyst as they would in any other unsuitable host. Like ascaridids, anisakids have 3 distinct lips at the anterior end, but differ in the configuration of the excretory system.

All anisakids have an indirect life cycle involving aquatic intermediate hosts. Eggs leave with the faeces. The first one or 2 (accounts vary) larval moults occur within the egg. If eggs falling in water are eaten by small planktonic invertebrates, such as copepods, the third stage larva develops in the haemocoel. If this host is eaten by a larger crustacean, squid or bony fish the larva is transferred and re-encysts in the body cavity or muscles of the new host. The larva can be transferred to new hosts several times. If the third stage larva within its intermediate host is consumed by a suitable (usually piscivorous) vertebrate host, the larva moults twice and matures in the stomach or intestine. Humans usually acquire infections of anisakids by feeding upon raw, lightly marinated or inadequately cooked marine bony fishes (infection by consuming raw squid and raw marine crustaceans is also possible). Infection can be prevented by cooking fish properly or by the freezing of fish or fish products intended for consumption raw or marinated. Fish inspection may eliminate heavily infected fish and evisceration immediately following netting may prevent the migration of larvae to the muscles, but it is not possible to prevent the infection of wild marine fishes without a heavy culling of marine mammals.

Although the worms may moult once in humans, they tend to penetrate the gut wall in an attempt to re-encyst; whether this is in the stomach or intestine may depend upon the size of the food bolus. Symptoms of infection can mimic gastric or duodenal ulcers. Repeated infections are more serious, and worms may have to be removed by surgery. In Japan, where this has been an important parasite of humans because of local fish-eating habits, the presence of these worms has been linked to cases of gastric and intestinal cancer. (See Chapter 34.)

SUPERFAMILY DRACUNCULOIDEA STILES, 1907

Family Dracunculidae Stiles, 1907

Main features. Dracunculoidea. With considerable sexual dimorphism. Head end rounded, bilaterally symmetrical. Lips and pseudolabia absent. Buccal capsule weakly developed, reduced to cuticular ring. Oesophagus apparently undivided. Oesophageal glands usually uninucleate. Anus atrophied in adult. Male tail without caudal bursa. Body of female long, cylindrical. Vulva normally in middle of body. Viviparous. Transmission indirect; copepods acting as intermediate hosts. Usually in tissues and tissue spaces of reptiles, birds and mammals.

One genus, *Dracunculus* Reichard, 1759, infects the subcutaneous tissues of humans, the species involved also occurring in a variety of mammals, especially dogs. These worms resemble filarioids in being tissue parasites, but they have a different life cycle, which involves an aquatic intermediate host, and they do not release microfilariae into the blood.

Fully developed female worms migrate to the skin and produce a blister which bursts, permitting the rupturing of the worm and its uterus when contact is made with water. First stage larvae eaten by copepods enter the haemocoel and moult twice. Vertebrates become infected with these parasites when they drink water containing copepods harbouring the third stage larva. The larvae penetrate the gut wall and enter connective tissue within the body, where they moult twice. After mating the females develop in the subcutaneous regions. Humans become infected by drinking water containing infected copepods. The parasite is readily controlled by the filtering of drinking water or by using water sources, such as springs or deep wells, where contact with animal skin is not possible and copepods are absent.

Migrating worms in the subcutaneous regions may cause some tenderness, but the presence of the parasite may not be apparent until the blister forms. The blister may be painful and cause considerable inflammation, a large ulcer and, when secondary infections are involved, an abscess. (See Chapter 35.)

SUPERFAMILY FILARIOIDEA WEINLAND, 1858

Family Onchocercidae Leiper, 1911

Main features. Filarioidea. Body long, cylindrical. Head bilaterally symmetrical. Lips and pseudolabia absent. Buccal cavity usually relatively small; not greatly cuticularized. Oesophagus usually with anterior muscular region and posterior glandular region; sometimes regions difficult or impossible to differentiate. Male tail without caudal bursa; caudal alae usually narrow or apparently absent. Vulva in anterior half of body but posterior to nerve ring. Ovoviviparous or viviparous; eggs thin-shelled, with poorly differentiated larvae (microfilariae). Microfilariae appear in blood, lymph or skin of host. Transmission indirect; with blood-feeding insects acting as intermediate hosts. In tissues and tissue spaces of amphibians, reptiles, birds and mammals.

Several genera of filarioid are parasitic in humans, the more important of which are *Brugia* Buckley, 1958, *Dipetalonema* Diesing, 1861, *Dirofilaria* Railliet and Henry, 1910, *Loa* Stiles, 1905, *Mansonella* Faust, 1929, *Onchocerca* Diesing, 1841 and *Wuchereria* Silva Araujo, 1877. These tissue parasites are usually found in the lymphatic system, subcutaneous connective tissue or other connective tissues. They differ from dracunculids in that their life cycle is terrestrial and they produce larvae (**microfilariae**) which are found in the blood, skin, etc. A generic key to microfilariae, which are more likely to be seen than the adult worms, was produced in French by Bain and Chabaud (1986).

The life cycle is indirect, involving a biting insect as an intermediate host. Mature female worms release first or second stage larvae surrounded by their first stage cuticle into the blood. These often exhibit a diurnal periodicity which brings them into the peripheral circulation during the period when blood-feeding insects, such as mosquitoes and blackfly, are likely to feed. When taken in by a suitable insect, they pass into the haemocoel, grow, moult into the infective third stage and migrate to the region of the insect's mouthparts. The worm is than injected into a new host when the insect next feeds. After entering a suitable host the larvae migrate to the lymphatic system or connective tissue, moult twice and mature. Humans, therefore, become infected when they are bitten by insects, and some control can be achieved by reducing the numbers of vectors by the drainage of marshes, use of insecticides, etc.

Human infection (filariasis) causes various symptoms, depending upon the species and site of the parasite; elephantiasis caused by inflammation in the lymphatic system in various parts of the body is the most extreme. In some cases symptoms are few and in others subcutaneous swellings or nodules occur which can result in abscesses if the worm dies; such infections are often accompanied by rashes and intense itching. Microfilariae may also cause problems when they become lodged in regions such as the central nervous system or eyes. (See Chapters 32, 33.)

SUPERFAMILY GNATHOSTOMATOIDEA RAILLIET, 1895

Family Gnathostomatidae Railliet, 1895

Main features. Gnathostomatoidea. Body long, cylindrical or stout; often armed with spines. Head bilaterally symmetrical; with 2 large, trilobed, lateral pseudolabia. Collar region may be enlarged to form cephalic bulb, which may be covered with transverse rows of recurved hooks. Inner face of pseudolabia folded into rounded, tooth-like formations which interlock with those on opposite interlabium. Buccal cavity normally relatively uncuticularized. Oesophagus with anterior muscular region and longer posterior glandular region. Male tail without caudal bursa. Transmission indirect; with cope-

pods and vertebrates acting as intermediate hosts. In anterior gut of vertebrates.

Several species of the genus, *Gnathostoma* Owen, 1836, occur occasionally as accidental parasites of humans in their larval form. These worms normally occur as adults in the stomach, usually in nodules in the stomach wall, of carnivorous mammals and pigs. They are recognizable by the presence of regular rows of spines on the body; on an inflated cephalic bulb these spines are larger and flattened.

The life cycle normally involves 2 intermediate hosts. Eggs leave leave the body in the faeces. In water these develop and hatch to release a larva which has moulted once. When eaten by a suitable copepod the larva penetrates the haemocoel; if the copepod is then eaten by a suitable freshwater fish or frog, the larva moults into the infective third stage. Fish, snakes, rodents, chickens and humans which may eat these hosts can act as paratenic hosts. The definitive host becomes infected by feeding upon the second intermediate or a paratenic host. Worms found in humans, normally the third stage larva, are obtained through eating raw or poorly cooked fish (occasionally, perhaps, chicken). Prevention involves the cooking or freezing of freshwater fish and fish products.

In humans larvae penetrate the gut wall and migrate via the liver to the subcutaneous regions. Their penetration of the gut wall can cause some pain and presence in the subcutaneous regions results in swelling and symptoms similar to the cuticular larva migrans of some ascaridids. More serious problems and even death can be caused if worms reach more sensitive areas of the body, such as the eyes or central nervous system. (See Chapter 34.)

SUPERFAMILY METASTRONGYLOIDEA LEIPER, 1908

Family Angiostrongylidae Böhm and Gebauer, 1934

Main features. Metastrongyloidea. Longitudinal cuticular ridges on body absent. Cephalic vesicle (cuticular inflation) absent. Buccal cavity absent or reduced and weakly cuticularized. Mouth unarmed; not surrounded by lips or comb-like leaf-crown(s). Oesophagus cylindrical; not divided into 2 regions. Male with caudal bursa supported by rays; bursa often reduced. Vulva near anus. Larvae in molluscs. Adults in respiratory system, and, occasionally, blood system and other organs, of marsupials, insectivores, rodents and carnivores.

One metastrongyloid genus, *Angiostrongylus* Kamensky, 1905 (includes *Parastrongylus* Baylis, 1928) occurs in humans. Metastrongyloids are commonly called **lungworms**. Angiostrongylids capable of infecting humans normally parasitize the lungs or blood system of rodents. They are recognizable by the presence in the male of a caudal bursa supported by rays, in conjunction with their site of infection, i.e. the respiratory or blood systems.

Eggs produced by worms in the pulmonary or mesenteric vessels of rodents, etc., release first stage larvae into the intestine (those in the lungs are swallowed with mucus) which are voided with the faeces. If these larvae penetrate or are eaten by certain snails, slugs or, less frequently, crabs and land planarians, they penetrate the tissues and moult twice. When an infected mollusc is eaten by a suitable mammal, the third stage larvae penetrate the gut wall and migrate in the blood system or lymphatic system, moulting twice (sometimes in the central nervous system) prior to maturing in the pulmonary or mesenteric arteries. Humans presumably become infected with these worms by eating raw or poorly cooked snails, or accidentally consuming molluscs on salad and other raw plant material. Prevention involves the cooking or freezing of snails, the careful washing of salad material and rodent control.

The migration of these worms to the central nervous system is potentially serious, producing symptoms resembling meningitis, paralysis and blindness; occasionally this results in death. Pulmonary symptoms may not be apparent, but worms in vessels associated with the intestine can cause inflammation, granulomata, thrombosis and necrosis, especially in the region of the appendix. (See Chapter 34.)

SUPERFAMILY OXYUROIDEA COBBOLD, 1864

Family Oxyuridae Cobbold, 1864

Main features. Oxyuroidea. Body short and stout. Buccal cavity absent or weakly developed. Oesophagus relatively short; not divided into anterior muscular and posterior glandular regions but with posterior muscular bulb. Male tail with wide caudal alae which may resemble caudal bursa, but supported by arrangement of usually similar pedunculate papillae rather than assortment of rays. Usually one spicule. Eggs often flattened on one side; with relatively thick shells; usually embryonated on deposition; 2 larval moults occurs within egg. Life cycle direct. In intestine of mammals.

Only one genus, *Enterobius* Leach, 1853 (commonly known as 'threadworm' or 'pinworm'), regularly occurs in humans and other primates, although *Syphacia* Seurat, 1916, a rodent parasite, has been reported as an accidental infection in humans. Oxyurids are small, intestinal parasites with a direct life cycle and recognizable by the presence of a large posterior bulb on the oesophagus.

Gravid female worms leave the body through the anus, depositing eggs in the perianal region. They eject eggs in huge numbers as their bodies dehydrate and burst, which cause an itch. Two larval moults occur within the egg. Humans are reinfected by swallowing the eggs, which become accidentally attached to food or lodged under fingernails following scratching of the perianal region. Once swallowed, the eggs hatch and the third stage larvae moult and develop into adults in the intestine. Autoinfection of humans is common. Prevention involves improvements in personal hygiene, in terms of both individuals and the entire population, and especial care in relation to food preparation.

The presence of these worms generally does little harm, apart from discomfort related to an itching of the perianal regions, although penetration of the gut wall has been observed, resulting in non-proven links with appendicitis and other complaints. Gravid

females which migrate into the vagina may cause a mucoid discharge. (See Chapter 29.)

SUPERFAMILY PHYSALOPTEROIDEA RAILLIET, 1893

Family Physalopteridae Railliet, 1893

Main features. Physalopteroidea. Body cylindrical; without lateral rows of spines. Head bilaterally symmetrical. Pseudolabia 2; unlobed; armed with denticles (teeth) on free border. Cuticle posterior to pseudolabia often expanded to form cephalic collar. Buccal cavity usually relatively small; not greatly cuticularized. Oesophagus with anterior muscular region and longer posterior glandular region. Male tail without caudal bursa; but caudal alae often wide. Transmission indirect; with arthropods acting as intermediate hosts. Adults in gut of all vertebrate groups and occasionally crustaceans.

Only one physalopteroid, a species of the genus *Physaloptera* Rudolphi, 1819 which normally occurs in the intestine of primates, has been reported from humans. Other species of *Physaloptera* occur in birds of prey and insectivorous or carnivorous mammals. Important diagnostic features of physalopterids include the presence of 2 large, symmetrical, unlobed pseudolips armed with teeth and a cephalic collar (an expansion of the cuticle immediately posterior to the pseudolips).

Physalopterids have an indirect life cycle, normally involving an arthropod intermediate host and often a vertebrate paratenic host. Eggs of these gut parasites leave with the faeces; if eaten by insects, such as cockroaches, other beetles and crickets, the third stage larva develops. The final host becomes infected by feeding upon insects or, especially in the case of carnivores, upon insectivorous vertebrates such as frogs and rodents. Humans presumably become infected by feeding (usually accidentally) on insects. Accidental infection can presumably be avoided by keeping food in a meat safe, refrigerator, etc.

Little is known about the pathogenicity of the worm, but infections are likely to be light. Some damage to the intestinal wall may be caused by the armed mouthparts, as species in animals do appear to feed on the gut wall and erode the mucosa, leaving bleeding wounds behind them as they browse.

SUPERFAMILY RHABDITOIDEA ÖRLEY, 1880

Family Rhabditidae Örley, 1880

Main features. Rhabditoidea. Small, slender worms. Head with 6 lips (or 3 double lips). Buccal cavity long, cylindrical; with chitinized thickenings in wall. Oesophagus long, narrow, with prominent posterior valved bulb. Caudal alae of male form bursa. Mainly free-living, saprophagous forms; occasionally accidental parasites of vertebrates.

Rhabditids are free-living worms which are often swallowed accidentally or become associated with human faeces, the most frequently recorded examples being of the genus *Rhabditis* Dujardin, 1844. Some species of the genus *Pelodera* Schneider, 1866 are known to infect human skin in rare cases, producing symptoms similar to cutaneous larva migrans. Humans presumably become infected by soil contamination of existing wounds. The occurrence of these parasites in the skin is so rare that preventative measures are not worthwhile.

Family Strongyloididae Chitwood and McIntosh, 1928

Main features. Rhabditoidea. Parasitic stage usually a parthenogenetic female (alternates with free-living sexual generation, with oesophagus bearing 2 swellings). Small, slender worms. Buccal cavity reduced or well developed, but not long. Oesophagus long, narrow, lacking prominent valved bulb posteriorly. Vulva in posterior quarter of body. In alimentary canal of terrestrial vertebrates.

This is a group with an irregular alternation of generations, a parasitic parthenogenetic female alternating with a free-living sexual generation. One genus, *Strongyloides* Grassi, 1879, occurs in humans. The parasitic females found in humans are small, slender worms which live in the intestinal mucosa. They can be confused with trichinellids in gross morphology, but the long, cylindrical oesophagus is quite different, lacking the large gland cells of the latter.

Several life cycle pathways are possible, both direct and indirect, the latter involving alternation of generations. Eggs laid in the mucosa or submucosa of the intestine release first stage larvae which escape into the intestine and are voided with the faeces. These larva feed in the soil and moult twice. The third stage larvae can: (1) continue to develop into male and female worms capable of continuing to produce free-living generations (and thus more third stage larvae), especially in warmer climates; or (2) penetrate the skin of a terrestrial vertebrate, migrate via the blood stream to the lungs, escape into the alveoli where they moult twice to become a parthenogenetic female, pass up the trachea and are swallowed. Variations on the pulmonary migration route may be possible. Once in the intestine the worms enter the mucosa and submucosa. Humans become infected by contamination with infected soil or faeces; autoinfection is also possible as, in some cases, larvae can reinfect the same host be re-invading the gut wall and migrating via the pulmonary route or penetrating the skin in the perianal region. Prevention involves improvements in sewage disposal and personal hygiene.

Symptoms of intestinal infection vary from none to severe enteritis, although diarrhoea is most common. Very heavy infections may result in damage to the mucosa. Penetration of the skin by larvae may cause a rash and symptoms similar to a cutaneous larva migrans, and the passage through the lungs may result in a cough or pneumonia. Autoinfection may cause the disease to last for many years. Hyperinfestation can occur in immunosuppressed patients. (See Chapter 30.)

SUPERFAMILY SPIRUROIDEA ÖRLEY, 1885
Family Gongylonematidae Hall, 1916

Main features. Spiruroidea. Body covered with large verruciform thickenings. Head bilaterally symmetrical. Mouth octagonal. Pseudolabia absent. Buccal cavity cuticularized;

short. Oesophagus divided into anterior muscular and posterior glandular regions. Caudal alae present in male. Adult in mucosa of anterior alimentary canal of birds and mammals.

A species of *Gongylonema* Molin, 1957, the 'gullet worm' of domestic ruminants, has been recorded in humans as an accidental parasite. These worms usually occur in the oesophagus or stomach of various mammals embedded in the mucosa or submucosa. They are readily recognized by the verruciform cuticular thickenings on the surface of the body.

The life cycle is indirect. Eggs of these worms are voided with the faeces and hatch once they have been swallowed by an insect, such as a coprophagous beetle. The final host becomes infected by feeding upon beetles harbouring the third stage larva. Once in the new host the worms moult twice and penetrate the surface layers of the anterior parts of the alimentary canal, where they reside. Humans, where infections are usually sited in the mucosa and submucosa of the buccal cavity, presumably become infected by accidentally eating beetles. Prevention can be helped by a regular de-worming of farm animals and careful washing of food items.

Although the worms may be quite large, their presence tends to cause little in the way of symptoms apart from some local irritation and inflammation. (See Chapter 34.)

SUPERFAMILY STRONGYLOIDEA BAIRD, 1853
Family Chabertiidae Popova, 1952

Main features. Strongyloidea. Mouth round or oval; usually surrounded by well-developed comb-like leaf-crown (single or double) or lips. Buccal cavity cuticularized. Oesophagus claviform; not divided into 2 regions. Male with caudal bursa supported by rays; dorsal ray usually with 2 branches on each side of median fissure. In alimentary canal of mammals.

Strongyloid nematodes are occasional accidental parasites of humans. Chabertiids usually occur in the intestine of various herbivorous mammals, including farm animals, where they often cause nodules in the intestinal wall. Species of the genus *Oesophagostomum* Molin, 1861 and, less frequently, *Ternidens* Railliet and Henry, 1909 which parasitize primates, have been reported in humans. They are recognized by the presence of a double crown of leaf-like spines which surround the mouth, a cuticular buccal capsule and by the wide caudal bursa of the male which is supported by rays.

The life cycle is direct. Eggs laid in the intestine pass out with the faeces; the first stage larva emerges from the egg and feeds, developing into an infective third stage larva. The host, usually a herbivore, acquires the worms when feeding upon vegetation; the larvae penetrate the intestinal mucosa, grow and moult, prior to returning to the intestine, moulting once again and maturing. Humans presumably become infected by accidentally ingesting larvae with vegetation from the vicinity of primate populations. In some situations the parasite can be passed between humans.

When the larvae penetrate the gut wall they become encapsulated in a cyst which forms a fibrous nodule. The rupturing of the nodule, which occurs when the worm returns to the lumen, may result in dysentery or even peritonitis. These nodules are sometimes misinterpreted as other diseases, such as carcinomas. The worms can also occur in subcutaneous cysts in humans, but how they arrive in this position is not known. (See Chapter 34.)

Family Syngamidae Leiper, 1912

Main features. Strongyloidea. Mouth hexagonal; leaf-crown and lips rudimentary or absent. Buccal cavity cuticularized; hexagonal in cross-section; with teeth at base. Oesophagus claviform; not divided into 2 regions. Male with caudal bursa supported by rays. Vulva usually near mid-body. Usually in respiratory system of birds and mammals or urinary system of pigs.

One genus of syngamid, *Mammomonogamus* Ryzhikov, 1948, is occasionally reported from humans in the tropics. These are usually parasitic in the respiratory system (trachea and bronchi) of domesticated ruminants and infect humans only accidentally. Syngamids are recognizable in that the male and larger female are usually joined together in a Y formation; they differ considerably from other lungworms (the metastrongyloids) in the presence of a large, cuticular buccal cavity.

The life cycle of syngamids may be direct, similar to that of the chabertiid strongyloids, or indirect and involve paratenic hosts. Eggs produced in the respiratory tract are swallowed with mucus and voided with the faeces. Development in the soil is similar to that of chabertiids, except that the larvae may be eaten by a variety of invertebrate hosts, such as earthworms, snails, slugs and arthropods, which act as paratenic hosts. If the third stage larva or its paratenic host is eaten by a suitable vertebrate, the larvae penetrate the gut lining and migrate to the lungs via the blood system. Here they moult and develop to maturity in the respiratory tract. Humans become infected by accidentally ingesting the larvae or its paratenic host. Some prevention is possible by the careful washing of salad material and other vegetation.

Worms in the trachea, larynx and bronchi may cause irritation and a cough.

SUPERFAMILY THELAZIOIDEA SKRJABIN, 1915

Family Thelaziidae Skrjabin, 1915

Main features. Thelazioidea. Body often small, cylindrical; unspined. Head bilaterally symmetrical. Pseudolabia absent. Mouth hexagonal or oval. Buccal cavity cuticularized; variable, sometimes long and cylindrical. Oesophagus may or may not be visibly divided into anterior muscular region and longer posterior glandular region. Male tail without caudal bursa; caudal alae usually absent. Transmission indirect; with invertebrates (but not copepods) and vertebrates acting as intermediate hosts. In orbit of birds and mammals.

One thelaziid genus, *Thelazia* Travassos, 1918, normally parasitic in domesticated animals such as dogs and farm animals, has occasionally been reported in the eye of humans. Thelaziids can be recognized by their location in the eye, the possession of a cuticularized buccal cavity and the absence of pseudolabia.

Thelaziid worms usually occur in the orbit, conjunctival sac or lachrymal glands. First stage larvae occur in eye secretions. If ingested by a fly, they moult twice in its tissues, migrate to the mouth parts and are transmitted to the mammalian host, and presumably to humans, when the fly feeds upon eye secretions. Two final moults occur in the eye. There seem to be no practical control measures.

Symptoms caused by the presence of these worms include excessive tear formation, itching and some discomfort. In animals, conjunctivitis and some damage to the eye tissues may occur, but the worms are not generally very pathogenic.

SUPERFAMILY TRICHOSTRONGYLOIDEA LEIPER, 1908

Family Trichostrongylidae Leiper, 1908

Main features. Trichostrongyloidea. Body usually not coiled. Longitudinal cuticular ridges present or absent. Cephalic vesicle absent. Male with caudal bursa supported by rays; dorsal ray usually short and not deeply divided. Life cycle direct. In mammals such as lagomorphs and ruminants; occasionally in birds.

Numerous trichostrongyloid genera, common stomach parasites of domesticated ruminants, have been reported as accidental parasites of humans. These include *Ostertagia* Ransom, 1907, *Nematodirus* Ransom, 1907, *Haemonchus* Cobb, 1898, *Marshallagia* Orloff, 1933 and, by far most frequently, *Trichostrongylus* Looss, 1905; with the exception of the molineid *Nematodirus*, these are all trichostrongylids. Trichostrongylid are generally recognizable by the presence of series of longitudinal cuticular ridges which run along the body, a caudal bursa supported by rays in the male and their presence in the stomach or intestine.

The life cycle is direct. Eggs are passed out with the faeces, hatch on the ground and release a first stage larva which feeds and develops in the soil. After 2 moults the infective third stage larva can be transmitted to a suitable herbivore on vegetation. Within the gut the worms moult twice prior to maturing as adults. Humans presumably become infected by feeding upon raw vegetation harbouring the larvae. Some level of prevention is possible by the cooking or careful washing of vegetables and other plant material.

Light infections pose no problem, but diarrhoea and some abdominal pain have been reported. Limited damage at the site of attachment may occur as the head of the worms tends to penetrate the mucosa. (See Chapter 34.)

4 PHYLUM ACANTHOCEPHALA

Acanthocephalans, or 'thorny-headed worms', represent a phylum of parasites of uncertain affinities. Like the tapeworms, members of this group are so well adapted to parasitism that they have lost their digestive system and reduced their muscular, nervous and excretory systems, but they differ in that they are dioecious worms with a body cavity. The body is composed of a large trunk and a retractable anterior proboscis armed with a regular array of hooks used for attachment to the gut wall (Fig. 24.4). Like tapeworms, they are intestinal parasites and absorb nutrients through their body-wall. Movement of the proboscis and its armature is complex, involving retractor muscles, a muscular proboscis receptacle and fluid-filled sacs (lemnisci). The body wall is a syncytium with large, often fragmented nuclei, comprises a complex outer tegument and an inner layer of muscles, and contains a lacunar system of interconnecting canals which may serve as a circulatory system. The males contain 2 testes and a series of accessory glands called cement glands. In the females the ovary breaks down early in development to form ovarian balls; the body cavity of mature females is usually full of eggs.

The life history of acanthocephalans is remarkably constant relative to that of other helminth groups. All have the same larval stages and all utilize arthropods as intermediate hosts. Essentially, female worms in the intestine produce eggs which are voided with the faeces. If eaten by a suitable arthropod, the egg releases a larva armed with hooks, called an **acanthor**, which enters the haemocoel. This develops into a stage called an **acanthella** within which the internal organs of the adult begin to develop. When the proboscis develops it usually invaginates into the body and the larva becomes encysted; this resting stage is called a **cystacanth** (Fig. 24.4). The final host becomes infected either by feeding directly upon an arthropod harbouring the cystacanth larva or a vertebrate paratenic host harbouring a juvenile form which is basically a re-encysted cystacanth. Once in the intestine of a suitable final host the parasites attach to the gut wall and develop to maturity. In some cases, where the final host does not normally feed upon arthropods, the paratenic host becomes a necessary part of the life history.

The different classes of acanthocephalans are not readily distinguished using gross morphology, their systematics being based upon internal details which are often difficult to elucidate. At the specific level the armature of the proboscis, in terms of the number of rows of hooks and the number of hooks per row, is the most important criterion.

No acanthocephalans are primarily human parasites. Data on their pathogenicity are limited, as records in humans tend to be scarce. However, since the proboscis with its armature of hooks does penetrate the gut wall, some local inflammation and abdominal pain is to be expected; but, as the worms do not feed upon the gut wall and their location tends to be semipermanent, this may not persist. Nevertheless, in some cases, especially when the juvenile parasite finds the human gut unsuitable for development, it may pass right through and perforate the intestine with a consequent possibility of causing peritonitis.

The classification presented in Table 24.5 is based on Schmidt (1972) and Amin (1985).

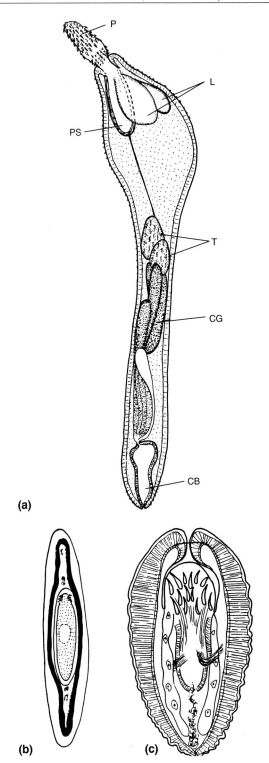

Fig. 24.4 Acanthocephalans: (a) Male *Corynosoma* (Polymorphidae) (the body cavity of the female is usually full of eggs, apart from which it contains no other useful taxonomic features not present in the male); (b) Egg of *Bolbosoma* (Polymorphidae) containing acanthor larva; (c) Cystacanth larva of *Macracanthorhynchus* (Oligacanthorhynchidae) with withdrawn proboscis. *Abbreviations*: CB, copulatory bursa; CG, cement glands; L, lemnisci; P, proboscis; PS, proboscis sac; T, testes. (Adapted from: (a), Yamaguti 1963; (b), Meyer 1933; (c), Van Cleave, 1947).

Table 24.5 Classification of acanthocephalans found in humans

Class	Order	Family
Archaeacanthocephala	Moniliformida	Moniliformidae
	Oligacanthorhynchida	Oligacanthorhynchidae
Palaeacanthocephala	Echinorhynchida	Echinorhynchidae
	Polymorphida	Polymorphidae

4.1 Class Archiacanthocephala Meyer, 1931

Main features. Acanthocephala. Relatively large worms. Spines on body trunk absent. Main longitudinal vessels of lacunar system dorsal or dorsal and ventral. Subcuticular nuclei few; elongate, branched or with residual fragments situated close together. Cement glands of male usually 8; uninucleate. Insects (and millipedes) act as intermediate hosts. Adults in intestine of terrestrial vertebrates.

ORDER MONILIFORMIDA SCHMIDT, 1972
Family Moniliformidae Van Cleave, 1924

Main features. Moniliformida. Body medium-sized to long; usually with pseudosegmented wall. Proboscis cylindrical; with long, straight rows of hooks. Proboscis receptacle with double-layered wall, retractor muscles piercing its posterior end and cerebral ganglion positioned posteriorly. Protonephridial organs absent. Eggs oval; with sculptured surface. In birds and mammals.

The order Moniliformida has only one family containing a single genus, *Moniliformis* Travassos, 1915. This genus, which normally occurs in rodents, has been reported on rare occasions in humans. It is recognizable by a pseudosegmentation of the body (i.e. a series of annular thickenings of the body wall) and its cylindrical proboscis. The larger females can reach more than 20 cm in length.

Eggs of these intestinal worms are passed in the faeces. When eaten by an insect, normally a beetle (especially grain beetles) or a cockroach, the cystacanth larva develops in the haemocoel. If the arthropod host is eaten by a rodent, the worms excysts in the gut, the proboscis evaginates and the worm attaches to the intestinal wall and develops to maturity. Humans become infected by accidentally ingesting beetles with food. Prevention can presumably be effected by rodent control and keeping food intended to be eaten cold in beetle-proof containers.

Since the proboscis of these worms does penetrate the gut lining, it is likely to produce some local inflammation. Symptoms such as abdominal pain and diarrhoea have been reported, but data on the effect of these parasites in humans are few.

ORDER OLIGACANTHORHYNCHIDA PETROCHENKO, 1956
Family Oligacanthorhynchidae Southwell and MacFie, 1925

Main features. Oligacanthorhynchida. Body medium-sized to very long. Proboscis subspherical; with short, straight rows of small numbers of hooks. Sensory papilla present at apex of proboscis and each side of neck. Proboscis receptacle with thick, single-layered wall, retractor muscles piercing it dorsally and cerebral ganglion positioned on ventral inner surface. Protonephridial organs present. In birds and mammals.

These parasites are especially common in pigs, but also occur in a wide range of terrestrial mammals. They are commonly covered in transverse wrinkles but lack any regular pseudosegmentation; the females especially reach a large size, sometimes more than 40 cm. One genus, *Macracanthorhynchus* Travassos, 1917, occurs on rare occasions in humans.

The life cycle is similar to that of moniliformids, except that, although a range of beetles, cockroaches, etc. can harbour the parasite, the main intermediate hosts would appear to be dung beetles which become infected when they feed upon manure. Humans acquire the parasite by ingesting beetles as food, accidentally with food or as a cure for ailments. The keeping of food intended to be eaten cold in beetle-proof containers should help prevent accidental infection.

The worms cause inflammation and a granuloma at the site of attachment; but abdominal pain and perforation of the bowel have been reported and, in pigs, death from peritonitis does occasionally occur.

4.2 Class Palaeacanthocephala Meyer, 1931

Main features. Acanthocephala. Small to medium-sized worms. Spines present or absent on trunk. Proboscis shape variable. Main longitudinal canals of lacunar system lateral. Subcuticular nuclei numerous, fragmented; occasionally limited to anterior region of trunk. Cement glands of male separate; tubular to globular. In intestine of aquatic vertebrates.

ORDER ECHINORHYNCHIDA SOUTHWELL AND MACFIE, 1925
Family Echinorhynchidae Cobbold, 1876

Main features. Echinorhynchida. Body not spined. Normally in intestine of bony fishes and amphibians.

Two echinorhynchid genera, *Acanthocephalus* Koelreuter, 1771 and *Pseudoacanthocephalus* Petrochenko, 1956, have been reported as occurring accidentally in humans. These genera normally occur in the intestine of fishes or amphibians. Humans presumably acquire the parasite by feeding upon freshwater crustacean intermediate hosts harbouring the cystacanth larvae or a vertebrate host which had ingested the cystacanth. They are unlikely to have any great pathogenic effect, although there is one report of a young worm having penetrated the gut wall and ended up on the peritoneum.

ORDER POLYMORPHIDA PETROCHENKO, 1956

Family Polymorphidae Meyer, 1931

Main features. Polymorphida. Body spined. Normally in intestine of aquatic birds and marine mammals.

Two polymorphid genera, *Corynosoma* Lühe, 1904 and *Bolbosoma* Porta, 1908, are occasionally reported from humans. These are normally parasitic in marine mammals, usually whales and dolphins in the case of *Bolbosoma* and seals in the case of *Corynosoma*. In addition to their marine link, these worms are recognizable by the presence of spines on the trunk of the body and, in the case of *Bolbosoma*, by a large expansion of the neck region posterior to the proboscis.

The basic life history of these marine polymorphids is similar to that of the terrestrial forms, but the eggs are voided with the faeces into water and the arthropod host harbouring the infective cystacanth larva is a crustacean rather than an insect. Furthermore, bony fishes, which feed upon infected crustaceans, act as paratenic hosts, the cystacanth larva passing through the fish's gut wall and re-encysting as a juvenile worm. Marine mammals become infected by feeding upon these fishes, which, in cases where the definitive host does not feed upon crustaceans, represent a necessary step in the life cycle. Humans become infected by feeding upon raw or poorly cooked marine fishes. It seems unlikely that the worms can mature in humans. The proper cooking or freezing of fish would kill the parasite.

There is little information on the pathogenicity of these worms; but they are known to begin to develop in humans, so penetration of the gut wall by the proboscis will elicit local inflammation and symptoms of abdominal pain (which is sometimes acute). There is one reported case of perforation of the intestine.

REFERENCES

Abuladze KI, 1964, Taeniata of animals and man and diseases caused by them (in Russian), *Osnovy Tsestodologii*, vol. 4, ed Skrjabin KI, Nauka, Moscow.

Amin O, 1985, Classification, *Biology of the Acanthocephala*, eds Crompton DWT, Nickol BB, Cambridge University Press, Cambridge, 27–72.

Anderson RC, Chabaud AG, Willmott S, eds, 1974–1983, *CIH Keys to the Nematode Parasites of Vertebrates*, Vols 1–10, Commonwealth Agricultural Bureaux, Farnham Royal.

Bain O, Chabaud AG, 1986, Atlas des larves infestantes de Filaires, *Trop Med Parasitol*, **37**: 301–40.

Brooks DR, 1989, The phylogeny of the Cercomeria (Platyhelminthes: Rhabdocoela) and general evolutionary principles, *J Parasitol*, **75**: 606–16.

Brooks DR, O'Grady RT, Glen DR, 1985, Phylogenetic analysis of the Digenea (Platyhelminthes: Cercomeria) with comments on their adaptive radiation, *Can J Zool*, **63**: 411–43.

Brooks DR, Bandoni S et al., 1989, Aspects of the phylogeny of the Trematoda Rudolphi, 1808 (Platyhelminthes: Cercomeria), *Can J Zool*, **67**: 2609–24.

Caballero y C. E, 1944, Estudios Helminthologicos de la Region Onchocercosa de Mexico y la Republica de Guatemala. Nematoda. Prima Parta. Filarioidea. I, *An Inst Biol Univ Mex*, **15**: 87–105.

Chitwood M, Lichtenfels JR, 1972, Identification of parasitic Metazoa in tissue sections, *Exp Parasitol*, **32**: 407–519.

Coombs I, Crompton DWT, 1991, *A Guide to Human Helminths*, Taylor and Francis, London.

Cooper DW, 1988, The preparation of serial sections of platyhelminth parasites, with details of the materials and facilities required, *Syst Parasitol*, **12**: 211–29.

Cort WW, 1919, The cercaria of the Japanese blood fluke, *Schistosoma japonicum* Katsurada, *Univ Calif Publs Zool*, **18(17)**: 485–507.

De Clercq D, Rollinson D et al., 1994, Schistosomiasis in Dogon country, Mali: identification and prevalence of the species responsible for infection in the local community, *Trans R Soc Trop Med Hyg*, **88**: 653–6.

Fuhrmann O, 1931, Dritte Klasse des Cladus Plathelminthes. Cestoidea, vol. II(2), eds Kükenthal W, Krumbach T, *Handbuch der Zoologie*, Walter de Gruyter, Berlin, 141–16.

Garcia LS, Bruckner DA, 1993, *Diagnostic Medical Parasitology*, 2nd edn, American Society for Parasitology, Washington DC.

Gibson DI, Bray RA, 1994, The evolutionary expansion and host-parasite relationships of the Digenea, *Int J Parasitol*, **24**: 1213–26.

Hugot JP, Tourte-Schaefer C, 1985, Morphological study of the two pinworms parasitic in man: *Enterobius vermicularis* and *E. gregorii*, *Ann Parasit Hum Comp*, **60**: 57–64.

Khalil LF, Jones A, Bray RA, eds, 1994, *Keys to the Cestode Parasites of Vertebrates*, CAB International, Wallingford, Oxon.

Lightowlers MW, Gottstein B, 1995, Echinococcosis/hydatidosis: antigens, immunological and molecular diagnosis, *Echinococcus and Hydatid Disease*, eds Thompson, RCA, Lymbery AJ, CAB International, Wallingford, Oxon, 355–410.

Meyer A, 1933, Acanthocephala, *Klassen und Ordnungen Teirreichs*, vol IV(2,2), ed Bronn HG, Akademisches Verlagsgesellschaft, Leipzig, 333–582.

Moravec F, 1982, Proposal for a new systematic arrangement of nematodes of the family Capillariidae, *Folia Parasitol*, **29**: 119–32.

Muller R, 1975, *Worms and Diseases. A Manual of Medical Helminthology*, Heinemann Medical, London.

Pearson JC, 1992, On the position of the digenean family Heronimidae: an inquiry into a cladistic classification of the Digenea, *Syst Parasitol*, **21**: 81–166.

Schell SC, 1985, *Handbook of Trematodes of North America*, Idaho University Press.

Schmidt GD, 1972, Revision of the class Archiacanthocephala Meyer, 1931 (Phylum Acanthocephala), with emphasis on Oligacanthorhynchidae Southwell et Macfie, 1925, *J Parasitol*, **58**: 290–7.

Thienpont D, Rochette F, Vanparijs OFJ, 1986, *Diagnosing Helminthiasis by Coprological Examination*, Janssen Research Foundation, Beerse, Belgium.

Van Cleave HJ, 1947, A critical review of the terminology for immature stages in acanthocephalan life histories, *J Parasitol*, **33**: 118–25.

Vogel H, 1934, Der Entwicklungzyklus von *Opisthorchis felineus* (Riv.) nebst Berkungen über die Systematik und Epidemiologie, *Zoologica (Stuttgart)*, **33(86)**: 1–103.

Wright CA, Ross GC, 1980, Hybrids between *Schistosoma haematobium* and *S. mattheei* and their identification by isoelectric focusing of enzymes, *Trans R Soc Trop Med Hyg*, **74**: 326–32.

Yamaguti S, 1963, *Systema Helminthum. III. Nematodes of Vertebrates*, Interscience, New York.

Yorke W, Maplestone PA, 1926, *The Nematode Parasites of Vertebrates*, Churchill, London.

Chapter 25

SCHISTOSOMES

S Kojima

1 The parasites	2 Clinical and pathological aspects of infection

1 THE PARASITES

Schistosomes are the causative agents of the disease **schistosomiasis**. Over 200 million people in 74 countries and territories in the world are affected and 500–600 million are at risk, according to the estimation of the World Health Organization (WHO 1996). Hierographics in the papyrus of Kahun refer to haematuria, a typical sign of urinary schistosomiasis which is mentioned 50 times in various medical papyri (Contis and David 1996), indicating that people in endemic areas were aware of the disease in ancient times. In the middle of the nineteenth century Daijiro (Yoshinao) Fujii (1847), a physician of the late Edo era in Japan, gave precise descriptions of clinical symptoms observed among peasants in Katayama District which clearly refer to schistosomiasis, although the disease was then of unknown aetiology.

In Cairo in 1851, Theodor Bilharz found a trematode in the blood of mesenteric veins of a young man on autopsy. It was not hermaphrodite, as were other flukes known at that time, but had separate sexes. He named the worm *Distomum haematobium* and described this as the cause of haematuria, based on the presence of terminal-spined eggs in the urine, although he considered lateral-spined eggs to belong to the same species. In 1859, Cobbold used a new genus name *Bilharzia* for the worm he found in the portal vein of a sooty monkey, although the name *Schistosoma* (meaning split body) had already been used by Weinland in 1858. In 1864, Harley found eggs with a terminal spine, but not those with a lateral spine, in the urine of patients with haematuria living in South Africa. In 1902, Manson found lateral-spined ova in a stool sample of a British patient with anaemia, instead of the hookworm eggs that he had expected, but no ova were detected in the urine of this patient, who had spent 15 years in the West Indies. He suggested the possible existence of 2 species of *Bilharzia*, one with terminal-spined eggs, the other depositing lateral-spined eggs

in the rectum; in 1907 Sambon designated the latter as *Schistosoma mansoni*.

Meantime, in Japan, as early as 1888 a peculiar parasite ovum was detected at autopsy by Majima in the liver of a patient who had ascites and systemic oedema. On 26 May 1904 Fujiro Katsurada discovered the anterior half of a male worm in the portal vein of a female cat kept for more than 10 years as a pet of a physician in Kofu Valley, Yamanashi Prefecture, where a serious endemic disease with abdominal swelling or abdominal fluid had been noted. Two months later, Katsurada found 24 males and 8 females from another cat and described the worms as *Schistosomum japonicum* (Katsurada 1904). The fact that this was a human parasite was confirmed by Akira Fujinami by an autopsy of a farmer from Katayama District carried out on 30 May of the same year (Fujinami 1904). It was also in 1904 that Catto in Singapore independently discovered worms of the same type in a Chinese man from Fukien who had died from cholera, and Blanchard named the parasite *Schistosoma cattoi*. This work was published in 1905 but later the parasite was found to be identical with one described by Katsurada. Using cows for experimental infections, Fujinami and Nakamura (1909) found that the infection was acquired by the percutaneous route. In 1913, Miyairi and Suzuki were able to determine that an amphibious snail, *Oncomelania nosophora*, was the intermediate host of this parasite. This discovery had a strong influence on the work of Leiper (1916), who was able to find the snail intermediate hosts of schistosomiasis in Egypt and to differentiate definitively between *S. haematobium* and *S. mansoni* on the infectivity to snails of miracidia derived respectively from terminal-spined or lateral-spined eggs.

The presence of human schistosomiasis has been known in the lower Mekong river basin since the late 1950s, and direct evidence of endemicity in Khong Island, Laos, was obtained by Iijima and Garcia (1967) (cited in Iijima, Lo and Ito 1971) who demonstrated that 8.6% of 547 inhabitants of the island were positive for *S. japonicum*-like eggs. Iijima, Lo and Ito (1971) reported that the Mekong schistosome differed from the Japanese strain of *S. japonicum*: the ovary was larger, the variation in number of the testes was greater and the eggs were smaller. Harinasuta et al. (1972) identified an aquatic snail, now known as *Tricula* (currently *Neotricula*) *aperta* (Davis 1980), as the intermediate host. Voge, Bruckner and Bruce (1978) concluded that the Mekong schistosome was a new species, *S. mekongi*.

Further historical details of studies on schistosomes and schistosomiasis are provided by Grove (1990).

1.1 Classification

The human schistosomes or blood flukes are digenetic trematodes belonging to the superfamily Schistosomatoidea of the suborder Strigeata. They differ from other trematodes in that (1) the adult are dioecious, being either male or female; (2) the adult worms parasitize blood vessels; (3) they lack a muscular pharynx; (4) they produce nonoperculate eggs; and (5) the cercaria, with a bifurcated tail, invades the final host percutaneously. Four species, *S. japonicum*, *S. mekongi*, *S. mansoni* and *S. haematobium*, are important agents of human schistosomiasis, although other species such as *S. intercalatum*, *S. bovis* and *S. mattheei* parasitic in other mammalian hosts may produce infections in humans (Table 25.1).

1.2 Morphology and structure

The adult forms of all schistosomes infective to humans basically resemble one another.

SCHISTOSOMA JAPONICUM

The male of *S. japonicum* measures about 15 mm in length by 0.5 mm in breadth; the female is long and slender like a nematode, measuring about 22 mm × 0.3 mm. The body surface of the male looks smooth under light microscopy, but scannning electron microscopy demonstrates folded protrusions with semi-spherical sensory organs that posess a small process in the centre (Sakamoto and Ishii 1977). The surface of the female is covered with minute spines. Near the anterior end of the body there are 2 suckers, oral and ventral. Following a short oesopahgus, the intestine divides at the level of the ventral sucker into 2 parallel gut caeca that rejoin behind the gonads to form a blind caecum ending near the posterior end of the body. In the male, 7 testes are usually present on the dorsal side just below the ventral sucker. The vas efferens from each of the testes leads to the common vas deferens which runs via a small seminal vesicle to the genital pore situated posterior to the ventral sucker. On the ventral side, the body is flattened and folded to form a groove, the **gynecophoric canal**, in which the female is held firmly (Fig. 25.1). In the female, the ovary is located near the posterior union of the lateral gut caeca about halfway along the body. The **vitelline glands** surround the caecum from the

Table 25.1 Schistosomes that may parasitize humans

Schistosome species	Final hosts	Intermediate hosts	Geographical distribution
S. haematobium	Human, monkey, baboon, chimpanzee	*Bulinus globosus*, *B. truncatus*	Africa, Middle East
S. mansoni	Human, monkey, baboon, chimpanzee, dog, rodent	*Biompalaria alexandrina*, *B. sudanica*, *B. pfeifferi*, *B. glabrata*	Africa, South America, Caribbean islands
S. japonicum	Human, dog, cat, rodent, cow, pig, sheep, goat, horse	*Oncomelania nosophora*, *O. hupensis*, *O. quadrasi*, (*O. formosana*)[a]	China, Philippines, Celebes (Taiwan)[a]
S. mekongi	Human, dog	*Neotricula aperta*	Laos, Cambodia, Thailand
S. intercalatum	Human	*Bulinus globosus*, *B. africanus*	West/Central Africa
S. bovis	Cattle, sheep, goat, equine, baboon, human?	*Bulinus truncatus*, *B. africanus*	Southern Europe, Africa, Iraq
S. mattheei	Horse, sheep, cow, zebra, antelopes, baboon, human	*Bulinus africanus*, *B. globosus*	Southern Africa

[a]Zoophilic strain, not infective to humans.

extreme end of the body up to the level of the posterior end of the ovary. The oviduct runs forward from the end of the ovary and joins the vitelline duct to form the **ootype**, where ova are fertilized, provided with vitelline materials and shells, and then passed into the uterus. The uterus is a long straight tube and opens behind the ventral sucker; 50–150 eggs develop in utero at one time. Ova deposited in tissues develop to the larval stage, the **miracidium**, within a week. Passage of the eggs through the vein wall and tissues to the lumen of the intestine is aided by the release through micropores in the shell of histolytic enzymes secreted by the miracidium. The eggs discharged in faeces are ovoid (70–100 × 50–65 μm) with a small spinose process near one end, but without an operculum (Fig. 25.2).

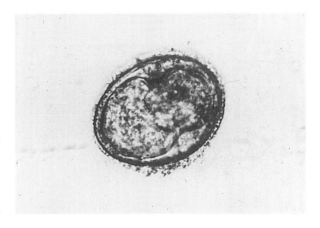

Fig. 25.2 *Schistosoma japonicum* ovum.

SCHISTOSOMA MEKONGI

Adult worms of this schistosome closely resemble those of *S. japonicum* in all aspects of size, shape, internal structure and body surface, except that the ovary is larger (Iijima, Lo and Ito 1971). Embryonated eggs of *S. mekongi* are also quite similar in shape and structure to those of *S. japonicum*, but are smaller, measuring 61.7 × 51.2 μm (Iijima, Lo and Ito 1971).

SCHISTOSOMA MANSONI

The adult worms of *S. mansoni* are slightly smaller than those of *S. japonicum*; the male is 6–12 mm long and the female 7–17 mm (Fig 25.3). The dorsal surface of the male is covered with many tubercles, each of which possesses fine spines on its surface. The tubercles are numerous in the region behind the ventral sucker but sparse in the posterior regions. Numerous pits are observed between the tubercles, and ciliated sensory organelles are also present on the surface. According to McLaren (1980), the gynaecophoric canal is formed by the folding of the lateral edges of the body, and a wide band of large spines of the dorsal surface of the inner fold may interlock with a narrower band of spines on the ventral surface of the outer fold. In addition, the surface of the canal bears many blunt spines suitable for holding the female in position without damaging her surface, and posteriorly the canal bears many finely pointed, anteriorly directed, elongate spines that prevent the female from slipping out backwards. The male has 4–13 (usually 7–8) testes. In the female, the ovary is in the anterior third of the body and the rest of the body is occupied centrally by the reunited caeca and laterally by the vitellaria. The uterus is very short and contains a few eggs at the most. The eggs have a yellowish-brown transparent shell with a distinct lateral spine and measure 114–175 × 45–68 μm (Fig. 25.4).

SCHISTOSOMA HAEMATOBIUM

The male worm measures 10–15 × 0.75–1 mm. The body surface is covered with minute wart-like projec-

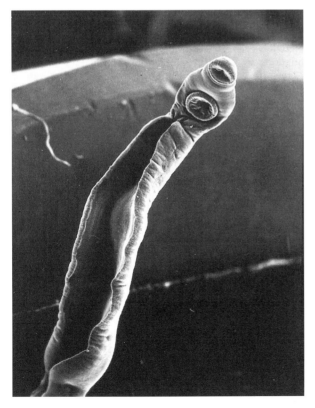

Fig. 25.1 Scanning electron micrograph of a male worm of *Schistosoma japonicum*, showing the gynecophoric canal.

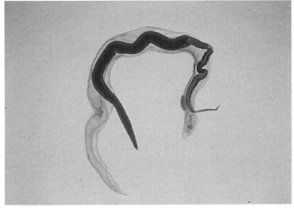

Fig. 25.3 Adult worms of *Schistosoma mansoni*.

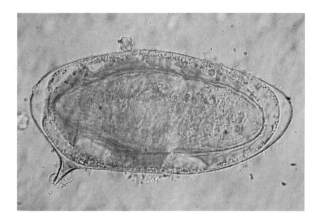

Fig. 25.4 *Schistosoma mansoni* ovum. See also Plate 25.4.

tions and 4 or 5 testes are present. The female is long and slender, measuring 16–26 × 0.25 mm. The ovary is situated in the posterior third of the body and the uterus is long, containing up to 100 eggs at one time. Mature eggs, usually discharged in the urine, have a yellowish-brown transparent shell with a prominent terminal spine and measure 112–170 × 40–70 μm (Fig. 25.5).

1.3 Location in host and general biology

The adult worms of *S. japonicum*, *S. mekongi* and *S. mansoni* inhabit the mesenteric veins, whereas the adult *S. haematobium* lives primarily in the veins of the vesical and pelvic plexuses, less commonly in the portal vein and its mesenteric branches. The adult worm is covered by a syncytial tegument approximately 4 μm in thickness, in which surface pits form deep, tortuous channels which may be branched and interconnected, thereby increasing the effective surface by a factor of as much as 10 (Hockley 1973). The physiological role of the pits is yet unknown.

The external surface of the tegument is a plasma membrane composed of 2 lipid bilayers (Hockley and McLaren 1973), of which the outer may fuse with foreign lipid membranes of host neutrophils and eosinophils (Caulfield et al. 1980), probably as a result of the production of mono-

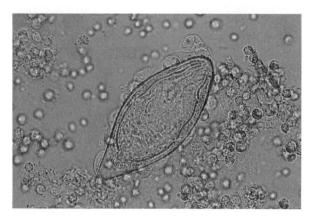

Fig. 25.5 *Schistosoma haematobium* ovum.

palmitoylphosphatidylcholine by the parasite (Furlong and Caulfield 1989). Since the parasite cannot synthesize essential lipids *de novo*, lipids, particularly free fatty acids, bound to serum proteins such as albumin, are potential sources of lipids for the parasite. The parasite also has receptors for serum lipoproteins on the outer bilipid membrane, by which the parasite may acquire another source of lipids from the host (Rumjanek, McLaren and Smithers 1983, Rogers et al. 1990). The outer bilipid membrane is shed continuously and replaced by products of organelles transported through a channel originated from the tegumental cells which are located under the circular and longitudinal muscle layers.

Schistosomes absorb glucose from the host plasma through the tegument (Fripps 1967, Rogers and Beuding 1975, Uglem and Read 1975). Glucose must be transported to internal cells across several membranes such as the 2 lipid bilayers and the basal membrane of the tegument as well as the plasma membranes of internal cells, a transport system that is unique to schistosomes. Indeed, 2 cDNA clones encoding the proteins SGTP1 and SGTP4, with features conserved in the facilitated diffusion glucose transporter family, have been identified by screening an adult *S. mansoni* cDNA library (Skelly et al. 1994). Immunolocalization studies have revealed the presence of SGTP4 in both of the lipid bilayers that cover the tegumental surface of adults and schistosomula, and also in the discoid and multilamellar bodies in adults as well as in the membranous bodies in schistosomula (Jiang et al. 1996), while SGTP1 is present in the basal membrane of the tegument (Zhong et al. 1995). These results suggest that SGTP4 may be responsible for transporting glucose from plasma into the tegument, whereas SGTP1 may function to transport free glucose from the tegument into the extracellular matrix beneath the tegument as well as into the muscle (Jiang et al. 1996, Zhong et al. 1995). These proteins are homologues of GLUT-1, the human glucose transporter protein (Mueckler et al. 1985).

Absorbed glucose is metabolized through the Embden–Meyerhof pathway and the Krebs cycle. Studies on the mode of action of anti-schistosomal drugs have demonstrated the importance of the key enzymes involved in these pathways as the target of chemotherapy. For example, compounds of antimony, though no longer used for treatment because of their side effects, inhibit phosphofructokinase activity at concentrations 70–80 times lower than those inhibiting the isozyme of the host, while praziquantel, the most effective drug currently available, affects the transport of calcium ions across cell membranes, which may result in tegumental vacuolization and disruption (Mehlhorn et al. 1981, 1983).

Adult worms also ingest red blood cells through the mouth and utilize haemoglobins as well as serum globulins as nutrients after cleaving by proteolytic enzymes. Binding of the proteolytic enzymes to haemoglobin is optimal at pH4.0 in lumen of the gut. Since their digestive system ends in a blind caecum, residual black haematin is regurgitated together with the proteolytic enzyme to the circulation, from where it is taken up by phagocytic cells in the liver and spleen of the host. Meanwhile, the enzyme–haemoglobin complex dissociates owing to the change of pH, resulting in release of the enzyme in the plasma as a circulating antigen that in turn sensitizes hosts, inducing immediate-type hypersensitivity reactions to the enzyme (Senft and Maddison 1975).

It is likely that the female may obtain supplementary nutrients through the intimate contact with the male ventral tegument. This may be related to the fact that unisexual infections usually fail to induce sexual maturation of females, although certain lipid metabolites such as ecdysteroids and dolichols have been suggested to act as promotors for sexual development and egg production by adult worms, respectively (Furlong 1991, Fried and Haseeb 1991).

1.4 Life cycle

The life cycle of all species follows a common pathway from the sexual generation of adult schistosomes within the vascular system of the definitive host to asexual generations in the intermediate host of freshwater snails, and a return to the definitive host by skin penetration of infective larval stages (Fig. 25.6).

When embryonated eggs discharged in faeces or urine enter fresh water, miracidia hatch from the eggs, rapidly swim by means of cilia that cover the body surface except the apical papilla, and penetrate the exposed surface of the body of snail intermediate hosts. The attachment and penetration of the miracidium are assisted by secretions from the anterior penetration glands which open anterolaterally via ducts to the base of the apical papilla.

The intermediate hosts differ from species to species of schistosome (Table 25.2). Moreover, differences in host specificity may exist among species or strains of the snail intermediate hosts in terms of infectivity of geographically different strains of schistosomes.

The intermediate hosts of *S. japonicum* are a complex of amphibious snails of *Oncomelania hupensis* (Fig. 25.7), of which there are 6 subspecies: *O. h. hupensis* in mainland China; *O. h. quadrasi* in the Philippines; *O. h. nosophora* in Japan; *O. h. lindoensis* in Sulawesi, Indonesia; *O. h. formosana* in Taiwan where a zoophilic strain of *S. japonicum* exists; finally, experimental infection with the strain has been demonstrated in *O. h. chiui*, another subspecies found in Taiwan. Recent studies suggest that these subspecies should be elevated to specific status like *O. hupensis* or *O. quadrasi* (Sturrock 1993). These oncomelanid snails have conical or subconical dextral shells of 4–8 whorls with a height of less than 10 mm. *O. quadrasi* is more aquatic than the other species, which may crawl out of water on nearby vegetation and mud surface and can survive for at least a few months of a dry season in natural conditions. *S. mekongi* is transmitted by the α, β and γ races of *Tricula* (currently *Neotricula*) *aperta* (Sornmani 1976), of which the β race is the most susceptible to infection (Liang and Kitikoon 1980).

S. mansoni is transmitted by planorbid snails of the genus *Biomphalaria*. These snails are widely distributed throughout Africa and parts of the Arabian peninsula, and also in the New World, in Caribbean islands on and the South American continent in Venezuela, Surinam, French Guiana and Brazil. In the New World, *B. glabrata*, *B. tenagophila*, and *B. straminea* are the natural host of *S. mansoni*, although several other species of *Biomphalaria* have been proved experimentally infective. Among these species, *B. glabrata* (Fig. 25.8) is highly susceptible and produces a large number of cercariae for a prolonged period of time, although recent studies have suggested that this species is being replaced locally by a susceptible strain of *B. straminea* in northeast Brazil and by susceptible *B. tenagophila* in southeast Brazil (Sturrock 1993). *B. straminea* is widely spread from several Caribbean islands through Panama and Costa Rica in the central American isthmus to Paraguay and Argentina and has been proposed as a competitor species for the biological control of *S. mansoni*, although it is obvious that the deliberate introduction of this species is not recommended because of the appearance of susceptible strains in Brazil (Sturrock 1993).The African *Biomphalaria* species are classified into 4 major groups.

1 The *pfeifferi* group is distributed widely in Africa south of the Sahara, the Malagasy Republic, and extends into Aden, Yemen and southwest Saudi Arabia.
2 The *choanomphala* group is restricted to certain of the great natural lakes including Lake Victoria.
3 The *alexandrina* group is distributed from Egypt and Libya in the Nile Delta to Israel and northern Sudan. This group also includes *B. angulosa* which has a scattered distribution in mountain areas from southern Tanzania to South Africa and has been proved to be a natural host in Malawi (Teesdale 1982).
4 The *sudanica* group has a distribution limited to an equatorial band across tropical Africa.

The intermediate hosts of *S. haematobium* are pulmonate snails of the genus *Bulinus*, although its classification is still a matter of debate and snails are roughly divided into 4 species groups (Fig 25.9).

1 The *africanus* group includes 10 species, among which are the species susceptible to *S. intercalatum*. *B. globosus* belongs to this group and is distributed throughout most of subsaharan Africa, whereas *B. africanus* is spread throughout east, central and southern Africa.
2 The *forskali* group includes 5 species transmitting *S. haematobium*: *B. forskali* distributed throughout most of tropical Africa, *B. beccarii* in Aden and Saudi Arabia, *B. camerunensis* in Cameroon, *B. cernicus* in Mauritius and *B. senegalensis* in the Gambia, Senegal and Mauritania.
3 The *reticulatus* group includes *B. reticulatus* and *B. wrighti*, which are distributed focally from Ethiopia to South Africa, and in Aden and Arabia, respectively.
4 The *truncatus/tropicus* complex, the species of medical importance as natural intermediate hosts of *S. haematobium*, includes *B. truncatus*, *B. rohlfsi* and *B. guerni*. *B. trucatus* is the principal intermediate host in Africa north of the Sahara and also in Arabia, whereas *B. rohlfsi* plays an important role in the transmission in West African countries, including Cameroon, Mali, Mauritania, Nigeria and Ghana. The construction of the Akosombo Dam and the creation of the man-made Lake Volta in Ghana led to a spread of breeding sites for *B. rholfsi* and caused an epidemic of urinary schistosomiasis (Klumpp and Chu 1977).

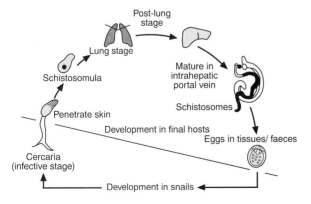

Fig. 25.6 Life cycle of *Schistosoma japonicum*, as a representative of all schistosomes.

Post-lung stage

Lung stage

Schistosomula

Penetrate skin

Cercaria (infective stage)

Mature in intrahepatic portal vein

Schistosomes

Development in final hosts

Eggs in tissues/ faeces

Development in snails

After penetration into the intermediate host, the mira-

Table 25.2 Intermediate hosts of human schistosomes[a]

Schistosome species	Intermediate hosts	Geographical distribution
S. japonicum	Oncomelania hupensis	
	O. h. hupensis	Mainland China
	O. h. nosophora	Japan
	O. h. quadrasi	Philippines
	O. h. lindonensis	Sulawesi
S. mekongi	Neotricula aperta	Laos, Cambodia
S. mansoni	Biomphalaria	
	B. glabrata	Caribbean islands, Venezuela, Brazil, Argentina
	B. straminea	Caribbean islands, Central and South America
	B. tenagophila	Southeast Brazil
	B. pfeifferi group	
	B. pfeifferi	All subsaharan Africa
	B. rhodesiensis	East/Central to South Africa
	B. ruepelli	Yemen to East Africa
	B. arabica	Arabian peninsula
	B. choanomphala group	
	B. choanomphala	Central African lakes
	B. alexandrina group	
	B. alexandrina	Nile valley from North Sudan
	B. angulosa	Mountain areas from East to South Africa
	B. sudanica group	
	B. sudanica	Eastern tropical Africa
	B. camerunensis	Western tropical Africa
	B. salinarum	Southwest Africa
S. haematobium	Bulinus	
	B. africanus group	
	B. abyssinicus	Somalia, Ethiopia
	B. africanus	East, Central and Southern Africa
	B. globosus	Most of subsaharan Africa
	B. jousseaumei	West Africa
	B. nasutus	East Africa
	B. obtusispira	Madagascar
	B. forskali group	
	B. beccarii	Aden
	B. camerunensis	West Cameroon crater lakes
	B. cernicus	Mauritius
	B. forskali	Most of tropical Africa
	B. senegalensis	Mauritania, Senegal, Gambia
	B. reticulatus group	
	B. reticulatus[b]	Focal from Ethiopia to South Africa
	B. wrighti	Saudi Arabia, Oman, Yemen
	B. truncatus/tropics complex	
	B. guernei	West Africa
	B. liratus	Madagascar
	B. rohlfsi	West Africa
	B. truncatus	Mediterranean, south to Mauritania and Malawi, east to Iran

[a]Adapted from Sturrock (1993).
[b]Experimentally infected with a strain of *S. haematobium*.

cidium loses the ciliated surface and develops into mother and daughter sporocysts, and then produces fork-tailed cercariae in the course of several weeks (4 weeks in the case of *S. mansoni* under favourable conditions but longer in other species, especially in *S. japonicum*) (Fig. 25.10). As a result of asexual multiplication within mother and daughter sporocysts, thousands of cercariae, all of the same sex, are produced from a single miracidium. The cercariae measure around 400 μm in length including the tail, the ter-

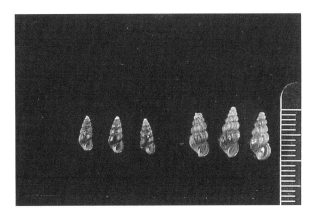

Fig. 25.7 Intermediate snail hosts of *Schistosoma japonicum*: left, *Oncomelania hupensis nosophora* collected from Yamanashi, Japan; right, *Oncomelania hupensis hupensis* collected from Jian-xi Province, China.

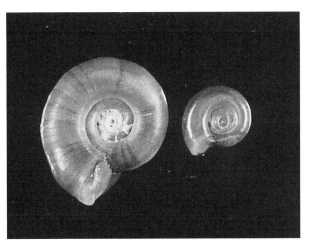

Fig. 25.8 *Biomphalaria glabrata*, the intermediate host of *Schistosoma mansoni*.

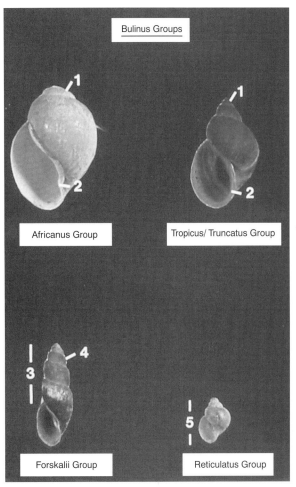

Fig. 25.9 Four species groups of the intermediate snail hosts of *Schistosoma haematobium* (see also Table 25.2). (WHO Slide Set Series; Snail hosts, Schistosomiasis).

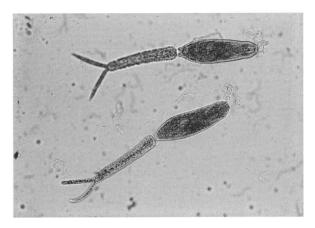

Fig. 25.10 Cercariae, the infective larval stage.

minal one-third of which is bifurcated. Their surface and internal structures are essentially identical among schistosome species. They have a muscular oral sucker occupying about one-third of the body and a small ventral sucker or acetabulum. The cercariae infect the definitive host by penetrating the skin, aided by proteolytic enzymes secreted from the penetration glands, losing their tails out and transforming to the next larval stage, the **schistosomulum**. During the whole penetration process, drastic morphological and physiological changes take place in the larvae. Thus, the cercarial glycocalyx is lost and replaced by a double bilayer; this is marked by a change from a trilaminate appearance to a heptalaminate membrane.

After penetration schistosomula migrate into the lungs via the venous circulation. This migration route seems to be essential for their development and is associated with the acquisition of biological differences, since schistosomula recovered from the lungs are not only elongated but are more resistant than newly transformed schistosomula to antibody-dependent cell-mediated cytotoxicity, although the mechanisms are as yet unknown (see section 2.3). The schistosomula break out from the lungs through the pulmonary capillaries and are carried through the left heart into the systemic circulation, finally reaching the portal system. It takes 3–4 days for *S. japonicum* schistosomula to migrate into the lungs after skin penetration, followed by another 3–4 days stay in the lungs; *S. mansoni* reaches the lungs and leaves for the final destination at least 2 days earlier than *S. japonicum* (Usawattanakul, Kamijo and Kojima 1982). Some schistosomula may take another route through the diagphragm to reach the liver. In the intrahepatic portal circulation, feeding begins and further growth occurs. The lateral gut caeca grow posteriorly and eventually unite behind the ventral sucker and the developing gonads. Within several weeks, pairing of the worms take place on sexual maturation, and they migrate to the mesenteric veins, or to the vesical plexus (probably via anastomoses in the umbilical plexus in the case of *S. haematobium*), where the females lay eggs. The prepatent period between penetration by cercariae and the first appearance of eggs in the excreta is around 35 days for *S. japonicum* and *S. mansoni* and about 70 days for *S. haematobium*, despite the fact that the worms of this species reach sexual maturity by day 31 and that it takes some 6–10 days for eggs to reach the lumen of the gut or bladder (Sturrock 1993).

1.5 Transmission and epidemiology

As is obvious from the life cycle of schistosomes, human infections depend absolutely on the presence of intermediate snail hosts in bodies of water which may be contaminated with human faeces and excreta as a result of insanitary habits or polluted with excreta from reservoir hosts, which have to be considered in disease control, especially in the case of *S. japonicum* infection. Thus, transmission is influenced by biological, economic and sociocultural factors such as (1) the distribution, biology and population dynamics of the intermediate hosts, (2) the patterns and extent of environmental contamination with human excreta through insanitary conditions and utilization as fertilizer, or with excreta from domestic animals in the case of *S. japonicum*, (3) human water contact activities, patterns and duration, (4) water development projects including extension of irrigation systems and construction of dams, and most seriously (5) people's knowledge of the disease itself and their attitudes towards, or practices for, avoiding the infection.

Despite its public health importance in many tropical and subtropical areas, which is second only to that of malaria, schistosomiasis has been ignored and given a low priority in health policy mainly because of the low socioeconomic status of developing countries, and the tendency to give economic development priority over health and welfare. Thus, water development projects, particularly construction of dams, artificial lakes and irrigation canals, often associated with dynamic population resettlement, have become a major factor in the spread and intensification of the disease.

Schistosomiasis also may be categorized as one of the emerging and re-emerging diseases. A typical example is a recent outbreak of intestinal schistosomiasis in the delta of the Senegal river basin where the presence of the disease has never been reported. In the 1980s the Diama dam was constructed at the mouth of the river to avoid a backward flow from the sea. A year and a half after it became operational (in

August 1986), a first case of *S. mansoni* infection was detected at Richard-Toll. The prevalence of *S. mansoni* infection rapidly increased from 1.9% in 1988 to 71.5% in late 1989, with a total of 49.4% positive cases out of 3926 stool examinations. *B. pfeifferi* was found to be the major intermediate host in this area (Talla et al. 1990). Another example of schistosomiasis as a re-emerging disease occurred in Japan where endemic schistosomiasis was observed among dairy cows pastured along the bank of the Tone river in Chiba Prefecture, and also involved some inhabitants in the infection. This was 15 years after the disease ceased to be considered endemic (Yokogawa et al. 1971, 1973).

Community-based epidemiological studies of schistosomiasis demonstrate that prevalence (expressed as the percentage of the population found infected at a given point of time) and intensity of infection (expressed in terms of egg output in excreta) are usually higher among younger age groups than in older age groups. A typical example obtained from a study of urinary schistosomiasis in a defined area of southern Ghana is shown in Fig. 25.11, indicating that the peak prevalence and intensity occur in children aged 10–14 years, accompanied by a gradual decline in prevalence and intensity in older age groups (Aryeetey et al., unpublished data). This phenomenon is more marked in *S. haematobium* than in *S. mansoni*, but in *S. japonicum* infection the reduction in prevalence and intensity in older age groups may not be observed. The decline in egg output in community based studies may reflect the development of immunity to reinfection, or alternatively the possibility of reduced water contact in the older age groups (see section 2.4).

Thus, the control of schistosomiasis apparently involves many factors and requires a long-term effort with a complex of strategies. So far, there are only 3 countries – Japan, Montserrat and Tunisia – where the transmission of the disease is considered to have ceased (WHO 1993). In Japan, beginning in 1947, a programme to control the disease in previously known endemic areas was undertaken by the Japanese Ministry of Health and Welfare and other institutions in collaboration with the United States 406th Medical General Laboratory. Voluntary organizations, composed of staff from local governments, physicians' associations, teachers' associations and representatives from endemic communities, made a major contribution to the intensive control programme, which included snail control and improvement of environmental and sanitary conditions, since they had been actually established before World War II. Based on these activities, the government carried out massive surveys in 1973 and 1978 on inhabitants, *Oncomelania* snails and reservoir hosts throughout endemic areas. Although 2 snail colonies still exist, including a new habitat found recently in a limited area which has no relation to former endemic areas (Kojima et al. 1988), schistosomiasis japonica is considered to have been eradicated from Japan by 1978 (Hunter and Yokogawa 1984).

Further details on the epidemiology of schistoso-

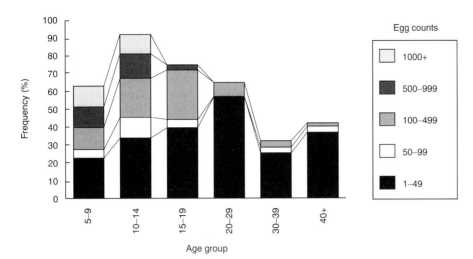

Fig. 25.11 Prevalence and intensity of *Schistosoma haematobium* infection in southern Ghana (Aryeetey et al., unpublished data).

miasis are given in an outstanding review by Jordan and Webbe (1993)

2 CLINICAL AND PATHOLOGICAL ASPECTS OF INFECTION

Clinical symptoms and pathological changes caused by schistosome infections may reflect migratory routes and developmental stages of the parasites after their penetration from the skin. In general, an acute infection is not apparent from the symptoms among people living in endemic areas, unless they are exposed to a massive infection for a special reason such as flooding. Pathological changes are caused mainly by schistosome eggs deposited in various tissues. Host immune responses to antigens excreted from embryonated eggs, which are now the focus of cytokine studies, result in formation of granulomas that lead eventually to fibrotic changes in the tissues involved in chronic infections. Thus, the lesions produced by the infections are essentially the same among the 3 major species of schistosomes.

2.1 Clinical manifestations

Clinical manifestations may reflect developmental stages of the parasites and host responses to toxic or antigenic substances derived from the parasites and eggs.

The initial manifestations may appear following penetration of cercariae and migration of schistosomula from the skin to lungs. Table 25.3 summarizes the symptoms of Chinese and Japanese patients who were infected with *S. japonicum* in the floods that occurred in the Yangtze river in 1945 and the Tone river in 1926, indicating that cercariae may induce dermatitis with slight exanthema and itch upon their penetration. Dermatitis usually disappears within a week and migration of schistosomula into the lungs provokes cough with association of a mild fever and dullness. Anaemia may be observed among one fifth of patients (Table 25.3).

After a latent period of about a month, the acute

Table 25.3 Symptoms observed among people with acute schistomiasis japonica (figures are percentages)

Symptoms	Chinese cases (200 cases)[a]	Japanese cases (75 cases)[b]
Initial phase		
Dermatitis	44.0	67.0
Prepatent phase		
Malaise/fatigue		67.0
Cough	63.0	
Bloody sputum	5.5	
Anorexia	88.0	38.6
Abdominal pain	41.0	(+)
Anaemia	23.0	24.0
Oviposition phase		
Chill	78.0	77.3
Fever	100.0	77.3
Sweat	72.0	73.3
Diarrhoea	51.0	5.3
Dysentery	10.0	(−)
Hepatomegaly	96.5	85.3
Splenomegaly	62.5	22.7
Ascites	8.5	9.3

[a]Ling, Cheng and Chung (1949).
[b]Kashiwado et al. (1927).

phase of disease may suddenly start with a high fever accompanied by rigors, termed **Katayama fever** after the Katayama District in Hiroshima Prefecture, Japan, where Yoshinao Fujii originally described the acute onset of the illness (see section 1, p. 1). Among the Japanese patients described in Table 25.3, the majority had such an onset 31–50 days after the infection. The onset corresponds to the start of oviposition by mature female worms. In the case of *S. japonicum* and *S. mansoni*, female worms lay eggs in the mesenteric branches of the portal vein along the intestinal wall and although a relatively large part of the eggs are carried into the liver and other organs by the blood flow, the remainder of them may stay in the small venules until the embryos they contain develop to miracidia within 10 days. Antigenic substances excreted from miracidia diffuse out through submicroscopic pores in the egg-shell and elicit an acute inflammation in the surrounding tissues, resulting in the rupture of the vascular wall and escape of the eggs from the venules through the intestinal submucosa and mucosa into the intestinal lumen. Typical egg granulomas formed in the liver are shown in Fig. 25.12. The inflammation causes recurrent daily fever, abdominal pain and enlarged tender liver and spleen, and discharge of eggs into the intestinal canal is accompanied by dysentery or diarrhoea (Table 25.3). Blood chemistry may reveal a transient elevation of glutamic pyruvic transaminase, glutamic oxaloacetic transaminase and alkaline phosphatase 5–6 weeks after infection. Eosinophilia may be observed in most of the patients with or without increase of leukocyte counts. Serum levels of IgE may increase as observed in other helminth infections (Kojima, Yokogawa and Tada 1972). These symptoms characterize **intestinal schistosomiasis**. In *S. haematobium* infection, Katayama fever is much less commonly reported: the major complaints are haematuria, burning sensation or pain on micturition and suprapubic discomfort. Proteinuria and microscopic haematuria are especially common among children in endemic areas in Africa.

The chronic phase of manifestations in *S. japonicum* and *S. mansoni* infections is characterized by hepato-splenomegaly and may therefore be called **hepato-splenic schistosomiasis**, although development of polyps or mucosal proliferation of the intestine may also be observed in most cases. Egg granulomas are replaced by fibrotic tissues, which are prominent in the periportal areas and lead to the development of pipestem fibrosis (von Lichtenberg et al. 1971) (Fig. 25.13). In association with liver dysfunction, diagnostic techniques such as computed tomography or ultrasonography may reveal pathological changes with characteristic reticulate or hexagonal patterns in patients with chronic schistosomiasis (Fig. 25.14a, b). The liver gradually decreases in size but increases in hardness as fibrosis is gradually extended into the parenchyma, resulting eventually in liver cirrhosis in severe cases (Fig. 25.15). The enlarged spleen may reach

the level of the umbilicus or even at times expand to fill most of the abdomen. Portal hypertension and hypoalbuminaemia may induce ascites (Fig. 25.16). Dilatation of abdominal collateral veins (Fig. 25.16) and oesophagogastric varices are observed in advanced cases, and bleeding from the varices may cause sudden death. Anaemia is more noticeable than in the previous stages. Acute or chronic cerebral involvement may occur in schistosomiasis japonica due to embolism of eggs or heterotopic parasitism of female worms, causing headache, Jacksonian epileptic seizures, paraesthesia and poor vision (Ariizumi 1963). Hepatic coma may occur as a complication, although its frequency is far less than that of liver cirrhosis. Another complication in *S. mansoni* infection is schistosomal cor pulmonale which is caused by vascular peripheral obstruction resulting in increased intrapulmonary artery hypertension. Symptoms are fatigue, palpitations, exertional dyspnoea and cough with occasional haemoptysis.

In urinary schistosomiasis, the main complaint is recurrent painless haematuria resulting from ulcers of the bladder mucosa. A burning sensation on micturition, frequency and suprapubic discomfort or pain may precede or be associated. The bladder wall may

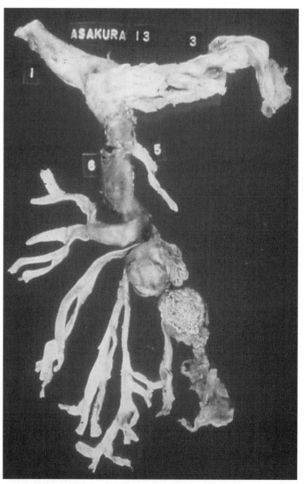

Fig. 25.13 Pipestem fibrosis in a Japanese patient with schistosomiasis japonica.

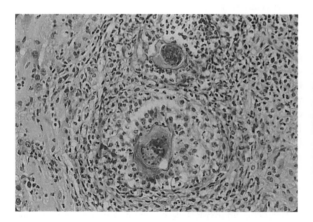

Fig. 25.12 Granuloma formation around newly deposited eggs of *Schistosoma japonicum*. See also Plate 25.12.

(a)

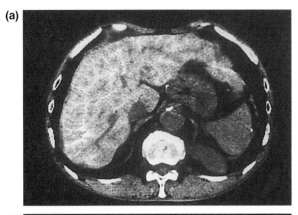

(b)

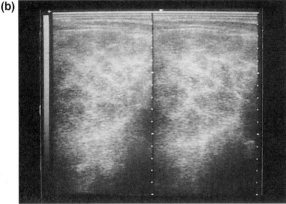

Fig. 25.14 Hepatic fibrosis in a patient with chronic schistosomiasis japonica: (a) computed tomography; (b) ultrasonography. Note the characteristic reticulate or hexagonal patterns.

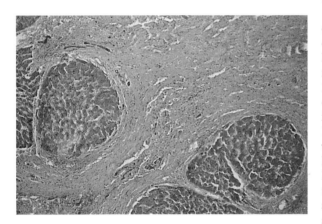

Fig. 25.15 Liver cirrhosis due to *Schistosoma japonicum* infection. A case found in Yamanashi Prefecture, Japan. See also Plate 25.15.

be thickened, with a papillary proliferation of the mucosa that is reversible if appropriate chemotherapy is carried out (Fig 25.17a,b). In chronic cases, however, hydronephrosis may result from obstruction of the urinary tract, causing renal parenchymal dysfunction (Fig. 25.18). Coexistence of bacteriuria may accelerate damage of kidney function. *Escherichia coli* is the most common organism, although *Pseudomonas* spp., *Klebsiella* spp. and *Salmonella* spp. are also found in

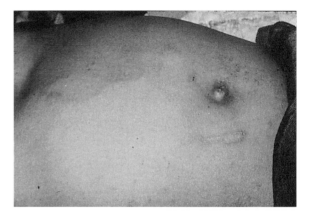

Fig. 25.16 The abdomen of a patient with chronic schistosomiasis japonica, showing ascites and dilatation of abdominal collateral veins.

complicated cases. Obstructive uropathy has been reported to predispose to caliculi (Cheever et al. 1978). The association of bladder cancer with *S. haematobium* infection has been discussed in the context of the involvement of urinary tract infections by species of nitrate-reducing bacteria. The urine of patients infected with *S. haematobium* contained higher levels of nitrosamines, in association with nitrate-reducing bacteria, than the urine of either Egyptian or German controls, and this may result in the endogenous formation of carcinogenic *N*-nitrosocompounds in the urine (Mostafa, Badawi and O'Connor 1995).

The involvement of gynaecological organs may be observed in *S. haematobium* infection. As a disease entity, female genital schistosomiasis has been neglected, despite the fact that vaginal schistosomiasis was reported from Egypt as early as in 1899 (Madden 1899). It has generally been considered that the presence of *S. haematobium* eggs is not as common in female genital organs as in male genital organs (Farid 1993), although in the female lesions are found in the vulva, vagina, cervix, and less commonly the ovaries, Fallopian tubes or uterus (Wright, Chiphangwi and Hutt 1982). However, *S. haematobium* may migrate through the network of female pelvic vasculature, and adaptive changes in the vasculature during puberty and especially during pregnancy make 'ectopic' localization of the parasites possible (Feldmeier et al. 1995). Since sexually transmitted diseases increase the probability of HIV transmission, presumably through lesions in the genital mucosa, female genital schistosomiasis may be an important risk factor for transmission of HIV (Feldmeier, Krantz and Poggensee 1994). From published data there seems to be pathophysiological, immunological and epidemiological evidence for an association between genital ulcer due to *S. haematobium* and HIV infection in women (Feldmeier et al. 1995). If so, control of urinary schistosomiasis should be seriously tackled to prevent further widespread dissemination of HIV infection.

(a)

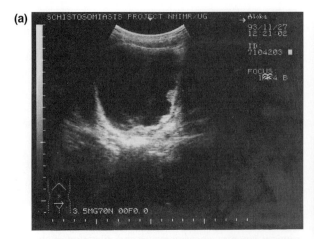

(b)

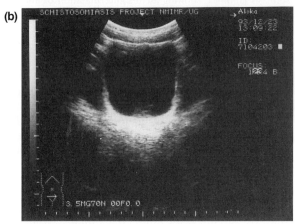

Fig. 25.17 Ultrasonography of a 12 year old boy with urinary schistosomiasis: (a) before chemotherapy with praziquantel; (b) one month after the chemotherapy (courtesy of Dr Yukiko Wagatsuma).

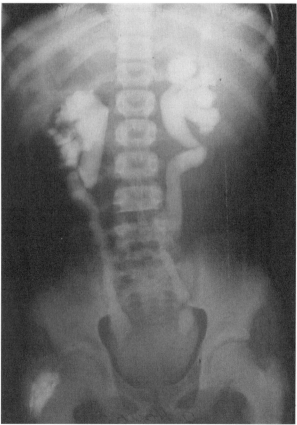

Fig. 25.18 Hydronephrosis due to *Schistosoma haematobium* infection (courtesy of Dr Yukiko Wagatsuma).

2.2 Pathogenesis and pathology

As mentioned above (section 2.1, p. 487), the pathologic changes in schistosome infections are caused mainly by the deposition of the eggs into various tissues and organs where granulomas or pseudotubercles are formed around them. In primary infections, the granuloma is composed of aggregations of mononuclear phagocytes, neutrophils, lymphocytes, plasma cells and fibroblasts (Fig. 25.12). Giant cells are also frequently observed in the granulomas. Granulomas may vary in size and cellular components with the immune status of the host; in experimental infections in immunized animals, a dominant cellular infiltration of eosinophils and lymphocytes is observed around the eggs, and the egg granuloma is smaller.

Granuloma formation around schistosome eggs has been considered to be the result of delayed-type hypersensitivity reactions mediated through a T cell mediated immune response to soluble egg antigens (Warren, Domingo and Cowan 1967). However, recent studies have demonstrated that there exist at least 2 subsets of T helper cells with a CD4[+] phenotype, termed Th1 and Th2 cells, which can be distinguished from each other by their cytokine productions (Mosmann and Coffman 1989). The cytokines derived from Th1 cells, such as IL (IL)-2, interferon-γ, or tumour necrosis factor (TNF)-β, may be responsible for activation of macrophages and cell-mediated immunity, whereas IL-4 or IL-5, the cytokine produced by Th2 cells, stimulates IgE production or eosinophilia, respectively (Mosmann and Coffman 1989; Takatsu, Takaki and Hitoshi 1994) (see Chapter 4).

Thus, cytokine production from T helper subsets has been studied to gain new insights into granuloma formation in murine schistosomiasis mansoni. Surprisingly, the production of Th2 cytokines was found to correspond to the onset of egg deposition (Gryzch et al. 1991). In another experiment, lymphocytes from mice vaccinated with irradiated cercariae or from infected animals were compared for their ability to produce interferon-γ and IL-2 as compared with IL-4 and IL-5. After stimulation with specific antigen or mitogen, T cells from vaccinated mice or prepatently infected animals responded primarily with Th1 cytokines, whereas lymphocytes from patently infected mice instead produced Th2 cytokines. The Th2 response in infected animals was shown to be induced by schistosome eggs and directed largely against egg antigens, whereas the Th1 reactivity in vaccinated mice was triggered primarily by larval antigens. Interestingly, Th1 responses in mice carrying egg-producing infections were found to be profoundly down-regulated. Moreover, the injection of eggs into vaccinated mice resulted in a reduction of antigen and mitogen-stimulated Th1 function accompanied by a coincident expression of Th2 responses (Pearce et al. 1991).

Cheever et al. (1992a) were able to demonstrate that in vivo treatment of infected mice with anti-IL-2 antibodies significantly diminished the size of circumoval granulomas in the liver, resulting in decrease of hepatic fibrosis to half that in untreated mice. Antibody-treated animals also displayed a marked reduction in both peripheral blood and tissue eosinophilia while IgE levels were unchanged or increased. Spleen cell cytokine production in response to antigen or mitogen stimulation was selectively altered by in vivo anti-IL-2 administration. IL-5 responses were dramatically reduced, whereas IL-4, IL-2 and interferon-γ responses were not consistently changed. These findings suggest a role for IL-2 in egg-induced pathology but indicate that the primary function of this cytokine in schistosome-infected mice may be in the generation of Th2- rather than Th1-associated responses (Cheever et al. 1992a).

By using a synchronized granuloma development model in the lung (von Lichtenberg 1962), it has been demonstrated that although the effects of neutralization of interferon-γ or IL-2 were variable, in vivo treatment of egg-injected mice with either anti-IL-2 or anti-IL-4 antibodies dramatically diminished the size of egg granulomas in the lungs (Chensue et al. 1992, Wynn et al. 1993). Both groups of antibody-treated animals displayed a marked reduction in IL-4 as well as IL-5 mRNA expression, although interferon-γ and IL-2 mRNA levels were unchanged or slightly increased. The up-regulation of mRNA expression of the IL-4 and IL-5 genes was also shown to be greater than that of Th1 cytokine genes in the granulomatous liver at 8 weeks postinfection (Henderson et al. 1991; Wynn et al. 1993).

Further studies in which mice were treated with anti-IL-4 before egg deposition demonstrated decreased IL-4, IL-5, and IL-10 production in response to in vitro antigenic stimulations as well as decreased IL-5 and IL-13 mRNA levels in the liver (Cheever et al. 1994). It was found that non-B, non-T cells were a major source of IL-4 in infected mice treated with control monoclonal antibody, and that the diminished IL-4 response in anti-IL-4-treated animals was caused, at least in part, by a reduction in the number of these cells, as well as by decreased secretion of IL-4 per cell. In contrast, production of the Th1 cytokines IL-2 and interferon-γ was elevated in anti-IL-4-treated infected mice in vitro, and the corresponding mRNAs in the liver increased. Anti-IL-4 treatment did not consistently reduce the size of hepatic granulomas around *S. mansoni* eggs, but markedly inhibited granuloma formation in the lungs of the same animals after intravenous egg injection. Nevertheless, anti-IL-4-treatment showed consistent and marked reductions in hepatic collagen deposition at 8 weeks in *S. mansoni*-infected mice (Cheever et al. 1994). Similarly, hepatic fibrosis was markedly diminished in anti-IL-4-treated mice at 10 weeks after infection with *S. japonicum* (Cheever, Finkelman and Cox 1995). These findings suggested that IL-4 plays a major role in the development of the Th2 response in murine schistosomiasis and contributes to the pathogenesis of hepatic fibrosis. Moreover, the administration of cytokines themselves into infected mice has also been shown to modulate the granuloma formation. According to Yamashita and Boros (1992), chronically infected mice treated with 10–1000 U of recombinant IL-4 showed significantly enhanced liver granulomatous responses compared with untreated animals and the augmented granulomas contained more enlarged macrophages and connective tissue matrix.

Quite recently, however, controversial results have been reported on the role of IL-4 in granuloma formation. When mice in which the IL-4 gene had been deleted (IL-4$^{-/-}$ mice)

were infected with *S. mansoni*, at 8 and 16 weeks after infection, liver pathology was similar to that in wild-type animals in terms of the size, cellularity, cellular composition, and collagen content of granulomas. However, when compared to normal mice, smaller granulomatous responses were observed in IL-4$^{-/-}$ mice only when eggs were injected intravenously to form granulomas in the lungs, despite the fact that Th1 cytokine production seemed to be dominant in lymphoid cells of IL-4 deficient mice stimulated with soluble egg antigen (Pearce et al. 1996). These results suggest that IL-4 is not necessary for hepatic granuloma formation.

On the other hand, IL-10, another cytokine produced by Th2 cells, was shown to down-regulate Th1 responses by working synergistically with IL-4 (Oswald et al. 1992). IL-10 decreases egg antigen-specific Th cell responses by down-regulating MHC class II as well as B7 costimulatory molecule expression on accessory cells (Flores-Villanueva, Reiser and Stadecker 1994). Systemic administration of IL-10 significantly inhibited delayed-type hypersensitivity reactions to egg antigen as well as primary and secondary granuloma formation to eggs embolized in the lung. However, significant inhibition of hepatic granuloma formation associated with the natural infection required the use of an IL-10/Fc fusion protein with a prolonged in vivo half-life. Lymph node cells from IL-10/Fc-treated mice produced less IL-2 and interferon-γ and more IL-4 and IL-10 than control cells, suggesting that reduced egg granuloma formation resulted primarily from down-regulation of Th1 responses. These results indicate that suitable administration of exogenous IL-10 can be effective in ameliorating immunopathologic damage associated with schistosomiasis (Flores-Villanueva et al. 1996).

Administration of recombinant interferon-γ or IL-12 can also inhibit granuloma formation (Wynn et al. 1994). IL-12 is a key cytokine that promotes NK cell activity and Th1 responses. It has been demonstrated that the Th1-related cytokine, interferon-γ, augments endotoxin-stimulated IL-12 production in oil-elicited macrophages, whereas the Th2 cytokines, IL-4 and especially IL-10, are profoundly inhibitory. Thus, there exixts a positive feedback stimulation of IL-12 production by interferon that is regulated by IL-10 and IL-4 in vivo (Wynn et al. 1994). Further experiments have revealed that sensitization with eggs plus IL-12 partly inhibits granuloma formation and dramatically reduces the tissue fibrosis induced by natural infection with *S. mansoni*. These results may provide an example of a vaccine against parasites which acts by preventing pathology rather than infection (Wynn et al. 1995).

Thus, granulomatous inflammation in schistosomiasis mansoni seems to be a complexly regulated consequence of T cell-mediated hypersensitivity to soluble egg antigen (SEA). Thus, 3 consecutive independent chromatographic procedures have been carried out to fractionate and identify SEA recognized by schistosome-specific cloned murine, CD4$^+$ Th1-type lymphocytes, which had previously been shown to be capable of mediating granuloma formation in vivo when adoptively transferred to normal syngeneic hosts challenged with an intravenous injection of eggs. The stimulatory activity resided in 2 acidic egg molecules, with apparent molecular masses of 64–68 kDa and 38–42 kDa, each of which ran as a single band on SDS–PAGE after purification. Fast performance liquid chromatography and SDS–PAGE performed under reducing conditions suggested that the 2 molecules are related and that the 38–42 kDa molecule is a subunit of the 64–68 kDa molecule. Polyclonal lymphoid cells from schistosome-infected mice were similarly stimulated by the purified 64–68 kDa and 38–42 kDa molecules, implying that these are sensitizing antigens in the natural disease (Chikunguwo et al. 1993). This kind of identification of the molecules among crude SEA seems to be important for further studies on the identification of vaccine candidates that might regulate granuloma formation.

Antibody-mediated modulation of granulomas may occur in cases of schistosomiasis japonica, in which IgG1 antibodies are involved (Olds and Stavitsky 1986). Mitchell, Tiu and Garcia (1991) have discussed similarities and differences between *S. mansoni* and *S. japonicum* infections from various aspects of biology as well as immune responses, and also suggested that differences may exist even among geographical isolates or strains of the latter species.

An important aspect of granuloma formation is the nature of the cellular components. Infiltration of eosinophils is one of the conspicuous cellular responses observed. IL-5 is essential for granuloma eosinophilia, since treatment of mice with anti-IL-5 monoclonal antibody suppressed the eosinophil response (Cheever et al. 1992b). The granuloma eosinophils make substance P, a cytokine with immunoregulatory properties, which belongs to a family of hormones called tachykinins. This substance may modulate interferon-γ production through interaction with a substance P-like receptor expressed on CD4$^+$ granuloma T lymphocytes (Cook et al. 1994). Other prominent cellular components in granulomas are macrophages and fibroblasts. Macrophages produce macrophage inflammatory protein 1α (MIP-1α), a 6–8 kDa protein which is lipopolysaccharide inducible and monocyte- and neutrophil-chemotactic, and it has been shown that this protein contributes to cellular recruitment during schistosome egg granuloma formation (Lukacs et al. 1993). Moreover, IL-1, interferon-γ, and IL-10, cytokines found within the granuloma, were able to induce significant production of MIP-1 by granuloma fibroblasts, whereas the constitutive expression of monocyte chemoattractant protein-1 (MCP-1) was demonstrated in both unstimulated and cytokine-stimulated granuloma fibroblasts. Interestingly, normal noninflammatory fibroblasts from uninfected mice showed no significant production of MIP-1 or MCP-1 in response to these cytokines. These results suggest that granuloma fibroblasts may be phenotypically altered compared with normal fibroblasts and have a significant role in leukocyte recruitment, granuloma growth and maintenance of the egg-induced lesions (Lukacs et al. 1994a).

Recent studies have demonstrated a crucial role for tumour necrosis factor (TNF) during inflammatory granuloma formation. In addition, TNF has been shown to up-regulate adhesion molecules that participate in cellular recruitment and lymphocyte activation. The mechanism of TNF activation during *S. mansoni* egg granuloma formation and its relationship to the expression of ICAM-1 have been studied in some detail. Firstly, high affinity human soluble TNF receptor (TNFR) coupled to the Fc portion of an Ig (sTNFR:Fc construct) could effectively diminish granuloma formation and lymphocyte activation in vivo. Secondly, increased steady state ICAM-1 mRNA expression was observed in primary egg granulomas when compared with normal lung and foreign body (Sephadex bead) granulomas, which suggests a role for ICAM-1 in antigen-induced lesion formation. Subsequent studies have demonstrated that sTNFR:Fc treatment down-regulated granuloma formation and ICAM-1 expression, whereas anti-ICAM-1 decreased SEA-specific T cell proliferation in vitro. In addition, passive immunization of mice with anti-ICAM-1 monoclonal antibody during primary granuloma formation resulted in an attenuation of lesion development as compared with lesion development in a control antibody-treated group. The proliferative response to SEA was also significantly reduced in ex vivo experiments that used spleen cells from the anti-ICAM-1 treated mice. These data demonstrate that both TNF and ICAM-1 participate in lymphocyte activation and granuloma formation and suggest that one mechanism of TNF in granuloma development is through TNF-induced ICAM-1 expression (Lukacs et al. 1994b).

Thus, it is evident from these observations that cell–cell interactions through cytokine production and their responses to these cytokines, including expression of adhesion molecules, are essential for the development of egg granulomas. It might therefore be possible in future that immunomodulation with cytokines or antibodies to key molecules involved in the granuloma formation may be applied for clinical use in the prevention or treatment of tissue damage due to schistosome eggs. In addition, it should not be overlooked that cytokines secreted from non-Th cells may also be important in regulating egg granuloma formation.

2.3 Immune responses

In the preceding section, immune responses mainly to SEA were discussed from the pathological point of view, whereas this section focuses on immunity to schistosomiasis.

It has been assumed from epidemiological studies in endemic areas that age-dependent immunity may develop against infection, or against reinfection after treatment, with *S. mansoni* (Butterworth et al. 1985; Dessein et al. 1988) or *S. haematobium* infection (Hagan et al. 1991) (for review, see Butterworth 1994; Gryseels 1994). Using a mathematical model, it has also been shown that predicted patterns of variation in age-related changes in the intensity and prevalence of *S. haematobium* infection are consistent with the epidemiological effects of acquired immunity (Woolhouse et al. 1991). At present, however, there is no effective vaccine against schistosomiasis or any other human parasitic disease. In order to develop such vaccines, it is obviously important to elucidate mechanisms involved in protective immunity at the cellular and molecular levels because of the complex life cycles and stages of parasites which occur in the human body.

To better understand effector mechanisms in immunity to schistosomiasis, animal models may be useful at least for the initial steps of analysis, although there are apparent limitations in that results observed in animals do not always parallel those in humans. There are 2 experimental models for the induction of immunity to schistosome infections in vivo; the concomitant immunity model and the attenuated vaccine model. **Concomitant immunity** is so called after the immunity developed to a second tumour graft in animals that already carry the same tumour; thus animals (originally rhesus monkeys) carrying an initial infection of adult schistosomes show partial but significant protection to a cercarial challenge infection (Smithers and Terry 1967). Although this model may reflect more closely the immunity observed in humans, it has been replaced by the **attenuated vaccine** model in which animals are immunized with irradiated cercariae that can migrate into the lungs or liver but cannot mature. In the former model much of the parasite attrition appears to be closely linked to the pathology induced by the prior infection (Dean et al. 1978; Wilson, Coulson and McHugh 1983; von Lichtenberg 1985) rather than to immunologically specific antiparasite mechanisms.

As in other parasitic infections, cellular and humoral immune responses are observed in schistosomiasis against antigens derived from various developmental stages of schistosomes, although the responses to SEA play a major role in the pathology of this disease as described above. Responses may be observed against stage specific antigens or alternatively crossreactive antigens common to various stages. Immune responses may vary due to genetic difference in the class I and class II molecules of the major histocompatibility complexes (MHC), although the complexity of parasite antigens usually conceals such clear-cut regulation of the responses. These class I and class II molecules participate in the presentation of antigens by antigen-presenting cells to T cells. T cells with the CD8 marker on the surface may directly destroy cells infected with pathogens in the context of self recognition (i.e. the recognition of antigens complexed with an autologous class I molecule), whereas CD4 T cells (Th cells) recognize antigens complexed with a class II molecule and assist in immune responses by producing cytokines.

Recent work using murine models has clarified the involvement of Th cells in protective immunity to various parasitic infections including schistosomiasis. For example, interferon-γ has been shown to play a role in resistance to *S. mansoni* infection, whereas Th2 cytokines such as IL-4, IL-10 and IL-13 seem to be involved in determining susceptibility to parasitic infections or exaggerating pathological changes due to the infections by down-regulating Th1 responses and/or Th1-related cytokines such as IL-12 (Sher et al. 1992).

In addition to antigen presentation through the interaction of the processed antigen within a 'cradle' of the MHC molecule and the T cell receptor, stimulation of B cells or macrophages by activated T cells requires the interaction of other co-stimulatory molecules such as CD40 expressed on antigen-presenting cells, which may up-regulate another co-stimulatory signal such as B7, and their corresponding ligands, CD40 ligand (CD40L) or CD28, respectively, expressed on activated T cells (Yang and Wilson 1996; Grewal et al. 1996). The interaction between CD40 on macrophages or dendritic cells and CD40L on activated T cells has been shown to play a critical role in the accumulation of mRNA for a subunit p40 of IL-12 and bioactive IL-12 production (Kato et al. 1996). Moreover, further studies have revealed that the CD40–CD40L interaction may transduce some signal(s) so as to activate NF-κB which is transported into the nucleus and binds to the promoter region of the gene encoding for p40 (Nariuchi, personal communication). Since the production of IL-12 may result in the generation of Th1 responses, the involvement of this CD40–CD40L interaction may be expected in protection to *S. mansoni* infection, if interferon-γ plays a role in resistance by stimulating macrophages to produce IL-12 or in activating the cells to produce nitric oxide which contributes to resistance.

In humans, however, epidemiological surveys carried out in areas endemic for schistosomiasis mansoni or urinary schistosomiasis have suggested that there is a good correlation between the development of IgE antibodies, resulting from Th2 responses, and age-dependent resistance to reinfection (Hagan et al. 1991, Hagan 1992, Butterworth 1994). Indeed, parasite antigen-specific and -nonspecific IgE production and eosinophilia or eosinophil infiltration in parasitized local tissues are characteristic Th2 responses to helminth infections but not to viral, bacterial or protozoan infections.

The production and differentiation of eosinophils are controlled by at least 3 haemopoietic cytokines – GM-CSF, IL-3, and IL-5 – for each of which eosinophils have high-affinity receptors. IL-5 is considered the most important cytokine, being selectively involved in the production and maturation of eosinophils from bone marrow progenitors as well as in their prolonged survival and activation (Lopez et al. 1988; Chihara et al. 1990) (for reviews, see Takatsu, Takaki and Hitoshi 1994; Wardlaw, Moqbel and Kay 1995). The role of eosinophils as parasite-killer cells has been described by Mahmoud, Warren and Peters (1975) using anti-eosinophil serum in vivo and by Butterworth et al. (1975) who used an in vitro technique to determine release of chromium-51 from schistosomula damaged by blood eosinophils from normal individuals in the presence of patients' sera. The activity in sera from infected individuals was associated with an IgG fraction and could be removed on IgG-specific immunoadsorbent (Butterworth et al. 1977).

In human and rat systems, eosinophils have been shown to be the effector cells involved in antibody- or complement-dependent damage to various parasites including *S. mansoni* (Mackenzie et al. 1977; Capron et al. 1978; Ramalho-Pinto, McLaren and Smithers 1978;

Anwar, Smithers and Kay 1979). In the rat sysytem, Capron et al. (1978) demonstrated that IgG2a is the isotype responsible for promoting the adherence. The adherence of eosinophils to schistosomula, followed by movement of secretion granules toward the basal region of the cell interacting with the parasite surface, is a critical step for mediating the killing activity, the fusion of granules forming small vacuoles, the contents of which are released on to the surface of schistosomula (McLaren 1980). Using a slow-motion movie camera, these steps were also observed in antibody-dependent cell-mediated cytotoxicity (ADCC) against schistosomula of *S. japonicum* by a human eosinophilic leukaemia cell line, EoL-3, when the activity of the cells was enhanced by pretreatment with recombinant TNF (Fig. 25.19) (Janecharut et al. 1992). This was consistent with previous results demonstrating that TNF has no direct effect on the parasite but enhances human eosinophil cytotoxicity to *S. mansoni* larvae in a dose-dependent fashion (Silberstein and David 1986). In another experiment, TNF was reported to exhibit direct toxicity to schistosomula at high concentrations or at lower concentrations in the presence of interferon-γ (James et al. 1990).

Eosinophil granules contain several basic proteins such as a major basic protein (MBP) in the electron-dense crystalline core, or eosinophil cationic protein (ECP), eosinophil-derived neurotoxin (EDN), eosinophil protein X (EPX), and eosinophil peroxidase (EPO) in the less electron-dense matrix, and some of these are known to be toxic to parasites (Gleich and Adolphson 1986). However, it has been claimed that the precise regulatory and functional roles of eosinophils in protective immunity as well as in the pathology of human helminthiases are still unclear, because information in humans is largely limited to measurements of blood and tissue eosinophilia and IgE during the migration of helminths in various tissue sites (Wardlaw, Moqbel and Kay 1995). Another reason for the argument against the protective roles of eosinophils in ADCC is that the precise molecular structure

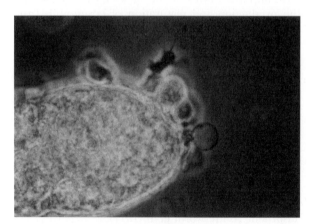

Fig. 25.19 Antibody-dependent cytotoxicity of EoL-3 cells against schistosomula *of Schistosoma japonicum*. An observation with a slow-motion camera, showing that granules and other contents of the cells are concentrated toward the surface of schistosomula (Janecharut et al. 1992).

of receptors reported to be expressed on eosinophils has not yet been well characterized, and there is controversy particularly concerning the exact nature of the interaction between IgE and eosinophils (Wardlaw, Moqbel and Kay 1995), even though the presence of a high affinity IgE receptor has been described not only on mast cells or basophils but also on human eosinophils (Gounni et al. 1994).

To examine the roles of IgE antibodies in protection, a hybridoma that produces a monoclonal IgE antibody to *S. japonicum* has been established (Kojima, Kanazawa and Niimura 1987). This monoclonal antibody (SJ18ε.1) recognized a 97 kDa antigen and the antibody was shown to be protective when it was passively transferred into mice during the early phase of the infection or used in ADCC in the presence of macrophages or rat eosinophils (Kojima, Kanazawa and Niimura 1987; Janecharut, Hata and Kojima 1991; Janecharut et al. 1992) The antibody reacted with a single protein of the same size extracted from *S. mansoni* that had been identified as paramyosin (Fig. 25.20), a muscle protein unique for invertebrates, by gene cloning and analysis of the deduced amino acid sequence (Laclette et al. 1991). By using SJ18ε.1 to screen a cDNA library obtained from adult *S. japonicum*, the gene coding for the target molecule has been cloned to confirm that the target of this monoclonal antibody is paramyosin (Nara et al. 1994). It has also been demonstrated that paramyosin localizes in the tegument and postacetabular glands as well as in the muscle tissues of schistosomula (Nara et al. 1994), although the localization of the molecule in tissues other than the muscles, even in isolated teguments, is argued to be questionable (Schmidt et al. 1996). Contrary to the argument, however, a comparative immunolocalization study among schistosome adults, cercariae and lung schistosomula by electron microscopy has revealed that paramyosin is localized within the muscle layer of all 3 developmental stages, within granules of the postacetabular glands of cercariae, and within the tegument matrix and surface of lung schistosomula (Gobert et al. 1977). *S. japonicum* paramyosin is composed of some 866 amino acids and is thought to have an α-helical conformation. If compared with the amino acid sequences of paramyosin demonstrated for other helminths, *S. japonicum* shares 96% homology with *S. mansoni* (Laclette et at. 1991), and 72% with *Echinococcus granulosus* (Muhlschlegel et al. 1993), but only around 35% with a parasitic or non-parasitic nematode, *Dirofilaria immitis* (Limberger and McReynolds 1990) or *Caenorhabditis elegans* (Kanagawa et al. 1989), indicating that the sequence of paramyosin is well conserved among platyhelminths.

Since ADCC in the presence of IgE antibodies has been shown to be involved in immunity to schistosome infections (Kojima, Nimura and Kanazawa 1987, Janecharut, Hata and Kojima 1991, Janecharut et al. 1992, Capron and Capron 1994), determination of the B cell epitope of paramyosin responsible for protection is important for the development a peptide vaccine for schistosomiasis. The epitope recognized by SJ18ε.1 was examined using a series of deletion mutants expressed in *Escherichia coli* and it was found that the antibody reacted with recombinant paramyosin containing 113 amino acids (Glu[301]–Ala[413]) but not with a shorter peptide (Glu[301]–Asp[343]). Thus, the epitope recognized by this antibody was expected to exist within 71 amino acid residues (Asp[343]–Ala[413]). Further analysis was carried out by a multi-pin system using heptameric peptides synthesized sequentially from these 71 amino acids of paramyosin and the result demonstrated significant binding of SJ18ε.1 to a

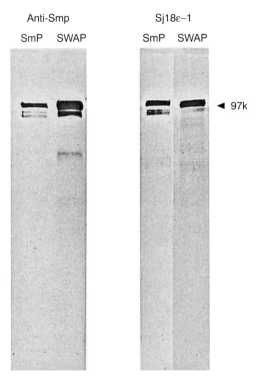

Anti-Smp   Sj18ε–1

SmP SWAP   SmP SWAP

◄ 97k

Fig. 25.20 SJ18ε.1 recognizes paramyosin of *Schistosoma mansoni*. SWAP, soluble worm antigen preparation of *S. mansoni*; SmP, paramyosin purified from SWAP; Anti-SmP, rabbit antiserum specific to SmP; SJ18ε.1, a mouse monoclonal IgE antibody (in collaboration with Dr Isabella Oswald and Dr Alan Sher.)

sequence consisting of 4 amino acid residues (Ile^{359}-Arg-Arg-Ala^{362}). The target epitope of SJ18ε.1 was common to paramyosins of *S. mansoni*, *Taenia solium* and *Echinococcus granulosus* but not to nematode paramyosins, suggesting that the epitope is specific for platyhelminths (Nara et al. 1997).

Paramyosin is a muscle protein of invertebrates and Pearce et al. (1988) have demonstrated that vaccination of mice with this molecule is effective in induction of resistance to *S. mansoni* infection. When administered intradermally with BCG at total doses of only 4–40 µg per mouse, both the native molecule and a recombinant expression product containing approximately 50% of the whole paramyosin were found to confer significant resistance (26–33%) against challenge infection, whereas 2 mg of an unfractionated complex soluble worm antigen preparation (SWAP) was required to induce similar levels of protection. In addition, paramyosin was shown to stimulate T lymphocytes from vaccinated mice to produce lymphokines such as interferon-γ that activate macrophages to kill schistosomula. Neither schistosome myosin nor a heterologous paramyosin from a different invertebrate genus was protective, indicating a requirement for specific epitopes in the immunization. That the protection induced by paramyosin involves a T-cell-mediated mechanism was supported by the failure of anti-paramyosin antibodies to transfer significant resistance to infection to recipient mice. Lymphocytes from mice vaccinated with paramyosin

were found to produce interferon-γ in response to living schistosomula, suggesting that during challenge infection of vaccinated hosts, paramyosin (a nonsurface antigen, according to Pearce et al. 1988) may elicit a protective T-cell response as a consequence of its release from migrating parasite larvae. These results suggest that the induction of T-cell-dependent cell-mediated immunity against soluble nonsurface antigens may be an effective strategy for immunization against multicellular parasites and also, in the case of schistosomes, identify paramyosin as a candidate vaccine immunogen in this category (Pearce et al. 1988). However, it is known that paramyosin is recognized by IgG antibodies in sera from patients with chronic schistosomiasis japonica (Kojima, Niimura and Kanazawa 1987) and elevated levels of antibody responses to paramyosin have been reported in *S. mansoni* infection among cured individuals after treatment with praziquantel (Correa-Oliveira et al. 1989). Therefore, it may be possible to induce an antibody-dependent cell-mediated immunity to human schistosomiasis by immunization with paramyosin, although at present the critical role of induction of Th1 responses in protection to human schistosomiasis cannot be excluded.

The other vaccine candidates for schistosomiasis are summarized in Table 25.4 and Fig. 25.21. Among them, the 23 kDa molecules of *S. japonicum* (Sj23) or *S. mansoni* (Sm23) are integral membrane proteins (Rogers et al. 1988) and the molecules share an 84% amino acid homology (Davern et al. 1991). Hydrophobicity analyses for both molecules suggest the presence of transmembrane regions arranged as 3 consecutive regions at the N-terminus followed by a relatively hydrophilic domain with a fourth domain at the C-terminus (Wright, Henkel and Mitchell 1990). Using antibodies, this protein has been detected in all stages of the parasite found in the human host, notably the lung stage, and therefore is of interest as a vaccine candidate. It is of particular significance that Sm23 (composed of 218 amino acids) was strikingly similar, with respect to both amino acid sequence (36% identity) and putative domain structure, to ME491, a human stage-specific melanoma-associated antigen (Wright, Henkel and Mitchell 1990). Sm23 and Sj23 also show a strong homology with a family of membrane proteins including the lymphocyte-expressed surface molecules CD37 and TAPA-1 and have therefore been suggested to play a role in cellular proliferation and parasite growth, because these membrane proteins are considered to be involved in cell proliferation (Davern et al. 1991). Thus, Sm23 and Sj23 have been shown to be members of a proposed new superfamily of membrane proteins whose structures do not conform to the previously known classifications. To date the other members include CD9 (p23), CD53, MRC OX-44, CO-029, MRP-1, L6, the gene product of TI-1, the target of monoclonal antibody AD-1. Most of these molecules, except for Sm23 and Sj23, are found in membranes of haemopoietic and/or malignant cells, although their function is not yet clear. In regard to schistosomes dwelling in the blood, however, this homology may be considered as an example of molecular mimicry, in which the parasite might have evolved a host-like molecule in an attempt to escape from host immune responses. Nevertheless, Sm23 has been shown to be a major antigen recognized by sera from animals vaccinated with irradiated cercariae (Richter and Harn 1993). The 2 predicted external hydrophilic domains were found to be highly immunogenic and contained several B-cell epitopes. There were at least 4

T-cell epitopes in the large hydrophilic domain. One segment of 23 amino acids contained both a T-cell and a B-cell epitope as well as the putative glycosylation site. This particular segment was recognized by immune sera and cells of every mouse strain tested. The elucidation of these epitopes demonstrates the immunogenic nature of this molecule and raises questions as to the role of Sm23 in the host–parasite relationship (Reynolds, Shoemaker and Harn 1992). However, it is still obscure whether these molecules are able to induce protection to human schistosomiasis, although a monoclonal antibody to Sj23 has been successfully used in immunodiagnostic assays to detect *S. japonicum* infection in Filipino patients (Davern et al. 1991). By using full-length Sm23 prepared with the baculovirus expression system, and the N-terminal 133 amino acids and the 85 C-terminal amino acids expressed by means of the prokaryotic vector pGEX, a total of 70 sera from patients from Sudan and Egypt were examined by ELISA or western blot analysis (Koster, Hall and Strand 1993). The anti-Sm23 antibody titres in infected patients varied widely and were not correlated with egg counts or age of the individuals. Most of the seroreactivity was directed against the C-terminal polypeptide.

Parasite enzymes have also been identified as vaccine candidates. The triose-phosphate isomerase (TPI) of *S. mansoni* was first described as a 28 kDa target antigen recognized by a monoclonal antibody (M.1) generated from mice immunized with membrane enriched extracts of mechanically transformed schistosomula (Harn et al. 1985). The monoclonal antibody M.1 passively transfers partial resistance (41–49%) to cercarial challenge in naive mice. Thus, the 28 kDa antigen recognized by M.1 is a putative vaccine candidate. Purified native 28 kDa antigen from adult parasites was shown to function enzymatically in a manner analogous to yeast and mammalian TPI in the reverse reaction. Addition of M.1 antibody to the enzyme reaction altered the catalytic activity of schistosome TPI. To determine the immunologic cross-reactivity of this vaccine candidate with mammalian TPI,

western blot analysis was performed and demonstrated that M.1 was immunologically specific for the schistosome enzyme (Harn et al. 1992). Amino acid sequence analysis of the purified native antigen revealed a significant homology to the human glycolytic enzyme, triose-phosphate isomerase (D-glyceraldehyde-3-phosphate ketol-isomerase, EC 5.3.1.1). The complete coding DNA for *S. mansoni* TPI was isolated and it was confirmed that this cDNA encodes the 28 kDa antigen recognized by M.1. The complete cDNA has been expressed within an *Escherichia coli* host to produce high levels of soluble recombinant *S. mansoni* TPI protein. The product was purified by the M.1 antibody and a functional TPI was obtained with an intrinsic specific activity comparable to that of rabbit and yeast TPI (Shoemaker et al. 1992). Further studies by Reynolds, Dahl and Harn (1994) have demonstrated that schistosome TPI is a potent inducer of IL-2 and interferon-γ production, driving production of these cytokines in the same cell populations of infected animals that have high Th2 responses directed at other SEA. With the goal of synthetic peptide vaccine design, recombinant TPI was used to determine specific T-cell and B-cell epitopes recognized by 2 strains of mice representing high and moderate responders (C57Bl/6J and CBA/J). All epitopes were selected from non-conserved regions of TPI and were thus parasite-specific. The investigators defined minimal size immunoreactive epitopes and synthesized 4-armed multiple antigenic peptides (MAP) consisting of T-cell and B-cell epitopes that could be recognized by both strains of mice in the same molecule. Characterization of the immunoreactivity of the MAP showed that higher antibody recognition of the MAP was attained when the B-cell epitope was placed on the N-termini relative to the T-cell epitope, whereas equivalent immunoreactivity occurred for the T-cell epitopes when located at either position. Most interesting was the finding that one of the minimal T-cell epitopes, when incorporated into the MAP, required enlarging to retain immunoreactivity. Finally, both the full-length TPI molecule and the final

Table 25.4 Vaccine candidates for schistosomiasis

Identity of antigen	Size (kDa)	Stage	Function/ localization	Protection (%) (mouse)	Reference
Paramyosin (Sm97) (Sj97)	97	Schistosomula Adult worms	Muscle protein	30	Pearce et al. (1988)
			Muscle, tegument	20–60	Unpublished, Kojima, Niimura and Kanazawa (1987), Nara et al. (1994)
Sj23/Sm23	23	All stages	Tegument		Reynolds, Shoemaker and Harn (1992)
TPI	28	All stages	Enzyme	30–60	Shoemaker et al. (1992), Reynolds, Dahl and Harn (1994)
GAPDH	37	Schistosomula Adult worms	Enzyme		Dessein et al. (1988)
GST (Sj26/Sj28) (Sm26/Sm28)	26/28	Schistosomula Adult worms	Enzyme	30–70	Balloul et al. (1987b)
IrV-5	200	Schistosomula	Muscle	32–75	Soisson et al. (1992)
IrV-1	90	All stages	Tegument		Hawn, Tom and Strand (1993)
FABP (Sm14)	14	Schistosomula	Tegument	67	Tendler et al. (1996)

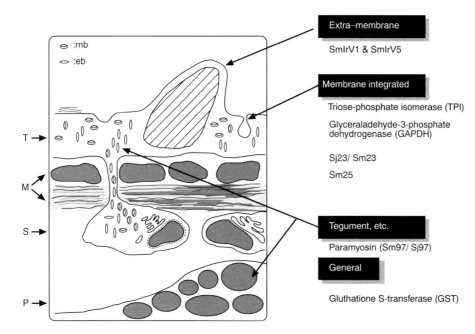

Extra–membrane

SmIrV1 & SmIrV5

Membrane integrated

Triose-phosphate isomerase (TPI)

Glyceraladehyde-3-phosphate
dehydrogenase (GAPDH)

Sj23/ Sm23

Sm25

Tegument, etc.

Paramyosin (Sm97/ Sj97)

General

Gluthatione S-transferase (GST)

Fig. 25.21 Localization of vaccine candidates for schistosomiasis.

version of the MAP were found to be immunogenic to T cells in naive animals and these molecules induced cross-recognition in the form of IL-2 and interferon-γ production (Reynolds, Dahl and Harn 1994).

Glyceraldehyde-3-phosphate dehydrogenase (GAPDH) was first identified as a 37 kDa molecule of schistosomula recognized by Brazilian children resistant to *S. mansoni* infection (Dessein et al. 1988). The cDNA for this antigen was cloned by screening a schistosome cDNA expression library with antibodies against the purified protein. The amino acid sequence of the encoded polypeptide shows 72.5% positional identity with human GAPDH. Antibodies against the recombinant protein identified the 37 kDa molecule on the larvae (Goudot-Crozel et al. 1989). Since a number of conserved proteins have been found to be major targets of host-protective immunity against *S. mansoni*, it is interesting to note, as suggested by these authors, that genetic restriction of the immune response to these antigens may occur in heterogeneous human populations because of the limited number of T-cell epitopes carried by these host-like proteins and that such genetic effects might allow parasite transmission through non-responder (susceptible) individuals.

Other candidates of an enzymatic nature are the glutathione *S*-transferases (GST) that consist of at least 2 isoenzymes of 26 kDa and 28 kDa for both *S. japonicum* and *S. mansoni* (Sj26, Sj28, Sm26 and Sm28) (Tiu et al. 1988). Mice of the inbred strain 129/J (WEHI 129/J) relatively resistant to chronic infection with *S. japonicum* were shown to be high responders to Sj26 (Smith et al. 1986). The cDNA sequence encoding Sj26, Sj28, Sm26 and Sm28 has been isolated and expressed in *E. coli* (Smith et al. 1986; Ballol et al. 1987; Henkle et al. 1990; Trottein et al. 1990). Despite their immunological cross-reactivity using rabbit antisera, Sj28 is weakly immunogenic relative to Sm28 in mouse immunization experiments using GSTs purified from adult worms. The difference in immunogenicity is also observed during schistosome infection in mice. Using surface-labelled living *S. japonicum* worms, evidence was obtained for a surface location of Sj28 comparable to that reported for the *S. mansoni* molecule. The nucleotide and deduced amino acid sequences of cDNA clones corresponding to Sj28 and Sm28 have been compared. Despite obvious homology (77% identity), differences were found in regions known to contain T-cell epitopes in the *S. mansoni* protein, which may be an explanation for the striking differences in immunogenicity in regard to antibody production in mice. The 26 kDa GSTs (Sj26 and Sm26) are also closely related on the basis of nucleotide and deduced amino acid sequences, with 82% identity in the putative coding regions. When the amino acid sequences of Sj28 and Sm28 were compared with those of Sj26 and Sm26, the overall sequence identity was approximately 20%. However, a relatively conserved region was identified in otherwise structurally different molecules which may participate in common properties of these enzymes (Henkle et al. 1990). A study of the tissue distribution of the cloned Sm26 by immunoelectron microscopy demonstrated similarities to Sm28 in that they are present in the tegument and in subtegumentary parenchymal cells. However, a major difference was observed in the protonephridial region in which Sm26 was present in the cytoplasmic digitations localized in the apical chamber delineated by the flame cell body, suggesting that Sm26 may be actively excreted by adult worms (Trottein et al. 1990). Experimental vaccination of rats, hamsters and monkeys with a recombinant fusion protein induced a strongly cytotoxic antibody response. Immunization of rats and hamsters with Sm28 resulted in significant protection against a natural challenge infection with live cercariae (Ballol et al. 1987). Moreover, the antibody response raised against this protein was able to kill *S. mansoni* schistosomula in in vitro cytotoxicity assays in the presence of rat eosinophils. The inhibition of this cytotoxic activity by an aggregated myeloma IgG2a indicated that one of the major isotypes involved in this in vitro model is IgG2a. The passive transfer of Sm28 antisera induced a significant level of protection against experimental infection. Vaccination of Fischer rats and BALB/c mice with purified 28 kDa protein resulted in a marked decrease (up to 70%) in the parasite burden in both experimental infection models (Balloul et al. 1987b). However, immunization with recombinant Sj26 was not sufficient to induce consistent immunity and maximum resistance was approximately 50%, while no protection was obtained in BALB/c mice, known low responders to Sj26. Although only Freund's complete adjuvant was used, the data indicated that satisfactory levels of resistance to *S. japonicum* may not be attained by vaccination with Sj26 alone. The requirement for other antigens, including the additional GST isoenzyme of Sj28, has been suggested to establish whether Sj26 will be an important component of a defined multivalent vaccine against schistosomiasis japonica (Mitchell et al. 1988).

An interesting molecule has been shown as a schistosome vaccine candidate by Strand and her colleagues (Soisson et al. 1992). Mice exposed to radiation-attenuated cercariae of *S. mansoni* are highly resistant to challenge infection, and sera from these mice can confer partial resistance when transferred to naive recipients. These sera recognize antigens present in schistosomula and adult worms, among them an 200 kDa antigen. A cDNA encoding a 62 kDa portion of this antigen was cloned and the deduced amino acid sequence of this cDNA clone was found to share homology with myosins of other species. To assess the immunoprophylactic potential, vaccination trials were carried out in mice using the recombinant polypeptide expressed as a fusion protein with β-galactosidase presented in the form of proteosome complexes with the outer membrane protein of meningococcus. The level of protection achieved was 32%, and this could be increased to 75% by removal of those amino acids included in the fusion protein that were derived from the vector to yield a polypeptide, designated rIrV-5. A similar level of protection was achieved when mice were immunized with the same dose of rIrV-5 in the form of protein complexes but without outer membrane protein, suggesting that protection did not require the use of adjuvant. However, at least 3 immunizations were necessary to achieve protection. Using monoclonal antibodies and sera from mice vaccinated with rIrV-5, the native protein recognized by antibodies against rIrV-5 was found to be a 200 kDa protein that was expressed on the surface of newly transformed schistosomula (Soisson et al. 1992). A further vaccination trial has been carried out in baboons with the rIrV-5 or radiation-attenuated cercariae. rIrV-5 was presented either in the form of protein micelles or complexed with the outer membrane protein of meningococcus to form proteosomes. The level of protection achieved in these groups ranged from 0 to 54%, with a mean of 27.7%, whereas in baboons exposed to radiation-attenuated cercariae the level of protection was very high, with a mean of 84%. The resistance observed after vaccination with rIrV-5 or radiation-attenuated cercariae was reflected in the overall histopathology. Vaccination of baboons with rIrV-5 or radiation-attenuated cercariae elicited an antibody response against epitopes exposed on the surface of newly transformed schistosomula. Analysis of individual baboon sera by ELISA demonstrated that there was a direct correlation between the anti-rIrV-5 titre and resistance to challenge worm burden, suggesting that the immunoprotective mechanism is antibody-dependent (Soisson et al. 1993).

Furthermore, in relation to SmIrV5, the molecular cloning and sequencing of SmIrV1, another candidate antigen recognized by immune sera raised in mice vaccinated with irradiated cercariae, has been performed (Hawn, Tom and Strand 1993). SmIrV1 contained a deduced amino acid sequence of 582 residues with similarity to 3 proteins: calnexin, calreticulin, and OvRal1 (a surface antigen of the filarial nematode *Onchocerca volvulus*). SmIrV1 was divided into 3 regions: a neutral N-terminal region with a putative signal sequence, followed by a proline- and tryptophan-rich P region in which 2 sets of sequences are repeated 4 times and a C-terminal region which is highly acidic with an isoelectric point of 4.7. The P and C regions of SmIrV1 reacted with sera of immunized as well as chronically infected mice.

Immunoprecipitation studies with antibodies raised against a portion of recombinant IrV1 demonstrated its presence in cercariae, schistosomula and adult worms with an apparent molecular mass on SDS–PAGE of 90 kDa. There was an approximate 6-fold increase in protein expression level during the transformation from cercariae to schistosomula. Consistent with a potential role as a molecular chaperone, IrV1 was associated with several metabolically labelled proteins in co-immunoprecipitation studies with the adult worm tegumental fraction. Similar to calnexin, IrV1 was metabolically labelled with phosphorus-32 on serine and threonine residues in adult worms and was one of the major phosphoproteins of this stage. This phosphorylation was developmentally regulated and coincided with the transformation of cercariae into schistosomula. The localization was also stage-specific as IrV1 was transported from internal regions of cercariae to the outer tegumental layer of schistosomula. Since the presence of IrV1 on the surface of schistosomula is an unprecedented localization for this family of endoplasmic reticulum proteins, further studies of the immunoprophylactic potential of this molecule are anticipated (Hawn and Strand 1994).

Relevant to the vaccine model with radiation-attenuated cercariae, another approach has been tried for the identification of candidate vaccine antigens (Richter and Harn 1993). To optimize recognition of a wide spectrum of antigens, several factors that may influence the level of protection in this model have been taken into consideration. The factors include the effect of single versus multiple vaccinations with irradiated cercariae, the dose of irradiation (150 or 500 Gy) administered to the cercariae, and the genetic background of mouse strains, high-responder (C57BL/6J) versus moderate-responder (CBA/J) mice. Results indicated that the number of vaccinations did not alter antibody specificity but modified the relative antibody titres against particular antigens, that the dose of irradiation used to attenuate the immunizing cercariae had a similar effect on antibody titres but in addition influenced antibody specificity, i.e only mice that had been vaccinated with moderately irradiated cercariae recognized cathepsin B (Sm31) and Sm32 and, interestingly, that when vaccinated mice of the C57BL/6J and CBA/J strains were compared, differences in antibody responses to particular antigens were observed. Both strains recognized the integral membrane protein Sm23, GST and cathepsin B, whereas Sm32 and paramyosin were recognized only by CBA/J mice, and heat shock protein (HSP) 70 was recognized exclusively by C57BL/6J mice. Thus, this study conclusively identified 6 distinct antigens that are specifically recognized by the humoral immune response of vaccinated mice. Interestingly, a distinct cellular immune response to paramyosin as well as to HSP70 was associated with high levels of resistance in C57BL/6J mice vaccinated with 15 krad (150 Gy)-irradiated cercariae (Richter, Harn and Matuschka 1995), suggesting the importance of T-cell involvement in induction of resistance to the infection.

More recently, Harn and his colleagues have also demonstrated that carbohydrate epitopes are major targets of sera from C57BL/6J and CBA/J mice vaccinated with 150 or 500 Gy (15 or 50 krad) irradiated cercariae of *S. mansoni* (Richter, Incani and Harn 1996). Antibody titres to carbohydrate epitopes increased with the number of vaccinations and were considerably higher in C57BL/6J mice than in CBA/J mice. The specificity of this anti-carbohydrate response was determined by measuring antibody binding to defined oligosaccharide residues known to be present on the parasite. A predominant target of the humoral anti-carbohydrate response of vaccinated mice was lacto-*N*-fucopentaose III, a molecule relevant to cell trafficking. There was no binding to its non-fucosylated homologue, lacto-*N*-neotetraose, or to oligosaccharides present on keyhole limpet haemocyanin. The strongest antibody response to lacto-*N*-fucopentaose III was observed for C57BL/6J and CBA/J mice repeatedly vaccinated with 150 Gy-irradiated cercariae, which also achieve the highest levels of protection. The predominant antibody class binding to lacto-*N*-fucopentaose III was IgM. From these results, the authors have concluded that in the irradiated cercariae vaccine model, C57BL/6J and CBA/J mice produce anti-carbohydrate antibodies against various stages of *S. mansoni* and that the oligosaccharide lacto-*N*-fucopentaose III is one target of this response. Lacto-*N*-fucopentaose III and its specific antibodies may profoundly affect host resistance and parasite homing.

Finally, a fatty acid binding protein was shown to form the basis of the protective immune crossreactivity between the parasitic trematode worms *Fasciola hepatica* and *S. mansoni* (Tendler et al. 1995). A recombinant form of the *S. mansoni* antigen, rSm14, protected outbred Swiss mice by up to 67% against challenge with *S. mansoni* cercariae in the absence of adjuvant and without provoking any observable autoimmune response. The same antigen also provided complete protection against challenge with *F. hepatica* metacercariae in the same animal model. The results suggest that it may be possible to produce a single vaccine that would be effective against at least 2 parasites, *F. hepatica* and *S. mansoni*, which are of veterinary and human importance respectively (Tendler et al. 1996).

Because there is a complex of cytokine networks and pathways of signal transduction, the development of vaccines against schistosomiasis must be carefully designed in order to focus particular effectors against specific target stages or molecules. In addition, further studies are urgently required in humans to elucidate immune effector mechanisms. Vaccines that can reduce schistosomiasis morbidity and mortality by lowering intensity of the infection should be adopted for practical use, when they become available, even if they are not effective in inducing complete elimination of parasites. Other factors such as the technical feasibility of production, the prospects of passage through existing regulatory bodies, and the ease of incorporation into existing immunization programmes, must be taken into account (Bergquist 1995).

2.4 Diagnosis

Specific diagnosis of schistosomiasis can be made by detection of the characteristic eggs in the stools or urine under microscopic examination. Biopsy at rectoscopy or cystoscopy may reveal eggs in the mucosa. For quantitative determination, which is necessary for evaluation of the success of chemotherapy or control operations, the Kato–Katz smear technique (though semiquantitative) or urine filtration technique may be used for intestinal or urinary schistosomiasis, respectively.

Indirect methods for the diagnosis depend on clinical symptoms and signs, and biochemical or immunological analyses. Especially for urinary schistosomiasis, haematuria is a suggestive sign and microhaematuria or proteinuria may correlate well with the intensity of infection in endemic areas (Savioli and Mott 1989). Immunodiagnosis may be useful for demonstration of active or chronic schistosomiasis. A unique immuno-

logical method for the diagnosis of schistosomiasis is the circumoval precipitin (COP) test in which precipitate is formed around the eggs containing live miracidia after incubation in the serum of infected individuals (Fig. 25.22).

The enzyme-linked immunosorbent assay (ELISA) is also widely used in diagnosis. Furthermore, ELISAs for the detection of circulating anodic antigen (CAA) and circulating cathodic antigen (CCA) in serum and urine have been developed and applied as an epidemiologic tool in a recent, intense focus of *S. mansoni* in Senegal (Polman et al. 1995). CAA and CCA in serum and CCA in urine were found in 94%, 83% and 95%, respectively, of the population, of which 91% were positive on stool examination. Circulating antigens were also detectable in sera and urine of most egg-negative individuals. The sensitivities of the urine CCA and serum CAA ELISA were substantially higher than that of a single egg count, and increased with egg output. The CAA and CCA levels correlated well with egg counts and with each other. The age-related evolution of antigen levels followed a similar pattern to egg counts, providing supplementary evidence for a genuine reduction of worm burden in adults in spite of the supposed absence of acquired immunity in this recently exposed community.

The selection and application of any diagnostic method used for field studies must correspond to the type of information sought by the public health officer or epidemiologist, based on operational and financial constraints, and such constraints and drawbacks must be taken into consideration for interpretation of test results (Feldmeier and Poggensee 1993).

2.5 Chemotherapy, prevention and control

There have been great advances in chemotherapy of schistosomiasis during the past 2 decades. Compared to antimonials, which were the only available chemotherapeutic agents for schistosomiasis from the 1920s to the 1960s, new drugs are more consistently effective, less toxic and applicable to oral rather than parenteral administration, thereby making field trials of mass chemotherapy feasible.

The drug of choice is praziquantel, which is effec-

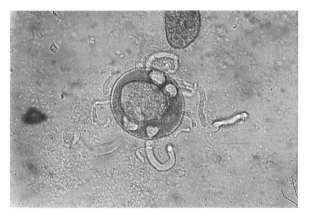

Fig. 25.22 *Circum oval precipitin (COP) test.*

tive against all species of schistosomes, although the precise mechanism by which it kills the parasites remains to be clarified (Redman et al. 1996). In vitro treatment of *S. japonicum* with praziquantel resulted in contraction of the parasite and the vacuolization of the tegument within 5 min after exposure to 1 mg praziquantel ml^{-1} in medium TC 199 (Mehlhorn et al. 1983). Praziquantel induces an influx of calcium ions across the tegument, causing an immediate muscular contraction (Mehlhorn et al. 1981). Praziquantel-induced contraction was found to be biphasic in normal parasites when incubated in high-magnesium medium, although only the larger, second contraction was observed in worms of which the tegument had been removed (Blair, Bennet and Pax 1994). These observations may suggest the presence of praziquantel-sensitive sites in the tegument (Redman et al. 1996). For schistosomiasis japonica, oral administration of praziquantel in 3 doses each of 20 mg kg^{-1} at 4 h intervals may result in 80% cure. At this dosage, about a half of the individuals receiving the treatment may complain of side effects such as abdominal discomfort, drowsiness, headache, backache, fever, sweating, and dizziness, although these are usually mild and transient. For schistosomiasis mansoni and haematobia, treatment with praziquantel is effective in a single dose of 40 mg kg^{-1}.

Recently, however, the possible existence of an *S. mansoni* isolate insusceptible to praziquantel has been reported from Senegal where the parasitologic cure rate 12 weeks after treatment was as low as 18%, although the frequency of egg counts with more than 1000 eggs g^{-1} faeces decreased to 5%, and the mean egg count of those remaining positive was reduced by 86% (Stelma et al. 1995). The low cure rates may be due to intense transmission and/or undeveloped immune responses in this recently exposed population. However, reduced drug susceptibility of the parasite isolate has now been confirmed by laboratory experiments in which groups of mice were infected with cercariae from the Senegalese isolate, or with laboratory-maintained Kenyan or Puerto Rican isolates. In 2 separate experiments, praziquantel was less effective against the parasite from Senegal than against the 2 other geographic isolates (Fallon et al. 1995). The insusceptibility of the Senagalese isolate to praziquantel may be defined as **tolerance**, indicating an innate insusceptibility of a parasite to a drug to which it has never been previously exposed (Fallon et al. 1996), whereas a genetically transmitted loss of susceptibility in a parasite population that was previously susceptible to a given schistosomicidal drug has been termed **resistance** (Cioli, Pica-Mattoccia and Archer 1993). Indeed, recent work carried out in Egypt, where praziquantel has been extensively used, has demonstrated that a small percentage (1–2.4%) of villagers may harbour parasites which cannot be killed even after repeated administration of high doses of praziquantel (Ismail et al. 1996) and when isolates obtained from these uncured individuals were examined in the mouse model, the ED$_{50}$ values of the isolates were found to be 3 times higher than that of

one reference control isolate (Fallon et al. 1996). The reduced susceptibility of *S. mansoni* to praziquantel in infected human populations has important implications for current schistosomiasis control programmes.

In relation to the efficacy of praziquantel, it has been suggested that the chemotherapeutic effect of the drug may depend on the host immune response (Sabah et al. 1985). Further studies have revealed that this is an antibody-dependent phenomenon (Brindley and Sher 1987, Doenhoff et al. 1987), and that the target antigen is a 200 kDa glycoprotein abundant in the tubercles and parenchyma of adult worms of *S. mansoni* (Brindley et al. 1989). Praziquantel is known to insert readily into lipid bilayers (Harder, Goosens and Andrews 1988, Schepers et al. 1988), causing rearrangement of the lipid molecules in the tegument and thereby leading to the influx of calcium ions into the schistosome and eventually resulting in the exposure of the previously masked target molecules (Brindley et al. 1989).

Another drug of choice for the treatment of schistosomiasis mansoni is oxaminiquine, which is given orally at 15 mg kg^{-1} body weight as a single dose for adults and 20 mg kg^{-1} for children with 2 divided doses. The dose may vary with geographic origin of the infection. Oxaminiquine is not effective against *S. haematobium* infection. Instead, metrifonate, an organophosphorus cholinesterase inhibitor, is used for the treatment of urinary schistosomiasis. Three doses at 5–15 mg kg^{-1} body weight are given at 2 week intervals.

Since immature (2–4 week old) worms are less susceptible to praziquantel than are larval (1–2 week old) worms or adult (5 week old or older) worms (Fallon et al. 1996) and some isolates of *S. mansoni* have been shown to be insusceptible to praziquantel, it is important to find new drugs for schistosomiasis. Quite recently, it has been reported that artemether, a derivative of artemisinin, is not only effective against malaria but also therapeutically effective against schistosomes, and that artemether is more effective against 7 day old schistosomules than other developmental stages of schistosomes (Xiao and Catto 1989). When artemether was administered intragastrically to mice on day 7 after infection with *S. japonicum* cercariae at a single dose of 300 mg kg^{-1} body weight, and the same dose of artemether was repeated at 1–3 week intervals 1–4 times after the first dosing, most of the female worms were killed before oviposition, with female worm reduction rates of 70–90%, resulting in protection of the host from damage induced by schistosome eggs. When rabbits and dogs were treated intragastically with artemether at 10 mg kg^{-1} on day 7 after infection, followed by 1–4 repeated weekly doses, the worm reduction rates were 85–99%. Moreover, some parameters related to acute schistosomiasis, such as temperature, eosinophil count and eggs in the faeces, were negative, and low specific antigen and antibody levels in serum were seen. Further study showed that the appropriate regimens of artemether were also effective in early treatment of reinfection

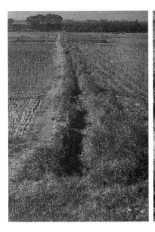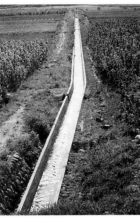

Fig. 25.23 Cement lining of irrigation ditches for control of *Oncomelania* snails (Courtesy of Yamanashi Prefectural Institute of Public Health).

with cercariae. Histopathological examination of the livers showed that early treatment with artemether exhibited a promising protective effect in dogs and rabbits. Based on these results, these authors concluded that early treatment with artemether could be recommended for field trials for controlling acute schistosomiasis, reducing infection rate and intensity of infection (Xiao et al. 1995).

Control of schistosomiasis is not an easy task. Even after successful treatment, reinfection easily takes place in most of endemic areas, unless transmission is cut off somewhere between the intermediate hosts

and the final hosts in the life cycle of the parasites. Control of schistosomiasis japonica is complicated by the existence of reservoir hosts, mainly domestic animals such as cows, pigs, sheeps and goats in China and dogs, cats, and water buffaloes in the Philippines, in addition to wild rats. Use of human night soil for fertilizer should be avoided in endemic areas. The snail hosts constitute a key factor in the control of schistosomiasis. In Japan, a periodical distribution of molluscicides such as sodium pentachlorophenate, Yurimin and later B-2 (sodium 2,5-dichloro-4-bromophenol), was applied in combination with cement lining of irrigation ditches in endemic areas for control of *Oncomelania* snails (Fig. 25.23). However, these measures can hardly be applied in such huge endemic areas as in China, and molluscicides are not suitable for application into water sources where aquatic snail hosts are abundant and on which people's daily life depends. Therefore, improvements of environmental sanitation and safety of supply water are essential for control. The successful control accomplished in Japan by 1978 indicates that to achieve the goal of control, the organization of voluntary associations including mothers' groups, and groups of medical doctors and workers, in cooperation with national and local government, may be important for self education and motivation of people themselves, although Japan has undergone rapid socioeconomic development resulting in drastic changes in agriculture or living styles, land reclamation projects, and increased awareness of schistosomiasis (Hunter and Yokogawa 1984).

REFERENCES

Anwar ARE, Smithers SR, Kay AB, 1979, Killing of schistosomula of *Schistosoma mansoni* coated with antibody and/or complement in preferential killing by eosinophils, *J Immunol*, **122**: 628–37.

Ariizumi M, 1963, Cerebral schistosomiasis japonica. Report of one operated case and fifty clinical cases, *Am J Trop Med Hyg*, **12**: 40–55.

Balloul JM, Gryzch JM et al., 1987a, A purified 28,000 dalton protein from *Schistosoma mansoni* adult worms protects rats and mice against experimental schistosomiasis, *J Immunol*, **138**: 3448–53.

Balloul JM, Sondermeyer P et al., 1987b, Molecular cloning of a protective antigen of schistosomes, *Nature* (London), **326**: 149–53.

Bergquist NR, 1995, Controlling schistosomiasis by vaccination: a realistic option?, *Parasitol Today*, **11**: 191–4.

Blair KL, Bennett JL, Pax RA, 1994, *Schistosoma mansoni*: myogenic characteristics of phorbol ester-induced muscle contraction, *Exp Parasitol*, **78**: 302–16.

Butterworth AE, 1994, Human immunity to schistosomes: some questions, *Parasitol Today*, **10**: 378–80.

Butterworth AE, Capron M et al., 1985, Immunity after treatment of human schistosomiasis mansoni. II. Identification of resistant individuals, and analysis of their immune responses, *Trans R Soc Trop Med Hyg*, **79**: 393–408.

Butterworth AE, Remold HG et al., 1977, Antibody-dependent eosinophil-mediated damage to 51Cr-labeled schistosomula of *Schistosoma mansoni*: mediation by IgG, and inhibition by antigen-antibody complexes, *J Immunol*, **118**: 2230–6.

Butterworth AE, Sturrock RF et al., 1975, Eosinophils as mediators of antibody-dependent damage to schistosomula, *Nature* (London), **256**: 727–9.

Capron M, Capron A, 1994, Immunoglobulin E and effector cells in schistosomiasis, *Science*, **264**: 1876–7.

Capron M, Capron A et al., 1978, Eosinophil-dependent cytotoxicity in rat schistosomiasis. Involvement of IgG2a antibody and role of mast cells, *Eur J Immunol*, **8**: 127–33.

Caulfield JP, Korman G et al., 1980, The adherence of human neutrophils and eosinophils to schistosomula: evidence for membrane fusion between cells and parasites, *J Cell Biol*, **86**: 46–63.

Cheever A, Finkelman FD et al., 1992a, Treatment with anti-IL-2 antibodies reduces hepatic pathology and eosinophilia in *Schistosoma mansoni*-infected mice while selectively inhibiting T cell IL-5 production, *J Immunol*, **148**: 3244–8.

Cheever AW, Finkelman FD, Cox TM, 1995, Anti-interleukin-4 treatment diminishes secretion of Th2 cytokines and inhibits hepatic fibrosis in murine schistosomiasis japonica, *Parasite Immunol*, **17**: 103–9.

Cheever AW, Kamel IA et al., 1978, *Schistosoma mansoni* and *S. haematobium* infections in Egypt. III. Extrahepatic pathology, *Am J Trop Med Hyg*, **27**: 55–7.

Cheever AW, Williams ME et al., 1994, Anti-IL-4 treatment of *Schistosoma mansoni*-infected mice inhibits development of T cells and non-B, non-T cells expressing Th2 cytokines while decreasing egg-induced hepatic fibrosis, *J Immunol*, **153**: 753–9.

Cheever AW, Xu Y et al., 1992b, The role of cytokines in the pathogenesis of hepatic granulomatous disease in *Schistosoma mansoni* infected mice, *Mem Inst Oswaldo Cruz*, **4**: 81–5.

Chensue SW, Ruth JH et al., 1995, In vivo regulation of macrophage IL-12 production during type 1 and type 2 cytokine-mediated granuloma formation, *J Immunol*, **155**: 3546–51.

Chensue SW, Terebuh PD et al., 1992, Role of IL-4 and IFN-γ

in *Schistosoma mansoni* egg-induced hypersensitivity granuloma formation. Orchestration, relative contribution, and relationship to macrophage function, *J Immunol*, **148**: 900–6.

Chihara J, Plumas J et al., 1990, Characterization of a recptor for interleukin-5 (IL-5) on human eosinophils: variable expression and induction by granulocyte/macrophage colony stimulating factor (GM-CSF), *J Exp Med*, **172**: 1347–51.

Chikunguwo SM, Quinn JJ et al., 1993, The cell-mediated response to schistosomal antigens at the clonal level. III. Identification of soluble egg antigens recognized by cloned specific granulomagenic murine CD4+ Th1-type lymphocytes, *J Immunol*, **150**: 1413–21.

Cioli D, Pica-Mattoccia L, Archer S, 1993, Drug resistance in schistosomes, *Parasitol Today*, **9**: 162–6.

Contis G, David AR, 1996, The epidemiology of bilharzia in ancient Egypt: 5000 years of schistosomiasis, *Parasitol Today*, **12**: 253–5.

Cook GA, Elliott D et al., 1994, Molecular evidence that granuloma T lymphocytes in murine schistosomiasis mansoni express an authentic substance P (NK-1) receptor, *J Immunol*, **152**: 1830–5.

Correa-Oliveira R, Pearce EJ et al., 1989, The human immune response to defined immunogens of *Schistosoma mansoni*: elevated antibody levels to paramyosin in stool-negative individuals from two endemic areas in Brazil, *Trans R Soc Trop Med Hyg*, **83**: 798–804.

Davern KM, Wright MD et al., 1991, Further characterisation of the *Schistosoma japonicum* protein Sj23, a target antigen of an immunodiagnostic monoclonal antibody, *Mol Biochem Parasitol*, **48**: 67–75.

Davis GM, 1980, Snail hosts of Asian Schistosoma infecting man: evolution and coevolution, *The Mekong Schistosome*, Malacological Review, Michigan, 195–238.

Dean DA, Minard P et al., 1978, Resistance of mice to secondary infection with *Schistosoma mansoni*. II. Evidence for a correlation between egg deposition and worm elimination, *Am J Trop Med Hyg*, **27**: 957–65.

Dessein AJ, Begley M et al., 1988, Human resistance to *Schistosoma mansoni* is associated with IgG reactivity to a 37-kDa larval surface antigen, *J Immunol*, **140**: 2727–36.

Fallon PG, Sturrock RF et al., 1995, Short report: diminished susceptibility to praziquantel in a Senegal isolate of *Schistosoma mansoni*, *Am J Trop Med Hyg*, **53**: 61–2.

Fallon PG, Tao L-F et al., 1996, Schistosome resistance to praziquantel: fact or artifact?, *Parasitol Today*, **12**: 316–20.

Farid Z, 1993, Schistosomes with terminal-spined eggs: Pathological and clinical aspects, *Human Schistosomiasis*, eds. Jordan P., Webbe G, Sturrock RF, CAB International, Wallingford, Oxon, 159–93.

Feldmeier H, Krantz I, Poggensee G, 1994, Female genital schistosomiasis as a risk-factor for the transmission of HIV, *Int J Std Aids*, **5**: 368–72.

Feldmeier H, Poggensee G, 1993, Diagnostic techniques in schistosomiasis control. A review, *Acta Tropica*, **52**: 205–20.

Feldmeier H, Poggensee G et al., 1995, Female genital schistosomiasis. New challenges from a gender perspective, *Trop Geogr Med*, **47** (**Suppl. 2**): 2–15.

Flores-Villanueva PO, Reiser H, Stadecker MJ, 1994, Regulation of T helper cell responses in experimental murine schistosomiasis by IL-10. Effect on expression of B7 and B7–2 costimulatory molecules by macrophages, *J Immunol*, **153**: 5190–9.

Flores-Villanueva PO, Zheng XX et al., 1996, Recombinant IL-10 and IL-10/Fc treatment down-regulate egg antigen-specific delayed hypersensitivity reactions and egg granuloma formation in schistosomiasis, *J Immunol*, **156**: 3315–20.

Fried B, Haseeb MA, 1991, Role of lipids in *Schistosoma mansoni*, *Parasitol Today*, **7**: 204.

Fripps PJ, 1967, The site of (1–14C) glucose assimilation in *Schistosoma haematobium*, *Comp Biochem Physiol*, **23**: 893–8.

Fuji Y, 1847, Katayama-ki, *Chugai Iji Shimpo*, **691**: 55–6 (redescription by Fujinami A, Chinese).

Fujinami A, 1904, Wetere Mitteilung uber die pathologische Anatomie der sog. 'Katayama-Krankheit' und der Krankheitserreger derselben, *Kyoto Igaku Zassi*, **1**: 201–13 (Japanese, with German abstract).

Fujinami A, Nakamura H, 1909, Infection route, development of the parasite, and infectivity of animals in Katayama disease (schistosomiasis japonica) in Hiroshima Prefecture, *Kyoto Igaku Zassi*, **6**: 224–52 (Japanese).

Furlong ST, 1991, Unique roles for lipids in *Schistosoma mansoni*, *Parasitol Today*, **7**: 59–62.

Furlong ST, Caulfield JP, 1989, *Schistosoma mansoni*: synthesis and release of phospholipids, lysophospholipids, and neutral lipids by schistosomula, *Exp Parasitol*, **69**: 65–77.

Gleich GJ, Adolphson CR, 1986, The eosinophilic leukocyte: structure and function, *Adv Immunol*, **39**: 177–253.

Gobert GN, Stenzel DJ et al., 1997, *Schistosoma japonicum*: immunolocalization of para myosin during development, *Parasitology*, **114**: 45–52.

Goudot-Crozel V, Caillol D et al., 1989, The major parasite surface antigen associated with human resistance to schistosomiasis is a 37-kD glyceraldehyde-3P-dehydrogenase, *J Exp Med*, **170**: 2065–80.

Gounni AS, Lamkhioued B et al., 1994, High-affinity IgE receptor on eosinophils is involved in defence against parasites, *Nature* (London), **367**: 183–6.

Grewal IS, Foellmer HG et al., 1996, Requirement for CD40 ligand in costimulation induction, T cell activation, and experimental allergic encephalomyelitis, *Science*, **273**: 1864–7.

Grove DI, 1990, *A History of Human Helminthology*, CAB International, Wallingford, Oxon, 187–295.

Gryseels B, 1994, Human resistance to *Schistosoma* infections: age or experience?, *Parasitol Today*, **10**: 380–4.

Grzych JM, Pearce E et al., 1991, Egg deposition is the major stimulus for the production of Th2 cytokines in murine schistosomiasis mansoni, *J Immunol*, **146**: 1322–7.

Hagan P, 1992, Reinfection, exposure and immunity in human schistosomiasis, *Parasitol Today*, **8**: 12–6.

Hagan P, Blumenthal UJ et al., 1991, Human IgE, IgG4 and resistance to reinfection with *Schistosoma haematobium*, *Nature*, **349**: 243–5.

Harinasuta C, Sornmani S et al., 1972, Infection of aquatic hydrobiid snails and animals with *Schistosoma japonicum*-like parasites from Khong Island, Southern Laos, *Trans R Soc Trop Med Hyg*, **66**: 184–5.

Harn DA, Gu W et al., 1992, A protective monoclonal antibody specifically recognizes and alters the catalytic activity of schistosome triose-phosphate isomerase, *J Immunol*, **148**: 562–7.

Harn DA, Mitsuyama M et al., 1985, Identification by monoclonal antibody of a major (28 kDa) surface membrane antigen of *Schistosoma mansoni*, *Mol Biochem Parasitol*, **16**: 345–54.

Hawn TR, Strand M, 1994, Developmentally regulated localization and phosphorylation of SmIrV1, a *Schistosoma mansoni* antigen with similarity to calnexin, *J Biol Chem*, **269**: 20083–9.

Hawn TR, Tom TD, Strand M, 1993, Molecular cloning and expression of SmIrV1, a *Schistosoma mansoni* antigen with similarity to calnexin, calreticulin, and OvRal1, *J Biol Chem*, **268**: 7692–8.

Henderson GS, Conary JT et al., 1991, In vivo molecular analysis of lymphokines involved in the murine immune response during *Schistosoma mansoni* infection. I. IL-4 mRNA, not IL-2 mRNA, is abundant in the granulomatous livers, mesenteric lymph nodes, and spleens of infected mice, *J Immunol*, **147**: 992–7.

Henkle KJ, Davern KM et al., 1990, Comparison of the cloned genes of the 26- and 28-kilodalton glutathione S-transferases of *Schistosoma japonicum* and *Schistosoma mansoni*, *Mol Biochem Parasitol*, **40**: 23–34.

Hockley DJ, 1973, Ultrastructure of the tegument of *Schistosoma*, *Adv Parasitol*, **11**: 233–305.

Hockley DJ, McLaren DJ, 1973, *Schistosoma mansoni*: changes in the outer membrane of the tegument during development from cercariae to adult worm, *Int J Parasitol*, **3:** 13–25.

Hunter GW III, Yokogawa M, 1984, Control of schistosomiasis japonica in Japan. A review – 1950–1978, *Jpn J Parasitol*, **33:** 341–51.

Iijima T, Garcia R, 1967, *WHO/Bilh/67.64*, WHO Assignment Report, WHO, Geneva.

Iijima T, Lo C-T, Ito Y, 1971, Studies on schistosomiasis in the Mekong Basin. I. Morphological observation of the schistosomes and detection of their reservoir hosts, *Jpn J Parasitol*, **20:** 24–33.

Ismail M, Metwally A et al., 1996, Characterization of isolates of *Schistosoma mansoni* from Egyptian villagers that tolerate high doses of praziquantel, *Am J Trop Med Hyg*, **55:** 214–8.

James SL, Glaven J et al., 1990, Tumour necrosis factor (TNF) as a mediator of macrophage helminthotoxic activity, *Parasite Immunol*, **12:** 1–13.

Janecharut T, Hata H, Kojima S, 1991, Effects of heterologous helminth infections on passive transfer of immunity using a mouse monoclonal IgE antibody against *Schistosoma japonicum*, *Parasitol Res*, **77:** 668–74.

Janecharut T, Hata H et al., 1992, Effects of recombinant tumour necrosis factor on antibody-dependent eosinophil-mediated damage to *Schistosoma japonicum* larvae, *Parasite Immunol*, **14:** 605–616.

Jiang J, Skelly PJ et al., 1996, *Schistosoma mansoni*: the glucose transport protein SGTP4 is present in tegumental multilamellar bodies, discoid bodies, and the surface lipid bilayers, *Exp Parasitol*, **82:** 201–10.

Jordan P, Webbe G, 1993, Epidemiology, *Human Schistosomiasis*, eds. Jordan P, Webbe G, Sturrock RF, CAB International, Wallingford, Oxon, 87–158.

Kagawa H, Gengyo K et al., 1989, Paramyosin gene (unc-15) of *Caenorhabditis elegans*. Molecular cloning, nucleotide sequence and models for thick filament structure, *J Mol Biol*, **207:** 311–33.

Kashiwado T, Ishijima F et al., 1927, Clinical report on the outbreak of schistosomiasis japonica in the Sakura region, *J Chiba Med Soc*, **5:** 1473–528.

Kato T, Hakamada R et al., 1996, Induction of IL-12 p40 messenger RNA expression and IL-12 production of macrophages via CD40-CD40 ligand interaction, *J Immunol*, **156:** 3932–8.

Katsurada F, 1904, *Schistosomum japonicum*, ein neuer menschlicher Parasit, durch welchen eine endemische Krankheit in verschiedenen Gegenden Japans verursacht wird, *Annot Zool Japan*, **5:** 147–60.

Klumpp RK, Chu KY, 1977, Ecological studies of *Bulinus rohlfsi*, the intermediate host of *Schistosoma haematobium* in the Volta Lake, *Bull WHO*, **55:** 715–30.

Kojima S, Kanazawa T et al., 1988, Epidemiologic studies on schistosomiasis japonica in a newly found habitat of *Oncomelania* snails in Japan, *Am J Trop Med Hyg*, **38:** 92–6.

Kojima S, Niimura M, Kanazawa T, 1987, Production and properties of a mouse monoclonal IgE antibody to *Schistosoma japonicum*, *J Immunol*, **139:** 2044–9.

Kojima S, Yokogawa M, Tada T, 1972, Raised levels of serum IgE in human helminthiases, *Am J Trop Med Hyg*, **21:** 913–8.

Koster B, Hall MR, Strand M, 1993, *Schistosoma mansoni*: immunoreactivity of human sera with the surface antigen Sm23, *Exp Parasitol*, **77:** 282–94.

Laclette JP, Landa A et al., 1991, Paramyosin is the *Schistosoma mansoni* (Trematoda) homologue of antigen B from *Taenia solium* (Cestoda), *Mol Biochem Parasitol*, **44:** 287–95.

Leiper RT, 1916, On the relation between the terminal-spined and lateral-spined eggs of *Bilharzia*, *Br Med J*, **i:** 411.

Liang Y-S, Kitikoon V, 1980, Susceptibility of *Lithoglyphopsis aperta* to *Schistosoma mekongi* and *Schistosoma japonicum*, *The Mekong Schistosome*, Malacological Review, 53–60.

Limberger RJ, McReynolds LA, 1990, Filarial paramyosin: cDNA sequences from *Dirofilaria immitis* and *Onchocerca volvulus*, *Mol Biochem Parasitol*, **38:** 271–80.

Ling CC, Cheng WJ, Chung HL, 1949, Clinical and diagnostic features of schistosomiasis japonica. A review of 200 cases, *Chinese Med J*, **67:** 347–66.

Lopez AF, Sanderson, CJ et al., 1988, Recombinant human interleukin 5 is a selective activator of human eosinophil function, *J Exp Med*, **167:** 219–24.

Lukacs NW, Chensue SW et al., 1994a, Production of monocyte chemoattractant protein-1 and macrophage inflammatory protein-1 α by inflammatory granuloma fibroblasts, *Am J Pathol*, **144:** 711–18.

Lukacs NW, Chensue SW et al., 1994b, Inflammatory granuloma formation is mediated by TNF-α-inducible intercellular adhesion molecule-1, *J Immunol*, **152:** 5883–9.

Lukacs NW, Kunkel SL et al., 1993, The role of macrophage inflammatory protein 1 α in *Schistosoma mansoni* egg-induced granulomatous inflammation, *J Exp Med*, **177:** 1551–9.

Mackenzie CD, Ramalho-Pinto FJ et al., 1977, Antibody-mediated adherence of rat eosinophils to schistosomula of *Schistosoma mansoni* in vitro, *Clin Exp Immunol*, **30:** 97–104.

Madden FC, 1899, A case of bilharzia of the vagina, *Lancet*, **i:** 1716.

Mahmoud AAF, Warren KS, Peters PA, 1975, A role for the eosinophil in acquired resistance to *Schistosoma mansoni* infection as determined by anti-eosinophil serum, *J Exp Med*, **142:** 805–13.

Martin LK, Beaver PC, 1968, Evaluation of Kato thick-smear technique for quantitative diagnosis of helminth infections, *Am J Trop Med Hyg*, **17:** 382–91.

McLaren DJ, 1980, Schistosoma mansoni: *The Parasite Surface in Relation to Host Immunity*, Research Studies Press, Chichester, 1–229.

Mehlhorn H, Becker B et al., 1981, In vivo and in vitro experiments on the effects of praziquantel on *Schistosoma mansoni*. A light and electron microscopic study, *Arzneimittel Forsch*, **31:** 544–54.

Mehlhorn H, Kojima S et al., 1983, Ultrastructural investigations on the effects of praziquantel on human trematodes from Asia: *Clonorchis sinensis*, *Metagonimus yokogawai*, *Opisthorchis viverrini*, *Paragonimus westermani* and *Schistosoma japonicum*, *Arzneimittel Forsch*, **33:** 91–8.

Mitchell GF, Garcia EG et al., 1988, Sensitization against the parasite antigen Sj26 is not sufficient for consistent expression of resistance to *Schistosoma japonicum* in mice, *Trans R Soc Trop Med Hyg*, **82:** 885–9.

Mitchell GF, Tiu WU, Garcia EG, 1991, Infection characteristics of *Schistosoma japonicum* in mice and relevance to the assessment of schistosome vaccines, *Adv Parasitol*, **30:** 167–200.

Miyairi K, Suzuki M, 1913, On the development of *Schistosoma japonicum*, *Tokyo Iji Shinshi*, **No. 1836:** 1–5 (in Japanese).

Mosmann TR, Coffman RL, 1989, Heterogeneity of cytokine secretion patterns and function of helper T cells, *Adv Immunol*, **46:** 111–47.

Mostafa MH, Badawi AF, O'Connor PJ, 1995, Bladder cancer associated with schistosomiasis, *Parasitol Today*, **11:** 87–9.

Mueckler M, Caruso C et al., 1985, Sequence and structure of a human glucose transporter, *Science*, **229:** 941–5.

Muhlschlegel F, Sygulla L et al., 1993, Paramyosin of *Echinococcus granulosus*: cDNA sequence and characterization of a tegumental antigen, *Parasitol Res*, **79:** 660–6.

Nara T, Matsumoto N et al., 1994, Demonstration of the target molecule of a protective IgE antibody in secretory glands of *Schistosoma japonicum* larvae, *Int Immunol*, **6:** 963–71.

Nara T, Tanabe K et al., 1997, The B cell epitope of paramyosin recognized by a protective monoclonal IgE antibody to *Schistosoma japonicum*, *Vaccine*, **15:** 79–84.

Olds GR, Stavitsky AB, 1986, Mechanisms of in vivo modulation of granulomatous inflammation in murine schistosomiasis japonica, *Infect Immunity*, **52:** 513–18.

Oswald IP, Gazzinelli RT et al., 1992, IL-10 synergizes with IL-4 and transforming growth factor-β to inhibit macrophage cytotoxic activity, *J Immunol*, **148:** 3578–82.

Pearce EJ, Casper P et al., 1991, Downregulation of Th1 cytokine production accompanies induction of Th2 responses by a parasitic helminth, *Schistosoma mansoni*, *J Exp Med*, **173**: 159–66.

Pearce EJ, Cheever A et al., 1996, *Schistosoma mansoni* in IL-4-deficient mice, *Int Immunol*, **8**: 435–44.

Pearce EJ, James SL et al., 1988, Induction of protective immunity against *Schistosoma mansoni* by vaccination with schistosome paramyosin (Sm97), a nonsurface parasite antigen, *Proc Natl Acad Sci USA*, **85**: 5678–82.

Peters PAS, Mahmoud AAF et al., 1976, Field studies of a rapid, accurate means of quantifying *Schistosoma haematobium* eggs in urine samples, *Bull Wld Hlth Org*, **54**: 159–62.

Polman K, Stelma FF et al., 1995, Epidemiologic application of circulating antigen detection in a recent *Schistosoma mansoni* focus in northern Senegal, *Am J Trop Med Hyg*, **53**: 152–7.

Ramalho-Pinto FJ, McLaren DJ, Smithers SR, 1978, Complement-mediated killing of schistosomula of *Schistosoma mansoni* by rat eosinophils in vitro, *J Exp Med*, **147**: 147–56.

Redman CA, Robertson A et al., 1996, Praziquantel: an urgent and exiting challenge, *Parasitol Today*, **12**: 14–20.

Reynolds SR, Dahl CE, Harn DA, 1994, T and B epitope determination and analysis of multiple antigenic peptides for the *Schistosoma mansoni* experimental vaccine triose-phosphate isomerase, *J Immunol*, **152**: 193–200.

Reynolds SR, Shoemaker CB, Harn DA, 1992, T and B cell epitope mapping of SM23, an integral membrane protein of *Schistosoma mansoni*, *J Immunol*, **149**: 3995–4001.

Richter D, Harn DA, 1993, Candidate vaccine antigens identified by antibodies from mice vaccinated with 15- or 50-kilorad-irradiated cercariae of *Schistosoma mansoni*, *Infect Immunity*, **61**: 146–54.

Richter D, Harn DA, Matuschka F-R, 1995, The irradiated cercariae vaccine model: looking on the bright side of radiation, *Parasitol Today*, **11**: 288–93.

Richter D, Incani RN, Harn DA, 1996, Lacto-*N*-fucopentaose III (Lewis x), a target of the antibody response in mice vaccinated with irradiated cercariae of *Schistosoma mansoni*, *Infect Immunity*, **64**: 1826–31.

Rogers MV, Davern KM et al., 1988, Immunoblotting analysis of the major integral membrane protein antigens of *Schistosoma japonicum*, *Mol Biochem Parasitol*, **29**: 77–87.

Rogers MV, Henkle KJ et al., 1989, Identification of a multispecific lipoprotein receptor in adult *Schistosoma japonicum* by ligand blotting analyses, *Mol Biochem Parasitol*, **35**: 79–88.

Rogers SH, Beuding E, 1975, Anatomical localization of glucose uptake by *Schistosoma mansoni* adults, *Int J Parasitol*, **5**: 369–71.

Rumjanek FD, McLaren DJ, Smithers SR, 1983, Serum-induced expression of a surface protein in schistosomula of *Schistosoma mansoni*: a possible receptor for lipid uptake, *Mol Biochem Parasitol*, **4**: 337–50.

Sabah AA, Fletcher C et al., 1985, *Schistosoma mansoni*: reduced efficacy of chemotherapy in infected T-cell-deprived mice, *Exp Parasitol*, **60**: 348–54.

Sakamoto K, Ishi Y, 1977, Scanning electron microscope observations on adult *Schistosoma japonicum*, *J Parasitol*, **63**: 407–12.

Savioli L, Mott KE, 1989, Urinary schistosomiasis on Pemba Island: low-cost diagnosis for control in a primary health care setting, *Parasitol Today*, **5**: 333–7.

Schmidt J, Bodor O et al., 1996, Paramyosin isoforms of *Schistosoma mansoni* are phosphorylated and localized in a large variety of muscle types, *Parasitology*, **112**: 459–67.

Senft AW, Maddison SE, 1975, Hypersensitivity to parasite proteolytic enzyme in schistosomiasis, *Am J Trop Med Hyg*, **24**: 83–9.

Sher A, Gazzinelli R et al., 1992, Role of T-cell derived cytokines in the downregulation of immune responses in parasitic and retroviral infection, *Immunol Rev*, **127**: 183–204.

Shoemaker C, Gross A et al., 1992, cDNA cloning and functional expression of the *Schistosoma mansoni* protective antigen triose-phosphate isomerase, *Proc Natl Acad Sci USA*, **89**: 1842–6.

Silberstein DS, David JR, 1986, Tumor necrosis factor enhances eosinophil toxicity to *Schistosoma mansoni* larvae, *Proc Natl Acad Sci USA*, **83**: 1055–9.

Skelly PJ, Kim JW et al., 1994, Cloning, characterization and functional expression of cDNAs encoding glucose transporter proteins from the human parasite, *Schistosoma mansoni*, *J Biol Chem*, **269**: 4247–53.

Smith DB, Davern KM et al., 1986, Mr 26,000 antigen of *Schistosoma japonicum* recognized by resistant WEHI 129/J mice is a parasite glutathione S-transferase, *Proc Natl Acad Sci USA*, **83**: 8703–7.

Smithers SR, Terry RJ, 1967, Resistance to experimental infection with *Schistosoma mansoni* in rhesus monkeys induced by the transfer of adult worms, *Trans R Soc Trop Med Hyg*, **61**: 517–33.

Soisson LA, Reid GD et al., 1993, Protective immunity in baboons vaccinated with a recombinant antigen or radiation-attenuated cercariae of *Schistosoma mansoni* is antibody-dependent, *J Immunol*, **151**: 4782–9.

Soisson LM, Masterson C P et al., 1992, Induction of protective immunity in mice using a 62-kDa recombinant fragment of a *Schistosoma mansoni* surface antigen, *J Immunol*, **149**: 3612–20.

Sornmani S, 1976, Current status of research on the biology of Mekong Schistosoma, *Southeast Asia J Trop Med Publ Hlth*, **7**: 208–213.

Stelma FF, Talla I et al., 1995, Efficacy and side effects of praziquantel in an endemic focus of *Schistosoma mansoni*, *Am J Trop Med Hyg*, **53**: 167–70.

Sturrock RF, 1993, The intermediate hosts and host-parasite relationships, *Human Schistosomiasis*, eds. Jordan P, Webbe G, Sturrock RF, CAB International, Oxon, 33–85.

Takatsu K, Takaki S, Hitoshi Y, 1994, Interleukin-5 and its receptor system: implications in the immune system and inflammation, *Adv Immunol*, **57**: 145–90.

Takatsu K, Takaki S, Hitoshi Y, 1994, Interleukin-5 and its receptor system: implications in the immune system and inflammation, *Adv Immunol*, **57**: 145–90.

Talla I, Kongs A et al., 1990, Outbreak of intestinal schistosomiasis in the Senegal River Basin, *Ann Soc Belge Med Trop*, **70**: 173–80.

Teesdale CH, 1982, *Biomphalaria angulosa* Mandahl-Barth as an intermediate host of *Schistosoma mansoni* in Malawi, *Ann Trop Med Parasitol*, **76**: 373.

Tendler M, Brito CA et al., 1996, A *Schistosoma mansoni* fatty acid-binding protein, Sm14, is the potential basis of a dual-purpose anti-helminth vaccine, *Proc Natl Acad Sci USA*, **93**: 269–73.

Tendler M, Vilar MM et al., 1995, Vaccination against schistosomiasis and fascioliasis with the new recombinant antigen Sm14: potential basis of a multi-valent anti-helminth vaccine?, *Mem Inst Oswaldo Cruz*, **90**: 255–6.

Tiu WU, Davern KM et al., 1988, Molecular and serological characteristics of the glutathione S-transferases of *Schistosoma japonicum* and *Schistosoma mansoni*, *Parasite Immunol*, **10**: 693–706.

Trottein F, Kieny MP et al., 1990, Molecular cloning and tissue distribution of a 26-kilodalton *Schistosoma mansoni* glutathione S-transferase, *Mol Biochem Parasitol*, **41**: 35–44.

Uglem GL, Read CP, 1975, Sugar transport and metabolism in *Schistosoma mansoni*, *J Parasitol*, **61**: 390–7.

Usawattanakul W, Kamijo T, Kojima S, 1982, Comparison of recovery of schistosomula of *Schistosoma japonicum* from lungs of mice and rats, *J Parasitol*, **68**: 783–90.

Voge M, Bruckner D, Bruce JI, 1978, *Schistosoma mekongi* sp. n. from man and animals, compared with four geographic strains of *Schistosoma japonicum*, *J Parasitol*, **64**: 577–84.

von Lichtenberg F, 1962, Host response to eggs of *S. mansoni*. I. Granuloma formation in the unsensitized laboratory mouse, *Amer J Pathol*, **41**: 711–31.

von Lichtenberg F, 1985, Conference on contended issues of immunity to schistosomes, *Am J Top Med Hyg*, **34:** 78–85.

von Lichtenberg F, Sadun EH et al., 1971, Experimental infection with *Schistosoma japonicum* in chimpanzees. Parasitologic, clinical, serologic, and pathological observations, *Am J Trop Med Hyg*, **20:** 850–93.

Wardlaw AJ, Moqbel R, Kay AB, 1995, Eosinophils: biology and role in disease, *Adv Immunol*, **60:** 151–266.

Warren KS, Domingo EO, Cowan RBT, 1967, Granuloma formation around schistosome eggs as a manifestation of delayed hypersensitivity, *Amer J Pathol*, **51:** 735–56.

WHO, 1993, *The Control of Schistosomiasis (WHO Expert Committee)*, World Health Organization, Geneva, 15, 18 and 79.

WHO, 1996, *The World Health Report 1996: fighting disease, fostering development*, World Health Organization, Geneva, 39.

Wilson RA, Coulson PS, McHugh SM, 1983, A significant part of the concomitant immunity of mice to *Schistosoma mansoni* is a consequence of a leaky hepatic portal system, not immune killing, *Parasite Immunol*, **5:** 595–601.

Woolhouse ME, Taylor P et al., 1991, Acquired immunity and epidemiology of *Schistosoma haematobium*, *Nature* (London), **351:** 757–9.

Wright ED, Chiphangwi J, Hutt M, 1982, Schistosomiasis of the female genital tract. A histopathological study of 176 cases from Malawi, *Trans R Soc Trop Med Hyg*, **76:** 822–9.

Wright MD, Henkle KJ, Mitchell GF, 1990, An immunogenic Mr 23,000 integral membrane protein of *Schistosoma mansoni* worms that closely resembles a human tumor-associated antigen, *J Immunol*, **144:** 3195–200.

Wynn TA, Cheever AW et al., 1995, An IL-12-based vaccination method for preventing fibrosis induced by schistosome infection, *Nature* (London), **376:** 594–6.

Wynn TA, Eltoum I et al., 1993, Analysis of cytokine mRNA expression during primary granuloma formation induced by eggs of *Schistosoma mansoni*, *J Immunol*, **151:** 1430–40.

Wynn TA, Eltoum I et al., 1994, Endogenous interleukin 12 (IL-12) regulates granuloma formation induced by eggs of *Schistosoma mansoni* and exogenous IL-12 both inhibits and prophylactically immunizes against egg pathology, *J Exp Med*, **179:** 1551–61.

Yamashita T, Boros DL, 1992, IL-4 influences IL-2 production and granulomatous inflammation in murine schistosomiasis mansoni, *J Immunol*, **149:** 3659–64.

Yang Y, Wilson JM, 1996, CD40 ligand-dependent T cell activation: requirement of B7-CD28 signaling through CD40, *Science*, **273:** 1862–4.

Yokogawa M, Sano M et al., 1971, An outbreak of *Schistosoma* infection among dairy-cows in the Tone River Basin in Chiba Prefecture (1), *Jpn J Parasitol*, **20:** 507–11.

Yokogawa M, Sano M et al., 1973, Epidemiological survey for schistosomiasis among the inhabitants in Tone river basin, Chiba Prefecture and snail control by burning, *Jpn J Parasitol*, **22:** 116–25.

Zhong C, Skelly PJ et al., 1995, Immunolocalization of a *Schistosoma mansoni* facilitated diffusion glucose transporter to the basal, but not the apical, membranes of the surface syncytium, *Parasitology*, **110:** 383–94.

LUNG AND LIVER FLUKES

M R Haswell-Elkins and D B Elkins

1 The parasites	2 Clinical and pathological aspects of infection

1 THE PARASITES

An estimated 70–100 million people harbour food-borne trematodes globally (Anon 1982). This large group of parasites includes the **liver flukes**, *Opisthorchis viverrini*, *Clonorchis sinensis*, *O. felineus*, *Fasciola hepatica* and *F. gigantica* and 9 or more species of the **lung fluke**, *Paragonimus* (Beaver, Jung and Cupp 1984, Toscano et al. 1995). A third group of food-borne trematodes found in humans, not detailed here, are the **intestinal flukes** (a wide variety including *Fasciolopsis*, *Echinostoma* and *Heterophyes*). Schistosomes, or **blood flukes,** are also trematodes, but are acquired by skin penetration, not via contaminated food (see Chapter 25).

Fasciola hepatica (Fig. 26.1a) was first referred to by de Brie in 1379 in sheep with 'liver rot', 500 years before the discovery and formal description of trematodes that infect humans. The parasite was named by Linnaeus in 1758, just before its discovery in a human by Pallas in 1760. *F. gigantica* was found in a giraffe and named by Cobbold in 1855. The life cycle of *Fasciola* was the first to be elucidated for a trematode; this was achieved concurrently but independently by Leuckart and Thomas in the 1880s and Lutz in 1892 (Beaver, Jung and Cupp 1984).

F. hepatica and *F. gigantica* are parasites of global veterinary importance, causing huge productivity losses in sheep, goats and cattle. The 2 species are difficult to differentiate morphologically, although they utilize different snail hosts. Their relative importance to veterinary and human health is debated. The less studied *F. gigantica* may be the more important veterinary species in the tropics, while *F. hepatica* predominates in cooler regions. Human fascioliasis is uncommon but distributed globally (Chen and Mott 1990).

Paragonimus westermani (Fig. 26.2a) was first discovered in the lungs of Bengal tigers by Kerbert in 1878. Shortly after, the worm was found at human autopsy and eggs were found in sputum by Ringer, Manson and Baelz in Taiwan and Japan. Kobayashi, S. Yokogawa and other Japanese investigators revealed the complete life cycle. There is debate regarding the number and relative importance of individual *Paragonimus* species infecting humans. Until recently, *P. wes-*

termani was thought to be the only agent of human infection, but at least 9 species are now known to be involved (Miyazaki 1982, Yokogawa 1982, Toscano et al. 1995).

C. sinensis was discovered by McConnel in 1874 at the autopsy of a Chinese carpenter in Calcutta, and the parasite was subsequently named by Cobbold in 1875. *O. felineus* was first reported in a cat, while in 1892 Winogradoff reported the first human infection in Siberia. *O. viverrini* (Fig. 26.3a) was first described in cats in 1886 by Poirier, then infection was discovered in a resident of Chiangmai, Northern Thailand by Kerr. Leiper identified the worms as a species distinct from *O. felineus* in 1915. These parasites have lived with humans for millennia; *Clonorchis* eggs have been found in a corpse from the West Han dynasty in China dated 278 BC (cited in Chen et al. 1994). Recently the liver flukes have attracted considerable interest because of their close association with bile duct cancer. *O. viverrini* infection was classified as a human carcinogen by the International Agency for Research on Cancer, and *C. sinensis* infection was judged a probable carcinogen (IARC 1994).

1.1 Classification

The liver and lung flukes belong to the Phylum Platyhelminths (flatworms), Class Trematoda and Subclass Digenea (Beaver, Jung and Cupp 1984). The latter term (digenetic trematodes) is often used to indicate the indirect life cycle involving several morphological stages and at least one intermediate host. The medically important food-borne flukes were once classified under a single genus, Distoma, referring to their 2 conspicuous suckers. Later it became clear that distomate flukes comprised a large and complex group of parasites, as indicated by today's classification into several superfamilies.

Fasciola, along with intestinal flukes *Fasciolopsis* and *Echinostoma*, belongs to the superfamily Echinostomatoidea. *Paragonimus* is a member of the superfamily Plagiorchioidea; whereas *Opisthorchis* and *Clonorchis* fall within the superfamily Opisthorchioidea. These orders are differentiated on the basis of life cycle (intermediate hosts), morphological structure (especially of the excretory bladder), the suckers in the adult worm and spines in intermediate stages, and size and maturity of eggs when laid.

Most food-borne trematodes are zoonotic, i.e. usual parasites of non-human animals which 'accidentally' infect

(a)

5.0 mm

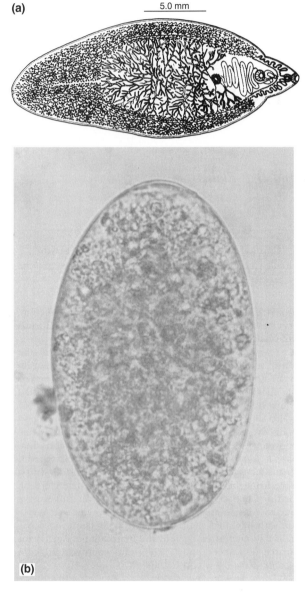

(b)

Fig. 26.1 The adult (a) and egg (b) of the liver fluke, *Fasciola hepatica*. (Drawn by S. Kaewkes, reproduced with permission.)

people. There are several species, for example of *Dicrocelium, Opisthorchis* and *Eurytrema*, which infect birds, livestock and mammalian wildlife and have been reported rarely in humans (Beaver, Jung and Cupp 1984).

1.2 Morphology and structure

The adult flukes are elongated, often described as 'leaf shaped' and bilaterally symmetrical with 3 body layers, but have no true body cavity (Schmidt and Roberts 1994, Rim 1986). They are covered with a non-ciliated integument which is not simply a secreted sheath: it is composed of complex, living tissue often containing invaginations and spines. *Fasciola* and *Paragonimus* species are covered with large spines. Muscles lie subcutaneously below the integument enveloping

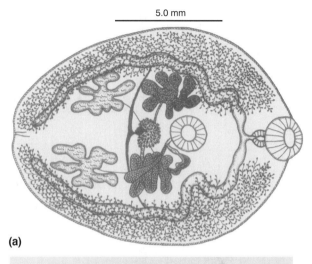

(a)

5.0 mm

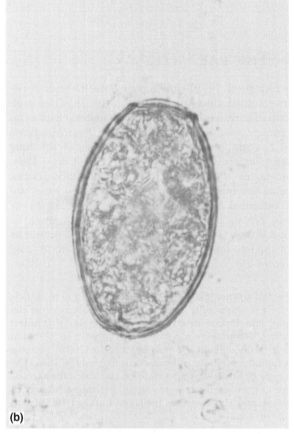

(b)

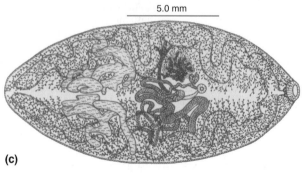

(c)

5.0 mm

Fig. 26.2 The adult (a) and egg (b) of the lung fluke, *Paragonimus westermani* and adult worm of *P. heterotremus* (c) (Drawn by S. Kaewkes, reproduced with permission.)

(a)

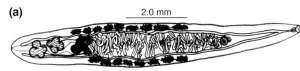

2.0 mm

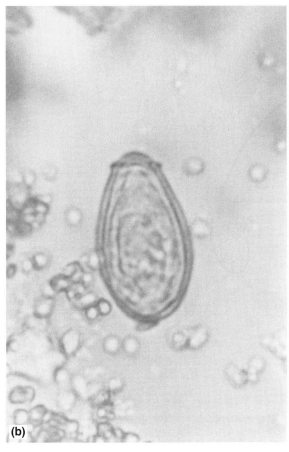

(b)

2.0 mm

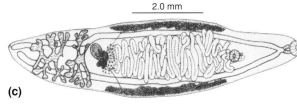

(c)

Fig. 26.3 The adult (a) and egg (b) of the. liver fluke, *Opisthorchis viverrini* and adult worm of *Clonorchis sinensis* (c) (Drawn by S. Kaewkes, reproduced with permission.)

the body, while specialized structures, such as the oesophagus and suckers, possess radial muscle fibres.

As mentioned above, the oral (surrounding the mouth) and ventral suckers are located in the anterior end, while the digestive system ends blindly with no rectum or anus. A specialized group of cells called solenocytes, or flame cells, join into an excretory bladder which exits through an excretory pore at the posterior end. This system probably carries out excretory functions and controls water balance. There is no circulatory system. The nervous system comprises an oesophageal commissure with ladder like pairs of nerve trunks running in each plane of the body ending in sensory processes. Eyespots may occur on free-swimming larval stages, but not on the adults.

A special feature of food-borne trematodes is their hermaphroditic (monoecious) reproductive system, that is, each individual worm produces both eggs and sperm. This contrasts with the schistosome trematodes which are dioecious (the sexes are separate) but in very close physical association (see Chapter 25). Most of the reproductive organs are positioned posteriorly to the ventral sucker, with their external opening (genital pore) often in close proximity to the ventral sucker.

The largest of the human liver and lung flukes is *Fasciola gigantica* (up to 75 mm long by 12 mm wide), followed by *F. hepatica* (30 mm × 13 mm) (see Figs 26.1a, 26.4). Both possess 'shoulders' and a conical anterior end. No single morphological feature definitively separates the 2 species, although genetic differences have been described (Blair and McManus 1989). *F. gigantica* tends to be more oblong with a longer, rounded posterior end, as compared to the short and more angular posterior end of *F. hepatica*. The testes of *F. gigantica* are located closer toward the anterior end, and its ventral sucker is larger than that of *F. hepatica*.

The intestinal caeca, testes and vitelline follicles of *Fasciola* are extensively branched. The eggs (Fig. 26.1b) are large, ovoid, yellowish brown with a small operculum and contain an immature larva, the miracidium. The eggs of *F. gigantica* (190 μm) tend to be consistently larger than those of *F. hepatica*, which are 140–150 μm long (Beaver, Jung and Cupp 1984).

Paragonimus (see Fig. 26.2a) is roughly half the size of *Fasciola*, measuring up to 16 mm long and 8 mm wide, oval-shaped and reddish brown in colour with an integument covered with scale-like spines (Miyazaki 1982). The ventral sucker is located toward the middle of the body and is of similar size to the oral sucker on the anterior end. The fluke possesses a large excretory bladder. Various morphological and life cycle differences in the adult worms distinguish the many species capable of infecting humans (e.g. *P. heterotremus*, Fig. 26.2c). The yellowish brown *Paragonimus* eggs are oval, measure 90 × 55 μm and have a flattened operculum (Fig. 26.2b). They are unembryonated when laid.

In humans, *Clonorchis* measures up to 20 mm long and 5 mm wide (see Fig. 26.3c), whereas the *Opisthorchis* species are somewhat smaller (see Figs 26.3a; 26.5; Komiya 1966, Rim 1986, Sadun 1955). The ventral sucker is smaller than the oral and located within the anterior half of the worm. Like *Fasciola*, the adult worm morphologies do not provide definitive separation, but the flame cell patterns on cercariae are distinct (Wykoff et al. 1965). The number and shape of testicular lobes, their location and the appearance of vitelline glands vary between, but also within, the species.

The genital pore through which eggs pass is located near the ventral sucker, with the large, coiled uterine glands filling most of the body. Eggs (Fig. 26.3b) are small (approximately 25 × 15 μm), yellowish brown, contain fully developed miracidia when laid, and have a knob at the posterior end and a distinct operculum on the anterior end. Measurements and shape vary

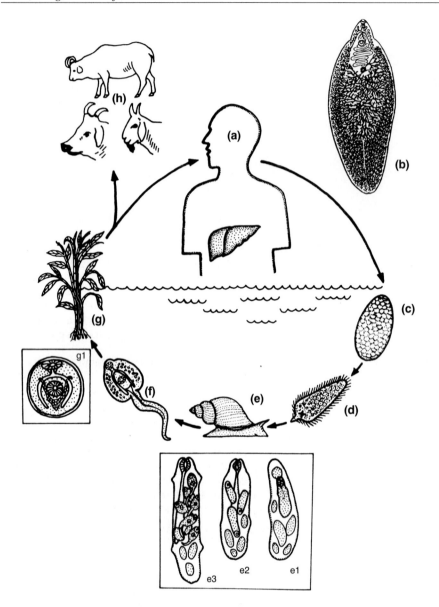

Fig. 26.4 The life cycle of *Fasciola hepatica.* (a) Definitive host: human; (b) The adult worm; (c) Unembryonated egg; (d) Miracidium; (e) First intermediate host: *Lymnaea* sp. Intramolluscan stages: el, sporocyst; e2, mother redia; e3, daughter redia; (f) Cercaria; (g) Second intermediate host: aquatic plants. Aquatic plant stage: gl, metacercaria; (h) Reservoir hosts: sheep, cattle, goat. (Drawn by S. Kaewkes, reproduced with permission.)

within and between species (Sadun 1955, Kaewkes et al. 1991, Ditrich et al. 1992).

1.3   General biology

Movement is a very important feature of trematodes. Their complex life cycle requires finding and entering appropriate hosts and extensive migration from the duodenum to the appropriate site of maturation within the final host (Schmidt and Roberts 1994). Flukes also undergo remarkable physiological adjustment in order to tolerate and function in their highly varied environments, from fresh water to invertebrate host to mammalian tissue. The fact that trematodes successfully utilize these extremely complex routes to achieve adulthood and reproduction reflects complex evolutionary development to maximize transmission.

Hou (1955) described the movement of *Clonorchis* by means of attachment and detachment of its 2 suckers combined with extension and contraction of the body. The 2 suckers, together with a collar of spines

on the immature worm, are presumably used to migrate up the biliary tract, against the flow of bile (Apinhasmit et al. 1993). Mature worms probably move short distances within the ducts. Attachment is secured by the ventral sucker adhering to the biliary epithelium, leaving the oral sucker free for feeding.

The nutritional supply of human trematodes is not precisely understood. Initially it was postulated that *Clonorchis* feeds on red blood cells, bile and epithelial cells. Hou (1955), however, suggested that the parasite lives on protein, oxygen and glycogen derived from mucin and tissue fluid entering the lumen following desquamation. *Fasciola* feeds on blood and hepatic tissue as it transverses the parenchyma during the migration phase, and its food supply in the bile duct may be similar to that of *Clonorchis*. The biliary flukes live in conditions of very low oxygen tension, and anaerobic glycolysis of glycogen to glucose is the major energy pathway (Schmidt and Roberts 1994). Ammonia, urea and amino acids are excreted. Among the amino acids released by *Fasciola* are remarkably

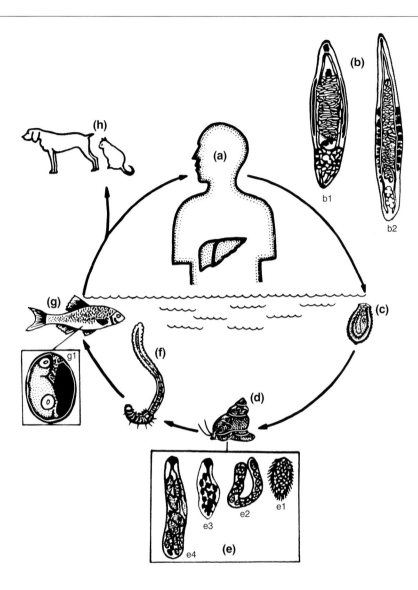

Fig. 26.5 The life cycle of human liver flukes: (a) Definitive host: human; (b) The adult worm. b1, *Clonorchis sinensis;* b2, *Opisthorchis viverrini;* (c) Embryonated egg; (d) First intermediate host: *Bithynia* sp.;(e) Intramolluscan stages. e1, miracidium; e2, sporocyst; e3, mother redia; e4, daughter redia; (f) Cercaria; (g) Second intermediate host: cyprinoid fish. Stage in fish: g1, metacercaria; (h) Reservoir hosts: dog, cat and other mammals. (Drawn by S. Kaewkes, reproduced with permission.)

high levels of proline (Isseroff, Tunis and Read 1972) produced by a parasite-derived enzyme, ornithine transaminase (Ertel and Isseroff 1974). The excess proline is implicated in pathogenesis (see section 2.2).

1.4 Life cycle

The life cycles of food-borne trematodes are complex, involving one or more intermediate hosts (the first always a snail), several morphological stages and distinct generations. These stages are similar between liver and lung flukes, and although intermediate host species vary, all are freshwater not marine.

DETAILS OF THE PARASITES IN HUMANS AND OTHER DEFINITIVE HOSTS

The infective stages of these flukes are called **metacercariae**. Humans become infected with *Opisthorchis* and *Clonorchis* by consuming raw or undercooked fish containing encysted metacercariae (Fig. 26.5). *Paragonimus* is acquired by eating metacercariae in raw crabs (Fig. 26.6), whereas *Fasciola* metacercariae encyst on aquatic plants (see Fig. 26.4). Ingested

metacercariae excyst in the duodenum, releasing larvae.

Newly excysted *Opisthorchis* and *Clonorchis* larvae migrate through the ampulla of Vater and the extra-hepatic bile ducts to the smaller, intrahepatic ducts where they mature. Within one month, adult worms begin producing an average of 10 000 eggs per day which exit the bile ducts and are excreted in the faeces (Sithithaworn et al. 1991).

Paragonimus larvae undergo systemic migration. Upon ingestion, the larvae are released in the duodenum, penetrate the intestine and enter into the abdominal cavity. The parasites enter and remain in the abdominal wall for some days, then continue migration through the diaphragm into the pleural cavity and lungs. When they reach the terminal alveoli or under the pleura, they become encapsulated by the host's inflammatory response and produce eggs. Eggs are expelled in the sputum or may be dislodged by coughing, swallowed and excreted in the faeces.

Fasciola metacercariae excyst in the duodenum, and the immature worms migrate through the duodenal wall, into the body cavity. They then burrow through

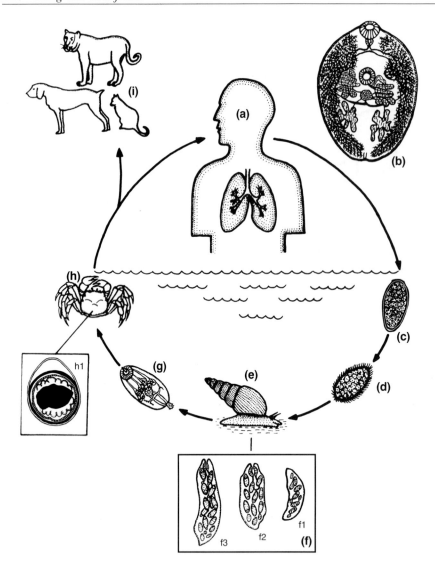

Fig. 26.6 The life cycle of *Paragonimus westermani*: (a) Definitive host: human; (b) The adult worm; (c) Unembryonated egg; (d) Miracidium; (e) First intermediate host: Thiarid snail; (f) Intramolluscan stages. f1, sporocyst; f2, mother redia; f3, daughter redia; (g) Cercaria; (h) Second intermediate host: crustaceans. Stage in crustacean: h1, metacercaria; (i) Reservoir hosts: dog, cat, tiger. (Drawn by S. Kaewkes, reproduced with permission.)

Glisson's capsule and across the hepatic parenchyma to the proximal bile ducts and gallbladder where they mature. This migration takes 6–7 weeks. The adult worms begin producing eggs which exit in the faeces 3–4 months after ingestion of metacercariae.

The worms may live many years. The maximum reported life span of *Clonorchis* in the absence of reinfection is 26 years from a Chinese emigrant, and average life span in endemic areas is about 10 years (Atwood and Chou 1978, Chen et al. 1994). Similarly *Paragonimus* is thought to live a maximum of 20 years and an average of 6 years; and *Fasciola* probably lives around 10 years (Chen and Mott 1990).

O. viverrini, *C. sinensis* and *O. felineus* infect pigs, cats, civets, rats, dogs and other mammals. *Fasciola* infections are maintained in domestic livestock, e.g. sheep, goats and cattle. *Paragonimus* infection can be carried by tigers and cats, rats, wolves, dogs and foxes. Although infection cannot occur by consuming adult worms or eggs within livers of infected animals, *Paragonimus* may establish through consumption of incompletely cooked pig or wild boar meat containing lung fluke larvae (Miyazaki 1982).

Patterns of infection in reservoir hosts are not always closely linked with those in humans, since these are determined by distributions of intermediate hosts, whereas human infection is further limited by eating behaviour (Sadun 1955, Rim 1986). However, reservoir hosts may be particularly important where human infections are uncommon or sporadic, and human egg excretion is inefficient (e.g. *Fasciola*, *Paragonimus*), or blocked by sanitation or anthelmintic treatment (*Opisthorchis* and *Clonorchis*).

DEVELOPMENTAL STAGES OF THE PARASITES

Freshwater bodies (small ponds, streams and rivers, flooded rice fields, and large reservoirs) or (for *Fasciola hepatica*) submerged grass become contaminated with eggs from the faeces and sputum (for *Paragonimus*) of infected people or reservoir hosts. The parasites must enter an appropriate snail. Species of *Bithynia*, *Melanoides*, *Parafossarulus* and *Assiminea* are important first intermediate hosts of *Opisthorchis* and *Clonorchis*. These snails become infected by ingesting eggs which already contain a fully mature miracidial larvae. In contrast, *Paragonimus* eggs develop and hatch in water after approximately 3 weeks. The released miracidia must find and penetrate a permissible species of snail; the major ones are of the genera *Semisulcospira*, *Thiara* and *Oncomelania*. *F. hepatica* miracidia develop and hatch within 2 weeks and swim until finding an appropriate snail of the genus *Lymnaea*. *F. gigantica* requires aquatic species of *Lymnaea*.

Inside the snail, the miracidia develop into **sporocysts** and **rediae**, which undergo parthenogenetic reproduction, finally giving birth to **cercariae**. Cercariae emerge and swim to find an appropriate site for transformation into **metacercariae**. Nearly 100 species of cyprinoid fish serve as the second intermediate host of *Opisthorchis* or *Clonorchis* (Komiya 1966, Vichasri, Viyanant and Upatham 1982). *Paragonimus* cercariae penetrate gills and muscles of freshwater mitten crabs (*Potamon*, *Sesarma*, *Eriocher*) or crayfish (*Astacus*); 53 crustacean species have been reported to serve as second intermediate hosts (Toscano et al. 1995). The cercariae transform into metacercariae in the viscera, muscles or gills. *Fasciola* encysts on green water vegetation, e.g. watercress; it does not enter a second intermediate host.

These life cycles require at least 4 months to complete and may be prolonged by winter hibernation of snails (Rim 1986). Seasonal variation in transmission, water temperature, densities of intermediate and reservoir hosts and human sanitation and eating behaviour govern life cycle completion and the prevalence of human infection.

1.5 Transmission and epidemiology

Geographic distribution

Crude estimates of the global number of human liver fluke infections is in the order of 30 million, made up of 19 million with *Clonorchis*, 9 million with *O. viverrini* and 1.2 million *O. felineus* infections (Rim 1986, Jongsuksantigul et al. 1992, Iarotski and Be'er 1993). Countries with endemic human liver fluke infection are Thailand and Laos (*O. viverrini*), Korea, China, Taiwan, (formerly Japan) and Vietnam (*C. sinensis*), and the Russian Federation and possibly eastern Europe (*O. felineus*). Approximately one-third of the 20 million mainly Laos-descendent people of northeast Thailand are infected with *O. viverrini*. Infections in China are also ethnically and geographically associated. Cantonese, notably Hakka people, are most frequently infected in the southern provinces of Guangdong and Guangxi, while infections in northeast China occur among the Korean national minority who migrated there (Chen et al. 1994). Infection in Hong Kong is probably acquired from eating fish imported alive from southern China.

The human lung flukes, which comprise approximately 9 species of *Paragonimus*, infect an estimated 22 million people globally (Miyasaki 1982, Yokogawa 1982, Toscano et al. 1995); with approximately 10 million in China alone. China harbours 3 species infecting humans, *P. westermani*, *P. heterotremus* and *P. skrjabini*. Other Asian countries with endemic *Paragonimus* infection include Philippines, Korea, Thailand and Laos. Peru and Ecuador report large areas endemic for *P. mexicanus*, while Cameroon and

Nigeria report *P. africanus* and *P. uterobilateralis*. Scattered reports have come from parts of India, Japan, Latin America, Liberia, Guinea and some Pacific countries.

Fasciola infections are much less numerous but even more globally widespread than *Paragonimus*. The World Health Organization reviewed numbers of cases of human *Fasciola hepatica* reported in the scientific literature and public health reports between 1970 and 1990 (Chen and Mott 1990). A total of 2594 reported cases were found in 42 countries; those reporting the most cases include France, the UK, Portugal, Spain and the former USSR (Tadzhikstan), Peru, Cuba and Egypt. This undoubtedly represents an underestimation because few community-based epidemiological studies have been performed. Furthermore, infection is often asymptomatic or without specific symptoms, diagnosis is problematic and reporting is incomplete. Little is known about the extent of human *F. gigantica* infection except that it has been reported in Africa, Asia, Hawaii, the former USSR, Vietnam and Iraq.

In addition to the endemic areas for all of these flukes, regional and global migration of people has sometimes broadened their distribution. Since life cycles usually do not become established, this has limited epidemiological relevance. Given the potential severity of resulting disease, however, it is of clinical importance that physicians recognize these infections (Chan and Lam 1987). The World Health Organization is concerned about the spreading of human trematode infections via the increasing international trade in fresh aquatic foods from countries in which such infections are endemic (Maurice 1994).

Social factors related to transmission

Raw or undercooked freshwater fish and crab are prepared in many different ways and these dishes are often of considerable cultural, medicinal and nutritional significance, making change difficult. This is aggravated by frequently held beliefs that marination in various sauces or consumption with alcohol kills the parasites. Transmission can also occur via contamination of utensils, hands and surfaces used first to prepare crabs, fish or vegetables for cooking and then for other foods taken raw. *Fasciola* and *Paragonimus* infection through contaminated water may be possible, but of lesser importance than through food.

Traditionally in southern China and among the Cantonese of Hong Kong, raw fish containing *Clonorchis* metacercariae is eaten by dipping in rice porridge or kongee (Chen et al. 1994). Large fish may be sliced and eaten raw with ginger and garlic. In some areas, children become infected by catching and incompletely roasting fish during play. Koreans eat raw fish soaked in vinegar, red-pepper mash or hot bean paste with rice wine at social gatherings (Choi 1984, Rim 1986). Vietnamese people reportedly eat raw fish in salads (Chen et al. 1994). Infection in Japan, which is now very rare, came from eating slices of large raw fish with vinegar or soya bean paste (Komiya 1966). Sushi and other uncooked sea fish eaten in Japan today do not carry *Clonorchis*.

In northeast Thailand and Laos, preparations may contain fresh (*koi pla*), partially fermented *(som pla)* or fully fermented *(pla ra)* uncooked fish which contain *Opisthorchis* metacercariae. *Koi pla* is probably the most important source of infection (Bunnag and Harinasuta 1984). People in western Siberia and other areas of the former USSR endemic for *O. felineus* enjoy eating uncooked fish frozen, salted or smoked with condiments. In addition to some groups of aboriginal people, migrants to endemic areas also become infected (Iarotski and Be'er 1993).

Raw crabs also carry important medical and social significance in some areas. For example in Korea, raw crayfish juice was used as a treatment for childhood measles (Choi 1990, Cho 1994), and young Bakossi women in Cameroon ate raw crabs to increase fertility (Kum and Nchinda 1982). Both practices have apparently become rare. Crabs and crayfish are also caught and eaten raw or incompletely roasted by children and workers in rice fields (Cabrera 1984). Traditional dishes often involve raw crab or crayfish meat or juice mixed with lemon juice (*ceviche* in Peru), brine, soya sauce (Korean *ke-jang*), alcohol (drunken crabs, China) or vinegar (Laos).

The consumption of watercress has been implicated in most human *F. hepatica* infections, especially in Europe (Hardman, Jones and Davies 1970, Jones et al. 1977). Morning glory and other water plants may be important vehicles of *F. gigantica* in Asia (Tesana, Pamarapa and Sae Sio 1989).

DISTRIBUTION OF INFECTION IN HUMAN COMMUNITIES

Local patterns of infection within endemic communities are partially determined by social customs and attitudes toward raw foods. This is especially true where these foods are thought to have medicinal or fertility-enhancing properties, where catching and eating raw foods is part of children's play or where the foods accompany certain social activities, such as drinking parties. Infection patterns may also reflect differential effectiveness of health education efforts in endemic countries.

Levels of *Opisthorchis* and *Clonorchis* infection vary greatly between communities, but age-related patterns are generally similar. The youngest ages show low prevalence and intensity, while these increase in the pre- and early teens and often reach a plateau in the late teen age groups (e.g. 15–19) or continue to rise. Prevalence and intensity either do not differ, or are higher, among males compared to females; sex differences tend to be greater in areas endemic for *Clonorchis* (Upatham et al. 1984, Rim 1986, Haswell-Elkins et al. 1991). The population of *O. viverrini*, and probably of all the liver and lung flukes, is highly aggregated within a small minority of heavily infected people.

There have been very few community-based studies of *Paragonimus* and *Fasciola* infections, so that their distribution is not well characterized. Studies in the 1950s and 1960s in Korea revealed prevalences of *Paragonimus* infection of up to 45% (according to skin testing) in endemic communities and as high as 13% nationwide. Recently, however, the occurrence of areas of high prevalence has dropped dramatically (Choi 1990, Cho 1994). In other endemic countries, e.g. China, Thailand, Laos, Cameroon, Nigeria, Peru and China, infections tend to occur at low prevalences (under 10%) in defined areas.

Mountainous areas with unpolluted water are favourable for *Paragonimus* transmission, and the availability of native freshwater fish and incomplete sanitation may determine *Opisthorchis* and *Clonorchis* prevalence in areas where these are eaten raw. *Fasciola* infection occurs mainly in rural areas and is most common among sheep and cattle herders. Outbreaks within communities and households are frequent, owing to the sharing of contaminated aquatic vegetables.

1.6 Location in host

Opisthorchis and *Clonorchis* locate within the small, intrahepatic bile ducts; in heavy infections, adult worms may also be found in the extrahepatic bile ducts, pancreatic ducts and gallbladder (Hou 1955, Sithithaworn et al. 1991). Infection is confined to the hepatobiliary tract lumen; there is no tissue migration phase (Sun, Chou and Gibson 1968). *Fasciola* also finally dwells in the bile duct, but its migration out of the duodenum and through the hepatic parenchyma causes much more tissue trauma and acute inflammation than that of *Clonorchis* and *Opisthorchis*. *Paragonimus* are found within fibrotic capsules in the terminal alveoli or under the pleura in the lungs after going through a similarly complex migratory process.

In addition to these usual migratory routes, some worms of *Fasciola* and *Paragonimus* may become lodged in ectopic sites. Ectopic sites of *Paragonimus* include the liver, brain, mesenteric lymph nodes, intestinal wall and subcutaneous tissue of the groin. *Fasciola* may locate in the liver parenchyma, blood vessels, lungs, subcutaneous tissue and the brain. Thus, as discussed below, clinical manifestations of this infection may be due to their accumulation in their 'normal' site or due to one worm which becomes encapsulated in a sensitive, ectopic site.

2 CLINICAL AND PATHOLOGICAL ASPECTS OF INFECTION

Although these infections are not considered numerous enough to be among the top tropical parasitic diseases according to the World Health Organization, there is no question that they are highly pathogenic and cause significant human disease. The very important clinical aspect of *Opisthorchis viverrini*, and to a lesser extent of *Clonorchis* infection, is the extreme susceptibility of infected people to bile duct cancer (IARC 1994). This cancer has a very poor prognosis, and few patients live longer than 6 months after diagnosis. Thus mortality due to complications of this fluke infection is very high in the endemic area of northeast Thailand, which reports the world's highest incidence of liver cancer (Vatanasapt et al. 1990, 1993).

Very importantly, in endemic areas, these infections are usually asymptomatic or may contribute to a high background level of non-specific illness that is difficult to distinguish from other causes. For example, the haemoptysis of *Paragonimus* requires parasitological and bacteriological differentiation from that of the more prevalent tuberculosis in co-endemic areas (Toscano et al. 1995). Similarly, the abdominal pain reportedly occurring in *Opisthorchis* infection is difficult to differentiate from that due to other causes. However, particularly in the case of the liver flukes associated with cholangiocarcinoma, the absence of symptoms does not indicate a medically unimportant infection. In fact, the typical lack of specific clinical signs and symptoms (or pain and discomfort) makes treatment and prevention even more difficult.

2.1 Clinical manifestations

The likelihood and types of clinical manifestations associated with these fluke infections are dependent on the location of the parasite in the liver, lungs or ectopic site, the species of fluke, number of worms harboured, duration of infection and, possibly, nutritional status and the individual's pattern of immune responses to parasite antigens.

O. VIVERRINI, C. SINENSIS, O. FELINEUS

The frequency and types of clinical disease seem to differ between the 3 closely related species. Most notably, there many reports in the *O. felineus* and *C. sinensis* literature detailing specific signs and symptoms accompanying well defined clinical stages of opisthorchiasis, from acute to chronic (Bronshtein 1986, Chen et al. 1994). Acute infection, characterized by chills and high fever, abdominal pain and distension, hepatitis-like symptoms and eosinophilia, is frequently reported in *O. felineus*. In contrast there are fewer reports of acute clonorchiasis (Koeningstein 1949, Chen et al. 1994) and none for *O. viverrini*. This difference may be due to the large number of migrants entering endemic areas of *O. felineus* who first become infected as adults (Iarotski and Be'er 1993); which may be a rare occurrence regarding the other 2 species.

Studies in 2 communities with very high levels of *O. viverrini* infection reported significantly increased frequencies of hepatomegaly, abdominal pain in the right upper quadrant, flatulence, dyspepsia and weakness associated with increasing intensity of infection (Upatham et al. 1984). An estimated 5–10% of the community had mild symptoms attributable to the infection. Hospital-based studies on patients with *Opisthorchis* and *Clonorchis* infection (lacking comparison with uninfected controls) have reported much higher frequencies of signs and symptoms. In addition to the above mentioned symptoms, eosinophilia, anorexia, dizziness, weight loss, diarrhoea, anaemia, oedema, neuropsychiatric symptoms and retardation of growth

and sexual maturity have been reported (Bunnag and Harinasuta 1984, Chen et al. 1994).

Stones in the gallbladder, liver and bile ducts have been linked to liver fluke infection. Eggs or worm fragments are often found in the nidus (Teoh 1963, Riganti et al., 1988). Hepatolithiasis is considered a major clinical manifestation of *Clonorchis* infection. An increase in gallbladder stone frequency with increasing intensity of *Clonorchis* infection was found by ultrasonography among Hakka people in Taiwan, from 4.2% in uninfected subjects to over 14% of those with heavy infections (Hou et al. 1989). Epidemiological associations with stones, however, are weaker for *O. viverrini* infection.

Ascending cholangitis, obstructive jaundice, portal hypertension, ascites and gastrointestinal bleeding are severe complications of liver fluke infection. However, only 88 cases of severe disease were reported among 15 243 infected people who presented to a Bangkok hospital for praziquantel treatment (Pungpak et al. 1985). Furthermore, these disease presentations are also typical of cholangiocarcinoma which may have been present in some patients.

Studies using ultrasonography have shown very strong relationships between gallbladder enlargement, wall irregularities and sludge and intensity of infection (Lim 1990, Mairiang et al. 1992). These abnormalities were not accompanied by clinical signs and symptoms and recovered 11 months after praziquantel treatment (Mairiang et al. 1993).

As mentioned above, the most important clinical manifestation of opisthorchiasis, also occurring in clonorchiasis, is bile duct cancer. People with heavy *O. viverrini* infection face at least a 14-fold increased risk of cholangiocarcinoma over uninfected people from the same communities (Haswell-Elkins et al. 1994a). This cancer is a major cause of death in the endemic area of northeast Thailand, where age-standardized incidences are 84.6 and 36.8 per 100 000 males and females, respectively (Vatanasapt et al. 1993). This compares to 2–4 cases per 100 000 typically arising in non-endemic areas. Areas endemic for *Clonorchis* infection also report higher frequencies of bile duct cancer (Rim 1986, IARC 1994). The average age of patients is 50 years, and due to an absence of early symptoms, those affected present to hospital in the late stages of the disease. Prognosis with or without surgery is poor.

FASCIOLA HEPATICA AND *F. GIGANTICA*

As with opisthorchiasis and clonorchiasis, fascioliasis is often asymptomatic, especially in light or chronic infection. Reported symptoms are grouped into 3 phases, depending on where the parasites are in their migration (Chen and Mott 1990).

First, the acute or invasive stage occurring when the flukes are in migration through the liver parenchyma may be accompanied by fever, mild to severe abdominal pain, gastrointestinal disturbances, urticaria, dermatographia and cough (Hardman, Jones and Davies 1970, Chen and Mott 1990, Patrick and Isaac-Renton 1992). Clinical signs may include hepatomegaly and splenomegaly, ascites containing eosinophils and other leucocytes, mild to moderate anaemia with its accompanying symptoms, pulmonary signs, eosinophilia and jaundice.

The latent phase of infection, during which the flukes are in the bile ducts, is generally asymptomatic, perhaps involving gastrointestinal symptoms; it can last for years. Some individuals progress to the obstructive phase of infection with chronic cholecystitis and cholangitis, which may be accompanied by biliary colic, epigastric pain, jaundice, nausea, pruritis and right upper quadrant pain precipitated by fatty foods. Gallbladder enlargement and stones are frequently found in these patients.

Ectopic *Fasciola* infections leading to pulmonary, cardiac, gastric, caecal, cerebral and neurological disorders have all been reported. These appear to be rare, although the frequency with which parasitic origins of such diseases are missed is unknown.

PARAGONIMUS WESTERMANI AND OTHER LUNG SPECIES

Because of interspecies differences in migratory behaviour and extent of pulmonary pathology, clinical manifestations vary between the various *Paragonimus* species infecting humans (Miyazaki 1982).

In general, however, the clinical manifestations of *Paragonimus* infection are often misdiagnosed as tuberculosis (Beaver, Jung and Cupp 1984, Toscano et al. 1995). Non-specific symptoms, e.g. diarrhoea, abdominal and chest pain, allergic reactions, fever and chills may be present during the migration phase. Once the worms establish, the most common symptoms are cough and haemoptysis which may be accompanied by night sweats and general malaise (Yokogawa 1982). Up to 50 ml of gelatinous, rusty brown sputum containing traces of blood and parasite eggs may be expectorated daily during paroxysmal coughing. Severe infections might progress to pleurisy, persistent rales, clubbed fingers and pneumothorax. The severity of pulmonary lesions viewed by chest roentgenograms is associated with intensity of egg output and duration of infection with *P. heterotremus* in Thailand (Vanijanonta, Bunnag and Harinasuta 1984).

Symptoms of ectopic infection occur after those in the lungs. If parasites lodge in the brain or spinal cord, which happens more frequently in children, severe disease may result (Miyazaki 1982, Bunnag and Harinasuta 1984, Jaroonvesama 1988). Symptoms may include headache, fever, paralysis, visual disturbances and (sometimes fatal) convulsive seizures. Recovery may be spontaneous, but symptoms may recur. Lesions are visualized by computed tomography or cerebral angiography.

Migration of worms under the skin leads to the formation of migratory swellings containing the parasites and eggs. Intestinal paragonimiasis which manifests as multiple granulomatous nodules or ulcers can be mistaken for gastric or abdominal tumours.

2.2 Pathogenesis and pathology

Although the role of immune responses in protection against infection is debated in all of these parasites, it is clear that these play an important role in pathogenesis and may determine whether clinically significant disease results.

PARAGONIMUS

Juvenile *Paragonimus* which migrate successfully to the lungs elicit insignificant pathology. However, adult worms and trapped eggs in the pulmonary parenchyma stimulate inflammation and granuloma formation, consisting mainly of eosinophils and neutrophils (Miyazaki 1982). These granulomas develop into fibrous capsules 1.5–5 cm in diameter usually surrounding a pair or triplet of worms, eggs and blood streaked fluid. Leakage of fluid into the bronchioles causes paroxysmal coughing, haemorrhage and blood in the sputum. Flukes which lodge in ectopic sites, e.g. the brain, spinal cord, intestine and heart, invoke similar inflammatory responses leading to ulcerations and abscesses which cause severe damage in sensitive sites.

O. VIVERRINI , O. FELINEUS AND C. SINENSIS

The acute phase of disease appears to result from acute inflammatory reactions to parasite antigens met for the first time (Chen et al. 1994). Typically light, chronic infections show minimal pathological change. In heavier infections, the liver may be enlarged with localised dilatation of slightly thickened, fibrosed peripheral bile ducts (Hou 1955, Tansurat 1971, Rim 1986). Histopathological changes (see Fig. 26.7) include proliferation and desquamation of bile duct epithelial cells, glandular formation, goblet cell metaplasia, inflammatory infiltration by lymphocytes, monocytes and eosinophils and severe fibrosis (Pairojkul et al. 1991). Although pathological changes are most frequent in the small ducts where the flukes reside, the gallbladder is commonly enlarged and its function affected, leading to bile stasis. In some cases, the extrahepatic bile ducts may also become inflamed and fibrosed, leading to strictures and stagnant bile. This might facilitate bacterial infection, leading to abscess formation and acute cholangitis (Chen et al. 1994).

Parasite products, mechanical or obstructive changes and the immune response all play a role in chronic pathogenesis, as well as in the carcinogenesis associated with infection. Based on experimental evidence, some authors suggest that the bile duct epithelial proliferation during chronic infection increases susceptibility to carcinogens, especially N-nitrosodimethylamine, in the diet (Thamavit et al. 1978, Migasena 1982). However, others have shown that infection also increases endogenous generation of nitric oxide and nitrosamines (Srivatanakul et al. 1991, Haswell-Elkins et al. 1994b). Furthermore, infection induces the enzyme cytochrome P450 2A6 which may be capable of transforming both endogenous and dietary nitrosamines to DNA-damaging agents (Kirby et al. 1994).

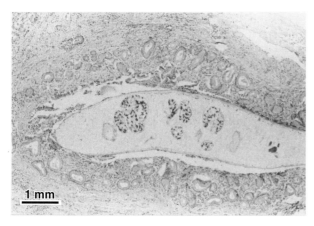

Fig. 26.7 Pathology of liver flukes: mature liver fluke, *Opisthorchis viverrini*, residing in the lumen of the human intrahepatic bile duct. Epithelial desquamation, adenomatous hyperplasia, periductal fibrosis and inflammatory infiltration are seen in the bile duct wall. Bar = 1 mm. (Photograph by B. Sripa, reproduced with permission.)

Fasciola hepatica and *F. gigantica*

Although *Fasciola* inhabits the bile duct and stimulates chronic inflammation and fibrosis, like *Opisthorchis* and *Clonorchis*, it has not been associated with biliary carcinoma. The pathological lesions are more similar to those of *Paragonimus*. This includes granulomatous inflammation encompassing eggs and abscess formation around the adult worms appearing grossly as multiple yellow nodules. Track-like inflammatory lesions appear along the migration route of the worms (Chen and Mott 1990). The cells initially involved are mainly polymorphonuclear leucocytes, histiocytes and lymphocytes. Later lesions contain lymphocytes and plasmocytes with fibrosis and calcification. Similarly, ectopically located parasites, mostly found in subcutaneous tissue, may form abscesses.

The pathogenesis of *Fasciola* therefore involves acute and chronic immune responses leading to granulomas, abscess and hepatic fibrosis. Direct parasite products and movement play a well defined role in pathology as the parasites eat their way through the liver to the bile ducts undergoing considerable growth. In addition, large amounts of proline produced and excreted by the flukes may be directly responsible for bile duct hyperplasia and dilatation and collagen deposition (Wolf-Spengler and Isseroff 1983).

2.3 Immune responses, nature and source of antigen

Whether the immune responses which develop in humans in response to liver and lung fluke infections confer protective immunity against the currently held parasites or newly acquired flukes remains unclear, and very little attention has been given toward vaccine development for humans (Sirisinha 1984, Spithill 1992).

Because of the economic and veterinary importance of fascioliasis, the immunology of *Fasciola* has been extensively studied in sheep, cattle and rodents. Differing degrees of acquired resistance are seen among these animals (Smithers 1976). Cattle and most rodents develop resistance to reinfection, but sheep and goats do not and may die in the face of continued exposure and accumulation of worms. Humans *Fasciola* infections are usually self-limiting and only few migrating larvae achieve establishment. However, this may not be related to immune responses.

Experimental vaccine trials against *Fasciola* in livestock have demonstrated that significant protection (up to 98%) can be conferred with irradiated larval vaccines (Spithill 1992). Vaccines targeting important individual antigens have been partially successful. For example, immunization with a recombinant glutathione *S*-transferase of *F. hepatica* has conferred over 50% protection against worm establishment in sheep.

Epidemiological patterns reveal little evidence of, but also do not rule out, protective immunity in humans exposed to *Opisthorchis* and *Clonorchis* (Sirisinha 1984). There is no decline in prevalence or intensity of infection among individuals exposed to decades of infection, and reinfection may occur rapidly following treatment in areas of heavy infection (Upatham et al. 1984, 1988). The parasites clearly survive in the face of high levels of parasite-specific IgG, IgA and IgE in both serum and bile (Wongratanacheewin et al. 1988), and of T cell reactivity to parasite antigens as demonstrated by delayed type hypersensitivity responses following skin testing (Rim 1986). Recently, however, Akai et al. (1994) have proposed that IgA antibodies to a 38 kDa antigen and IgM antibodies against a 42 kDa antigen of adult worms may confer protective immunity.

Even less is known about acquired immunity in human *Paragonimus* infection. However, the use of skin testing and antibody tests as diagnostic tools (see below) indicates that people mount strong cellular and humoral immune responses to parasite antigens. These do not appear to be protective.

2.4 Diagnosis

Similarities in egg morphology and cross-reactive antigens between intestinal flukes and liver flukes complicate both parasitological and immunological diagnosis. *Fasciola* eggs are indistinguishable from those of human *Fasciolopsis* and *Echinostoma* species, and *Opisthorchis* and *Clonorchis* eggs look similar to minute intestinal fluke eggs. Food-borne parasites often present in mixed infections and have overlapping endemic areas (Lee et al. 1984, Radomyos, Bunnag and Harinasuta 1984, Kaewkes et al. 1991). Nevertheless, diagnosis of lung and liver fluke infections is reliably and frequently based on the observation of eggs in the stool (all of the parasites) or sputum (*Paragonimus* only). Stoll's dilution method, formalin–ether (or formalin–ethyl acetate) concentration method (FECT) and AMS III are the most sensitive methods for processing specimens for egg examination (Chen and Mott 1990, Sithithaworn et al. 1991,

Toscano et al. 1995). *Fasciola* and *Paragonimus* infection pose a problem of diagnosis in the migratory phase, or in ectopic infection, when no eggs are passed.

Immunodiagnostic tests based on antibody detection are considered supplementary tools, rather than definitive diagnostic assays (Rim 1986, Sirisinha 1986). These tests cannot differentiate between current and past infection. Furthermore, the low sensitivity of antibody tests in detecting light infections and cross-reactions between trematodes are problematic (Chen et al. 1987, Ditrich et al. 1991, Elkins et al. 1991). Despite this, antibody tests are necessary in *Fasciola* and *Paragonimus* infections because of the need for diagnosis of prepatent infection. A variety of immunological tests have been used, with enzyme linked immunosorbent assay (ELISA) being sensitive and practical (Shaheen et al. 1989, Itoh and Sato 1990). Skin testing using extracts of adult *C. sinensis* or *P. westermani* antigens were widely used in Korea and China as epidemiological tools, but require confirmation for individual diagnosis (Komiya 1966, Rim 1986, Cho 1994). Immunoassays which detect parasite antigen (as opposed to host antibodies) may be the ideal diagnostic tools. Monoclonal antibodies to an 89 kDa antigen of *O. viverrini* antigens used in a faecal-based diagnostic ELISA are sensitive and specific (Sirisinha et al. 1995). Similar methods are reported for *Clonorchis* (Chen et al. 1987).

Clinical, pathological and radiological information clearly plays an important role in diagnosis as well as in determining the extent of pathological change that has occurred. Evidence of *Paragonimus* infection may be shown on radiographs as patchy foci of fibrotic change, with a characteristic 'ring shadow' (Bunnag and Harinasuta 1984, Toscano et al. 1995). Ultrasound diagnosis reveals abnormalities associated with liver flukes, e.g. gallbladder enlargement, stones and bile duct tumours (van Beers et al. 1990, Lim 1990, Mairiang et al 1992). Parasite fragments and eggs can sometimes be seen in surgical tissue or biopsies, revealing the unsuspected cause of the disease.

2.5 Control

The main tools for control of liver and lung flukes have been anthelmintic treatment, sanitation improvement and health education. The rationale is that treatment is required to eliminate the long-lived parasites immediately, sanitation interrupts transmission from human faeces to snails, and health education stops people from eating raw foods and becoming reinfected after treatment. Alternative strategies, such as freezing and irradiating fish (Song 1987, Lee et al. 1989, Iarotski and Be'er 1993), biological agents to destroy cercariae (Intapan, Kaewkes and Maleewong 1992) and treating reservoir hosts have been suggested but not widely implemented. Improving sanitation through latrines and stopping night-soil use on fields and fish ponds have been widely implemented to prevent liver fluke infection. Furthermore, environmental changes, the use of pesticides and pollution of river systems by industrial effluents, have also reduced intermediate host populations (Komiya 1966, Cho 1994).

A single dose of praziquantel is generally used at 40 mg/kg body weight for *O. viverrini* and *C. sinensis* in Korea, while higher, multiple doses (3×25 mg/kg for 1–3 days) are used in China. *Paragonimus* is also effectively killed by praziquantel at a dose of 25 mg/kg 3 times a day for 3 days. Side effects are transient and relatively minor. Published efficacy of praziquantel at these doses is over 90% (Chen et al. 1983, Viravan et al. 1986, Sui, Shu-hua and Catto 1988). *Fasciola* is not sensitive to praziquantel and treatment remains problematic (Patrick and Isaac-Renton 1992). Drugs currently used or proposed for this infection are dehydroemetine, bithionol and triclabendazole (Farag et al. 1988, Chen and Mott 1990). The latter drug may be the most promising (Wessely et al. 1988).

Despite the value of treatment, reinfection can and does occur in the case of *Opisthorchis* and *Clonorchis*. Complete success in control has been hampered by the difficulty in changing human behaviour. Health education campaigns have focused primarily on providing information about the disease, rather than on prevention. Since raw food consumption is often culturally specific, it often holds great importance for the identity of minorities, e.g. the Laos-descendent Thais of the northeastern region, the Korean minority of northeastern China, the aboriginal people of Siberia. Community participation and culturally appropriate health education messages are a vital element of long-term success (Sornmani 1987, Keittivuti, Keittivuti and Srithong 1986).

REFERENCES

Akai PS, Pungpak S et al., 1994, Possible protective immunity in human opisthorchiasis, *Parasite Immunol*, **16:** 279–88.

Anonymous, 1982, Introduction 'The wormy world', *Parasitic Zoonoses*, CRC Handbook Series in Zoonoses, vol III section C, eds Hillyer GV, Hopla CE, CRC Press, Boca Raton, FL, 1–16.

Apinhasmit W, Sobhon P et al., 1993, *Opisthorchis viverrini*: changes of the tegumental surface in newly excysted juvenile, first week and adult flukes, *Int J Parasitol*, **23:** 829–39.

Attwood HD, Chou ST, 1978, The longevity of *Clonorchis sinensis*, *Pathology*, **10:** 153–6.

Beaver PC, Jung RC, Cupp EW, 1984, *Clinical Parasitology*, 9th edn, Lea and Febiger, Philadelphia, PA, 406–81.

Beers B van, Pringot J et al., 1990, Hepatobiliary fascioliasis: non-invasive imaging findings, *Radiology*, **174:** 809–10.

Blair D, McManus DP, 1989, Restriction enzyme mapping of ribosomal DNA can distinguish between fasciolid (liver fluke) species, *Mol Biochem Parasitol*, **36:** 201–8.

Bronshtein AM, 1986, Morbidity from opisthorchiasis and diphyllobothriasis in the aboriginal population of the Kyshik village in the Khanty-Mansy Autonomous Region, *Med Parazitol (Mosk)*, **3:** 44–8 (in Russian).

Bunnag D, Harinasuta T, 1984, Opisthorchiasis, clonorchiasis, and paragonimiasis, *Tropical and Geographic Medicine*, eds McGraw RP, McIvor D, McGraw-Hill, New York, 461–9.

Cabrera BD, 1984, Paragonimiasis in the Phillipines: current status, *Arzneimittel Forsch*, **34:** 1188–92.

Chan CW, Lam SK, 1987, Diseases caused by liver flukes and cholangiocarcinoma, *Bailliere's Clinical Gastroenterology*, **1**: 297–318.

Chen MG, Hua XJ et al., 1983, Praziquantel in 237 cases of clonorchiasis sinensis, *Chin Med J*, **96**: 935–40.

Chen MG, Mott KE, 1990, Progress in assessment of morbidity due to *Fasciola hepatica* infection: a review of recent literature, *Trop Dis Bull*, **87**: R1–R38.

Chen MG, Lu Y et al., 1994, Progress in assessment of morbidity due to *Clonorchis sinensis* infection: a review of recent literature, *Trop Dis Bull*, **91**: R7–R65.

Chen YT, Liu YH et al., 1987, Detection of circulating antigen in sera from clonorchiasis sinensis patients by ELISA double sandwich method, *Chin Med J*, **101**: 92–7.

Cho S-Y, 1994, Epidemiology of paragonimiasis in Korea, *Collected Papers on Parasite Control in Korea*, eds Chai J-Y, Cho S-Y et al., The Korean Association of Health, Seoul, 51–7.

Choi DW, 1984, *Clonorchis sinensis*: life cycle, intermediate hosts, transmission to man and geographical distribution in Korea, *Arzneimittel Forsch*, **34**: 1145–51.

Choi DW, 1990, *Paragonimus* and paragonimiasis in Korea, *Korean J Parasitol*, **28**: 79–102.

Ditrich O, Giboda M et al., 1992, Comparative morphology of eggs of the Haplorchiinae (Trematoda: Heterophyidae) and some other medically important heterophyid and Opisthorchiid flukes, *Folia Parasitol*, **39**: 123–32.

Ditrich O, Kopacek P et al., 1991, Serological differentiation of human small fluke infections using *Opisthorchis viverrini* and *Haplorchis taichui* antigens, *Southeast Asian J Trop Med Public Health*, **22 (Supplement)**: 174–8.

Elkins DB, Sithithaworn P et al., 1991, *Opisthorchis viverrini*: relationships between egg counts, worms recovered and antibody levels within an endemic community in Northeast Thailand, *Parasitology*, **102**: 283–8.

Ertel J, Isseroff H, 1974, Proline in fascioliasis: 1. Comparative activities of ornithine-L-transaminase and proline oxidase in *Fasciola* and mammalian livers, *J Parasitol*, **60**: 574–7.

Farag HF, Salem A et al., 1988, Bithionol (Bitin) treatment in established fascioliasis in Egyptians, *J Trop Med Hyg*, **91**: 240–5.

Hardman EW, Jones RLH, Davies AH, 1970, Fascioliasis – a large outbreak, *Br Med J*, **3**: 502–5.

Haswell-Elkins MR, Elkins DB et al., 1991, Distribution patterns of *Opisthorchis viverrini* within a human community, *Parasitology*, **103**: 97–101.

Haswell-Elkins MR, Mairiang E et al., 1994a, Cross-sectional study of *Opisthorchis viverrini* infection and cholangiocarcinoma in communities within a high-risk area in Northeast Thailand, *Int J Cancer*, **59**: 505–9.

Haswell-Elkins MR, Satarug S et al., 1994b, Liver fluke infection and cholangiocarcinoma: model of endogenous nitric oxide and extragastric nitrosation in human carcinogenesis, *Mutat Res*, **305**: 241–252.

Hou MF, Ker CG et al., 1989, The ultrasound survey of gallstone diseases of patients infected with *Clonorchis sinensis* in Southern Taiwan, *J Trop Med Hyg*, **92**: 108–11.

Hou PC, 1955, The pathology of *Clonorchis sinensis* infestation of the liver, *J Pathol Bacteriol*, **70**: 53–68.

IARC Working Group, 1994, *Schistosomes, Liver Flukes and Helicobacter pylori*, IARC Monographs on the Evaluation of Carcinogenic Risks to Humans, vol. 6., International Agency for Research on Cancer, Lyon, 121–75.

Iarotski LS, Be'er SA, 1993, *Epidemiology and control of opisthorchiasis in the former USSR*, Unpublished document SCH/SG/93/WP.12, WHO, Geneva.

Intapan P, Kaewkes S, Maleewong W, 1992, Control of *Opisthorchis viverrini* cercariae using the copepod *Mesocyclops leuckarti*, *Southeast Asian J Trop Med Public Health*, **23**: 348–9.

Isseroff H, Tunis M, Read CP, 1972, Changes in amino acids of bile in *Fasciola hepatica* infections, *Comp Biochem Physiol*, **41B**: 157–63.

Itoh M, Sato S, 1990, Multi-dot enzyme-linked immunosorbent assay for serodiagnosis of trematodiasis, *Southeast Asian J Trop Med Pub Health*, **21**: 471–4.

Jaroonvesama N, 1988, Differential diagnosis of eosinophilic meningitis, *Parasitol Today*, **88**: 262–6.

Jones EA, Kay JM et al., 1977, Massive infection with *Fasciola hepatica* in man, *Am J Med*, **63**: 836–42.

Jongsuksantigul P, Chaeychomsri W et al., 1992, Study on prevalence and intensity of intestinal helminthiasis and opisthorchiasis in Thailand, *J Trop Med Parasitol*, **2**: 80–95 (in Thai).

Kaewkes S, Elkins DB et al., 1991, Comparative studies on the morphology of the eggs of *Opisthorchis viverrini* and lecithodendriid trematodes, *Southeast Asian J Trop Med Public Health*, **22**: 623–30.

Keittivuti A, Keittivuti B, Srithong Y, 1986, Control of liver fluke infections through community and voluntary participation at Kalasin province, Thailand, *Proceedings of the Second International Symposium on Public Health in Asia and the Pacific Basin*, Faculty of Public Health, Mahidol University, Bangkok, Thailand, 204–16.

Kirby GM, Pelkonen P et al., 1994, Association of liver fluke (*Opisthorchis viverrini*) infestation with increased expression of CYP2A and carcinogen metabolism in male hamster liver, *Mol Carcinog*, **11**: 81–9.

Koenigstein RP, 1949, Observations on the epidemiology of infections with *Clonorchis sinensis*, *Trans R Soc Trop Med Hyg*, **42**: 503–6.

Komiya Y, 1966, *Clonorchis* and clonorchiasis, *Adv Parasitol*, **4**: 53–106.

Kum, PN, Nchinda, TC, 1982, Pulmonary paragonimiasis in Cameroon, *Trans R Soc Trop Med Hyg*, **76**: 768–772.

Lee SH, Hwang SW et al., 1984, Comparative morphology of eggs of heterophyids and *Clonorchis sinensis* causing human infections in Korea, *Korean J Parasitol*, **22**: 171–80.

Lee SH, Park YH et al., 1989, The effects of gamma irradiation on the survival and development of *Clonorchis sinensis* metacercariae, *Korean J Parasitol*, **27**: 187–95.

Lim JH, 1990, Radiologic findings in clonorchiasis, *Am J Radiol*, **155**: 1001–8.

Mairiang E, Elkins DB et al., 1992, Relationship between intensity of *Opisthorchis viverrini* infection and hepatobiliary disease detected by ultrasonography, *J Gastroenterol Hepatol*, **7**: 17–21.

Mairiang E, Haswell-Elkins MR et al., 1993, Reversal of biliary tract abnormalities associated with *Opisthorchis viverrini* infection following praziquantel treatment, *Trans R Soc Trop Med Hyg*, **87**: 194–7.

Maurice J, 1994, Is something lurking in your liver?, *New Scientist*, **19 March**: 26–31.

Migasena P, 1982, Liver flukes relationship to dietary habits and development programs in Thailand, *Adverse Effects of Foods*, eds Patrice Jellife EF, Jellife DB, Plenum, New York, 307–11.

Miyazaki I, 1982, Paragonimiasis, *Parasitic Zoonoses*, CRC Handbook Series in Zoonoses vol III section C, eds Hillyer GV, Hopla CE, CRC Press, Boca Raton, FL, 143–64.

Pairojkul C, Sithithaworn P et al., 1991, Risk groups for opisthorchiasis-associated cholangiocarcinoma indicated by a study of worm burden-related biliary pathology, *Kan-Tan-Sui*, **22**: 111–20.

Patrick KM, Isaac-Renton J, 1992, Praziquantel failure in treatment of *Fasciola hepatica*, *Can J Infect Dis*, **3**: 33–6.

Pungpak S, Riganti M et al., 1985, Clinical features in severe opisthorchiasis viverrini, *Southeast Asian J Trop Med Pub Health*, **16**: 405–9.

Radomyos P, Bunnag D, Harinasuta T, 1984, Worms recovered in stools following praziquantel treatment, *Arzneimittel Forsch*, **34**: 1215–17.

Riganti M, Pungpak S et al., 1988, *Opisthorchis viverrini* eggs and adult flukes as nidus and composition of gallstones, *Southeast Asian J Trop Med Pub Health*, **19**: 633–6.

Rim HJ, 1986, The current pathobiology and chemotherapy of clonorchiasis, *Korean J Parasitol*, **24 (supplement)**: 1–141.

Sadun EH, 1955, Studies on *Opisthorchis viverrini* in Thailand, *Am J Hyg*, **2:** 81–115.

Schmidt GD, Robert LS, 1994, *Foundations of Parasitology*, 5th edn, Mosby Year Book, St. Louis, MO, 227–259.

Shaheen HI, Kamal KA et al., 1989, Dot-enzyme-linked immunosorbent assay (Dot-ELISA) for the rapid diagnosis of human fascioliasis, *J Parasitol*, **75:** 549–52.

Sirisinha S, 1984, Some immunological aspects of opisthorchiasis, *Arzneimittel Forsch*, **34:** 1170–2.

Sirisinha S, 1986, Immunodiagnosis of human liver fluke infections, *Asian Pacific J Allergy Immunol*, **4:** 81–8.

Sirisinha S, Chawengkirttikul et al., 1995, Evaluation of a monoclonal antibody-based enzyme linked immunosorbent assay for the detection of *Opisthorchis viverrini* infection in an endemic area, *Am J Trop Med Hyg*, **52:** 521–4.

Sithithaworn P, Tesana S et al., 1991, Relationship between faecal egg count and worm burden of *Opisthorchis viverrini* in human autopsy cases, *Parasitology*, **102:** 277–81.

Smithers SR, 1976, Immunity to trematode infection with special reference to schistosomiasis and fascioliasis, *Immunology of Parasitic Infections*, eds Cohen S, Sadun E, Blackwell Scientific Publications, Oxford, 297–332.

Song SB, 1987, Larvicidal action of liquid nitrogen against metacercariae of *Clonorchis sinensis*, *Korean J Parasitol*, **25:** 129–40.

Sornmani S, 1987, Control of opisthorchiasis through community participation, *Parasitol Today*, **3:** 31–3.

Spithill TW, 1992, Control of tissue parasites. III. Trematodes, *Animal Parasite Control Utilizing Biotechnology*, ed Yong WK, CRC Press, Boca Raton, FL, 199–219.

Srivatanakul P, Ohshima H et al., 1991, Endogenous nitrosamines and liver fluke as risk factors for cholangiocarcinoma in Thailand, *Int J Cancer*, **48:** 821–5.

Sui F, Shu-hua X, Catto BA, 1988, Clinical use of praziquantel in China, *Parasitol Today*, **4:** 312–5.

Sun T, Chou ST, Gibson JB, 1968, Route of entry of *Clonorchis sinensis* to the mammalian liver, *Exp Parasitol*, **22:** 346–51.

Tansurat P, 1971, Opisthorchiasis, *Pathology of Protozoal and Helminthic Diseases*, ed Marcial-Rojas E, Williams and Wilkins, Baltimore, MD, 536–545.

Teoh TB, 1963, A study of gall-stones and included worms in recurrent pyogenic cholangitis, *J Pathol Bacteriol*, **86:** 123–9.

Tesana S, Pamarapa A, Sae Sio O-T, 1989, Acute cholecystitis and *Fasciola* sp. infection in Thailand: report of two cases, *Southeast Asian J Trop Med Pub Health*, **20:** 447–52.

Thamavit W, Bhamarapravati N et al., 1978, Effects of dimethyl-nitrosamine on induction of cholangiocarcinoma in *Opisthorchis viverrini*-infected Syrian golden hamsters, *Cancer Res*, **38:** 4634–9.

Toscano C, Hai YS et al., 1995, Paragonimiasis and tuberculosis – diagnostic confusion: a review of the literature, *Trop Dis Bull*, **92:** R1–R27.

Upatham ES, Viyanant V et al., 1984, Relationship between prevalence and intensity of *Opisthorchis viverrini* infection, and clinical symptoms and signs in a rural community in northeast Thailand, *Bull WHO*, **62:** 451–61.

Upatham ES, Viyanant V et al., 1988, Rate of re-infection by *Opisthorchis viverrini* in an endemic Northeast Thai community after chemotherapy, *Int J Parasitol*, **18:** 643–9.

Vanijanonta S, Bunnag D, Harinasuta T, 1984, Radiological findings in pulmonary paragonimiasis heterotremus, *Southeast Asian J Trop Med Pub Health*, **15:** 122–8.

Vatanasapt V, Martin N et al., 1993, *Cancer in Thailand 1988–1991*, IARC Technical Report No. 16, International Agency for Research on Cancer, Lyon, 57–92.

Vatanasapt V, Uttaravichien T et al., 1990, Northeast Thailand: A region with a high incidence of cholangiocarcinoma, *Lancet*, **1:** 116–17.

Vichasri S, Viyanant V, Upatham ES, 1982, *Opisthorchis viverrini*: intensity and rates of infection in cyprinoid fish from an endemic focus in Northeast Thailand, *Southeast Asian J Trop Med Pub Health*, **13:** 138–41.

Viravan C, Bunnag D et al., 1986, Clinical field trial of praziquantel in opisthorchiasis in Nong Ranya Village, Khon Kaen Province, Thailand, *Southeast Asian J Trop Med Pub Health*, **17:** 63–6.

Wessely K, Reischig HL et al., 1988, Human fascioliasis treated with triclabendazole (Fasinex) for the first time, *Trans R Soc Trop Med Hyg*, **82:** 743–5.

Wolf-Spengler ML, Isseroff H, 1983, Fascioliasis: bile duct collagen induced by proline from the worm, *J Parasitol*, **69:** 290–4.

Wongratanacheewin S, Bunnag D et al., 1988, Characterization of humoral immune response in the serum and bile of patients with opisthorchiasis and its application in immunodiagnosis, *Am J Trop Med Hyg*, **38:** 356–62.

Wykoff DE, Harinasuta C et al., 1965, *Opisthorchis viverrini* in Thailand – the life cycle and comparison with *O. felineus*, *J Parasitol*, **51:** 207–14.

Yokogawa M, 1982, Paragonimiasis, *Parasitic Zoonoses*, CRC Handbook Series in Zoonoses, vol III Section C, eds Hillyer GV and Hopla CE, CRC Press, Boca Raton, FL, 123–42.

INTESTINAL TAPEWORMS

J Andreassen

1 THE PARASITES

1.1 Introduction and historical perspective

Intestinal tapeworms are among the earliest known human parasites. They have been known since prehistoric times and are referred to in the Papyrus Ebers from about 1500 BC (Hoeppli 1956). As early as the second century Galen recognized *Taenia*, but it was not until 1592 that Dunas discovered *Diphyllobothrium*, the broad tapeworm. The first illustration of a tapeworm (*Taenia*) was the *pittoresce* picture made by Andry in 1700. In 1782, the connection between tapeworms and hydatids was found by Goeze, who also found differences between the 2 human species of *Taenia*. In 1790, Abildgaard demonstrated that plerocercoid larvae from sticklebacks became adult tapeworms in ducks to which they were fed, but it was not until 1845 that Dujardin showed adult *Taenia* in humans to arise from cysticerci in meat. Six years later the life cycle of *Taenia saginata* was established by Küchenmeister, but it was not until 1917 that the complex life cycle of *D. latum* was found by Janicki (Grove 1990, Smyth 1990, Saklatvala 1993). As late as 1993 a new human species, *Taenia asiatica*, was described (Eom and Rim 1993), although it is now questioned whether this is a separate species or a subspecies of *T. saginata* (McManus and Bowles 1994) (see section 3.2).

Until the early 1960s tapeworms were said to have a more or less inert outer cuticle thought to prevent the worm being digested by the host's intestinal enzymes. However, at the same time, the worms had to absorb all nutrients through this surface, because tapeworms have no gut. By electron microscopy, it was then shown that the surface was a living structure, a tegument (see section 1.3, 'Morphology and structure'), which at the same time could absorb nutrients (see section 1.4, 'Feeding') and have mech-

anisms to inhibit host enzymes from digesting the worms (see section 1.4, 'Physiology').

The exact prevalence of human intestinal tapeworms is not known, but it has been estimated that as many as 100 million people worldwide may be infected with either *T. solium* or *T. saginata* (FAO 1991), and about 20 million with the dwarf tapeworm, *Hymenolepis nana*. None of the intestinal tapeworm infections is really life threatening, but the presence of the adult pig tapeworm, *T. solium*, increases the risk of acquiring cysticercosis by the uptake of infective eggs, and an infection with the broad tapeworm, *D. latum*, may give rise to pernicious anaemia (see section 3.6, 'Clinical and pathological aspects of infection').

The geographical distribution of intestinal tapeworm infections in humans corresponds to the distribution of their intermediate hosts, and, since the cyclophyllid tapeworms, such as species of *Taenia* and *Hymenolepis*, have intermediate hosts living in close contact to humans, they are worldwide, while the pseudophyllid species of *Diphyllobothrium* have a more restricted distribution because they need certain freshwater fishes as intermediate hosts.

1.2 Classification

All tapeworms belong to the class Cestoda and the subclass Eucestoda, which is made up of a number of orders. Tapeworm species which may infect humans belong to 6 families from 2 orders (Khalil, Jones and Bray 1994). (See Table 27.1.)

1.3 Morphology and structure

Human adult tapeworms are flat worms (Plathelminths) with a length ranging from a few centimetres (*Hymenolepis nana*) up to several metres (e.g. *Taenia* species). They are white or greyish to yellow. Calcareous corpuscles are present in tissues filling the

Table 27.1 Classification of human tapeworms

Order: Cyclophyllidea	Scolex with 4 round suckers and mostly armed with hooks. Development through 2 larval stages
Family: Taeniidae	Species: *Taenia saginata, T. saginata asiatica, T. solium*
Family: Hymenolepididae	Species: *Hymenolepis nana, H. diminuta*
Family: Dipylididae	Species: *Dipylidium caninum*
Family: Mesocestoididae	Species: *Mesocestoides corti*
Family: Anoplocephalidae	Species: *Bertiella* e.g. *studeri, Inermicapsifer madagascariensis*
Order: Pseudophyllidea	Scolex has 2 elongated slit-like suckers. Development through 3 larval stages
Family: Diphyllobothridae	Species: *Diphyllobothrium latum*
	A number of zoonotic animal species of *Diphyllobothrium* may sporadically infect humans, e.g. *D. dendriticum, D. nihonkaiense, D. pacificum, D. cordatum, D. hians, D. houghtoni, D. orcini, D. scoticum, D. ursi, D. yonagoense*

spaces between internal organs. Yellow colouration comes from eggs in the posterior part of the worms.

Tapeworms found in the small intestine of humans are adults in different developmental stages. The adult worm always consists of a head (**scolex**) and a neck region (the growth region), and if time and conditions allow, the neck continues in a series of **proglottides** (segments), which together form a **strobila**. The scolex has muscular suckers which function as holdfast organs and are used in locomotion. There are either 4 round suckers (**acetabula**), as in the cyclophyllids, or 2 elongated grooves (**bothria**), as in the pseudophyllids. On the scolex, some species also have small hooks, which can be inserted into the intestinal epithelium and thereby help the worm to maintain its position in the gut. The hooks are often situated in one or 2 circles (2 in *T. solium* and one in *H. nana*) on a retractable rostellum (cone) between the suckers on the anterior end of the scolex. From the narrow neck region, the width of the worm increases and folds of the body wall are made at regular intervals along its length, forming the proglottides, and giving the tapeworm an appearance like a segmented worm (Fig. 27.1).

The body wall (see Fig. 27.2) is called a **tegument** and consists of a syncytial distal cytoplasm with connections (cytoplasmic tubules) to a perinuclear cytoplasm lying beneath the basal lamella and circular and longitudinal muscles. The surface of the tegument is made up of microvillus-like structures called **microthriches** (**microthrix** in the singular). The microthriches have an electron-dense bent tip and are, like microvilli on most other absorptive cells, covered by a thin layer of glycoproteins and mucopolysaccharides called a **glycocalyx**.

Beneath the tegumental basal lamella lies 2 layers of muscles: an outer circular layer and an inner longitudinal one, allowing the worms to move. Special muscles run to the suckers, where bands of criss-cross fibres help improve the function of the suckers. Radial muscles may go to inner organs such as, the cirrus, uterus and vagina.

The nervous system consists of a brain-like structure in the scolex built up of a central ganglion, and lateral and rostellar ganglia connected by a central nerve ring. From the ganglia, nerves run to the suckers and rostellum. Lateral and median longitudinal nerves run from the ring all the way back to the posterior end of the tapeworm. There are transverse commissures between the longitudinal nerves and connections to inner organs and sensory organs in the body wall.

The excretory system is a typical protonephridial system, as in other platyhelminths, consisting of 2 lateral canals in each side (dorsal and ventral) connected in the scolex. The 2 ventral, lateral canals are connected with a transverse canal in the posterior of each proglottid. The excretory canals are build up of terminal cells (**flame cells**) connected to canal cells; flow through the system is made by a bundle of cilia in these terminal cells. The excretory fluid is carried to the scolex in the dorsal canals and back through the ventral canals which open to the exterior at the terminal proglottid. Around the cilia in the flame cells is a lattice-like system of projections from the flame cell and the canal cells. Ultrafiltration takes place at the basal lamina through gaps in the latticelike system.

Tapeworms are acoelomate, lacking not only a body cavity (coelom) but also a circulatory system.

The reproductive system is a typical hermaphroditic system, where the male and female organs differentiate progressively from the anterior region. The reproductive organs are repeated, with one set in each of the proglottides. Proglottides are considered mature when the reproductive organs found in them are sexually mature. Copulation then takes place and fertilized eggs are formed. When the eggs are mature, i.e. contain first stage larva, the proglottid is said to be gravid. Male organs typically consists of a few large or many small testes from which spermatozoa are passed via vasa efferentia to a common vas deferens and then via a seminal vesicle to a long muscular and protrusible cirrus surrounded by a cirrus sac. The female organs normally consist of a single bilobed ovary, an ootype, where egg composition and wall formation start, a vagina leading to a common genital pore and a compact or dispersed vitellarium from which vitelline cells are brought to the ootype to participate in the formation of a capsule (normally called an **eggshell**), as in the case of pseudophyllids, or in nourishment of the fertilized egg cell. In the cyclophyllids the capsule is absent or poorly developed, while the **embryophore** (the inner

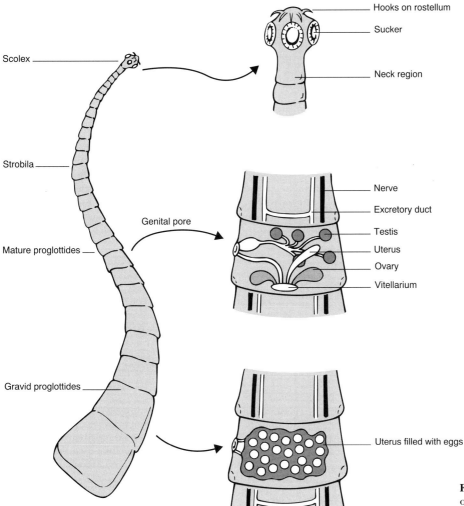

Scolex

Strobila

Mature proglottides

Gravid proglottides

Genital pore

Hooks on rostellum

Sucker

Neck region

Nerve

Excretory duct

Testis

Uterus

Ovary

Vitellarium

Uterus filled with eggs

Fig. 27.1 The organization of an adult tapeworm. (Based on *Taenia.*)

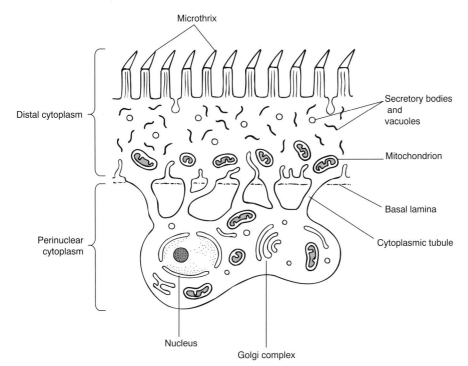

Microthrix

Distal cytoplasm

Perinuclear cytoplasm

Secretory bodies and vacuoles

Mitochondrion

Basal lamina

Cytoplasmic tubule

Nucleus

Golgi complex

Fig. 27.2 The tegument of an adult tapeworm.

envelope) forms a shell. In the cyclophyllid *Hymenolepis*, only one vitelline cell takes part in egg formation. Eggs are then passed into the uterus, which may or may not extend to the common genital pore. In some species, such as *Diphyllobothrium*, the eggs are operculate, as in most digeneans.

A fertilized egg cell develops to the first larval stage, called either an **oncosphere** (ball with hooks) or **hexacanth** (larva with 6 hooks), inside an eggshell. (See Fig. 27.3.)

1.4 General biology

Usually, only one or a very few of the large human tapeworms are present in a patient, but up to 28 worms *(T. saginata)* have been recorded in humans, indicating an aggregated distribution of the parasite in the human population. In infections of the dwarf tapeworm *(H. nana)*, many worms may be present in a human intestine. Individuals heavily infected with intestinal nematodes, often called **wormy people**, have been shown to be predisposed to this condition (Anderson 1986). Whether this situation also exists in humans infected with tapeworms is not known.

The large human tapeworms are capable of living for many years, in some cases up to 20 years (Wright 1984), but perhaps as long as the host. It has been shown that the rat tapeworm, *H. diminuta*, can live as long as the host, and, if repeatedly transplanted into the duodenum of young rats, can survive for at least 14 years (Read 1967).

When only a single tapeworm is present, it has been shown that self-insemination, i.e. transfer of sperm within the same segment or between segments in the same strobila, takes place. When multiple tapeworms are present, both self-insemination and cross-insemination take place (Nollen 1983).

MOVEMENT

The tapeworm utilizes its suckers and, if present, the hooks found on the scolex, to hold on to the villi of the intestine. Movement about the intestine is carried out by means of the suckers and the subtegumental musculature. Prepatent and diurnal movements are discussed below (see section 1.7, 'Location in host').

FEEDING

Since tapeworms have no mouth, all food has to be absorbed through the tegument. The microthriches help to increase the absorbant area of the tegument. A functional amplification factor for tapeworms has been shown to vary from slightly less than 2 to about 12, compared to about 26 for a mouse small intestine (Threadgold and Robinson 1984).

Tapeworms are normally in close contact to the intestinal mucosa (see section 1.7, 'Location in host'), which may be important for absorption of food. Small molecules, such as amino acids and glucose, have been shown to be taken up through the tegument via diffusion or active transport, but pinocytosis (endocytosis) of larger molecules such as proteins is still controversial.

Although the energy metabolism of tapeworms mainly involves carbohydrates, amino acids play a major role in the high protein synthesis necessary for the large egg production. Since the worms cannot synthesize long chain fatty acids and lipids such as cholesterol, the absorption of these compounds is essential. It has been shown that bile salts are required for this transport across the tegument. The uptake of purine and pyrimidine is highly complex. For further details see Pappas and Read (1975).

PHYSIOLOGY

Excretion of waste products must take place through the tegument by exocytosis or through the excretory system.

Tapeworms have no special breathing organs and no vascular system: all exchange of oxygen and carbon dioxide has to take place over the tegument. The mitochondria in the tegument have few cristae, indicating that the metabolism of tapeworms is largely anaerobic.

There were few investigations of the physiology and biochemistry of the nervous system of cestodes until the development of immunocytochemical techniques. These techniques have demontrated a number of neuropeptides which probably function as either neurotransmitters or neuromodulators and are responsible for coordinating behavioural responses (see reviews by Gustafsson 1985 and Halton et al. 1990).

BIOCHEMISTRY

The main constituents of cestodes normally show a rather high level of carbohydrates (especially glycogen) and lipids and a relatively low level of proteins.

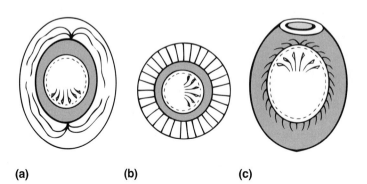

(a)   **(b)**   **(c)**

Fig. 27.3 Representative tapeworm eggs (not to scale): (a) hymenolepid; (b) taeniid; (c) *Diphyllobothrium*.

Mucopolysaccharides or complexes with proteins, such as mucoproteins or glycoproteins, are the main components of the surface glycocalyx. It has been suggested that this surface glycocalyx protects the worms from being digested by the host's proteolytic enzymes (Robertson and Cain 1984). On the other hand, digestion of nutrients to a state available for absorption can be made by enzymes bound to the glycocalyx, which has a turnover time of about 6 h. These enzymes may be of parasitic origin (intrinsic) or derived from their host (extrinsic).

Several neurotransmitters have been found in cestodes, e.g. acetylcholine, serotonin (5-hydroxytryptamine), noradrenaline (norepinephrine), dopamine and octopamine. Serotonin is regarded as the main excitatory neurotransmitter of motor activity and acetylcholine as the main inhibitory neurotransmitter.

1.5 Life cycle

Not only a final host (a human being) but also at least one intermediate host is necessary for the completion of the life cycle of a cestode. For pseudophyllids, at least 2 intermediate hosts are necessary. Only one human tapeworm, *H. nana*, can complete its life cycle without an intermediate host. All larval stages are passed on to the next host via the oral route (for details see under the individual species). Humans become infected with an adult tapeworm by eating an infected intermediate host or infected organs from an intermediate host. When an infective larva is eaten by a human, excystation occurs if the larva is encysted, and, if the scolex is 'retracted' it will be 'inverted'; growth then commences from the neck region. In pseudophyllids, growth does not commence until everything except the scolex and neck has been shed from the plerocercoid larva. This active process takes about 60 h in golden hamsters.

1.6 Transmission and epidemiology

Human tapeworm infections caused by *T. saginata* and *T. solium*, commonly called taeniosis or taeniasis, are cosmopolitan. Prevalence is normally low but very much dependent on cultural factors and the level of hygiene and veterinary control. In some African countries, prevalences above 10% have been reported. In contrast to these low levels in the final host, the prevalence of cysticercus infections in the intermediate hosts may in some regions be very high.

The total production of tapeworm eggs per infected human is an important epidemiological factor, which, for the large human tapeworms, is probably negatively correlated with the total number of tapeworms present per host, so that the fewer tapeworms per person, the more eggs are produced.

1.7 Location in host

All adult human tapeworms live in the lumen of the small intestine, but, dependent on the species, in different parts of the small intestine. The 2 species of *Taenia* live in the upper part of the jejunum, while *Diphyllobothrium* and *H. nana* normally live in the

upper two-thirds of the ileum. The scolex is found deeply embedded in the villi, while the strobila lies with its flat side close to the mucosa, sometimes in a spiral along the intestine.

The rare human tapeworm, *Hymenolepis diminuta*, which has rats as final hosts, has been shown to migrate in the small intestine of rats both during its prepatent period and diurnally. The newly excysted worm establishes itself about 30–40% down the small intestine. During the second week, the worm migrates anteriorly, stopping in the upper 10–20% of the small intestine. If many worms are present, they can be found spread over a larger part of the small intestine. Circadian migratory behaviour has also been found for *H. diminuta* in rats, where the worms are found more anteriorly in the small intestine in the morning and more posteriorly in the evening. This migration of the worms has been shown to be dependent on the host's feeding rhythm (see review by Arai 1980). Whether these migrations take place for the large human tapeworms are not known, but it is likely.

2 CLINICAL AND PATHOLOGICAL ASPECTS OF INFECTION

Generally, intestinal tapeworms are considered to be minimally pathogenic, causing no or very slight symptoms as compared to many other human parasitic diseases. However, they do utilize some of the food consumed by the host. Normally, sufficient food supplies are available and the host is not affected. In cases of malnutrition, tapeworm infections may have a deleterious effect on the infected person. The amount of energy taken from the host by tapeworms has been investigated for *Hymenolepis diminuta* in rats and shown to be 0.8%, which is comparable to carnivore predation on a prey population (Bailey 1975).

The effect of the broad tapeworm (*Diphyllobothrium latum*) on vitamin B_{12} and cobalamin absorption is discussed later (see section 3.6, 'Clinical and pathological aspects of infection').

2.1 Clinical manifestations

The large human tapeworms may disturb gastrointestinal motility. Although no specific symptoms for any of the human intestinal tapeworms are known, patients may experience abdominal pain, nausea, weakness, loss of weight, increased appetite, headache, constipation, dizziness, diarrhoea, pruritis ani, excitation and even vomiting and anorexia. Both nausea and abdominal pain may be explained as a result of extension, or spasm, of the intestine caused by the movement of the tapeworms. The mechanisms of the other symptoms mentioned are obscure.

2.2 Pathogenesis and pathology

Our knowledge of specific changes in the human intestinal environment and intestinal absorption caused by tapeworms is rare (see review by Rees 1967). However, in rats infected with *H. diminuta*, the worms cause a decrease in pH (perhaps because they excrete fatty acids), an increase in pCO_2 and pO_2 and a reduction to about half the number of intestinal microorganisms, when compared to uninfected rats (Mettrick 1971).

Blood eosinophilia, commonly found in many other human helminth infections, has also been described in some cases, as have inflammatory reactions in the intestinal mucosa. However, only in experimental models with rats and mice have changes in the small intestine in the number of eosinophils, mast cells and goblet cells been followed during a tapeworm infection. Peripheral eosinophilia, combined with pruritis, urticaria or asthma, have been described in human taeniasis and are indicative of an allergic reaction stimulated by the tapeworms. Human self-infections with the tapeworm *H. diminuta* also showed pronounced eosinophilia, along with an increase in plasma viscosity, but circulating IgE was not detected (Turton, Williamson and Harris 1975).

Complications may occur when proglottides move into new locations, such as the appendix or the uterine cavity or, after vomiting, into the cavities connecting with the oral cavity.

2.3   Immune responses

Although antibodies in sera from humans infected with adult tapeworms have been demonstrated in many cases, almost nothing is known about functional immunity to adult tapeworms in humans; our knowledge is mainly confined to animal models. Turton, Williamson and Harris (1975) made self-infections with *H. diminuta* and found increases in specific IgG and IgM, but not in IgE. However, the IgE is produced against intestinal tapeworm infections in dogs (Williams and Perez-Esandi 1971), mice (Moss 1971) and rats (Harris and Turton 1973), as in human intestinal nematode infections. It has also been shown, using the macrophage migration inhibition test, that humans infected with adult *Taenia saginata* develop a delayed-type hypersensitivity reaction (Boro'n-Kaczmarska et al. 1978).

In few cases, spontaneous cure has been observed in *T. saginata* infections, but it is not known whether this is caused by a direct immunological reaction or through a non-specific cross-reaction caused by another parasite, e.g as a result of increased plasma leakage to the gut lumen caused by hookworms.

The reason why only one or a few of the large human tapeworms are found at a time is not known, but the possibility exists that it is a result of **concomitant immunity** (previously called **premunition**), i.e. the host cannot get rid of existing worms but at the same time is in some way immune to new infections. The resistance to new infections is not a result of crowding effects from the present worms, as has been shown in rats infected with *H. diminuta*. The greater the biomass of primary worms present in the intestine, the greater the biomass of the superimposed worms. This indicates that the adverse effect on the superimposed worms comes from the host, i.e. it is immunologically

mediated and not just an effect caused by the present primary worms (Andreassen 1991).

Human taeniid tapeworms are found not only together with other tapeworm species, but also with other intestinal worms, especially nematodes (large roundworms and hookworms), and protozoans. The interspecific interactions between these species are not known, but it is obvious that the presence of other parasites in the intestine will interfere with the presence of tapeworms and with the host's reactions against them. It is known from experimental infections in mice and rats with the tapeworm *H. diminuta* that the immunologically mediated expulsion of existing intestinal nematodes will at the same time, expel a new infection of the tapeworm and destrobilate an existing tapeworm population (Behnke, Bland and Wakelin 1977, Christie, Wakelin and Wilson 1979). These experiments indicate that adult tapeworms are more resistant to non-specific host reactions than newly excysted worms. In vitro experiments have indeed shown that newly excysted cysticercoids of *H. diminuta* are completely lysed in fresh normal rat serum, while the scolex and neck region of older worms are more resistant (Christensen, Bøgh and Andreassen 1986).

Protozoan infections, such as trypanosomes in the blood and flagellates such as *Giardia* in the gut, are often immunosuppressive and may increase the survival time of tapeworms in humans. Other immunosuppressive infections, special situations such as pregnancy and lactation, and immunosuppressive treatments will probably be favourable to a human tapeworm infection.

The antigens stimulating immune reactions in the final host probably come from the surface of the tapeworm and from gland secretions. It has been suggested (Elowni 1982) that the scolex and the germinative (neck) region of intestinal tapeworms are the main source of protective antigens. This is very likely, because these parts of the tapeworm are in the closest contact with the host's mucosa. Furthermore, the scolex has a rostellar gland, and antibodies have been shown to be produced in the host against secretions from this gland (Hoole, Andreassen and Birklund 1994).

2.4   Diagnosis

An intestinal tapeworm infection as such can be diagnosed by finding proglottides or cestode eggs in the patient's faeces. Several techniques for detecting eggs are available, e.g. thick and thin smears and concentration techniques using sedimentation or flotation. Anal swabs may also be effective. If only eggs are present, it is not possible to differentiate *T. saginata* from *T. solium*. To diagnose these species the scolex or those stages of proglottides showing species characteristics (see descriptions of individual parasites in sections 3 and 4) are needed.

Serological diagnosis of human intestinal tapeworms has been carried out using different antigen preparations in precipitation, complement fixation, skin hypersensitivity, agglutination and ELISA tests but with variable results. A single serological test can determine the presence of antibodies, but cannot differentiate between a present and a past infection.

Recently, methods have been developed to detect coproantigens of *Taenia* species in human faecal samples by means of a coproantigen ELISA (Allan et al. 1992). Diagnostic identification of a tapeworm proglottid or a fraction of it has been carried out with *T. saginata* using the polymerase chain reaction to amplify extracted genomic DNA and electrophoresis to identify a 0.55 kb DNA fragment (Gottstein et al. 1991). This is a highly sensitive, specific and easy technique for identification of *T. saginata* proglottides and eggs; a single egg should be enough to make a species identification (Gottstein and Mowatt 1991).

2.5 Control

From a human health point of view, the tapeworms *T. solium* and *D. latum* are particularly important: *T. solium* because of the risk of cysticercosis (see Chapter 28, Larval tapeworms) and *D. latum* because of the risk of pernicious anaemia due to vitamin B_{12} deficiency.

CHEMOTHERAPY

Two compounds, the older niclosamide and the newer praziquantel, act against adult intestinal worms (WHO 1995), but other drugs have been or still are in use, including extracts of certain seeds from locally grown plants. Niclosamide is a very safe drug because minimal amounts are absorbed in the gastrointestinal tract; in contrast, praziquantel is extensively absorbed by the host. Praziquantel has been shown also to have some effects against cysticerci of *T. solium*. Normally, a single dose is highly effective (at least 80%). Niclosamide functions by blocking glucose absorption by the adult tapeworm. Adult worms treated with praziquantel rapidly contract and disintegrate in the intestine.

PROPHYLAXIS

For human consumers, prophylaxis depends on the tapeworm species concerned (see descriptions of individual parasites in sections 3 and 4). Generally speaking, humans can avoid tapeworm contamination by avoiding food which has not been properly prepared. Meat or fish should be heated to a minimum of 57°C at the centre, deep frozen at −10°C for 10 days or pickled in a 25% salt solution for 5 days before being eaten. To reduce the risk of infected meat being eaten by humans, it is important to have an adequate veterinary meat inspection before meat is released for consumption, although a veterinary inspection can never be 100% effective. The dwarf tapeworm, *H. nana*, needs special control measures (see section 3.4).

TRANSMISSION

To avoid infection of intermediate hosts, it is important that human faecal material is kept away from these animals. Safe disposal of sewage is important in minimizing the transmission; water from sewage plants should not be used to water grasslands

grazed by cattle or pigs. Viable tapeworm eggs can also reach grasslands and cattle grazing along rivers and lakes via effluent from sewage plants. Viable eggs in proglottides taken up by birds can pass through them and be dispersed on to fields, where the intermediate host can be infected or its feed contaminated. Under natural conditions, desiccation is normally the most important factor reducing the survival of the eggs: hot, dry summers will kill more eggs than cold, wet winters. Health education, not only of consumers, but also of people involved in every step in the life cycle, is important to prevent transmission of human tapeworms.

3 SPECIES AFFECTING HUMANS

3.1 *Taenia saginata* (beef tapeworm)

The name beef tapeworm comes from the fact that beef is the main source of infection. *T. saginata* has a cosmopolitan distribution wherever inadequately cooked beef is eaten.

Stoll (1947) estimated that about 39 million people were infected. Although present data are not sufficient to make a new estimate, it seems justified to multiply Stoll's number by the increase in the total global population, giving about 60 million people currently infected with *T. saginata*.

The economic loss due to taeniasis or cysticercosis in cattle is very high in some countries. The cost due to medical treatment of people is only a small proportion of the loss due to cysticercosis, which varies from region to region, not only in total loss, but also in loss per animal.

MORPHOLOGY AND STRUCTURE

The mature tapeworm, which can reach a length of 4–6 m or even more, has 1000–2000 proglottides. In the proglottides the genital pore is seen laterally but irregularly alternating from one side to the other. The scolex has 4 suckers but no hooks. Because of the lack of hooks, the species has also been named *Taeniarhynchus saginatus*.

GENERAL BIOLOGY

The maximum size of the worm is reached when only one tapeworm is present. When 2 or more are present, the individual length decreases, to about 2 m when 8 worms are present (Tesfa-Yohannes 1990), and as little as 50–80 cm when 16 worms are present (Altmann and Bubis 1959). An increasing number of worms present in the small intestine of humans coincides with a decrease in the number of proglottides; an increase from 1 to 8 worms shows a decrease in the number of proglottides from about 600 to 350. This is a typical example of the effect of crowding, but, in parasites (unlike free-living animals), not only do the worms themselves interfere with each other and compete for space and food, but also the immunological reactions from the host have an influence on the growth of the worms.

LIFE CYCLE

In the life cycle (see Fig. 27.4) humans are the only final host and infections are acquired by eating raw or undercooked meat, e.g. by eating a 'rare' steak containing the cysticercus stage in a host capsule. When the cysticercus or bladder worm (previously named as a separate species, *Cysticercus bovis*) reaches the stomach, proteolytic enzymes start dissolving the capsule. In the small intestine, the cysticercus is stimulated to evaginate. The scolex attaches to the intestinal mucosa by means of the 4 suckers and starts growing into a mature tapeworm. Maturity is reached after about 10–14 weeks. The gravid proglottides contain up to about 80 000 mature eggs each and an average of 6–9 proglottides may be expelled in 24 h, giving a total daily egg output of about 600 000 eggs. Meat from domestic cattle is the main source, but water buffaloes are also known as intermediate hosts. Unhooked cysticerci have also been reported in meat and livers from wild ruminants in Africa, but the significance of these observations needs further investigation. Llamas in South America and reindeer in the northern hemisphere have also been reported as intermediate hosts. A dozen cases of hookless cysticerci found in humans and described as *T. saginata* cysticercosis have been reported, but these require confirmation. The intermediate hosts become infected by eating mature eggs or gravid proglottides filled with eggs. The proglottides, which are quite mobile after being deposited, may migrate out of the faecal pat and thereby be more easily eaten by cattle. During the migrations, most eggs leave the proglottis. The eggs hatch in the small intestine, and the free oncospheres then penetrate the gut wall and reach the muscles via the blood. In the intramuscular connective tissue they develop to a cysticercus, which, in the mature stage after about 10–15 weeks, is a greyish white bladder about 5–9 mm with an opaque invaginated scolex and neck.

TRANSMISSION AND EPIDEMIOLOGY

The beef tapeworm is an important infection of both humans and cattle throughout the beef-eating world, but especially in the tropics, where cattle-grazing areas are more often contaminated with human faeces. It is important from the point of view both of human health and of economics, especially in potentially beef-exporting African countries with a high incidence of cysticercosis in cattle (see section 2.5, 'Control'). Under ideal conditions, the eggs may survive in the field for up to 6 months.

Gravid proglottides from infected humans living in areas with water closets accumulate in sewage plants. When sewage sludge is used as fertilizer on grazing pastures, cattle may become infected. Pastures may also be contaminated with eggs from sewage plants when treated effluent (still containing viable cestode eggs) is released into rivers running through grazing areas. Cattle may then become infected by drinking or eating along the rivers or by farmers watering pastures with water from the contaminated rivers. A more 'sophisticated' way to contaminate pastures is through droppings from gulls which have eaten proglottides at open sewage plants or at places where human faeces are deposited directly in water. Cattle may also be infected through human activities such as camping, where human faeces are deposited on grassland. A farmer may also risk a cysticercus 'storm' in his cattle if he empties septic tanks, mixes the content with slurry and sprays it over the pastures as a fertilizer.

Another parameter of special epidemiological interest is the longevity of infective cysticerci. This is quite variable, even in the same host. Cysts in some organs are killed, yet remain alive in others. Cysticerci have been shown to be viable for a maximum of 3 years in their intermediate host.

LOCATION IN HOST

The mature tapeworm has been shown to attach mainly to the upper jejunum, with the posterior part of the body down in the ileum. However, the tapeworm is mobile in the intestinal lumen (Prévot, Hornbostel and Dorken 1952).

CLINICAL AND PATHOLOGICAL ASPECTS OF INFECTION

Clinical manifestations

Infected humans are not always aware of having a beef tapeworm, but the observation of moving proglottides in the anal region, in the underclothing or on the stool normally brings the patient to the doctor. Infected persons often complain of having abdominal discomfort (epigastric pain), nausea, weakness, loss of weight, increased or decreased appetite and headache. Constipation, dizziness, diarrhoea, pruritis ani and excitation are also noted, while vomiting is an infrequent symptom.

Pathogenesis and pathology

Occasionally obstructive appendicitis or cholangitis occurs in *T. saginata* infections due to aberrant migration of segments, which have been found also in the uterine cavity. After vomiting, proglottides may, in very rare cases, obstruct the respiratory tract, enter the middle ear through the eustachian tube or localize in the adenoid tissue of the nasopharynx. Symptoms such as abdominal pain and nausea suggest that the tapeworm has an irritative action, and biopsies of the intestinal mucosa taken from infected patients often show slight inflammatory reactions. Moderate eosinophilia has been reported in varying percentages of infected persons, but an increase in IgE has not yet been demonstrated.

Immunity

Acquired immunity against *T. saginata* infections in humans after elimination of an infection has not been demonstrated and is probably of little importance; in contrast, concomitant immunity may be important.

Diagnosis

If only gravid proglottides are present for diagnosis, normally as apolytic discharge in faeces, the presence of a vaginal sphincter muscle, which can be seen on

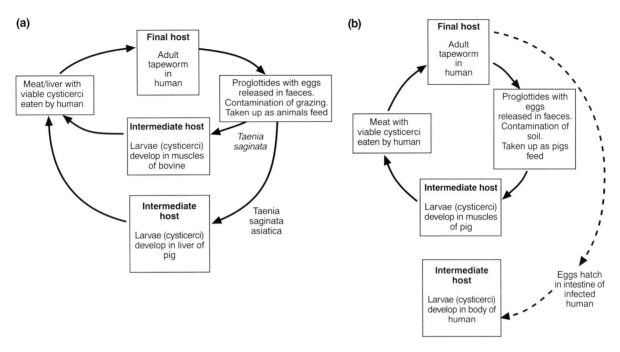

Fig. 27.4 Life cycles of the human tapeworms: (a) *T. saginata* and *T. saginata asiatica*; (b) *T. solium*.

cleared specimens, can identify it as *T. saginata* and distinguish it from *T. solium* (Fig. 27.5).

The presence of 2 ovarian lobes is also species specific for *T. saginata*. If the scolex is recovered after therapy, the absence of hooks is a characteristic of *T. saginata*; the pork tapeworm (*T. solium*) has hooks on the rostellum (see Verster 1967). The 2 species overlap in the number of uterine branches in gravid proglottides, which therefore can only be used when the number on each side of the stem is >16 (*T. saginata*) or <10 (*T. solium*).

For detecting eggs (Fig. 27.3), anal swabs are superior to methods using faeces (thick smears and concentration or flotation methods). However, eggs cannot be used for species determination.

Control

Details of chemotherapy, prophylaxis and transmission are given in Table 27.2 (see also section 2.5, 'Chemotherapy'). Although it seems simple to break the life cycle of *T. saginata*, (humans being the only final host), both human and animal infections are in fact very difficult to control. To control cattle infections, contact with human faeces should be avoided. Cattle should be kept away from pastures where there is risk of contamination. Humans should not eat undercooked or raw meat unless it has been properly frozen, meat should be controlled by veterinarians and infected people should be treated in order to break the parasite life cycle.

Eggs of *T. saginata* can survive for a long period of time, depending on temperature and moisture. Higher temperatures and lower humidity result in shorter egg survival times. To prevent establishment of viable cysticerci in cattle, immunization may be a

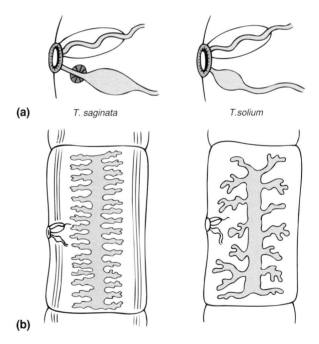

Fig. 27.5 Diagnostic feature of T. saginata and T. solium: (a) genital atria; (b) gravid proglottides.

possibility. Although an effective vaccine has been produced, no commercial vaccine is yet available.

3.2 *Taenia saginata asiatica* (Asian *Taenia*)

This human tapeworm was described by Eon and Rim (1993) as a new species, *T. asiatica*. Some authors still regard it as a separate species (Galan-Puchades and Mas-Coma 1996), although most consider it as a subspecies of *T. saginata*

Table 27.2 Control measures against taeniasis (taeniosis)

Prophylaxis
Reduction of human consumption of raw infected meat
Cook properly and/or freeze meat from cattle and pigs and other intermediate hosts
Veterinary meat inspection
Reduction of intermediate hosts becoming infected
Keep human faeces away from cattle and pigs and other intermediate hosts

Therapy	
Chemotherapy (drugs)	
Against intestinal tapeworms in humans	Praziquantel, niclosamide
Against larval stages in the intermediate host	(see Chapter 28)
Vaccination	
Against adult intestinal tapeworms	Not yet possible
Against larval stages in the tapeworms' intermediate hosts	(see Chapter 28)

(MaManus and Bowles 1994, Fan et al. 1995). It has been characterized genetically by Bowles and McManus (1994). According to Fan (1988) it has been present in Taiwan since at least 1915. It is now found in Korea, Taiwan, Indonesia and Thailand but probably occurs also in other Asian countries such as Burma (Myanmar) and the Philippines (Ito 1992).

MORPHOLOGY AND STRUCTURE

The morphology of the adult tapeworm is very similar to that of *T. saginata*, but the scolex generally has a larger diameter and the cysticercus is different in morphology, development and species of intermediate host; for further details see Fan (1988), Eom and Rim (1993) and Fan et al. (1995).

LIFE CYCLE

The life cycle differs from that of *T. saginata* in that the intermediate hosts are pigs rather than cattle, and the preferred location in the pig is the liver, rarely the omentum, serosa or muscles (Fan et al. 1995). Pigs, calves, goats and monkeys have successfully been infected experimentally with eggs of *T. saginata asiatica*. Fully mature cysticerci are developed within 4 weeks, whereas it takes 10–12 weeks for *T saginata* in cattle (Fig. 27.4) .

TRANSMISSION AND EPIDEMIOLOGY

To understand the transmission and epidemiology of this new strain of *T. saginata* we require more knowledge of the prevalence and egg production of the adult tapeworms in the human population. Furthermore, it is important to know not only which animals are confirmed intermediate hosts, along with the corresponding prevalence and infection intensity, but also the potential intermediate hosts in the area concerned.

CLINICAL AND PATHOLOGICAL ASPECTS OF INFECTION

See under *T. saginata*.

Diagnosis

When a human tapeworm infection is diagnosed as *T. saginata* (see section 3.1), only identification of the source of infection, i.e. whether the patient has eaten undercooked beef or raw pig liver, may indicate if the infection is caused by the Asian subspecies *T. saginata asiatica*.

3.3 *Taenia solium* (pork tapeworm)

The name pork tapeworm relates to the fact that pork is the main source of human infection. It has a worldwide distribution except among Muslims and Jews, who do not eat pork, or where strict veterinary inspection and treatment of human cases have caused its eradication. *T. solium* is especially common in Latin America.

MORPHOLOGY AND STRUCTURE

The mature tapeworm normally reaches a length of about 2–4 m (sometimes more), and contains about 800–1000 proglottides. The scolex has 4 suckers and a small rostellum with a double crown of 25–30 small hooks.

LIFE CYCLE

Humans can act not only as final host, as for *T. saginata*, but also as intermediate host (Fig. 27.4), which is the more serious situation (see Chapter 28, Larval tapeworms). The source of infection to humans functioning as final host is meat from domestic pigs or wild boar containing the cysticercus stage, previously named as a separate species (*Cysticercus cellulosae*). When this is eaten, development to the adult stage is as described for *T. saginata* (see section 3.1). Pigs, wild boar and occasionally other mammals become infected by eating mature eggs or gravid proglottides filled with up to 40 000 eggs. The proglottides, which, unlike those of *T. saginata*, are only slightly mobile after being deposited in human faeces, are in certain places easily eaten by pigs, which will quite happily eat human faeces. In pigs the development to an infectious cysticercus is essentially as for *T. saginata* in cattle, except that the invaginated scolex has hooks on the rostellum and the developmental time is shorter, 7–9 weeks.

TRANSMISSION AND EPIDEMIOLOGY

In some areas the prevalence in pigs may reach 25%, and in heavily infected pigs (so-called **measly pork**) the infection can be detected by the presence of cysts in the tongue of the living pig. Such levels of infection are not uncommon in countries where pigs live in close proximity to humans who defaecate in places where the pigs can eat the faeces.

LOCATION IN HOST

The mature tapeworm has been shown to attach mainly to the upper jejunum, as in *T. saginata*.

CLINICAL AND PATHOLOGICAL ASPECTS OF INFECTION

Clinical manifestations

Unlike those of *T. saginata*, the gravid proglottides of *T. solium* are released in groups and are not as active as those of *T. saginata*. Therefore, infected persons do not recognize the infection as easily. Otherwise the clinical manifestations are as described for *T. saginata* (see section 3.1).

Pathogenesis and pathology

See 'Pathogenesis and pathology' (section 2.2) and *T. saginata* (section 3.1).

Immunity

See 'Immune responses' (section 2.3) and *T. saginata* (section 3.1).

Diagnosis

Adult *T. solium* worms can be identified by the presence of hooks on the scolex, unlike *T. saginata*. For species characteristics in the proglottides, see *T. saginata*.

CONTROL

See Table 27.2 and Pawlowski (1990) for more details and references.

Prophylaxis

To prevent infection, veterinary inspection and thorough cooking of pork are essential. In most parts of the world, these are easier and cheaper than the measures necessary for prohibiting porcine access to human faeces or food contaminated with eggs of *T. solium*.

Chemotherapy

Praziquantel is the drug of choice for *T. solium* because it not only kills the adult tapeworm in a single dose, but, when taken in high doses over 3–7 days, also kills the cysticerci, thus offering a cure for cysticercosis (see Chapter 28, Larval tapeworms). As for *T. saginata*, treatment with a single dose of 4 tablets (each of 500 mg) of niclosamide chewed thoroughly after a small meal is also effective against the adult worm in the intestine.

When treating patients, it is important that nausea and especially vomiting is avoided; should proglottides with eggs or eggs alone come into the stomach and later into the small intestine, the patient may acquire cysticercosis. A purgative should therefore be given 1–2 h after the anthelmintic treatment.

Transmission

Theoretically, transmission to humans may also be inhibited by vaccination of pigs against oncospheres from *T. solium* eggs. However, a commercial vaccine is not yet available (see Chapter 28, Larval tapeworms).

3.4 *Hymenolepis nana* (dwarf tapeworm)

Hymenolepis nana infects not only humans but also rodents such as mice and rats. In rodents the tapeworm is regarded by some as a special strain (*H. nana* var. *fraterna*), but cross-infections in both directions are possible. This means that *H. nana* is a zoonosis, where the infection can be maintained in animals and accidentally infect humans. Stoll (1947) estimated that about 20 million people were infectd and this number has probably increased since then.

MORPHOLOGY AND STRUCTURE

The adult tapeworm is small, as the name indicates, reaching only 4–5 cm in length. The scolex has 4 cup-shaped suckers and a retractable, prominent and movable rostellum with a ring of small hooks.

LIFE CYCLE

This tapeworm has an indirect life cycle with an insect as the intermediate host. It is exceptional among tapeworms in also being able to use the final host for development directly from the egg containing the oncosphere larva (Fig. 27.6).

Intermediate hosts include grain- and flour-eating beetles such as species of *Tribolium* and *Tenebrio*, fleas such as *Pulex irritans*, *Xenopsylla cheops* and *Ctenocephalides canis*, and moths. The indirect life cycle begins when these insects or their larvae eat an infective *H. nana* egg. They crush the eggshell, and enzymes in the gut then stimulate the oncosphere to free itself from the enclosing membranes. When free in the gut lumen, the oncosphere penetrates the gut wall by means of its 6 hooks and glandular secretions. In the

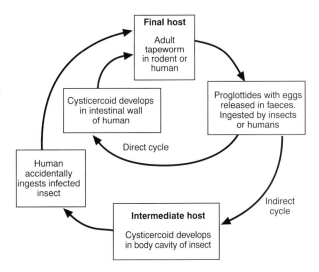

Fig. 27.6 Life cycle of the human dwarf tapeworm, *Hymenolepis nana*.

body cavity of the insect, the oncospheres transform and grow into the second larval stage, the **cysticercoid**, which is infective to the final host. After an infected insect is eaten by humans (chiefly children), bile salts in the small intestine stimulate the emergence and liberation of the young tapeworm from the cysticercoid. In humans the tapeworm grows to patency within 3–4 weeks. The direct life cycle of *H. nana* takes place when infective eggs are ingested. In the lumen of the small intestine a free oncosphere penetrates an intestinal villus and grows to the cysticercoid stage in about 96 h. Thereafter, the villus ruptures, the cysticercoid becomes free in the lumen of the small intestine and grows to an adult tapeworm. It is said that in heavy infections eggs may hatch in the intestine before passing out with the faeces resulting in autoinfection, but the importance of this is questionable.

Transmission and epidemiology

Transmission takes place directly from hand to mouth, by contaminated food and drinking water, or in rare cases, by infected insects. Infection is most prevalent where hygiene is insufficient. e.g. in young children and inhabitants of institutions. Although humans are the main source of infection, infected rodents are always a potential source. This tapeworm is present throughout the world, with overall prevalences ranging from nearly zero to about 4% in some countries and as high as 16% in children.

Location in host

In humans the adult tapeworms are said to be found in the upper two-thirds of the ileum, whereas in mice they are found in the posterior part of the ileum.

Clinical and pathological aspects of infection

Clinical manifestations

The presence of low numbers of these tapeworms causes no symptoms, but, if as many as 1000–2000 worms are present in children, there may be abdominal pain, lack of appetite, eventual diarrhoea or dizziness.

Pathogenesis, pathology and immunity

In heavy infections enteritis may be produced. Nothing seems to be known about immune reactions in human infections, although there is considerable knowledge of experimental infections in mice and rats (see review by Ito and Smyth 1987).

Diagnosis

Free eggs or proglottides filled with eggs may be found in faeces. The egg with the characteristic 2 groups of polar filaments is species specific.

Control

Chemotherapy

The drug of choice is praziquantel, of which a single dose is highly effective. A second choice is niclosamide. When a person is found to be infected, treatment should include the entire household.

Prophylaxis

Sanitary improvements, uncontaminated food supplies and rodent control in houses and nearby surroundings are important in prevention of this infection, but the hygienic status of children and inhabitants of institutions is the most important. Because of the direct life cycle and the zoonotic status of this infection, this tapeworm is difficult to control and impossible to eradicate.

3.5 *Hymenolepis diminuta*

Morphology and structure

The scolex of this species has no hooks on its rostellum, unlike *H. nana*. Furthermore, *H. diminuta* is a larger than *H. nana*, reaching a length of at least 1 m in single infections in rats, and perhaps more in human infections.

Life cycle

The life cycle of this tapeworm is identical to the indirect life cycle of *H. nana* (see section 3.4) and always needs an intermediate host. The prepatent period in man is about 3 weeks. It has been shown in rats that, when only a few tapeworms are present, they may live as long as the host (see section 1.4, 'General biology') In a self-induced infection with 30 cysticercoids and a superimposed infection with 100 cysticercoids on day 22, Turton, Williamson and Harris (1975) did not find any eggs in faeces and concluded that the worms were expelled before patency.

Transmission and epidemiology

In order to be infected with an adult *H. diminuta*, humans have to ingest larvae (cysticercoids) from the body cavity of an insect. Since the tapeworm is very rare in humans, the source of infection must come from infected rats expelling gravid proglottides in their faeces, from where the insects eat infective eggs. This infection is therefore a true zoonosis: infected rats must be present in order to infect insects, which in turn are consumed by humans. Poor sanitary conditions are a requirement for occurrence of this parasite.

Clinical and pathological aspects of infection

Since infected rats and insects, functioning as final and intermediate hosts, respectively, may live worldwide, this is a cosmopolitan zoonosis. However, few (200–300) cases have been reported (Levi et al. 1987, Millon, Berbineau and Barale 1994). It is found mainly in children under 3 years of age, but surveys have also found infected adults. Because of the few human cases reported and small pathological effects of the adult tapeworms, this parasite is of little medical importance.

Clinical manifestations

Although diarrhoea, anorexia, nausea, headache and dizziness have been reported, no clinical symptoms were observed in the only experimental human infection (Turton, Williamson and Harris 1975). However, this was in a healthy adult, and a different picture might possibly be detected in children naturally infected with this tapeworm.

Pathogenesis, pathology and immune responses

In the experimental infection referred to above eosinophilia was observed but there was no evidence of anaemia or change in serum transaminases, indicating an absence of tissue damage, although there was an increase in plasma viscosity (Turton, Williamson and Harris 1975). Parasite-specific antibodies were detected using a fluorescent antibody technique at a titre of 1:160 on day 21 after an infection with 30 cysticercoids. On day 22, another 100 cysticercoids were ingested. The antibody titre remained at 160 after the second infection and, since no tapeworm eggs were found using saline flotation techniques, the authors concluded that the infection was established but the tapeworms were expelled before reaching maturity. The reason for this spontaneous cure could be host immune reactions caused by the rather high infection doses. A year later, the same person infected himself with 200 cysticercoids on days 0, 6, 13 19 and 21 and was treated with niclosamide 7 times between day 24 and 31. These infections caused pronounced eosinophilia and an increase in parasite-specific IgM and IgG, but not IgE.

Diagnosis

In faecal samples, this species can easily be differentiated from *H. nana* by the larger size of proglottides or the absence of polar filaments on the inner membrane of the eggs.

CONTROL

Chemotherapy and prophylaxis

Treatment is as for *H. nana*. Good sanitary conditions, reduced rodent populations (especially rats) and avoidance of close rodent contact with humans or human food supplies will reduce the risk of infection.

3.6 *Diphyllobothrium latum* (human broad tapeworm or fish tapeworm)

The name fish tapeworm relates to the fact that a fish is the source of infection to humans, and the name broad (*latum*) to the fact that the proglottides are much wider than they are long, unlike the *Taenia* species.

This tapeworm is mainly known globally in temperate zones, and has been very common in parts of Europe where freshwater fishes are a common part of the diet; especially where certain lightly salted fish are eaten as delicacies. In Europe, the Baltic countries, Russia and especially Finland have been pointed out as having a high prevalence of human fish tapeworms. However, it is also present in tropical Africa and parts of Asia. In North and South America it is believed to have been introduced by immigrants. *Diphyllobothrium*

latum is the subject of a monograph by Von Bonsdorff (1977).

MORPHOLOGY AND STRUCTURE

D. latum is the longest tapeworm found in man, reaching up to 10 m or more, with over 3000 proglottides.

LIFE CYCLE

Fertilized eggs (50 × 60–70 μm in size) are released from mature proglottides through the uterus pore and can be found free in the faeces. After the liberation of the eggs, groups of proglottides then detach and degenerate; this is known as **pseudoapolysis**. The fertilized egg starts development in a suitable environment outside the host and time of embryonation is dependent on the temperature. When the first larva, the **coracidium**, has developed, it is ciliated, containing an oncosphere. It hatches from the operculated egg only when exposed to light. When freely suspended in freshwater, its food reserves enable it to swim around for about 12 h or until eaten. In order to complete its life cycle (Fig. 27.7), the coracidium must be eaten by suitable species and stages of small copepods, mainly of the genus *Diaptomus*, but also *Cyclops*. In the intestine of the copepod, the ciliated embryophore is shed and the oncosphere (hexacanth) penetrates the intestine into the hemocoele. Here it develops to an infective **procercoid** larva, where the 6 hooks of the hexacanth are confined to a small constricted posterior part called a **cercomer**. When copepods with infective procercoid larvae about 0.5 mm in length are eaten by a suitable second intermediate host (a freshwater fish) the procercoid penetrates the intestine of the fish and grows to the final larval stage, the **plerocercoid**. This lies freely in the body cavity or in the gut wall, or migrates to the muscles or the ovaries. The elongated plerocercoid (10–20 mm × 2–3 mm), which is not encysted or encapsulated, has a well-developed and normally contracted, partly invaginated scolex. Only certain species of freshwater fishes are suitable intermediate hosts, and they vary from location to location. If a small infected fish is eaten by a larger suitable fish host, the plerocercoids are, to some degree, able to penetrate the intestine of this second host and survive without further development; i.e. this host is a **paratenic** host in which the infective stage may accumulate. Secretions of enzymes from glands in the scolex are probably assisting the penetration of the intestinal wall. Humans become infected when they eat undercooked, raw, or lightly salted meat or roe from infected freshwater fishes. The adult, egg-producing stage is reached after about 4 weeks.

TRANSMISSION AND EPIDEMIOLOGY

Humans are the main final host and contribute most to the spread of the infection, but dogs, cats and foxes and, in some places, bears and pigs may be possible final hosts. Depending on the geographical location several different species of both copepods and freshwater fishes may act as first and second intermediate hosts, respectively. In Europe, the most important second intermediate hosts are pike, perch and turbot.

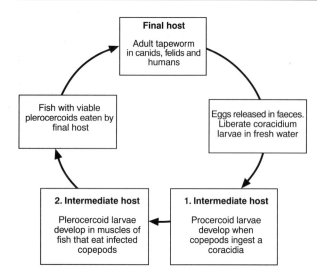

Final host

Adult tapeworm in canids, felids and humans

Fish with viable plerocercoids eaten by final host

Eggs released in faeces. Liberate coracidium larvae in fresh water

2. Intermediate host

Plerocercoid larvae develop in muscles of fish that eat infected copepods

1. Intermediate host

Procercoid larvae develop when copepods ingest a coracidia

Fig. 27.7 Life cycle of the human fish tapeworm, *Diphyllobothrium latum.*

LOCATION IN HOST

The tapeworm is usually found in the ileum or jejunum.

CLINICAL AND PATHOLOGICAL ASPECTS OF INFECTION

The number of human carriers of *D. latum*, which was estimated as about 10 million by Stoll (1947), has decreased in countries like Finland, where it is endemic and has caused many cases of pernicious anaemia. Although there are no recent data on the prevalence of *D. latum* infections, this infection is probably still frequent in countries where much freshwater fish is eaten.

Clinical manifestations

Most human infections are with only one tapeworm and cause no or very vague ill effects. Minor clinical manifestations such as fatigue, weakness, diarrhoea and numbness of the extremities may occur. It has been shown that worm carriers have a significantly higher frequency of these symptoms than controls (Saarni et al. 1963). In a few cases pernicious anaemia may develop due to manifest vitamin B_{12} deficiency (deficiency of cobalamins in general). Clinical diagnosis of this tapeworm-induced pernicious anaemia is made not only by a decreased vitamin B_{12} level in serum (around 100 pg/ml), but also by the presence of macrocytic megaloblastic anaemia in conjunction with leukopaenia, thrombocytopaenia and increased haemolysis. Furthermore, symptoms involving the central nervous system, such as paraesthesia, disturbances of motility and co-ordination and impairment of deep sensibility are also clinical criteria of tapeworm-induced pernicious anaemia.

Pathogenesis and pathology

D. latum, which contains more than 50 times as much vitamin B_{12} as *T. saginata*, has been shown to absorb as much as 80–100% of a single oral dose of vitamin

B_{12}, thereby competing with the host for this important vitamin. The size of the tapeworm and its proximity to the stomach will influence the amount of B_{12} absorption by the parasite: large worms in close proximity to the stomach reduce B_{12} availability to the host, greatly enhancing the probability of parasite-induced pernicious anaemia. In fact, it has been indicated that the anaemia may be relieved, if the tapeworm is forced further back in the intestine. However, other factors such as a relative deficiency in intrinsic factor due to endogenous or exogenous damage to the gastric mucosa, an inadequate supply of vitamin B_{12} in the diet or an increased requirement of vitamin B_{12} may contribute to the development of tapeworm-induced pernicious anaemia.

Immunity

Practically nothing is known about immune reactions in humans against *D. latum*, and there is no evidence of acquired immunity.

Diagnosis

Diagnosis of diphyllobothriasis is impossible from purely clinical symptoms. Confirmation of pernicious anaemia in a patient coming from an endemic area and known to have a diet of raw fish are relatively good indications. Evidence of the characteristic eggs of *D. latum* in faecal examinations is a reliable diagnosis, although eggs may be overlooked at routine examinations in about 5% of worm carriers. In suspected cases, several faecal specimens must be examined.

CONTROL

Chemotherapy

The broad tapeworm is more easily expelled than the *Taenia* species. Several drugs have been used, but niclosamide or praziquantel are the drugs of choice. Since the cure is not always 100%, examination for eggs in faecal samples should be performed 3 weeks after treatment.

Prophylaxis

It is very difficult, and in practice impossible, for sewage plants to remove 100% of eggs present in waste water. Adequate heating of fish dishes for a minimum of 10 min at 50°C (bone deep), or deep freezing (at least −10°C for 24 h) of fish or roe intended to be eaten raw or semi-raw is another prophylactic control measure. Brining of infected fish or roe should be very strong (10–12% NaCl) in order to kill plerocercoid larvae. However, this does not generally suit the taste of people eating the fish. In certain endemic areas, education of the public about the danger and how to avoid it should be given high priority.

Transmission

Because of uncontrolled defaecation, many *D. latum* eggs are often transferred directly to freshwater lakes, where first and second intermediate hosts are present. Therefore, control of this infection must cover chemotherapy of infected humans (removal of adult worms)

and control of human faeces (reducing risk of fresh-water contamination). Even if infected persons are found and treated and the egg-removal efficacy of sewage plants is improved to 100%, fish infections may still be maintained through infections of wild mammals.

4 SPORADIC ZOONOTIC ANIMAL TAPEWORMS THAT MAY INFECT HUMANS

Species are listed in alphabetical order of genus and species name.

4.1 *Bertiella* spp.

Species of *Bertiella* are found in primates and have been described as incidental zoonotic infections in humans in the tropics. *Bertiella studeri*, a common parasite in non-human primates in Africa, has been reported in a number of human cases. The life cycle of these tapeworms is not yet completely known but mites are suspected to be the infective intermediate host. Recently, human cases of *B. studeri* have been described in India (Panda and Panda 1994) and Indonesia (Kagei, Purba and Sakamoto 1992).

4.2 *Diphyllobothrium dendriticum*

This tapeworm, which is found in adult form in the intestine of many fish-eating birds, has also been shown to be infective to humans. The plerocercoid is found encysted on the entrails of many salmonid fishes. Because these are normally removed from the fish before preparation for human consumption, it is a rare human infection.

4.3 *Diphyllobothrium nihonkaiense*

This tapeworm, a close relative of *D. latum*, is described in Japan (Ohnishi and Murata 1994), where the number of cases have increased (Nishiyama 1994).

4.4 *Diphyllobothrium pacificum*

This species, which is adult in sea lions, has been described as a human tapeworm acquired from marine fishes. It has been found in Peru (Baer et al. 1967, Baer 1969), Japan (Tsuboi, Torii and Hirai 1993) and Equador (Gallegos and Brousselle 1991).

4.5 Other *Diphyllobothrium* species

A number of *Diphyllobothrium* species naturally occurring in free-living animals have been reported in a single or very few human cases. *Diphyllobothrium cordatum*, which occurs in seals, walruses and dogs, has been reported in humans in Greenland and Iceland; *D. hians* has been reported from Japan; *D. houghtoni*, a canine and feline tapeworm, has been found in humans in China; *D. orcini* and *D. scoticum* in Japan; *D. ursi*, a tapeworm of North American bears, has infected one person in British Columbia, Canada; *D. yonagoense* has been described from Japan. Some of these species may not be identified correctly.

4.6 *Dipylidium caninum* (the double-pored tapeworm)

This is a very common tapeworm in dogs and cats. Human infections are rare and normally restricted to young children, because infected fleas from cats or dogs must be ingested in order to acquire the infective cysticercoid stage (Gleason 1962). However, it has been suggested that infected fleas may be crushed in the dog's mouth, thereby releasing the cysticercoids, and these may be transmitted to children in the dog's saliva (Chappell 1991). This infection, which seldom causes any symptoms, can easily be diagnosed by the presence of active barrel-shaped proglottides. Furthermore, packets of about 15 eggs can be seen microscopically in the proglottides. Recently, cases have been described in Austria (Brandstetter and Auer 1994), USA (Raitiere 1992) and Japan (Watanabe, Horii and Nawa 1993).

4.7 *Mesocestoides* spp.

Species of this tapeworm are common in carnivorous mammals, such as foxes. Mites are probably the infective intermediate host. Incidental intake of infected mites has resulted in a few human cases published in Japan and the United States (Schultz et al. 1992). *Mesocestoides lineatus* has been recently found in humans in China (Jin, Yi and Liu 1991) and Korea (Eom, Kim and Rim 1992).

4.8 *Inermicapsifer madagascariensis*

This small (about 5 cm long) tapeworm, has been reported in humans from the eastern hemisphere, but also in children in Cuba and South America. It is common in rodents and hyraxes, and human cases have been reported from Madagascar and Mauritius and several countries in South and East Africa, where it is suspected to be more common than records indicate (Nelson, Pester and Rickman 1965). It was found in a 10 month old girl in Kenya (Chunge, Kabiru and Mugo 1987).

REFERENCES

Allan JC, Craig PS et al., 1992, Coproantigen detection for immunodiagnosis of echinococcosis and taeniasis in dogs and humans, *Parasitology*, **104**: 347–55.

Altmann G, Bubis JJ, 1959, A case of multiple infection with *Taenia saginata*, *Israel Med J*, **18**: 35.

Anderson RM, 1986, The population dynamics and epidemiology of intestinal nematode infections, *Trans R Soc Trop Med Hyg*, **80**: 686–96.

Andreassen J, 1991, Immunity to adult cestodes: Basic knowledge and vaccination problems. A review, *Parassitologia*, **33**: 45–53.

Arai HP, 1980, Migratory activity and related phenomena in *Hymenolepis diminuta*, *Biology of the Tapeworm* Hymenolepis diminuta, Academic Press, New York, 615–37.

Baer JG, 1969, *Diphyllobothrium pacificum*, a tapeworm from sea lions endemic in man along the coastal area of Peru, *J Fish Res Bd (Canada)*, **26**: 717–23.

Baer JG, Miranda CH et al., 1967, Human diphyllobothriasis in Peru, *Z Parasitenkd*, **28**: 277–89.

Bailey GNA, 1975, Energetics of a host-parasite system: A preliminary report, *Int J Parasitol*, **5**: 609–13.

Behnke JM, Bland PW, Wakelin D, 1977, Effect of the expulsion phase of *Trichinella spiralis* on *Hymenolepis diminuta* infection in mice, *Parasitology*, **75**: 79–88.

Boro'n-Kaczmarska A, Machicka-Roguska B et al., 1978, Untersuchungen über das Verhalten des Macrophagenmigrations-hemmtestes mit dem Polysaccharidantigen 'C' von *Taenia sag-*

inata in der menschlichen Täniase, *Zbl Bakt Hyg, IAbt Orig A*, **240**: 538–41.

Bowles J, McManus DP, 1994, Genetic characterization of the Asian *Taenia*, a newly described taeniid cestode of humans, *Am J Trop Med Hyg*, **50**: 33–44.

Brandstetter W, Auer H, 1994, *Dipylidium caninum*, ein seltener Parasit des Menschen, *Wiener Klin Wochen*, **106**: 115–16.

Chappell CL, 1991, Misinformation about *Dipylidium*. In reply, *Ped Infect Dis J*, **10**: 169.

Christensen JPB, Bøgh HO, Andreassen J, 1986, *Hymenolepis diminuta*: The effect of serum on different ages of worms *in vitro*, *Int J Parasitol*, **16**: 447–53.

Christie PR, Wakelin D, Wilson MM, 1979, The effect of the expulsion phase of *Trichinella spiralis* on *Hymenolepis diminuta* infection in rats, *Parasitology*, **78**: 323–30.

Chunge RN, Kabiru EW, Mugo BM, 1987, A human case of infection with a rodent cestode (*Inermicapsifer*) in Kenya, *East African Med J*, **64**: 424–27.

Elowni EE, 1982, *Hymenolepis diminuta*: the origin of protective antigens, *Exp Parasitol*, **53**: 157–63.

Eom KS, Rim H-J, 1993, Morphologic description of *Taenia asiatica* sp. n., *Korean J Parasitol*, **31**: 1–6.

Eom K, Kim SH, Rim HJ, 1992, Second case of human infection with *Mesocestoides lineatus* in Korea, *Korean J Parasitol*, **30**: 147–50.

Fan PC, 1988, Taiwan *Taenia* and taeniasis, *Parasitol Today*, **4**: 86–88.

Fan PC, Lin CY et al., 1995, Morphological description of *Taenia saginata asiatica* (Cyclophyllidea: Taeniidae) from man in Asia, *J Helminth*, **69**: 299–303.

FAO, 1991, *Report of the FAO expert consultation on helminth infections of livestock in developing countries (AGA, 815)*, FAO, Rome, 16–17.

Gallegos R, Brousselle C, 1991, Parasitoses intestinales chez les habitants d'un archipel Equatorien, *Bull Soc Franç Parasitol*, **9**: 219–223.

Galán-Puchades MT, Mas-Coma S, 1996, Considering *Taenia asiatica* at species level, *Parasitol Today*, **12**: 123.

Gleason NN, 1962, Records of *Dipylidium caninum*, the double-pored tapeworm, *J Parasitol*, **48**: 812.

Gottstein B, Deplazes P et al., 1991, Diagnostic identification of *Taenia saginata* with the polymerase chain reaction, *Trans R Soc Trop Med Hyg*, **85**: 248–49.

Gottstein B, Mowatt MR, 1991, Sequencing and characterization of an *Echinococcus multilocularis* DNA probe and its use in the polymerase chain reaction (PCR), *Mol Biochem Parasitol*, **44**: 183–94.

Grove DI, 1990, *A History of Human Helminthology*, CAB International, Wallingford, Oxon, 355–438.

Gustafsson MK, 1985, Cestode neurotransmitters, *Parasitol Today*, **1**: 72–75.

Halton DW, Fairweather L et al., 1990, Regulatory peptides in parasitic platyhelminths, *Parasitol Today*, **6**: 284–90.

Harris WG, Turton JA, 1973, Antibody response to tapeworm (*Hymenolepis diminuta*) in the rat, *Nature* (London), **246**: 521–22.

Hoeppli R, 1956, The knowledge of parasites and parasitic infections from ancient times to the 17th century, *Exp Parasitol*, **5**: 398–419.

Hoole D, Andreassen J, Birklund D, 1994, Microscopical observations on immune precipitates formed *in vitro* on the surface of hymenolepid tapeworms, *Parasitology*, **109**: 243–48.

Ito A, 1992, Cysticercosis in Asian-Pacific regions, *Parasitol Today*, **8**: 182.

Ito A, Smyth JD, 1987, Adult cestodes – Immunology of the lumen-dwelling cestode infections, *Immune responses in Parasitic Infections: Immunology, Immunopathology and Immunoprophylaxis. vol II: Trematodes and Cestodes*, ed. Soulsby EJL, CRC Press, Boca Raton, FL, 115–63.

Jin LG, Yi SH, Liu Z, 1991, (The first case of human infection with *Mesocestoides lineatus* (Goeze, 1782) in Jilin Province) In Chinese with English summary, *J Norman Bethune Univ Med Sci*, (No. 4): 360–1.

Kagei N, Purba Y, Sakamoto O, 1992, Two cases of human infection with *Bertiella studeri* in North Sumatra, Indonesia, *Jpn J Trop Med Hyg*, **20**: 166–68.

Khalil LF, Jones A, Bray RA, 1994, *Keys to the Cestode Parasites of Vertebrates*, CAB International, Wallingford, Oxon.

Levi MH, Raucher BG et al., 1987, *Hymenolepis diminuta*: one of three enteric pathogens isolated from a child, *Diagnostic Microbiol Infect Dis*, **7**: 255–9.

McManus DP, Bowles J, 1994, Asian (Taiwan) *Taenia*: species or strain?, *Parasitol Today*, **10**: 273–275.

Mehlhorn H, Becker B et al., 1981, On the nature of the proglottids of cestodes: light and electron microscope study of *Taenia*, *Hymenolepis* and *Echinococcus*, *Z Parasitenkde*, **65**: 243–59.

Mettrick DF, 1971, Effect of host dietary constituents on intestinal pH and the migratory behaviour of the rat tapeworm, *Hymenolepis diminuta*, *Can J Zool*, **49**: 1513–25.

Millon L, Berbineau L, Barale T, 1994, *Hymenolepis diminuta* chez l'enfant. À propos de 2 cas, *Bull Soc Franç Parasitol*, **12**: 157–60.

Moss GD, 1971, The nature of the immune response of the mouse to the bile duct cestode, *Hymenolepis microstoma*., *Parasitology*, **62**: 285–94.

Nelson GS, Pester FRN, Rickman R, 1965, The significance of wild animals in the transmission of cestodes of medical importance in Kenya, *Trans R Soc Trop Med Hyg*, **59**: 507–24.

Nishiyama, T, 1994, Environmental changes and tapeworm diseases in Japan – special reference to diphyllobothriasis nihonkaiense (diphyllobothriasis latum) (In Japanese with English summary), *Jpn J Parasitol*, **43**: 471–6.

Nollen PM, 1983, Patterns of sexual reproduction among parasitic platyhelminths, *Parasitology*, **86**: 99–120.

Ohnishi K, Murata M, 1994, Praziquantel for the treatment of *Diphyllobothrium nihonkaiense* infections in humans, *Trans R Soc Trop Med*, **88**: 580.

Panda DN, Panda MR, 1994, Record of *Bertiella studeri* (Blanchard, 1891), an anoplocephalid tapeworm, from a child, *Ann Trop Med Parasitol*, **88**: 451–52.

Pappas PW, Read CP, 1975, Membrane transport in helminth parasites: a review, *Exp Parasitol*, **37**: 469–530.

Pawlowski ZS, 1990, Perspectives on the control of *Taenia solium*, *Parasitol Today*, **6**: 371–3.

Prévot R, Hornbostel H, Dorken H, 1952, Lokalisationsstudien bei *Taenia saginata*, *Klin Wochenschr*, **30**: 78–80.

Raitiere CR, 1992, Dog tapeworm (*Dipylidium caninum*) infestation in a 6-month-old infant, *J Fam Prac*, **34**: 101–2.

Read CP, 1967, Longevity of the tapeworm, *Hymenolepis diminuta*, *J Parasitol*, **53**: 1055–6.

Rees G, 1967, Pathogenesis of adult cestodes, *Helminth Abstr*, **36**: 1–23.

Robertson NP, Cain GD, 1984, Glycosaminoglycans of tegumental fractions of *Hymenolepis diminuta*, *Mol Biochem Parasitol*, **12**: 173–83.

Saklatvala T, 1993, Milestones in parasitology, *Parasitol Today*, **9**: 347–48.

Saarni M, Nyberg W et al., 1963, Symptoms in carriers of *Diphyllobothrium latum* and in non-infected controls, *Acta Med Scand*, **173**: 147–54.

Schultz LJ, Roberto RR et al., 1992, *Mesocestoides* (Cestoda) infection in a California child, *Ped Infect Dis J*, **11**: 332–4.

Smyth JD, 1990, Peter Abildgaard: forgotten pioneer of parasitology, *Parasitol Today*, **6**: 337–39.

Stoll N, 1947, This wormy world, *J Parasitol*, **33**: 1–18.

Tesfa-Yohannes T-M, 1990, Effectiveness of praziquantel against *Taenia saginata* infections in Ethiopia, *Ann Trop Med Parasitol*, **84**: 581–85.

Threadgold LT, Robinson A, 1984, Amplification of the cestode surface: a stereological analysis, *Parasitology*, **89**: 523–35.

Tsuboi T, Torii M, Hirai K, 1993, Light and scanning electron microscopy of *Diphyllobothrium pacificum* expelled from a man, *Jpn J Parasitol*, **42:** 422–8.

Turton JA, Williamson JR, Harris WG, 1975, Haematological and immunolological responses to the tapeworm, *Tropenmed Parasitol*, **26:** 196–200.

Verster AJM, 1967, Redescription of *Taenia solium* Linnaeus, 1758 and *Taenia saginata* Goeze, 1782, *Z Parasitenkde*, **29:** 313–28.

Von Bonsdorff B, 1977, *Diphyllobothriasis in Man*, Academic Press, London.

Watanabe T, Horii Y, Nawa Y, 1993, A case of *Dipylidium caninum* in an infant – first case found in Miyazaki prefecture, Japan, *Jpn J Parasitol*, **42:** 234–6.

Williams JF, Perez-Esandi MV, 1971, Reaginic antibodies in dogs infected with *Echinococcus granulosus, Immunology*, **20:** 451–55.

WHO, 1995, *Model prescribing information – Drugs used in parasitic diseases*, 2nd edn, WHO, Geneva, 91–8.

Wright EP, 1984, Human infestation by *Taenia saginata* lasting over 20 years, *Postgrad Med J*, **60:** 495–6.

Larval cestodes

A Flisser

1 The parasites	2 The diseases

1 THE PARASITES

1.1 Introduction, classification and history

Larval cestodes belong to the phylum Platyhelminthes, which are acoelomate metazoa with an elongated dorsoventrally flattened body in their adult stage and a vesicular bladder in their larval stage. The most important human parasites of this group belong to the class Cestoda, subclass Eucestoda, order Cyclophyllidea, family Taeniidae and genera *Taenia*, *Hymenolepis*, *Diphyllobothrium* and *Echinococcus*. Except for *Echinococcus*, these parasites lodge in the human intestine in their adult stage. *Taenia solium*, *Echinococcus granulosus*, *E. multilocularis* and *E. vogeli* also parasitize humans in their larval stage. The metacestode of *T. solium* is known as a **cysticercus** and that of *Echinococcus* as a **hydatid cyst**. The general term for the disease caused by the cysticercus is termed **cysticercosis** and, depending of the site where these parasites lodge, is also known as neurocysticercosis, ophthalmocysticercosis or muscular cysticercosis. In the case of hydatid cyst, there are 3 types of **echinococcosis**: cystic echinococcosis due to *E. granulosus*, alveolar echinococcosis due to *E. multilocularis* and polycystic echinococcosis due to *E. vogeli*. The first is the most frequent of the 3, the second one is the most aggressive and the third is very rare.

Human cysticercosis is considered a public health problem in many developing countries of Latin America, non-Islamic Asia and Africa and it is clearly associated with lack of education and proper sanitary conditions (Flisser 1988). Cystic echinococcosis is of cosmopolitan distribution but concentrated in the major sheep-raising and pastoral areas. Alveolar echinococcosis has been reported in Alaska, China, parts of Europe and throughout Russia, but since the life cycle involves foxes and field mice, exposure to humans is relatively less common. Polycystic echinococcosis has been identified in humans in Brazil, Colombia, Ecuador, Panama and Venezuela because *E.*

vogeli is native to the humid tropical forests of South America (D'Alessandro et al. 1979, Kammerer and Schantz 1993).

Tapeworms in human faeces were first recognized by the Egyptians. The species was probably *Taenia saginata* since Egyptians did not eat pork. Hippocrates, Aristotle and Threophrastus called them 'flatworms' meaning band or ribbon worm, whereas Romans, such as Celsus, Pliny the Elder and Galen, named them 'lumbricus latus', meaning broad or wide worm. Only many centuries later were cysticerci discovered in human beings. They were first reported by Rumler in 1558, but the disease was not identified as parasitic until in 1697 Malpighi discovered the animal nature of cysticerci. Goeze recognized their helminthic essence in 1784 and Leuckart (1886) defined them in great detail. Tyson in 1683 detailed the head of tapeworms and later in 1691 described the hydatides that he found in 'rotten sheep'. Goeze in 1782 described the scolices of echinococcal cysts and indicated their similarity to the heads of tapeworms; he concluded that echinococci were alive, verminous in nature and related to tapeworms.

The life cycle of *T. solium* was defined by van Beneden in 1854 who fed a pig with eggs from a human *T. solium* and found numerous cysts in muscles, and by Kuchenmeister, who in 1855 discovered adult tapeworms in the intestines of convicts who ate pork infected with cysticerci some time before execution (Grove 1990). In 1933 Yoshino ingested swine cysticerci in order to obtain a reliable source of eggs to infect pigs and studied with great histological detail the early development of cysticerci. He also reported that, following his own infection, 1–5 gravid proglottids were expelled per day for 2 years (Yoshino 1933). The name 'Cysticercus cellulosae' was given by Zeder and by Rudolphi at the beginning of last century, but was abolished when cysticerci were shown to be larval stage of *Taenia*.

The life cycle of *Echinococcus* was demonstrated by von Siebold in 1853 when he infected dogs with hydatid cysts from sheep and 27 days later discovered intestinal worms, consisting of a head and 3 segments containing reproductive organs and eggs, which he called *Taenia echinococcus*. Leuckart in 1867 infected suckling pigs with ova of *T. echinococcus* and was able to study the resulting cysts at intervals after infection. Naunyn in 1863 infected dogs with hundreds of scolices obtained after autopsy of a patient with a large hepatic cyst. The dog, when killed after 5 weeks, had mature small tapeworms identical to *Taenia echinococcus*. Thus Naunyn not only confirmed that hydatid cysts of human origin undergo the same development as cysts of animal origin but, in demonstrating that the adult worms obtained from the 2 sources were similar, also showed that there was only a single species. Naunyn concluded that the *Echinococcus* from man is the bladder worm stage of *T. echinococcus* living in the intestine of the dog. These results were confirmed soon afterwards by Krabbe and Finsen in Iceland in 1866 and by Thomas in Australia in 1883, all of whom used hydatid cysts obtained from humans (Grove 1990).

1.2 Morphology and structure

The body of an adult tapeworm has a head (**scolex**), a neck, and a chain of segments (**strobila**). The scolex is the size of a pinhead, while the strobila may be several metres long, as in *Taenia*, containing more than 1000 proglottids. In *Echinococcus* there are only 2–5 segments and the strobila measures only a few millimetres. The scolex has 4 suckers and a rostellum with a double crown of hooks (Figs 28.1a–c).

The most conspicuous features of tapeworms are the lack of a mouth or digestive cavity and the presence of repeated units or proglottids at different developmental stages. The proximal proglottids are immature, i.e. have not yet developed sexual organs, the mature proglottids contain functional hermaphroditic sexual organs, where fertilization occurs and the terminal proglottids are gravid, being little more than sacs full of eggs (see Chapter 27).

Eggs are spherical and range in size from 20 to 50 μm. They have a radial appearance under light microcopy because the embryophore that surrounds the embryo (**oncosphere**) is formed by contiguous blocks. The eggs of *Taenia* and *Echinococcus* are morphologically indistinguishable at the light microscope level.

The embryophore protects the oncosphere while the egg is in the external environment, making eggs extremely resistant and enabling them to disperse and withstand a wide range of environmental temperatures (Gemmell and Lawson 1986, Torgerson et al. 1995, Veit et al. 1995).

When the eggs are released from the definitive host they are, or quickly become, fully embryonated and infective to a suitable host. When eggs are ingested by the intermediate host, the cementing substance that joins the embryophoric blocks is digested and the oncosphere is released in the small intestine (Flisser 1994).

The liberated and activated oncosphere is mobile and uses its hooks to penetrate into the mucosa, reaching the lamina propria within 3–120 min after hatching. Penetration is presumably assisted by secretions from the penetration glands, but may be purely mechanical, involving hook and body movements (Thompson 1995).

After penetration, larvae are transported through blood vessels into the tissues, where they develop into the metacestode, specifically named **cysticercus** (*Taenia*) or **hydatid cyst** (*Echinococcus*). Macroscopic *T. solium* cysticerci measuring around 0.3 mm were seen in liver, brain and skeletal muscles of pigs 6 days after infection, and after 60–70 days cysticerci had fully developed scolices and measured 6–9 mm. Full development of cysticerci (to a size of 8–15 mm) takes 2–3 months in pigs (Yoshino 1933). Several in vivo and in vitro studies have demonstrated that *Echinococcus* oncospheres rapidly undergo a series of reorganizational events during the first 14 days, involving cellular proliferation, degeneration of oncospheral hooks, muscular atrophy, vesicularization, central cavity formation and development of both germinal and

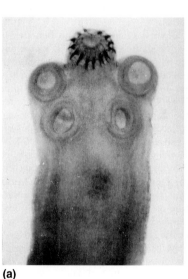

(a)

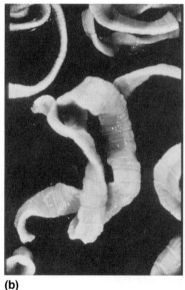

(b)

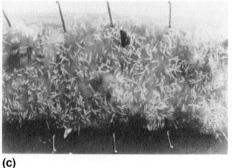

(c)

Fig. 28.1 (a) *Taenia solium* scolex showing the double crown of hooks and one sucker; (b) *Taenia solium* strobila with immature proglottids (upper left) and mature proglottids; (c) Multiple *Echinococcus granulosus* adult parasites in the intestine of a dog. (By courtesy of Professor P Craig).

laminated layers (Rausch 1954, Heath and Lawrence 1976). The minimum time required for the development of protoscolices inside cysts within the human host is not known, in pigs it takes 10–12 months and in sheep 10 months to 4 years, although protoscolices can be formed in cysts that measure 0.5–2 cm. The cysticercus is formed by one scolex, while each hydatid cyst contains multiple protoscolices formed by asexual budding processes of the bladder's germinal layer. The metacestode and the adult worm are macroscopic and have the same scolex, but eggs and oncospheres are microscopic.

There are 2 morphological types of cysticerci: cellulose and racemose (see Fig. 28.2). Cellulose cysticerci are small, spherical or oval, white or yellow, vesicles that measure 0.5–1.5 cm and have a translucent bladder wall, through which the scolex can be seen as a small solid eccentric granule. Usually this stage grows no further. This type of cysticercus is frequently separated from the host tissue by a thin collagenous capsule, within which it remains alive. The racemose cysticercus either appears as a large, round or lobulated bladder circumscribed by a delicate wall or resembles a cluster of grapes. It measures up to 10 or even 20 cm and may contain 60 ml fluid. The scolex cannot be seen; in some cases only detailed histological studies will reveal its remains. Neuropathological observations of human brain suggest that parasites lodged in spacious areas are able to grow and transform into racemose cysticerci, since a parasite with a bilobulated aspect was found (Rabiela, Rivas and Flisser 1989). In support of this hypothesis is the finding that experimental infections with *T. serialis* in mice demonstrated an aberrant large cysticercus devoid of scolex in the peritoneal cavity (Lachberg, Thompson and Lymberry 1990). Alternatively, growth of cysticerci might be controlled by the immune response of the host, as suggested by in vitro experiments which showed that the presence of the inflammatory capsule that surrounds *T. solium* cysticerci inhibits their evagination (Ostrosky et al. 1991, Flisser and Madrazo 1996).

The fully developed *E. granulosus* hydatid cyst is typically unilocular, subspherical in shape and fluid filled. The cyst consists of an inner germinal nucleated layer supported externally by a tough, elastic, acellular laminated layer of variable thickness, surrounded by a host-produced fibrous adventitial layer. Asexual proliferation takes place in the germinal layer and brood capsule formation is entirely endogenous; within each capsule several protoscolices are found. Occasionally cysts may adjoin and coalesce, forming groups of clusters of small cysts of different size. In humans, the slowly growing hydatid cysts may attain a volume of many litres and contain many thousands of protoscolices. With time, internal septae and daughter cysts may form within the primary cyst, disrupting the unilocular pattern (Schantz 1994, Thompson 1995). (See Fig. 28.3.)

The metacestode of *E. multilocularis* is the most complex and develops quite differently from that of *E. granulosus*. The size of the parasites varies from less than 1 mm to 20 mm, but the lesions caused by the metacestodes vary from minor foci (a few millimetres in diameter) up to large areas of infiltration. The metacestode is a multivesicular infiltrating structure with no limiting host–parasite barrier (adventitial layer). The larval mass usually contains a semisolid matrix rather than fluid and is formed by numerous small vesicles embedded in a dense stroma of connective tissue. The metacestode consists of a network of filamentous solid cellular protrusions of the germinal layer which are responsible for infiltrating growth, transforming into tube-like and cystic structures where proliferation occurs both endogenously and exogenously (see Fig. 28.4.)

Detachment of germinal cells from infiltrating cellular protrusions and their subsequent distribution via the lymph or blood can give rise to the distant metastatic foci characteristic of alveolar echinococcosis. In rodents, the natural intermediate hosts, the larval mass proliferates rapidly by exogenous budding of germinative tissue and produces an alveolar-

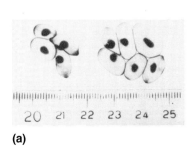

(a)

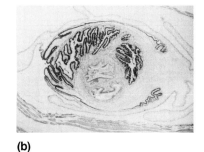

(b)

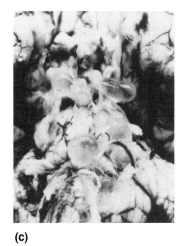

(c)

Fig. 28.2 (a) Cellulose type *Taenia solium* cysticerci from pig muscle. (By courtesy of Dr D. Correa); (b) Histological section of a cellulose type cysticercus in host muscle showing the spiral canal and the bladder wall (By courtesy of Dr AS de Aluja); (c) Racemose type *Taenia solium* cysticerci in the base of a human brain. (By courtesy of Dr MT Rabiela).

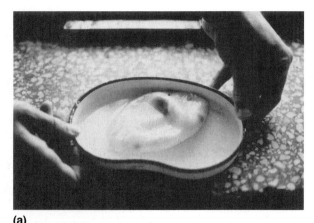

(a)

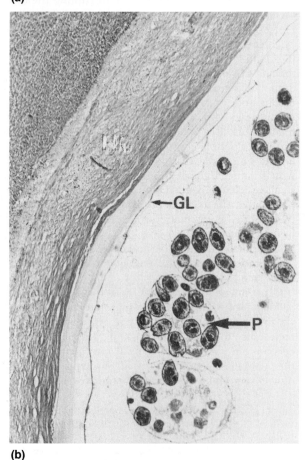

(b)

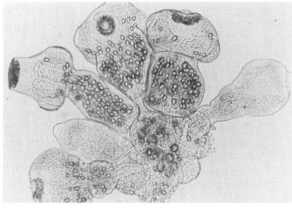

(c)

Fig. 28.3 Continued.

Fig. 28.3 (a) *Echinococcus* cyst from the liver of a patient in Urumqi, China. (By courtesy of Professor P Craig); (b) Histologic section of an *Echinococcus granulosus* cyst with many protoscolices (P) and the germinal layer (GL). (By courtesy of Dr P Schantz); (c) *Echinococcus granulosus* protoscolices seen under light microscopy, partly evaginated. (By courtesy of Prof. P Craig).

like pattern of microvesicles filled with protoscolices, but in humans the larval mass resembles a malignancy in appearance and behaviour because it proliferates continuously by exogenous budding and invades the surrounding tissues. Protoscolices are rarely observed in infections of humans. (Wilson and Rausch 1980, Ali-Khan et al. 1983).

The metacestode of *E. vogeli* exhibits developmental and structural characteristics considered intermediate to those of *E. granulosus* and *E. multilocularis,* with sizes that range from 2 to 80 mm. It may occur singly, in small groups, or occasionally in dense aggregations in which each cyst is enclosed by its separate adventitial layer. It has internal division of fluid-filled cysts to form multichambered growths due to endogenous proliferation and convolution of both germinal and laminated layers, leading to the formation of secondary subdivisions of the primary vesicle with production of brood capsules and protoscolices in the resultant chambers, which are often interconnected (D'Alessandro et al. 1979 Rausch, D'Alessandro and Rausch 1981).

Cystic hydatid cysts develop in 6 months in mice, 10 months in sheep and 1 year in swine. Alveolar cysts develop in 2–4 months in mice. Development of any of these metacestodes in humans is not known because it is impossible to define the time of infection. The life span of these parasites can be as long as 4 or more years in sheep, up to 16 years in horses and, impressively, several decades in humans (Dixon and Lipscomb 1961, Spruance 1974, Rabiela et al. 1982).

1.3 General biology

Studies on the biochemistry of Platyhelminthes are sparse. The first contributions dealing with tapeworms, from Read (1952), related to anaerobic metabolism in the rat tapeworm and the role of carbohydrates in cestode biology, and these stimulated work on the biochemistry of protoscolices of *E. granulosus.* More recently it was shown that cysticerci use either aerobic or anaerobic pathways according to oxygen availability in the environment (Cervantes-Vazquez et al. 1990), oxygen uptake being a useful measurement of their viability (Correa et al. 1987, Flisser et al. 1990a).

Larval cestodes obtain nutrients by diffusion through their bladder wall which bears plasma-membrane bounded microvilli covered by a loose glycocalyx. The syncytial tegument is filled with ellipsoidal vesicles of different sizes and is connected by cytoplasmic processes to the underlying nucleated cell bodies. The excretory or protonephridial system consists of flame cells which form a dense network attached to excretory ducts. The bladder wall also contains

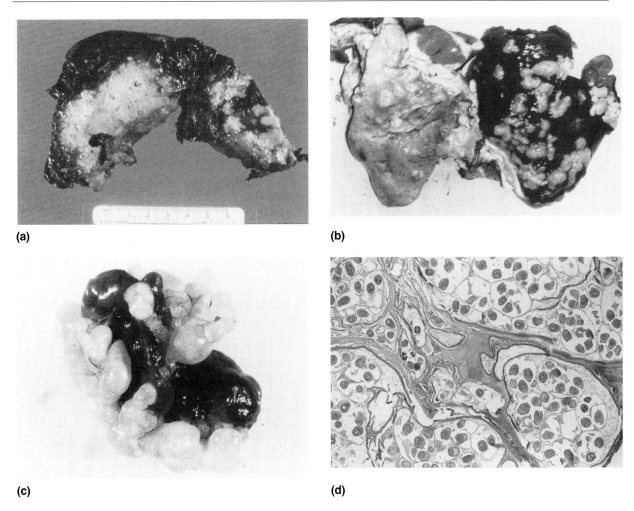

(a)

(b)

(c)

(d)

Fig. 28.4 (a) *Echinococcus multilocularis* in the liver of a 61 year old female from Minnesota, USA. (By courtesy of Dr P Schantz); (b) *Echinococcus multilocularis* in the liver and lungs of a sheep. (By courtesy of Professor RAC Thompson); (c) *Echinococcus multilocularis* in the liver of a cotton rat 4 months after infection . (By courtesy of Professor P Craig); (d) Histological section of *Echinococcus multilocularis* showing multiple vesicle filled with protoscolices. (By courtesy of Dr P Schantz).

a network of nerve-like cells. Immunohistochemical studies on protoscolices of *E. granulosus* have identified serotonin in nerve cell bodies in the lateral ganglia and in association with the lateral longitudinal nerve cords as well as in the central nerve ring, the rostellar nerves and the nerve plexus of the suckers; some peptidergic nerve elements were also detected (Fairweather et al. 1994).

Several glycoproteins have been detected on the tegumentary surface of the bladder wall of *T. solium* cysticerci: the most abundant (of 55 kDa) was found to be the heavy chain of the host's IgG and one of 180 kDa was also present on proglottid surface of several taeniids (Landa et al. 1994). The excretory–secretory molecule designated *T. solium* antigen B, initially identified as an immunodominant antigen (Flisser, Woodhouse and Larralde 1980), has received great interest. It has been purified and characterized as a glycoprotein (Guerra et al. 1982) which has a significant homology with paramyosin from *Schistosoma mansoni* (Laclette et al. 1991) and it inhibits the C1 component of the complement system (Laclette et al. 1992). Paramyosin from *E. granulosus* shows 71% identity with *S. mansoni* paramyosin and a significant homology with *T. solium* paramyosin (Muhlschlegel et al. 1993). Cholinesterases and cysteine and aspartic, but not serine, protease activities have been identified in *T. solium* cys-

ticerci (White et al. 1992). In *E. granulosus* several enzymes have been demonstrated in the tegument that may have a digestive or absorptive function (McManus and Bryant 1995). At least 5 proteolytic enzymes have been detected in the cyst fluid (Marco and Nieto 1991) and gluthathione *S*-transferase has been isolated from protoscolices (Fernandez and Hormaeche 1994). The chemical composition of hydatid cysts from different geographic and host origins has been studied in detail (Sanchez and Sanchez 1971, Frayha and Haddad 1980) and has revealed basic differences between the UK horse and sheep strains of *E. granulosus* and between these and *E. multilocularis* (McManus and Smyth 1978). A subsequent study of the biochemical composition of *E. granulosus* in Kenya indicates differences between protoscolices of cattle, goat, camel and sheep origin but similarities between the sheep and human parasites (McManus 1981).

Many different molecular biological techniques have been applied with great success to the characterization of *E. granulosus* strains. Biological criteria indicate that distinct horse–dog and sheep–dog forms of *E. granulosus* occur in UK (reviewed by Thompson and Lymbery 1988) and this has been confirmed by a variety of molecular techniques (Bowles and McManus 1993). These studies also indicate that the sheep strain is genetically uniform and cosmopolitan in its geographical distribution and that the horse strain is genetically similar to that infecting equines in other countries. DNA sequence data show that the sheep and horse strain parasites do not interbreed despite the fact that they use the same definitive host and occur sympatrically. Based on this and many other data, the sheep and horse strains of *E. granulosus* should probably be regarded as different species (McManus and Bryant 1995).

1.4 Life cycle

The life cycle of larval cestodes involves only 2 hosts, one definitive and one intermediate, and 3 developmental stages: the adult tapeworm in the definitive host, eggs in the environment and the metacestode in the intermediate host (see Figs 28.5 and 28.6). The cycle is simple in principle: the adult stage develops in the intestine after the host ingests the metacestode lodged in the tissue of the intermediate host. The metacestode develops in muscle, liver or lungs after the intermediate host ingests eggs from the environment. Eggs or proglottids are released into the environment from the adult intestinal parasite. In *T. solium*, the adult stage occurs only in human beings, whereas dogs and other canids are the hosts of the adult *Echinococcus* . Intermediate hosts for *T. solium* are mainly pigs, although hydatid cysts can occur in a great variety of mammals. Cysticerci can develop in other mammals but have no epidemiological relevance. The importance of *T. solium* and *Echinococcus* is that humans can also harbour the larval stage which may cause severe disease (see Figs 28.5 and 28.6).

Depending on the geographical location and the intermediate hosts, 2 biological forms of *E. granulosus* have been recognized, the northern and the European biotypes. The northern biotype is maintained in the tundra and taiga by a predator–prey relationship between the wolf and large deer (elks, reindeer and other cervids) but may also occur in humans where reindeer are domesticated, as in western Alaska and Eurasia, being acquired from dogs used in herding or from eggs dispersed by wolves. Coyotes may also become infected from scavenging. The intermediate hosts of the European biotype include camels, cattle, goat, horses, pigs and sheep; buffalo, wild boar, llama, kangaroo, wallaby, gazelle, giraffe and impala, among others, have also been reported to have hydatid cysts. The European biotype is almost cosmopolitan, as a result of the introduction of domestic animals and their helminths by Europeans in colonizing other regions from the early sixteenth century onwards. The adult stage occurs mainly in dogs but also in foxes, dingoes, jackals and hyenas (Rausch 1995).

The adult stage of *E. multilocularis* is found mainly in foxes, rarely in wolves, regionally in coyotes, and also in cats, black bear and lynx. Only 8 families of rodents have been reported to be infected with the metacestodes, these include voles and lemmings, hamsters and gerbils, rats and mice, squirrels, shrews, moles and pikas.

E. vogeli is a neotropical species maintained in the bush dog and the paca. Other mammals can be easily infected, as was seen in Los Angeles Zoo where several young animals were housed near a bush dog captured in Colombia. During the following 10 years 7 orangutans, 3 chimpanzees, 2 gibbons and a siamang died or were killed with terminal disease; thereafter 3 gorillas died and 2 survivors had advanced disease (Howard and Gendron 1980).

1.5 Location in the host

Characteristically, *T. solium* cysticerci lodge in the central nervous system, the eye, subcutaneous tissue and striated muscle (see Fig. 28.7). It is not known why

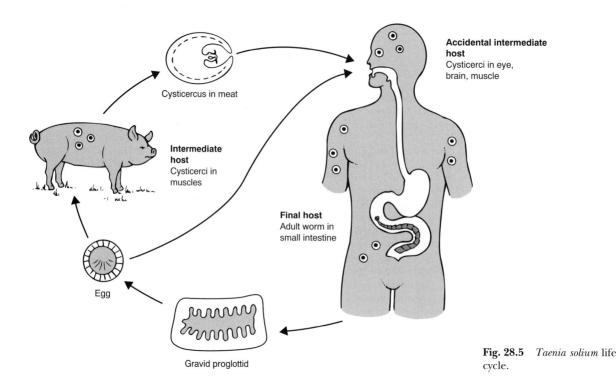

Cysticercus in meat

Accidental intermediate host
Cysticerci in eye, brain, muscle

Intermediate host
Cysticerci in muscles

Final host
Adult worm in small intestine

Egg

Gravid proglottid

Fig. 28.5 *Taenia solium* life cycle.

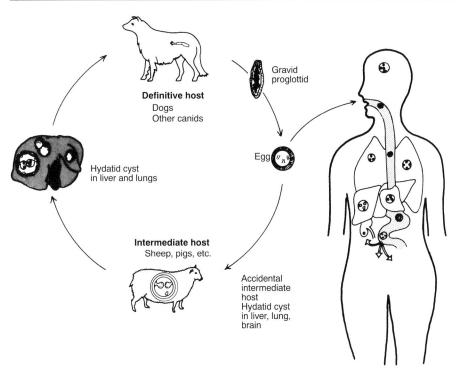

Fig. 28.6 *Echinococcus* life cycle.

cysticerci develop primarily in these tissues; cysticerci have exceptionally been found many other organs and tissues, most probably as a result of severe immuno-suppression. The location of parasites in 2188 cases of cysticercosis collected from several Latin American countries was: central nervous system 82%, eye and annexes 17%, subcutaneous tissue 7%, muscle 5%, other organs 6%, generalized 1%. In the central nervous system cysticerci are more frequently found in subarachnoidal spaces, and less often in parenchyma and ventricles (Rabiela et al. 1982, Escobar 1983). From 161 neurosurgical cases, 89 had cysticerci in the fourth ventricle, 20 in the third ventricle 17 in the lateral ventricle, 27 were subarachnoidal and 8 were spinal (Madrazo and Flisser 1992). The cellulose type is the most frequent cysticercus in human brain, although in 9–13% of studied cases, cysticerci of both types coexisted in the same brain (Rabiela et al. 1982). Racemose cysticerci are only found in spacious areas of the brain such as ventricular cavities and some subarachnoidal spaces, mainly the basal meningeal cisternae (Rabiela, Rivas and Flisser 1989); they are found only in human brain and not in swine. Studies of ocular infections indicate that 46% of cysticerci are found in vitreous humour, 37% are subretinal, 12% are subconjuntival, 2% occur in the orbit, 2% are subcutaneous and 1% occur in the anterior chamber (Puig-Solanes 1974, Gomez-Leal 1989). In ocular, muscular and subcutaneous cysticercosis only cellulose cysticerci are found.

Most primary infections of *E. granulosus* in humans consist of a single cyst; however, 20–40% of patients have multiple cysts or multiple organ involvement. The liver is the most common site, followed by the lungs. The frequency of *E. granulosus* cysts recorded in the Australian Hydatid Registry was: liver 63%, lungs 25%, muscles 5%, bones 3%, kidney 2%, spleen 1%, brain 1% and exceptionally other organs. Similar figures were recorded in Switzerland. Cysts may be very big (one reported in 1928 contained 48 l of fluid) but at the time of diagnosis most cysts measure 1–10 cm. In contrast to cysticercosis, where parasites do not change in size, except when racemose cysts are formed, hydatid cysts do grow. A study performed in 265 Turkana patients showed that average growth was 9 cm per year, 16% of cysts did not expand, 30% grew slowly (1–5 mm per year), 42% showed a moderate growth rate (6–15 mm per year) and 11% increased rapidly in size (31 mm in average per year), with a maximum growth in one case of 160 mm per year (Ammann and Eckert 1995).

The primary location of alveolar hydatid is the liver, but the capacity for tumour-like proliferation and the potential for metastasis means that development can also occur in lung, brain, bone or other organs (Eckert, Thompson and Mehlhorn 1983, Ammann and Eckert 1995). Distant metastases were found in 13% of 70 Swiss patients and in 10% of 152 Japanese patients (Mesarina-Wicki 1991, Sato et al. 1993). Polycystic echinococcosis has characteristics intermediate between the cystic and alveolar forms (D'Alessandro et al. 1979, Meneghelli et al. 1992). The relatively large cysts are filled with liquid and contain brood capsules with numerous protoscolices. The primary location is the liver, but cysts may spread to contiguous sites.

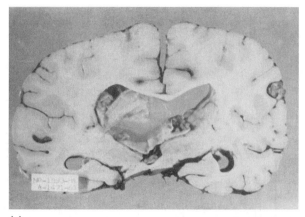

(a)

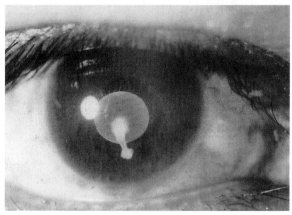

(b)

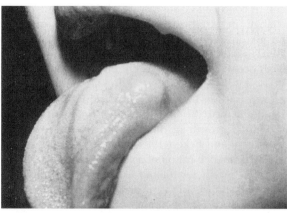

(c)

Fig. 28.7 (a) Brain section showing a huge ventricular cysticercus and a small subarachnoidal parasite. (By courtesy of Dr J Olvera); (b) *Taenia solium* cysticercus in the anterior chamber of the eye: interestingly, it is evaginated. (By courtesy of Dr D Lozano); (c) Tongue of child with a cysticercus in the muscle. (By courtesy of Dr A Martuscelli).

2 THE DISEASES

2.1 Clinical manifestations and pathology

Neurocysticercosis is characterized by its great diversity of signs and symptoms. It is a complex disease with major manifestations depending on the number,

location and type of parasites lodged in the CNS and meninges as well as by the extent of the inflammatory response (Earnest et al. 1987, Takayanagui and Jardim 1983, del Brutto and Sotelo 1988). Seizures are the most frequent clinical manifestation, occurring on average in 70% of cases (Flisser 1994) and late onset epilepsy shows a strong association with cysticercosis (Vazquez and Sotelo 1992, Garcia et al. 1993). Patients with seizures caused by parenchymal calcified or cellulose single cysticerci have a mild disease as compared to those that have hydrocephalus as a consequence of meningeal arachnoiditis, which is frequently fatal (see Fig. 28.8).

Racemose cysticerci elicit a more intense inflammatory reaction and frequently produce severe mass effects. Progressive inflammation is elicited when the parasite is in contact with the meninges and causes scar tissue proliferation that gives rise to mechanical obstruction of CSF circulation and intracranial hypertension due to hydrocephalus. Acute stages of the disease produce intracranial hypertension due to intense oedema induced by numerous developing cysticerci (most commonly found in young patients), ependymitis or arachnoiditis (Rabiela et al. 1982, Escobar 1983, Rabiela, Rivas and Flisser 1989, Puri et al. 1991, Madrazo and Flisser 1992). Idiopathic epilepsy, multiple intracranial space-occupying lesions, chronic meningitis, some bacterial and parasitic infections as well as primary and secondary malignancies affecting the central nervous system can mimic neurocysticercosis (Rodriguez-Carbajal and Boleaga-Duran 1982, Almeida-Pinto et al. 1988, Puri et al. 1991). A similar picture of clinical heterogeneity is also found in ocular cysticercosis (Puig-Solanes 1974, Gomez-Leal 1989). Cysticerci in the subcutaneous tissue and muscles are usually asymptomatic or well tolerated (Botero et al. 1993) probably because they are found in small numbers. Muscular pseudohypertrophy due to cysticercosis has been reported in cases that have many parasites and marked muscle enlargement and pain (Zhipiao et al. 1980, Rim and Joo 1989). In 2188 patients with neurocysticercosis from several Latin American countries, 68% were between 20 and 49 years of age, only 19% were detected below 20 years, and 13% were above 50 years. In contrast, in 30 Mexican cases of ocular cysticercosis 38% were under 20 years, 58% were between 20 and 49 years and 4% were above 50 years (Cardenas et al. 1989) probably indicating that cysticerci in the eyes are easily seen and thus diagnosed at a younger age, and that neurological symptoms start several years after infection.

Symptomatology in cystic echinococcosis is usually related to parasite burden. Because of the slowly growing nature of echinococcal cysts, most cases of liver and lung cysts are diagnosed in adult patients and symptoms are related to tumour-like lesions. Only 10–20% of cases are diagnosed in patients less than 16 years, primarily where cysts are located in the brain or eye, the latter being similar to cysticercosis. Clinical manifestations are variable and determined by the site, size, and condition of the cysts, for example, 67% of 297 patients with cysts > 5 cm diameter had symp-

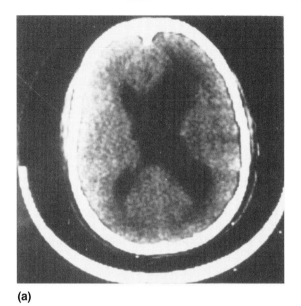

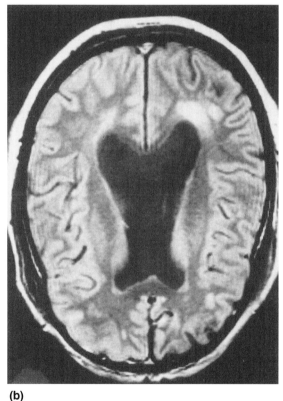

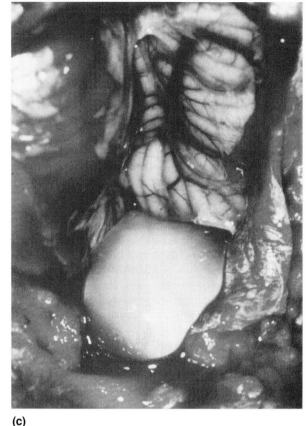

(c)

Fig. 28.8 Continued.

Fig. 28.8 Hydrocephalus due to CSF blockage caused by a racemose type cysticercus seen in CT (a), MR (b) and during surgery (c). (By courtesy of Dr I Madrazo).

toms, as compared to 48% of 123 cases with cysts < 5 cm; overall 38% were asymptomatic. The signs and symptoms of hepatic echinococcosis may include hepatic enlargement, with or without a palpable mass, liver abscesses, calcified lesions, epigastric pain, nausea, and vomiting, portal hypertension, inferior vena cava compression or thrombosis, secondary biliary cirrhosis, biliary colic-like symptoms, biliary peritonitis or fistula formation. If a cyst ruptures, the sudden release of its contents may precipitate allergic reactions ranging from mild to fatal anaphylaxis, bacterial infection may occur and there is spread of protoscolices, which may result in a multiple secondary echinococcosis disease (Kammerer and Schantz 1993, Ammann and Eckert 1995). Clinical symptoms of pulmonary cystic echinococcosis are tumour-like chest pain, chronic cough, fever, haemoptysis pneumothorax, pleuritis, lung abscess, eosinophilic pneumonitis, lung embolism and sometimes expectoration of cyst content (Schantz and Okello 1990). Nearly 40% of patients with pulmonary hydatidosis have liver involvement as well (Little 1976). Cysts in other locations such as the heart, spine and brain and even bone also generate tumour-like symptomatology (Ammann and Eckert 1995). Brain hydatid cysts may be confused with neurocysticercosis because of similar images in tomography. In these cases, the epidemiological history is the best way of confirming diagnosis, together with specific immunological tests (Flisser 1988).

Infection of the liver with *E. multilocularis*, the primary location in humans, closely mimics hepatic carcinoma or cirrhosis. Clinical cases are characterized by a chronic course of the disease lasting for weeks, months or years. Lesions consist of a central necrotic cavity filled with a white amorphous material that is covered with a thin peripheral layer of dense fibrous tissue (Wilson and Rausch 1980, Rausch et al. 1987).

Focal areas of calcification exist, as does extensive infiltration by proliferating vesicles. The initial symptoms of alveolar hydatid disease are usually vague. Mild upper quadrant and epigastric pain with hepatomegaly may progress to obstructive jaundice. Occasionally, the initial manifestations are related to metastases to the lungs or brain. The mortality in progressive, clinically manifest cases may be 50% to 75% (Wilson and Rausch 1980, Kammerer and Schantz 1993) and much higher figures (up to 100%) have been recorded in untreated or inadequately treated patients. Radiographic or serologic screening of high-risk patients results in detection of early-stage disease, improving prognosis through earlier application of therapy (Kammerer and Schantz 1993). Spontaneous death of alveolar hydatid cysts was clearly documented in 5 asymptomatic individuals in Alaska; lesions were circumscribed and calcified with a mineralized wall and a cavity filled with amorphous necrotic material, in some cases also with folded parasite membranes, suggesting that death at early stages is probably not uncommon (Rausch et al. 1987). Alveolar echinococcosis is typically seen in persons of advanced age, the average age being > 50 years as compared to < 40 in cystic echinococcosis.

2.2   Immune response

Immune responses in patients with neurocysticercosis have been studied mainly because of the need to standardize immunological methods for diagnosis (Flisser, Woodhouse and Larralde 1980, Flisser and Larralde 1986, Richards and Schantz 1991). Anti-cysticercus antibodies of several immunoglobulin isotypes have been detected, although the most frequently found are IgG antibodies in serum, cerebrospinal fluid and saliva. Interestingly IgG anti-cysticercus antibodies are not found in all compartments of the same patient (Cho et al. 1986, Espinoza et al. 1986, Feldman et al. 1990, Wilson et al. 1991). The presence of IgG confirms that the disease is usually chronic and long-term. A few reports indicate an increase in total or specific IgE (Goldberg et al. 1981, Gorodezky et al. 1987, Short et al. 1991), IgM is less frequently found in CSF than IgG, and IgA antibodies have been reported in few cases although not in saliva. Antibodies have been detected in 94% of cases with 2 or more parasites, but only 28% of cases with single lesions, and in most cases with undamaged parasites, but in only 44% of cases with calcified cysticerci (Espinoza et al. 1986, Baily et al. 1988, Chang et al. 1988, Michault et al. 1990, Michel et al. 1990, Wilson et al. 1991). Differences have also been found between benign and malignant cysticercosis, the later state being more antigenic.

As in cysticercosis, the humoral immune response in patients with hydatid disease has been used widely to diagnose infection or disease and the main emphasis has been characterization of parasite antigens (Lightowlers et al. 1993, Lightowlers and Gottstein 1995). Experimental studies indicate that antibodies to antigen 5 are among the first detected following infection with *E. granulosus* (Conder, Andersen and

Schantz 1980) but are also found in patients with neurocysticercosis or alveolar echinococcosis (Varela-Diaz, Coltorti and D'Alessandro 1978, Schantz and Gottstein 1986, Moro et al. 1992). ELISA and western blotting are usually performed with anti-human IgG as this is the main isotype in human hydatid disease. The demonstration of parasite-specific IgE has attracted particular attention but, as in human neurocysticercosis, has no signficant immunodiagnostic advantage in cystic echinococcosis. In contrast, 68% of patients with alveolar echinococcosis tested positive for parasite-specific IgE by ELISA and between 50% and 88% by the radioallergosorbent test (Vuitton et al. 1988, Gottstein 1992, Liu, Lightowlers and Rickard 1992, Moro et al. 1992, Lightowlers and Gottstein 1995). Strain variation in the parasite, geographical origin of the patient and differences in the host–parasite relationship may significantly affect the serological response.

The main antigen recognized by patients in both diseases is antigen B. However, *T. solium* antigen B is different from *E. granulosus* antigen B. The first is a glycoprotein of 110 kDa (Guerra et al. 1982) while the second is a lipoprotein of 120–160 kDa (Oriol and Oriol 1975). Both are immunodominant; 85% of patients with neurocysticercosis have sera that react with *T. solium* antigen B (Flisser, Woodhouse and Larralde 1980, Espinoza et al. 1986) and 86% of patients with hydatid disease recognize *E. granulosus* antigen B (Williams, Pérez-Escandi and Oriol 1971). Immunological and biochemical assays have demonstrated that immunodominant antigen B, antigen 5 and arc 5 from *Echinococcus* seem to be the same. *T. solium* antigen B is non-specific; it is found in many platyhelminthes, and sera from patients with hydatid disease cross-react with this antigen (Olivo, Plancarte and Flisser 1988). *E. granulosus* antigen B, antigen 5 and arc 5 have been extensively studied (reviewed in Lightowlers and Gottstein 1995) mainly in order to ascertain their identity, and as these authors suggest 'it would be valuable for these antigens to be compared between the different laboratories involved, in order to clarify whether the molecules are indeed one and the same'.

For diagnosis of cysticercosis, antigenic extracts are usually prepared from *T. solium* cysticerci from infected pigs (Flisser and Larralde 1986). Alternatively, antigens from other sources such as *T. crassiceps*, *T. hydatigena* and *T. saginata*, or obtained by genetic engineering (McManus et al. 1989) have also been used. Cyst fluid, protoscolices and cyst membranes of *E. granulosus* from a variety of hosts are the sources of antigen for diagnostic tests of hydatid disease. Fluid from fertile cysts contains higher concentrations of antigens than from sterile cysts, although viable non-fertile cysts also contain suitable antigens, while fluid from sheep and human liver cysts also contain higher concentration of 2 major antigens than that of cattle and pig cysts. In general, hydatid cyst fluid is a better source of antigen than protoscolices and cyst membranes. *T. hydatigena* and *T. ovis* have also been evaluated as source of antigens (Yong, Heath and van Knapen 1984), enabling successful antigen preparation from heterologous taeniid parasite species.

Because crude antigen extracts generate cross-reactions, the use of purified or semi-purified antigens will increase specificity. Characterization of *T. solium* and *E. granulosus* antigens has changed from gel diffusion and immuno-electrophoresis to western blot, immunoprecipitation, chromatofocusing, lentil-lectin chromatography, monoclonal antibodies and recombinant DNA technology (reviewed in Flisser 1994 for cysticercosis and in Lightowlers and Gottstein 1995 for hydatid disease). In cysticercosis the use of a crude electrophoretic extract gave no clear specific band patterns in western blots (Espinoza and Flisser 1986, Larralde et al. 1989); however, a similar assay using a semi-purified antigenic fraction identified 7 specific glycoproteins (Gp50, Gp42–39, GP24, GP21, GP18, GP14 and GP13), the 3 with highest molecular weights reacting most frequently with sera from clinical cases (Tsang, Brand and Boyer 1989, Feldman et al. 1990, Wilson et al. 1991) and population samples (Schantz et al. 1994, Thais et al. 1994). Further progress has been made by recombinant DNA techniques, using *E. granulosus* clones that react with sera from patients with cystic hydatid disease (see for example. Ferreira and Zaha 1994), and clones from *E. multilocularis* immunoreactive with sera from patients with alveolar hydatid disease (see for example Hemmings and McManus 1989).

Data on cellular immune responses are limited but, interestingly, show similarities in both larval cestode diseases: an increase in CD8[+] lymphocytes (Allan et al. 1981, Flisser et al. 1986, Vuitton et al. 1989, Molinari et al. 1990, Craig 1994), a decrease in γ-interferon (Suntsov et al. 1990a,b, Ostrosky-Zeichner et al. 1996), and polyclonal activation of B lymphocytes (Craig 1994). Parasite molecules with immunosuppressive effects have also been reported (Molinari et al. 1990). Nevertheless, a systematic and focused analysis of the relationship between cytokine effects and the outcome of larval cestode diseases is still needed.

The mechanisms by which established larval cestodes survive in hosts resistant to reinfection remain unknown. Evidence exists for a variety of immune-evasion mechanisms. Three have been described in cysticercosis (Flisser 1989): survival of parasites lodged in 'immunologically privileged sites', masking of cysticerci by host immunoglobulins and suppression of host responses. In hydatid disease, studies in experimental models have focused attention on the influence of the parasite on the specific and non-specific immune responses of the host, such as pathological alterations in the architecture of lymphoid organs, inhibition of cellular immune responses to specific antigens and of leucocyte chemotaxis; in human hydatid disease, reduced blastoid transformation and auto-antibodies against a variety of antigens have been demonstrated. The impact of AIDS on the susceptibility of endemic populations for cysticercosis and hydatid disease could result in a significant terminal disease (Heath 1995), as an example, huge brain cysticerci have been found in 2 HIV patients (Ostrosky-Zeichner and Soto 1996).

Few studies have been undertaken to determine factors which regulate innate susceptibility to larval cestode infections. Host age, sex, strain and physiological state have marked influences in determining innate resistance to infection (reviewed by Flisser 1994).

Intermediate hosts develop specific humoral and cellular responses to the parasites which confer a significant level of resistance to reinfection. The contribution of these immune responses to the destruction of the parasite after initial establishment is less clear. A proportion of cysticerci and of hydatid cysts die some time after initial establishment, so that calcified lesions can be observed together with viable and with dead parasites. Although it is not known whether immunity is responsible for the death of these parasites, there is evidence, for example, that the inflammatory response is associated with restricting the growth and metastasis of the cyst mass in hosts refractory to infection with *E. multilocularis* (Ali-Khan and Siboo 1980) and that in experimental treatment of pigs with cysticercosis, cestocidal drugs damage cysticerci but eosinophils, lymphocytes and macrophages destroy them (see Fig. 28.9) (Flisser et al. 1990b, Torres et al. 1992). Nevertheless despite the development of specific immune responses, viable cysts frequently persist for long periods.

Several aspects of the immunobiology of larval cestode infections in the intermediate host have provided the framework for research on vaccination. Many studies have been performed in order to evaluate protection against cysticercosis and against hydatid disease (Mitchell 1990, Rickard et al. 1995). The immune response against larval cestodes may be divided into 2 phases, the first directed against recently hatched oncospheres attempting to penetrate the gut mucosa and establish themselves in host tissues, and the second aimed at the established metacestode. Immune effector mechanisms of the first phase are more successful in destroying the parasites than those of the second phase because established metacestodes have evolved highly effective mechanisms to evade the host's defences, described above. Early oncospheres are highly vulnerable to immune attack, but only briefly, and thus there is a race between parasite development and the generation of the host immune response in the critical first few days of infection.

For vaccination most studies have used crude antigens obtained from oncospheres, metacestodes or adult tapeworms; predictably, living oncospheres or oncospheral antigens are the most effective. Recombinant vaccines have been used successfully against *T. solium* in pigs (Manoutcharian et al. 1996) and *T. ovis* in sheep (Johnson et al. 1989).

2.3 Diagnosis

In the past, the pleomorphic symptomatology of neurocysticercosis has required the use of a variety of diagnostic procedures. Most of these have now been replaced by imaging techniques such as computed tomography (CT) and magnetic resonance (MR) (Suss, Maravilla and Thompson 1986, Almeida-Pinto et al. 1988, Jena et al. 1988, Rodacki et al. 1989, Teitelbaum et al. 1989). As alternative or complementary diagnostic procedures, immunological assays are used to detect anti-cysticercus antibodies in CSF or serum. Enzyme-linked immunosorbent assays (ELISA)

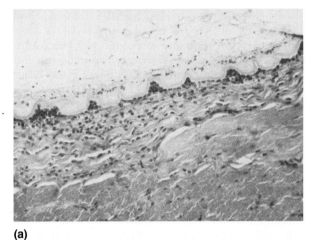

(a)

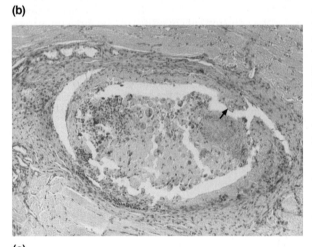

(b)

(c)

Fig. 28.9 Effect of treatment of pigs with praziquantel on cysticerci: eosinophils (a) and lymphocytes (b) surround the parasite and macrophages phagocytose cell debris (c). The arrow in (c) indicates a larval hook. (By courtesy of Dr AS de Aluja).

and western blotting (WB) are currently used for clinical support of symptomatic patients in several countries (Espinoza et al. 1986, Gottstein, Zinni and Schantz 1986, Pammenter, Rossoun and Epstein 1987, Michault et al. 1989, Tsang, Brand and Boyer 1989, Zinni, Farrell and Wadee 1990, Wilson et al. 1991).

Their high positivity facilitates diagnosis of neurocysticercosis, especially when CT or MR are not available or not conclusive.

CT and MR are used to identify cysticerci in the brain and thus confirm the aetiology of the disease and define the number, stage, location and extent of lesions. Because of their vesicular structure, living cysticerci are seen as hypodense or low signal intensity images, the scolex giving a hyperdense or high signal intensity, usually eccentric, inside the vesicle (see Fig. 28.10).

Isolated cysticerci detected in brain parenchyma by imaging techniques are frequently seronegative whereas multiple or subarachnoidal cysticerci are usually seropositive (Wilson et al. 1991). Cysticerci in ventricles can also be detected, especially by MR. Imaging techniques also show vasculitis, inflammation and oedema surrounding the parasite, ring-like enhancement being associated with an acute infection (cysticercotic encephalitis) and indicating an active inflammatory process. Hydrocephalus is a common finding associated with intraventricular and/or basal cysticerci, and imaging techniques are very helpful non-invasive techniques for following the outcome, especially after a shunt has been introduced. In long-term disease, parasites of different sizes can be seen with diverse tomographic pictures of brain response (Flisser et al. 1988). Calcified cysticerci are seen in CT as hyperdense dots but are usually not detected by MR because of the lack of signal from calcifications. In countries where cysticercosis is endemic, clinicians usually consider this aetiology in the initial diagnosis of cases that have mass occupying lesions, enhancing nodules, hydrocephalus, or other images that might be associated with neurocysticercosis. More consideration should be given to it in developed countries, where cases of neurocysticercosis are currently being diagnosed or misdiagnosed (Michael, Levy and Paige 1990). Cysticerci in eyes are easily diagnosed when parasites are viable but can easily be misdiagnosed when there are inflammatory reactions or involution of the parasite (Gómez-Leal 1989). Subcutaneous and muscle cysticerci may be detected by palpation and diagnosed by biopsy.

Immunodiagnosis has the great advantage of lower cost than CT or MR, and the presence of specific anticysticercus antibodies may confirm the disease. ELISA has clearly improved immunodiagnosis and is being used routinely for confirmation of clinical diagnosis when imaging techniques are not available or are not conclusive. It has a high sensitivity, between 75% and 90% with serum, and lumbar CSF gives better results. The main disadvantage of ELISA is cross-reactivity with other helminth infections since the antigen employed is a crude homogenate of cysticerci or vesicular fluid. Western blotting overcomes cross-reactivity because it employs an enriched fraction of glycoproteins (Gp). In addition the technique separates the antigens present in the Gp fraction during electrophoresis prior to the antigen–antibody reaction. The presence of 1–7 specific Gp bands is considered diagnostic of *T. solium* infections. When 2 or more cysticerci are

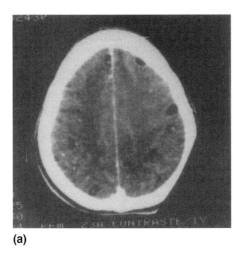

(a)

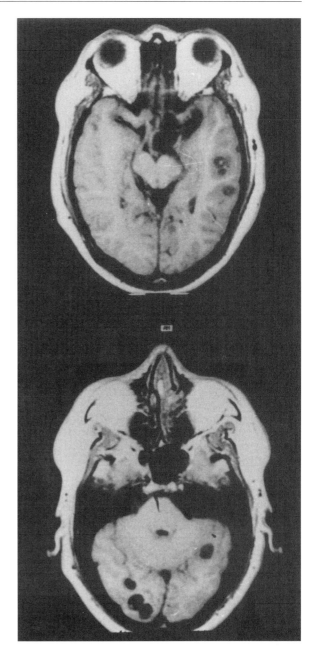

(b)

Fig. 28.10 Multiple small cysticerci seen by CT (a), MR (b) and in anatomical section of the brain (c). The scolex can be seen in some parasites. (By courtesy of Drs I Madrazo and J Olvera).

present blotting is 100% specific and has 100% sensitivity with serum samples and 95% with CSF. Antigens can be detected in CSF, or in semi-purified fractions of CSF, by ELISA using monoclonal antibodies (Correa et al. 1989, Choromanski, Estrada and Kuhn 1990, Chen et al. 1991). Although the sensitivity of antigen detection is lower than that of antibody detection, positive cases confirm the presence of the parasite without the need of other diagnostic procedures.

The presence of a cyst-like mass in a person with a history of exposure to sheepdogs in areas in which *E. granulosus* is endemic supports the diagnosis of cystic echinococcosis. However, hydatid cysts must be differentiated from benign cysts, cavitary tuberculosis, mycoses, abscesses, and benign or malignant neoplasms. A non-invasive confirmation of the diagnosis can usually be accomplished by the use of ultrasonography, CT, MR or radiography (Ammann and Eckert 1995). The liver is the most frequently involved organ and 60–85% of the cysts are located in the right lobe. Ultrasonography, CT and MR are useful in diagnosing deep-seated lesions in all organs and defining the extent and condition of avascular fluid-filled cysts (Fig. 28.11) (von Sinner 1991, Choji et al. 1992, Amman and Eckert 1995).

Images of *E. granulosus* hydatid disease typically show round, solitary or multiple, sharply contoured cysts, measuring from 1 to over 15 cm, these represent about 38–48% of all cysts. In 29– 46% of all cysts the presence of internal daughter cysts produces structures comparable to a cartwheel. Thin, crescent or ring-shaped calcifications of variable degree located in the cyst wall occur in about 10% of the cysts, giving an eggshell pattern; these require about 5–10 years to develop (Fig. 28.11a,b). CT allows measurement of the size of the parasites, which is useful for chemotherapeutic follow-up and gives a correct diagnosis in a high proportion of cases (60–90%). The usual CT image of *E. multilocularis* infection is that of indistinct solid tumours seen as heterogeneous hypodense

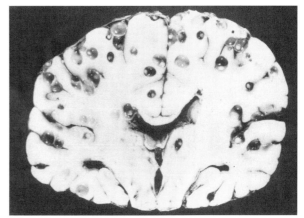

(c)

Fig. 28.10 Continued.

masses often associated with central necrotic areas and calcifications, lesion contours are irregular without a well-defined wall (Fig. 28.11c,d).

Frequently the lesion extends beyond the liver, which can cause compression or obstruction of other structures such as the inferior vena cava, hepatic veins and portal branches (Ammann and Eckert 1995). Clusters of microcalcifications or irregular plaque-like calcified foci are often found in central or peripheral parts of the lesions. The lungs may be involved either by direct extension of the liver process or by parasite metastases seen as multiple small solid foci located usually eccentrically at the periphery of the lobes. Serologic tests are usually positive at high titres; purified *E. multilocularis* antigens are highly specific, and comparing a patient's titres to both purified-specific and shared antigens permits serologic discrimination between patients infected with *E. multilocularis* and those infected with *E. granulosus*.

Diagnostic puncture should be avoided because of the risk of secondary echinococcosis due to spillage of viable protoscolices or of metastases in the site of injection from germinative tissue adhering to the needle. There is also the risk of anaphylactic reactions from leakage of cyst fluid (Ammann and Eckert 1995). The availability of immunodiagnostic tests for confirmation of US, CT or MR images reduces the need of puncture for diagnosis, although puncture is presently being used as an alternative therapeutic treatment (PAIR; see section 2.4, p. 553).

Virtually every serodiagnostic technique devised for any disease has been evaluated for hydatid diagnosis, often with considerable discrepancies between laboratories (Craig 1994). As Schantz and Gottstein (1986) discuss, selection of a particular immunodiagnostic test involves consideration of the sensitivity and specificity of the techniques, the purpose for which they will be used, available technical expertise and cost. Sensitivity and specificity vary according to the technique used, the quality of antigens and the characteristics of the groups of hydatid patients and controls used in the study. ELISA, indirect hemagglutination, latex agglutination and indirect immunofluorescence have a high sensitivity (60–90%) although some

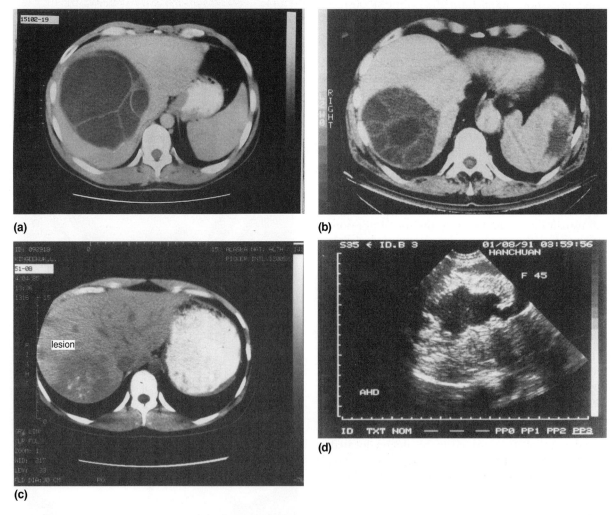

(a)

(b)

(c)

(d)

Fig. 28.11 (a) CT showing a solitary *Echinococcus granulosus* human liver cyst. (By courtesy of Dr P Schantz); (b) CT showing an *Echinococcus granulosus* human liver cyst with a cartwheel appearance. (By courtesy of Dr P Schantz); (c) CT showing an *Echinococcus multilocularis* liver cyst showing plaque-like calicified foci (By courtesy of Dr P Schantz); (d) Ultrasonography of a liver from a patient from Gansu, China with alveolar echinococcosis. (By courtesy of Professor P Craig).

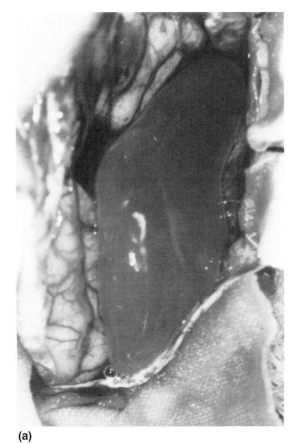

(a)

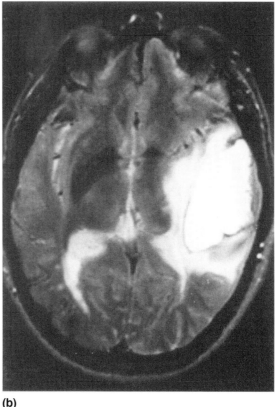

(b)

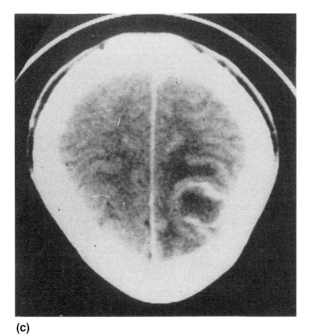

(c)

Fig. 28.12 Surgical removal of a huge brain cysticercus (a) that can be seen to have a similar size in MR (b) and as the end of the vesicle surrounded by an inflammatory reaction in CT (c). (By courtesy of Dr G Zenteno).

patients do not develop a detectable immune response. Hepatic cysts are more likely to elicit an immune response than pulmonary cysts, but about 10% of patients with hepatic cysts and 40% with pulmonary cysts do not produce detectable serum antibodies and give false negative results, which may result in a dangerous puncture of a hydatid cyst (Ammann and Eckert 1995). ELISA, which is now used routinely, has a similar sensitivity to the indirect hemagglutination test and thus both are procedures of choice for the initial screening of sera. Specific confirmation of reactivity can be obtained by demonstrating antibodies to antigen 5 (arc 5) by immunodiffusion or immunoelectrophoresis or to the 8–12 kDa band in western blot. Eosinophilia is present in fewer than 25% of infected persons and hypergammaglobulinaemia in about 30% of the patients with cystic echinococcosis (Ammann and Eckert 1995). Techniques useful for diagnosing cystic or alveolar hydatid disease are also of value in diagnosing polycystic hydatid disease since these parasites have common antigens.

2.4 Therapy

Treatment is based on palliative drugs to control symptoms and inflammation, placement of ventricular shunts that drain CSF to the peritoneal cavity, or surgery to remove brain cysticerci or hydatid cysts from liver and lungs. The advent of cestocidal drugs has improved prognosis of many cases (Earnest et al. 1987, Kammerer and Schantz 1993, Ammann and Eckert 1995).

Antiepileptic drugs are the treatment of choice in neurocysticercotic patients with calcifications, in which seizures are the only manifestation of the disease and there is no imaging evidence of living parasites. Ventricular shunting is the most common neurosurgical approach to control hydrocephalus caused by cysticerci in the ventricles, periventricular or basal cisternae, or by ependimitis, inflammatory scarring, arachnoiditis or adhesive basilar meningitis. Patients with hydrocephalus always require a ventricular shunt before other measures are attempted. CSF shunting is a relatively simple surgical technique used to treat intracranial hypertension due to blockage of CSF circulation, but complications may arise from the high protein levels in CSF (which can cause blockage), from bacterial infections or from surgical inexperience (Colli et al. 1986, Madrazo and Flisser 1992). A ventriculoperitoneal shunt with a new design based on the rate of CSF production and shunt resistance, rather than on ventricular pressure, has recently been evaluated with promising results (Sotelo, Rubalcava and Gómez-Llata 1995). In an hospital study of 632 cases subjected to ventriculoperitoneal shunting, 77% were resolved with one operation, but 11% needed 3 or more shunt placements (Mateos and Zenteno 1987). In another study 68% of 69 cases were readmitted to the hospital one or more times for shunt revision (Colli et al. 1986). Removal of solitary brain cysticerci is often followed by prompt improvement and excellent recovery (Colli et al. 1994). In a series of 27 cases with cysticerci in the fourth ventricle submitted for direct surgical removal of the parasite, 81% had excellent results but the remaining cases had poor results owing to severe arachnoiditis found at surgery (Loyo, Kleriga and Estañol 1980) (Fig. 28.12)

Parasites in the intraspinal subarachnoidal space require surgery because the compression causes spinal cord dysfunction. Neurocysticercosis can involve any cranial nerve; surgery is the most frequent indication for optic nerve involvement and removal of arachnoiditic tissue surrounding nerves will produce different degrees of clinical benefit (Escobedo 1988, Madrazo and Flisser 1992). Treatment of ocular cysticercosis usually involves removal of parasites from vitreous or subretinal locations. In some cases photocoagulation with a laser beam is used and in severe inflammation extrusion of the eye is recommended (Santos, Dalma and Ortiz 1979, Kruger-Leite et al. 1985, Cárdenas et al. 1992). Muscle and subcutaneous cysticerci are efficaciously eliminated by cestocidal treatment (Rim and Joo 1989).

Surgical removal of cystic echinococcosis, which can be performed in about 90% of patients, has few complications and the best prognosis. It is the preferred treatment when cysts are large (> 10 cm diameter), secondarily infected, or located in the brain or the heart. The aim of surgery is total removal of the cyst while avoiding the adverse consequences of spilling its contents. Pericystectomy is the usual procedure but resection of the involved organ may be used depending on the location and condition of the cyst. Although surgery provides cure in a high percentage of cases there may be 2–25% recurrence (Kammerer and Schantz 1993, Amman and Eckert 1995). Postoperative complications may occur in 10% to 25% of cases and mortality is around 2% but may increase considerably with further operations. Surgical resection of the infected liver segment and of alveolar hydatid cyst lesions from other affected organs is indicated in all operable cases even though it is impossible to know whether an operation has removed all parasite tissue. It is now common practice for postoperative chemotherapy to be routinely carried out for at least 2 years after radical surgery, with careful monitoring of the patient during a minimum of 10 years for possible recurrence (Ammann and Eckert 1995). Because alveolar hydatid disease is often not diagnosed until the disease is advanced, the lesion is then inoperable.

Cestocidal treatment is based on praziquantel (a synthetic acylated isoquinoline-pyrazine) and albendazole (a benzimidazole derivative). Pharmacokinetic and toxicological studies of both drugs indicate rapid absorption and in general no toxicological effects (Marriner et al. 1986, Frohberg 1989). Both drugs are useful for eliminating living cysticerci located in brain parenchyma and the subarachnoidal space (Cruz, Cruz and Horton 1991) but the proper dosages have not yet been precisely defined. Praziquantel is usually used at 50 mg/kg body weight in 3 daily doses given with meals during 15 days, with improvement in 70–96% of patients with cysticerci in brain parenchyma; longer or shorter treatment, even for 1 day, has also been successful (Bittencourt et al. 1990, Corona et al. 1996). Albendazole was initially used at 15 mg/kg for 1 month but in later protocols this was reduced to 8 days. Efficacy of cestocidal treatment is measured by the reduction in number and/or size of cysticerci seen by imaging techniques, clinical improvement, withdrawal of corticoid or anti-epileptic treatment and disappearance of ventricular dilatation. Steroids should be used in patients who show exacerbation of neurological symptoms or develop adverse reactions not related to drug toxicity. These effects are seemingly due to a strong inflammatory reaction and can be considered as a reliable indicator of drug effectiveness. Headache, nausea and seizures are common during treatment, but are usually transient and can be ameliorated with analgesic, antiemetic or antiepileptic drugs when reactions are mild, or with steroids when severe (Sotelo et al. 1985, del Brutto and Sotelo 1988). The need for cestocidal drugs has been questioned mainly because children appear not to warrant antiparasitic drug therapy (Mitchell and Snodgrass 1985, Mitchell and Crawford 1988). However, there are several reasons why cestocidal treatment should always be considered: intraparenchymal single lesions can mimic neoplastic or other infectious brain diseases; drugs are efficacious and well tolerated, and side effects can be controlled; and some cases are seronegative even with the highly sensitive western blot. Subarachnoidal cysticerci in the cerebral convexity or in the cisternas of the skull base should be surgically treated only when cestocidal or anti-inflammatory treatment has failed, especially when there is secondary hydrocephalus or diagnostic doubt (Madrazo and Flisser 1992).

Albendazole and mebendazole in relatively high doses and over prolonged periods, can severely damage or kill protoscolices and cysts of *E. granulosus* in animals (Perez-Serrano et al. 1994, Taylor and Morris 1988). When surgery is not recommended because of the patient's general condition and the extent and location of the cysts, cestocidal treatment should be used. Both albendazole (10 mg/kg body weight per day) and mebendazole (40–50 mg/kg) are effective; however, because of its superior intestinal absorption and penetration into the cysts, albendazole is slightly more efficacious. Adverse reactions (neutropenia, liver toxicity, alopecia, and others), reversible upon cessation of treatment, have been noted with both drugs. A minimum period of treatment is 3 months, but the long-term prognosis in individual patients is difficult to predict, therefore, prolonged follow up with ultrasound or other imaging procedures is needed to determine the eventual outcome. Recent trials have shown that, with both drugs, success rates are variable; 20–70% of patients improved, but this included high proportions of inoperable and severe cases (Davis, Dixon and Pawlowski 1989, Todorov et al. 1992, Craig 1994). In general approximately one-third of patients treated with benzimidazole drugs have been cured of their disease, as seen by complete and permanent disappearance of cysts, and an even higher proportion have responded with significant regression of cyst size and alleviation of symptoms. Small (< 7 mm diameter) isolated cysts, surrounded by minimal adventitial reaction, respond best, whereas complicated cysts with multiple compartments and daughter cysts, or with thick or calcified surrounding adventitial reactions, are relatively refractory to treatment. Echinococcal disease responds more readily to chemotherapy in children than it does in adults (Goccmen, Toppare and Kiper 1993, Kammerer and Schantz 1993, Ammann and Eckert 1995). The few available results of praziquantel treatment of cystic echinococcosis do not yet allow conclusions (Craig 1994, Ammann and Eckert 1995). The use of cyclosporin A for postoperative control of secondary cystic echinococcosis has been suggested (Hurd, Mackenzie and Chappell 1993).

Long-term treatment with mebendazole (50 mg/kg per day) or albendazole (10 mg/kg) inhibits growth of larval *E. multilocularis*, reduces metastasis, and enhances both the quality and length of survival; prolonged therapy may eventually be larvicidal in some patients, but recurrence of the disease also occurs (Ammann et al. 1993). Liver transplantation has been employed successfully on otherwise terminal cases. Because the lesions due to *E. vogeli* are so extensive, surgical resection is always difficult and usually incomplete and a combination of surgery with albendazole is most likely to be successful (Kammerer and Schantz 1993). The principles of management of cystic and alveolar echinococcosis also apply to polycystic echinococcosis.

Combinations of cyst puncture, aspiration and drainage, with or without injection of chemicals (called percutaneous aspiration-injection-reaspiration, PAIR), have also been evaluated. Percutaneous puncture is performed under sonographic guidance, followed by aspiration of the liquid contents, instillation of a protoscolicidal agent (95% ethanol or 20% sodium chloride solution) and reaspiration (Filice et al. 1990, Khuroo et al. 1993). To avoid sclerosing cholangitis, this procedure must not be performed in patients whose cysts have biliary communication; the presence of the latter can be determined by testing the cyst fluid for presence of bilirubin or by intraoperative cholangiogram. The possibility of secondary echinococcosis resulting from accidental spillage during this procedure can be minimized by concurrent treatment with albendazole; indeed, combining PAIR and chemotherapy may improve the results of either treatment alone. Recently hydatid cysts in infected gerbils were injected with ivermectin and found severely damaged and with no viable protoscolices between 44 and 58 days postinjection (Ochieng-Mitula and Burt 1996).

2.5 Transmission, epidemiology and prophylaxis

Human cysticercosis is a disease related to underdevelopment. It is present in countries that lack proper sanitary infrastructure and hygiene as well as insufficient health education (Gemmell et al. 1983) as exemplified by the emergence of neurocysticercosis in 1978 in West New Guinea where it became a disaster among the Ekari population, to whom the disease was unknown prior to the entrance of cysticercotic pigs as official gifts. Some 18–20% of the population acquired cysticercosis. The disease was detected by an epidemic of severe burns resulting from convulsions manifested while the people were sleeping around house fires. Individuals also had subcutaneous nodules (Muller et al. 1987). Human cysticercosis is still endemic in Brazil, Colombia, Ecuador, Guatemala, Mexico, Peru, China, India, New Guinea, South Africa, West Africa, Zimbabwe, Ile de la Reunion and Madagascar. Cases are also reported in the USA, Honduras, Panama, Portugal, Spain and the UK (detailed references are found in Flisser 1994).

Several epidemiological studies have shown a correlation between human cysticercosis, taeniosis and epilepsy and between seropositive people, infected pigs and disposal of faeces (Michault et al. 1990, Sarti et al. 1992, 1994, Garcia et al. 1995). The results of surveys have identified community, behavioural and environmental practices that must be modified to prevent continued transmission of cysticercosis and taeniosis. Most importantly, these studies have shown that the main risk factor is the presence of a *Taenia* carrier in the immediate environment. Treatment of known carriers of intestinal tapeworms will have a direct influence on transmission within the community (Cruz et al. 1989, Pawlowski 1990, Diaz-Camacho et al. 1991).

The greatest prevalence of cystic echinococcosis is in temperate countries, including southern South America, the entire Mediterranean littoral, the southern and central parts of the former Soviet Union, central Asia, China, Australia, and parts of Africa. In the USA, most infections are seen in immigrants from countries in which the disease is highly endemic. Sporadic autochthonous transmission is currently recognized in Alaska, California, Utah, Arizona, and New Mexico. Geographic strains of *E. granulosus* exist with different host affinities. The northern or sylvatic strain is maintained in wolves and wild cervids (moose and reindeer) in northern Alaska, Canada, Scandinavia, and Eurasia. Pastoral strains are maintained in dogs and domestic ungulates throughout the world. Populations of *E. granulosus* in different assemblages of hosts (dog–sheep, dog–horse, dog–pig, and dog–cattle) differ morphologically, developmentally, biochemically, and possibly in infectivity and pathogenicity to humans. For example, the dog–sheep strain, the most widespread of the variants, is relatively pathogenic in humans in comparison to the northern sylvatic strain that occurs in wolf–wild cervid hosts. There is much evidence that the strain adapted to the dog–horse cycle, occurring in parts of Europe and the Middle East, rarely, if ever, infects humans. Probes characterizing the nuclear and mitochondrial DNA of the variant populations provide reliable genetic markers to distinguish them. Globally, sheep are the most important intermediate hosts, but swine, cattle, goats, horses and camels are more important in certain regions. Certain human activities, such as the widespread rural practice of feeding the viscera of home-butchered sheep to dogs, facilitate transmission of the sheep strain and consequently increase the risk that humans will become infected. Dogs infected with *Echinococcus* tapeworms pass eggs in their faeces, and humans become infected through faecal–oral contact, particularly in the course of playful and intimate contact between children and dogs. Eggs adhere to hairs around the infected dog's anus and are also found on the muzzle and paws. Indirect transfer of eggs, either through contaminated water and uncooked food or through the intermediary of flies and other arthropods, may also result in infection of humans. In endemic areas, personal preventive measures include careful hygiene, strict dietary regulation of pet dogs to preclude ingestion of sheep offal, and avoidance of dogs that are not so regulated. Periodic prophylactic treatment of pet dogs for intestinal echinococcosis may sometimes be necessary. Control measures applicable in communities include health education, regulation of livestock slaughtering in abattoirs and on farms, control of dogs, and periodic mass treatments of dogs with praziquantel (5 mg/kg) to reduce the prevalence of *E. granulosus* below levels necessary for continued transmission (reviewed in Rausch 1995). A targeted campaign of education and surveillance based on specific antibody detection in dogs as an indicator of exposure to *E. granulosus* is now in progress in Western Australia (Thompson et al. 1993).

The life cycle of *E. multilocularis* involves foxes and their rodent prey in ecosystems generally separate from humans, although there is ecological overlap with humans, because domestic dogs or cats may become infected when they eat infected wild rodents. As a result, exposure of humans to *E. multilocularis* is relatively less common than exposure to *E. granulosus*. Alveolar hydatid disease has been reported in parts of central Europe, much of Russia, the Central Asian republics, and western China, the northwestern portion of Canada and western Alaska. The incidence appears to be increasing in central North America. Hunters, trappers, and persons who work with fox fur are often exposed to alveolar hydatid disease. Hyperendemic foci have been described in some Eskimo villages of the North American tundra and in China where local dogs regularly feed on infected commensal rodents; the epidemiology of alveolar echinococcosis in China remains one of the major challenges in temperate areas with human prevalences of 2–5% in some communities (Craig 1994). Eliminating *E. multilocularis* from its wild animal hosts is impractical; therefore, contact with dogs and foxes in areas where the infection is endemic should be avoided. Preventing infections in humans depends on education to improve hygiene and sanitation. Infections in dogs and cats prone to eat infected rodents can be prevented by monthly treatments with praziquantel (Kammerer and Schantz 1993, Rausch 1996).

Very little is known about the circumstances associated with polycystic hydatid disease due to *E. vogeli*. Bush dogs are rare and avoid human beings and therefore probably play little role in transmission to humans. In endemic areas, infections are probably acquired from the faeces of domestic dogs that have been fed on viscera of infected pacas, a practice that has been reported commonly by patients (Meneghilli et al. 1992).

REFERENCES

Ali-Khan Z, Siboo R, 1980, Pathogenesis and host response in subcutaneous alveolar hydatidosis. I. Histogenesis of alveolar cyst and a qualitative analysis of the inflammatory infiltrates, *Z Parasitenk*, **62**: 241–4.

Ali-Khan Z, Siboo R et al., 1983, Cystolytic events and the possible role of germinal cells in metastasis in chronic alveolar hydatidosis, *Ann Trop Med Parasitol*, **77**: 497–512.

Allan D, Jenkins P et al., 1981, A study of immunoregulation of BALB/c mice *by Echinococcus granulosus equinus* during prolonged infection, *Parasite Immunol*, **3**: 137–42.

Almeida-Pinto J, Veiga-Pires JA et al., 1988, Cysticercosis of the brain. The value of computed tomography, *Acta Radiol*, **29**: 625–8.

Ammann R, Eckert R, 1995, Clinical diagnosis and treatment of echinococcosis in humans, Echinococcus *and Hydatid Disease*, eds Thompson RCA, Lymbery AJ, CAB International, Wallingford, Oxon, 411–51.

Ammann R, Ilitsch N et al., 1993, Effect of chemotherapy on the larval mass and on the long-term course of alveolar echinococcosis, *Hepatology*, **19**: 735–42.

Baily GG, Mason PR et al., 1988, Serological diagnosis of neuro-cysticercosis: evaluation of ELISA tests using cyst fluid and other components of *Taenia solium* cysticerci as antigens, *Trans R Soc Trop Med Hyg*, **82:** 295–9.

Bittencourt PRM, Gracia CM et al., 1990, High-dose praziquantel for neurocysticercosis: efficacy and tolerability, *Eur Neurol*, **30:** 229–34.

Botero D, Tanowitx HB et al., 1993, Taeniasis and cysticercosis, *Parasitic Dis*, **7:** 683–97.

Bowles J, MacManus DP, 1993, Molecular variation in *Echino-coccus*, *Acta Trop (Basel)*, **53:** 291–305.

Cardenas F, Palcarte A et al., 1989, *Taenia crassiceps:* experimental model of intraocular cysticercosis, *Exp Parasitol*, **69:** 324–9.

Cardenas F, Quiroz H et al., 1992, *Taenia solium* ocular cysticercosis: findings in 30 cases, *Ann Ophthalmol*, **24:** 25–8.

Cervantes M, Gonzalez-Angulo A, Marquez-Monter H, 1986, Anatomia bioquimica del *Cisticercus celulosae*.I. Estudio histoquimico y analisis por energia dispersiva de rayos X: acidos mucopolisacaridos, glucogeno, grasa, ADN, calcio y fierro, *Patologia (Mex)*, **24:** 209–18.

Cervantes-Vazquez M, Correa D et al., 1990, Respiratory changes associated with the in vitro evagination of *Taenia solium* cysterci, *J Parasitol*, **76:** 108–12.

Chang KH, Kim WS et al., 1988, Comparative evaluation of brain CT and ELISA in the diagnosis of neurocysticercosis, *AJNR*, **9:** 125–30.

Chen JP, Zhang XY et al., 1991, Determination of circulating antigen in cysticercosis patients using McAb-based ELISA, *Chung Kuo Chin Sheng Chung Hsueh Yu Chi Sheng Chung Ping Tsa Chih*, **9:** 122–5.

Cho SY, Kim SI et al., 1986, Evaluation of enzyme-linked immunosorbent assay in serological diagnosis of human neurocysticercosis using paired samples of serum and cerebrospinal fluid, *Korean J Parasitol*, **24:** 25–41.

Choji K, Fujita N et al., 1992, Alveolar hydatid disease of the liver: computed tomography and transabdominal ultrasound with histopathological correlation, *Clin Radiol*, **46:** 97–103.

Choromanski L, Estrada JJ, Kuhn RE, 1990, Detection of antigens of larval *Taenia solium* in the cerebrospinal fluid of patients with the use of HPLC and ELISA, *J Parasitol*, **76:** 69–73.

Colli BO, Martelli N et al., 1986, Results of surgical treatment of neurocysticercosis in 69 cases, *J Neurosurg*, **65:** 309–15.

Colli BO, Martelli N et al., 1994, Cysticercosis in the central nervous system, *Arq Neuropsiquiatr*, **52:** 166–86.

Conder GA, Andersen FL, Schantz PM, 1980, Immunodiagnostic tests for hydatidosis in sheep: an evaluation of double diffusion, immunoelectrophoresis, indirect hemagglutination and intradermal tests, *J Parasitol*, **66:** 577–84.

Corona T, Lugo R et al., 1996, Single day praziquantel therapy for neurocysticercosis, *N Engl J Med*, **334:** 125.

Correa D, Dalma D et al., 1985, Heterogeneity of humoral immune components in human cysticercosis, *J Parasitol*, **71:** 533–41.

Correa D, Laclette JP et al., 1987, Heterogeneity of *Taenia solium* cysticerci obtained from different naturally infected pigs, *J Parasitol*, **73:** 443–5.

Correa D, Sandoval MA et al., 1989, Human neurocysticercosis: comparison of enzyme-immunoassay capture techniques based on monoclonal and polyclonal antibodies for the detection of parasite products in cerebrospinal fluid, *Trans R Soc Trop Med Hyg*, **83:** 814–16.

Craig PS, 1994, Current research in echinococcosis, *Parasitology Today*, **10:** 209–11.

Cruz I, Cruz ME et al., 1994, Human subcutaneous *Taenia solium* cysticercosis in an Andean population with neurocysticercosis, *Am J Trop Med Hyg*, **51:** 405–407.

Cruz M, Davis A et al., 1989, Operational studies on the control of *Taenia solium* taeniasis/cysticercosis in Ecuador, *Bull WHO*, **67:** 401–7.

Cruz M, Cruz I, Horton J, 1991, Albendazole versus praziquantel in the treatment of cerebral cysticercosis: clinical evaluation, *Trans R Soc Trop Med Hyg*, **85:** 224–47.

D'Alessandro A, Rausch RL et al., 1979, *Echinococcus vogeli* in man, with a review of polycystic hydatid disease in Colombia and neighbouring countries, *Am J Trop Med Hyg*, **28:** 303–17.

Davis A, Dixon H, Pawlowski ZS, 1989, Multicentre clinical trial of benzimidazole-carbamates in human cystic echinococcosis. *Bull WHO*, **67:** 503–8.

del Brutto OH, Sotelo J, 1988, Neurocysticercosis: an update, *Rev Infect Dis*, **6:** 1075–87.

Dixon HBF, Lipscomb FM, 1961, Cysticercosis: an analysis and follow up of 450 cases, *Privy Council Med Res Special Rep Ser*, **229:** 1–58.

Diaz-Camacho S, Candil A et al., 1991, Epidemiological study of *Taenia solium* taeniasis/cysticercosis in a rural village of Mexico, *Am J Trop Med Hyg*, **45:** 522–31.

Earnest MP, Reller LB et al., 1987, Neurocysticercosis in the United States: 35 cases and a review, *Rev Infect Dis*, **9:** 961–79.

Eckert J, Thompson RCA, Mehlhorn H, 1983, Proliferation and metastases formation of larval *Echinococcus multilocularis*. I. Animal model, macroscopical and histological findings, *Z Parasitenk*, **69:** 737–48.

Escobar A, 1983, The pathology of neurocysticercosis, *Cysticercosis of the Central Nervous System*, eds Palacios E, Rodriguez-Carbajal J, Taveras JM, Thomas, Springfield IL, 27–54.

Escobedo F, 1988, Neurosurgical aspects of neurocysticercosis, *Operative Neurosurgical Techiques*, 2nd edn, eds Schmidek H, Sweet W, Grune and Stratton, Orlando, FL, 93–102.

Espinoza B, Flisser A, 1986, Antigenos especificos y de reaccion cruzada de helmintos parasitos, *Arch Invest Med (Mex)*, **17:** 299–311.

Espinoza B, Ruiz-Palacios G et al., 1986, Characterization by enzyme linked immunosorbent assay of the humoral immune response in patients with neurocysticercosis and its application in immunodiagnosis, *J Clin Microbiol*, **24:** 536–41.

Fairweather Y, McMullan MT et al., 1994, Serotoninergic and peptidergic nerve elements in the protoscolex of *Echinococcus granulosus* (Cestoda, Cyclophyllidea), *Parasitol Res*, **80:** 649–56.

Feldman M, Placarte A et al., 1990, Comparison of two assays (EIA and EITB) and two samples (saliva and serum) for the diagnosis of neurocysticercosis, *Trans R Soc Trop Med Hyg*, **84:** 559–62.

Fernández C, Hormaeche CE, 1994, Isolation and biochemical characterisation of a glutathione S-transferase from *Echinococcus granulosus* protoscoleces, *Int J Parasitol*, **24:** 1063–6.

Ferreira HB, Zaha A, 1994, Expression and analysis of the diagnostic value of an *Echinococcus granulosus* antigen gene clone, *Int J Parasitol*, **24:** 863–70.

Filice C, Pirola F, et al., 1990, A new therapeutic approach for hydatid liver cysts. Aspiration and alcohol injection under sonographic guidance, *Gastroenterology*, **98:** 1366–8.

Flisser A, 1988, Neurocysticercosis in Mexico, *Parasitol Today*, **4:** 131–7.

Flisser A, 1989, *Taenia solium* cysticercosis: some mechanisms of parasite survival in immunocompetent hosts, *Acta Leiden*, **57:** 259–63.

Flisser A, 1994, Taeniasis and cysticercosis due to *Taenia solium*, *Progress in Clinical Parasitology*, ed Tsieh Sun, CRC Press, Boca Raton, FL, 77–116.

Flisser A, Espinoza B et al., 1986, Host–parasite relationship in cysticercosis: immunologic study in different compartments of the host, *Vet Parasitol*, **20:** 95–202.

Flisser A, Gonzalez D et al., 1990a, Praziquantel treatment of brain and muscle porcine *Taenia solium* cysticercosis. 2. Immunological and cytogenetic studies, *Parasitol Res*, **76:** 640–2.

Flisser A, Gonzalez D et al., 1990b, Praziquantel treatment of porcine brain and muscle *Taenia solium* cysticercosis. 1. Radiological, physiological and histopathological studies, *Parasitol Res*, **76:** 263–9.

Flisser A, Larralde C, 1986, Cysticercosis, *Immunodiagnosis of Parasitic Diseases*, eds Walls KW, Schantz PM, Academic Press, Orlando, FL, **109–61**.

Flisser A, Madrazo I et al., 1988, Comparative analysis of human and porcine neurocysticercosis by computed tomography, *Trans R Soc Trop Med Hyg*, **82:** 739–42.

Flisser A, Madrazo I, 1996, Evagination of *Taenia solium* in the fourth ventricle, *N Engl J Med*, **335:** 753–4.

Flisser A, Woodhouse E, Larralde E, 1980, Human cysticercosis: antigens, antibodies and non-responders, *Clin Exp Immunol*, **39:** 27–37.

Frayha GJ, Haddad R, 1980, Comparative chemical composition of protoscoleces and hydatid cyst fluid of *Echinococcus granulosus* (Cestoda), *Int J Parasitol*, **10:** 359–64.

Frohberg H, 1989, The toxicological profile of praziquantel in comparison to other anthelminthic drugs, *Acta Leiden*, **57:** 201–15.

García HH, Gilman R et al., 1993, Cysticercosis as a major cause of epilepsy in Peru, *Lancet*, **341:** 197–9.

García HH, Gilman RH et al., 1995, Factors associated with *Taenia solium* cysticercosis: Analysis of 946 Peruvian neurologic patients, *Am J Trop Med Hyg*, **52:** 145–8.

Gemmell MA, Lawson JR, 1986, Epidemiology and control of hydatid disease, *The Biology of Echinococcus and Hydatid Disease*, ed Thompson RCA, Allen and Unwin, London, 189–216.

Gemmell M, Matyas Z et al., 1983, *Guidelines for surveillance, prevention and control of taeniasis/cysticercosis*. VPH/83.49, World Health Organization, Geneva.

Goccmen A, Toppare MF, Kiper N, 1993, Treatment of hydatid disease in childhood with mebendazole. *Eur Resp J*, **6:** 253–7.

Goldberg AS, Heiner DC et al., 1981, Cerebrospinal fluid IgE and the diagnosis of cerebral cysticercosis, *Bull Los Angeles Neurol Soc*, **46:** 21–5.

Gomez-Leal A, 1989, Cisticercosis del globo ocular y sus anexos, *Cisticercosis Humana y Porcina, su Conocimiento e Investigacion en Mexico*, eds Flisser A, Malagon F, Limusa-Noriega; Mexico DF, 129–139.

Gorodezky C, Diaz ML et al., 1987, IgE concentration in sera of patients with neurocysticercosis, *Arch Invest Med (Mex)*, **18:** 225–7.

Gottstein B, 1992, Molecular and immunological diagnosis of echinococcosis, *Clin Microbiol Rec*, **5:** 248–61.

Gottstein B, Zinni D, Schantz PM, 1986, Species specific immunodiagnosis of *Taenia solium* cysticercosis by ELISA and immunoblotting, *Trop Med Parasitol*, **38:** 299–303.

Grove DI, 1990, *A History of Human Helminthology*, CAB International, Wallingford, Oxon, 355–83.

Guerra G, Flisser A et al., 1982, Biochemical and immunological characterization of antigen B purified from cysticerci of *Taenia solium, Cysticercosis. Present State of Knowledge and Perspectives*, eds Flisser A et al., Academic Press, New York, 437–51.

Heath DD, 1995, Immunology of *Echinococcus* infections, *Echinococcus and Hydatid Disease*, eds Thompson RCA, Lymbery AJ, CAB International, Wallingford, Oxon, 183–200.

Heath DD, Lawrence SB, 1976, *Echinococcus granulosus*: development in vitro from oncosphere to immature hydatid cyst, *J Parasitol*, **73:** 417–23.

Hemmings L, McManus DP, 1989, The isolation and differential antibody screening of *Echinococcus multilocularis* antigen gene clones with potential for immunodiagnosis, *Mol Biochem Parasitol*, **33:** 171–82.

Howard EB, Gendron AP, 1980, *Echinococcus vogeli* infection in higher primates at the Los Angeles Zoo, *The Comparative Pathology of Zoonosis Animals*, eds Montali RJ, Migaki G, Smithsonian Institution Press, Washington, DC, 379–82.

Hurd H, Mackenzie KS, Chappell LH, 1993, Anthelmintic effects of cyclosporin A on protoscoleces and secondary hydatid cysts of *Echinococcus granulosis* in the mouse, *Int J Parasitol*, **23:** 315–20.

Jena A, Sanchetee PC et al., 1988, Cysticercosis of the brain shown by magnetic resonance imaging, *Clin Radiol*, **39:** 542–6.

Johnson KS, Harrison GBL et al., 1989, Vaccination against ovine cysticercosis using a defined recombinant antigen, *Nature* (London), **338:** 585–7.

Kammerer WS, Schantz PM, 1993, Echinococcal disease, *Parasitic Dis*, **7:** 605–18.

Khuroo MS, Dar MY, et al., 1993, Percutaneous drainage versus albendazole therapy in hepatic hydatidosis: A prospective, randomised study, *Gastroenterology*, **104:** 1452–9.

Kruger-Leite E, Jalkh AE et al., 1985, Intraocular cysticercosis, *Am J Ophthalmol*, **99:** 252–7.

Kuchenmeister F, 1855, Offeness sendschreiben an die k.k. Gesellschaft der Aertze zu Wien. Experimenteller nachweis, dass *Cysticercus cellulosae* innerhalb des menschlichen darmkanales sich in *Taenia solium* unwandelt (translated in Kean, BH, Mott JE, Russell AJ 1978 eds *Tropical Medicine and Parasitology Classic Investigations*, Cornell University Press, Ithaca, NY, 677), *Wien Med Wochenschr*, **5:** 1–4.

Lachberg S, Thompson RCA, Lymbery AJ, 1990, A contribution to the etiology of racemose cysticercosis, *J Parasitol*, **76:** 592–4.

Laclette JP, Landa A et al., 1991, Paramyosin is the *Schistosoma mansoni* (trematoda) homologue of antigen B from *Taenia solium* (cestoda), *Mol Biochem Parasitol*, **44:** 287–96.

Laclette JP, Shoemaker C et al., 1992, Paramyosin inhibits complement C1, *J Immunol*, **148:** 124–8.

Landa A, Merchant MT et al., 1994, Purification and ultrastructural localization of surface glycoproteins *of taenia solium* (Cestoda) cysticerci, *Int J Parasitol*, **24:** 265–9.

Larralde C, Montoya RM et al., 1989, Deciphering western blots of tapeworm antigens (*Taenia solium, Echinococcus granulosus* and *Taenia crassiceps*) reacting with sera from neurocysticercosis and hydatid disease patients, *Am J Trop Med Hyg*, **40:** 282–90.

Leuckart R, 1879, *Die Parasiten des Menschen und die von ihnen herruhrenden Krankheiten. Ein Hand- und Lehrbuch fur Naturforscher und Aertze*. CF Winter'sche Verlangshandlung, Leipzig, Vol 1, 1009, *The Parasites of Man and the Diseases which Proceed from them. A Textbook for Students and Practitioners*, transl Hoyle WE, Young J (1886), Pentland, Edinburgh, 771.

Lightowlers MW, Gottstein B, 1995, Echinococcosis/hydatidosis: antigens, immunological and molecular diagnosis, *Echinococcus and Hydatid Disease*, eds Thompson RCA, Lymbery AJ, CAB International, Wallingford, Oxon, 355–93.

Lightowlers MW, Mitchell GF, Rickard MD, 1993, Cestodes, *Immunology and Molecular Biology of Parasitic Infections*, 3rd edn, eds Warren KS, Agabian N, Blackwell Scientific, Oxford, 436–70.

Little JM, 1976, Hydatid disease at Royal Prince Alfred Hospital. 1964 to 1974, *Med J Aust*, **1:** 903–8.

Liu D, Lightowlers MW, Rickard MD, 1992, Evaluation of a monoclonal antibody-based competition ELISA for the diagnosis of human hydatidosis, *Parasitology*, **104:** 357–61.

Loyo M, Kleriga E, Estanol B, 1980, Fourth ventricular cysticercosis, *Neurosurgery*, **7:** 456–8.

Madrazo I, Flisser A, 1992, Parasitic infestations of the cerebrum. Cysticercosis, *Brain Surgery. Complication Avoidance and Management*, ed Appuzo JML, Churchill Livingston, Edinburgh, 1419–30.

Manoutcharian K, Rosas G et al., 1996, Cysticercosis: identification and cloning ofprotective recombinant antigens, *J Parasitol*, **82:** 250–4.

Marco M, Nieto A, 1991, Metalloproteinases in the larvae of *Echinococcus granulosus*, *Int J Parasitol*, **21:** 743–6.

Marriner SE, Morris DL et al., 1986, Pharmacokinetics of albendazole in man, *Eur J Clin Pharmacol*, **30:** 705–8, 413–422.

Meneghilli VG, Martinelli ALC et al., 1992, Polycystic hydatid dusease (*Echinococcus vogeli*): Clinical laboratory, and morphological findings in nine Brazilian patients, *J Hepatol*, **14:** 203–10.

McManus DP, 1981, A biochemical study of adult and cystic

stages of *Echinococcus granulosus* of human and animal origin from Kenya, *J Helminthol*, **55:** 21–7.

McManus DP, Bryant C, 1995, Biochemistry, physiology and molecular biology of *Echinococcus*, *Echinococcus and Hydatid Disease*, eds Thompson RCA, Lymbery AJ, CAB International, Wallingford, Oxon, 135–71.

McManus DP, Garcia-Zepeda E et al., 1989, Human cysticercosis and taeniasis: molecular approaches for specific diagnosis and parasite identification, *Acta Leiden*, **57:** 81–91.

McManus DP, Smyth JD, 1978, Differences in the chemical composition and carbohydrate metabolism of *Echinococcus granulosus* (horse and sheep strains) and *E. multilocularis*, *Parasitology*, **77:** 103–9.

Mateos JH, Zenteno GH, 1987, Neurocisticercosis. Analisis de mil casos consecutivos, *Neurol Neuropsiq Psiquiat (Mex)*, **27:** 53–5.

Mesarina-Wicki B, 1991, Long-term course of alveolar echinococcosis in 70 patients treated by benzimidazole derivatives (mebendazole and albendazole) (1976–1989), Medical dissertation, University of Zurich.

Michault A, Duval G et al., 1990, Etude seroepidemiologique de la cysticercose a l'ile de la Réunion, *Bull Soc Path Exot Filiales*, **83:** 82–92.

Michault A, Leroy D et al., 1989, Diagnostic immunologique dans le liquide cephalo-rachidien et le serum de la cysticercose encephalique evolutive, *Path Biol (Paris)*, **37:** 249–253.

Michael AS, Levy JM, Paige ML, 1990, Cysticercosis mimicking brain neoplasm: MR and CT appearance, *J Comput Assist Tomogr*, **14:** 708–11.

Michel P, Michault A et al., 1990, Le serodiagnostic de la cysticercose par ELISA et western blot. Son interet et ses limites a Madagascar, *Arch Inst Pasteur Madagascar*, **57:** 115–42.

Mitchel GF, 1990, Vaccines and vaccination strategies against helminths, *Parasites. Molecular Biology, Drug and Vaccine Design*, eds Agabian N, Cerami A, Wiley-Liss, New York, 349–63.

Mitchell GW, Crawford RO, 1985, Intraparenchymal cerebral cysticercosis in children: a benign prognosis, *Pediatrics*, **82:** 76–82.

Mitchell GW, Snodgrass SR, 1988, Intraparenchymal cerebral cysticercosis in children: diagnosis and treatment, *Pediatr Neurol*, **1:** 151–6.

Molinari JL, Tato P et al., 1990, Depresive effect of a *Taenia solium* cysticercus factor on cultured human lymphocytes stimulated with phytohemaglutinin, *Ann Trop Med Parasitol*, **84:** 205–8.

Moro PL, Gilman RH et al., 1992, Immunoblot (western blot) and double immunodiffusion (DD5) tests for hydatid disease cross-react with sera from patients with cysticercosis, *Trans R Soc Trop Med Hyg*, **86:** 422–3.

Mühlschlegel F, Sygulla L et al., 1993, Paramyosin of *Echinococcus granulosus*: CDNA sequence and characterization of a tegumental antigen, *Parasitol Res*, **79:** 660–6.

Muller R, Lillywhite J et al., 1987, Human cysticercosis and intestinal parasitism amongst the Ekari people of Irian Jaya, *J Trop Med Hyg*, **90:** 291–6.

Ochieng-Mitula PJ, Burt MDB, 1996, The effects of ivermectin on the hydatid cyst of *Echinococcus granulosus* after direct injection at laparotomy, *J Parasitol*, **82:** 155–7.

Olivo A, Plancarte A, Flisser A, 1988, Presence of antigen B from *Taenia solium* cysticercus in other platyhelminthes, *Int J Parasitol*, **18:** 543–5.

Oriol C, Oriol R, 1975, Physicochemical properties of a lipoprotein antigen of *Echinococcus granulosus*, *Am J Trop Med Hyg*, **24:** 96–100.

Ostrosky L, Correa D et al., 1991, *Taenia solium*: inhibition of spontaneous evagination of cysticerci by the host inflammatory capsule, *Int J Parasitol*, **21:** 603–4.

Ostrosky-Zeichner L, Garcia E et al., 1996, Humoral and cellular immune response within the subarachnoid space of patients with neurocysticercosis, *Arch Med Res*, (in press).

Ostrosky-Zeichner L, Soto JL, 1996, Neurocysticercosis and HIV infection, report of two cases and review, *Surg Neurol*, (in press).

Pammenter MD, Rossouw EJ, Epstein SR, 1987, Diagnosis of neurocysticercosis by enzyme-linked immunosorbent assay, *S Afr Med J*, **71:** 512–14.

Pawlowski ZS, 1990, Perspectives on the control of *Taenia solium*, *Parasitol Today*, **6:** 371–3.

Pérez-Serrano J, Casado N et al., 1994, The effects of albendazole and albendazole sulphoxide combination-therapy on *Echinococcus granulosus* in vitro, *Int J Parasitol*, **24:** 219–24.

Puig-Solanes M, 1974, Consideraciones clinico-patologicas acerca de la cisticercosis intraocular: cisticerco viable y cisticerco en involucion, *Arch Soc Española Oftalmol*, **34:** 341–64.

Puri V, Sharma DK et al., 1991, Neurocysticercosis in children, *Indian J Pediatr*, **28:** 1309–17.

Rabiela MT, Rivas A, Flisser A, 1989, Morphological types of *Taenia solium* cysticerci, *Parasitol Today*, **5:** 357–9.

Rabiela MT, Rivas A et al., 1982, Anatomopathological aspects of human brain cysticercosis, *Cysticercosis: Present State of Knowledge and Perspectives*, eds Flisser A, Willms K, Laclette JP, Larralde C, Ridaura C, Beltran F, Academic Press, New York, 179–200.

Rausch RL, 1954, Studies on the helminth fauna of Alaska. XX. The histogenesis of the alveolar larva of *Echinococcus* species, *J Infec Dis*, **94:** 178–86.

Rausch RL, 1995, Life cycle patterns and geographic distribution of *Echinococcus* species, *Echinococcus and Hydatid Disease*, eds Thompson RCA, Lymbery AJ, CAB International, Wallingford, Oxon, 89–119.

Rausch RL, D'Alessandro A, Rausch VR, 1981, Characteristics of the larval *Echinococcus vogeli* Rausch and Bernstein, 1972 in the natural intermediate host, the paca, *Cuniculus paca* L (Rodentia: Dasyproctidae), *Am J Trop Med Hyg*, **30:** 1043–52.

Rausch RL, Wilson JF et al., 1987, Spontaneous death of *Echinococcus multilocularis* cases diagnosed serologically (by Em2 ELISA) and clinical significance, *Am J Trop Med Hyg*, **36:** 576–85.

Read CP, 1952, Contributions to cestode enzymology. 1. The cytochrome system and succinic dehydrogenase in *Hymenolepis diminuta*, *Exp Parasitol*, **1:** 353–62.

Rim HJ, Joo KH, 1989, Clinical evaluation of the therapeutic efficacy of praziquantel against human cysticercosis, *Acta Leiden*, **57:** 235–45.

Richards F, Schantz PM, 1991, Laboratory diagnosis of cysticercosis, *Clin Lab Med*, **11:** 1011–28.

Rickard MD et al., 1995, *Taenia ovis* recombinant vaccine – 'quo vadit', *Parasitology*, **110:** S5–S9.

Rodacki MA et al., 1989, CT features of cellulosae and racemosus neurocysticercosis, *J Comput Assist Tomogr*, **13:** 1013–16.

Rodriguez-Carbajal J, Boleaga-Duran B, 1982, Neuroradiology of human cysticercosis, *Cysticercosis: Present State of Knowledge and Perspectives*, eds Flisser A, Willms K, Laclette JP, Larralde C, Ridaura C, Beltran F, Academic Press, New York, 139–62.

Sanchez FA, Sanchez AC, 1971, Estudio de algunas propiedades físicas y componentes químicos del líquido y pared germinativa de quistes hidatídicos de diversas especies y de diferente localización, *Rev Ibér Parasitol*, **31:** 347–66.

Santos R, Dalma A, Ortiz E, 1979, Management of subretinal and viteous cysticercosis: Role of photocoagulation and surgery, *Ophthalmology*, **86:** 1501–04.

Sarti E, Schantz PM et al., 1992, Prevalence and risk factors for *Taenia solium* taeniasis and cysticercosis in humans and pigs in a village in Morelos, Mexico, *Am J Trop Med Hyg*, **46:** 677–84.

Sarti E, Schantz PM et al., 1994, Epidemiologic investigation of *Taenia solium* taeniasis and cysticercosis in a rural village of Michoacan State, Mexico, *Trans R Soc Trop Med Hyg*, **88:** 49–52.

Sato N, Aoki S et al., 1993, Clinical features, *Alveolar Echinococcosis of the Liver*, eds Uchino J, Sato N, Hokkaido University School of Medicine, Sapporo, 63–68.

Schantz PM, 1994, Larval cestodiases. Infection of the digestive glands, *Infectious Diseases. A Treatise of Infectious Processes*, 4th edn, eds Hoeprich PD, Jordan MC, Ronald AR, JB Lippincott, Philadelphia, 850–60.

Schantz PM, Gottstein B, 1986, Echinococcosis (hyuaditidosis), *Immunodiagnosis of Parasitic Diseases*, Vol. 1. Helminthic Diseases, eds Walls KW, Schantz PM, Academic Press, Orlando, FL, 69–107.

Schantz PM, Okelo GBA, 1990, Echinococcosis (Hydatidosis), *Tropical and Geographical Medicine*, 2nd edn, eds Warren KS, Mahmoud AAF, University Hospitals of Cleveland, 504–18.

Schantz PM, Sarti E et al., 1994, Community-based epidemiological investigations of cysticercosis due to *Taenia solium*: comparison of serological screening tests and clinical findings in two populations in Mexico, *Clin Infect Dis*, **18**: 879–85.

Short JA, Heiner DC et al., 1991, Immunoglobulin E and G4 antibodies in cysticercosis, *J Clin Microbiol*, **28**: 1635–9.

Sotelo J, Rubalcava MA, Gomez-Llata S, 1995, A new shunt for hydrocephalus that relies on CSF production rather than on ventricular pressure: initial clinical experiences, *Surg Neurol*, **43**: 324–32.

Sotelo J, Torrs B et al., 1985, Praziquantel in the treatment of neurocysticercosis: long-term follow-up, *Neurology*, **35**: 752–5.

Spruance SL, 1974, Latent period of 53 years in a case of hydatid cyst disease, *Arch Intern Med*, **134**: 741–2.

Suntsov S, Ozeretskovskaya N et al., 1990a, Status of interferon during helminthiases. Communication 1. Human unilocular hydatidosis, *Med Parazitol (Mosk)*, **6**: 27–9.

Suntsov S, Ozeretskovskaya N et al., 1990b, Interferon status during helminthiases. Communication 2. Multilocular hydatidosis, *Med Parazitol (Mosk)*, **6**: 43–4.

Suss RA, Maravilla KR, Thompson J, 1986, MR Imaging of intracranial cysticercosis: comparison with CT and anatomopathologic features, *AJNR*, **7**: 235–41.

Takayanagui OM, Jardim E, 1983, Aspectos clinicos da neurocisticercose. Analise de 500 casos, *Arq Neuro-Psiquiatr*, **41**: 50–63.

Taylor DH, Morris DL, 1988, In vitro culture of *Echinococcus multilocularis*: protoscolicidal action of praziquantel and albendazole sulphoxide, *Tran R Soc Trop Med Hyg*, **82**: 265–7.

Teitelbaum GP, Otto RJ et al., 1989, MR imaging of neurocysticercosis, *Am J Roentgenol*, **153**: 857–66.

Thais JH, Goldsmith RS et al., 1994, Detection by immunoblot assay of antibodies to *Taenia solium* cysticerci in sera from residents of rural communities and from epileptic patients in Bali, Indonesia, *Southeast Asian J Trop Med Public Health*, **25**: 464–8.

Thompson RCA, 1995, Biology and systematics of *Echinococcus*, *Echinococcus and Hydatid Disease*, eds Thompson RCA, Lymbery AJ, CAB International, Wallingford, Oxon, 1–37.

Thompson RCA, Lymbery AJ, 1988, The nature, extent and significance of variation within the genus *Echinococcus*, *Adv Parasitol*, **27**: 210–63.

Thompson RCA, Robertson ID et al., 1993, Hydatid disease in Western Australia: a novel approach to education and surveillance, *Parasitol Today*, **9**: 431–3.

Todorov T, Mechkov G, et al., 1992, Factors influencing the response to chemotherapy in human cystic echinococcosis, *Bull WHO*, **70**: 347–58.

Torgerson PR, Pilkington J et al., 1995, Further evidence for the long distance dispersal of taeniid eggs, *Int J Parasitol*, **25**: 265–7.

Torres A, Plancarte A et al., 1992, Praziquantel treatment of porcine brain and muscle *Taenia solium* cysticercosis. 3. Effect of 1-day treatment, *Parasitol Res*, **78**: 161–4.

Tsang VCW, Brand AJ, Boyer AE, 1989, An enzyme-linked immunoelectrotransfer blot assay by glycoprotein antigens for diagnosing human cysticercosis (*Taenia solium*), *J Infect Dis*, **159**: 50–9.

van Beneden PJ, 1854, Note sur des experiences relatives au developpement des cysticerques, *Ann Sci Nat*, **1**: 104.

Varela-Díaz VM, Coltorti EA, D'Alessandro A, 1978, Immunoelectrophoresis tests showing *Echinococcus granulosus* arc 5 in human cases of *Echinococcus vogeli* and cysticercosis-multiple myelona, *Am J Trop Med Hyg*, **27**: 554–7.

Vázquez V, Sotelo J, 1992, The course of seizures after treatment of cerebral cysticercosis, *N Engl J Med*, **327**: 696–701.

Veit P, Bilger B et al., 1995, Influence of environmental factors on the infectivity of *Echinococcus multilocularis* eggs, *Parasitology*, **110**: 79–86.

von Sinner WN, 1991, New diagnostic signs in hydatid disease: radiography, ultrasound, CT and MRI correlated to pathology, *Eur J Radiol*, **12**: 150–9.

Vuitton DA, Bresson HS et al., 1988, IgE-dependent humoral immune response in *Echinococcus multilocularis* infection: circulating and basophil-bound specific IgE against *Echinococcus* antigens in patients with alveolar echinococcosis, *Clin Exp Immunol*, **71**: 247–52.

Vuitton D, Bresson HS et al., 1989, Cellular immune response in *Echinococcus multilocularis* infection in humans. II Natural killer cell activity and cell subpopulations in the blood and in the periparasitic granuloma of patients with alveolar echinococcosis, *Clin Exp Immunol*, **78**: 67–74.

White AC, Molinari JL et al., 1992, Detection and preliminary characterization of *Taenia solium* metacestode proteases, *J Parasitol*, **78**: 281–7.

Williams JF, Pérez-Escandi MV, Oriol R, 1971, Evaluation of purified lipoprotein antigens of *Echinococcus granulosus* in the immunodiagnosis of human infection, *Am J Trop Med Hyg*, **20**: 575–9.

Wilson JF, Rausch RL, 1980, Alveolar hydatid disease. A review of clinical features of 33 indigenous cases of *Echinococcus multilocularis* infection in Alaskan Eskimos, *Am J Trop Med Hyg*, **29**: 1340–55.

Wilson M, Bryan RT et al., 1991, Clinical evaluation of the cysticercosis enzyme-linked immunoelectrotransfer blot in patients with neurocysticercosis, *J Infect Dis*, **164**: 1007–9.

Yong WK, Heath DD, van Knapen F, 1984, Comparison of cestode antigen in an enzyme-linked immunosorbent assay for the diagnosis of *Echinoccus granulosus*, *Taenia hydatigena* and *T. ovis* infections in sheep, *Res Vet Sci*, **36**: 24–31.

Yoshino K, 1933, Studies on the post-embryonal development of *Taenia solium*. Part III. On the developmento of cysticercus cellulosae within the definite intermediate host, *J Med Ass Formosa*, **32**: 166–9.

Zhipiao XB, Yvequing Z et al., 1980, Muscular pseudohypertrophy due to cysticercosis cellulosa. Report of 3 cases, *Chin Med J*, **93**: 4853.

Zini D, Farrell VJR, Wadee AA, 1990, The relationship of antibody levels to the clinical spectrum of human neurocysticercosis, *J Neurol Neurosurg Psychiatry*, **53**: 656–61.

Gastrointestinal nematodes — Ascaris, hookworm, Trichuris and Enterobius

D W T Crompton

Nearly 200 species of helminth have been found associated with the human alimentary tract (Coombs and Crompton 1991), many of these probably being the result of accidental or spurious infections. Of the habitual parasites, the pinworm or threadworm *Enterobius vermicularis* (L, 1758) and four species of soil-transmitted nematodes, the roundworm *Ascaris lumbricoides* L, 1758, hookworms *Ancylostoma duodenale* (Dubini, 1843) Creplin, 1845 and *Necator americanus* (Stiles, 1902) Stiles, 1903 and the whipworm *Trichuris trichiura* (L. 1771) Stiles, 1901 are some of the commonest infections on earth (Table 29.1).

The origins of these human–helminth relations are intriguing and might perhaps be traced to human activities leading to the domestication of animals. A qualitative survey indicates that humans share surprisingly few intestinal helminth infections with the other 180 or so species of primate (see Coombs and Crompton 1991, Macdonald 1984). *E. vermicularis* may well have evolved with humans from our primate ancestors, but the soil-transmitted species might perhaps be traced to human activities leading to the domestication of animals. Humans do, however, seem to have in common either the same or similar types of infection to those found in domesticated animals, especially dogs (Beaver 1954) and pigs (Bell, Palmer and Payne 1988). Perhaps human *A. lumbricoides*, if it

really is a species in its own right (see Crompton 1989), might have been acquired from porcine *A. suum* or its ancestor after the last ice age. Pigs were probably domesticated in several places (Clutton-Brock 1987), but China is likely to have been one of the first and there remains an intimate relationship today between Chinese people and their pigs (Peng, Zhou and Crompton 1995).

The domestication of the very few species of mammal that humans now rely on for food, clothing and transport began about 9000 years BP (Clutton-Brock 1987) when the human population was about 10 million (Lewin 1989). Evidence from early writings (Bryan 1930, Ebbell 1937), from mummified bodies (see Cockburn and Cockburn 1980) and from archaeological digs (Fry and Moore 1969, Bundy and Cooper 1989) indicates that pinworm, roundworm, hookworm and whipworm were well established in humans a few thousand years ago. Today the human population is over 5 billion and by the year 2010 is likely to be 7 billion with around 80% of the people living in the countries currently identified as less developed (Bulatao et al. 1990). Pinworms are the only species that is common in temperate countries; pinworms and the soil-transmitted species are widely distributed in countries with warmer climates, often occurring concurrently in individuals. It has been estimated that

Table 29.1 Features of *Ascaris*, hookworms and *Trichuris* in human hosts

	Ascaris lumbricoides	*Ancylostoma duodenale*	*Necator americanus*	*Trichuris trichiura*
Phylum	Nematoda	Nematoda	Nematoda	Nematoda
Class	Secernentea	Secernentea	Secernentea	Adenophorea
Order	Ascaridida	Strongylida	Strongylida	Enoplida
Family	Ascarididae	Ancylostomatidae	Ancylostomatidae	Trichuridae
Genus	*Ascaris*	*Ancylostoma*	*Necator*	*Trichuris*
Species	*lumbricoides*	*duodenale*	*americanus*	*trichiura*
Trivial name	Roundworm	Hookworm	Hookworm	Whipworm
No. species/subspecies in genus[a]	16	23	8	71
No. species infecting humans[b]	2	7	3	3
Global no of infections[c]	1470×10^6	135×10^6	735×10^6	1300×10^6
Estimate of cases of morbidity[d]	$120–215 \times 10^6$	$27–39 \times 10^6$	$63–91 \times 10^6$	$90–130 \times 10^6$

[a]Yamaguti (1961).
[b]See Table 130.2 and Coombs and Crompton (1991).
[c]Bundy (1994).
[d]Chan *et al.* (1994). The estimates for the separate species of hookworm are based on the assumption that 30% are due to *A. duodenale* and 70% to *N. americanus* (Crompton and Stephenson 1990).

around a billion people are infected with *A. lumbricoides*, *A. duodenale*, *N. americanus* and *T. trichiura*, often concurrently (Crompton 1989); this means that 4 out of every 10 people in much of Africa, Asia and South America harbour worms.

The notion that humans may have acquired the soil-transmitted nematodes during the domestication of a few species of wild mammal over a period of a few thousand years should not be discarded too lightly without further consideration. The human host has undergone about 400 generations and a vast social and technical evolution during the last 10 000 years while *A. lumbricoides* has undergone about 20 000 generations which, coupled with its prodigious fecundity, could have created the circumstances for an explosive evolution.

The history of human helminth infections has been carefully documented by Grove (1990). Although 3 of these intestinal species (*Ascaris, Enterobius* and *Trichuris*) were known to Linnaeus in the 18th century, and *Ancylostoma* was identified in the early 19th century, details of their life histories did not become known until much later. A fundamental observation in the case of *A. lumbricoides* was made by Koino (1922) who courageously swallowed about 2000 eggs and subsequently passed 667 worms after taking an anthelmintic drug. He was extremely ill during the course of this experimental infection at a time when the larvae would have been occupying his lungs. Looss (1901) published the results of an experiment which proved that hookworm larvae penetrate skin. He placed a drop of water containing infective larvae of *A. duodenale* on the skin of a leg awaiting amputation. An hour later, when the surgery had been completed, Looss retrieved samples of skin and found the larvae beneath the skin. Calandrucci in 1886, having confirmed over a period of 6 months that he was free

from infection with *T. trichiura*, swallowed infected eggs of the helminth and found eggs in his stools 27 days later. This result was published by Grassi (1887) who may not have given Calandrucci sufficient credit for his effort (Grove 1990). These studies are of great importance because they established the nature of the helminths' life cycles and the routes of transmission to human hosts.

1 CLASSIFICATION

In this chapter, the 5 species of helminth are assumed to belong to the phylum Nematoda as advocated by Maggenti (1982) rather than a class of the phylum Aschelminthes as adhered to by Hyman (1951). Much work needs to be done before we have a secure understanding of the phylogeny of these ubiquitous animals which thrive as free-living, plant-parasitic and animal-parasitic organisms (Andrassy 1976, Maggenti 1982, Poinar 1983). A simple classification for soil transmitted nematodes, based mainly on Anderson, Chabaud and Willmott (1974) is set out in Table 29.1. Although the ecology and general biology of *A. lumbricoides*, *A. duodenale*, *E. vermicularis*, *N. americanus* and *T. trichiura* have much in common, the latter species has major morphological differences from the others. Most noticeably, it lacks phasmids (paired, glandular sensory organs) at its caudal end and is equipped with a stichosome oesophagus. Taxonomists have used the presence or absence of phasmids as a basic feature in the systematic organization of nematodes.

If adult worms, either alive or in a good state of preservation are available, an investigator should have no difficulty in identifying the genera under discussion. The keys prepared by Yamaguti (1961) and Anderson et al. (1974) are recommended together with the biological and clinical descriptions published by Beaver and Jung (1985). Problems are likely to be encountered, if only morphological evidence is available, in trying to distinguish from each other, for example, all the 7 species of *Ancylostoma* reported from humans (Tables 29.1, 29.2). Adult *A. lumbricoides* and adult *A. suum* remain virtually indistinguishable on morphological grounds (see Crompton 1989) as are *T. trichiura* and the other species of *Trichuris* found in non-human primates and pigs.

2 MORPHOLOGY AND STRUCTURE

Detailed accounts of the anatomy, functional morphology and structure of animal-parasitic nematodes, including the species considered here, *Trichuris*, have been published by Chitwood and Chitwood (1974), Gibbons (1986) and Bird and Bird (1991) among others. Each of these treatises deals comparatively with different features such as the cephalic region and the nervous system rather than presenting descriptions of individual species. The brief accounts given below for the 4 species of soil-transmitted nematode under review in this chapter cover features not highlighted in the definitive works cited above. Inevitably, some of the details are based on extrapolation from the results of studies on *A. suum*, *Anc. caninum* and *T. suis* from animal hosts.

2.1 *Ascaris lumbricoides*

The eggs of *A. lumbricoides* are seen in human stool samples in 2 general forms: unfertilized eggs (Fig. 29.1a) and fertilized eggs which may or may not possess a cortical layer (Figs 29.1b,c). Typically eggs in stools appear to be brown in colour, probably because they become stained by bile pigments while in the gastrointestinal tract. The eggshell of a fertilized egg (50–70 × 40–50 μm) consists of an inner lipid layer responsible for selective permeability (Perry and Clark 1982), a chitin–protein layer responsible for structural strength and an outer vitelline layer (Foor 1967, Wharton 1980). The inner layer contains a remarkably resilient lipoprotein, known as ascaroside, which explains how the eggs with enclosed infective larvae can survive formaldehyde, disinfectants and other destructive chemicals. The fertilized egg is frequently observed to have an uneven deposit of mucopolysaccharide (the cortical layer) on its outer surface (Fig. 29.1b). This deposit is obtained when the egg is passing through the uterus of the female worm (Foor 1967) and is responsible for its adhesive properties (Kagei 1983).

The first stage larva of *A. lumbricoides* develops inside the eggshell, moults there and forms the second stage larva. Soon after hatching, second stage larvae have a typical filariform appearance and measure about 250 × 14 μm (Nichols 1956). Just before the second moult in the lungs, they measure about 560 × 28 μm in length. After the fourth (final) moult in the small intestine, growth is rapid. Freshly recovered adult male and female *A. lumbricoides* are often observed to be a pinkish cream in colour and to measure 200–300 mm in length. A male, which is usually smaller than a female of the same age, has a curved posterior tail which accommodates the copulatory apparatus. Skryabin, Shikhobalova and Mozgovoi (1991) describe adult *A. lumbricoides* as having a mouth surrounded by 3 well-developed lips, rows of small 'teeth' (= denticles of Sprent 1952) on the lips, a cuticle with transverse striations, a didelphic uterus and the vulva in the anterior half of the body. The morphology of these denticles is a character widely used by workers who seek to distinguish *A. lumbricoides* from *A. suum* (Maung 1973).

Table 29.2 Zoonotic infections of humans with species of *Ascaris, Ancylostoma, Necator* and *Trichuris*

Genus and species	Non-human hosts	Observations on infection in human hosts	References
Ascaris suum	Pig	Sexually mature; in small intestine	Davies and Goldsmith (197?)
Ancylostoma brasiliense	Cat, dog	Cutaneous larva migrans (CLM)[a]	Yoshida et al. (1974)
A. caninum	Dog	CLM; adult worm in small intestine	Croese et al. (1994)
A. ceylanicum	Cat, dog	Adult in small intestine	Carroll and Grove (1986)
A. japonica	Unresolved	Reported once from human in Japan	Barriga (1982a)
A. malayanum	Bear	No information	Yorke and Maplestone (1926)
A. tubaeforme	Cat	CML	Muller (1975)
Necator argentinus	Unresolved	Reported once from human	Yoshida (1973)
N. suillus	Pig	Reported at least once from human	Barriga (1982a)
Trichuris suis	Pig	Adult in large intestine	Barriga (1982b)
T. vulpis	Dog	Sexually mature adult in appendix	Kenney and Eveland (1978)

[a]For a full discussion of CLM see Beaver (1956).

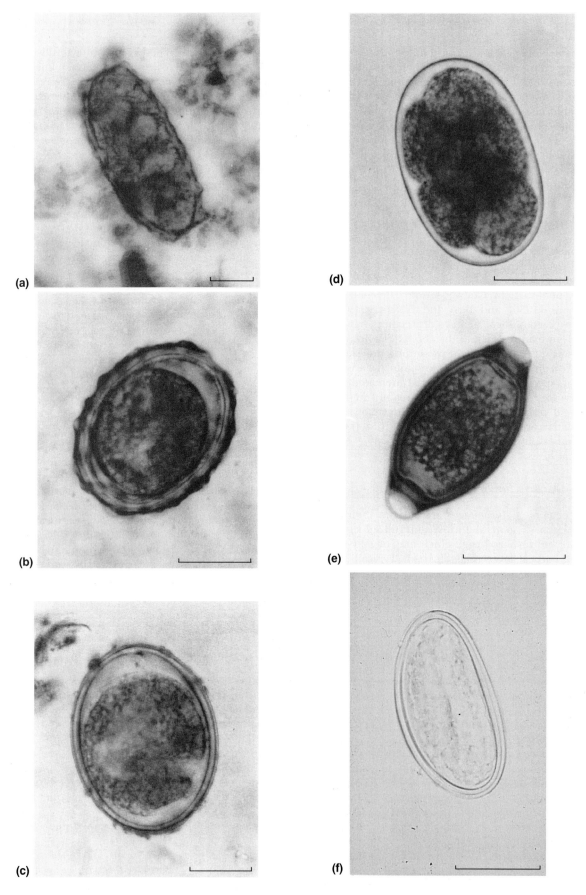

Fig. 29.1 Photomicrographs of eggs of soil-transmitted nematodes as seen in human stool samples: (a) unfertilized egg of *Ascaris lumbricoides*; (b) fertilized egg of *A. lumbricoides* with cortical layer; (c) fertilized egg of *A. lumbricoides* with cortical layer; (d) egg of a hookworm; (e) egg of *Trichuris trichiura*; (f) egg of *Enterobius vermicularis*. Scale represents 25 μm. (a–e), from WHO (1994); (f), courtesy of R. Muller.

The cuticle of *A. lumbricoides* under natural circumstances is only ever exposed to the conditions prevailing in the host. Collagen, stabilized by disulfide links, forms the main structural protein of the adult cuticle which becomes more complex with each moult (Bird and Bird 1991). Collagen is now known to be the principal protein in the cuticles of all adult nematode species investigated to date. An investigation into the composition of the cuticles of developmental stages of *A. suum* from pigs revealed that the proteins extracted with 2-mercaptoethanol from third and fourth stage larvae and from adult worms were readily digested on incubation with bacterial collagenase (Fetterer, Hill and Urban 1990). A significant amount of the cuticle from second stage larvae was not affected by 2-mercaptoethanol and was not digested by bacterial collagenase. Presumably the same results may apply to *A. lumbricoides*, with the differences detected in the second stage larval cuticle being an adaptation either to survival outside the host or the infection process or both events.

2.2 *Ancylostoma duodenale* and *Necator americanus*

When seen in human stools (Fig 29.1d), the eggs of these 2 species are indistinguishable, being characteristically barrel-shaped with a thin shell and measuring about $60 \times 75 \times 36$–$40 \mu m$ (WHO 1994). If hookworm eggs alone are available, identification of the species cannot be made without first using the Harada–Mori technique to culture the newly-hatched larvae to the third stage when morphological differences become apparent (WHO 1981).

Descriptions of the morphology of the larval stages of hookworms are available through the experimental studies of Nichols (1956) and observations summarized by Pawlowski, Schad and Stott (1991). The first stage larvae which escape from the eggs measure about $200 \mu m$ in length. They feed on organic debris and moult, and the resulting second stage larvae measure up to $500 \mu m$. After another moult, the infective third stage larvae measure from 500–$700 \mu m$, those of *Ancylostoma* being generally longer than those of *Necator* (WHO 1981).

The most detailed description of the morphology of adult *A. duodenale* is to be found in the classic account by Looss (1905). For both species, male worms (5–11 mm) are shorter than females (9–13 mm) and *A. duodenale* is generally longer and more sturdily built than *N. americanus*. Proof of identity is obtained by comparing the morphologies of the buccal capsule (Fig. 29.2). The term 'hookworm' derives from the prominent curve to the anterior end of specimens of *N. americanus* (Pawlowski, Schad and Stott 1991).

2.3 *Enterobius vermicularis*

Pinworm eggs are ovoid, measuring 50–54 $\mu m \times 20$–27 μm. They are asymmetrically flattened on one side, and appear colourless when recovered from the perianal skin (Fig. 29.1f). The outer layer of the eggshell

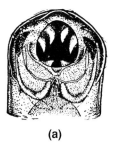 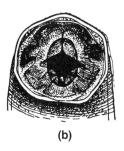

(a)   **(b)**

Fig. 29.2 Buccal capsules of (a) adult *Ancylostoma duodenale* and (b) adult *Necator americanus*.

is albuminous and sticky, enabling the egg to adhere readily. When laid the egg contains an immature first stage larva, but this develops rapidly. When swallowed the eggs hatch in the small bowel and the larvae pass down into the large bowel, where they complete their moulting and development. Adult worms, which measure about 10×0.5 mm (female) and 2.5×0.2 mm (male), live primarily in the caecum, in close contact with the mucosa. Males are rarely seen, but the gravid females can sometimes be seen as white or yellowish worms around the anus. Such worms have prominent uteri filled with eggs.

2.4 *Trichuris trichiura*

The eggs of *T. trichiura* are lemon-shaped with a characteristic plug at each end (Fig. 29.1e). They are usually brown in a human stool sample and measure from 57–58 $\times$ 26–30 μm. As with eggs of *Ascaris* spp. and hookworms, it is virtually impossible to distinguish eggs of *T. trichiura* from those of *T. suis* and *T. vulpis* (Kenney and Yermakov 1980, Yoshikawa et al. 1989). According to studies by Wharton and Jenkins (1978) the eggs of *T. suis* have a shell similar in structure to that of *A. lumbricoides*, an observation which explains the survival of the enclosed infective larva under adverse environmental conditions (see Bundy and Cooper 1989). Apparently, there is a higher proportion of chitin in the plugs at the poles of an egg of *T. trichiura* than elsewhere in the eggshell. Wharton and Jenkins have suggested that this may facilitate the hatching process if the activated larva releases chitinase (see Rogers 1960). On hatching in the intestine, the second stage larval *T. trichiura* measures about 260 $\times$ 15 μm in length (Beck and Beverley-Burton 1968). These larvae, if they behave as do those of other species of *Trichuris*, burrow into the intestinal mucosa, and it is Bundy and Cooper's view that *Trichuris* spp. are essentially tissue parasites. There is some confusion about where the intestinal penetration takes place and whether or not the larvae migrate along the intestinal tissues to reach the large intestine. During this prepatent phase (Table 29.3), *T. trichiura* must complete the series of 4 moults and is found as an adult intimately associated with the wall of the large intestine.

Adult whipworms have a highly characteristic shape from which the trivial name is derived. The long, thin anterior end lies in a burrow in the mucosa while the

Table 29.3 Some features of the life histories of *Ascaris,* hookworms and *Trichuris*[a]

	Ascaris lumbricoides	*Ancylostoma duodenale*	*Necator americanus*	*Trichuris trichiura*
Longevity in host (years)	1–2	1	3–5	1–3
Location of adult worms	Jejunal lumen	Jejunal mucosa	Jejunal mucosa	Tissue of large intestine
Reproductive strategy	Dioecious	Dioecious	Dioecious	Dioecious
Fecundity (eggs/O/day)	c. 240 000	10 000–25 000	5000–10 000	14 000–20 000
Prepatent period (days)	67–76	53	49–56	60–90
Patent period (days)	c. 300–650	c. 300	c. 1050–1775	c. 300–1000
Embryonation (days)	12 ± 2 days, 31°C			28 days, 25°C
Infective stage	L2 in eggshell[b]	Free L3	Free L3	L2 in eggshell
Max. survival of infective stage	Up to 15 years			Up to 6 years[c]
Usual transmission route	Oral	Skin/oral	Skin	Oral
Tissue migration	Liver and lungs	Not necessary	Lungs	
Arrested development		+[d]		..

[a]Abstracted mainly from Hoagland and Schad (1978), Bundy and Cooper (1989), Crompton (1994).
[b]L, larva; L1, L2, L3, L4 refer in the text to the first, second, third and fourth larval (juvenile) stages, there being a moult after each stage has completed its contribution to the life history.
[c]Based on observations made on *T. suis* by Hill (1957).
[d]Discovered by Schad *et al.* (1973).

thicker end, which contains the reproductive tract extends into the intestinal lumen. The worms are white in colour and the males (30–45 mm) are not only shorter than the females (30–50 mm), but also have a coiled posterior end when viewed in vitro. The most characteristic morphological feature of species of *Trichuris* and their relatives is the stichosome which is a glandular structure encircling the slender oesophagus in the thin, anterior half of the worms (Beck and Beverley-Burton 1968).

Although *Enterobius* occurs throughout the world, it is usually perceived as important only in temperate countries, primarily because it is the only common intestinal nematode there. Many characterisitcs of pinworms, e.g. their relatively low pathogenicity and their biology and mode of transmission (which is directly contaminative and not dependent on initial faecal dissemination into the environment) differentiate them from the other parasites covered in this chapter. *Ascaris,* hookworms and *Trichuris* are more pathogenic, they often occur together, their modes of transmission are facilitated by similar environmental and socioeconomic factors, and they are studied epidemiologically as a coherent group. For these reasons the soil-transmitted species will be considered together and separately from *Enterobius*.

3 SOIL-TRANSMITTED NEMATODES: BIOLOGY AND FEEDING

Comprehensive summaries of current knowledge and assumed knowledge of specific aspects of the biology of *A. lumbricoides, A. duodenale, N. americanus* and *T. trichiura* are available in reviews by Miller (1978), Crompton, (1989 1994), Bundy and Cooper (1989), Schad and Warren (1990) and Misegna and Gilles (1987). We may assume that moulting, energy metabolism, excretion and reproduction occur as described for animal-parasitic nematodes generally by Bird and Bird (1991), Barrett (1981), Lee and Atkinson (1976) and Adiyodi and Adiyodi (1983). Their feeding activities merit special consideration, partly because little is understood about how they obtain nutrients and energy while living as larval parasites and partly because of the role of the feeding of the adult stages in pathogenesis and chronic disease. Feeding is based on the development of the muscular oesophagus to pump fluids or materials in suspension along a simple gut (Bennet-Clark 1976).

3.1 *Ascaris lumbricoides*

During the development of the eggs, the parent worm must supply the zygote with nutrients sufficient to ensure progression to the infective second stage larva and subsequent survival. After hatching in the human gut, the larvae must either carry with them or obtain, through direct feeding on host tissues and metabolites, enough food and energy to ensure a successful migration back to the gut and a series of development moults. The tissue migrations of parasitic larvae have remained an enigma: are the parasites reliving their life cycles in a once intermediate but now definitive host? (Smyth 1994). Given that *A. lumbricoides* starts its association with its host in the gut and then returns there, perhaps natural selection would have been expected to have eliminated the migratory phase, with its exposure to the host's full array of immunological mechanisms, unless there were some compensatory benefits for the parasite (Read and Skorping 1995). Read and Skorping found that helminths which migrated grew relatively larger than those that did not. Nematode fecundity is linked to worm size, so a benefit for the survivors of the tissue migration becomes apparent.

Once *A. lumbricoides* is established in the lumen of the host's small intestine it feeds on digestion products by pumping chyme through its own gut. In doing so, adult *A. lumbricoides* are likely to swallow bacteria including some which may be pathogenic to the worms, such as *E. coli* and *S. aureus* (Adedeja and Ogunba 1991). Wardlaw, Forsyth and Crompton (1994) found that the pseudocoelomic fluid of *A. suum* contained potent bactericidal activity which was not due to lysozyme. Antibacterial defence mechanisms would be expected to be present in an organism adapted to live in the intestine and feed on its intestinal contents.

Davey (1964), after examining *A. suum* obtained within half an hour from freshly slaughtered pigs, observed many pig intestinal epithelial cells in the parasites' guts. He estimated that whereas the concentration of free epithelial cells in the pig's gut would be expected to be about $6 \times 10^4 / mm^3$, the concentration in the anterior part of the gut of the worms was about $4 \times 10^6 / mm^3$. This finding suggests that *A. suum* may either selectively feed on discharged epithelial cells or even browse on the mucosa in addition to ingesting chyme. There is no doubt that the mucosal surface of a pig harbouring intestinal stages of *A. suum* shows histological damage (Martin et al. 1984), a finding commensurate with the observed maldigestion of lactose in *Ascaris*-infected pigs (Forsum, Nesheim and Crompton 1981) and children (Carrera, Nesheim and Crompton. 1984).

3.2 *Ancylostoma duodenale* and *Necator americanus*

Hatched larval hookworms feed voraciously on bacterial and organic matter until the non-feeding third stage larvae are formed. Presumably these contain suf-ficient stored energy to support skin penetration. It is not known whether newly penetrated third stage larvae feed in the host or whether the next moult must occur and then the fourth stage larva will feed actively. Third stage larvae of *A. duodenale* entering the host by the oral route appear not to undergo a tissue migration (Pawlowski, Schad and Stott 1991). Those larvae of *A. duodenale* that penetrate skin and migrate through tissue must need much more food and energy than those entering the oral route. The third stage larva of *N. americanus* must always penetrate skin and undergo tissue migration to reach the gut.

The intestinal stages of hookworms feed on blood obtained by puncturing the capillary network in the mucosa. Host blood is then pumped along the worm's gut and nutrient molecules absorbed from the host's plasma. Feeding by both *A. caninum* and *A. duodenale* involves the release of an anticoagulant secreted at the time of feeding (Hotez and Cerami 1983). Probably much of the blood taken by a hookworm as it feeds passes through its body into the host's gut lumen (Crompton and Whitehead 1993). When the worm bites into the mucosa at a second site, the lacerations at the first site together with residual anticoagulant activity mean that further blood loss occurs. From an experimental study of *A. caninum* in dogs, Wang et al. (1983) concluded that an individual female worm pumped about 0.043 ± 0.04 ml of host blood per day and that a further 0.046 ± 0.019 ml was lost as a haemorrhage from the abandoned feeding site. Female worms cause more blood loss than males.

3.3 *Trichuris trichiura*

Despite current interest in the biology of whipworms, largely stimulated by the work of Bundy and colleagues (see Bundy and Cooper 1989), there remains some controversy about their feeding activities. Do the worms suck blood, a view supported by Beck and Beverley-Burton (1968), or do they digest host tissues by releasing proteolytic enzymes (see Watson 1962)? Burrows and Lillis (1964) clearly demonstrated that *T. vulpis* feeds on dog blood. They found dog blood in the guts of *T. vulpis* and by direct observation described how the worms, through a series of rapier-like slashing movements, could lacerate capillaries and then pump released blood into their guts. They also found blood in the gut of *T. trichiura*. The structure of the buccal apparatus with its piercing stylet also suggests that blood-feeding is its probable purpose. Furthermore, rectal bleeding and iron-deficiency anaemia are characteristics of some patients suffering from trichiuriasis (Fisher and Cremin 1970, Lotero, Tripathy and Bolanos 1974, Bundy and Cooper 1989). The aetiology of iron deficiency anaemia is complex and may not arise directly from the feeding activity of *T. trichiura*; the nutritional status of the hosts and polyparasitism are 2 of the factors which must be accounted for. Nevertheless, whipworms undoubtedly ingest host blood obtained from the mucosa of the large intestine.

4   SOIL-TRANSMITTED NEMATODES: LIFE HISTORIES

The direct life history patterns of *A. lumbricoides, A. duodenale, N. americanus* and *T. trichiura* are well understood in general terms and can be represented diagrammatically in the form of a flow chart (Fig. 29.3). This scheme is important because it focuses attention on the fact that a soil-transmitted nematode exists in 2 populations; a free-living cohort based on the eggs and related early larval stages and an endoparasitic cohort based on the later larval stages and the adult worms in the gut. More detailed information about the life histories is summarized in Table 29.3, and much recent information is available in articles edited by Crompton, Nesheim and Pawlowski (1985, 1989) and Schad and Warren (1990) and in the review by Bundy and Cooper (1989). Aspects of the life histories are treated in some detail in the sections dealing with transmission and with epidemiology.

5   SOIL-TRANSMITTED NEMATODES: TRANSMISSION AND ESTABLISHMENT OF INFECTION

5.1   *Ascaris lumbricoides*

Infective second stage larvae of *A. lumbricoides* must usually be swallowed by the human host in order to initiate the establishment of an infection. The larvae escape from the egg, presumably in response to the same stimuli identified by Rogers (1960) for the hatching *in vitro* of eggs of *A. suum,* pass through the intestinal wall and reach the liver via the hepatic portal system. If the time course for *A. lumbricoides* in humans is the same as that for *A. suum* in pigs, mice and rabbits, the larval stages spend about 4 days in the liver and about 14 days in the lungs and then begin to re-enter the gut via the bronchi and trachea. At least 65

days must pass after infection before eggs are first detected in the stools (Table 29.3; Takata 1951).

The eggs of *A. lumbricoides* are produced in vast numbers (Table 29.3) and, although many will either perish during embryonation due to exposure to ultraviolet radiation or become inaccessible to humans through the activities of earthworms and seepage into the soil during rainfall, enough survive to ensure the persistence of the infections. In a recent experimental study carried out with eggs of *A. suum* contaminating soil in Poland, Mizgajska (1993) found that 0.1–4.5% of the eggs retained infectivity (observed larval movements) for 17 months and most of these had remained with the top 50 mm of the soil. During this period, some eggs had reached a depth of 210 mm in the soil. Any community lacking facilities for the safe disposal of human faeces will remain vulnerable to infection with *A. lumbricoides,* and use of untreated night-soil as a fertilizer for vegetables will probably increase the risk of infection. The complex eggshells of *A. lumbricoides* (Wharton 1980) protect the larvae from mechanical, chemical and physical damage, and the external mucopolysaccharide ensures that the eggs adhere to objects. In areas where infection is endemic, infective eggs have been found adhering to cooking and eating utensils, money, furniture, door handles, fruit, vegetables and fingers (Kagei 1983) as well as contaminating the soil in households, gardens and public parks (Morishita 1972, Yadav and Tandon 1989, Wong and Bundy 1990). Some evidence suggests that the eggs can become airborne and be inhaled in dust, thus gaining access to the alimentary tract (Bidinger, Crompton and Arnold 1981, Kroeger et al. 1992).

Although there need be no doubt that transmission nearly always depends on swallowing eggs from a contaminated environment, other routes of transmission may also exist. For example, 3 case studies indicate that *A. lumbricoides* may occasionally pass the placenta (Chu et al. 1972, Rathi et al. 1981, da Costa-Macedo and Rey 1990) and, since larval *Ascaris* can be transplanted between hosts experimentally, there is even the slight chance that infections may be established inadvertently through organ-transplant surgery.

5.2   *Ancylostoma duodenale* and *Necator americanus*

The third stage larvae of hookworms are responsible for transmission and the establishment of infections. Hoagland and Schad (1978) have concluded that *A. duodenale* is an opportunistic species, partly because the third larval stages (Table 29.3) can penetrate skin or enter via the oral route. Recent evidence from China indicates that larval *A. duodenale* may pass from the mother to infect the fetus *in utero;* transmammary infection with *A. duodenale* cannot be ignored (see Banwell and Schad 1978).

Under favourable conditions, first stage larvae hatch from hookworm eggs within about 24 h of faeces being deposited on the soil. One of the factors which explains why *A. duodenale* is not confined to tropical

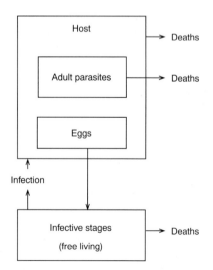

Fig. 29.3   Life history pattern of soil-transmitted nematodes.

and subtropical countries is the ability of its eggs to survive at 7°C even if embryonation is not occurring (Beaver and Jung 1985). Hookworms flourish particularly in rural communities where there are long-established traditions of the daily use of defaecation fields. The rhabditiform larvae feed on bacteria and organic debris, moult and continue to feed as second stage larvae. These moult in turn to form third stage filariform larvae, which no longer feed, but wait for the conditions facilitating skin contact and penetration. Hookworm larvae which fail to make contact with a susceptible host probably die from desiccation within a few days. According to Schad, even under the most favourable survival conditions of shade, moisture and soil texture, probably less than 1% of a batch of infective larvae will live for more than a month (see Banwell and Schad 1978).

Skin penetration by hookworms has been studied in most detail using a hamster-adapted strain of *N. americanus*. Based on earlier work which showed that larval enzymes were involved (Matthews 1982), Salafsky, Fusco and Siddiqui (1990) developed an artificial membrane which the larvae would attack and penetrate. They found that the presence of human essential fatty acids in the membrane significantly increased the ability of the larvae to penetrate in vitro and that these acids, especially linoleate, influenced the secretion of eicosanoid compounds by the larvae. Eicosanoids affect T cells and B cells and so may modulate the host's immune response during skin penetration (Salafsky, Fusco and Siddiqui 1990).

Hoagland and Schad (1978) took the view that *N. americanus* was less of an opportunist than *A. duodenale* with less flexibility in the infection process. *Ancylostoma duodenale* can function as a food-borne infection (Schad, Nawalinski and Kochar, 1983).

5.3 *Trichuris trichiura*

The transmission and establishment of an infection of *T. trichiura* has much in common with that of *A. lumbricoides*, being dependent on the ingestion of an infective egg from a contaminated environment. The overall success of the process depends on the numbers of infective eggs, their accessibility to humans and their survival characteristics, these being related to climatic and soil conditions (see Bundy and Cooper 1989).

6 SOIL-TRANSMITTED NEMATODES: EPIDEMIOLOGY AND POPULATION BIOLOGY

Knowledge of the epidemiology and population biology of soil-transmitted nematodes has advanced rapidly during the last decade. Recognition of the need to quantify the public health significance of the infections together with the development of a mathematical approach to study how these infections survive have given impetus to this work. The theoretical aspects of the population biology of the helminths have also led to the development of models (1) for

the control of soil-transmitted helminth infections by means of chemotherapy (Anderson 1989), (2) for evaluating the effects of control measures (Medley, Guyatt and Bundy 1993), (3) for estimating the morbidity attributable to the infections (Guyatt and Bundy 1991, Lwambo, Bundy and Medley 1992, Chan et al. 1994) and (4) for simulating host immune responses (Anderson 1994). Some workers have expressed concern about the lack of validation of some of the models and the fact that they are generally based on limited data (Hoffman 1994). This view does, however, not detract from their value in helping to understand the relationships between humans, roundworms, hookworms and whipworms.

The 4 common species of soil-transmitted nematode are particularly amenable to study and the following epidemiological generalizations apply: (1) Accurate diagnosis can be made by the detection of eggs in the stools. (2) Counts of eggs in defined quantities of stool can give a useful comparative indirect measure of the intensity of infection, assuming that the egg count increases as the number of female worms in the gut increases. (3) In practice, density-dependent constraints apply to the individual fecundity of female worms; after a certain worm burden has been reached, individual egg production will decline. (4) The life histories are direct and the population of worms in a host does not increase unless new infective stages are acquired. (5) The distribution of numbers of worms per host is overdispersed or aggregated so that in a given population of hosts a few will tend to harbour most of the worms. (6) Individual hosts appear to be predisposed to a particular infection intensity.

Detailed treatments of the principles underlying the epidemiology and population biology of soil-transmitted nematodes are documented and developed by Bundy (1986, 1988), Anderson and May (1985, 1991) and Scott and Smith (1994). Perhaps Croll and Ghadirian's (1981) research on 'wormy persons', which dealt with infections on *A. lumbricoides*, *A. duodenale*, *N. americanus* and *T. trichiura* was the catalyst for much of the endeavour which has been applied to understanding soil-transmitted nematodes. In this section of this chapter, the 4 species are treated together since their population biology has so much in common and they often occur together in the same community or individual.

6.1 Global distribution and abundance

Crompton (1989) reckoned that human infections with *A. lumbricoides* were occurring in 150 of the world's countries; some national situations were trivial but others were probably of considerable public health significance. The same global pattern of infection probably applies to the hookworms and to *T. trichiura*. Of the hookworms, *N. americanus* prevails in tropical and subtropical regions whereas *A. duodenale* tends to occur in the cooler and somewhat drier regions (Pawlowski, Schad and Stott 1991). Mixed infections of hookworms also exist especially in northern India and the middle of China. Bundy and Cooper (1989) pointed out that while *T. trichiura* overlaps with *A. lumbricoides* in its distribution, it is also still a problem in some temperate countries. Estimates of the numbers of cases of infection with the 4 species of soil-transmitted helminth are given in Table 29.1. Overall, at least a fifth of the world's population is infected. The recent collaboration of scientists between China and other countries has enabled new estimates to be made of the numbers of cases of *A. lumbricoides* in that country. Chan et al. (1994) estimated 568 million cases and Peng, Zhou and Crompton (1995) have calculated the number to be 538 million, indicating that the national prevalence of *A. lumbricoides* infection in China is about 47%. A national prevalence figure, however, belies the fact that infections like *A. lumbricoides* in humans are not distributed evenly between communities (Crompton 1989, Yu 1994, Peng, Zhou and Crompton 1995). Climate, local economies, social customs and ethnicity influence the distribution.

6.2   Prevalence

The results of surveys to estimate the prevalence of these infections are of limited usefulness. They identify locations where infections occur and provide information about the numbers of cases; they contribute little to assessments of the extent of morbidity. Apart from providing information about the number of cases, the most useful aspect of prevalence data is to examine the relationship between prevalence and host age. Typical patterns are shown diagrammatically for *A. lumbricoides*, hookworm and *T. trichiura* (Fig 29.4). These relationships have been detected in many surveys carried out in many countries (Bundy and Cooper 1989, Anderson and May 1991, Crompton 1994). The data are generally obtained by examining stool samples for the presence of helminth eggs, the stools having been obtained during cross-sectional surveys. The conduct of a survey is often complex and the reader is recommended to consult the protocol described by Thein Hlaing (1989).

The relationship between prevalence and age reveals that *A. lumbricoides* and *T. trichiura* become established in infants, soon after weaning (Fig 29.4a,c). Maximum prevalence values are attained in most cases when children reach the age of 10 and then a gradual decline with age is observed. The age–prevalence pattern is somewhat different in the case of hookworm infections, there being a more gradual rise in the number of cases with plateau values being observed as people reach young adulthood (Fig 29.4b).

6.3   Intensity

The population biology and public health significance of soil-transmitted nematodes cannot be understood and strategies for their control cannot be developed without reliable information about the intensities of infection. Intensity in this context is defined as the number of worms per infected host and it can be measured directly by counting worms expelled with stools

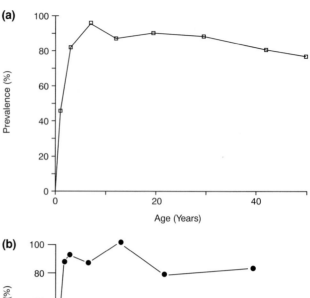

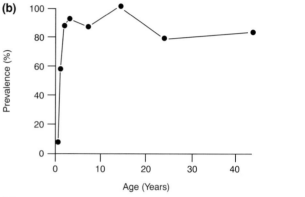

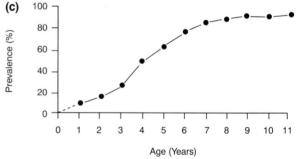

Fig. 29.4   Diagrammatic representations of the age–prevalence pattern between human hosts and soil-transmitted nematodes: (a) *Ascaris lumbricoides*; (b) *Trichuris trichiura*; (c) hookworm. Redrawn from (a) Elkins et al. (1985); (b) Bundy (1986); (c) Nawalinski et al (1978).

after anthelmintic chemotherapy or indirectly by counting eggs in known amounts of stool.

Provided there is good compliance, expulsion chemotherapy is the preferred method for measuring intensity, but it relies on highly effective anthelmintic drugs. Ideally all the worms present in the host's intestine should be expelled within 24 h so that relatively few stools have to be examined. This is generally the case for *A. lumbricoides*. Hookworms and *T. trichiura* being much smaller than *A. lumbricoides* are much harder to find in the stools. Furthermore, more than one dose of drug and more than one stool collection may be required to release and recover all the *T. trichiura* from the large intestine (Bundy and Cooper 1989). Although quantitative egg counts are much easier to perform and many more subjects can be investigated in an intensity survey as a result, the information is inevitably less accurate than that obtained from the expulsion method. Egg counts may fail to give information about intensity if the infection consists of male or immature worms only or if there are density dependent constraints on female worm fecundity (Thein Hlaing et al. 1984). Generally, egg counts using the Kato Katz method (WHO 1994) do provide a useful estimate of intensity with the number of eggs per gram of stool being observed to increase as the worm burden increases (Forrester and Scott 1990).

The typical relationship between infection intensity and host age is shown diagrammatically in Figs 29.5 for *A. lumbricoides*, hookworms and *T. trichiura*. During childhood, the age–intensity profile for *A. lumbricoides* and *T. trichiura* mirrors that for the age–prevalence profile, there being a rapid acquisition of worms. In later life, the intensity of these 2 species declines (Fig. 29.5a,c); due to the development of some degree of immunity, to changes in behaviour or to a combination of these factors. The intensity of hookworm infections follows the same trend as the age–prevalence relationships (Fig 29.5b) with adults tending to carry the greater worm burdens. These age–intensity relationships determine which sections of the population will be most at risk of morbidity, which will be responsible for most contamination of the environment with transmission stages and which will be most in need of treatment if resources become available.

6.4 Frequency distribution of numbers of worm per host

Prevalence and intensity data reveal that soil-transmitted nematodes are not distributed randomly in host populations; most infected hosts harbour a few worms each while a few hosts harbour most of the worms (Anderson 1986, Bundy 1986, Crompton 1994). The observed pattern (Fig 29.6) is best described by the negative binomial distribution and the worms are said to be aggregated or overdispersed. When the negative binomial model is fitted to worm frequency distribution data the aggregation constant (k) is usually found to be <1, indicating aggregation (Anderson 1986). Similarly if the ratio of the variance to mean number of worms in the population under study ($S^2/\bar{x}$) is >1, aggregation or overdispersion is also confirmed (Anderson and Gordon 1982).

6.5 Predisposition to intensity of infection

Predisposition, in the context of soil-transmitted nematodes, is the term used to describe the observation that after anthelmintic chemotherapy, individuals seem to acquire worm burdens similar to those they harboured before treatment. The observation appears to be secure whether expelled numbers of worms or egg counts are used as measures of intensity.

Predisposition was recognized by Schad and Anderson (1985) during a study of hookworm populations in West Bengal in 1968 to 1970. They found statisti-

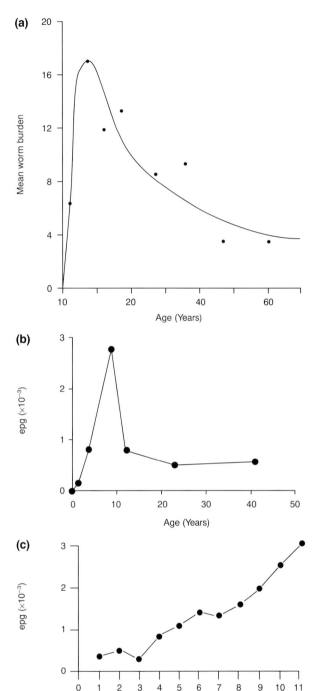

Fig. 29.5 Diagrammatic representations of the age–intensity patterns between human hosts and soil-transmitted nematodes: (a) *Ascaris lumbricoides*; (b) *Trichuris trichiura*; (c) hookworm. Redrawn from (a) Thein-Hlang (1985); (b) Bundy (1986); (c) Schad and Anderson (1985)

cally significant positive associations in individual pre- and post-treatment levels of infection intensity. Reinfections occurred rapidly after treatment and people who were heavily infected initially were found to reacquire significantly heavier than average infections (p <0.001). It is equally interesting to note that in the case of infection with *A. lumbricoides*, some individuals

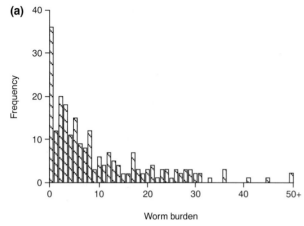

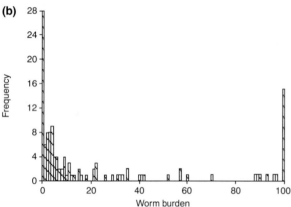

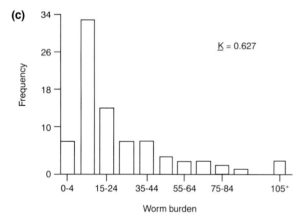

Fig. 29.6 Diagrammatic representations of the frequency distribution of numbers of worms per host: (a) *Ascaris lumbricoides*; (b) *Trichuris trichiura*; (c) hookworm. Redrawn from (a) Elkins et al. (1985); (b) Bundy (1986); (c) Schad and Anderson (1985).

appear to be predisposed not to acquire an infection despite being exposed to as many infective stages as those who do (Holland et al. 1989).

Predisposition is now accepted as a normal feature of the host–parasite relationship between humans and *A. lumbricoides*, hookworms and *T. trichiura*. It has been observed for *A.lumbricoides* in India (Haswell-Elkins, Elkins and Anderson 1987), Myanmar (Thein Hlaing, Than Saw and Myint Lwin 1987), Nigeria (Holland et al. 1989) and Malaysia (Chan, Kan and Bundy 1992).

It has been studied for *T. trichiura* by Bundy (1986), Haswell-Elkins, Elkins and Anderson (1987) and Chan, Kan and Bundy (1992) and has been demonstrated for *A. lumbricoides* and *T. trichiura* together in a community in Thailand (Upatham et al. 1992). Predisposition is not likely to arise by chance; genetic, ecological and behavioural factors probably control the process (see Keymer and Pagel 1990). That individuals may be predisposed not to acquire infections despite as much exposure as those who do (Holland et al. 1992) indicates a strong host influence in the process.

7 SOIL-TRANSMITTED NEMATODES: CLINICAL MANIFESTATIONS, MORTALITY AND MORBIDITY

Many of the millions of people infected with soil-transmitted nematodes may show no signs or symptoms of any ill health. Clinical problems are generally related to the intensity of infection and so only the relatively few hosts who carry the heavy worm burdens will be expected to be ill. Nevertheless diseased individuals will not be numerically rare (Bundy and Cooper 1989). Chan et al. (1994) have estimated that there may be 120–215 million cases of morbidity due to *A. lumbricoides*, 90–130 due to hookworm and 60–100 million due to *T. trichiura*.

The difficulties encountered in estimating morbidity rates include: (1) the problem of deciding what constitutes a clinical case (see Pawlowski 1982); (2) the possibility that the infections exacerbate existing problems rather than cause them; and (3) the scarcity of accurate records and reporting, particularly in the regions where the infections are highly endemic. In such regions, growth stunting should be considered as a feature of chronic ascariasis, hookworm disease and trichuriasis, iron deficiency anaemia as a feature of hookworm disease and sometimes of trichuriasis, and rectal prolapse and chronic dysentery as features of trichuriasis. These conditions, the mechanisms by which they arise and the related pathology have been summarized by Miller (1978), Holland (1987a,b), Stephenson (1987), Bundy and Cooper (1989) and Tomkins and Watson (1989). The impact of each infection invariably has its main effect on a different section of the population and the threshold burden responsible for causing disease may vary depending on local conditions.

Mortality rates are even more difficult to estimate although people regularly die as a result of soil-transmitted nematode infections. Pawlowski and Davies (1989) considered that perhaps 100 000 people die annually from ascariasis and Pawlowski, Schad and Scott (1991) suggested that 60 000 die from hookworm disease.

7.1 Ascariasis

The illness associated with *A. lumbricoides* infection occurs in acute and chronic forms (Table 29.4). The acute forms may arise either from the larval migration through the lungs, from allergic responses or from complications involving the adult worms.

Larval migration leading to acute pulmonary ascariasis is associated with fever, skin rash, pneumonitis, substernal pain and eosinophilia (Stephenson 1987). The problem appears to be more serious in regions like Saudi Arabia where climatic conditions ensure that *A. lumbricoides* is transmitted seasonally (Gelphi and Mustafa 1967). Stephenson pointed out that larval *A. lumbricoides* will remain as associated with respiratory complications rather than being identified as a causative agent. However, the deliberate self-infection

by Koino (1922) and the malicious contamination of a festive meal with infective eggs of *A. suum* described by Warren (1972) indicate that the larval stages initiate acute pulmonary disease.

Larval and adult *A. lumbricoides* and *A. suum* secrete allergens which elicit the production of IgE by the host leading to hypersensitivity and histamine release (Pawlowski 1982, Coles 1985). Hypersensitivity may be induced in uninfected laboratory workers studying the worms. In its most serious form, a sensitized person will collapse with bronchospasms. There is little quantitative information about the extent of this aspect of the biology of *A. lumbricoides*. In both infected and uninfected people, the presence of *Ascaris* appears to either stimulate or complicate asthma but more research is needed to clarify this problem. Experimental infections of rhesus monkeys with eggs of *A.*

Table 29.4 Features of morbidity due to ascariasis (based on Stephenson, 1987a)

Stage	Event	Clinical features	Outcome
Larval migration	Migration of larvae through liver and lungs	Pneumonitis, asthma, dyspnea, cough, substernal pain	?Decrease food intake
Maturation, oviposition	Presence of juveniles and patent adult worms in small intestine	Abdominal pain, abdominal distention, colic, nausea, vomiting, intermittent diarrhoea, anorexia, restlessness, anal itching, enterocolitis Disordered small bowel pattern, jejunal mucosal abnormalities	Decrease food intake Increase nutrient loss Malabsorption: protein malabsorption, fat malabsorption, D-xylose and lactose malabsorption, vitamin A malabsorption
Allergic reaction	Exposure to *Ascaris* allergen at any stage of life cycle[a]	Hypersensitivity reactions including asthma, conjunctivitis, facial oedema, urticaria abdominal pain, heartburn, diarrhoea	Decrease food intake Increase nutrient loss
Complications	Migration or aggregation of adult *Ascaris* in intestine	Intestinal obstruction, intussusception, volvulus Invasion of bile duct (producing obstructive jaundice, gallstones, cholangitis, or liver abscesses) Acute pancreatitis, acute appendicitis, intestinal perforation, peritonitis, upper respiratory tract obstruction.	Life-threatening illnesses which all decrease food intake and may increase nutrient requirements (due to fever) and nutrient losses (due to diarrhoea)

[a]Person need not be infected.

suum induces an IgE-mediated pathology in the lungs (Patterson and Harris 1985).

Acute ascariasis involving adults presents as a variety of obstructions and surgical complications (Table 29.5) Among children, intestinal obstruction caused by a bolus of worms appears to be the commonest problem and may lead to tissue necrosis and perforation of the intestinal wall. From the data summarized in Table 29.5, it would appear that girls suffer more intestinal obstructions than boys. Louw (1966) drew attention to the importance of *A. lumbricoides* as a cause of abdominal complications by recording that 100 (12.8%) of the 731 abdominal emergencies in children (aged 1–12 years) admitted between 1958 and 1962 to a hospital in Cape Town, South Africa, were due to *A. lumbricoides*. Of the 100 cases, 68 proved to be intestinal obstructions. Among adults, complications involving the biliary system appear to be the commonest acute complication due to *A. lumbricoides* (Table 29.5). Presumably, the adult worms migrate from small intestine up the common bile duct where they may remain or may move on to the liver or to the pancreas. It is not known why adult worms leave the intestine; in some cases larval worms may have reached unusual sites during the natural tissue migratory phase. That might explain how *A. lumbricoides* has been recovered from sites such as the middle ear (Berkowitz, Sochet and Packirisamy 1980). Details of the diagnosis and management of cases of acute ascariasis due to adult worms have been given by Pinus (1985) and Erdener et al. (1992) among others.

Chronic ascariasis (Table 29.4) has been extensively studied in children in many locations during the past 20 years (Crompton 1992, Thein Hlaing 1993). Given that the study design is adequate and there is good compliance in the study population (Crompton and Stephenson 1985), convincing circumstantial evidence can be obtained to show that infection with *A. lumbricoides* interferes with the growth and development of children, especially during the period of 2–10 years of age. This conclusion is based on a study design in which the nutritional status (height and weight for age) was compared before and after intervention with an effective anthelmintic drug. The adverse contribution of chronic ascariasis to childhood nutritional status has been demonstrated in various countries worldwide (Gupta et al. 1977, Stephenson et al. 1980, Thein Hlaing et al. 1992; see Tomkins and Watson 1989), although not every investigation has detected this effect.

Various experimental studies of ascariasis in pigs and clinical investigations of ascariasis in humans have shown that the presence of adult worms in the small intestine is associated with some degree of crypt hyperplasia and villous atrophy (Tripathy et al. 1972, Stephenson et al. 1980, Martin et al. 1984). Under certain conditions, maldigestion and malabsorption occur (Forsum, Nesheim and Crompton 1981, Carrera, Nesheim and Crompton 1984) with recovery being observed following anthelmintic treatment (Taren et al. 1987). Probably the most serious aspect of an *Ascaris* infection is a reduction in food intake, which has been well documented for *A. suum* infections in pigs (see Nesheim 1985) and has been demonstrated ·more recently by Fasli Jalal (1991) in rural children in Indonesia.

Currently, ascariasis (and hookworm disease and trichuriasis) should be considered as contributors to different degrees of childhood malnutrition. Infections with soil-transmitted nematodes have also been convincingly linked to impaired cognitive performance in young children (Nokes et al. 1992, Nokes and Bundy 1994, Simeon et al. 1994) It may be wiser to view these infections as one of the many interacting socioeconomic determinants which impair cognitive performance (see Connolly and Kvalsvig 1993).

7.2 Hookworm disease

Not all the people infected with hookworms suffer from iron deficiency anaemia, but many do and many of them are at risk because the intestinal stages feed on blood and cause a loss of blood into the intestinal lumen (Roche and Layrisse 1966). Anaemia is defined as a reduction in blood haemoglobin concentration below expected values for age and sex (WHO 1972). In physiological terms, in an anaemic individual, the circulating number of red blood cells becomes insufficient to meet the oxygen needs of the body and the symptoms of a severe hookworm infection mimic those of anaemia: breathlessness, lassitude, headache, palpitations, apathy and depression. Often occult

Table 29.5 Complications of acute ascariasis related to adult *Ascaris lumbricoides* in relation to patient age and gender (Crompton, 1994)

	Age			Gender		Deaths	
	All cases	**Child**	**Adult**	**Male**	**Female**	**Child**	**Adult**
Biliary system	1124	380	374	92	117	4	23
Gastrointestinal tract	3408	2149	73	572	716	85	9
Hepatic abscess	100	52	6	17	15	13	1
Pancreatitis	67	28	26	11	15	1	2
Miscellaneous complications	94	77	15	50	41	9	3
Totals	4793	2686	494	742	964	112	38

The cases recorded in this table were abstracted from 230 reports published between 1971 and 1992.
The cases described were from 54 countries. Often reports were found to be incomplete, with no information given about the age or gender of the patients.

blood is found in the stools (Holland 1987a). Studies from many countries including India, Kenya, Thailand and Venezuela have detected the relationship depicted in Fig 29.7 (Hill and Andrews 1942). Blood haemoglobin concentration in adults is observed to fall in a non-linear manner in relation to increasing hookworm infection intensity. A values of 100 mg/ml in an adult is judged to indicate anaemia (WHO 1972).

Whether anaemia develops or not during the course of a hookworm infection depends not only on the intensity of the infection and species of hookworm (*A. duodenale* takes more blood than *N. americanus*), but also on the iron status and physiological needs of the host, the quality and quantity of the daily iron intake and the bioavailability of the iron for absorption from the small intestine. This complex relationship has been discussed in detail by Holland (1987a), Crompton and Stephenson, (1990) and Crompton and Whitehead (1993). Maintaining the required number of circulating red blood cells probably has a high priority for iron metabolism, so hookworm-infected individuals who are not clinically anaemic may have a deteriorating iron status and latent iron deficiency. Measurements of plasma ferritin concentration, transferrin saturation and erythrocyte protoporphyin would probably indicate that clinically non-anaemic individuals with hookworm infections are under iron stress, as has been demonstrated by Mansour, Francis and Farid (1985) for people suffering from schistosomiasis mansoni.

Since many features of hookworm disease indicate iron deficiency anaemia, it is to be expected that women and girls of child-bearing age, pregnant women and people engaged in heavy manual labour will be most at risk from the adverse effects of infec-

tion. On average, menstruating females lose about 1.5 mg iron per day, about the same amount as is absorbed from the gut under optimal conditions (Crompton and Whitehead 1993). Although there is no menstrual loss (0.7 mg iron per day) during pregnancy and lactation, the mother must meet all the iron requirements of the developing fetus and the suckling infant. H Torlesse (personal communication 1994) has recently estimated that at any given time about 30 million are currently pregnant and infected with hookworm. Many of these people must be experiencing acute anaemia exacerbated by the demands of pregnancy and the blood loss due to hookworms. The birth of underweight children is a major consequence of anaemia during pregnancy, and in developing countries the deaths of about 200 000 women can be ascribed to anaemia as a complication of childbirth or the early postpartum period (Viteri 1994). As many as 1 in 25 pregnant women die in some developing countries due to complications associated with the pregnancy and birth (WHO 1995).

Worker productivity in relation to anaemia has attracted considerable research attention. Study designs have sought to examine the cost:benefit ratios in financial terms of expenditure to relieve anaemia (iron supplements and antiparasite drugs) compared with the increased revenue from increased productivity by the non-anaemic workers. The results have shown that anaemic sugar cane cutters (Viteri and Torun 1974), road builders (Brookes, Latham and Crompton 1979, Wolgemuth et al. 1982), rubber tappers (Basta, Soekirman and Scrimshaw 1979) and tea pickers (Gardner et al. 1977) do not have the same work output as either non-anaemic controls or those given treatment to relieve the anaemia. Vigorous physical work is difficult to carry out and sustain once blood haemoglobin concentration has fallen to a value of 7 mg/ml (see Fig. 29.7). In developing countries, where productivity depends largely on manual labour, widespread hookworm infections may make a substantial contribution to the depressed economies of some countries (Holland 1987a).

Iron deficiency anaemia is a factor which reduces cognitive performance; on measures of achievement at school, anaemic children usually show lower scores than non-anaemic counterparts (see Connolly and Kvalsvig 1993). According to Pollitt (1990) there is sufficient evidence to conclude that iron deficiency anaemia is linked to impaired educational performance. Again hookworm infections, with their contribution to iron loss, must contribute to this problem. It should be noted that reduced appetite and loss of nutrients including zinc (Migasena et al. 1984) through plasma leakage into the gut, together with malabsorption, which also occurs in some cases, are likely to affect school performance as well as growth (Holland 1987a) and physical fitness (Stephenson et al. 1993).

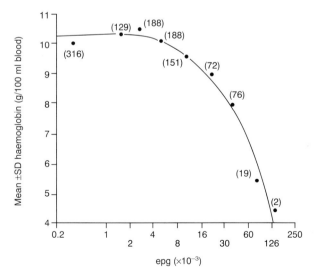

Fig. 29.7 The relationship between declining blood haemoglobin concentration and increasing hookworm intensity, expressed as egg-count classes, obtained from a study of 1141 residents of South Georgia, USA. The egg counts have been corrected to a formed-stool basis. (Data from Hill and Andrews 1942.)

7.3 Trichuriasis

The pathology of an infection with *T. trichiura* involves chronic inflammation of the mucosa of the large intestine associated with the intimate contact that the worms make with the mucosa. The degree of inflammation may extend from the distal part of the small intestine to the rectum depending on the intensity of the infection (Bundy and Cooper 1989). Since the infection is confined largely to the large intestine, malabsorption of digestion products is not likely to be a serious consequence. However, the lacerations caused by the feeding activities of the worms may enable secondary bacterial infections to become established. Secondary bacterial establishment has been demonstrated in experimental infections of *T. suis* in pigs (Hall, Rutter and Beer 1976) which developed dysentery. It is frequently observed that children with heavy infections of *T. trichiura* often suffer from chronic dysentery (see Holland 1987b).

Rectal prolapse is the most striking lesion associated with trichuriasis. Apparently, the surface tissue of the rectum becomes extremely oedematous and the prolapsing occurs as the patient strains to defecate. Bundy and Cooper (1989) suggests that the mechanism of the prolapse is similar to that intussusception and that remission often occurs within a few days of effective anthelmintic chemotherapy.

Rectal bleeding occurs during trichuriasis (Fisher and Cremin 1970, Lotero, Tripathy and Bolanos 1974) and this has prompted a vigorous debate about the contribution of the worms to the development of iron deficiency anaemia. Infected people undoubtedly lose blood during an infection from both the feeding activities of the worms and the extensive damage to the mucosa of the large intestine. Iron lost into the gut lumen from this tissue would essentially represent a net loss to the host. After a critical review of an extensive literature, Holland (1987b) and Bundy and Cooper (1989) independently concluded that trichuriasis contributed significantly to iron deficiency anaemia. Recently, Ramdath et al. (1995) compared the blood picture of 264 *Trichuris*-infected children with that of 157 matched, uninfected children. Children judged to have heavy infections (> 10 000 eggs/g) had significantly lower ($p < 0.05$) blood haemoglobin concentrations and mean cell volumes than uninfected children or those with lower infection intensities. Also 33% of the heavily infected children were diagnosed as anaemic compared with 11% of the rest of those in the study.

Several studies have shown that trichuriasis, like ascariasis and often in combination with it, is a factor involved in growth-stunting in children (Bowie et al. 1978, Holland 1987b; Simeon et al. 1994). For example, Gilman et al. (1983) found that the nutritional status of children increased significantly following anthelmintic expulsion of *T. trichiura* ($p < 0.05$). The children in this study who were judged to be heavily infected also showed blood in their stools and some degree of anaemia and dysentery. Twelve percent of the children presented with finger clubbing; this lesion is a curious thickening at the ends of the fingers and toes and is associated with other illnesses besides trichuriasis. In a cross-sectional survey of 260 children in St Lucia, Cooper and Bundy (1986) found a strong association between measures of impaired rates of growth and infection intensities greater than 20 000 epg. More recently, Cooper et al. (1990) have linked the observed growth depression in children with heavy infections to the dysentery syndrome which is a feature of trichuriasis. Nineteen Jamaican children, ranging in age from 2 to 10 years and known to be suffering from heavy *T. trichiura* infections, were studied. Nutritional status was assessed and blood haemoglobin concentrations ($\bar{x} = 7.0 \pm 2.5$ mg/ml) measured. The growth rates of 11 of these children were calculated, following anthelmintic treatment, for a period of 6 months, and a remarkable rate of catch-up growth was detected despite the absence of any food supplementation other than the provision of oral ferrous sulfate to correct the iron-deficiency anaemia. Cooper et al. (1990) proposed that the chronic inflammation of the large intestine which persists during *T. trichiura* infections was in some way linked to the growth deficits detected in these heavily infected children.

8   SOIL-TRANSMITTED NEMATODES: IMMUNITY

Extensive experimental work has contributed greatly to our understanding of host immune responses, both protective and allergic, to intestinal nematode infections in mammalian hosts. Studies have been carried out with rats and *Nippostrongylus brasiliensis*, with rats and mice and *Trichinella spiralis* and with mice and *Heligmosomoides polygyrus* and *Trichuris muris*. A full introduction to the relevant literature has been compiled by Behnke (1990). Although laboratory strains of hosts and helminths have been involved in this work and the use of host strains has been crucial to identifying genetic aspects of immune responses (Wakelin 1978), we can be confident of the significance of the results because, as Holland (1983) described for wild rats and *N. brasiliensis*, natural infections do occur. Knowledge of human immune responses to *A. lumbricoides*, *Anc. duodenale*, *N. americanus* and *T. trichiura* is somewhat diffuse, often being based on either interpretations of epidemiological data or extrapolation of results from closely related host–parasite relationships.

The species of worms in question fall into Anderson and May's (1979) category of macroparasites which rarely elicit protective immunity in their hosts, even after numerous exposures. When strong immunity does develop, it is likely to decline unless further exposure occurs. The response to parasite antigens is likely, through hypersensitivity, to damage the host as much as the parasite. There is, however, strong circumstantial evidence to show that protective host immune responses operate, albeit in a heterogeneous manner, during an intestinal nematode infection. How can the observed overdispersed frequency distribution of numbers of worms per host be explained without recourse to the host immune response (Fig 29.6; Crompton, Keymer and Arnold 1984)? How can the decline in intensity of *A. lumbricoides* infection with host age (Fig 29.5a) be fully explained unless some immunity develops? How can predisposition to a particular intensity of infection be explained without predicting a role for the immune response (Keymer and Pagel 1990, Holland et al. 1992)? Having reviewed much experimental work, Wakelin (1988) concluded, 10 years after his seminal review of the genetic control of susceptibility and resistance to infection (Wakelin 1978), that it seems reasonable to conclude that humans show distinct genetic differences in ability to respond to and resist infections with gastrointestinal nematodes.

Difficulties are encountered in studying human immune responses to soil-transmitted nematodes for a variety of reasons. First, the worms are remarkably host specific; there are no convenient laboratory hosts such as rats or mice which will sustain the life history in an appropriate time frame. Even if such hosts did exist, extrapolation of results would be risky. There are some closely related infections from which useful results may be obtained even though the problem of extrapolation remains. *Ascaris lumbricoides*, *A. suum*, *T. trichiura* and *T. suis* will develop in non-human primates and in pigs. *Ancylostoma caninum*, which is closely related to *Anc. duodenale*, develops naturally in dogs. Although results on how *Anc. caninum* feeds (see section 3.2) may reasonably be applied to how *A. duodenale* feeds, it seems imprudent to assume that the immunology of the 2 host–parasite relationships will be the same. Work with non-human primates, pigs and dogs is expensive and is always open to public concern and criticism.

The 4 species of nematode elicit antibody responses of which an increase in helminth species-specific IgE and a potentiation of non-specific IgE are features (Wakelin, Harnett and Parkhouse 1993). In the case of *A. lumbricoides*, IgE increase would account for much of the observed hypersensitivity including mast cell degranulation, transient urticaria and respiratory problems (Coles 1985). Recently, Kennedy and colleagues have isolated and characterized from both *A. lumbricoides* and *A. suum* an allergenic molecule (ABA-1) with a molecular weight of 14 kDa (Kennedy and Qureshi 1986, Kennedy et al. 1986). Interestingly, Tomlinson et al. (1989) discovered that in mice there is MHC-associated genetic control of IgE recognition of ABA-1 and then Kennedy et al. (1990) found considerable variation between the degree of recognition of individual humans to the same molecule.

A balance perhaps exists between the degree of protection and the amount of hypersensitivity elicited by exposure to the mixture of immunogens and allergens released during the course of an *A. lumbricoides* infection. Experiments some years ago demonstrated that pigs develop some immunity to *A. suum* (Taffs 1968). Although many epidemiological patterns cannot be explained without invoking an immunological component, some results remain perplexing. Recently, Palmer et al. (1995) measured the antibody responses of a group of Bangledeshi children to antigens prepared from adult and larval *A. lumbricoides*. The children came from an area where the infection was highly endemic and their worm burdens had been measured on 4 occasions by expulsion chemotherapy. Children with repeated heavy infections generally had higher concentrations of antibody isotypes to antigens of *A. lumbricoides*, as assessed by ELISA, than did children with lighter burdens. The isotypes IgG1, IgG4 and IgE occurred in significantly higher concentrations in the heavily infected children. Palmer et al. (1995) concluded that these responses, when related to worm burdens which averaged 39, 45, 26 and 30 over the 4 rounds of treatment in the heavily infected children compared with 7, 6, 6 and 12 in others, played no major part in protecting against heavy infections. However, perhaps without these responses, worm burdens would have been even higher and hosts and parasites could have perished together.

There is good evidence of the development in dogs of solid protective immunity to the hookworm *Anc. caninum* and a canine hookworm vaccine became available for a period (Miller 1978). Miller was convinced, from the available epidemiological data and from experimenting on himself, that immunity in human–hookworm infections would be similar to that elucidated for dogs and *A. caninum* (Miller 1979). However, hookworm infections of humans, especially with *N. americanus*, are comparatively long lasting, suggesting that the parasites may be able to interfere with the potentially protective host response.

As with *A. lumbricoides*, the immune response to *T. trichiura* is likely to be heterogeneous, not fully protective and a contributing factor to the complex pathology described by Bundy and Cooper (1989). The reader is directed to volumes compiled and edited by Wakelin and Blackwell (1988) and Behnke (1990) for a full introduction to host–helminth immunological interactions.

9 SOIL-TRANSMITTED NEMATODES: DIAGNOSIS

For epidemiological surveys, operational research programmes and control activities, the diagnosis of soil-transmitted nematode infections continues to rely on the collection and examination of stool samples for helminth eggs or larvae (Fig 29.1) and the method to be used depends on the purpose of the study or survey (Thein Hlaing 1989). A useful summary of those available is given by Theinpont, Rochette and Vanparijs (1986). The procedure now recommended by the World Health Organization (WHO 1994) is that known universally as the Kato Katz method which gives reliable information about infection intensities. Despite the efforts to develop serological tests to aid diagnosis and techniques to detect antigens and metabolites in faeces, coprological examination remains the method best suited to the resources and skills available in developing countries where the infections are endemic (Wakelin, Harnett and Parkhouse 1993).

In modern hospitals and clinics, other diagnostic

techniques are available, but not for mass application. For example, in the case of acute ascariasis, real-time ultrasound (Cremlin 1982), radiography (Choudhuri, Saha and Tandon 1986) and endoscopic retrograde cholangiopancreatography (Khan, Raj and Visvanathan 1993) are regularly employed. Fibre optics may be used; Cooper and Bundy (1987) describe the use of a flexible fibre optic colonoscope to study infections of *T. trichiura*.

10 SOIL-TRANSMITTED NEMATODES: PROSPECTS OF PREVENTION AND CONTROL

Every public health expert would agree with Evans and Stephenson (1995) that a significant reduction in disease due to soil-transmitted intestinal nematodes will not occur until poverty is reduced and living conditions, sanitation and water supplies have improved. There are, however, compelling reasons for targeting anthelmintic treatment against particular groups in communities where the infections are highly endemic (Savioli, Bundy and Tomkins 1992). Children attending primary schools offer the most convenient group for the application of this control measure for the following reasons: (1) Epidemiological surveys and computer simulations of models of the population dynamics of *A. lubricoides* and *T. trichiura* indicate that children of this age group are more heavily infected than adults (see Anderson and May 1991). They are also acquiring hookworms, although these infections tend to be relatively less common in urban than rural communities (Crompton and Savioli 1993). (2) High quality, effective, safety-tested anthelmintic drugs are now available (WHO 1987) and guidance for their use in the community is available (Fig. 29.8; Anderson 1989). (3) Schools serve as a gathering point for drug delivery and administration, which can be undertaken by school teachers, and schools are the focus of education in the community so that health education can

be reinforced. (4) Most importantly, the children suffer much of the morbidity as well as impairments to their growth and general development (Evans and Stephenson 1995). Targeted treatment is directed at reducing the intensity of infection in the community, not seeking eradication.

Whether control measures are adopted or not depends on the needs and resources of the people involved. Where governments have taken action based on political decisions as in Japan, Israel and South Korea, there has been marked success in reducing the occurrence of ascariasis (see Crompton, Nesheim and Pawlowski 1985, 1989). It is not appropriate, however, for the staff of agencies based away from areas of high endemicity to argue that control programmes must be established. That decision can only be made by the authorities in charge of the resources which are usually extremely meagre and insufficient for the range of problems needing health care. The World Health Organization has now advised that children need treatment to relieve them from the effects of intestinal helminth infections (Tomkins and Watson 1989), but this advice is given knowing that such measures as may be adopted will need to fit into the prevailing system of primary health care.

We may write about the need to adopt affordable and sustainable measures to control intestinal nematode infections. What does this mean, and can it be brought about? In many systems of primary health care, local communities, on the basis of the best information available to them and with consideration of their own real and perceived needs, must decide on priorities. The available actions may be minimal; modern drugs may be available, traditional medicines may be employed, education may be strengthened. Perhaps communities may be advised to integrate anti-worm actions with other forms of health care as has successfully been done with family planning and nutrition programmes by the Japanese Organization for International Co-operation in Family Planning

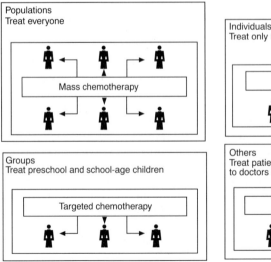
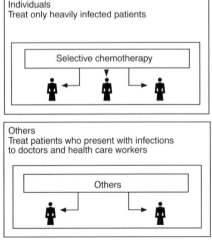

Fig. 29.8 Proposals for the use of anthelmintic drugs. (Based on Anderson 1989 and Crompton 1991).

(Kunii 1983). A wide range of control strategies is now available (WHO 1987, Crompton, Nesheim and Pawlowski 1989, Savioli, Bundy and Tomkins 1992) and some progress against intestinal worms can be made if local people can be helped to organize and control their community health affairs.

11 ENTEROBIUS: BIOLOGY, TRANSMISSION AND EPIDEMIOLOGY

11.1 Biology

Infection occurs as a result of ingesting fully developed. infective eggs. After hatching in the small bowel subsequent development takes place entirely within the intestine, there being no systemic migration similar to that undertaken by *Ascaris*, and worms mature within about 5 weeks. The adults are found primarily in the large bowel, lying closely applied to the mucosal surface. On the basis of studies made with rodent pinworm it can be assumed that the worms feed on material present in the lumen and possibly on the cellular debris that accumulates on the epithelium and in the crypts. The worms are mobile and move within the large bowel, the females also migrate down the rectum to the anus at night to release eggs. Males live for some 7 weeks, females 5–13 weeks (Cook 1995).

Unlike the soil-transmitted species considered above, the eggs of *Enterobius* are not released into the intestinal lumen, but are released on the perianal skin after the females have migrated to the anal region. Hence diagnosis of pinworm infection cannot be made reliably through faecal smears or similar techniques. Egg release occurs through the female reproductive opening or when the worm dies and disintegrates on the surface of the skin, each female releasing an estimated 10 000 eggs (Faust, Russell and Jung 1970). Movement to the anal region causes local irritation and itching. When laid the eggs already contain immature larvae and these complete development very rapidly, maturing within 6 h at body temperature (Cook 1995). The eggs are 'sticky' and readily adhere, but, being light, are also easily dispersed. If the local environmental conditions are not too dry they can survive for considerable periods.

11.2 Transmission

The characteristics of the eggs, and the way in which they are released from females favours several routes of transmission. In children, the itching associated with the presence of female worms on the perianal skin prompts scratching, as a result of which eggs adhere to the hands and fingers, from where they are easily transferred to the mouth. Contamination of nightclothes or bedding can also result in eggs being transferred to the hands. The lightness of the eggs results in a wide dispersal in bedrooms and houses, and accidental transmission to other family members can occur from these sources. In one school, counts of eggs present on the wall of the lavatory showed some 5000 per square foot (0.093 m^2) (BMJ, 1974). Eggs can become airborne when clothes, bedding or dust are disturbed. They may then contaminate food or the hands of people in the vicinity, but it has also been suggested that airborne eggs can be inhaled and then swallowed.

11.3 Epidemiology

Pinworm infections are most frequent in school age children, but can occur in any age group. They are the commonest worm parasites in temperate, developed countries, where prevalence figures in young children can reach 80–90%, but infections are distributed globally, and *Enterobius* often accompanies the soil-transmitted nematodes in the warmer, less developed parts of the world (reviewed by Haswell-Elkins *et al.* 1987). Data on prevalence can be misleading, as some figures have been based on detection of eggs in stool samples, which frequently fails to detect infections. Haswell-Elkins *et al.* (1987) determined prevalence in an Indian village by recovering worms after chemotherapy and recorded overall figures of 70.8% (74.3% in males, 67.5% in females) with a mean intensity of 25.8 worms. By the age of 4 years 60% of children were infected. Eleven months after initial treatment the population was sampled again, when prevalence and intensity were found to be significantly higher (87.1% and 40.2 worms). Infections were markedly aggregated in the host population: for example, in the second study the heaviest infection recorded was 2152 worms.

12 ENTEROBIUS: CLINICAL MANIFESTATIONS

In most cases *Enterobius* infections are asymptomatic. The commonest symptom is the itching associated with movement of the female worms to the anal regions (anal and perineal pruritus), although it has been suggested that these symptoms reflect the existence of other dermatological problems (Ganor 1987). Infected children may show irritability, enuresis and weight loss. The worms normally cause only minor pathology in the intestine. Unlike the other intestinal nematodes, *Enterobius* infection is not associated with a pronounced eosinophilia. or with elevated IgE (Jarrett and Kerr 1973). In girls worms may migrate into the vagina, causing a vaginitis. Urinary infections in children have been associated with such migratory behaviour and adult women may also be affected in this way. The presence of *Enterobius* in the appendix (2.7% of 1419 appendices removed during a 5 year period in Bristol, England, Budd and Armstrong 1987; 2.5% of 2921 appendices in India, Gupta, Gupta and Keswant 1989) has suggested a link with appendicitis, but this is considered rare.

Infections can lead occasionally to more severe complications, if the worms find their way into the peritoneum, either via intestinal perforations or following migration through the female reproductive tract. Dead worms and eggs have been identified in granulomata in several sites (vagina, cervix, fallopian tubes, omentum, peritoneum, even the liver, kidneys and lungs (Cook 1995).

13 *ENTEROBIUS*: DIAGNOSIS AND CONTROL

Infection can be diagnosed directly by observing worms in the perianal region or on the surface of the stool. More commonly diagnosis requires the detection of eggs. These occur on the perianal skin and can be collected onto the surface of an adhesive transparent tape, pressed on to the skin. The tape can then be transferred to a slide, with a clearing agent (e.g. toluene, cedar oil) for microscopic examination. Such examination is best performed in the morning when the patient first wakes, and repeated examination (3–6 tests) may be necessary to ensure positive diagnosis. Commercial detection kits are available. Eggs can sometimes be found in stools, but diagnosis is very unreliable. If infection is confirmed in one individual

in a household, other family members should also be examined and treated.

Pinworms are easily removed by anthelmintic treatment. The use of piperazine compounds has been standard for many years but requires treatment daily for 7 days. Pyrantel compounds are effective in a single (10 mg/kg) dose, as are the benzimidazoles mebendazole (100 mg tablet) and albendazole (400 mg tablet). Where *Enterobius* occurs with other intestinal nematodes, use of the benzimadazoles has the additional benefit of eliminating the other species as well.

Although treament is effective, reinfection occurs readily unless steps are taken to minimize contact with infective eggs. Personal hygiene is important, particularly hand washing, fingernail cleaning and regular bathing. Infected children can be made to wear gloves in bed to prevent contamination of their hands. Heavily infected areas such as bedrooms must be kept scrupulously clean and dust free, and bed linen and night clothes should be changed and laundered frequently. In practice, elimination of eggs in this way is very difficult and to be effective these approaches must be accompanied by repeated chemotherapy to remove the adult worms.

REFERENCES

Adedeja SO, Ogunba EO, 1991, Bacterial flora of *Ascaris suum* (Goeze 1782) and its relationship to the host flora, *Trop Vet*, **9:** 123–9.

Adiyodi KG, Adiyodi RG, eds, 1983, *Reproductive Biology of Invertebrates*, (6 volumes beginning in 1983), John Wiley, Chichester.

Anderson RC, Chabaud AG, Willmott S, eds, 1974, *CIH Keys to the Nematode Parasites of Vertebrates*, Commonwealth Agricultural Bureaux, Farnham Royal, UK.

Anderson RM, 1986, The population dynamics and epidemiology of intestinal nematode infections, *Trans R Soc Trop Med Hyg*, **80:** 686–96.

Anderson RM, 1989, Transmission dynamics of *Ascaris lumbricoides* and the impact of chemotherapy, *Ascariasis and its Prevention and Control*, eds Crompton DWT, Nesheim MC, Pawlowski ZS, Taylor and Francis, London, 253–73.

Anderson RM, 1994, Mathematical studies of parasitic infection and immunity, *Science*, **264:** 1884–6.

Anderson RM, Gordon DM, 1982, Processes influencing the distribution of parasite numbers within host populations with special emphasis on parasite-induced host mortalities, *Parasitology*, **85:** 373–98.

Anderson RM, May RM, 1979, Population biology of infectious diseases: Part 1, *Nature* (London), **280:** 361–7.

Anderson RM, May RM, 1985, Helminth infections of humans: mathematical models, population dynamics, and control, *Adv Parasitol*, **24:** 1–101.

Anderson RM, May RM, 1991, *Infectious Diseases of Humans. Dynamics and Control*, Oxford University Press, Oxford.

Andrassy I, 1976, *Evolution as a Basis for the Systematization of Nematodes*, Pitman, London.

Banwell JG, Schad GA, 1978, Hookworms, *Clin Gastroenterol*, **7:** 129–56.

Barrett J, 1981, *Biochemistry of Parasitic Helminths*, Macmillan, London.

Barriga OO, 1982a, Ancylostomiasis, *CRC Handbook Series in Zoonoses Section C: Parasitic Zoonoses* , vol. II, ed Schulz MG, CRC Press, Boca Raton, FL, 3–24.

Barriga OO, 1982b, Trichuriasis, *CRC Handbook Series in Zoonoses*

Section C: Parasitic Zoonoses, vol. II, ed. Schultz MG, CRC Press, Boca Raton, FL, 339–45.

Basta SS, Soekirman KD, Scrimshaw NS, 1979, Iron deficiency anaemia and productivity of adult males in Indonesia, *Am J Clin Nutr*, **32:** 916–25.

Beaver PC, 1954, Parasitic diseases of animals and their relation to public health, *Small Anim Pract*, **49:** 199–205.

Beaver PC, 1956, Larva migrans, *Exp Parasitol*, **6:** 587–621.

Beaver PC, Jung RC, eds, 1985, *Animal Agents and Vectors of Human Disease*, 5th edn, Lea and Febiger, Philadelphia, PA.

Beck JW, Beverley-Burton M, 1968, The pathology of *Trichuris*, *Capillaria* and *Trichinella* infections, *Helminthol Abstr*, **37:** 1–26.

Behnke JM, ed, 1990, *Parasites: Immunity and Pathology*, Taylor and Francis, London.

Bell JC, Palmer SR, Payne JM, 1988, *The Zoonoses. Infections Transmitted from Animals to Man*, Edward Arnold, London.

Bennet-Clark HC, 1976, Mechanics of nematode feeding, *The Organization of Nematodes*, ed Croll NA, Academic Press, London, 313–42.

Berkowitz FE, Sochet E, Packirisamy G, 1980, *Ascaris* in the middle ear, *S Afr Med J*, **58:** 680.

Bidinger PD, Crompton DWT, Arnold SE, 1981, Aspects of intestinal parasitism in villages from rural peninsular India, *Parasitology*, **83:** 373–80.

Bird AF, Bird J, 1991, *The Structure of Nematodes*, 2nd edn, Academic Press London.

BMJ, Children's worms (Editorial), *Br Med J*, 1974, **4:** 3.

Bowie MD, Morison A et al., 1978, Clubbing and whipworm infestation, *Arch Dis Child*, **53:** 411–13.

Brooks RM, Latham MC, Crompton DWT, 1979, The relationship of nutrition and health to worker productivity in Kenya, *East Afr Med J*, **56:** 413–21.

Bryan CP, 1930, *The Papyrus Ebers*, Geoffrey Bles, London.

Budd JS, Armstrong C, 1987, Role of *Enterobius vermicularis* in the aetiology of appendicitis, *Br J Surg*, **74:** 748–9.

Bulatao RA, Bos E et al., 1990, *World Population Projections*, Johns Hopkins University Press, Baltimore, MD.

Bundy DAP, 1986, Epidemiological aspects of *Trichuris* and trichuriasis in Caribbean communities, *Trans R Soc Trop Med Hyg*, **80:** 706–18.

Bundy DAP, 1988, Population ecology of intestinal helminth infections in human communities, *Phil Trans R Soc B*, **321**: 405–20.

Bundy DAP, Cooper ES, 1989, *Trichuris* and trichuriasis in humans, *Adv Parasitol*, **28**: 107–73.

Burrows RB, Lillis WG, 1964, The whipworm as a blood sucker, *J Parasitol*, **50**: 675–80.

Carrera E, Nesheim MC, Crompton DWT, 1984, Lactose maldigestion in *Ascaris*-infected pre-school children, *Am J Clin Nutr*, **39**: 255–64.

Carroll SM, Grove DI, 1986, Experimental infections of humans with *Ancylostoma ceylanicum*: clinical, parasitological, haematological and immunological findings, *Trop Geogr Med*, **38**: 38–45.

Chan L, Kan SP, Bundy DAP, 1992, The effect of repeated chemotherapy on age-related predisposition to *Ascaris lumbricoides* and *Trichuris trichiura*, *Parasitology*, **104**: 371–7.

Chan MS, Medley GF et al., 1994, The evaluation of potential global morbidity attributable to intestinal nematode infections, *Parasitology*, **109**: 373–87.

Chitwood BG, Chitwood MB, 1974, *Introduction to Nematology*, University Park Press, Baltimore, MD.

Choudhuri G, Saha SS, Tandon RK, 1986, Gastric ascariasis, *Am J Gastroenterol*, **81**: 788–90.

Chu W-G, Pen P-M et al., 1972, Neonatal ascariasis, *J Pediatr*, **81**: 783–5.

Clutton-Brock J, 1987, *A Natural History of Domesticated Mammals*, Cambridge University Press, Cambridge; BM (NH), London.

Cockburn A, Cockburn E, eds, 1980, *Mummies, Disease and Ancient Cultures*, Cambridge University Press, Cambridge.

Coles GC, 1985, Allergy and immunopathology of ascariasis, *Ascariasis Audits Public Health Significance*, eds Crompton DWT, Nesheim MC, Pawlowsky ZS, Taylor and Francis, London, 167–84.

Connolly KJ, Kvalsvig JD, 1993, Infection, nutrition and cognitive performance in children, *Parasitology*, **107**: S187–S200.

Cook GC, 1995, *Enterobius vermicularis* infection, Enteric Infection 2. *Intestinal helminths*, eds Farthing MJG, Keusch GT, Wakelin D, Chapman & Hall, London, 213–23.

Coombs I, Crompton DWT, 1991, *A Guide to Human Helminths*, Taylor and Francis, London.

Cooper ES, Bundy DAP, 1987, Trichuriasis, *Intestinal Helminthic Infections*, ed. Pawlowski ZS, Baillière Tindall, London.

Cooper ES, Bundy DAP et al., 1990, Growth suppression in the *Trichuris* dysentery syndrome, *Eur J Clin Nutr*, **44**: 285–91.

Cremlin BJ, 1982, Real-time ultrasound in paediatric biliary ascariasis, *S Afr Med J*, **61**: 914–16.

Croese J, Loukas A et al., 1994, Occult enteric infection by *Ancylostoma caninum*: a previously unrecognized zoonosis, *Gastroenterology*, **106**: 3–12.

Croll NA, Ghadirian F, 1981, Wormy persons: contributions to understanding the nature and patterns of overdispersion with *Ascaris lumbricoides*, *Ancylostoma duodenale*, *Necator americanus* and *Trichuris trichiura*, *Top Geogr Med*, **33**: 241–8.

Crompton DWT, 1989, Biology of *Ascaris lumbricoides*, *Ascariasis and its Prevention and Control*, eds Crompton DWT, Nesheim MC, Pawlowski ZS, Taylor and Francis, London, 9–44.

Crompton DWT, 1991, The challenge of parasitic worms, *Trans Nebraska Acad Sci*, **18**: 73–86.

Crompton DWT, 1992, *Ascaris* and childhood malnutrition, *Trans R Soc Trop Med Hyg*, **86**: 577–9.

Compton DWT, 1994, *Ascaris lumbricoides*, *Parasitic and Infectious Diseases*, eds Scott ME, Smith G, Academic Press, London, 175–96.

Crompton DWT, Keymer AE, Arnold SE, 1984, Investigation over-dispersion: *Moniliformis moniliformis* (Acanthocephala) and rats, *Parasitology*, **88**: 317–31.

Crompton DWT, Nesheim MC, Pawlowski ZS, eds, 1985, *Ascaris and its Public Health Significance*, Taylor and Francis, London.

Crompton DWT, Nesheim MC, Pawlowski ZS, eds, 1989, *Ascariasis and its Prevention and Control*, Taylor and Francis, London.

Crompton DWT, Savioli L, 1993, Intestinal parasitic infections and urbanization, *Bull WHO*, **71**: 1–7.

Crompton DWT, Stephenson LS, 1985, Ascariasis in Africa, *Ascariasis and its Public Health Significance*, eds Crompton DWT, Nesheim MC, Pawlowski ZS, Taylor and Francis London, 185–202.

Crompton DWT, Stephenson LS, 1990, Hookworm infection, nutritional status and productivity, *Hookworm Disease*, eds Schad GA, Warren KS, Taylor and Francis, London, 231–64.

Crompton DWT, Whitehead RR, 1993, Hookworm infections and human iron metabolism, *Parasitology*, **107**: S137–S145.

da Costa-Macedo LM, Rey L, 1990, Ascaris lumbricoides in neonate evidence of congenital transmission of intestinal nematodes, *Rev Inst Med Trop Sao Paulo*, **32**: 351–4.

Davey K, 1964, The food of *Ascaris*, *Canad J Zool*, **42**: 1160–1.

Davies NJ, Goldsmid JM, 1978, Intestinal obstruction due to *Ascaris suum* infection, *Trans R Soc Trop Med Hyg*, **72**: 107.

Ebbell B, 1937, The Papyrus Ebers: The Greatest Egyptian Medical Document, Levin and Munksgaard, Copenhagen.

Elkins DB, Haswell-Elkins M, Anerson RM, 1985, The epidemiology and control of intestinal helminths in the Pulicat Lake region of Southern India. 1. Study design and pre- and post-treatment observations on Ascaris lumbricoides infection, *Trans R Soc Trop Med Hyg*, **80**: 774–92.

Erdener A, Ozok G et al., 1992, Abdominal complications of *Ascaris lumbricoides* in children, *JAMA*, **42**: 73–4.

Evans AC, Stephenson LS, 1995, Not by drugs alone: the fight against parasitic helminths, *World Health Forum*, **16**: 258–61.

Fasli Jalal, 1991, Effects of deworming, dietary fat, and carotenoid rich diets on vitamin A status of preschool children infected with *Ascaris lumbricoides* in West Sumatera Province, Indonesia, PhD Dissertation, Cornell University, New York.

Faust EC, Russell PF, Jung RC, 1970, Craig and Faust's Clinical Parasitology, 8th edn, Lea & Fabinger, Philadelphia, PA.

Fetterer RH, Hill DE, Urban JF, 1990, The cuticular biology in developmental stages of *Ascaris suum*, *Acta Trop (Basel)*, **47**: 289–95.

Fisher RM, Cremin BJ, 1970, Rectal bleeding due to *Trichuris trichiura*, *Br J Radiol*, **43**: 214–15.

Foor WE, 1967, Ultrastructural aspects of oocyte development and shell formation in *Ascaris lumbricoides*, *J Parasitol*, **53**: 1245–61.

Forrester JE, Scott ME, 1990, Measurement of *Ascaris lumbricoides* infection intensity and the dynamics of expulsion following treatment with mebendazole, *Parasitology*, **100**: 303–8.

Forsum E, Nesheim MC, Crompton DWT, 1981, Nutritional aspects of *Ascaris* infection in young protein-deficient pigs, *Parasitology*, **83**: 497–512.

Fry GH, Moore JG, 1969, *Enterobius vermicularis*: 10,000 year-old human infection, *Science*, **166**: 1620.

Ganor S, 1987, In whom does pinworm infection itch?, *Int J Dermatol*, **26**: 667.

Gardner GW, Edgerton RV et al., 1977, Physical work capacity and metabolic stress in subjects with iron deficiency anaemia, *Am J Clin Nutr*, **30**: 910–17.

Gelphi AP, Mustafa A, 1967, Seasonal pneumonitis with eosinophilia: a study of larval ascariasis in Saudi Arabs, *Am J Trop Med Hyg*, **16**: 646–57.

Gibbons LM, 1986, *SEM Guide to the Morphology of Nematode Parasites of Vertebrates*, CAB International, Farnham Royal, Slough.

Gilman RH, Chong YH et al., 1983, The adverse consequences of heavy *Trichuris* infection, *Trans R Soc Trop Med Hyg*, **77**: 432–8.

Grassi B, 1887, *Trichocephalus* und Ascarisentwicklung. Preliminararnot, *Zentralbl Bakteriol Parasitenkunde*, **1**: 131–2.

Grove DJ, 1990, *A History of Human Helminthology*, CAB International, Wallingford, Oxon.

Gupta MC, Mithal S et al., 1977, Effect of periodic deworming on nutritional status of Ascaris-infected pre-school children receiving supplementary food, *Lancet*, **2**: 108–10.

Gupta SC Gupta AK, Keswani NK, 1989, Pathology of tropical appendicitis, *J Clin Pathol*, **42:** 1169–72.

Guyatt HL, Bundy DAP, 1991, Estimating the prevalence of morbidity due to intestinal helminths: prevalence of infection as an indicator of prevalence of disease, *Trans R Soc Trop Med Hyg*, **85:** 778–82.

Hall GA, Rutter JM, Beer RJ, 1976, A comparative study of the histopathology of the large intestine of convenionally reared, specific pathogen free and gnotobiotic pigs infected with *Trichuris suis, J Comp Pathol*, **86:** 285–92.

Haswell-Elkins MR, Elkins DB, Anderson RM, 1987, Evidence for predisposition in humans to infection with *Ascaris,* hookworm, *Enterobius* and *Trichuris* in a South Indian fishing community, *Parasitology*, **95:** 323–37.

Haswell-Elkins MR, Elkins DB et al., 1987, The distribution and abundance of *Enterobius vermicularis* in a South Indian fishing community, *Parasitology*, **95:** 339–54.

Hill AW, Andrews J, 1942, Relation of hookworm burden to physical status in Georgia, *Am J Trop Med*, **22:** 499–506.·

Hill CH, 1957, The survival of swine whipworm eggs in hog lots, *J Parasitol*, **43:** 104.

Hoagland KE, Schad GA, 1978, *Necator americanus* and *Ancylostoma duodenale*: life history parameters and epidemiological implications of two sympatric hookworms of humans, *Exp Parasitol*, **44:** 36–49.

Hoffman SL. Quoted in Goodman B, 1994, Models aid understanding, help control parasites, *Science*, **264:** 1862–3.

Holland C, 1983, Interactions between three species of helminth in the small intestine of rats, PhD Dissertation, University of Cambridge.

Holland C, 1987a, Hookworm infection, *Impact of Helminth Infections on Human Nutrition*, Taylor and Francis, London, 128–60.

Holland C, 1987b, Neglected infections-trichuriasis and strongyloidiasis, *Impact of Helminth Infections on Human Nutrition*, Taylor and Francis, London, 161–201.

Holland CV, Asaolu SO et al., 1989, The epidemiology of *Ascaris lumbricoides* and other soil-transmitted helminths in primary school children in Ile-Ife, Nigeria, *Parasitology*, **99:** 275–85.

Holland CV, Crompton DWT et al., 1992, A possible genetic factor influencing protection from infection with *Ascaris lumbricoides* in Nigerian children, *J Parasitol*, **78:** 915–16.

Hotez PJ, Cerami A, 1993, Secretion of a proteolytic anticoagulant by *Ancylostoma duodenale* hookworms, *J Exp Med*, **157:** 1594–603.

Hyman LH, 1951, *The Invertebrates: Acanthocephala, Aschelminthes, and Entoprocta*, vol. III, McGraw-Hill, New York.

Jarrett EEE, Kerr JW, 1973, Threadworms and IgE in allergic asthma, *Clin Allergy*, **3:** 203–7.

Kagei N, 1983, Techniques for the measurement of environmental pollution by infective stages of soil-transmitted helminths, *Collected Papers on the Control of Soil-transmitted Helminthiases*, vol. 2, 24–46.

Kennedy MW, Gordon AMS et al., 1986, Genetic (major histocompatibility complex?) control of the antibody repertoire to the secreted antigens of Ascaris, *Parasite Immunol*, **9:** 269–73.

Kennedy MW, Qureshi F, 1986, Stage-specific secreted antigens of the parasite larval stages of the nematode Asaris, *Immunology*, **58:** 512–22.

Kennedy MW, Tomlinson LA et al., 1990, The specificity of antibody response to internal antigens of *Ascaris*: heterogeneity in infected humans, and MHC(H-2) control of the repertoire in mice, *Clin Exp Immunol*, **80:** 219–24.

Kenney M, Eveland LR, 1978, Infection of man with *Trichuris vulpis*, the whipworm of dogs, *Am J Clin Pathol*, **69:** 199.

Kenney M, Yermakov V, 1980, Infection of man with *Trichuris vulpis*, the whipworm of dogs, *Am J Trop Med Hyg*, **29:** 1205–8.

Keymer A, Pagel M, 1990, Predisposition to helminth infection, *Hookworm Disease*, eds Schad GA, Warren KS, Taylor and Francis, London, 177–209.

Khan TTF, Raj SM, Visvanathan R, 1993, Spectrum of cholangitis

in a rural setting in North-eastern Peninsular Malaysia, *Trop Doct*, **23:** 117–18.

Koino S, 1922, Experimental infections on the human body with ascarides, *Jpn Med World*, **15:** 317–20.

Kroeger A, Schulz B et al., Helminthiasis and cultural change in the Peruvian rainforest, *J Trop Med Hyg*, **95:** 104–13.

Kunii C, 1983, *Humanistic Family Planning Approaches: The Integration of Family Planning and Health Goals*, United Nations Fund for Population Activities, New York.

Lee DL, Atkinson H, 1976, *Physiology of Nematodes*, 2nd edn, Macmillan, London.

Lewin R, 1989, *Human Evolution*, 2nd edn, Blackwell Scientific Publications, Oxford.

Looss A, 1901, Über das Eindrigen der Ankylostomalarven in die menschliche Haut, *Zentralbl Bakteriol Parasitenkunde*, **29:** 733–9.

Looss A, 1905, The anatomy and life history of *Ankylostoma duodenale* Dub. Pt I. The anatomy of the adult worm, *Records of the Egyptian Government, School of Medicine*, vol. III, National Printing Department, Cairo, 1–158.

Lotero H, Tripathy K, Bolanos O, 1974, Gastrointestinal blood loss in *Trichuris* infection, *Am J Trop Med Hyg*, **23:** 1203–4.

Louw JH, 1966, Abdominal complications of *Ascaris lumbricoides* infestation in children, *Br J Surg*, **53:** 510–21.

Lwambo NJS, Bundy DAP, Medley GFH, 1992, A new approach to morbidity assessment in hookworm endemic countries, *Epidemiol Infect*, **108:** 469–81.

Macdonald D, ed, 1984, *The Encyclopaedia of Mammals*, Unwin Hyman, London.

Maggenti A, 1982, Nemata (nematodes), *Synopsis and Classification of Living Organisms*, vol. 1, ed Parker SP, McGraw-Hill, New York.

Mansour MM, Francis WM, Farid Z, 1985, Prevalence of latent iron deficiency in patients with chronic *S. mansoni* infection, *Trop Geogr Med*, **37:** 124–8.

Martin J, Crompton DWT et al., 1984, Mucosal surface lesions in young protein-deficient pigs infected with *Ascaris suum* (Nematoda), *Parasitology*, **88:** 333–40.

Matthews BE, 1982, Skin penetration by *Necator americanus* larvae, *Z Parasitenkunde*, **68:** 81–6.

Maung M, 1973, *Ascaris lumbricoides* Linne, 1758 and *Ascaris suum* Goeze, 1782: morphological differences between specimens obtained from man and pig, *Southeast Asian J Trop Med Public Health*, **4:** 41–5.

Medley GFH, Guyatt HL, Bundy DAP, 1993, A quantitative framework for evaluating the effect of community treatment on the morbidity due to *Ascaris, Parasitology*, **106:** 211–21.

Migasena S, Sumetchotimaytha J et al., 1984, Zinc in the pathogenesis of hookworm anaemia, *Southeast Asian J Trop Med Public Health*, **15:** 206–8.

Miller TA, 1978, Industrial development and field use of the canine hookworm vaccine, *Adv Parasitol*, **16:** 333–42.

Miller TA, 1979, Hookworm infection in man, *Adv Parasitol*, **17:** 315–84.

Misegna S, Gilles HM, 1987, Hookworm infection, *Intestinal Helminthic Infections*, ed Pawlowski ZS, Baillière Tindall, London, 617–27.

Mizgajska H, 1993, The distribution and survival of eggs of *Ascaris suum* in six different natural soil profiles, *Acta Parasitol*, **38:** 170–4.

Morishita, K, 1972, Studies on the epidemiological aspects of ascariasis in Japan and basic knowledge concerning its control, *Progress of Medical Parasitology in Japan*, vol. 4, ed. Moroshita K et al., Meguro Parasitological Museum, Tokyo, 3–153.

Muller R, 1975, *Worms and Disease*, Heinemann Medical, London.

Nawalinski TA, Schad GA, Chowdhury AB, 1978, Population biology of hookworm in children in rural Bengal, I. General parasitological observations. *Am J Trop Med Hyg*, **27:** 1152–61.

Nesheim MC, 1985, Nutritional aspects of *Ascaris suum* and *A. lumbricoides* infection, *Ascaris and its Public Health Significance*, eds Crompton DWT, Nesheim MC, Pawlowski ZS, Taylor and Francis, London, 147–60.

Nichols RL, 1956, The aetiology of visceral larva migrans, II. Comparative larval morphology of *Ascaris lumbricoides, Necator americanus, Strongyloides stercoralis* and *Ancylostoma caninum, J Parasitol,* **42:** 363–99.

Nokes C, Bundy DAP, 1994, Does helminth infection affect mental processing and educational achievement?, *Parasitol Today,* **10:** 14–18.

Nokes C, Grantham-McGregor SM et al., 1992, Moderate to heavy infections of *Trichuris trichiura* affect cognitive function in Jamaican schoolchildren, *Parasitology,* **104:** 539–47.

Palmer DR, Hall A et al., 1995, Antibody isotype responses to antigens of *Ascaris lumbricoides* in a case-control study of persistently heavily infected Bangladeshi children, *Parasitology,* **111:** 385–93.

Patterson R, Harris KE, 1985, Parallel induction of immunoglobulin E-mediated *Ascaris* antigen airway responses and increased carbachol reactivity in rhesus monkeys by infection with *Ascaris suum, J Lab Clin Medicine,* **106:** 293–7.

Pawlowski ZS, 1982, Ascariasis: host-pathogen biology, *Rev Infect Dis,* **4:** 806–14.

Pawlowski ZS, Davis A, 1989, Morbidity and mortality in ascariasis, *Ascariasis and its Prevention and Control,* eds Crompton DWT, Nesheim MC, Pawlowski ZS, Taylor and Francis, London, 71–86.

Pawlowski ZS, Schad GA, Stott GJ, 1991, *Hookworm Infection and Anaemia,* World Health Organization, Geneva.

Peng Weidong, Zhou Xianmin, Crompton DWT, 1995, Aspects of ascariasis in China, *Helminthologia,* **32:** 97–100.

Perry RN, Clark AJ, 1982, Hatching mechanisms of nematodes, *Parasitology,* **83:** 435–49.

Pinus J, 1985, Surgical complications of ascariasis in Brazil, *Ascariasis and its Public Health Significance,* eds Crompton DWT, Nesheim MC, Pawlowski ZS, Taylor and Francis, London, 161–6.

Poinar GO, 1983, *The Natural History of Nematodes,* Prentice-Hall, Englewood Cliffs, NJ.

Pollitt E, 1990, *Malnutrition and Infection in the Classroom,* UNESCO, Paris.

Ramdath DD, Simeon DT et al., 1995, Iron status of schoolchildren with varying intensities of *Trichuris trichiura* infection, *Parasitology,* **110:** 347–51.

Rathi AK, Batra S et al., 1981, Ascariasis causing intestinal obstruction in a 45-day-old infant, *Indian Pediatr,* **18:** 751–2.

Read AF, Skorping A, 1995, The evolution of tissue migration by parasitic nematode larvae, *Parasitology,* **111:** 359–71.

Roche M, Layrisse M, 1966, The nature and causes of 'hookworm anaemia', *Am J Trop Med Hyg,* **15:** 1030–100.

Rogers WP, 1960, The physiology of infective processes of nematode parasites: the stimulus from the animal host, *Proc R Soc London B,* **152:** 367–86.

Salafasky B, Fusco AC, Siddiqui A, 1990, Necator americanus: factors influencing skin penetration by larvae, *Hookworm Disease,* eds Schad GA, Warren KS, Taylor and Francis, London, 329–39.

Savioli L, Bundy D, Tomkins A, 1992, Intestinal parasitic infections: a soluble health problem, *Trans R Soc Trop Med Hyg,* **86:** 353–4.

Schad GA, Nawalinski TA, Kochar V, 1983, Human ecology and the distribution and abundance of hookworm populations, *Human Ecology and Infectious Diseases,* Academic Press, London, 187–223.

Schad GA, Anderson RM, 1985, Predisposition to hookworm infection in humans, *Science,* **228:** 1537–40.

Schad GA, Chowdhury AB et al., 1973, *Science,* Arrested development in human hookworm infections, **180:** 502–4.

Schad GA, Warren KS, eds, 1990, *Hookworm Disease: Current Status and New Directions,* Taylor and Francis, London.

Scott ME, Smith G, eds, 1994, *Parasitic and Infectious Diseases,* Academic Press, London.

Simeon D, Callender J et al., 1994, School performance, nutritional status and trichuriasis in Jamaican school children, *Acta Paediatr,* **83:** 1188–93.

Skryabin KI, Shikhobalova NP, Mozgovoi AA, 1991, Oxyurata and Ascaridata, *Key to Parasitic Nematodes,* vol. 2, ed. Skryabin KI, E.J. Brill, Leiden.

Smyth JD, 1994, Introduction to Animal Parasitology, 3rd edn, Cambridge University Press, Cambridge.

Sprent JFA, 1952, Anatomical distinction between human and pig strains of *Ascaris, Nature* (London), **170:** 627–8.

Stephenson LS, 1987, *Impact of Helminth Infections on Human Nutrition,* Taylor and Francis, London.

Stephenson LS, Crompton DWT et al., 1980, Relationships between *Ascaris* infection and growth of malnourished preschool children in Kenya, *Am J Clin Nutr,* **33:** 1165–72.

Stephenson LS, Latham MC et al., 1993, Physical fitness, growth and appetite of Kenyan school boys with hookworm, *Trichuris trichiura* and *Ascaris lumbricoides* are improved four months after a single dose of albendazole, *J Nutr,* **123:** 1036–46.

Stephenson LS, Pond WG et al., 1980, *Ascaris suum:* nutrient absorption, growth, and intestinal pathology in young pigs experimentally infected with 15-day-old larvae, *Exp Parasitol,* **49:** 15–25.

Taffs LJ, 1968, Immunological studies on experimental infection of pigs with *Ascaris suum* Goeze. IV. The histopathology of the liver and lung, *J Helminthol,* **42:** 157–72.

Takata I, 1951, Experimental infection of man with *Ascaris* of man and the pig, *Kitasato Arch Exp Med,* **23:** 49–59.

Taren DL, Nesheim MC et al., 1987, Contributions of ascariasis to poor nutritional status of children from Chiriqui Province, Republic of Panama, *Parasitology,* **95:** 603–13.

Thein Hlaing, 1989, Epidemiological basis of survey design, methodology and data analysis for ascariasis, *Ascariasis and its Prevention and Control,* eds Crompton DWT, Nesheim MC, Powlowski ZS, Taylor and Francis, London, 351–368.

Thein Hlaing, 1993, Ascariasis and childhood malnutrition, *Parasitology,* **107:** S125–S136.

Thein Hlaing, Than Saw et al., 1984, Epidemiology and transmission dynamics of *Ascaris lumbricoides* in Okpo village, rural Burma, *Trans R Soc Trop Med Hyg,* **78:** 497–504.

Thein Hlaing, Than Saw, Myint Lwin, 1987, Reinfection of people with *Ascaris lumbricoides* following single 6-month and 12-month interval mass chemotherapy in Opko village, rural Burma, *Trans R Soc Trop Med Hyg,* **81:** 140–6.

Thein Hlaing, Thane Toe et al., 1992, A controlled chemotherapeutic intervention trial on the relationship between *Ascaris lumbricoides* infection and malnutrition in children, *Trans R Soc Trop Med Hyg,* **85:** 523–8.

Theinpont D, Rochette F, Vanparijs OFJ, 1980, *Diagnosing Helminthiasis through Coprological Examination,* Janssen Research Foundation, Beerse, Belgium.

Tomkins A, Watson F, 1989, Malnutrition and infection, *ACC/SCN Nutrition Policy Discussion Paper 5,* United Nations, New York.

Tomlinson LA, Christie JF et al., 1989, MHC restriction of the antibody repertoire to secretory antigens, and a major allergen of the nematode parasite, *Ascaris, J Immunol,* **143:** 2349–56.

Tripathy K, Duque E et al., 1972, Malabsorption syndome is ascariasis, *Am J Clin Nutr,* **25:** 1276–87.

Upatham ES, Viyanant V et al., 1992, Predisposition to reinfection by intestinal helminths after chemotherapy in south Thailand, *Int J Parasitol,* **22:** 801–6.

Viteri FE, 1994, The consequences of iron deficiency and anaemia in pregnancy on maternal health, the foetus and the infant, *SCN News,* **11:** 14–18.

Viteri FE, Torun B, 1974, Anaemia and physical work capacity, *Clin Haematol,* **3:** 609–26.

WHO, 1972, *Nutritional anaemias,* Technical Report Series 503, World Health Organization, Geneva.

WHO, 1981, *Intestinal protozoan and helminthic infections,* Technical Report Series 666, World Health Organization, Geneva.

WHO, 1987, *Prevention and control of intestinal parasitic infections,* Tehnical Report Series 749, World Health Organization, Geneva.

WHO, 1994, *Bench Aids for the Diagnosis of Intestinal Parasites,* World Health Organization, Geneva.

WHO, 1995, *Hookworm infection and anaemia in girls and women,* (WHO/CDS/IPI/95.1), World Health Organization, Geneva.

Wakelin D, 1978, Genetic control of susceptibility and resistance to parasitic infection, *Adv Parasitol,* **16:** 219–308.

Wakelin D, 1988, Helminth infections, *Genetics of Resistance to Bacterial and Parasitic Infection,* eds Wakelin D, Blackwell JM, Taylor and Francis, London, 153–224.

Wakelin D, Blackwell JM, eds, 1988, *Genetics of Resistance to Bacterial and Parasitic Infection,* Taylor and Francis, London.

Wakelin D, Harnett W, Parkhouse RME, 1993, Nematodes, *Immunology and Molecular Biology of Parasitic Infections,* 3rd edn, ed. Warren KS, Blackwell Scientific Publications, Oxford, 496–526.

Wang ZY, Wang XZ et al., 1983, Blood sucking activities of hookworms, *Chin Med J,* **96:** 281–6.

Wardlaw AC, Forsyth LMG, Crompton DWT, 1994, Bactericidal activity in the pig roundworm *Ascaris suum, J Appl Bacteriol,* **76:** 36–41.

Warren K, 1972, Ascaris – a practical joke?, *N Engl J Med,* **286:** 999–1000.

Watson JM, 1960, *Medical Helminthology,* Ballière, Tindall and Cox, London.

Wharton D, 1980, Nematode egg-shells, *Parasitology,* **81:** 447–63.

Wharton D, Jenkins, T, 1978, Structure and chemistry of the eggshell of a nematode (*Trichuris suis*), *Tissue and Cell,* **10:** 427–40.

Wolgemuth JC, Latham MC et al., 1982, Worker productivity and the nutritional status of Kenyan road construction laborers, *Am J Clin Nutr,* **32:** 68–78.

Wong MS, Bundy DAP, 1990, Quantitative assessment of contamination of soil by eggs of *Ascaris lumbricoides* and *Trichuris trichiura, Trans R Soc Trop Med Hyg,* **84:** 567–70.

Yadav AK, Tandon V, 1989, Prevalence of nematode eggs in the urban area of the city of Shilong, India – a public health problem, *Health Hyg,* **10:** 158–61.

Yamaguti S, 1961, *Systema Helminthum III. The Nematodes of Vertebrates,* vol. 1, Interscience Publishers, London.

Yorke W, Maplestone RA, 1926, *The Nematode Parasites of Vertebrates,* J and A Churchill, London.

Yoshida Y, 1973, Species of hookworms infecting man: patterns of development, *9th International Congress of Tropical Medicine and Malaria, Athens,* Abstract no. 255, 174.

Yoshida Y, Kondo K et al., 1974, Comparative studies on *Ancylostoma braziliense* and *Ancylostoma ceylanicum.* III. Life history in the definitive host, *J Parasitol,* **60:** 636–41.

Yoshikawa H, Yamada M et al., 1989, Variations in egg size of *Trichuris trichiura, Parasitol Res,* **75:** 649–54.

Yu S, 1994, Report on the first nationwide survey on the distribution of human parasites in China. 1. Regional distribution of parasite species, *Chin J Parasitol Parasitic Dis,* **12:** 241–7.

Chapter 30

STRONGYLOIDES AND CAPILLARIA

M Cappello and P J Hotez

STRONGYLOIDES

1 THE PARASITE

Nematodes belonging to the genus *Strongyloides* were first identified as a cause of intestinal disease by Normand in 1876, who discovered these worms in the faeces of French troops in Cochin-China. At autopsy, morphologically distinct worms were identified within the intestinal mucosa of those suffering from overwhelming disease. Bavay subsequently named the intestinal forms *Anguillula intestinalis* and the faecal forms *A. stercoralis* (1876). Soon after, it was determined that these represented different stages of development of the same parasite. The existence of an autoinfective cycle was suggested by Fuelleborn (1914), and later work by Nishigori (1928) demonstrated that first stage larvae could indeed develop into infective filariform larvae and invade the colonic mucosa, thereby initiating development within the same host.

1.1 Classification

Strongyloides belongs to the phylum Nematoda and the class Phasmidia, i.e nematodes containing phasmids or caudal chemoreceptors. Within this class, they are assigned to the order Rhabditida and the superfamily Rhabditoidea, which is composed of both free-living and parasitic worms. They are distinguished from the superfamily Rhabdiasoidea, also within the suborder Rhabditina, by the presence of a distinct oesophageal bulb. Two species cause disease in humans, *S. stercoralis* and *S. fuelleborni*.

1.2 Morphology and structure

Parasitic females, which reside in the mucosa of the small intestine, are small and thin, measuring approximately 2–3 mm in length and 30–50 μm in width (Fig. 30.1). The anterior portion is thicker than the posterior, and contains the oesophagus. The triradiate pharynx contains 2 subventral and one dorsal gland, which deposit their secretions into the intestinal lumen. The reproductive system contains a midline vulva and paired uteri leading anteriorly and posteriorly from the vagina. The spirally wound ovaries of *S. fuelleborni* help to distinguish it morphologically from *S. stercoralis*, whose ovaries are linearly aligned within the body of the worm. Little information is available about the sensory receptors in *Strongyloides*.

The existence of parasitic males has been debated over many years. Early observations by Faust (1933) that parasitic males exist, and that sexual reproduction may represent one route by which *Strongyloides* reproduces within the host, have

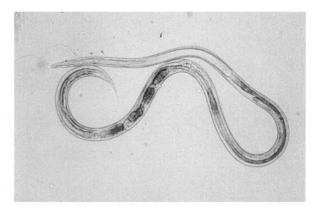

Fig. 30.1 *Strongyloides stercoralis* adult parasitic female (By courtesy of Dr Tom Nolan, University of Pennsylvania School of Veterinary Medicine).

not been confirmed by others. Part of the reason for the scepticism surrounding his findings may be the close morphological resemblance of the putative adult males to the free-living rhabditiform stage (Schad 1990).

The free-living adult female is approximately half the length of its parasitic counterpart (approximately 1.0 mm), although it is nearly twice as thick (80 μm). While the reproductive systems are morphologically similar, the uteri in the free-living adult female contain significantly more eggs. The free-living male is slightly smaller than the female, measuring approximately 50 μm in width. The reproductive system is composed of a tubular structure containing the testis, vas deferens and seminal vesicle. The copulatory spicules, which penetrate the female during copulation, are located on each side of the gubernaculum.

First stage rhabditiform larvae of *S. stercoralis* measure approximately 250 by 15 μm (Fig. 30.2). They are characterized by a muscular oesophagus, which comprises the anterior third of the body, and a short buccal cavity that distinguishes them from other nematodes, such as hookworms, which possess a more developed buccal tube. Third stage filariform, or infective, larvae are long and thin compared to the rhabditiform stages (Fig. 30.3). Paired alae on both sides of the worm offer structural stability during its movements along the ground. The mouth opening is small, and closed to the external environment, as the filariform stage is probably non-feeding. Recent work using electron microscopy with 3-dimensional reconstruction has delineated the location and structure of the amphidial neurons, highly specialized organs that may represent a means through which larvae sense environmental stimuli (Ashton et al. 1995).

The eggs of the parasitic female are deposited within the mucosa of the small intestine and usually hatch before reaching the lumen. As a result, they are rarely excreted in the faeces. Eggs from the free-living adult female are partially embryonated, and measure approximately 50–70 μm in length with an oval shape.

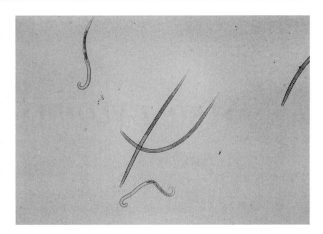

Fig. 30.3 *Strongyloides stercoralis* third stage (L3) filariform larvae (By courtesy of Dr Tom Nolan, University of Pennsylvania School of Veterinary Medicine).

1.3 General biology

Perhaps the most intriguing aspect of the biology of *Strongyloides* is its ability to alternate parasitic (**homogonic**) and free-living (**heterogonic**) life cycles. The factors that determine which route will be chosen have been studied for some species, and it appears that both internal, i.e. host specific, and external, e.g. environmental, conditions play a role in influencing developmental outcome (Moncol and Triantaphyllou 1978). In addition, certain geographic strains of *Strongyloides* may have a particular predilection for developing into one generation or the other (Neva 1986). It has also been observed that the free-living cycle develops most frequently in tropical climates with moist soil, while the parasitic life cycle may predominate in more temperate regions.

Rhabditiform first stage larvae deposited with faeces feed on bacteria and organic debris found in the surrounding soil. Those that develop into free-living adults continue to survive in this environment, whereas those that become filariform (i.e. infective third stage larvae) will ultimately cease to feed, while engaging in activities that might facilitate contact with a susceptible host. Filariform larvae have been shown to cluster in groups and stand on their tails, a behaviour called 'questing,' which is characteristic of the infective larval stage of parasitic nematodes.

1.4 Life cycle

Adult parasitic females, which reside within the crypts of the small intestine, deposit eggs that hatch prior to migrating into the lumen. The resulting first stage larvae are transported through the bowel, and excreted with the faeces. Larvae that are deposited on to moist, warm soil will develop either directly into infective filariform larvae or into free-living adult males and females, whose progeny will ultimately moult to become infective larvae. These infect their host by penetrating the skin, a process associated with the release of at least one hydrolytic enzyme (Brindley et

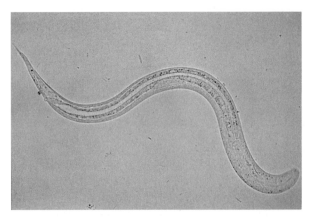

Fig. 30.2 *Strongyloides stercoralis* first stage (L1) rhabditiform larva (By courtesy of Dr Tom Nolan, University of Pennsylvania School of Veterinary Medicine).

al. 1995) that may function to degrade the extracellular dermal matrix. The traditionally accepted view of the life cycle of *S. stercoralis* maintains that, once within the dermis, larvae invade the venous circulation and are carried passively to the lungs, where they become trapped within capillaries and break through to the alveolar space. After migrating up the respiratory tree into the pharynx, the larvae are swallowed and travel to the small intestine. During this process, they moult to the fourth stage, probably during passage through the lungs. Recent work by Schad et al. (1989), however, has raised the possibility that this 'canonical route' represents only one of many potential pathways by which larvae may reach the small intestine.

Only females develop into adults within the intestine, where they reside and deposit eggs that have been produced by parthenogenesis. These eggs normally hatch within the epithelium, liberating first stage larvae into the lumen of the intestine. As a result, *Strongyloides* eggs are not routinely detected in the faeces of infected individuals. If the first stage larvae moult to the filariform stage during passage through the bowel, they may penetrate colonic mucosa or perianal skin, where they once again locate the venous circulation and begin the infective process anew. This autoinfection provides a means by which the parasite can multiply within the host, and explains how infections can be maintained for years after an individual leaves an endemic area. What regulates larval development in the intestine is not known, nor are the factors that sometimes trigger the explosive amplification of *Strongyloides* within the host called hyperinfection (see section 2.1, 'Clinical manifestations'), which can lead to the dissemination of parasites throughout various tissues.

1.5   Transmission and epidemiology

The predominant route of transmission of *S. stercoralis* is by skin contact with faecally contaminated soil. As a result, communities where close living conditions and poor sanitation facilities exist are frequently characterized by high prevalence rates of strongyloidiasis. These include both rural and urban areas in the developing world, as well as closed communities, such as institutions for the mentally handicapped (Braun et al. 1989). Zoonotic transmission of strongyloidiasis from asymptomatic dogs to animal workers has also been reported (Georgi and Sprinkle 1974).

The geographic distribution of *Strongyloides* is quite broad, and includes temperate as well as tropical climates. This undoubtedly is attributable to the remarkable phenotypic flexibility of the parasite, as it is able to adapt its life cycle and development to suit environmental conditions. Moreover, internal autoinfection allows for maintenance of the parasite within the host for years following initial exposure. Surveys of prisoners of war from World War II conducted more than 40 years later succeeded in identifying patent infections in up to 37% of those soldiers who were held captive in various parts of the Pacific (Hill 1988, Genta 1989). Since all infected individuals are at risk of hy-

perinfection and disseminated disease, the identification of those who may have acquired their infection in the distant past is of significant clinical importance.

Strongyloides hyperinfection is most frequently seen in those with underlying immune defects such as haematological malignancy, autoimmune disease or severe protein malnutrition. In addition, immunosuppressive therapy, particularly glucocorticoids, associated with any of the above conditions, as well as organ transplantation, may also precipitate hyperinfection and dissemination. Whether this is due to immunosuppression or a direct effect of steroids on the reproductive and developmental patterns of *Strongyloides* remains to be determined (Genta 1992). Coinfection with HIV, although reported in association with severe strongyloidiasis, is less common than might have been expected, given the significant overlap in the geographic distribution of these 2 diseases (Celedon et al. 1994, Gompels et al. 1991). In contrast to HIV, there is evidence that coinfection with HTLV-1 may be associated with more severe strongyloidiasis than that which is seen in HTLV-1 seronegative individuals (Robinson et al. 1994).

S. fuelleborni is also transmitted primarily by skin contact. However, epidemiological data from parts of Africa and Papua New Guinea suggest that this may not be the only route of infection. Investigations into the high prevalence of *S. fuelleborni* in African children led to the postpartum identification of larvae in the breast milk of a woman from Zaire (Brown and Girardeau 1977). In Papua New Guinea, high rates of infection (up to 65%) in children up to 3 months of age suggest that transmammary infection might also occur in this endemic area, although the parasite has not been identified in breast milk (Barnish and Ashford 1989, Ashford and Barnish 1990) In addition, *S. fuelleborni* has been identified as the causative agent of 'swollen belly syndrome', a fulminant and fatal enteritis that has been well documented among infants less than 6 months of age born in the highly endemic areas of Papua New Guinea (see section 2.1, 'Clinical Manifestations'). It has been suggested that transmammary infection followed by early external autoinfection from soiled nappies may result in the rapid multiplication of worms in these very young children (Ashford and Barnish 1990).

2   CLINICAL AND PATHOLOGICAL ASPECTS OF INFECTION

Strongyloidiasis can be divided into the following clinical categories: (1) asymptomatic carriage; (2) intestinal disease; and (3) hyperinfection with or without dissemination. Symptomatology is somewhat dependent on worm burden, which appears to be regulated by a delicate balance between the immune status of the host and the developmental tendencies of the parasite. In chronic strongyloidiasis, egg output remains relatively low and constant, proportionally few larvae undergoing internal autoinfection. In contrast, hyperinfection is associated with both an increase in the number of eggs produced as well as the proportion of larvae that develop internally to the filariform stage and reinvade the host.

2.1 Clinical manifestations

Chronic infection with *S. stercoralis* is most frequently asymptomatic (Milder et al. 1981, Neva 1986, Berk et al. 1987). When symptoms do present, they usually involve the gastrointestinal tract. Intermittent abdominal pain, distention, bloating and diarrhoea alternating with constipation are characteristic of intestinal disease. Children may develop a malabsorption syndrome caused by infection with *S. stercoralis*, characterized by growth stunting and failure to thrive (O'Brien 1975, Burke 1978). Pruritus and urticaria, particularly involving the perianal skin and buttocks, are also common symptoms of chronic *Strongyloides* infection. A serpiginous, pruritic eruption usually found on the trunk or buttocks, named **larva currens** (racing larva) by Arthur and Shelley (1958), may represent skin penetration by autoinfective filariform larvae in this area. This pathognomonic rash tends to progress and subside over a period of hours, and its intermittent nature often hinders the diagnosis of strongyloidiasis.

The most serious clinical manifestations of strongyloidiasis occur in the setting of hyperinfection, where the dramatic increase in the number of parasites within the host results in dissemination of larvae to various tissues. The increase in worm burden results from an increase in both the number of eggs produced by the female parasites in the intestine and the proportion of those larvae that undergo autoinfection. Usually associated with some underlying host immune defect, hyperinfection is most frequently associated with immunosuppressive therapy, particularly glucocorticoids, which are often used as part of the treatment of such conditions as haematological malignancies and autoimmune diseases, making it difficult to determine which is ultimately responsible for triggering the increase in parasite load. The reason for the close association between exogenous steroid therapy and hyperinfection is unclear, although it has been suggested that steroids mimic an endogenous hormone produced by the parasite that stimulates egg production and development (Genta 1992). Coinfection with HTLV-1 may also predispose to *Strongyloides* hyperinfection, perhaps due to a defect in effector IgE responses (Dixon et al. 1989, Robinson et al. 1994).

Patients with *Strongyloides* hyperinfection generally experience a worsening in abdominal symptoms, often accompanied by paralytic ileus (Cookson et al. 1990), gastrointestinal bleeding (Bhatt et al. 1990, Dees et al. 1990) and even perforation. In addition, the increase in the number of worms migrating through the lungs often results in wheezing, dyspnoea and occasionally pulmonary haemorrhage. Patchy infiltrates, diffuse interstitial pneumonitis, and bronchopneumonia may be detected by chest radiography (Meltzer et al. 1979, Berenson et al. 1987, Chu et al. 1990, Kramer et al. 1990).

During hyperinfection, filariform larvae may gain access to the arterial circulation, thereby allowing dissemination to numerous tissues and solid organs. In fact, filariform (and rarely rhabditiform) larvae have been recovered from biopsies of lymph nodes (Adam et al. 1973), endocardium (Neefe et al. 1973), pancreas (Kuberski et al. 1975), liver (Neefe et al. 1973), kidney (Civantos et al. 1969) and brain (Neefe et al. 1976), and have even been isolated from peripheral blood (Onuigbo and Ibeachum 1991). Involvement of the central nervous system can be associated with seizures and mental status changes (Igra-Siegman et al. 1981, Genta and Walzer 1989, Cappello and Hotez 1993), and is frequently accompanied by pyogenic abscess or meningitis caused by gram-negative bacteria, which may be carried from the gut by migrating larvae. Cutaneous manifestations of disseminated strongyloidiasis include petechiae and sometimes severe purpura (Kalb and Grossman 1986, Berenson et al. 1987, Genta et al. 1988, Ronan et al. 1989). Unlike the rash of chronic strongyloidiasis (larva currens), skin biopsies in disseminated disease often reveal filariform larvae.

Children suffering from swollen belly syndrome caused by *S. fuelleborni* usually present early in life (8–10 weeks of age) with protein-losing enteropathy, abdominal distention and respiratory distress (Ashford and Barnish 1990). Diarrhoea is generally not pronounced, and fever is absent. Severe hypoproteinaemia (without proteinuria) is a characteristic finding and leads to the development of peripheral oedema and ascites. Egg counts are often greater than 100 000/g faeces. Untreated, the condition is associated with significant mortality.

2.2 Pathogenesis and pathology

The intestinal pathology associated with *Strongyloides* infection is indicated by a variety of histological findings. The spectrum of damage, ranging from scattered petechiae with mild oedema to ulcerated, atrophic and fibrotic mucosa can occasionally coexist in a single patient. Parasites may be found in all layers of the intestinal wall, and infiltrates of mononuclear cells and neutrophils may be identified (Genta and Walzer 1989).

In disseminated disease, migrating larvae cause extensive tissue damage to the colon, lungs and other organs. Because of the association with immunosuppression, biopsy specimens containing these aberrantly migrating larvae may reveal only a mild inflammatory response surrounding the parasite. Invasion of the central nervous system can be associated with meningitis characterized by a predominance of either neutrophils or lymphocytes.

2.3 Immune responses

The immune responses that accompany *Strongyloides* infection are not well understood. To date, there have been numerous reports of elevated serum IgE in chronic strongyloidiasis. However, the diagnostic significance of this observation is unclear, since at least one study reported elevated serum IgE levels in less than 10% of chronically infected individuals (Willis and Nwokolo 1966). Recently, an association between HTLV-1 infection and faecal excretion of *Strongyloides* larvae was reported from Jamaica (Robinson et al. 1994). The authors found that HTLV-1 infected individuals with strongyloidiasis showed an age-related depression in serum IgE levels when compared to those seronegative for HTLV-1. These data suggest that serum IgE may confer some degree of protection against heavy infection with *Strongyloides*, and that this immune response is somehow inhibited by HTLV-1.

2.4 Diagnosis

The diagnosis of chronic strongyloidiasis is most reliably made by identifying rhabditiform (or rarely filariform) larvae in the faeces of an infected individual. However, the excretion of eggs in uncomplicated intestinal infection can be quite erratic, and multiple stool examinations may be required. Various stool concentration techniques and use of the Baermann method (by which motile larvae are extracted from stool specimens) may increase the diagnostic yield of faecal examination (Genta et al. 1987). An agar plate method that relies on the use of inverted microscopy to identify tracks made by motile *S. stercoralis* larvae has been shown to be more sensitive than some of these other techniques (Sukhavat et al. 1994).

Strongyloides larvae can also be detected in duodenal aspirates, either by endoscopy or by the use of the string test (Beal et al. 1970, Goldsmid and Davies 1978). The latter involves swallowing a gelatin capsule containing a coiled piece of string. The proximal portion of the string is attached externally, and approximately 4 h later, the string is removed. The duodenal fluid adhering to the string is then examined microscopically for the presence of larvae. The sensitivity of the string test is probably slightly higher than that of routine stool examination.

A variety of serological tests for strongyloidiasis have been developed, including indirect haemaglutination (Gam et al. 1987), indirect immunofluorescence (Dafalla 1972), and enzyme linked immunosorbent assay (ELISA) (Carroll et al. 1981, Genta et al. 1987). The most sensitive and specific of these is ELISA, which has been used to screen populations at risk for harbouring chronic *S. stercoralis* infection. Anyone with a positive serological test for *Strongyloides* should have a thorough stool examination to identify the presence of larvae and confirm the diagnosis.

During hyperinfection with dissemination, *Strongyloides* larvae can be detected in a variety of body fluids and tissues. The massive migration of parasites through the pulmonary circulation and into the lungs results in the frequent identification of larvae in sputum or bronchoalveolar lavage specimens (Berenson et al. 1987, Chu et al. 1990, Kramer et al. 1990). Eosinophilia, which is a frequent finding in chronic strongyloidiasis, is often absent in hyperinfection, in many cases because of exogenous corticosteroid therapy.

In contrast to *S. stercoralis*, the diagnosis of *S. fuelleborni* infection is made by identifying eggs in the faeces, rather than larvae. Children with swollen belly syndrome tend to have extremely heavy infections, and excrete large numbers of eggs daily.

2.6 Control

At present, thiabendazole remains the drug of choice for the treatment of chronic strongyloidiasis. It is administered orally at a dose of 25 mg/kg twice a day for 2 successive days. Although not extensively studied, this dose appears to be effective in children as well. Parasitological cure rates of 60–100% have been reported, although the length of follow up in these studies varied. The major drawback to thiabendazole therapy is compliance, since its use is associated with an extremely high occurrence of adverse side effects. These include nausea, dizziness, and neuropsychiatric symptoms, which have been reported in up to 89% of patients taking this drug (Grove 1982).

Ivermectin, a broad spectrum anthelmintic, has also been reported to be effective in the treatment of chronic strongyloidiasis (Naquira et al. 1989, Lyagoubi et al. 1992). Recently, a randomized trial in Southeast Asian refugees found that while both were equally successful at eradicating *S. stercoralis* infection, single-dose ivermectin was associated with significantly fewer side effects than a 3 day regimen of thiabendazole (Gann et al. 1994).

Follow up of patients after treatment for chronic strongyloidiasis should include periodic faecal examinations for larvae. In addition, the serum eosinophil count should return to normal within 1–3 months of successful therapy. The use of ELISA to monitor long-term treatment efficacy has also been suggested, particularly in those with an underlying immune defect or taking immunosuppressive drugs.

Successful treatment of *Strongyloides* hyperinfection requires prompt diagnosis and initiation of anthelmintic therapy. Treatment with thiabendazole (25 mg/kg twice a day) should be continued indefinitely, pending both clinical response and the eradication of larvae from stool, sputum and other body fluids. Concurrent bacterial infections, e.g. bronchopneumonia and meningitis, should be treated aggressively with antibiotics. Even with appropriate therapy, the mortality from disseminated strongyloidiasis approaches 50–75% (Genta and Walzer 1989). Ivermectin has also been used successfully to treat hyperinfection (Torres et al. 1994), and it may ultimately become a suitable alternative to thiabendazole. However, definitive data regarding its efficacy in *Strongyloides* hyperinfection are lacking at this time.

Thiabendazole treatment of children with swollen belly syndrome caused by *S. fuelleborni* appears to be effective, although reinfection is likely to occur in endemic areas (Ashford and Barnish 1990, Barnish and Barker 1987).

Because *Strongyloides* larvae can survive in warm,

moist environments for days, control of transmission within an endemic area requires proper disposal of human waste. In addition, outbreaks documented among animal care workers underline the importance of exercising caution when handling specimens from laboratory animals.

CAPILLARIA

3 THE PARASITE

3.1 Introduction and historical perspective

Human parasitic zoonoses caused by members of the genus *Capillaria* are uncommon, except in the Philippines and Thailand, where epidemics caused by the intestinal species *C. philippinensis* have been described. Since 1964, intestinal capillariasis has been recognized as an important cause of morbidity and mortality in these areas, with impressive outbreaks in Northern Luzon and Southern Leyte (Cross 1995). Unlike most other intestinal nematodes, *C. philippinensis* is associated with a substantial mortality during epidemics (Detels et al. 1969), and shares with *Strongyloides stercoralis* the unusual ability to undergo autoinfection and hyperinfection in humans. Much of our existing knowledge about human intestinal capillariasis derives from the earlier investigative work of Professor John H. Cross during his tenure at the U.S. Naval Medical Research Unit in the Philippines (Cross 1992).

In contrast to intestinal capillariasis, extraintestinal zoonotic capillariasis, caused by other members of the genus *Capillaria* (*C. hepatica*, *C. aerophila* and *C. plica*) is rare.

3.2 Classification

The Capillariinae is one of 3 subfamilies belonging to the superfamily Trichinelloidea. The Trichurinae (whipworms) and the Trichosomoidinae comprise the other 2 subfamilies. All members of the Trichinelloidea have a unique oesophageal structure that distinguishes them from other nematodes (see below). Anderson (1992) points out that the 'classification of the Capillariinae is one of the most difficult and unsatisfactory in the Nematoda'. Many investigators including Skrjabin et al. (1957) have assigned the 4 human parasites of the genus *Capillaria*, namely *C. philippinensis, C. hepatica, C. aerophilus* and *C. plica*, to other genera, including *Calodium, Eucoleus* and *Pearsonema* (Anderson 1992). Because these terms are usually unfamiliar to medical parasitologists and clinicians we will adopt the common usage term *Capillaria*.

3.3 Morphology and structure

Like all members of the Trichinelloidea, the adult *Capillaria* have a modified oesophageal gland called a **stichosome** comprised of unique gland cells called **stichocytes**. Each stichocyte communicates with the lumen of the ooesophagus by a single pore (Wright et al. 1985, Anderson 1992). Generally speaking, the

Trichinelloidea have a long narrow anterior end containing the stichosome, which broadens into a thickened posterior end. In the *Capillaria*, however, the differences in width between the anterior and posterior regions are much less exaggerated. The adult Capillariinae are also more delicate and smaller than the other Trichinelloidea subfamilies. Adult males of *C. philippinensis* measure 1.5–3.9 mm in length and females measure 2.3–5.3 mm in length (Chitwood et al. 1968, Cross 1995). Because it is difficult to recover and measure intact *C. hepatica* and *C. aerophila* from human tissue, there are no precise estimates of their length. From non-human hosts, lengths of 4–12 mm have been reported for *C. hepatica*, and 30–40 mm for *C. aerophila*.

The uterus of the female adult *C. philippinensis* contains thick-shelled eggs, thin-shelled eggs and larvae (Cross 1992). Eggs passed in the faeces are bipolar 'lemon-shaped' or 'barrel-shaped' and bear a superficial resemblance to those of the human whipworm *Trichuris trichiura* (see Fig. 30.4). They are, however, smaller (36–45 × 20 μm for *C. philippinensis* vs 50–54 × 22–23 μm for *T. trichiura*), more cylindrical in shape and have less prominent bipolar plugs which are somewhat flattened (Cross 1992). In contrast, the eggs of *C. aerophila* are large, measuring 59–80 × 30–40 μm (Soulsby 1982).

3.4 General biology

Humans are accidental hosts for all members of the genus *Capillaria*.

C. PHILIPPINENSIS

There is evidence to suggest that fish-eating birds are the natural definitive hosts of *C. philippinensis* (Cross and Basaca-Sevilla 1983). Humans become infected when they accidentally interrupt the fish–bird life cycle by eating infected, uncooked freshwater fish. *C. philippinensis* and *Strongyloides stercoralis* are the 2 major nematodes that can undergo autoinfection and hyperinfection in the human host.

C. HEPATICA

C. hepatica occurs in the liver of numerous rodent species worldwide, but will also infect at least 20 other mammals, including squirrel, muskrat, opossum and, rarely, humans (Borucinska and Nielsen 1993). *C. hepatica* has the unusual feature that all of its mammalian hosts are 'dead end' in that the eggs must be released from the liver by a predation (including cannibalism and scavenging).

C. AEROPHILA

C. aerophila is a worldwide parasite of wild carnivores where it lives in the upper and lower respiratory tree and parenchyma.

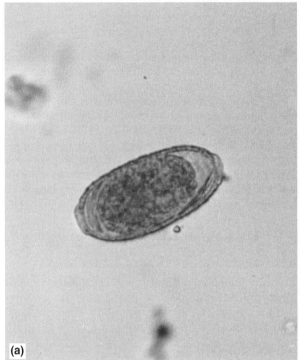

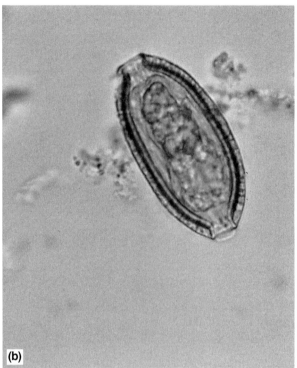

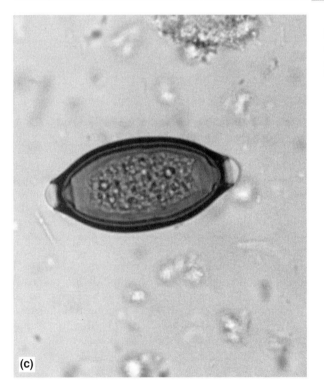

Fig. 30.4 Eggs of *Capillaria philippinensis* (a) and *C. hepatica* (b). Included for comparison is an egg from *Trichuris trichiura* (c). (By courtesy of Dr Dickson Despommier, Columbia University School of Public Health).

3.5 Life cycle

C. PHILIPPINENSIS

As Cross (1995) points out, the *C. philippinensis* life cycle is unique among human nematode parasites and was elucidated primarily by laboratory experimentation. Eggs from the faeces of infected patients embryonate in water at ambient temperatures in 5–10 days and develop further only if swallowed by small freshwater and brackish water fish. The bagsit (*Hypseleotris bipartita*) is a major intermediate fish host in the Philippines (Cross 1992). Upon ingestion the eggs hatch, giving rise to larval stages that grow in size. Humans become infected when they ingest larvae contained within the uncooked fish. The larvae become adults in the lumen and mucosa of the intestine. The length of time during which ingested larvae develop into adult male and oviparous adult female worms in humans is not known, although in experimental gerbil infections, the larvae develop into adults in 10–11 days (Cross 1992, 1995).

An unusual feature of *C. philippinensis* is its ability to cause autoinfection and hyperinfection in humans. The initial evidence for hyperinfection arose from studies with monkeys (*Macaca* spp.), in which 10 000–30 000 worms were recovered from monkeys infected with 30–50 larvae contained within fish (Cross et al. 1972, Cross 1992). This observation explains the extreme morbidity and relatively high mortality of intestinal capillariasis in humans. Autoinfection arises because the female adult worm is sometimes larviparous or can produce thin-walled eggs that hatch within the intestinal tract; these newborn larvae presumably can moult and re-invade the intestinal mucosa. Very heavy infections can develop as a result, as many as 200 000 worms having been recovered from 11 of human bowel fluid at autopsy (Cross 1992).

C. HEPATICA

The adult female resides in the liver, where it deposits groups of eggs. These develop larvae but remain encapsulated in the liver (Wright 1974). Therefore, for transmission to occur the embryonated eggs contained within infected livers must be eaten by animals or humans during cannibalism, predation or scavenging (Anderson 1992). In contrast, the unembryonated eggs will pass through the gut of so-called 'disseminator animals' and are then dispersed into the environment with the faeces (Anderson 1992). When infective eggs are ingested accidentally by humans, they hatch in the small intestine and produce larvae that migrate through the portal system to the liver (Gutierrez 1990). After approximately 4 weeks, the female adult worm begins to release eggs.

C. AEROPHILA

The adult female lives in the upper and lower respiratory tree (under the mucosa), where it produces eggs that are coughed and swallowed. Eggs passing out with the faeces will embryonate and enter a new host via contaminated food or water (Gutierrez 1990).

3.6 Transmission and epidemiology

C. PHILIPPINENSIS

The diet and eating habits of indigenous populations living in areas such as the Philippines and Thailand have been implicated in the transmission of intestinal capillariasis. For example, the Ilocanos of Northern Luzon use the intestinal juices from animals to season rice and typically consume whole freshwater fish uncooked (Cross 1992). Since the original reports of widespread intestinal capillariasis in the Philippines and in Thailand (Pradatsundararar et al. 1973), infection with *C. philippinensis* has been subsequently reported from other parts of Asia, including Japan (Nawa et al. 1988), Indonesia (Chichino et al. 1992, Bangs et al. 1994) and India (Kang et al. 1994), as well as from non-endemic areas such as Iran, Egypt and South America (Dronda et al. 1993).

C. HEPATICA

Probably because of its broad host specificity, there is a wide distribution of animal and human hepatic capillariasis. Cases have been reported from the Americas, Europe, Asia and Africa. Humans may be at high risk for *C. hepatica* infection in Zaire, Nigeria and other parts of West Africa where they consume the Gambian rat or cricetoma (Malekani et al. 1994).

C. AEROPHILA

Like *C. hepatica*, C. aerophila is a worldwide parasite of wild carnivores. Human infections have been reported primarily from Russia, although other cases have been reported from Morocco and Iran.

3.7 Location in host

C. PHILIPPINENSIS

In heavy infections, all stages of *C. philippinensis* can be found in the small intestine, particularly the jejunum. Extraintestinal *C. philippinensis* infection is a rare occurrence.

C. HEPATICA

The adult worms live in a host-derived capsule within the liver where they feed on cytoplasmic debris.

C. AEROPHILA

The adult worms live beneath the mucosa of the upper and lower respiratory tree.

4 CLINICAL AND PATHOLOGICAL ASPECTS OF INFECTION

C. philippinensis can be one of the most virulent helminthic pathogens of humans, with extremely high mortality rates during epidemics of intestinal capillariasis. Parasite virulence can be largely ascribed to the ability of the worm to cause hyperinfection.

Extraintestinal infections caused by other members of the genus *Capillaria* are relatively rare. Only about 30 cases of human hepatic capillariasis caused by *C. hepatica* have been reported, although the potential for transmission of this zoonosis may be high in some areas (Malekani et al. 1994). Zoonotic transmissions of *C. aerophila* and *C. plica* are probably very rare, as reflected by only a handful of case reports in the medical literature.

4.1 Clinical manifestations

C. PHILIPPINENSIS (INTESTINAL CAPILLARIASIS)

There is no evidence for asymptomatic intestinal capillariasis. Patients usually develop diarrhoea and abdominal pain that may progress in intensity. Borborygmi is a common presenting sign of intestinal capillariasis. Dehydration resulting from intestinal fluid losses is exacerbated by vomiting and anorexia. Infections lasting 2–3 months result in a severe protein-losing enteropathy characterized by cachexia, dehydration and anasarca. Death is often the outcome in patients who do not receive adequate fluid resuscitation, nutritional supplementation and anthelmintic chemotherapy. These patients often die from electrolyte disturbances that contribute to heart malfunction, as well as secondary bacterial superinfections and sepsis (Cross 1995).

C. HEPATICA (HEPATIC CAPILLARIASIS)

Heavy infections may cause an acute or subacute hepatitis accompanied by peritonitis, ascites and eosinophilia.

C. AEROPHILA (PULMONARY CAPILLARIASIS)

Heavy infections cause a tracheobronchitis accompanied by dyspnoea, dry cough, mild haemoptysis and pulmonary infiltrates (Gutierrez 1990).

4.2   Pathogenesis and pathology

C. PHILIPPINENSIS

The protein-losing enteropathy of intestinal capillariasis is a result of direct mucosal invasion by the adult worms, which is sometimes exacerbated by the host inflammatory response. Although the intestinal tract frequently has a gross normal appearance, a histopathological examination of the intestine from human autopsies reveals villus flattening and dilated crypts, with occasional inflammatory infiltrates (Cross 1995); numerous adult and larval worms can be identified in the intestinal mucosa where they are associated with ulcerative and degenerative changes. Nothing is known about the molecular and cellular events associated with *C. philippinensis* invasion, although the parasite may secrete bioactive molecules similar to those of *Trichuris*, which releases a proteolytic enzyme and a pore-forming protein from their stichosome (Drake et al. 1994).

C. HEPATICA

In hepatic capillariasis there is a remarkable degree of fibrosis in the liver (Attah et al. 1983). Histopathological examination reveals areas of focal destruction and numerous granulomata consisting of mononuclear cells and eosinophils. Many of these inflammatory changes occur at the site of worms and eggs. The adult worm is frequently identified by the characteristic presence of the stichosome on histological section. The eggs frequently appear in clusters.

C. AEROPHILA

A single case report of a biopsy in pulmonary capillariasis demonstrated numerous granulomas within the bronchiolar wall, producing marked airway destruction (Aftandelians et al. 1977). The parasite was identified in tissue sections (Gutierrez 1990).

4.3   Immune responses

Very little has been published on the immune responses to human capillariasis. Patients infected with *C. philippinensis* acquire humoral antibodies, including circulating immunoglobulin E (Rosenberg et al. 1970).

4.4   Diagnosis

C. PHILIPPINENSIS

In epidemic situations, patients who present with diarrhoea, borborygmi and abdominal pain are presumed to have intestinal capillariasis. The definitive diagnosis is usually made by identifying the characteristic-shaped eggs in the stool, although in severe hyperinfection it is not uncommon to also find larvae or even adult worms (Cross 1995). For lightly infected patients a number of concentration techniques are available in order to increase the sensitivity of faecal examination.

C. HEPATICA

The clinical manifestations of human *C. hepatica* infection can resemble those of visceral larva migrans caused by *Toxocara canis*. A definitive diagnosis can be made by demonstrating the presence of eggs, larvae or adults in liver biopsy specimens. Usually, there is extensive accompanying hepatic fibrosis (Gutierrez 1990).

C. AEROPHILA

Conceivably, parasite eggs may be demonstrated in sputum or faeces, although a pulmonary biopsy may be required to establish the diagnosis definitively (Aftandelians et al. 1977).

4.5   Control

C. PHILIPPINENSIS

Anthelmintics of the benzimidazole class, namely albendazole and mebendazole, are the treatments of choice for intestinal capillariasis. Mebendazole treatment usually requires 200 mg twice daily for 20 days, or albendazole 200 mg twice daily for 10 days (Medical Letter 1995). Relapses can occur with either agent, so that the patient must be followed and retreated for longer periods if necessary. Mebendazole is thought to be less active against the larval stages of the parasite and therefore may require longer treatment regimens (Cross 1995). Outpatient management of patients with intestinal capillariasis is often unsatisfactory because of the need for supporting therapy and the possibility of relapse following treatment. Cross (1995) points out that patients receiving specific anthelmintic therapy are often poorly compliant as outpatients, particularly with regard to receiving a full treatment course. Therapy must therefore be closely monitored, preferably in an in-patient setting. Patients need to be educated on the dangers of eating uncooked small fish, especially in endemic areas. The sanitary disposal of faeces will also reduce parasite transmission.

C. hepatica AND *C. aerophila*

Little is known about the efficacy of specific anthelmintic therapy for human infections with either of these 2 parasites. Because mebendazole is poorly absorbed outside the gastrointestinal tract, high doses would presumably be needed to achieve a therapeutic effect. Albendazole or thiabendazole may also be effective.

REFERENCES

Adam M, Morgan O et al., 1973, Hyperinfection syndrome with *Strongyloides stercoralis* in malignant lymphoma, *Br Med J*, **1:** 264–6.

Aftandelians R, Raafat F et al., 1977, Pulmonary capillariasis in a child in Iran, *Am J Trop Med Hyg*, **26:** 64–71.

Anderson RC, 1992, *Nematode Parasites of Vertebrates, Their Development and Transmission*, CAB International, Wallingford, Oxon, 544–50.

Arthur RP, Shelley WB, 1958, Larva currens: a distinct variant of cutaneous larva migrans due to *Strongyloides stercoralis*, *Arch Dermatol*, **78:** 186–90.

Ashford RW, Barnish, G, 1990, *Strongyloides fuelleborni* and similar parasites in animals and man, *Strongyloidiasis: A Major Roundworm Infection of Man*, ed Grove DI, Taylor and Francis, London, 271–86.

Ashton FT, Bhopale VM et al., 1995, Sensory neuroanatomy of a skin-penetrating nematode parasite: *Strongyloides stercoralis*. I. Amphidial neurons, *J Comp Neurol*, **357:** 281–95.

Attah EB, Nagarajan S et al., 1983, Hepatic capillariasis, *Am J Clin Pathol*, **79:** 127–30.

Bangs MJ, Purnomo, Andersen EM, 1994, A case of capillariasis in a highland community of Irian Jaya, Indonesia, *Ann Trop Med Parasitol*, **88:** 685–7.

Barnish G, Ashford RW, 1989, *Strongyloides fuelleborni* and hookworm in Papua New Guinea: patterns of infection within the community, *Trans R Soc Trop Med Hyg*, **83:** 684–8.

Barnish G, Barker J, 1987, An intervention study using thiabendazole suspension *against Strongyloides fuelleborni*-like infections in Papua New Guinea, *Trans R Soc Trop Med Hyg*, **81:** 60–3.

Bavay A, 1876, Sur l'anguillule stercorale, *C R Acad Sci, Paris*, **83:** 694–6.

Beal CB, Viens P et al., 1970, A new technique for sampling duodenal contents, *Am J Trop Med Hyg*, **19:** 349–52.

Berenson CS, Dobuler KJ, Bia, FJ, 1987, Fever, petechiae, and pulmonary infiltrates in an immunocompromised Peruvian man, *Yale J Biol Med*, **60:** 437–45.

Berk SL, Verghese A et al., 1987, Clinical and epidemiologic features of strongyloidiasis, *Arch Intern Med*, **147:** 1257–61.

Bhatt BD, Cappell MS et al., 1990, Recurrent massive upper gastrointestinal hemorrhage due *to Strongyloides stercoralis* infection, *Am J Gastroenterol*, **85:** 1034–6.

Borucinska JD, Nielsen SW, 1993, Hepatic capillariasis in muskrats (*Ondatra zibethicus*), *J Wildlife Dis*, **29:** 518–20.

Braun TI, Fekete T, Lynch A, 1989, Strongyloidiasis in an institution for mentally retarded adults, *Arch Intern Med 1*, **48:** 634.

Brindley PJ, Gam AA et al., 1995, Ss40: the zinc endopeptidase secreted by infective larvae *of Strongyloides stercoralis*, *Exp Parasitol*, **80:** 1–7.

Brown RC, Girardeau MHF, 1977, Transmammary passage of *Strongyloides* sp. larvae in the human host, *Am J Trop Med Hyg*, **26:** 215–19.

Burke JA, 1978, Strongyloides in childhood, *Am J Dis Child*, **132:** 1130–6.

Cappello M, Hotez PJ, 1993, Disseminated strongyloidiasis, *Sem Neurol*, **13:** 169–74.

Carroll SM, Karthigasu DT et al., 1981, Serodiagnosis of human strongyloidiasis by an enzyme-linked immunosorbent assay, *Trans R Soc Trop Med Hyg*, **75:** 706–9.

Celedon JC, Mathur-Waugh U et al., 1994, Systemic strongyloidiasis in patients infected with the human immunodeficiency virus, *Medicine*, **73:** 256–63.

Chichino G, Bernuzzi AM et al., 1992, Intestinal capillariasis (*Capillaria philippinensis*) acquired in Indonesia: a case report, *Am J Trop Med Hyg*, **47:** 10–12.

Chitwood MB, Valasquez C, Salazar NG, 1968, *Capillaria philippinensis* sp. n. (Nematoda: Trichinellida) from intestine of man in the Philippines, *J Parasitol*, **54:** 368–71.

Chu EC, Whitlock WL, Dietrich RA, 1990, Pulmonary hyperinfection syndrome with *Strongyloides stercoralis*, *Chest*, **97:** 1475–7.

Civantos F, Robinson MJ, 1969, Fatal strongyloidiasis following corticosteroid therapy, *Am J Dis Dis*, **14:** 643–51.

Cookson JB, Montgomery RD et al., 1990, Fatal paralytic ileus due to strongyloidiasis, *Br Med J*, **4:** 771–2.

Cross JH, 1992, Intestinal capillariasis, *Clin Microbiol Rev*, **5:** 120–9.

Cross JH, 1995, *Capillaria philippinensis* and *Trichostrongylus orientalis*, *Enteric Infection 2, Intestinal Helminths*, eds Farthing MJG, Keusch GT, Wakelin D, Chapman & Hall Medical, London, 151–64.

Cross JH, Basaca-Sevilla V, 1983, Experimental transmission of *Capillaria philippinensis* to birds, *Trans R Soc Trop Med Hyg*, **77:** 511–14.

Cross JH, Banzon TC et al., 1972, Studies on the experimental transmission of *Capillaria philippinensis* in monkeys, *Trans Roy Soc Trop Med Hyg*, **66:** 819–27.

Dafalla AA, 1972, The indirect fluorescent antibody test for the serodiagnosis of strongyloidiasis, *J Trop Med Hyg*, **75:** 109–11.

Dees A, Batenburg PL et al., 1990, *Strongyloides stercoralis* associated with a bleeding gastric ulcer, *Gut*, **31:** 1414–15.

Detels RL, Gutman L et al., 1969, An epidemic of human intestinal capillariasis: a study in a barrio in North Luzon, *Am J Trop Med Hyg*, **18:** 676–82.

Dixon AC, Yanaghihara ET et al., 1989, Strongyloidiasis associated with human T-cell lymphotropic virus type 1 infection in a nonendemic area, *West J Med*, **151:** 410–13.

Drake L, Korchev et al., 1994, The major secreted product of the whipworm *Trichuris*, is a pore-forming protein, *Proc R Soc London B*, **257:** 255–61.

Dronda F, Chaves F et al., 1993, Human intestinal capillariasis in an area of nonendemicity: case report and review, *Clin Infect Dis*, **17:** 909–12.

Faust EC, 1933, The development of *Strongyloides* in the experimental host, *Am J Hyg*, **18:** 114–32.

Fuelleborn F, 1914, Untersuchungen uber den Infektionsweg bei *Strongyloides* und *Ankylostomum* und die biologie dieser parasiten, *Arch Schiffs-u Tropenhyg*, **18, Beih. 5:** 26: 80.

Gam AA, Neva FA, Drotoski WA, 1987, Comparitive sensitivity and specificity of ELISA and IHA for serodiagnosis of strongyloidiasis with larval antigens, *Am J Trop Med Hyg*, **37:** 157–61.

Gann PH, Neva FA, Gam AA, 1994, A randomized trial of single and two-dose ivermectin versus thiabendazole for treatment of strongyloidiasis, *J Infect Dis*, **169:** 1076–79.

Genta RM, 1989, Global prevalence of strongyloidiasis: Critical review with epidemiologic insights into the prevention of disseminated disease, *Rev Infect Dis*, **11:** 755–67.

Genta RM, 1992, Dysregulation of strongyloidiasis: a new hypothesis, *Clin Microbiol Rev*, **5:** 345–55.

Genta RM, von Kuster LC, 1988, Cutaneous manifestations of strongyloidiasis, *Arch Dermatol*, **124:** 1826–30.

Genta RM, von Kuster LC, 1989, Cutaneous manifestations of strongyloidiasis, *Arch Dermatol*, **124:** 1826–30.

Genta RM, Walzer PD, 1989, Strongyloidiasis, *Parasitic Infections in the Compromised Host*, eds Walzer PD, Genta RM, Marcel Dekker, New York, 463–525.

Genta RM, Weesner R et al., 1987, Strongyloidiasis in US veterans of the Vietnam and other wars, *JAMA*, **258:** 49–52.

Georgi JR, Sprinkle CL, 1974, A case of human strongyloidiasis apparently contracted from asymptomatic colony dogs, *Am J Trop Med Hyg*, **23:** 899–901.

Goldsmid JM, Davies N, 1978, Diagnosis of parasitic infections of the small intestine by the enterotest duodenal capsule, *Med J Aust*, **1:** 519–20.

Gompels MM, Todd J et al., 1991, Disseminated strongyloidiasis in AIDS: uncommon but important, *AIDS*, **5:** 329–32.

Grove DI, 1982, Treatment of strongyloidiasis with thiabendazole: an analysis of toxicity and effectiveness, *Trans R Soc Trop Med Hyg*, **76:** 114–18.

Gutierrez Y, 1990, *Diagnostic Pathology of Parasitic Infections with Clinical Correlations*, Lea and Febiger, Philadelphia, PA.

Hill JA, 1988, Strongyloidiasis in ex-Far East prisoners of war, *Br Med J*, **296:** 753.

Igra-Siegman Y, Kapila R et al., 1981, Syndrome of hyperinfection with *Strongyloides stercoralis*, *Rev Infect Dis*, **3:** 397–407.

Kalb RE, Grossman ME, 1986, Periumbilical purpura in disseminated strongyloidiasis, *JAMA*, **256:** 1170–1.

Kang G, Mathan M et al., 1994, Human intestinal capillariasis: first report from India, *Trans R Soc Trop Med Hyg*, **88:** 204–5.

Kramer MR, Gregg PA et al., 1990, Disseminated strongyloidiasis in AIDS and non-AIDS immunocompromised hosts: diagnosis by sputum and bronchoalveolar lavage, *South Med J*, **83:** 1226–9.

Kuberski TT, Gabor EP, Boudreaux D, 1975, Disseminated strongyloidiasis: a complication of the immunosuppressed host West, *J Med*, **122:** 504–8.

Lyagoubi M, Datry et al., 1992, Chronic persistent strongyloidiasis cured by ivermectin, *Trans R Soc Trop Med Hyg*, **86:** 541.

Malekani M, Kumar V, Pandey VS, 1994, Hepatic capillariasis in edible *Cricetomys* spp. (Rodentia: Cricetidae) in Zaire and its possible public health implications, *Ann Trop Med Parasitol*, **88:** 569–72.

Medical Letter, 1995, Drugs for parasitic infections, *Medical Letter on Drugs and Therapeutics*, **37 (Issue 961).**

Meltzer RS, Singer C et al., 1979, Antemortem diagnosis of central nervous system strongyloidiasis, *Am J Med Sci*, **277:** 91–8.

Milder JE, Walzer PD et al., 1981, Clinical features of *Strongyloides stercoralis* infection in an endemic area of the United States, *Gastroenterology*, **80:** 1481–8.

Moncol DJ, Triantaphyllou AC, 1978, *Strongyloides ransomi*: factors influencing the in vitro development of the free living generation, *J Parasitol*, **64:** 220–5.

Naquira C, Jimenez G et al., 1989, Ivermectin for human strongyloidiasis and other intestinal helminths, *Am J Trop Med Hyg*, **403:** 304–9.

Nawa Y et al., 1988, A case report of intestinal capillariasis. The second case found in Japan, *Jpn J Parasitol*, **37:** 113–18.

Neefe LI, Pinilla O et al., 1973, Disseminated strongyloidiasis with cerebral involvement, *Am J Med*, **55:** 832–8.

Neefe LI, Owor R, Wamukota WM, 1976, A fatal case of strongyloidiasis with strongyloides larvae in the meninges, *Trans R Soc Trop Med Hyg*, **70:** 497–9.

Neva F, 1986, Biology and immunology of human strongyloidiasis, *J Infect Dis*, **153:** 397–406.

Nishigori M, 1928, The factors which influence the external development of *Strongyloides stercoralis* and on autoinfection with this parasite, *J Form Med Assn*, **276:** 1–56.

Normand A, 1876, Sur la maladie dite diarrhée de Cochin-Chine, *C R Acad Sci Paris*, **83:** 316–18.

O'Brien W, 1975, Intestinal malabsorption in acute infection with *Strongyloides stercoralis*, *Trans R Soc Trop Med Hyg*, **69:** 69–77.

Onuigbo MAC, Ibeachum GI, 1991, *Strongyloides stercoralis* larvae in peripheral blood, *Trans R Soc Trop Med Hyg*, **85:** 97.

Pradatsundarasar A, Pecharanond K et al., 1973, The first case of intestinal capillariasis in Thailand, *Southeast Asian J Trop Med Public Health*, **4:** 131–4.

Robinson RD, Lindo JF et al., 1994, Immunoepidemiologic studies of Strongyloides stercoralis and human T lymphotropic virus type I infections in Jamaica, *J Infect Dis*, **169:** 692–6.

Ronan SG, Reddy RL et al., 1989, Disseminated strongyloidiasis presenting as purpura, *J Am Acad Dermatol*, **21:** 1123–5.

Rosenberg EB, Whalen GE et al., 1970, Increased circulating IgE in a new parasitic disease – human intestinal capillariasis, *N Engl J Med*, **283:** 1148–9.

Schad GA, 1990, Morphology and life history of *Strongyloides stercoralis*, *Strongyloidiasis: A Major Roundworm Infection of Man*, ed DI Grove, Taylor and Francis, London, 85–104.

Schad GA, Aikens LM, Smith G, 1989, *Strongyloides stercoralis*: is there a canonical migratory route through the host?, *J Parasitol*, **75:** 740–9.

Skrjabin KE, Shikhobalova NP, Orlov IV, 1957 [1970], *Essentials of Nematology, Trichocephalidae and Capillariidae of Animals and Man and the Diseases Caused by them*, vol. VI, Academy of Sciences of the USSR, Israel Program for Scientific Translations, Jerusalem.

Soulsby EJL, 1982, Helminths, *Arthropods and Protozoa of Domesticated Animals*, 7th edn, Lea and Febiger, Philadelphia, PA.

Sukhavat K, Morakote N, Chaiwong P, Piangjai S, 1994, Comparative efficacy of four methods for the detection of *Strongyloides stercoralis* in human stool specimens, *Ann Trop Med Parasitol*, **88:** 95–6.

Torres JR, Isturiz R et al., 1994, Efficacy of ivermectin in the treatment of strongyloidiasis complicating AIDS, *Clin Infect Dis*, **17:** 900–2.

Willis AJ, Nwokolo C, 1966, Steroid therapy and strongyloidiasis, *Lancet*, **1:** 1396–8.

Wright KA, 1974, The feeding site and probable feeding mechanism of the parasitic nematode *Capillaria* hepatica (Bancroft, 1893), *Can J Zool*, **52:** 1215–20.

Wright KA, Lee DL, Shivers RR, 1985, A freeze-fracture study of the digestive tract of the parasitic nematode *Trichinella*, *Tissue Cell*, **17:** 189–98.

Chapter 31

TRICHINELLA AND TOXOCARA

D D Despommier

TRICHINELLA

1 THE PARASITE

Trichinella spiralis muscle larvae were first observed in 1835 by James Paget and Richard Owen at the British Museum using a borrowed microscope (Campbell 1983a). The muscle tissue was from a 51 year old mason who had died of tuberculosis, but who had also been infected with *T. spiralis* some years before his death. By the 1860s, its life cycle had been discovered by the famous German pathologist, Rudolph Virchow (Virchow 1859), and today most of its natural history and biology is known (see Campbell 1983b). Epidemiological and molecular biological studies (Pozio 1992) have given rise to the view that there is more than one species of trichinella, possibly as many as 5, and these studies represent a new avenue of interest for this now well-known worm. However, because of the low prevalance of these other related entities (e.g. *Trichinella pseudospiralis*; Andrews et al. 1994), only *T. spiralis* and its clinical consequences of infection will be emphasized in this chapter.

1.1 Morphology and structure

T. spiralis adult male and female worms can be distinguished by their morphology (Figs 31.1 and 31.2).

The female measures approximately 3 mm in length by 36 μm in diameter, while the male measures 1.5 mm in length by 36 μm in diameter. The male has a set of reproductive organs at its tail end termed claspers that it uses to hold on to the female worm during mating. Claspers can be easily seen and, in addition to size differences, provide an easy way to distinguish the sexes. The newborn larva (Fig. 31.3) measures 80 μm in length by 7–8 μm in diameter. Its oesophagus has a stylet (i.e. spear-like) organ (Fig. 31.4) which it

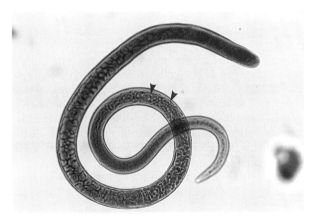

Fig. 31.1 Adult female *Trichinella spiralis*. Note the presence of numerous newborn larvae in her uterus (arrows). The parasite was fixed in osmium tetroxide, then dehydrated in a graded series of alcohols and embedded in epon. It measures 3 mm in length by 36 μm in diameter.

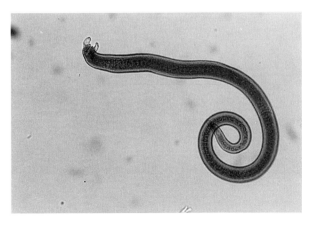

Fig. 31.2 Male adult *Trichinella spiralis*. This worm was prepared as described in Fig. 31.1. It measures 1.5 mm in length by 36 μm in diameter.

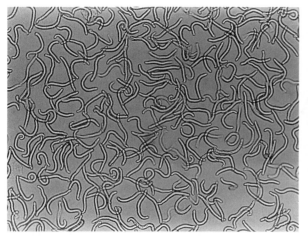

Fig. 31.3 Newborn larvae of *Trichinella spiralis* in maintenance culture. Each worm measures 80 μm in length by 7 μm in diameter. Unstained, living preparation.

uses to penetrate cells (Fig. 31.5). The infective muscle larva (Fig. 31.6) measures 1 mm in length by 36 μm in diameter.

1.2 General biology

Adult worms live in the upper part of the small intestine embedded in the cellular matrix of a row of epithelial cells. There they live as aerobic organisms, deriving nutrients from the host by an as yet unknown mechanism. They do not ingest host tissue directly, but probably transport small molecular weight nutrients across their cuticular surface or through their hypodermal gland cells.

The muscle larva (a precocious L1 stage worm) lives in an equally unique niche, inside a modified skeletal muscle cell, the Nurse cell (see Fig. 31.7). Thus, it, too, lives intracellularly, but carries out its metabolism as a strict anaerobe. Some details of its intermediary metabolism are known as the larvae are easy to obtain in large numbers (Stewart 1983).

Four larval stages of *T.spiralis* develop from the

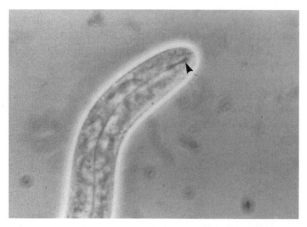

Fig. 31.4 The retracted stylet of the newborn larva (arrow). Phase contrast microscopy. Unstained, living preparation.

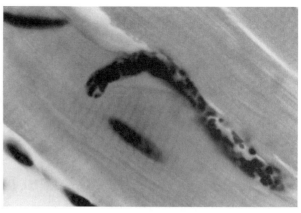

Fig. 31.5 A newborn larva of *Trichinella spiralis* penetrating a striated skeletal muscle fibre. The tissue was fixed in 10% formalin moments after the newborn larvae were injected into a mouse leg muscle bundle. Note the clean appearance of the entry hole and the separation of the contractile fibres adjacent to the larva. Judging by the deformation in the pattern of contractile elements in the above fibre, the larva most likely used it to push against in order to launch its penetration attack on the fibre below. Haematoxylin and eosin stain of a paraffin-embedded histological section.

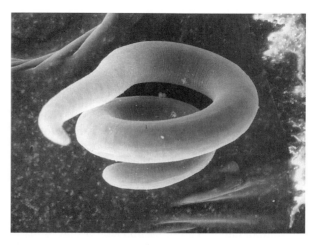

Fig. 31.6 Scanning electron micrograph of a fully grown L1 infective larva of *Trichinella spiralis*. It was isolated from an infected mouse by digestion in pepsin–HCl and had retained its spiral shape at the moment of fixation. This worm measures 1 mm in length by 36 μm in diameter.

ingested first stage muscle larva. All live in the small intestine but exist for only a short time (less than 30 h), transforming rapidly through each stage to adults in that niche. Morphogenic change is accompanied by a dramatic change in metabolism from anaerobic to aerobic in just 24 h. Throughout the process, they do not change their overall dimensions until they achieve adulthood, when they grow longer, but remain the same diameter. This feature alone makes this species unusual in the nematode world.

The newborn larva (Fig. 31.3) is the migratory stage of the infection. It travels from the small intestine to the muscle tissue, but also invades other tissues. For this reason, this stage is considered the most patho-

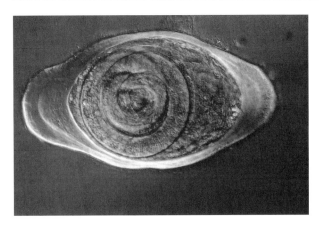

Fig. 31.7 The Nurse cell–parasite complex. The Nurse cell measures 200 µm. Nomarski-phase interference microscopy. (By courtesy of Eric Grave.)

genic, since it kills all cells it enters except striated skeletal muscle cells. For example, most of the significant clinical signs and symptoms of this parasite are induced by this stage (Capo and Despommier 1996). Its metabolism is anaerobic, but few studies on this aspect have been carried out on newborn larvae owing to the difficulty in obtaining them in large numbers.

1.3   Life cycle

When infected muscle tissue containing larvae in their Nurse cells is ingested, larvae are released in the stomach by the action of digestive enzymes, and the freed worms are transported to the upper two-thirds of the small intestine. There they penetrate into the epithelium, and after undergoing 4 moults during a 30 h period, mature to adults (see Fig. 31.8). Five days after infection, females begin depositing larvae (Fig. 31.9). Larvae are born continuously throughout the next 5 days, resulting in a total of more than 1000 newborns from each female worm. Intestinal trichinellosis can last up to 2–3 weeks, but ultimately adult worms are expelled by immune responses in which, at least in experimental animals, inflammatory responses play a central role. The protective immune mechanisms of humans are not known.

Newborn worms enter the lamina propria and from there penetrate the mesenteric lymphatics and blood stream (Wang and Bell 1986). All newborn worms ultimately find the general circulation and become distributed to all tissues. It is of interest that this stage of the infection is associated with bacteraemia caused by enteric flora, and deaths due to sepsis have been reported. Larvae emerge from capillaries and penetrate cells, and as a result those cells die. Remarkably, skeletal muscle fibres are the exception as they alone provide the proper conditions to support the growth and development of the parasite (Despommier 1990, Jasmer 1995). Within 20 days after entering the muscle cell, the larvae have altered their environment, creating the Nurse cell, which functions as a life support system for the parasite (Despommier 1993). Little is known regarding the molecular events leading to

Nurse cell formation, but it is thought that the worm interacts directly with the genome of the host through its secretions to produce this symbiotic relationship (Despommier et al. 1990). Larvae survive in their Nurse cells for months to years, but eventually most become calcified and die. Larvae that penetrate tissues other than striated skeletal muscle cannot induce this specialized cell and thus either re-enter the circulation or die.

1.4   Transmission and epidemiology

Eating meat is the usual way of acquiring infection with *Trichinella spiralis* (Campbell 1983). For this reason, most animals in nature have been found to harbour the infection in some form (i.e. either with *T. spiralis* itself or with related species). In humans, the current prevalence of infection with *T. spiralis* in North America, Europe and Asia cannot be estimated because there are no recent surveys, but sporadic epidemics occur with some regularity (Capo and Despommier 1996). Within the last 10–15 years, outbreaks have occurred in China, Japan, and the Middle East (Olaison and Ljungstrom 1992). Apparently, Puerto Rico and mainland Australia have no trichinella infections in either humans or in wild animals. *Trichinella pseudospiralis* is thought mainly to infect birds, but can also infect mammals. It has been isolated from Tasmania in the only remaining native carnivore, the Tasmanian Devil (Obendorf et al. 1990). A single human case has also been reported (Andrews et al. 1994).

Two other species of *Trichinella* have regional medical importance; *T. nativa* occurs in the Canadian Arctic where the major reservoir hosts are polar bears and walruses, and *T. nelsoni* causes trichinellosis in equatorial Africa with hyenas and large cats serving as reservoir hosts.

2   CLINICAL AND PATHOLOGICAL ASPECTS OF INFECTION

2.1   Clinical manifestations

ENTERIC STAGES

Trichinellosis is often mistaken for many other non-related clinical syndromes, and is thus frequently misdiagnosed. Nonetheless, specific signs and symptoms can help the physician make a proper diagnosis, even in early stages of the disease. For the duration of the 3 week period of the intestinal infection, patients can suffer many effects related to the damage that occurs there. Development of larvae to adults in the columnar epithelium is associated with enteritis. As newborn larvae are shed (i.e. 5–21 days after infection), mucosal inflammation intensifies, with inflammation consisting of eosinophils, neutrophils and lymphocytes. Antigen–antibody complexes develop in the surrounding tissues and probably also contribute to intestinal disease experienced by patients who have ingested large numbers of larvae.

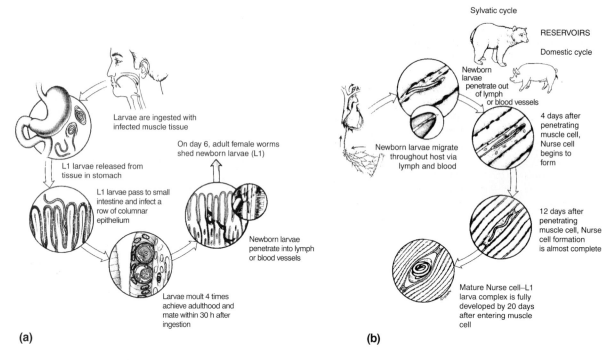

Fig. 31.8 Life cycle of *Trichinella spiralis*: (a) enteric stages; (b) parenteral stages.

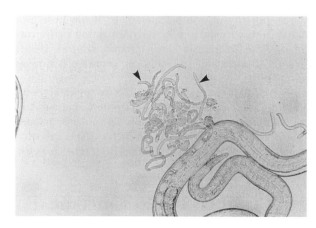

Fig. 31.9 A 'squash' preparation of a gravid female. Newborn larvae (arrows) were expressed from the worm's uterus.

PARENTERAL STAGES

Damage caused by larvae penetrating cells becomes serious when this occurs in cardiac and central nervous system (CNS) tissues. Myocarditis, sometimes severe enough to cause death, is transient as Nurse cells cannot form in heart tissue. In the CNS, larvae tend to stay and wander about, frequently causing significant damage even in mild infection.

In skeletal muscle fibres, parasite-secreted proteins and other antigens induce progressive infiltration of inflammatory cells. Myositis and tissue oedema develop on or about 14 days after penetration of the fibre. The amount of pathological change caused by the larvae is directly proportional to the number shed in the small intestine. However, there is much variation in the clinical presentation, related mostly to the type of muscle affected and the species of trichinella causing the damage. Lethal infection for most adults is of the order of 15 *T. spiralis* larvae per gram of diaphragmatic muscle, whereas as many as 1000 *T. nelsoni* parasites per gram of muscle are still well tolerated.

Heavy to moderate trichinellosis presents signs and symptoms in the early (intestinal), middle (systemic and tissue invasion), and late (convalescent) phases (Murrell and Bruschi 1994, Capo and Despommier 1996). Early intestinal distress (in. weeks 1–3) is associated with diarrhoea, abdominal pain, and vomiting. The systemic and tissue invasion phase (weeks 3–8) is accompanied by fever and myalgia, periorbital oedema, and haemorrhages in the nail beds and sclera of the eye, but can also seen in the mucous membranes. Oedema leads to muscle tenderness and pain. Photophobia is another consequence of heavy infection.

Progressive infection, in which larvae penetrate a variety of tissues, gives rise to even more serious and often confusing sequelae. Myocarditis occurs in nearly 20% of seriously ill patients and electrocardiographic changes are frequently noted during this phase. Dyspnoea is another complication of myositis. Neurological signs and symptoms vary greatly, but, coupled with other laboratory findings and a history of raw meat eating, should lead the alert physician to suspect infection with trichinella.

There is no evidence that long-term sequelae occur following even severe infection, at least with *Trichinella spiralis* (Feldmeier et al. 1991). However, from the worm's perspective there are long-term consequences, since numerous Nurse cells calcify and, as a result, the larvae inside them perish. This process usually takes place over several months to years following infection.

Whereas disease caused by other species of *Trichinella* present somewhat differently (Murrell and Bruschi 1994, Capo and Despommier 1996), details are unwarranted because of their low prevalence.

2.2 Pathogenesis and pathology

Most of the signs and symptoms (i.e. pathological consequences) of trichinellosis are caused by the migrating newborn larvae. Their ability to penetrate any cell and their non-specificity for various tissues in the body account for their pathogenicity. Cell death is associated with inflammation and subsequent granuloma formation which are the most significant pathological features of trichinellosis. Granulomata are composed of macrophages, neutrophils and eosinophils, and lymphocytes of various subsets (Wakelin and Denham 1983). The presence of these cells concentrated in a given region of a histological section of tissue should lead the pathologist to the parasite, even if the offending organism is not seen in that particular section of muscle (Fig. 31.10).

Symptoms caused by the enteric stages of the parasite (i.e. L1–L4 and the adult worm) presumably result from exposure of the host to the secretions of those stages. However, it is not known what pharmacological properties the secretions of the enteral stages possess that induce diarrhoeal disease (Despommier 1995), and this area represents a direction in research that parasitologists have yet to pursue. Damage to the enterocytes of the small intestine is transitory, yet some effects of the infection last well beyond the presence of the parasite, at least in experimental infections (Castro and Powell 1994). For example, animals infected with *T. spiralis* permanently lose their wheatgerm agglutinin binding sites along the brush border of the entire epithelium (Harari and Castro 1988), whereas other changes reverse completely (e.g. myenteric electric potential, peristalsis and secretory dysfunction; Castro and Powell 1994).

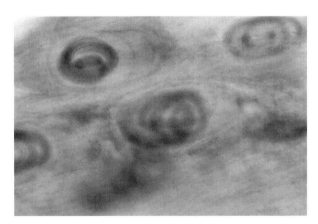

Fig. 31.10 A whole mounted biopsy of a piece of muscle containing numerous Nurse cell–parasite complexes. The maturity of each Nurse cell indicates that this is an old infection and is probably not the cause of the patient's current illness. Unstained preparation.

2.3 Immune responses

Most immune responses elicited during infection are non-protective and some even result in pathological changes and damage the host (Garside and Grencis 1992, Wakelin 1997). Each stage possesses unique secretory proteins which are highly antigenic (Silberstein 1983, Wakelin and Denham 1983, Gold et al. 1990) because of the presence of a unique sugar residue, tyvelose (Wisenewski, McNeil and Grieve 1993), and antigenic constitutive components, such as the cuticle (Despommier et al. 1967, Philipp et al. 1980). Immune responses are often intense and involve components of the humoral and cellular immune systems regulated by T helper lymphocytes (both Th 1 and Th 2) (Wakelin and Denham 1983, Despommier 1988, Curman, Pond and Nashold 1992, Murrell and Bruschi 1994, Capo and Despommier 1996) In consequence, many valid immunodiagnostic tests exist for this pathogen (Ljungstrom 1983).

In experimental animals, some forms of protective immunity (e.g. rapid expulsion in rats) are thought to result from a combination of responses, including eosinophils and antibodies of the IgE class (Ahmed, Wang and Bell 1991). This response, although well characterized, applies only to re-infection and is not the one responsible for adult worm expulsion from a primary infection. In the latter instance, adult worms are forced out of their multi-intracellular niche in the small intestine by changes that are possibly mediated by antibodies (Love, Ogilvie and McLaren 1976) and by inflammation and take up temporary residence in similar sites in the large intestine. This is followed shortly by their complete elimination from the host (Larsh 1952, 1970). Worms thus expelled are not killed by immunity, however, and are capable of re-infection if swallowed immediately by a naive animal.

2.4 Diagnosis

If trichinellosis is suspected, a positive diagnosis can be made as follows:

1 Demonstration of larvae in muscle by biopsy (Fig. 31.11). This is the most direct measure of infection, but larvae that have not yet developed fully are easily missed and light infections lead to low numbers of muscle larvae which can also be missed on biopsy. Digestion of the muscle tissue in 1% pepsin–1% HCl makes larvae easier to identify but young ones may be digested and thus are missed during microscopic examination.

2 Identification of a history of eating raw or undercooked meat of any kind, but particularly pork or pork products.

3 Consistent laboratory findings such as an elevated circulating eosinophilia (Murrell and Bruschi 1994, Capo and Despommier 1996) and antibody detected by enzyme-linked immunosorbent assay (ELISA) (Ljungstrom 1983).

Immunological tests can become positive as early as 2 weeks after infection. Counterimmunoelectrophoresis and ELISA can detect antibodies in some patients as

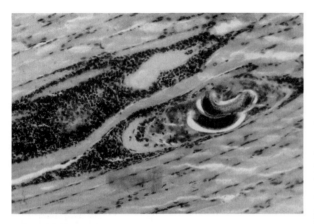

Fig. 31.11 Section through a piece of infected muscle tissue. A Nurse cell–parasite complex is seen in the middle of the photomicrograph, while an intense granulomatous response is noted around both it and in the muscle tissue above it. If another section through the tissue were to be made, most likely a worm would be observed in the upper granulomatous region, as well. Haematoxylin eosin stained section of a paraffin-embedded piece of infected muscle tissue.

early as 12 days after infection (Ljungstrom 1983). These tests remain positive for months to years after the patient has recovered, so a positive test alone is insufficient to rule in this parasite as the cause of the present illness. In patients with moderate to severe disease, muscle enzymes such as creatine phosphokinase and lactic dehydrogenase are released into the circulation causing an increase in their serum levels and their presence may be another clue to the presence of trichinella (Murrell and Bruschi 1994, Capo and Despommier 1996).

A laboratory finding that is nearly always associated with the infection is circulating eosinophilia (Gould 1970) which shows a pattern of rising (week 2–5), levelling off (week 4–8), and then falling (week 9–12) levels. Eosinophilia may be as high as 80–95% in severe cases (Kaljus 1936). Overall, the total white blood cell count is slightly elevated (i.e. 12 000–15 000 cells/mm^3). A history of ingesting raw or undercooked pork, or game animals such as bear, fox, opossum or raccoon 2 weeks or so earlier, accompanied by a bout of recent 'gastroenteritis' or 'flu-like illness' gives a clue to the diagnosis and should tell the physician to look further into the possibility of trichinellosis.

2.5 Control (therapy, prophylaxis, transmission)

Unfortunately, little is clinically available in the way of specific chemotherapy once the diagnosis is made. Removal of adult worms from the small intestine with thiabendazole (Gerwel, Pawlowski and Kocieka 1974) or mebendazole (Medical Letter on Drugs and Therapeutics 1993) may reduce the number of newborn larvae that reach the skeletal muscle, but diagnosis is usually made some time after the majority of larvae have

been produced (i.e. weeks 3–6 after infection). Mebendazole also reduces the worm burden in the muscle tissue in experimental animals, but its efficacy in humans is doubtful. Even if it did prove effective, it is of little clinical significance because the pathological consequences of infection are due largely to the migrating larvae which remain unaffected by that drug.

Prevention of *Trichinella* infection involves cooking all pork products at 59°C (137°F) for 10 min or freezing them at −20 °C for 3 days. At the community level, inspection of slaughtered pigs in some countries, for example the countries of the European Union, has greatly reduced the prevalence of infection. In other parts of the world, the United States and Asia, for example, meat is not inspected for *Trichinella*.

Prevention of outbreaks due to ingestion of game animals is more difficult because strains of *Trichinella* that infect wild animals may be resistant to freezing (Dick 1983). Furthermore, few hunters are aware of the risk of acquiring this infection from their bounty.

Strict herbivores are usually not infected with *Trichinella* but occasionally acquire it by accidentally eating an infected carcass (Bellani, Mantovani and Filppini 1978). An outbreak of trichinellosis in France, involving thousands of people (Ancelle et al. 1985), was traced back to a single horse imported from the United States and sold in Paris as 'steak' tartare.

TOXOCARA

3 THE PARASITES

Discovery of a larval nematode within the retinal granuloma of a child by Wilder in 1950 (Wilder 1950) led to the description of the condition known today as **visceral larva migrans** (VLM). Two years later, Beaver and colleagues (Beaver et al. 1952) described a number of infections, again in children, in which eosinophilia and severe multisystem disease was caused by migrating larvae of *Toxocara canis* and *Toxocara cati*, parasites whose definitive hosts are dogs and cats, respectively.

3.1 Morphology and structure

Both species of *Toxocara* are large pink round worms (Fig. 31.12), with the adults measuring 7–10 cm in length by 5–6 mm in width. The male has a curved posterior end, which distinguishes it from the straight-tailed female. Females lay large quantities of unembryonated eggs (Fig. 31.13) into the lumen of the small intestine, which then need to pass into the external environment in order to embryonate (Fig. 31.14).

3.2 General biology

Adult worms occupy the lumen of the small intestine and live unattached to the host. They maintain their

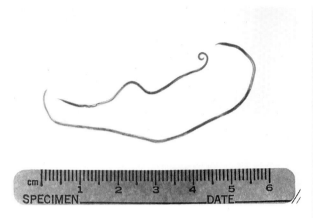

Fig. 31.12 Adult male and female *Toxocara canis*. The female is larger than the male and has a straight tail. Unstained, formalin fixed specimens.

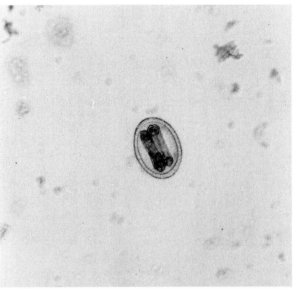

Fig. 31.14 The embryonated egg of *Toxocara canis*. Note the coiled L2 stage larva inside. This is the infectious stage. It is the same size as the unembryonated egg. Unstained preparation.

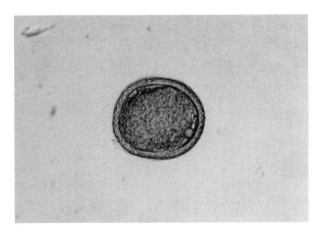

Fig. 31.13 The unembryonated egg of *Toxocara canis*. Note the striations on the eggshell and the absence of a larva inside. The egg measures about 90 μm in diameter at its widest point. Unstained preparation.

position in the lumen by serpentine movement against the flow of peristalsis. Worms ingest partially digested food of the host and process it through their gut. Little is known about the digestive physiology, but it is likely to be similar to that of *Ascaris lumbricoides*, i.e. to have the capability of digesting most foodstuffs and absorbing the resulting small molecular weight nutrients across the midgut microvilli. *Toxocara* is a facultative anaerobe and derives most of its energy from glycogen degradation (Gopinath and Keystone 1995). The pseudocoelom contains a special haemoglobin which presumably binds oxygen thus augmenting energy metabolism. The worms' pink colour is due to the presence of this substance.

3.3 Life cycle

Toxocara canis and *T. cati* have similar life cycles which resemble that of *Ascaris lumbricoides* in humans (Despommier and Karapelou 1987) (Fig. 31.15). Nonembryonated eggs are passed with the faeces into the environment and incubate in soil. Within 2 weeks, the eggs contain an infectious second stage larva (Fig.

31.14, arrow) that, if eaten by a dog (*T. canis*) or cat (*T. cati*), initiates infection by hatching in the small intestine. The freed larvae penetrates the small intestine and enter the general circulation. In the liver, they lodge in the presinusoidal capillaries because of their large diameter, and are stimulated to enter the parenchymal tissue where they feed on liver cells. They moult in the liver to the third stage, re-enter the general circulation and are carried to the lungs. Trapped by the alveolar capillaries, again because of their size, they penetrate into the alveolar space, crawl up the bronchioles into the trachea, bypass the epiglottis and are swallowed. In the small intestine, larvae moult for a fourth time, transforming into adult worms. Mating ensues soon thereafter and the females begin to pass unembryonated eggs, thus completing the life cycle in their definitive hosts.

Toxocara spp. cannot complete their life cycle in humans. Infection is initiated as in the dog or cat, namely by the ingestion of embryonated eggs. Larvae hatch in the small intestine but, as they do not receive the proper environmental cues (Castro 1982), begin their odyssey, wandering throughout the body, invading all organs and damaging tissue wherever they go. Larvae never mature and eventually die in situ. Death may occur soon after infection, but many worms can survive for several months, up to a year (Smith and Beaver 1953), without apparent side effects.

3.4 Transmission and epidemiology

A child who owns a pets, particularly a dog or cat, and who also has unexplained fever and eosinophilia, may well be infected with *Toxocara canis* or *T. cati*, and a history of pica makes visceral larva migrans a strong possibility (Hotez 1993). Ocular larva migrans (OLM)

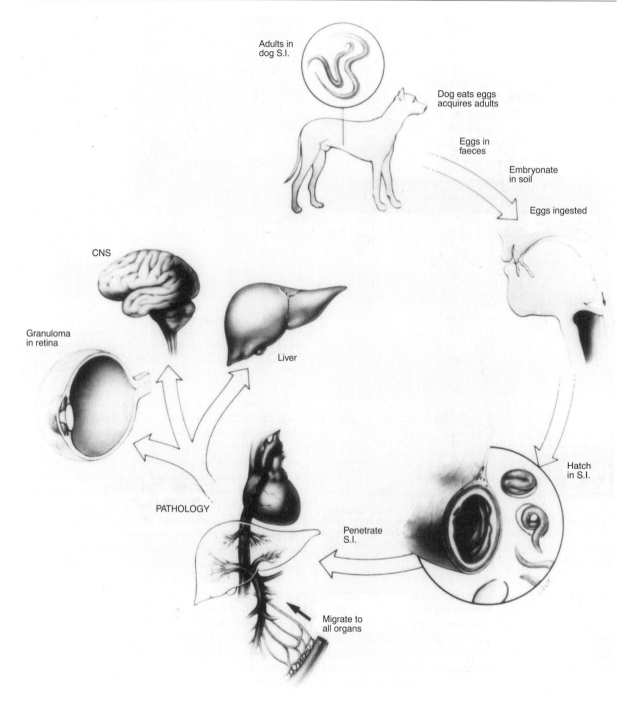

Fig. 31.15 Life cycle of *Toxocara canis*. (From Despommier, Gwadz and Hotez 1994).

should be suspected in anyone with unilateral vision loss and strabismus with a similar history of association with domestic animals (Despommier, Gwadz and Hotez 1995). Children living in rural settings such as farms are more likely to encounter toxocarid eggs than those living in cities. *Toxocara* spp. are found throughout the world and cause diseases similar to those described here.

4 CLINICAL AND PATHOLOGICAL ASPECTS OF INFECTION

The 2 recognized forms of *Toxocara* infection in humans are OLM and VLM (Schantz, 1989); both can be caused by either *Toxocara canis* or *T. cati*. The resultant clinical condition is thought to depend on the immune status of the infected individual as well as other related factors (Kazacos 1991).

4.1 Clinical manifestations

Ocular disease usually occurs in the absence of visceral disease and vice versa, and it has thus been suggested that the 2 manifestations of this infection be reclassified as **ocular larva migrans** (OLM) and **visceral larva migrans** (VLM) (Despommier et al. 1994).

VLM is mainly a disease of young children and its signs and symptoms include fever, respiratory distress, and hepatosplenomegaly (Gutierrez 1990). Myocarditis, nephritis, and CNS symptoms are not uncommon. CNS involvement may lead to seizures, psychiatric manifestations, or encephalopathy (Fortenberry, Kenney and Younger 1991).

OLM occurs primarily in older children and usually manifests as a unilateral vision disorder often accompanied by strabismus (Dinning et al. 1988). Invasion of the retina leading to granuloma formation is the most serious consequence of the infection (Gillespie et al. 1993) and occurs peripherally or in the posterior pole. These granulomata drag the retina creating distortion, heteropia, or macular detachment (Small et al. 1989). Diffuse endophthalmitis or papillitis with secondary glaucoma are other complications of larval migration and death. Blindness is common, but the degree of damage depends on the area affected.

4.2 Pathogenesis and pathology

Damage depends on the tissue invaded, with CNS, including the eyes, being most seriously affected (Fig. 31.16). Although tissue damage due to the migration of worms is a major cause of cell death, these insults are less harmful than the eosinophilic granulomata that are the hallmark of worm death. When the latter event occurs in the eye, it often resembles retinoblastoma (Despommier et al 1994). In the past, enucleation was performed in some unfortunate cases because of the unavailability of modern diagnostic tests. Granulomata induced by dying worms can be sufficiently intense to be responsible for the loss of sight in that eye.

4.3 Immune responses

The death of migrating larvae is accompanied by striking delayed-type and immediate-type hypersensitivity immune responses. Humoral responses include an extreme elevation in levels of both IgG and IgM, only some of which is specific for parasite components (Schantz, Meyer and Glickman 1979). Most antibody responses are against a unique cuticular-associated trisaccharide epitope that is shed by the worm during its migration throughout the tissues. This reagent, which can be collected in vitro, is useful in the immunodiagnosis of the infection. However, immune responses against this antigen appear not to be protective. Nothing is known regarding the immune mechanisms responsible for the death of the worm.

Cellular responses include elevated circulating levels of eosinophils which home in on dying worms in

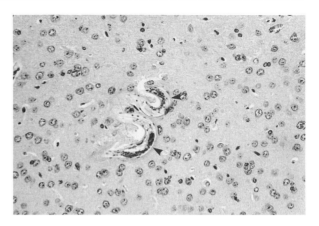

Fig. 31.16 A larva of *Toxocara canis* in the brain tissue of an experimentally infected mouse. Note the lack of any inflammatory response around the area of damage. The worm is approximately 20 μm in diameter. Haematoxylin and eosin stained section of paraffin-embedded tissue.

tissues. Granulomata consist of collections of eosinophils, lymphocytes, fibroblasts, epithelioid cells and giant cells. Remnants of larval tissue may be present in the centre of each granuloma (Fig. 31.16).

4.4 Diagnosis

Biopsy of liver or other tissues in which larvae are suspected is rarely positive, hence diagnosis depends primarily on indirect measures of the presence of the worm, such as immunological tests, particularly ELISA. Using antigens secreted by the third stage larvae, ELISA has sufficient specificity (approximately 92%) and sensitivity (approximately 78%) at a titre greater than 1:32 to be a useful adjunct to diagnosis (Schantz 1989). Elevated gammaglobulin and an elevated isohaemoagglutin titre (Despommier et al. 1994) also help the clinician confirm toxocariasis.

OLM is diagnosed on clinical criteria during an ophthalmologic examination. Serological tests for antibodies are not as reliable for OLM as they are for VLM. For example, only 45% of patients with OLM had antibody levels that correlated with the infection (Schantz, Meyer and Glickman 1979). Other laboratory findings include an elevated circulating eosinophilia sometimes approaching 70% (Snyder 1961), and hypergammaglobulinaemia of the IgM and IgG classes.

4.5 Control (therapy, prophylaxis and transmission)

Although diethylcarbamazine is listed in some references as an effective drug, its use is not recommended. In contrast, high doses of mebendazole (1 g 3 times a day) for 21 days were effective in treating an adult case of VLM (Bekhti 1984). Albendazole may also be efficacious (Medical Letter on Drugs and Therapeutics 1993). Corticosteroids suppress intense inflammation and thus relieve some of the more serious symptoms associated with worm migration and worm death. Most infected people recover within 3 months after infection regardless of which therapies are used. Treatments for OLM include surgery (vitrectomy), anthelmintic chemotherapy and corticosteroids.

REFERENCES

Ahmed A, Wang CH, and Bell RG, 1991, A role for IgE and intestinal immunity. Expression of rapid expulsion of *Trichinella spiralis* in rats infused with IgE and thoracic duct lymphocytes, *J Immunol*, **146:** 3563–70.

Ancelle T, Dupouy-Camet J et al., 1985, Outbreak of trichinosis due to horse meat in the Paris area, *Lancet*, **ii (21 September):** 660.

Andrews JRH, Ainsworth R, Abernathy D, 1994, *Trichinella pseudospiralis* in humans: description of a case and its treatment, *Trans R Soc Trop Med Hyg*, **88:** 200–3.

Beaver PC, Snyder CH et al., 1952, Chronic eosinophilia due to visceral larva migrans, *Pediatrics*, **9:** 7–19.

Bekhti A, 1984, Mebendazole in toxocariasis, *Ann Intern Med*, **100:** 463.

Bellani L, Mantovani A, Filippini I, 1978, Observations on an outbreak of human trichinellosis in northern Italy, *Trichinellosis*, eds Kim CW, Pawlowski Z, University Press of New England, Hanover, NH, 535–9.

Campbell WC, 1983a, Historical introduction, Trichinella *and* Trichinosis, ed Campbell WC, Plenum Press, New York, 1–28.

Campbell WC, 1983b, Epidemiology I. Modes of transmission, Trichinella *and Trichinosis*, ed Campbell WC, Plenum Press, New York, 425–44.

Capo V, Despommier DD, 1996, Clinical aspects of infection with *Trichinella* spp., *Clin Microbiol Rev*, **Jan:** 47–54.

Castro GA, 1982, Gastrointestinal physiology: environmental factors influencing infection and pathogenicity, *Cues that Influence Behavior of Internal Parasites*, ed Bailey WS, Agricultural Research Service, US Department of Agriculture, PO Box 53326, New Orleans, LA, 1–21.

Castro GA, Powell DW, 1994, The physiology of the mucosal immune system and immune-mediated responses in the gasrtointestinal tract, *Physiology of the Gastrointestinal Tract*, 3rd edn, ed Johnson LR, Raven Press, New York, 709–49.

Curman JA, Pond L, Nashold F, 1992, Immunity to *Trichinella spiralis* infection in vitamin A deficient mice, *J Exp Med*, **175:** 111–20.

Despommier DD, 1988, The immunobiology of *Trichinella spiralis*, *Immune Responses in Parasitic Infections: Immunology, Immunopathology, and Immunoprophylaxis.*, Vol I. Nematodes, ed Soulsby EJL, CRC Press, Boca Raton, FL, 43–60.

Despommier DD, 1990, The worm that would be virus, *Parasitol Today*, **6:** 193–5.

Despommier DD, 1993, *Trichinella spiralis* and the concept of niche, *J Parasitol*, **79:** 472–82.

Despommier DD, 1995, *Trichinella spiralis*, *Enteric Infection 2: Intestinal Helminths*, eds Farthing MJG, Keusch GT, Wakelin D, Chapman & Hall Medical, London, 107–16.

Despommier DD, Karapelou J, 1987, *Parasite Life Cycles*, 1st edn, Springer-Verlag, New York.

Despommier DD, Kajima M, Wostmann BS, 1967, Ferritin-conjugated antibody studies on the larva of *Trichinella spiralis*, *J Parasitol*, **53:** 618–24.

Despommier DD, Gold A et al., 1990, *Trichinella spiralis*: A secreted antigen of the infective L1 larva localizes to the cytoplasm and nucleoplasm of infected host cells, *Exp Parasitol*, **72:** 27–38.

Despommier DD, Gwadz RG, Hotez PJ, 1994, *Parasitic Diseases*, 3rd edn, Springer-Verlag, New York, 64–7.

Dick TA, 1983, Infectivity of isolates of *Trichinella* and the ability of the arctic strain to survive freezing temperatures in the raccoon, *Procyon lotor*, under experimental conditions, *J Wildlife Dis*, **19:** 333–6.

Dinning WJ, Gillespie SH et al., 1988, Toxocariasis: a practical approach to management of ocular disease, *Eye*, **2:** 580–2.

Feldmeier H, Biensle U et al., 1991, Sequelae after infection with *Trichinella spiralis*: a prospective cohort study, *Wien Klin Wochens*, **103:** 111–16.

Fortenberry JD, Kenney RD, Younger J, 1991, Visceral larva migrans producing static encephalopathy in an infant, *Pediatr Infect Dis*, **10:** 403–6.

Garside P, Grencis RK, 1992, T lymphocyte dependent enteropathy in murine *Trichinella spiralis* infection, *Parasite Immunol*, **14:** 217–55.

Gerwel C, Pawlowski Z, Kocieka W, 1974, Probable sterilization of *Trichinella spiralis* by thiabendazole: further clinical observation of human infection, *Trichinellosis*, ed Kim CW, Intext Educational, New York, 471–5.

Gillespie SH, Dinning WJ et al., 1993, The spectrum of ocular toxocariasis, *Eye*, **7:** 415–418.

Gold AM, Despommier DD, Buck SW, 1990, Partial characterization of two antigens secreted by the larva of *Trichinella spiralis*, *Mol Biochem Parasitol*, **41:** 187–96.

Gopinath R, Keystone JS, Ascariasis, trichuriasis, and enterobiasis, *Infections of the Gastrointestinal Tract*, eds Blaser MJ, Smith PD et al, Raven Press, New York, 1167–88.

Gould SE, 1970, B. Clinical pathology: diagnostic laboratory procedures, *Trichinosis in Man and Animals*, ed Gould SE, Charles C. Thomas, Springfield, Illinois, 191–221.

Gutierrez Y, 1990, Toxocara - visceral larva migrans, *Diagnostic Pathology of Parasitic Infections with Clinical Correlations*, ed Gutierrez Y, Lea and Febiger, Philadelphia, 262–72.

Harari Y, Castro GA, 1988, Evaluation of a possible functional relationship between chemical structure of the intestinal brush border and immunity to *Trichinella spiralis* in the rat, *J Parasitol*, **74:** 244–8.

Hotez PJ, 1993, Visceral and ocular larva migrans, *Semin Neurol*, **13:** 175–9.

Jasmer DP, 1995, *Trichinella spiralis*: Subversion of differentiated mammalian skeletal muscle cells, *Parasitol Today*, **11:** 185–88.

Kaljus WA, 1936, On the practical value of the intradermal reaction with the trichinelliasis antigen for the diagnosis of trichinelliasis in man, *Puerto Rico J Public Health*, **11:** 768–90.

Kazacos KR, 1991, Visceral and ocular larva migrans, *Semin Vet Med Surg (Small Anim)*, **6:** 227–35.

Larsh JE Jr, 1952, A study of the longevity and distribution of adult *Trichinella spiralis* in immunized and non-immunized mice, *J Elisa Mitchell Sci Soc*, **68:** 1–11.

Larsh JE Jr, 1970, Immunology, *Trichinosis in Man and Animals*, ed Gould SE, Charles C. Thomas, Springfield, IL, 129–46.

Ljungstrom, I, 1983, Immunodiagnosis in man, Trichinella *and Trichinosis*, ed Campbell WC, Plenum Press, New York, 403–24.

Love RJ, Ogilvie BM, McLaren DJ, 1976, The immune mechanism that expels the intestinal stage of *Trichinella spiralis* from rats, *Immunology*, **30:** 7–15.

Medical Letter on Drugs and Therapeutics, 1993, Drugs for parasitic infections, *The Medical Letter on Drugs and Therapeutics*, ed Abramowicz M, The Medical Letter, New York, **35 (Issue 911):** 9.

Murrell D, Bruschi F, 1994, Clinical trichinellosis, *Progress in Clinical Parasitology*, ed Tsien Sun, CRC Press, Boca Raton, FL, 117–50.

Obendorf DL, Handlinger JH et al., 1990, *Trichinella pseudospiralis* in Tasmanian wildlife, *Austr Vet J*, **67:** 108–10.

Olaison L, Ljungstrom I, 1992, An outbreak of trichinosis in Lebanon, *Trans R Soc Trop Med Hyg*, **86:** 658–60.

Philipp M, Parkhouse RME, Ogilvie BM, 1980, Changing proteins on the surface of a parasitic nematode, *Nature* (London), **287**: 538.

Pozio EG, La Rosa LK et al., Taxonomic revisions of the genus *Trichinella, J Parasitol*, 1992, **78**: 654–9.

Schantz PM, 1989, Toxocara larva migrans then and now, *Am J Trop Med Hyg*, **41(Suppl):** 21–34.

Schantz PM, Meyer D, Glickman LT, 1979, Clinical, serologic, and epidemiologic characteristics of ocular toxocariasis, *Am J Trop Med Hyg*, **28**: 24–8.

Silberstein DS, 1983, Antigens, Trichinella *and Trichinosis*, ed Campbell WC, Plenum Press, New York, 309–34.

Small, KW, McCuen BW et al., 1989, Surgical management of retinal retraction caused by toxocariasis, *Am J Ophthamol*, **108**: 10–14.

Smith MHD, Beaver PC, 1953, Persistence and distribution of *Toxocara* larvae in the tissues of children and mice, *Pediatrics*, **12**: 491–7.

Snyder CH, 1961, Visceral larva migrans – ten years experience, *Pediatrics*, **28**: 85–91.

Stewart GL, 1983, Biochemistry, Trichinella *and Trichinosis*, ed Campbell WC, Plenum Press, New York, 153–72.

Virchow R, Recherches sur le development du *Trichina spiralis*, *C R Acad Sci*, 1859, 660–2.

Wakelin D, 1997, Parasites and the immune system: conflict or compromise., *Bioscience*, **47**: 32–40.

Wakelin D, Denham DA, 1983, The immune response, Trichinella *and Trichinosis*, ed Campbell WC, Plenum Press, New York, 265–308.

Wang CH, Bell RG, 1986, *Trichinella spiralis*: migration of larvae in the rat, *Exp Parasitol*, **62**: 430–41.

Wilder HC, 1950, Nematode endophthalmitis, *Trans Am Acad Ophthalmol Otolaryngol*, **55**: 99–109.

Wisenewski N, McNeil M, Grieve RB, 1993, Characterization of novel fucosyl-containing and tyvelosyl-containing glycoconjugates from *Trichinella spiralis* muscle stage larvae, *Mol Biochem Parasitol*, **61**: 25–36.

C h a p t e r   3 2

LYMPHATIC FILARIASIS

R Muller and D Wakelin

1   THE PARASITE

1.1   Introduction and historical perspective

The filarial nematodes, of which some 8 species infect humans, are the major group of tissue-dwelling nematodes. They share a number of morphological and life cycle characteristics, in that all are long slender worms living in a variety of subcutaneous and lymphatic niches, with prolonged developmental cycles dependent upon vector transmission, but they cause a range of distinct pathologies. Adult female worms produce embryonic forms (microfilaria larvae) which are taken up by blood-sucking arthropods to produce the infective larval stages; these are then transmitted when the vectors next feed. Three species are of major significance, infecting large numbers of people over wide geographical areas – *Onchocerca volvulus*, *Wuchereria bancrofti* and *Brugia malayi*; *B. timori* is also pathogenic but has a restricted distribution. These species have been extensively studied and much is known of their pathology and their epidemiology. *O. volvulus* is associated primarily with a range of dermal and ocular conditions and is treated separately in chapter 083. The pathology associated with the other 3 species is primarily associated with acute and chronic changes in the lymphatic system and this group is therefore known as the **lymphatic filariae**. The other 4 species, *Loa loa*, *Mansonella ozzardi*, *M. perstans* and *M. streptocerca* are rather less well known, but do appear to be less important as causes of human disease. They invade a variety of body sites (Table 32.1) and are associated with relatively minor pathological changes.

This account focuses primarily on the 3 lymphatic filariae but also gives some account of the other species. Their distribution overlaps with *W. bancrofti*, and *B. malayi*, and differential diagnosis of infection is important. The biology of *Loa loa* is distinctive in that the adult worms actively migrate through the tissues, notably the eye.

The distinctive pathology associated with lymphatic infection, particularly the gross enlargement of limbs known as **elephantiasis**, has been known since antiquity (Sasa 1976, Grove 1990, Nelson 1996). It is recorded in the ancient medical literature of China, Egypt, India, Japan and Persia and was referred to as elephantiasis arabicum by Western physicians. The microfilarial stages were first discovered in hydroceles of a patient from Cuba in 1863. Wucherer reported microfilariae in the urine of an infected patient in 1866 and they were later (1872) found in the blood by Lewis. Adult worms were not reported until found in the abscess of a Chinese patient by Bancroft in Brisbane in 1876. The name *Filaria bancrofti* was proposed by Cobbold in 1877 and the generic name *Wuchereria* given in 1878.

The major contributions to understanding the life cycle of *W. bancrofti* were made by Manson working in South China. In 1878 he identified mosquitoes as vectors of infection, undertaking daily examinations of mosquitoes that had fed on the blood of an infected patient and eventually finding the developing larval stages. This was the first demonstration that arthropods could harbour an infective agent, and paved the way for the later identification of mosquitoes as vectors of diseases such as malaria and yellow fever (see chapter 1 for further details). Later, in 1881, Manson described the curious nocturnal periodicity of *W. bancrofti* – the microfilariae circulating in the peripheral blood at night, but then disappearing from the circulation during the day. The means of transmission from the mosquito was established by Bancroft in 1899 and Low in 1900, *Culex pipiens fatigans* (*C. quinquefasciatus*) being identified as an important vector species.

Identification of the other filariae was made much later. Microfilaria collected by Lichtenstein from northern Sumatra were examined by Brug, who realized that the larvae were not those of *W. bancrofti* (and indeed were unable to develop in *C. p. fatigans*) The name *Filaria malayi* was given in 1927 and altered by Buckley to *Brugia malayi* in 1960. The occurrence of

Table 32.1   Filarial nematodes infecting humans (other than *Onchocerca*)

Species	Vector insect	Primary pathology	Distribution
Wuchereria bancrofti	Mosquitoes	Lymphatic and lung	Asia, Africa, Australia, Pacific, South America
Brugia malayi	Mosquitoes	Lymphatic and lung	South-East Asia
B. timori	Mosquitoes	Lymphatic and lung	Indonesia
Loa loa	*Chrysops*	Allergic swellings	Africa
Mansonella ozzardi	Midges	Ill defined, allergic	Central and South America
M. perstans	Midges	Ill-defined, allergic	Africa, South America
M. streptocerca	Midges	Dermal	Africa

Loa loa in the eye had been reported during the eighteenth century in West African slaves transported to the New World and had probably been seen in the previous century. The worm was variously named *Filaria loa*, *F. lacrimalis* and *F. subconjunctivalis* until the genus *Loa* was finally established by Stiles in 1905. The species now included in *Mansonella* were identified at the end of the nineteenth century, Manson again playing a central role in their discovery. The generic names given to these species have gone through a number of changes, including *Filaria*, *Acanthocheilonema*, *Dipetalonema* and *Tetrapetalonema*.

1.2   Classification and morphology

Filarial nematodes belong to the phylum Nematoda, class Secernentea and superfamily Filarioidea. Their bodies are long, smooth (except in *Loa* and *Onchocerca*) and cylindrical, the females of the lymphatic species reaching some 80–100 mm × 0.25–0.30 mm. The head is simple, the mouth lacks lips and the buccal cavity is small. The mouth opens into the oesophagus, which has an anterior muscular region and a posterior glandular region. The tail of the male has no caudal bursa, but carries perianal papillae: these and the copulatory spicules can be useful in taxonomy. The vulva of the female is anterior and opens, via the vagina, into the long, coiled bifurcate uterus, that runs the length of the body. The females are ovoviviparous or viviparous, the uterus containing the microfilariae – embryos which develop within thin 'shells' that, in *W. bancrofti*, the *Brugia* species and *Loa*, are retained as 'sheaths' after the microfilariae are released. Other than *Loa*, the location of the adult worms in the body means that they are rarely seen intact, sometimes only in histological sections. In contrast, the microfilariae, which appear in the blood, are easily seen and provide a good basis for identification. They can be differentiated on the basis of size, the presence or absence of a sheath (Fig. 32.1), the distribution of nuclei in the caudal region of the larvae and the periodicity of their appearance in the peripheral blood (Table 32.1). Microfilariae of lymphatic filariae may also appear in hydrocele fluid and urine.

Microfilariae are, as their embryonic status implies, relatively undifferentiated. They measure 180–300 μm

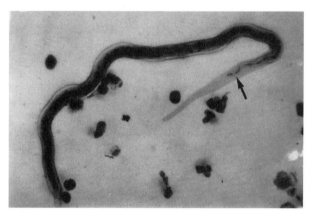

Fig. 32.1   Microfilaria of *Loa loa* in thick blood film stained in haematoxylin and eosin. Note sheath and tail with nuclei to tip (arrowed).

in length, depending on species, and about 3–10 μm in diameter. The body contains a number of nuclei, which may or may not extend into the caudal region, but there are no other morphologically detectable structures. In the sheathed forms (*W. bancrofti*, *B. malayi*, *B. timori*, *L. loa*) the sheath extends beyond the anterior and posterior ends of the larvae. The microfilariae of the unsheathed species (*M. ozzardi*, *M. perstans* and *M. streptocerca*) can be mistaken for those of *Onchocerca volvulus*, but do show a number of distinguishing features (see chapter 33, Fig. 33.3)

Relatively little detail is known of the biology of the human filariae, because most are highly host specific and will not complete their life cycles in conventional laboratory hosts. Some can develop in higher primates, and some stages of some species (e.g. *B. malayi*) can be established in laboratory rodents. The subperiodic strain of *B. malayi* occurs naturally in a number of wild animals including primates and felines. The closely related species *Brugia pahangi*, which can be maintained in cats, has been extensively used as an experimental model (Denham and Fletcher 1987) and much of our detailed knowledge of the biology of lymphatic filariae has come from this species.

All the filariae considered in this chapter are transmitted by blood-feeding arthropod vectors, a large number of insects acting in this capacity (Table 32.2).

Table 32.2 Genera of the insect vectors of filarial nematodes infecting humans (other than *Onchocerca*)

Species	Vector species	
Wuchereria bancrofti	Mosquitoes	*Culex, Anopheles, Aedes*
Brugia malayi	Mosquitoes	*Mansonia, Anopheles, Aedes*
B. timori	Mosquitoes	*Anopheles*
Loa loa	Tabanid	*Chrysops*
Mansonella ozzardi	Midges	*Culicoides, Simulium*
M. perstans	Midges	*Culicoides*
M. streptocerca	Midges	*Culicoides*

Microfilariae circulating in the peripheral blood are taken up as the insect feeds and pass into the midgut. Sheathed microfilariae lose their sheath at this stage. The larvae then penetrate the midgut wall, migrate into the haemocoel of the insect and then penetrate the thoracic flight muscles. Here they first develop into short thick 'sausage' forms and subsequently, over about 2 weeks, grow and undergo 2 moults to become filariform infective third stage (L3) larvae, measuring about 1–2 mm. These migrate out of the muscles into the insect's head region and escape from the mouthparts at the next blood meal, entering the wound made by the insect while feeding. Detail of the later development of the human filarial species is largely unknown. The L3 larvae of *B. pahangi* penetrate into lymphatics and migrate to the nearest lymph node. Here they spend about 3 weeks, undergoing a further moult, before moving back into the afferent lymphatic and completing the final moult to the adult stage. A proportion of the worms die at this stage, but the survivors may then live for several years, the adult females liberating microfilariae throughout this time. This pattern is likely to be representative of *W. bancrofti* and the human *Brugia* species, although the time scales are much greater. Figures for longevity for *W. bancrofti* of up to 10 years have been quoted, but a recent report suggests that 5 years is probably more accurate (Vanamail et al. 1996); the development and locations of the other human species are quite different from this pattern. The time taken for microfilariae to appear in the blood of infected humans, i.e. for the infection to became patent, can be considerable, probably as much as 12 months in the case of *W. bancrofti*, although less in the other species. This is because it is necessary for a minimum number of adult worms to be present in the body before there is a high probability of a mature female being fertilized by a mature male. Once released, the microfilariae may survive for many months.

1.3 Periodicity

It is characteristic of the lymphatic filariae that the appearance of the microfilariae in the peripheral blood shows marked periodicity. Manson's demonstration of this phenomenon in *W. bancrofti* showed that microfilariae appeared for about 1–2 h before and after midnight and then disappeared more or less completely for the rest of the 24 h period. This noctur-

nal pattern is true of *W. bancrofti* throughout much of its geographical range (Asia, Africa, Australia, South America), but in certain areas different patterns are seen. For example, in Pacific areas (e.g. Polynesia and the Philippines) a non-periodic (or slightly diurnally periodic) form is present in which microfilariae are present in the peripheral blood more or less constantly throughout much of the 24 h period. In South-East Asia there are subperiodic forms of *W. bancrofti*, in which, although microfilariae are present throughout the 24 h period, numbers in the blood are elevated at night. Periodic and subperiodic forms also exist in *B. malayi*. The nocturnally periodic form is common in coastal regions, open swamps and rice fields in India, Sri Lanka, Thailand, Malaysia, Korea and Japan, readily infects anopheline mosquitoes, can also be transmitted by *Mansonia* and *Aedes* mosquitoes, but does not establish easily in animal hosts. The subperiodic form occurs in freshwater swamps and forests in Malaysia, Thailand and the Phillipines, is highly infective for mansonian rather than anopheline mosquitoes and readily infects animal hosts. Confusingly, some periodic-form microfilariae may shed their sheaths during the processing of blood smear preparations; however, this can be useful diagnostically. Microfilaraemia in *B. timori* infections shows nocturnal periodicity. Of the other human filariae only *L. loa* shows periodicity, but this is distinctively diurnal, numbers of microfilariae peaking at about midday. Interestingly, a race of *Loa* that infects African primates shows nocturnal periodicity. When primates are infected with the human *Loa* this retains its nocturnal periodicity, suggesting that periodicity is genetically rather than host-determined (Duke 1964).

The biological rationale of periodicity is always explained in terms of accessibility of the parasite to vectors, the appearance of the microfilariae conciding with the periods of feeding activity in the arthropod, an adaptation that clearly has evolutionary and survival advantages for the worm. For example, periodic *W. bancrofti* is transmitted by night-biting mosquitoes and the subperiodic form by day-biting species. The diurnal *Loa* which infects humans is transmitted by a daytime biting species of *Chrysops*, whereas the nocturnal subspecies infecting primates is transmitted by nighttime feeders. Physiological explanations for periodicity were explored in great detail by Hawking (1967). In their simplest terms these pin-pointed differential respiratory gas tensions (oxygen and carbon dioxide) in pulmonary vessels as a decisive factor in triggering behavioural responses in the microfilariae. In mammals that are active during the day, the difference in gas tensions between the blood in pulmonary veins and arteries is greatest during the day and reduced at night. Microfilariae that show nocturnal periodicity accumulate in the lungs during the day, actively swimming against the blood flow to maintain their position. When the difference in gas tension is decreased at night the microfilariae pass through the lungs and circulate in the peripheral blood. Altering the daily activity patterns of the host can therefore alter the periodicity of the parasite, as has been demonstrated many times with *W. bancrofti* (Hawking 1967). However, this is not the only explanation and several other host-derived factors, including body temperature, have been implicated.

1.4 Transmission and epidemiology

All filariae infecting humans are insect transmitted, and a wide variety of species can act as vectors (Table 32.2). *W. bancrofti* and the *Brugia* species are mosquito transmitted, the *Mansonella* species are transmitted by *Culicoides* midges and *L. loa* uses *Chrysops*.

The life cycles of all mosqitoes involve an aquatic phase, the female laying eggs onto or into bodies of water. The larvae that hatch feed on particulate material and respire directly from atmospheric oxygen, breaking the surface film to acquire this, as do the active pupal stages. Only the adult female mosquitoes feed on blood, using their highly modified mouthparts to pierce the skin and probe until a capillary is located, the blood then being taken directly from the vessel. *Culex quinquefasciatus* is the most important vector of periodic *W. bancrofti*, being responsible for more than 50% of cases of lymphatic filariasis. It readily adapts to breeding in man-made environments, using bodies of water ranging from sewage and drainage channels to pools collecting in disused tyres and utensils. As a consequence urban filariasis, transmitted by these 'domestic' vectors, is a serious problem in many countries. In rural areas *Anophleles* species are the primary vectors (often transmitting malaria as well). Subperiodic *W. bancrofti* utilize *Anopheles* and *Aedes* mosquitoes. The larvae of the *Mansonia* mosquitoes that can transmit *B. malayi* obtain oxygen from the air spaces inside aquatic plants, using specialized siphons to pierce the tissues. *Mansonia* species are therefore rather more restricted ecologically than other groups and have been easier to control.

The *Chrysops* (mango flies) that transmit *Loa* to humans are very different insects from mosquitoes both in their biology and their feeding behaviour. These tabanids (horseflies) are large insects and the females have powerful mouthparts that can penetrate through clothing, feeding taking place outdoors during the daytime. Unlike mosquitoes, *Chrysops* feed from blood that forms pools at the site of the wound. Eggs are laid on vegetation overhanging small, muddy, rainforest streams and swamps. The larvae feed on

decaying organic matter in the water for up to a year, and pupate in the mud before emerging as adults.

Mansonella species are transmitted by tiny nocturnal midges belonging to the genus *Culicoides*. The insects have restricted activity ranges, often breeding in the locality of villages and entering houses to feed in the evening or at night. Breeding may occur in tree stumps or other suitable locations; some species breed in brackish water. Only females feed on blood, using their short mouthparts to create blood pools.

As with all vector-transmitted parasites, the epidemiology of the filarial diseases is determined by the distribution and behaviour of the insects concerned. An excellent example is the prevalence of *W. bancrofti* in urban environments, which is a direct consequence of the 'domestication' of the *Culex* vector. A further important factor concerns the numbers of larvae likely to be transmitted by a particular vector species and the consequences of infection upon the insect itself. In general, mosquitoes carry few infective larvae, thus the build-up of infections requires frequent bites from infective insects. *Culicoides* midges also carry very small numbers of larvae and, since vectors are numerous, *Mansonella* infections in humans are characteristically frequent but rather light. In contrast, individual *Chrysops* may carry large numbers of infective larvae of *Loa loa*, but the flies occur in smaller numbers. As a consequence levels of infection in humans are more variable but can be considerably heavier (see also page 617).

The 3 most important lymphatic filariae infect an estimated 118 million people (WHO 1995). The numbers known to be infected with *Loa* and the *Mansonella* species are much smaller, but accurate figures are probably not available, as these worms are considerably less pathogenic. The factors determining the epidemiology of the major infections and the relationships between infection and disease have received much attention (e.g. Denham and McGreevy 1977, Bundy, Grenfell and Rajagopalan 1991, Srividya et al. 1991, Grenfell and Michael 1992) as have the factors affecting uptake and transmission by vectors (e.g. Bryan and Southgate 1988a,b, Bryan, McMahon and Barnes 1990, Southgate 1992, Southgate and Bryan 1992 for *W. bancrofti*). An important influence on transmission is vector susceptibility. For example, some *Aedes aegypti* are genetically resistant to the development of *W. bancrofti* and *B. malayi* (Macdonald and Ramachandran 1965).

2 CLINICAL AND PATHOLOGICAL ASPECTS OF INFECTION

The disease caused by the lymphatic filariae follows rather variable courses in different individuals but, when populations are considered, a general pattern can be discerned. Infection is followed by a prepatent period, when no microfilariae are present in the blood, an apparently asymptomatic microfilaraemic stage, when the blood is positive, followed by acute and chronic stages. It is in the latter stage that the most severe gross changes, typified by elephantiasis, may occur and by this time the parasites are usually dead and degenerating. Some individuals develop atypical hypersensitivity responses, resulting in the condition known as **tropical pulmonary eosinophilia**. All of these pathological conditions are the consequences of the host's immune response to infection, the worms themselves being comparatively harmless in the absence of any response.

2.1 Clinical manifestations

Adult females of *Wuchereria* in the lymph vessels mature in about 7 months, and those of *Brugia* in about 2 months, and start producing microfilariae but it might take up to a year before these can be easily detected in the peripheral blood. A proportion of infected individuals continue to have microfilaraemia for many years without any symptoms of disease, although this situation can change suddenly at any time. However, even non-symptomatic persons show evidence of subclinical lymphatic disease when examined by lymphoscintigraphy (Dissanayake, Watawana and Piessens 1995) and there may possibly also be renal damage (WHO 1995). There can be a wide range of clinical manifestations, signs and symptoms varying from one endemic region to another. In many patients, acute attacks of 'filarial fever' ensue in a matter of a few months to many years after patency at the same time as microfilaraemia ceases. There is an intermittent recurrent fever lasting 3 to 15 days, with headache, general malaise, localized pain and tenderness with oedema and erythema above lymph vessels and glands, accompanied by acute lymphangitis and lymphadenitis of the groin or armpit regions. This stage is often accompanied by a high eosinophilia and there may be many attacks each year. These acute attacks start at about 6 years of age in many endemic regions and reach a peak at about the age of 25: with brugian filariasis they may commence in children as young as 2 years old.

Chronic disease usually takes 10–15 years to develop following repeated attacks of a retrograde adenolymphangitis with progressive residual damage in people exposed to repeated infections. In males, hydrocele, orchitis, funiculitis and epididymitis are common, and the development of lymph scrotum results in chyluria, with lymph getting into the urine. Hydrocele is a very common finding in some parts of the world, occurring in up to 50% of infected males in East Africa (Fig. 32.2).

Repeated leakage of lymph into tissues results first in lymphoedema, sometimes developing insidiously, then to elephantiasis of one or more limbs, breasts or scrotum, in which there is non-pitting oedema with growth of new adventitious tissue and thickened skin, often also with later verrucous growths and secondary bacterial and fungal infections (Fig. 32.3).

In India there are about 6 million attacks of acute filarial fever per year and over 15 million people have chronic lesions. In a survey about 11% of both sexes at risk developed lymphoedema (Srividya et al. 1991).

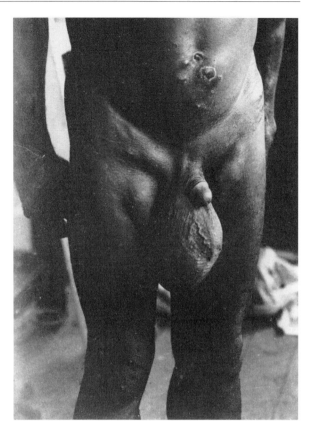

Fig. 32.2 Male patient with hydrocele and inguinal lymphadenopathy.

The incompetent lymphatics become fibrosed and the nodes eventually calcify. In the earlier stages oedema is reversible by raising or binding the affected part but this is no longer possible once elephantiasis has begun. On many Pacific islands filarial abscesses often break out on the inside of the upper thigh and this is also typical of infection with *B. timori*. The course of brugian filariasis is very similar to that of bancroftian filariasis but elephantiasis, when it occurs, is usually restricted to the legs and there is not the involvement of male genitalia.

Persons from non-endemic regions who become infected during a short intense period of exposure often have a hyper-responsive reaction, with repeated bouts of adenolymphangitis accompanied by general malaise continuing for about a year before the disease resolves without leading to elephantiasis; rarely do they become microfilaraemic. This course of infection was apparent in several thousand American servicemen stationed in the Pacific in World War II and in French troops in former Indochina.

Tropical pulmonary eosinophilia is caused by an abnormal host reaction to the presence of a lymphatic filarial infection. It occurs most commonly in southern India or in people of Indian descent. The symptoms are bouts of severe paroxysmal dry coughing, resembling an asthma attack, resulting from dense eosinophilic infiltration in the lungs and lasting for weeks or months. Patients are almost always amicrofilaraemic but have a strongly positive filarial serology. Another

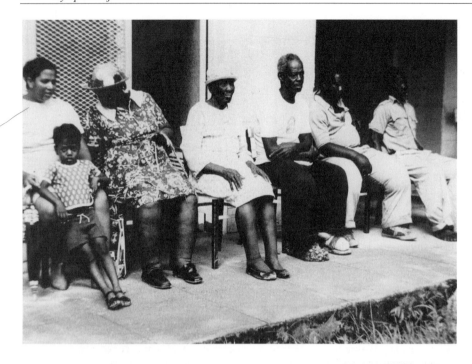

Fig. 32.3 Patients with elephantiasis caused by *W. bancrofti* attending a clinic. Note verrucous outgrowths on foot of patient (third from right) and that even advanced elephantiasis is not always superficially apparent in men.

manifestation of occult filariasis is the Meyers–Kouwenaar syndrome, found particularly in areas of the Pacific and the East Indies. In this syndrome microfilariae are again not present in the peripheral circulation, but there is a benign lymphadenitis with enlargement of the lymph nodes and spleen with many tissue eosinophils and granulomas. Histologically the lymph nodes are hyperplastic with aggregations of eosinophils and granulomas, often surrounding dead microfilariae. Both these conditions resolve rapidly after treatment with diethylcarbamazine at 10 mg kg^{-1} body weight for 5 days and this is diagnostic.

2.2 Pathogenesis and pathology

The principal pathology is associated with the presence of adult worms in the lymph nodes and vessels. Initially the sinus of the vessels increases in size, but when there have been repeated attacks of adenolymphangitis the lymph nodes progressively become enlarged, firm and fibrotic (Fig. 32.4).

The nodes become hyperplastic and microscopically show the presence of many lymphocytes, plasma cells, and polymorphs, particularly eosinophils, and there may be foci of necrosis. Sections of adult worms can be seen in the subscapular sinuses or in the lumen of the lymphatic vessels. The lymphatics are often invaded by bacteria but recent clinical studies (Dissayanake, Watawana and Piessens 1995) and experimental studies (Denham and McGreevy 1977, Denham and Fletcher 1987, Lawrence 1996) make this unlikely to be a primary cause of pathogenesis. The formation of lymphoid aggregates and larger germinal centres results in occlusion of the lumen. In chronic disease the nodes and vessels may contain dead worms surrounded by fibrotic and eventually calcified tissues. It is not known what triggers the

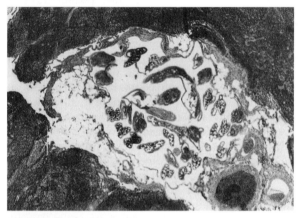

Fig. 32.4 Section of lymph node with adults of *W. bancrofti*. The lymphatic vessel is dilated and the endothelial lining is thickened with numerous inflammatory cells (haematoxylin and eosin stain).

initial inflammatory response to the living adult worms, although it may be associated with repeated reinfection pressure (e.g. in Calcutta each unprotected person will receive on average 1800 bites from infected mosquitoes per year).

In loiasis, adult *Loa* move through the connective tissues causing, usually painless, oedematous, Calabar swellings which disappear in a few days and reappear elsewhere. These are hypersensitivity reactions, probably to excretory products of the adults or perhaps to the microfilariae, and sometimes are accompanied by itching, erythema, fever and a generalized pruritis; the oedema is non-pitting. There is usually also a very high eosinophilia. The swellings measure about 5–10 cm in diameter and last for a few hours to a few days. They may occur anywhere on the body but are most common on the back of the hand or arm. Calabar swellings, which can be easily differentiated from onchocercal nodules because of their fugitive nature, appear 6–12 months after infection and reappear at intervals for another year or so before the adults move to the deeper tissues. Sometimes adult worms may wander slowly across the conjunctiva, causing some discomfort and oedema of the eyelid; they can be removed at this time with fine scissors and forceps before they disappear again (Fig. 32.5).

In heavy infections (more common than in other filariases because a single large sized *Chrysops* vector can contain 100 infective larvae) there may be very many microfilariae of *L. loa* in the peripheral blood during the day (up to 4000 per 50 mm³) and this raises the risk of microfilarial emboli blocking the capillaries of the brain, meninges or retina and causing associated symptoms. The risk of such emboli is increased enormously following treatment with diethylcarbamazine when many microfilariae are killed at one time and the resultant encephalitis can be fatal (Carme et al. 1991). High microfilaraemias have also been associated with endomyocardial fibrosis due to the degranulation of eosinophils.

Many patients with mansonelliasis are asymptomatic but each of the 3 species can have clinical manifestations. *M. perstans* and *M. ozzardi* infections have been associated with cutaneous itching, pruritis, articular pains, subcutaneous inflammation, enlarged inguinal lymph nodes and vague abdominal symptoms, accompanied by a high eosinophilia, typical of an allergic reaction. The microfilariae of *M. streptocerca* are found in the skin and symptoms of infection can include oedema and thickening of the skin, hypopigmented macules, pruritis and papules, mimicking mild onchocerciasis or leprosy.

2.3 **Immune responses**

Work with a number of experimental models, using a variety of filarial species in rodent hosts and *B. pahangi* in cats, has shown that infection can elicit strong immunity (Philipp et al. 1984, Denham and Fletcher 1987). Immunity may be seen as control of microfil-

araemia, killing of adult worms or a resistance to reinfection that operates against the infective L3 stage. The rodent models point to the central importance of T cell responses in mediating immunity and a major role for antibody-dependent cellular cytotoxic (ADCC) mechanisms in damaging the parasite. A great deal of attention has been paid recently to the involvement of T helper (Th) subsets in anti-filarial responses, and it is clear that there can be stage-specific differences in this respect (Lawrence 1996). Thus, in mice infected with *B. malayi*, it has been shown that adult worms (particularly females) and infective L3 elicit Th2 responses, with high IL-4 production and appearance of IgG1 and IgE antibodies, whereas exposure only to microfilariae elicits Th1 responses, characterized by high initial IFN-γ production and IgG2a antibody. However, chronic exposure to microfilariae can lead to Th2 responses and there is no Th1 response to microfilariae released from females *in situ*. These cytokine responses provide a functional basis for the involvement of eosinophils in ADCC mechanisms against infective L3 and for antibody (IgG2a)-mediated clearance of microfilariae.

Although the experimental systems developed for studying filarial infections in rodents have provided much valuable data, and have identified aspects of the immune response that can be directly related to immune phenomena in human filariasis, few are really close models in terms of the time course of infection or the resultant pathology. In many cases it is not possible to establish mature infections using infective L3, instead infections are established by implantation of adult worms or by direct injection of microfilariae. In contrast, infections with *B. pahangi* can be established in cats following exposure to L3 stages, and the data from this system offer useful parallels with the human disease. Unfortunately there is not the detailed immunological background for this host species that is available for rodents, and only random-bred (i.e. genetically heterogeneous) animals are available.

When cats are repeatedly infected with L3 of *B. pahangi* the majority (70%) become microfilaraemic and retain a high microfilaraemia for a considerable time – over 2 years – with large numbers of adult worms in their lymphatics. (Denham et al. 1992). The majority of the other 30% become microfilaraemic, but microfilariae then disappear from the blood, the time at which this occurs being very variable. In a small percentage of cats the amicrofilaraemic state occurs very early and after a small number of infections, in others loss of microfilariae does not occur until 1–2 years after initial infection. In some of the amicrofilaraemic cats the adult worms die, in others they remain alive. A very small percentage of cats never become microfilaraemic after infection. Pathological changes similar to those reported in humans (lymphadenitis, lymphangitis) occur in the infected cats and those that become amicrofilaraemic may also show lymphoedema. Cats exposed to repeated infections may eventually become resistant. This immunity is effective against the incoming infective L3 stages, and existing adults may continue to survive and repro-

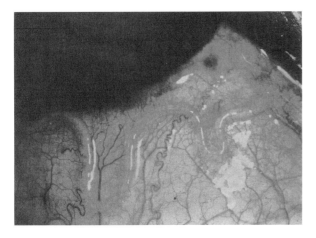

Fig. 32.5 Adult *Loa loa* migrating across the eye beneath the conjunctiva (photograph courtesy of Dr J Anderson, with permission).

duce, suggesting the existence of a state of concomitant immunity, as has been suggested for schistosomes (see chapter 25).

The value of these studies in the cat is that they provide a model of the spectrum of parasitological conditions seen in humans living in areas where lymphatic filariasis is endemic (King and Nutman 1991, Maizels and Lawrence 1991, Ottesen 1992). Four principal categories can be identified in such areas: (1) individuals who are parasitologically negative, showing no microfilaraemia, but are immunologically positive indicating exposure to infection; (2) those who are heavily infected, with many microfilariae in the blood, show little overt disease and low levels of anti-parasite immune responses; (3) those who are amicrofilaraemic, have severe disease and strong anti-parasite immune responses; (4) those who appear hyperresponsive to infection and present with conditions such as tropical pulmonary eosinophilia. Individuals in category 1 have been termed 'endemic normals' and have been presumed to be immune to infection. Whether these individuals are parasite-free has been debated. Day (1991) found that endemic normals in Papua New Guinea, where *W. bancrofti* was prevalent, not only had IgG4 anti-parasite antibodies, but also had circulating adult worm antigen in their sera, implying the presence of live worms. Thus the population shows a continuum, all individuals being infected but varying in the number of parasites, in the level of microfilaraemia and in the degree of pathology. The data observed in this study were consistent with the view that individuals acquire resistance as the result of repeated infection and that, as in the cat, there is the development of concomitant immunity, permitting existing adults to survive.

Considerable attention has been paid to the immunological mechanisms underlying resistance to infection, the low responsiveness of individuals who carry a heavy microfilaraemia and the existence of the different categories of infection status. Recent work has emphasized the importance of the balance between Th1- and Th2-mediated events in determining the outcome of infection (Ottesen 1992, King et al. 1993, Maizels et al. 1995). Filarial infections, like many helminth infections, are characterized by eosinophilia and elevated serum IgE, i.e. responses that are Th2 mediated. This particular combination of cells and antibody could play an important role in ADCC mechanisms that help to protect against incoming L3, but might also contribute to immunopathological responses such as tropical pulmonary eosinophilia. Individuals who are microfilaraemic, but lack major pathological changes, tend to have high levels of parasite-specific IgG4 antibody, sometimes contributing more than 90% of the total amount of filarial-specific antibody. In contrast, those who are amicrofilaraemic and who do have pathological lesions have higher levels of IgE and IgG$_3$. IgG4 antibodies that share antigen specificity with IgE can act as blocking antibodies and inhibit IgE-dependent allergic responses. IgE, IgG4 and eosinophilia are all Th2-dependent responses, but whereas amicrofilar-

aemic individals, like endemic normals, show high T cell responsiveness (as measured in vitro by antigen-specific proliferation), microfilaraemic individuals have reduced responses. Depression of overall T cell responses may correlate with reduced Th1 activity, arising from altered antigen presentation, disturbed IL-2 availability and function, or production of cytokines such as IL-10 that down regulate Th1 responses (Mahanty and Nutman 1995). As cytokines from Th1 cells can generate pro-inflammatory activity, depressed Th1 activity may explain in part the lack of pathology seen in this group. Although many of these explanations are speculative, data from experimental animal models and cytokine profiles from individuals in the various categories lend convincing support to these interpretations.

The reasons behind the altered immune responsiveness seen in categories of individuals in endemic regions remain unclear. It is likely that genetically different indivduals vary in their responses to given levels and frequency of infection, and it is possible that children born to infected mothers have altered responses to infection (Steel et al. 1994), but there is also good evidence that filarial worms release molecules that exert immunomodulatory effects on the host. Reduced T cell responsiveness is antigen specific, responses to non-parasite antigens being unaffected, and the depressed responsiveness seen in microfilaraemic individuals is lost when those individuals are treated (Piessens, Ratiwayanto and Piessens 1981). Direct evidence has also been obtained that parasite products depress lymphocyte responses in vitro (Lal et al. 1990). This complex relationship between host and parasite, and the possibilities of prenatal influences on the potential to respond protectively, create considerable practical difficulties in devising effective vaccines. Clearly a successful vaccine must include the antigens of the infective L3 stage in order to elicit an immunity that prevents the development of adult worms, thereby avoiding both the possibility of pathological responses and the likelihood of parasite-related immunomodulation.

2.4 Diagnosis

PARASITOLOGICAL DIAGNOSIS

Diagnosis depends on finding microfilariae in peripheral blood. In adults a drop of blood should be obtained from the ear or finger, in infants from the heel, just before or just after midnight for the periodic strains of *W. bancrofti* and *B. malayi*, and in the afternoon for the subperiodic strains and all the other filarial species. A thick blood film of at least 60 mm^3 should be made on a microscope slide (the thickness being such that the hands of a wrist watch can just be seen through it) and, after dehaemoglobinizing, drying and staining with standard blood stains, the film can be examined under the microscope for the presence of characteristic microfilariae (Fig. 32.6).

The microfilariae of *W. bancrofti*, *B. malayi* and *L. loa* measure 230–280 × 6–8 μm and all have a sheath. The sheath of *Loa*, however, stains with haematoxylin

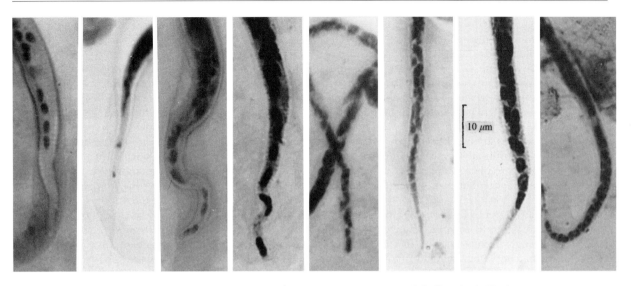

Fig. 32.6 Tails of human microfilariae (from Muller 1975 with permission). From left: Sheathed: *Wuchereria bancrofti*; *Brugia malayi*; *Loa loa* (stained in haematoxylin); *Loa loa* (stained in Giemsa, so sheath not apparent); Unsheathed: *Mansonella perstans*; *Mansonella ozzardi*; *Onchocerca volvulus* (from skin snip); *Mansonella streptocerca* (from skin snip).

but not with Giemsa or Wright's stain, while that of the periodic strain of *B. malayi* often becomes detached. The sheathed species can be differentiated by the graceful curves and lack of tail nuclei in the microfilariae of *W. bancrofti*, the 2 isolated nuclei in the tail of those of *B. malayi* and the presence of nuclei to the tip of the tail in those of *L. loa*. All the others lack a sheath and are smaller (170–230 × 3–4.5 μm), while those of *M. streptocerca* occur in the skin and will not be picked up by a blood film (they can be differentiated from those of *Onchocerca* while alive on a slide in a skin snip mounted in saline by their smaller size and 'shivering' type of motion). If very few microfilariae are expected, as in cases of symptomatic lymphatic filariasis, 10 ml of sequestrinated blood in a hypodermic syringe can be passed through a polycarbonate filter (e.g. Nuclepore, GEC, California) which can then be stained and examined on a microscope slide (Muller 1975). Blood can be preserved in 2% formalin with 10% teepol for later examination. A simple counting chamber can also be employed (Muller 1975).

CLINICAL DIAGNOSIS

Lymphangitis, lymphadenitis, or manifestations of lymph stasis in a patient in an endemic area, often with eosinophilia, are diagnostic of symptomatic lymphatic filariasis and in chronic cases calcified lymph nodes are often evident on radiography (Fig. 32.7).

IMMUNODIAGNOSIS

Circulating filarial antigen can be detected in a drop of blood with the use of monoclonal antibodies using a dot ELISA technique which can be carried out in an endemic country without sophisticated equipment (Hui-Jun et al. 1990). This test is very sensitive for diagnosis of lymphatic filariasis and should obviate the need for taking nighttime blood samples. It may not be very specific, however, so should be treated with

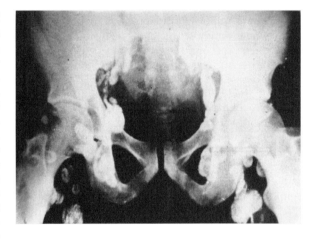

Fig. 32.7 Radiograph of pelvic region in a case of bancroftian filariasis. The incompetent calcified lymph nodes and vessels are radio-opaque.

caution in regions where other filariae may be present.

2.5 Control

Lymphatic filariasis has been identified recently as one of 6 potentially eradicable diseases (International Task Force 1993) and the World Health Organization is coordinating attempts to eliminate it as a major public health problem within the next few years (Taylor and Turner 1997).

The recent optimism expressed about the possibility of eliminating morbidity caused by lymphatic filariasis (International Task Force 1993, Ottesen and Ramachandran 1995) is due principally to advances in chemotherapy. Diethylcarbamazine (DEC) has been used for almost 50 years at a dose of 6 mg kg^{-1} body weight daily for 12 days. This treatment kills microfilariae and also appears to have some action against adult worms; however, it sometimes has to be repeated some months later and must be used with great care in areas of Africa where *O. volvulus* and *L. loa* infections may be present in the same individual. Treatment is also unlikely to be effective in the chronic stages of the disease. DEC will kill both the microfilariae and adults of *L. loa* when given at 2–6 mg kg^{-1} body weight daily for 2–4 weeks but very low test dosages must be given initially if microfilaraemia is high in order to avoid complications (Carme et al. 1991).

In the last few years it has been found that a single annual dose of 6 mg kg^{-1} body weight of DEC reduces the microfilarial density of *Wuchereria* and *Brugia* by 80–90% (WHO 1992). In addition, clinical trials have shown that a single annual dose of 400 µg kg^{-1} body weight of ivermectin (a macrocyclic lactone with very few side effects) will also completely clear blood microfilariae for long periods and the 2 drugs can be used in combination (WHO 1992, Moulia-Pelat et al. 1995). Recent trials indicate that additional treatment with albendazole has some macrofilaricidal action and can markedly reduce the recurrence of lymphangitis (Ottesen and Ramachandran 1995). These findings have greatly improved the prospects for worldwide mass chemotherapy campaigns. Such campaigns have already been successful in the past in countries where there has been a high level of compliance, such as Japan, Taiwan and South Korea. China is in the final stages of an elimination campaign through the use of DEC in cooking salt (1–4 g kg^{-1}). There are now reckoned to be about 1.65 million cases left in the whole country, mostly in the chronic stages; in 1950 there were about 30 million. It is possible that microfilarial rates in China (and in the Solomon Islands, which has had a similar campaign) are falling below a critical point for the continuation of anopheline transmission (Webber 1991).

Integrated control campaigns are likely to be the most successful and these will involve control of the vectors. *Culex quinquefasciatus* is the most important vector species of the *C. pipiens* complex for *W. bancrofti*

transmission in South America, the coastal region of East Africa and most of Asia. It is also spreading alarmingly in West Africa but is not so far able to act as an important vector there since its transmission potential is very low. Breeding sites are mostly associated with sewage or sullage and particularly with open drains, originally installed for storm water but later becoming choked and stagnant, and with pit latrines. Environmental control of this mosquito can best be achieved by adequate maintenance of open drains, septic tanks, soakage pits and flooded pit latrines. For the last, gauze traps can be placed over the vent pipe and squat hole to trap emerging mosquitoes and expanded polystyrene beads can be placed in the water to prevent larvae from obtaining air through their breathing tubes (Curtis 1990, Chang, Lian and Jute 1995). Spraying a film of oil over water surfaces has been used for many years, as has the addition of larvivorous fish to ponds. In rural areas the *Anopheles* vectors of *W. bancrofti* and periodic *B. malayi* breed in bodies of fairly clean water such as ponds, roadside pits and flood or irrigation water and these can sometimes be filled in. Larval insecticides are also widely used, although resistance to organochlorines and increasingly organophosphates is widespread (Curtis 1990).

In Sri Lanka and southern India periodic brugian filariasis has been virtually eliminated because the larval *Mansonia* vector has a breathing tube utilizing the roots of aquatic plants, such as water lettuce (*Pistia*), and these have been systematically removed from ponds.

Control of the *Aedes* vectors of subperiodic bancroftian filariasis in the South Pacific is more problematic since they breed in so many scattered and inaccessible sites and the adults do not rest inside houses. However, efforts are being made to involve local populations in removing man-made breeding sites such as old car tyres, tin cans and coconut shells.

Control of the vectors of *Loa* or *Mansonella* species is not at present feasible, because the former breed in inaccessible forest, swampy, areas and the latter in widely scattered small bodies of water.

REFERENCES

Bryan JH, McMahon P, Barnes A, 1990, Factors affecting transmission of *Wuchereria bancrofti* by anopheline mosquitoes. 3. Uptake and damage to ingested microfilariae by *Anopheles gambiae, An. arabiensis, An. merus* and *An. funestus* in East Africa, *Trans R Soc Trop Med Hyg*, **84:** 265–8.

Bryan JH, Southgate BA, 1988a, Factors affecting transmission of *Wuchereria bancrofti* by anopheline mosquitoes. 1. Uptake of microfilariae, *Trans R Soc Trop Med Hyg*, **82:** 128–37.

Bryan JH, Southgate BA, 1988b, Factors affecting transmission of *Wuchereria bancrofti* by anopheline mosquitoes. Damage to ingested microfilariae by mosquito foregut armatures and development of filarial larvae in mosquitoes, *Trans R Soc Trop Med Hyg*, **82:** 138–45.

Bundy DAP, Grenfell, BT, Rajagopalan PK, 1991, Immunoepidemiology of lymphatic filariasis: the relationship between infection and disease, *Immunoparasitology Today*, eds Ash C, Gallagher RB, Elsevier Trends Journals, A71–5.

Carme B, Boulesteix J, Boutes H, Purvehnce MF, 1991, Five cases of encephalitis during treatment of loiasis with diethylcarbamazine, *Am J Trop Med Hyg*, **44:** 684–90.

Chang MS, Lian S, Jute N, 1995, A small field-trial with expanded polystyrene beads for mosquito control in septic tanks, *Trans R Soc Trop Med Hyg*, **89:** 140–1.

Curtis CF (ed), 1990, *Appropriate Technology in Vector Control*, CRC Press, Boca Raton, FL.

Day KP, 1991, The endemic normal in lymphatic filariasis: a static concept, *Parasitol Today*, **7:** 341–3.

Denham DA, McGreevy PB, 1977, Brugian filariasis: epidemiological and experimental studies, *Adv Parasitol*, **15:** 243–308.

Denham DA, Fletcher C, 1987, The cat infected with *Brugia pahangi* as a model of human filariasis, *CIBA Foundation Symposium*, **127:** 225–35.

Denham DA, Medeiros F et al., 1992, Repeated infection of cats with *Brugia pahangi*: parasitological observations, *Parasitology*, **104:** 415–20.

Dissanayake S, Watawana L, Piessens WF, 1995, Lymphatic pathology in *Wuchereria bancrofti* microfilaraemic infections, *Trans R Soc Trop Med Hyg*, **89:** 517–21.

Duke BOL, 1964, Studies on loiasis in monkeys. IV. Experimental hybridization of the human and simian strains of *Loa*, *Ann Trop Med Parasitol*, **58:** 390–408.

Grenfell BT, Michael E, 1992, Infection and disease in lymphatic filariasis: an epidemiological approach, *Parasitology*, **104:** S81–90.

Grove DI, 1990, *A History of Human Helminthology*, CAB International, Wallingford, Oxon.

Hawking F, 1967, The 24-hour periodicity of microfilariae: biological mechanisms responsible for its production, *Proc R Soc London B*, **169:** 59–76.

Hui-Jun Z, Zheng-Hou T, Weng-Feng C, Piessens WF, 1990, Comparison of dot-ELISA with sandwich-ELISA for the detection of circulating antigens in patients with bancroftian filariasis, *Am J Trop Med Hyg*, **42:** 546–9.

International Task Force, 1993, *CDC Morbidity and Mortality Weekly Report*, **42:** 1–38.

King CL, Mahanty S et al., 1993, Cytokine control of parasite-specific anergy in human lymphatic filariasis. Preferential induction of a regulatory T helper type 2 lymphocyte subset, *J Clin Invest*, **92:** 1667–73.

King CL, Nutman TB, 1991, Regulation of the immune response in lymphatic filariasis and onchocerciasis, *Immunoparasitology Today*, eds Ash C, Gallagher RB, Elsevier Trends Journals, A54–8.

Lal RB, Kumaraswami V, Steel C, Nutman TB, 1990, Phosphorylcholine-containing antigens of *Brugia malayi* non-specifically suppress lymphocyte function, *Am J Trop Med Hyg*, **42:** 56–64.

Lawrence RA, 1996, Lymphatic filariasis: what mice can tell us, *Parasitol Today*, **12:** 267–71.

Macdonald WW, Ramachandran CP, 1965, The influence of the gene *fm* (filarial susceptibility, *Brugia malayi*) on the susceptibility of *Aedes aegypti* to seven strains of *Brugia*, *Wuchereria* and *Dirofilaria*, *Ann Trop Med Parasitol*, **59:** 64–73.

Mahanty S, Nutman TB, 1995, Immunoregulation in human lymphatic filariasis: the role of interleukin 10, *Parasite Immunol*, **17:** 385–92.

Maizels RM, Lawrence RA, 1991, Immunological tolerance: the key feature in human filariasis?, *Parasitol Today*, **7:** 271–6.

Maizels RM, Sartono E et al., 1995, T-cell activation and the balance of antibody isotypes in human filariasis, *Parasitol Today*, **11:** 50–6.

Moulia-Pelat JP, Glaziou P et al., 1995, Combination ivermectin plus diethylcarbamazine, a new effective tool for control of lymphatic filariasis, *Trop Med Parasitol*, **46:** 9–12.

Muller R, 1975, *Worms and Disease*, Heinemann Medical, London.

Nelson G, 1996, Lymphatic filariasis, *The Wellcome Trust Illustrated History of Tropical Diseases*, ed Cox FEG, Wellcome Trust, London, 294–303.

Ottesen EA, 1992, Infection and disease in lymphatic filariasis: an immunological perspective, *Parasitology*, **104:** S71–9.

Ottesen EA, Ramachandran CP, 1995, Lymphatic filariasis and disease: control strategies, *Parasitol Today*, **11:** 129–31.

Philip M, Worms MJ, Maizels RM, Ogilvie MB, 1984, Rodent models of filariasis, *Contemp Topics Immunobiol*, **12:** 275–321.

Piessens WF, Ratiwayanto S, Piessens PW, 1981, Effect of treatment with diethylcarbamazine on immune responses to filarial antigens in patients infected with *Brugia malayi*, *Acta Tropica*, **38:** 227–34.

Sasa M, 1976, *Human Filariasis: a Global Survey of Epidemiology and Control*, University Park Press, Tokyo.

Southgate BA, 1992, Intensity and efficiency of transmission and the development of microfilaraemia and disease: their relationship in lymphatic filariasis, *J Trop Med Hyg*, **95:** 1–12.

Southgate BA, Bryan JH, 1992, Factors affecting transmission of *Wuchereria bancrofti* by anopheline mosquitoes. 4. Facilitation, limitation, proportionality and their epidemiological significance, *Trans R Soc Trop Med Hyg*, **86:** 523–30.

Srividya A, Pani SP, Rajagopalan PK, Bundy DAP, 1991, The dynamics of infection and disease in bancroftian filariasis, *Trans R Soc Trop Med Hyg*, **85:** 255–9.

Steel C, Guinea A, McCarthy JS, Ottesen EA, 1994, Long-term effect of prenatal exposure to maternal microfilariaemia on immune responsiveness to filarial parasite antigen, *Lancet*, **343:** 8928–33.

Taylor MJ, Turner PF, 1997, Control of lymphatic filariasis, *Parasitol Today*, **13:** 85–6.

Vanamail P, Ramaaiah KD et al., 1996, Estimation of the fecund life span of *Wuchereria bancrofti* in an endemic area, *Trans R Soc Trop Med Hyg*, **90:** 119–21.

Webber RH, 1991, Can anopheline-transmitted filariasis be eradicated?, *J Trop Med Hyg*, **94:** 241–4.

WHO, 1992, *Lymphatic Filariasis: The Disease and its Control. Fifth Report of a WHO Expert Committee on Lymphatic Filariasis*, Technical Report Series 821, WHO, Geneva.

WHO, 1995, Lymphatic filariasis: ready now for global control, *Parasitol Today*, **11:** Part 4 (centrefold).

Chapter 33

ONCHOCERCIASIS

J Whitworth

1 The parasite	2 Clinical and pathological aspects of infection

1 THE PARASITE

1.1 Introduction and historical perspective

Onchocerciasis is caused by infection with *Onchocerca volvulus*, the only species in this genus that is a true human parasite. The parasite occurs naturally only in humans and gorillas, but can be transmitted experimentally to chimpanzees. Other species of *Onchocerca* are found in various animals, particularly bovines. Human infections with the cattle parasite *O. gutturosa* have occasionally been documented. These have presented as fibrous nodules containing infertile adult worms.

Adult worms, which live for about 8 years, are typically found in subcutaneous nodules where they are usually benign, apart from being a cosmetic blemish. Female worms produce millions of embryos (microfilariae) throughout their lives and a heavily infected carrier may harbour 50–200 million microfilariae. Microfilariae live for about 1 year in the skin and must be ingested by the correct species of the insect vector (the simulium black fly) if they are to develop further. Microfilariae that are taken up by a black fly migrate to its flight muscles, where they mature over the course of about 1 week into infective larvae. These enter another human via the bite wound made when the insect next feeds.

When those microfilariae that are not taken up by a vector die within skin and eye tissues, they provoke an immune response which, it is thought, leads to the inflammatory lesions and subsequent fibrosis that underlie the disease of onchocerciasis. This is a chronic progressive disease characterized by itchy and unsightly skin lesions and progressive eye damage, sometimes leading to blindness.

O. volvulus can only be transmitted by black flies of the genus *Simulium*. *Onchocerca* species that parasitize other animals may also be transmitted by black flies or by biting midges of the genus *Culicoides*. It is only the female black flies that bite humans, in order to obtain the blood necessary for egg development. They use their short, broad, rasping mouthparts, which cause a painful bite, but which are unable to penetrate clothing. The flies only bite during daylight hours. Because of the feeding and metabolic requirements of the larvae, black fly eggs are laid in well oxygenated waters. Transmission of infection therefore usually occurs close to

black fly breeding sites in fast flowing rivers, giving rise to the apt term 'river blindness' for this disease.

The first account of the microfilariae of *O. volvulus* was probably made by O'Neill (1875), who found them in the skin of 6 West African natives with papular skin rashes. He described the microfilaria as 'easily detectable...by its violent contortions. Thread-like in form, at one time undulating, and now twisted as if into an inexplicable knot, then, having rapidly untwined itself, it curls and coils into many loops'. This accurate and evocative description is readily recognized by those who have examined microfilariae emerging from skin fragments under a microscope. O'Neill also described the pointed tail, and reported the size of the microfilariae to be about 250 μm by 12 μm. As this is too long for *Mansonella perstans* and too wide for *M. streptocerca*, there can be little doubt that O'Neill was describing *O. volvulus*.

Prout (1901) described worms from a subcutaneous nodule removed from a Sierra Leone frontier policeman with vague rheumatic pains. He described the adult male and female worms and microfilariae (unsheathed with a sharp tail, central granular appearance, and a size of 250 μm by 5 μm), which he tentatively called *Filaria volvulus* after Leuckart (1893). Parsons (1908) also gave a description of nodules and commented that he suspected that the disease was more common than generally recognized and probably spread by a blood sucking insect.

Robles, working in Guatemala (1917), demonstrated an association between nodules and the skin lesions and anterior ocular features of onchocerciasis and suggested that black flies could transmit the infection. However, it was Blacklock, working in Sierra Leone, who provided definite evidence of transmission of onchocerciasis by *Simulium damnosum* (Blacklock 1926a, 1926b). He found microfilariae in 45% of skin snips taken from subjects with nodules. No definite evidence of skin or eye disease was noted. Blacklock showed that onchocercal larvae developed first in the gut, then the thorax of simuliids, subsequently invading the head and escaping from the proboscis through the membranous labrum.

The use of skin snips for diagnosis was first recorded in 1922 (Macfie and Corson 1922) when a needle and scissors were used to remove a 0.25 cm piece of skin from the lower back. The recognition of ocular onchocerciasis in Africa came from the work of Hissette (1932) in Zaire, who described punctate keratitis, sclerosing keratitis, iritis, retrobulbar neuritis and retinal lesions, whereas Bryant (1935) noted diffuse retinochoroiditis associated with optic atrophy in the Sudan. The definitive description of ocular onchocerciasis was published as a monograph in 1945 by Ridley, who was working in Ghana (Ridley 1945).

T003 ## 1.2 Classification

P009 Like all filarial worms of medical importance, the species *O. volvulus* belongs to the phylum Nematoda, superfamily Filarioidea, and family Dipetalonematidae. Adult female *O. volvulus* worms, at more than 35 cm, are exceptionally long for a member of the Filarioidea, which usually measure only 2–10 cm in length. Adult *O. volvulus* are normally found in characteristic fibrous nodules, distinguishing them from *Dracunculus medinensis* (superfamily Dracunculoidea), another long (about 100 cm) filarial human parasite found free in subcutaneous tissues.

T004 ## 1.3 Morphology and structure

P010 The adult worms are long and thin, tapering at both ends, although rounded at the anterior end. They are typically found subcutaneously in nodules or free in the tissues of humans. Both sexes exhibit sluggish movement. Microscopically the cuticle is seen to be raised in prominent transverse ridges and annular and oblique thickenings, which are more distinct posteriorly. In the male the cuticular annulations are more closely spaced and less conspicuous, and the cuticle contains more layers and is thinner than in females. The presence of 2 striae in the inner layer of the cuticle is a helpful diagnostic feature of *Onchocerca* in tissue sections. In females the prominence of the cuticular ridges diminishes with age and the thickness of the cuticle increases. As worms become older they become thicker and discoloured, changing from transparent white to yellowish to brown. They also exhibit more patches of calcification and cytoplasmic inclusions of iron granules, vacuoles and lipid droplets as they age.

P011 Adult male worms lengthen throughout their life and usually measure 2–4 cm in length by 0.15–0.20 cm in breadth. Morphologically, male worms are typical nematodes and considerably more mobile than females. Within nodules, males are usually found on the outside of the worm bundle, coiled around the anterior end of a female. The nerve ring is 140 μm from the anterior end. The alimentary canal is straight, ending close to the tip of the tail at the cloaca. The tail ends in a spiral and has a bulbous tip. There are 2 pairs of preanal and 2 postanal papillae, an intermediate large papilla and 2 unequal copulatory spicules which can protrude from the cloaca. The single reproductive tract runs centrally for almost the entire length of the worm. It consists of an anterior testis, a vas deferens and an ejaculatory duct leading to the cloaca (Fig. 33.1). Spermatogenesis is continuous and synchronized, so that only a single developmental stage is found in a particular transverse section.

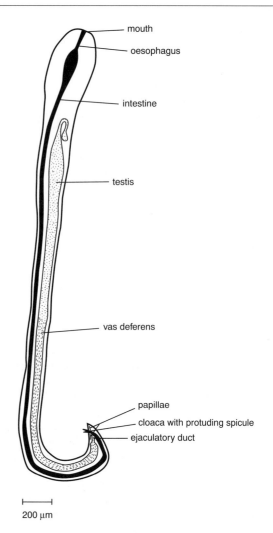

Fig. 33.1 Schematic representation of adult male *O. volvulus* worm.

P012 Adult female worms are highly modified nematodes, notable for their extreme length, wide lateral hypodermal chords, and their reduced muscle cells and intestinal lumen (Fig. 33.2). They measure 35–70 cm in length by about 400 μm in breadth. The nerve ring is 170 μm from the anterior end, and the anus is about 210 μm from the posterior end of the worm. The female reproductive tract runs from the posterior to anterior end of the worm and consists of the following: paired ovaries, one lying more posteriorly than the other; oviducts; seminal receptacles and uteri; and a single short vagina and vulva, found close to the anterior extremity. *O. volvulus* eggs (30–50 μm in diameter) have a striated shell with a pointed process at each end.

P013 The unsheathed, non-periodic microfilariae occur mainly in the skin (90%) and are also found in nodules. They are occasionally found in blood specimens, in most cases probably by dislodgement from the skin. They are also found in the tissues and chambers of the eye in heavy infections and have been reported in urine, sputum, cerebrospinal fluid and ascitic fluid, particularly after treatment with diethylcarbamazine.

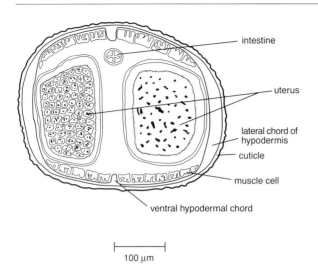

Fig. 33.2 Schematic representation of transverse section of mid-body of adult female *O. volvulus* worm.

Microfilariae are 200–360 μm long and 5–9 μm broad. They have a clear, swollen head with a cephalic space 7–13 μm long. The nuclei are well marked, with the anterior nuclei in rows and elongated terminal nuclei. The tail tapers to a sharp point with no nuclei in the caudal space, which measures 9–15 μm from the terminal nucleus to the tip of the tail. These features distinguish microfilariae of *O. volvulus* from those of the following unsheathed microfilariae that are possible sources of misdiagnosis of onchocerciasis in endemic areas: *M. perstans* (<200 μm long and no caudal space); *M. streptocerca* (180–240 μm long, a curved tail and no caudal space); and *M. ozzardi* (200–230 μm long and a fine attenuated hooked tail) (Fig. 33.3).

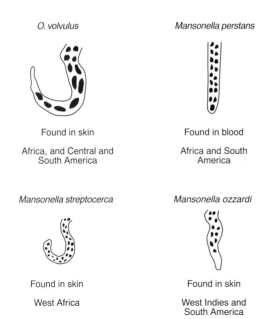

Fig. 33.3 Schematic representation of the tails of microfilariae of *O. volvulus* and other unsheathed human microfilariae.

1.4 General biology

The nodules (onchocercomata) containing the adult worms are usually less than 2 cm in diameter, firm, mobile and well defined, and neither tender nor painful. Each nodule typically contains one or 2 male worms and one or 2 female worms coiled in a mass, lying within a rim composed of vascularized and hyalinized scar tissue derived from the host. Occasionally, nodules may contain 10 or more adult worms and some contain liquefied or calcified necrotic worms. Nodules are well vascularized with fine vessels in close contact with worm coils. Interspersed among the worm bundle is material indicative of chronic inflammation: fibrin; plasma cells; neutrophilic and eosinophilic granulocytes; lymphocytes; and giant cells. Nodules lie subcutaneously in association with bony prominences, sometimes attached to the skin, or occasionally more deeply. The majority of nodules in African patients occur on the pelvic girdle (Albiez, Buttner and Duke 1988). In young children in Africa, relatively more nodules are found on the upper part of the body, especially the head. In Guatemala and Mexico nodules are more frequent on the head in all age groups, while in South America nodules are not common, but are mostly found on the lower half of the body. It is recognized that not all nodules are palpable and that not all adult worms are found within such nodules (Albiez 1983).

From the evidence that nodules normally contain more female worms than males (ratio 1:1.1 or 1.2) and that some nodules contain fertilized females, but no male worms, it is thought that the males are migratory, moving from nodule to nodule (Schulz-Key and Albiez 1977) whereas the female worms are generally sessile. Females have a cyclical reproductive pattern, requiring fertilization by males for each successive brood of embryos (Schulz-Key and Karam 1986). Primary oocytes mature as they pass down the length of the ovary and are released as individual cells into the oviduct and seminal receptacles where they are fertilized and begin dividing. Multicellular stages develop along the length of the uteri until, finally, they escape from the vulva as elongated microfilariae. Each reproductive cycle lasts about 2–4 months, development of an oocyte into a microfilaria taking about 3 weeks.

It has been suggested that the majority of microfilariae normally reside in the lymph vessels of dermal papillae, at which site they usually cause no host reaction, and that it is only extralymphatic microfilariae, particularly those that are dead or dying, which excite the host immune response thought to be responsible for the pathological features of onchocerciasis (Vuong et al. 1988). Adult worms do not directly contribute to the pathological features.

1.5 Life-cycle

The life-cycle of *O. volvulus* is shown in Fig. 33.4. Infective third-stage (L$_3$) larvae are introduced into the human host by biting female *Simulium damnosum* or other black fly vectors. There is no significant zoonotic cycle. Larvae undergo 2 moults before developing into adult worms. The first moult occurs close to the point of entry after 3–10 days and the second moult probably occurs about 1–2 months after the infective bite (Lok et al. 1984, Strote 1987, Bianco, Mustapha and Ham 1989, Duke 1991). The prepatent period from infection to production of detectable microfilariae is usually 12–15 months, with a range of 7–34 months (Prost 1980). Adult worms are long-lived; the average life span of female worms is estimated to be about 8 years, but can be as long as 15 years (Roberts et al. 1967).

P019 Microfilariae are produced by the female worms in large numbers (500–1500 per day) and migrate to the skin and eyes of infected subjects. They can survive in the body for 1–2 years (Eberhard 1986). When microfilariae are taken up with the blood meal by biting simuliids, some migrate from the gut of the vector into the thoracic muscles. There they moult twice and develop into infective larvae over a period of 6–8 days, increasing in length to 440–700 µm. These larvae then migrate to the head of the black fly where they may be transmitted to humans at the next blood meal by emerging through the membranous labrum of the mouthparts and penetrating into the wound.

T007
1.6 Transmission and epidemiology

T008
VECTORS OF *O. VOLVULUS*

P020 Adult black flies are small (under 4 mm long) Diptera found in all parts of the world, with the exception of a few islands. They are squat, heavy-bodied flies with a pronounced humped thorax. They are usually black and may have black, white or silvery hairs on the body. The wings are short and broad, with well developed anterior veins but otherwise membranous. In males the compound eyes occupy almost all of the head and meet anteriorly and dorsally (holoptic), whereas in females the eyes are separated on top (dichoptic). The rasp-like mouthparts are short and broad and do not penetrate deeply into the host's skin.

P021 The species of black fly acting as the main vector of onchocerciasis varies in different parts of the world as follows: members of the *Simulium damnosum* species complex in most of Africa and Arabia; members of the *S. naevei* complex in East Africa; *S. ochraceum* in Central America; *S. exiguum*, *S. metallicum*, *S. guianense*, and *S. oyapockense* in South America.

P022 Black flies lay their eggs on trailing vegetation in fast-flowing water. Each egg batch may contain 100–900 eggs which are laid with a secretion of mucus that is immediately wetted, thus cementing the eggs to the substrate. Eggs hatch after 1–2 days; the emerging larvae remain attached to the vegetation and filter the water for food. Larvae develop into pupae after 5–10 days, and adult flies emerge to the surface in a gas bubble 2 days later. Swarming and mating usually occur soon after emergence. Female black flies need mate only once during their life.

P023 All black flies feed on plant juices and sugar solutions. Only the female feeds on blood and this process has to be repeated for each ovarial cycle. For *S. damnosum*, feeding occurs in daylight, with biting activity peaking soon after sunrise, followed by a lesser peak in the late afternoon (Garms 1973). Host location is probably related to odour, CO_2 output, movement, colour or outline (Wenk 1981). In West Africa most black fly bites on humans are on the ankles and calves, with few bites more than 50 cm above the ground (Renz and Wenk 1983). In Central America most bites are on the head and shoulders. If these areas of the body are not exposed, the black fly will probably seek an alternative host. The relative efficiency of a species of black fly as a vector for *O. volvulus* thus depends partly on its degree of anthropophily, and the persistence with which a black fly will seek a blood meal from a human, rather than from an animal. *S. damnosum* normally takes 5 min to feed to full engorgement on humans (Crosskey 1962). The labrum

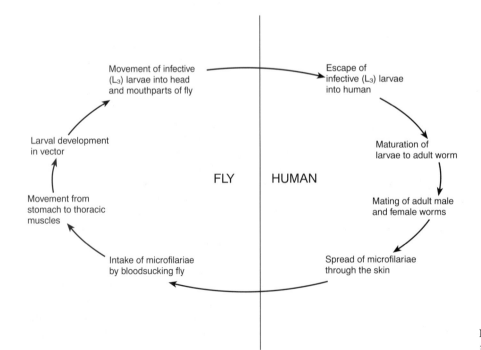

Fig. 33.4 Life cycle of *O. volvulus*.

stretches the skin, which is then penetrated by the maxillae and the rapid scissor-like action of the paired mandibles. These tear a ragged hole in the host's skin, to a depth of about 400 μm. Blood pools in the wound from ruptured capillaries and is then sucked up.

P024
Only a few of the ingested microfilariae will penetrate the mid gut wall and reach the flight muscles, so that the average number of infective larvae per infected fly is usually only 1 or 2. However, once larvae have started to develop their mortality is fairly low. The survival rate of the black fly is not adversely affected unless parasitized with more than 20 microfilariae (Duke 1962). The egg laying cycle of the fly is usually about 3–6 days, but development of *O. volvulus* takes 6–8 days. Thus a female black fly infected at her first blood meal cannot transmit larvae until her third meal. The longevity of black flies in the wild was originally estimated at about 15 days (Duke 1968a), with a theoretical maximum of 4 infective bites, but subsequent reports estimate the maximum life span at 4 weeks (WHO 1987). Studies of the movement of waves of migrating flies suggest that survival of individual black flies is possible for 7–10 weeks (Baker et al. 1990).

P025
There are normally major differences in the sizes of black fly populations in the dry and wet seasons related to the height of rivers and availability of breeding sites. Dispersal of black flies away from their riverine breeding sites does occur, especially in forested areas, but in general the risk of infection is highest close to rivers. Migration, as distinct from dispersal, of black flies is probably a mainly windborne phenomenon. In West Africa this may occur over long distances, up to 500 km (Baker et al. 1990), and may be crucial for the survival of *S. damnosum* populations during the dry season.

P026
Under field conditions only a small percentage of black fly populations is infected. Near to breeding sites the figure averages 3–5% of the total population and 6–10% of the parous population.

P009
EPIDEMIOLOGY

P027
Onchocerciasis is generally a cumulative infection, the severity of clinical features depending on the length of exposure to black fly bites and the density of microfilariae in the skin. Because of this, the disease tends to affect mainly the rural poor in sub-Saharan Africa, particularly West Africa. It is also endemic in Yemen and in parts of Central and South America. Onchocerciasis is an unpleasant disease, lasting many years and causing ever increasing disability to those afflicted. It has serious socioeconomic consequences for the most heavily affected communities in endemic areas. In such communities perhaps 70% of the population will be infected with microfilariae, and about half of these will have symptoms. About 15% will have serious skin or eye disease, and up to about 5% will be blind. Onchocerciasis is therefore one of the major causes of blindness in the world.

P028
The most important determinant of the burden of infection in a community is the infective density of the vector. The biting density of black flies can be measured by regular dawn to dusk catches using human bait at selected sites. This allows the calculation of the monthly biting rate (MBR), a theoretical estimate of the total number of bites an individual could receive if maximally exposed at that site.

$$MBR = \frac{\text{Number of black flies caught} \times \text{Number of days in month}}{\text{Number of catching days in month}}$$

P031
The annual biting rate (ABR) is the sum of 12 consecutive MBRs.

P032
The number of third stage infective larvae can be estimated by dissection. This permits the calculation of the monthly transmission potential (MTP), a theoretical estimate of the number of infective larvae that could be transmitted to a maximally exposed individual (Duke 1968b, Walsh et al. 1978).

$$MTP = \frac{MBR \times \text{Number of Onchocerca volvulus L3 larvae detected}}{\text{Number of flies dissected}}$$

P035
The annual transmission potential (ATP) is the sum of 12 consecutive MTPs.

P036
In practice, these indices give only a rough guide to the level of transmission, as a result of factors such as the following: 1. not all third stage larvae are truly infective; 2. only about 80% of L_3 larvae are transmitted during a blood meal; 3. no single individual is likely to be maximally exposed to bites; 4. the infective larvae of other *Onchocerca* species present in dissected black flies may be hard to distinguish from *O. volvulus*.

P037
Nevertheless, it has been shown that in the forest zone of West Africa the prevalence and intensity of infection and clinical features in humans are related to the numbers of biting flies and measured transmission potentials (Duke, Moore and Anderson 1972).

P038
It is thought that microfilariae show some geographical strain differences throughout their range. The pattern of clinical features of the disease shows geographical variation, which may be related to differences in parasite strain and vector parasite relationships. In West Africa there are 3 major strains of *O. volvulus*: a forest strain with low ocular pathogenicity associated with high nodule numbers and severe skin disease; a dry savanna strain with high ocular pathogenesis and an associated high rate of blindness; and a humid savanna strain with an intermediate pattern (Anderson et al. 1974b, Dadzie et al. 1989). Microfilariae are generally morphologically indistinguishable throughout their range, but in West Africa at least 4 different patterns of acid phosphatase staining are found, supporting the hypothesis that a number of biological strains exist. It has been reported that strain-specific DNA probes can distinguish *O. volvulus* parasites originating from forest and savanna areas of West Africa (Erttmann et al. 1987, Zimmerman et al. 1992). A possible mechanism to explain the evolution of these strains is that local populations of microfilariae became adapted to the specific sibling-species of vector in their area. This may then lead to incompatibility between parasite strains and vectors from different areas (Duke, Lewis and Moore 1966, WHO 1981).

T010   2   CLINICAL AND PATHOLOGICAL ASPECTS OF INFECTION

T011   2.1   Introduction

P039   The major features of the disease are ocular and dermatological pathologies. Communities where infection is common often suffer from socioeconomic depression. The disease is found in West, East and Central Africa, the Arabian Peninsula, and parts of South and Central America (Fig. 33.5). There are about 90 million people at risk of infection in the world, with about 18 million infected and at least 0.4 million blinded by the disease. The great majority of those infected, probably over 99%, live in Africa. These figures are generally accepted to underestimate the true situation (WHO 1987).

P040   Ocular disease is characterized by slowly progressive inflammatory changes in most parts of the eye leading in those most severely affected to visual impairment and blindness. It is also associated with increased levels of malnutrition and premature death. Skin disease often starts as an itchy papular dermatitis leading to irreversible skin changes.

T012   2.2   Clinical features of onchocerciasis

P041   The pattern and frequency of the clinical features of onchocerciasis vary according to duration and frequency of exposure, geographical location and individual variation (Manson-Bahr and Bell 1987). The most frequent symptom is itching. This may of be of any degree of severity and is sometimes incapacitating. It is usually generalized and often associated with excoriations. Other acute reactive dermal lesions include the following: papular eruptions anywhere on the body, reflecting intraepithelial abscesses; transient localized intradermal oedema; and lymphadenopathy, particularly of the inguinal and femoral glands. These lesions are typically firm and non-tender. Later skin lesions give the appearance of premature ageing associated with the following features: lichenoid change, hyperkeratosis, and exaggerated wrinkling of the skin; atrophy of the epidermis, with loose, redundant, thin

and shiny skin (Anderson et al. 1974a); depigmentation, often initially hyperpigmented macules, but more typically a spotty depigmentation of the shins which represents islands of repigmentation around hair follicles in areas of depigmentation. This is often termed 'leopard skin' (Buck 1974). Chronically enlarged lymph nodes and the surrounding fluid may become dependent leading to 'hanging groin' (Nelson 1958) and predisposing to hernia formation, lymphatic obstruction and mild elephantiasis. Some of these features are shown in Figs 33.6, 33.7, 33.8 and 33.9.

P042   The subcutaneous nodules containing adult worms are often visible and palpable, but they rarely cause any symptoms. Occasionally they may spontaneously rupture through the skin, cause local pressure symptoms or the contents may necrose, leading to abscess formation.

P043   Visual damage is the most serious clinical feature of

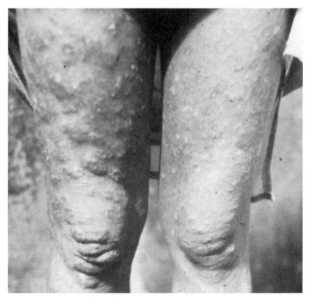

Fig. 33.6 Papular eruption (onchodermatitis) on the thighs of an adolescent girl in West Africa. Note the asymmetrical distribution. (Courtesy of Dr D Morgan.)

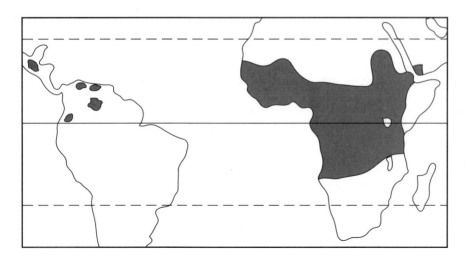

Fig. 33.5 Geographical distribution of onchocerciasis.

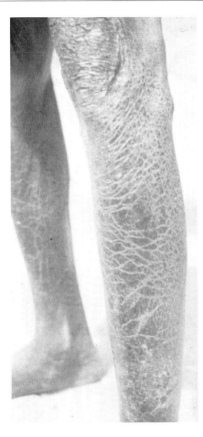

Fig. 33.7 Presbydermia (atrophic skin changes) on the leg of a young man. (Courtesy of Dr D Morgan.)

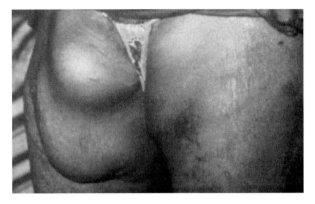

Fig. 33.9 Bilateral hanging groin and right inguinal hernia. (Courtesy of Dr D Morgan.)

onchocerciasis and may affect all tissues of the eye. Ocular lesions are usually seen only in those with moderate or heavy microfilarial loads. Two types of lesion affect the cornea: punctate keratitis and sclerosing keratitis (Anderson et al. 1974a). Punctate keratitis is caused by an acute inflammatory exudate surrounding dead and dying microfilariae in the cornea. These give rise to 'snowflake opacities' and resolve without sequelae. Sclerosing keratitis is a progressive exudative process with fibrovascular pannus formation that starts at the inferior or medial and lateral margins of the cornea and slowly becomes confluent. This may lead to irreversible visual damage and blindness if it encroaches on the visual axis. Anterior uveitis and iridocyclitis are usually mild, chronic and non-granulomatous conditions, but may cause anterior and posterior synechiae, leading to seclusio or oclusio pupillae and serious, potentially blinding, complications such as secondary cataract and glaucoma. Characteristic chorioretinal lesions are atrophy or hyperplasia of the retinal pigment epithelium, chronic non-granulomatous chorioretinitis and chorioretinal atrophy. These are typically widespread, unlike toxoplasmosis, and are usually first seen temporal to the macula. Postneuritic optic atrophy with constriction of visual fields is common in advanced disease, often associated with dense sheathing of retinal vessels.

Other clinical features such as weight loss, musculoskeletal pains and dizziness have been associated with onchocerciasis (Lamp 1967, Pearson et al. 1985, Burnham 1991), but the main clinical burden is due to the skin and eye lesions. In West Africa the prevalence of infection, as measured by the presence of skin microfilariae, increases with age up to 25 years, being generally higher in males than in females (Kirkwood et al. 1983a). The degree of visual damage is related to microfilarial density and the prevalence of visual loss increases with age. Males are 1.5 times more likely to be blind than females of the same age and microfilarial density. Visual damage is also significantly associated with blindness, poor nutritional status and increased risk of premature death (Prost and Vaugelade 1981, Kirkwood et al. 1983b). Other studies from villages in West African savanna regions suggest that blindness from onchocerciasis reduces

P044

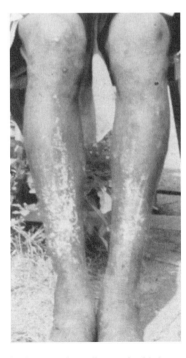

Fig. 33.8 Dispigmentation (leopard skin) on the shins. (Courtesy of Dr D Morgan.)

life expectancy by at least 13 years, and that if the prevalence of blindness in a community is 5%, almost half of adult males and one-third of females will become blind before they die (WHO 1987). Blindness strikes mainly at economically active adults in the prime of life. The development of onchocercal eye disease in an individual is therefore a catastrophe for himself and a burden for his family. At the community level, visual impairment can have serious socioeconomic consequences for the community, especially if villages are in an area of high transmission. Under these conditions heavy infections are acquired relatively early in life, so that there may be a considerable proportion of young, productive men with visual loss. It is in such situations that villages in fertile river valleys were abandoned in Burkina Faso and northern Ghana prior to the start of the WHO Onchocerciasis Control Programme.

T013

2.3 Pathology and pathogenesis of clinical features

P045 The majority of lesions of onchocerciasis are probably caused by the host's immune response to dead and dying microfilariae, with the production of small granulomatous reactions infiltrated with eosinophils. Immediate hypersensitivity, immune complex deposition, products of activated lymphoid cells, autoantibodies and cytotoxic T cells have also been implicated as contributory factors.

P046 Skin microfilariae are characteristically found in the upper dermis, usually without any surrounding host reaction. Early skin changes include the following: perivascular inflammatory infiltrates of eosinophils, plasma cells, histiocytes and lymphocytes; hyperkeratosis; acanthosis with increased melanin in the upper dermis; and dilated tortuous lymph and blood capillaries. Prolonged and heavy infections of the skin lead to loss of elastic fibres, fibrosis, scarring of the papillae, replacement of dermal collagen by hyalinized scar and, eventually, atrophy of the epidermis. Skin lesions may consequently show a wide range of histopathological appearances including acute exudative, granulomatous and fibrotic changes.

P047 Lymph node pathology in Africa tends to show scarring of lymphoid tissue with histological evidence of atrophy and fibrosis, chronic inflammatory infiltration and sinus histiocytosis (Gibson and Connor 1978). In the Yemen, follicular hyperplasia is a more common sign of the disease.

P048 Ocular lesions are also thought to be directly or indirectly related to invasion and local death of microfilariae. The snowflake opacities of punctate keratitis are focal collections of lymphocytes and eosinophils with some transient interstitial oedema around dead or dying microfilariae. Sclerosing keratitis, in contrast, consists of an inflammatory exudate mainly of lymphocytes and eosinophils, scarring and a fibrovascular pannus formation. Uveitis and chorioretinitis are usually low-grade indolent inflammatory processes.

2.4 Immunity

T014

P049

Although infection elicits strong immune responses, there is no good evidence of protective immunity to reinfection. Indeed, in endemic areas the density of microfilariae usually rises slowly throughout life. It may be that very heavy infections with onchocerciasis produce generalized depression of the immune system, although this hypothesis has not been confirmed.

P050 Increased titres of specific and non-specific antibodies, particularly IgG, IgM and IgE, are found in symptomatic subjects; some are specific for microfilariae, infective larvae and adult worms (Mackenzie 1980, Greene, Taylor and Aikawa 1981, Greene, Taylor and Aikawa 1985a, Ottesen 1985). There are also increased levels of circulating immune complexes of unknown significance. Cell-mediated immune responses are generally suppressed, at least in adults (Greene, Fanning and Ellner 1983, Gallin et al. 1988). Immune responsiveness appears to change with time of exposure to infection (Karam and Weiss 1985), with the IgG–IgE balance being an important determinant of microfilarial levels and clinical disease and, like the suppression of cell-mediated immunity, altering between the ages of 10 and 19 years. The intriguing features of immunoregulation in onchocerciasis are marked increases in polyclonal IgE and eosinophils, but the persistence of skin microfilariae with minimal host responsiveness (immunotolerance). There is some evidence of active and specific immune suppression by parasite antigens. Most people in endemic areas, although microfilaridermic, are asymptomatic and show reduced specific antibody levels and depressed B and T cell responses when these are tested in vitro (King and Nutman 1991). These authors suggest that at low antigen concentrations parasite-specific CD4+ T helper 2 (Th2) cells produce interleukin-4 (IL-4), whereas at higher antigen levels cells Th1 cells produce interferon-γ, probably under the stimulus of IL-12. The relative activity of these cytokines and cells controls the balance of IgE and IgG4. Indeed there is some evidence that individuals in endemic areas who appear to be immune to onchocerciasis produce high levels of IL-12 and have Th1 type responses. Additionally, IL-12 is able to reduce experimental keratitis induced by injection of *O. volvulus* antigen into the eye.

2.5 Diagnosis

T015

P051

The mainstay of diagnosis is the demonstration of microfilariae in skin snips. Bloodless skin snips (typically 2–6) are taken from both iliac crests and sometimes the calves in African or Yemeni cases and from the shoulders in American cases. The skin should be cleaned with spirit and allowed to dry before a piece of skin 2–3 mm in diameter and 0.5–1 mm deep is taken. The skin can be raised with a needle and the tip sliced off with a razor blade, or a corneoscleral punch (an obsolete ophthalmological surgical instrument) can be used. These punches enable snips to be taken easily and rapidly, but they are expensive, need regular setting and sharpening, and should be sterilized in cold glutaraldehyde between patients. The piece of skin should be placed in normal saline or distilled water on a slide or in the well of a microtitre plate for a fixed period (anything from 30 min to 24 h). About 60% of microfilariae will emerge after 30 min of incubation in normal saline, rising to over 75% after 24 h. Live microfilariae can be seen moving vigorously in the medium by direct microscopy. They can be distinguished from other species of microfilariae after staining with Giemsa or Mayer's haemalum.

052
In detailed community-based surveys in endemic areas the numbers of microfilariae are counted and the skin snip weighed. The community microfilarial load (CMFL) can then be derived as the geometric mean microfilarial count (per skin snip or per mg of skin) for a cohort of adults aged 20 years or older. This is an accurate measure of the endemicity of onchocerciasis in a community (Remme et al. 1986).

053
Rarely, onchocerciasis can be diagnosed during slit lamp examination by visualizing live microfilariae in the anterior chamber of the eye. The diagnosis can also be made by finding adult worms or microfilariae in surgically removed nodules.

054
A provocative diagnostic test – the Mazzotti test – is also possible. This is based on the reaction which is seen to some degree in virtually all onchocerciasis patients treated with diethylcarbamazine (DEC) (Mazzotti 1948). A single small oral dose of DEC (50 mg) is given, and a positive response is represented by the development of pruritus and rash within 24 h. Because of the dangers associated with Mazzotti reactions, this test should only be used for patients suspected of having onchocerciasis but with negative skin snips. This is because occasionally, particularly in heavily infected patients, severe side effects may occur such as headache, musculoskeletal pains, polyarthritis, large joint effusions, tender swollen lymph nodes, fever, tachycardia, hypotension and vertigo. Ocular reactions have also been reported, including conjunctival irritation, photophobia, punctate keratitis, acute uveitis, retinal pigment epithelial defects and optic neuritis. The mechanism of these reactions is not clearly understood, but is thought to be associated with inflammatory responses involving eosinophil degranulation related to microfilarial killing.

055
In non-endemic areas the combination of the presence of eosinophilia and typical clinical features is suggestive of onchocerciasis. Various serological tests have been described, but there is normally considerable cross-reactivity with antigens of other nematodes, limiting the usefulness of serological tests to screening in non-endemic areas. Recently, more specific ELISA tests have been described, as well as a diagnostic test based on the polymerase chain reaction (PCR), which detect microfilarial antigen in skin samples. These techniques are not yet in general use.

2.6   Control

T016
P056

The control of onchocerciasis can be approached in 2 main interrelated ways: identifying cases and reducing their morbidity, or reducing transmission of infection and thereby preventing new cases (Table 33.1). Currently the 2 main means of control involve reducing morbidity with the drug ivermectin, and interrupting transmission by the use of vector control.

VECTOR CONTROL

T017
P057

Once the life-cycle of *O. volvulus* and the role of black flies in transmitting infection had been established, it became clear that control of the disease might be feasible by attacking the vector. The history of vector control has been thoroughly reviewed by Davies (1994). The first report of successful vector control was made by Buckley (1951) who achieved control of *S. naevei* in a small focus in Kenya by removing all the shade trees along the rivers. However, most subsequent attempts to control the vector have been directed against the larvae, which are confined to a restricted and easily treated habitat. Garnham and McMahon (1947) successfully eradicated *S. naevei*, and eventually eliminated onchocerciasis from 4 isolated foci in Kenya, by using large doses of DDT at a few selected sites at 10–14 daily intervals. The insecticide was carried downstream, killing simuliid larvae over long stretches of river.

P058
Heartened by this success, several attempts to control *S. damnosum* were made in West Africa during the 1950s and 1960s (Taufflieb 1955, Davies, Crosskey and Johnston 1962, Le Berre 1968). All gave some success as long as the control activities were maintained, but black flies reinvaded when the control measures were stopped. However, it was felt that the disease could be controlled in the West African savanna by the use of larvicides if carried out on a large enough scale to prevent reinvasion by infected black flies. This led to the inception of the Onchocerciasis Control Programme (OCP) in 1974, a programme with an original expected duration of 20 years and with 2 objectives: to combat a disease that was widespread and

Table 33.1   Methods of control of onchocerciasis

Reduction of human/vector contact	Environmental means Protective clothing Insect repellents
Vector control	Regular larviciding at black fly breeding sites
Vaccine	A possibility for the future
Nodulectomy	Especially in central America (possibly for head nodules in African children)
Drugs	Microfilaricides ivermectin diethylcarbamazine (obsolete) Macrofilaricides suramin (obsolete)

severe in West Africa; and to remove a major obstacle to economic development (Walsh, Davies and Cliff 1981). The original area chosen for the OCP was the Volta river basin, tributaries of the Niger river and some smaller river valleys to the west. This area was to be controlled by the weekly application of insecticide, from fixed-wing aircraft and helicopters. The calculation of the dose of insecticide requires consideration of the flow rate and depth of water in the rivers, and these parameters may vary considerably at different times of year. Teams visit treated breeding sites weekly and record the presence of nulliparous females, pupae and late instar larvae. On the basis of the entomological and hydrological data, plans for larviciding are drawn up each week. The operations have been very successful, with *S. damnosum* virtually eliminated from large areas, and transmission generally being reduced to very low levels, almost always to less than 10% of pre-control figures. However, the programme has faced problems. First, the development of widespread insecticide resistance has necessitated the introduction of more expensive and toxic insecticides, and secondly, the invasion of the control area by infective black flies from the south-west made it necessary to extend the original control areas. OCP now covers some 1.3 million km² in 11 countries (Niger, Burkina Faso, Mali, Senegal, Guinea Bissau, Guinea, Sierra Leone, Ivory Coast, Ghana, Togo and Benin). The programme is estimated to have prevented 250 000 cases of blindness since 1974 and currently protects some 20 million people at a cost of less than 1 US$ per person per year. Five insecticidal compounds are now used routinely, sometimes in rotation, in an attempt to limit the development of resistance. The success of the programme is largely based on the high quality evaluation of the spraying operations and the potential for rapid response to evidence of treatment failure. The programme is due to continue until 2012, by which time it will have saved 13 million person years of labour that would otherwise have been lost to blindness.

NODULECTOMY

T018
P059

Systematic nodulectomy campaigns in Latin America were stimulated by the work of Robles in Guatemala and Mexico. In Guatemala, nodulectomy campaigns have been carried out since 1935 with over 250 000 nodules being removed. During this time the nodule carrier rate has fallen from 24% to 9%. It is not clear if this reduction has been wholly due to the campaign or whether other factors have contributed. Nevertheless, in one area with hyperendemic onchocerciasis the prevalence of blindness fell from 7% in 1934 to 0.5% in 1979 (WHO 1987). Nodulectomy has been less popular in Africa, with no systematic campaigns. Given the widespread distribution of onchocerciasis, the relatively poor state of African rural health services and the lack of any major documented impact of nodulectomy on the disease, mass nodulectomy campaigns are generally thought to be inappropriate in West Africa. However, since nodules on the head are associated with ocular complications (Anderson et al.

1975, Fuglsang and Anderson 1977), it may be reasonable to remove head nodules, particularly from children.

CHEMOTHERAPY

T019

Suramin

T020
P060

Suramin was the first successful drug for the treatment of onchocerciasis and, although no longer used, it remains the only true macrofilaricide. A dose of 6 g is sufficient to kill all adult worms, but significant side effects were reported in 10–30% of patients. This drug had to be given in a course of intravenous injections over several weeks and so treatment was restricted to hospital in-patients. It is clearly too toxic for general use, and treatment is occasionally fatal.

Diethylcarbamazine

T021
P061

The filaricidal action of diethylcarbamazine (DEC) was first reported by Hewitt et al. (1947). There was much hope that the drug would be useful for onchocerciasis, but, while DEC is an effective microfilaricidal drug, it does not kill adult *O. volvulus* and produces serious side effects. Treatment was therefore suppressive rather than providing radical cure. Severe systemic reactions were more common in heavily infected patients and DEC may aggravate ocular lesions or precipitate new ones. Treatment was oral, and usually a 5–7 day course of increasing doses was given to a total dose of 3.5 g, often in combination with corticosteroids, aspirin or antihistamines to control the side effects. Treatment with DEC has now been superseded by ivermectin.

Ivermectin

T022
P062

Ivermectin is a semi-synthetic product, being an 80:20 mixture of avermectins B_{1a} and B_{1b}, which are macrocyclic lactones synthesized by the actinomycete *Streptomyces avermectilis*. It is formulated as 6 mg tablets and given orally. The recommended dose is 150 μg kg^{-1} body weight taken annually. The manufacturer's exclusion criteria are as follows: children under 5 years of age or under 15 kg body weight; pregnant women; breast-feeding mothers within one week of delivery; and individuals with neurological disorders or severe intercurrent disease. The drug reaches a peak plasma concentration about 4 h after administration, is highly bound to albumin and is reported to have a wide tissue distribution. The precise mechanism of action is unknown, but the drug can act as an agonist of the neurotransmitter γ-aminobutyric acid (GABA), resulting in paralysis of microfilariae (Goa, McTavish and Clissold 1991).

Ivermectin was developed initially as a wide spectrum veterinary antihelminthic agent. It was first studied in man in Senegal by Aziz et al. (1982) and subsequent studies have found that ivermectin was as effective as DEC in reducing microfilarial counts, but had significantly fewer side effects (Greene et al. 1985b, Larivière et al. 1985, Diallo et al. 1986). The suppression of microfilarial levels lasts longer after ivermectin (at least 12 months) than DEC (6 months) (Awadzi et al. 1986, Taylor et al. 1986). Ivermectin

P063

does not kill adult worms but inhibits microfilarial release from female worms, with a consequent intra-uterine accumulation of degenerate microfilariae (Schulz-Key et al. 1985, 1986). Since ivermectin is only microfilaricidal, treatment is suppressive rather than curative and it may be necessary to take the drug for at least the life span of adult worms, i.e. up to 15 years (Whitworth 1992).

Community trials have shown that ivermectin is safe and well accepted and has important effects on the clinical morbidity of the disease, particularly on the ocular lesions (Whitworth et al. 1991b, Abiose et al. 1993). Ivermectin also has some useful activity against other nematode parasites including *Wuchereria bancrofti, Ascaris lumbricoides, Strongyloides stercoralis* (see Chapters 29, 30 and 32) and ectoparasites including head lice (Dunne, Malone and Whitworth 1991, Whitworth et al. 1991a). Caution should be applied in areas where *Loa loa* and *O. volvulus* coexist, as ivermectin can occasionally cause serious side effects in heavy infections of loiasis.

The risk of adverse reactions to ivermectin is related to the severity of infection. These have been reported in approximately 20% of individuals in hyperendemic areas, but the vast majority are mild and self-limiting. About 5% of patients have more severe reactions which affect the ability to work for a day or more. Commonly seen adverse reactions include: increased skin rash and itching; non-tender soft tissue swelling;

musculoskeletal pains; fever; lymph gland pain; and swelling. More serious reactions, which include severe postural hypotension, bronchospasm in asthmatics, abscesses and bullous eruptions, are rare. All of these respond to symptomatic treatment. Adverse reactions are much less common after subsequent doses of treatment, presumably because the microfilarial load has been reduced (Whitworth et al. 1991c).

Ivermectin is provided free by the manufacturers, and the cost of population-based distribution in endemic countries ranges from $0.29 per person to more than $2 per person, depending on the precise system that is used. There are now about 7 million people being treated under population-based distribution schemes, which are likely to be necessary for at least 10 years (WHO 1991). A rapid assessment technique based on the prevalence of palpable nodules has been developed to identify at-risk communities in areas where *S. damnosum* is the main vector (WHO 1992, Ngoumou and Walsh 1993).

In non-endemic areas, where infections are usually light, and patients are not exposed to further infection, ivermectin may be given at 3–6 monthly intervals as necessary, depending on the reappearance of skin microfilariae or recurrence of symptoms. About two-thirds of patients can be expected to relapse within 6 months of each dose of treatment (Churchill et al. 1994).

REFERENCES

Abiose A, Jones BR et al., 1993, A randomized, controlled trial of ivermectin for onchocerciasis: evidence for a reduction in the incidence of optic nerve disease, *Lancet*, **341**: 130–4.

Albiez EJ, 1983, Studies on nodules and adult *Onchocerca volvulus* during a nodulectomy trial in hyperendemic villages in Liberia and Upper Volta. I. Palpable and impalpable onchocercomata, *Tropenmed Parasitol*, **34**: 54–60.

Albiez EJ, Büttner DW, Duke BOL, 1988, Diagnosis and extirpation of nodules in human onchocerciasis, *Trop Med Parasitol*, **39**: 331–46.

Anderson J, Fuglsang H et al., 1974a, Studies on onchocerciasis in the United Cameroon Republic. I. Comparison of populations with and without *Onchocerca volvulus*, *Trans R Soc Trop Med Hyg*, **68**: 190–208.

Anderson J, Fuglsang H et al., 1974b, Studies on onchocerciasis in the United Cameroon Republic. II. Comparison of onchocerciasis in the rainforest and sudan-savanna, *Trans R Soc Trop Med Hyg*, **68**: 209–22.

Anderson J, Fuglsang H et al., 1975, The prognostic value of head nodules and microfilariae in the skin in relation to ocular onchocerciasis, *Tropenmed Parasitol*, **26**: 191–5.

Awadzi K, Dadzie KY et al., 1986, The chemotherapy of onchocerciasis XI. A double-blind comparative study of ivermectin, diethylcarbamazine and placebo in human onchocerciasis in Northern Ghana, *Ann Trop Med Parasitol*, **80**: 433–42.

Aziz MA, Diallo S et al., 1982, Efficacy and tolerance of ivermectin in human onchocerciasis, *Lancet*, **2**: 171–3.

Baker RHA, Guillet P et al., 1990, Progress in controlling the reinvasion of windborne vectors into the western area of the Onchocerciasis Control Programme in West Africa, *Phil Trans R Soc Lond*, **328**: 731–50.

Bianco AE, Mustapha MB, Ham PJ, 1989, Fate of developing larvae of *Onchocerca lienalis* and *O. volvulus* in micropore chambers implanted into laboratory hosts, *J Helminthol*, **63**: 218–26.

Blacklock DB, 1926a, The development of *Onchocerca volvulus* in *Simulium damnosum*, *Ann Trop Med Parasitol*, **20**: 1–48.

Blacklock DB, 1926b, The further development of *Onchocerca volvulus* Leuckart in *Simulium damnosum* Theobald, *Ann Trop Med Parasitol*, **20**: 203–18.

Bryant J, 1935, Endemic retino-choroiditis in the Anglo-Egyptian Sudan and its possible relationship to *Onchocerca volvulus*, *Trans R Soc Trop Med Hyg*, **28**: 523–32.

Buck AA, 1974, *Onchocerciasis. Symptomatology, Pathology, Diagnosis*, World Health Organization, Geneva, 80.

Buckley JJC, 1951, Studies on human onchocerciasis and Simulium in Nyanza province, Kenya. II. The disappearance of *Simulium naevei* from a bush-cleared focus, *J Helminthol*, **25**: 213–22.

Burnham GM, 1991, Onchocerciasis in Malawi. 2. Subjective complaints and decreased weight in persons infected with *Onchocerca volvulus* in the Thyolo highland, *Trans R Soc Trop Med Hyg*, **85**: 497–500.

Churchill DR, Godfrey-Faussett P et al., 1994, A trial of a three-dose regimen of ivermectin for the treatment of patients with onchocerciasis in the UK, *Trans R Soc Trop Med Hyg*, **88**: 242.

Crosskey RW, 1962, Observations on the uptake of human blood by *Simulium damnosum*: the engorgement time and size of the blood meal, *Ann Trop Med Parasitol*, **56**: 141–8.

Dadzie KY, Remme J et al., 1989, Ocular onchocerciasis and intensity of infection in the community. II. West African rainforest foci of the vector *Simulium yahense*, *Trop Med Parasitol*, **40**: 348–54.

Davies JB, 1994, Review of vector control. Sixty years of onchocerciasis vector control: a chronological summary with comments on eradication, reinvasion and insecticide resistance, *Annu Rev Entomol*, **39**: 23–45.

Davies JB, Crosskey RW, Johnston MRL, 1962, The control of *Simulium damnosum* at Abuja, Northern Nigeria, *Bull W H O*, **27**: 491–510.

Diallo S, Aziz MA et al., 1986, A double blind comparison of the efficacy and safety of ivermectin and diethylcarbamazine in a placebo controlled study of Senegalese patients with onchocerciasis, *Trans R Soc Trop Med Hyg*, **80**: 927–34.

Duke BOL, 1962, Studies on factors influencing the transmission of onchocerciasis. II. The intake of *Onchocerca volvulus* microfilariae by *Simulium damnosum* and the survival of the parasites in the fly under laboratory conditions, *Ann Trop Med Parasitol*, **56**: 255–63.

Duke BOL, 1968a, Studies on factors influencing the transmission of onchocerciasis. V. The stages of *Onchocerca volvulus* in wild 'forest' *Simulium damnosum*, the fate of the parasite in the fly and the age distribution of the biting population, *Ann Trop Med Parasitol*, **62**: 107–16.

Duke BOL, 1968b, Studies on factors influencing the transmission of onchocerciasis. VI. The infective biting potential of *Simulium damnosum* in different bioclimatic zones and its influence on the transmission potential, *Ann Trop Med Parasitol*, **62**: 164–70.

Duke BOL, 1991, Observations and reflections on the immature stages of *Onchocerca volvulus* in the human host, *Ann Trop Med Parasitol*, **85**: 103–10.

Duke BOL, Lewis DJ, Moore PJ, 1966, *Onchocerca-Simulium* complexes. I. Transmission of forest and sudan-savanna strains of *Onchocerca volvulus*, from Cameroon, by *Simulium damnosum* from various West African bioclimatic zones, *Ann Trop Med Parasitol*, **60**: 317–36.

Duke BOL, Moore PJ, Anderson J, 1972, Studies on factors influencing the transmission of onchocerciasis. VII. A comparison of the *Onchocerca volvulus* transmission potentials of *Simulium damnosum* populations in four Cameroon rain-forest villages and the pattern of onchocerciasis associated therewith, *Ann Trop Med Parasitol*, **66**: 219–34.

Dunne CL, Malone CJ, Whitworth JAG, 1991, A field study of the effects of ivermectin on ectoparasites in man, *Trans R Soc Trop Med Hyg*, **85**: 550–1.

Eberhard ML, 1986, Longevity of microfilariae following * removal of the adult worms, *Trop Med Parasitol*, **37**: 361–3.

Erttmann KD, Unnasch TR et al., 1987, A DNA sequence specific for forest form *Onchocerca volvulus*, *Nature* (London), **327**: 415–17.

Fuglsang H, Anderson J, 1977, The concentration of microfilariae in the skin near the eye as a simple measure of the severity of onchocerciasis in a community and as an indicator of danger to the eye, *Tropenmed Parasitol*, **28**: 63–7.

Gallin M, Edmonds K et al., 1988, Cell-mediated immune responses in human infection with *Onchocerca volvulus*, *J Immunol*, **140**: 1999–2007.

Garms R, 1973, Quantitative studies of the transmission of *Onchocerca volvulus* by *Simulium damnosum* in the Bong Range, Liberia, *J Tropenmed Parasitol*, **24**: 358–72.

Garnham PCC, McMahon JP, 1947, The eradication of *Simulium damnosum* Roubaud from an onchocerciasis area in Kenya colony, *Bull Entomol Res*, **37**: 619–28.

Gibson DW, Connor DH, 1978, Onchocercal lymphadenitis: clinicopathologic study of 34 patients, *Trans R Soc Trop Med Hyg*, **72**: 137–54.

Goa KL, McTavish D, Clissold SP, 1991, Ivermectin: a review of its antifilarial activity, pharmacokinetic properties and clinical efficacy in onchocerciasis, *Drugs*, **42**: 640–58.

Greene BM, Fanning MM, Ellner JJ, 1983, Non-specific suppression of antigen-induced lymphocyte blastogenesis in *Onchocerca volvulus* infection in man, *Clin Exp Immunol*, **52**: 259–65.

Greene BM, Taylor HR, Aikawa M, 1981, Cellular killing of microfilariae of *Onchocerca volvulus*: eosinophil and neutrophil-mediated immune serum-dependent destruction, *J Immunol*, **127**: 1611–18.

Greene BM, Gbakima AA et al., 1985a, Humoral and cellular immune responses to *Onchocerca volvulus* infection in humans, *Rev Infect Dis*, **7**: 789–95.

Greene BM, Taylor HR et al., 1985b, Comparison of ivermectin and DEC in the treatment of onchocerciasis, *N Engl J Med*, **313**: 133–8.

Hewitt RI, Kushner S et al., 1947, Experimental chemotherapy of filariasis. III. Effect of 1-diethylcarbamyl-1,4-methylpiperazine hydrochloride against naturally acquired infections in cotton rats and dogs, *J Lab Clin Med*, **32**: 1314–29.

Hissette J, 1932, Mèmoire sur l'*Onchocerca volvulus* 'Leuckart' et ses manifestations oculaires au Congo belge, *Ann Soc Belg Med Trop*, **12**: 433–529.

Karam M, Weiss N, 1985, Seroepidemiological investigations of onchocerciasis in a hyperendemic area of West Africa, *Am J Trop Med Hyg*, **34**: 907–17.

King CL Nutman TB, 1991, Regulation of the immune response in lymphatic filariasis and onchocerciasis, *Parasitol Today*, **7**: A54–8.

Kirkwood B, Smith P et al., 1983a, Variations in the prevalence and intensity of microfilarial infections by age, sex, place and time in the area of the Onchocerciasis Control Programme, *Trans R Soc Trop Med Hyg*, **77**: 857–61.

Kirkwood B, Smith P et al., 1983b, Relationships between mortality, visual acuity and microfilarial load in the area of the Onchocerciasis Control Programme, *Trans R Soc Trop Med Hyg*, **77**: 862–8.

Lamp HC, 1967, Musculoskeletal pain in onchocerciasis, *W Afr Med J*, **16**: 60–2.

Larivière M, Aziz M et al., 1985, Double-blind study of ivermectin and diethylcarbamazine in African onchocerciasis patients with ocular involvement, *Lancet*, **2**: 174–7.

Le Berre R, 1968, Bilan sommaire pour 1967 de lutte contre le vecteur de l'onchocercose, *Méd Afr Noire*, **15**: 71–2.

Leuckart R, 1893, *Filaria volvulus*. Skin diseases of tropical countries by Manson P, *Andrew Hope Davidson's Hygiene and Diseases of Warm Climates*, Pentland, Edinburgh, 963.

Lok JB, Pollack RJ et al., 1984, Development of *Onchocerca lienalis* and *O. volvulus* from the third to fourth larval stage in vitro, *Tropenmed Parasitol*, **35**: 209–11.

Macfie JWS, Corson JF, 1922, Observations on *Onchocerca volvulus*, *Ann Trop Med Parasitol*, **16**: 459–64.

Mackenzie CD, 1980, Eosinophil leucocytes in filarial infections, *Trans R Soc Trop Med Hyg*, **74, Suppl.**: 51–58.

Manson-Bahr PEC, Bell DR, 1987, *Manson's Tropical Diseases*, 19th edn, Baillière-Tindall, London, 373–87.

Mazzotti L, 1948, Possibilidad de utilizar como medio diagnostico en la onchocercosis, las reacciones alergicas consecutivas a la administracion de 'Hetrazan', *Rev Inst Salubr Enferm Trop (Mex)*, **9**: 235–7.

Nelson GS, 1958, 'Hanging groin' and hernia complications of onchocerciasis, *Trans R Soc Trop Med Hyg*, **52**: 272–5.

Ngoumou B, Walsh JF, 1993, *A manual for rapid epidemiological mapping of onchocerciasis*, World Health Organization, Geneva, TDR/TDE/ONCHO/93.4.

O'Neill J, 1875, On the presence of a filaria in craw-craw, *Lancet*, **1**: 265–6.

Ottesen EA, 1985, Immediate hypersensitivity responses in the immunopathogenesis of human onchocerciasis, *Rev Infect Dis*, **7**: 796–801.

Parsons AC, 1908, *Filaria volvulus* Leuckart, its distribution, structure and pathological effects,, *Parasitology*, **1**: 359–68.

Pearson CA, Brieger WR et al., 1985, Improving recognition of onchocerciasis in primary care – 1: non-classical symptoms, *Trop Doct*, **15**: 160–3.

Prost A, 1980, Latence parasitaire dans l'onchocercose, *Bull W H O*, **58**: 923–5.

Prost A, Vaugelade J, 1981, La surmortalite des aveugles en zone de savane ouest-africaine, *Bull W H O*, **59**: 773–6.

Prout WT, 1901, A filaria found in Sierra Leone. ?*Filaria volvulus* (Leuckart), *Br Med J*, **1**: 209–211.

Remme J, Ba O et al., 1986, A force of infection model for onchocerciasis and its applications in the epidemiological evaluation of the Onchocerciasis Control Programme in the Volta River basin area, *Bull W H O*, **64:** 667–81.

Renz A, Wenk P, 1983, The distribution of the microfilariae of *Onchocerca volvulus* in the different body regions in relation to the attacking behaviour of *Simulium damnosum* s.l. in the Sudan savanna of northern Cameroon, *Trans R Soc Trop Med Hyg*, **77:** 748–52.

Ridley H, 1945, Ocular onchocerciasis, including an investigation in the Gold Coast, *Br J Ophthalmol*, **10, Suppl.:** 58.

Roberts JMD, Neumann E et al., 1967, Onchocerciasis in Kenya 9, 11 and 18 years after elimination of the vector, *Bull W H O*, **37:** 195–212.

Robles R, 1917, Enfermedad nueva en Guatemala, *La Juventud Medica (Guatemala)*, **17:** 97–115.

Schulz-Key H, Albiez EJ, 1977, Worm burden of *Onchocerca volvulus* in a hyperendemic village of the rain forest in West Africa, *Tropenmed Parasitol*, **28:** 431–8.

Schulz-Key H, Karam M, 1986, Periodic reproduction of *Onchocerca volvulus*, *Parasitol Today*, **2:** 284–6.

Schulz-Key H, Kläger S et al., 1985, Treatment of human onchocerciasis: The efficacy of ivermectin on the parasite, *Trop Med Parasitol*, **36, Suppl. II:** 20.

Schulz-Key H, Greene BM et al., 1986, Efficacy of ivermectin on the reproductivity of female *Onchocerca volvulus*, *Trop Med Parasitol*, **37:** 89.

Strote G, 1987, Morphology of third and fourth stage larvae of *Onchocerca volvulus*, *Trop Med Parasitol*, **38:** 73–4.

Taufflieb R, 1955, Une campagne de lutte contre *Simulium damnosum* au Mayo Kebbi, *Bull Soc Pathol Exot Filiales*, **48:** 564–76.

Taylor HR, Murphy RP et al., 1986, Treatment of onchocerciasis. The ocular effects of ivermectin and diethylcarbamazine, *Arch Ophthalmol*, **104:** 863–70.

Vuong PN, Bain O et al., 1988, Forest and savanna onchocerciasis: comparative morphometric histopathology of skin lesions, *Trop Med Parasitol*, **39:** 105–10.

Walsh JF, Davies JB et al., 1978, Standardization of criteria for assessing the effect of *Simulium* control in onchocerciasis control programmes, *Trans R Soc Trop Med Hyg*, **72:** 675–6.

Walsh JF, Davies JB, Cliff B, 1981, World Health Organization onchocerciasis control programme in the Volta River Basin,, *Blackflies: The Future for Biological Methods in Integrated Control*, Academic Press, London, 85–103.

Wenk P, 1981, Bionomics of adult blackflies, *Blackflies: The Future for Biological Methods in Integrated Control*, Academic Press, London, 259–279.

Whitworth J, 1992, Drug of the month: ivermectin, *Trop Doct*, **22:** 163–164.

Whitworth JAG, Gilbert CE et al., 1991a, The effects of repeated doses of ivermectin on ocular onchocerciasis - results from a community based trial in Sierra Leone, *Lancet*, **338:** 1100–03.

Whitworth JAG, Morgan D et al., 1991b, A field study of the effect of ivermectin on intestinal helminths in man, *Trans R Soc Trop Med Hyg*, **85:** 232–4.

Whitworth JAG, Morgan D et al., 1991c, A community trial of ivermectin for onchocerciasis in Sierra Leone: adverse reactions after the first five treatment rounds, *Trans R Soc Trop Med Hyg*, **85:** 501–5.

World Health Organization, 1981, *Report of the WHO Independent Commission on the Long-term Prospects of the Onchocerciasis Control Programme*, WHO, Geneva, 77.

World Health Organization, 1987, WHO Expert Committee on Onchocerciasis, Third Report, Technical Report Series 752, WHO, Geneva, 167.

World Health Organization, 1991, *Strategies for Ivermectin Distribution Through Primary Health Care Systems*, WHO, Geneva, WHO/PBL/91.24.

World Health Organization, 1992, *Methods for Community Diagnosis of Onchocerciasis to Guide Ivermectin Based Control in Africa*, WHO, Geneva, TDR/TDE/ONCHO/92.2.

Zimmerman PA, Dadzie KY et al., 1992, *Onchocerca volvulus* DNA probe classification correlates with epidemiological pattern of blindness, *J Infect Dis*, **165:** 964–8.

Chapter 34

ANGIOSTRONGYLUS (PARASTRONGYLUS) AND LESS COMMON NEMATODES

K Yoshimura

ANGIOSTRONGYLUS CANTONENSIS (CHEN 1935) DOUGHERTY, 1946

1 INTRODUCTION

The genus *Angiostrongylus* includes c. 20 species infective to small mammals, of which 2 are pathogenic to humans. *A. cantonensis* is inherently neurotropic, causing eosinophilic meningoencephalitis, whereas *A. costaricensis* causes abdominal angiostrongyliasis. *A. mackerrase* may also cause eosinophilic meningitis in Australia. *A. malaysiensis* occurs in South East Asia and 3 cases of eosinophilic meningoencephalitis might have involved this species (Cross 1987). A comparative study of *A. cantonensis* and *A. malaysiensis* in monkeys revealed that the former was more pathogenic causing fatal infections.

A. cantonensis was first found in rats; a discovery made in China in 1935 and in Taiwan 2 years later. Human infection was first confirmed in Taiwan but its public health importance was not recognized until the parasite was found in the brain of a Filipino patient in Hawaii (Rosen et al. 1962).

2 CLASSIFICATION AND MORPHOLOGY

The genus *Angiostrongylus* belongs to the order Strongylida and the superfamily Metastrongyloidea. Although the genus has now been divided into 5 and *A. cantonensis, A. costaricensis, A. malaysiensis* and *A. mackerrase* placed in the new genus *Parastrongylus, Angiostrongylus* is used for classification here, because most parasitologists still use this terminology.

Adult males measure 20–25 mm × 0.32–0.42 mm. The buccal cavity has 2 lateral teeth but no lips. The oesophagus is club-shaped, and measures 0.31–0.32 mm long (Fig. 34.1). There is an excretory pore just posterior to the oesophagus. Spicules are slightly subequal in length, and range between 1.02 and 1.25 mm long. The gubernaculum is 0.095 mm long. The bursa and rays are well developed (Fig. 34.1).

Adult females measure 22–34 mm × 0.34–0.56 mm. The oesophagus is 0.35–0.46 mm long. The blood-filled intestine and white uterine tubules are spirally wound in a characteristic 'barber's pole' pattern. The vulva and anus open at distances of 0.19–0.27 mm and 0.04–0.06 mm respectively, from the tip of the tail (Fig. 34.1). Eggs measure c. 70 × 30 μm.

3 LIFE-CYCLE

The life-cycle in the rat was first described by Mack-erras and Sandars (1955). Adult worms live and lay eggs mainly in branches of the pulmonary artery, but sometimes in the right ventricle. Eggs are carried to the lung capillaries where they form emboli. They embryonate and hatch after about one week. First-stage (L_1) larvae enter alveoli, then migrate up the trachea. They are subsequently swallowed and passed out with faeces. In the intermediate host, larvae undergo 2 moults to the 2nd (L_2) and 3rd (L_3) stage, after 7–9 and 12–16 days respectively. The L_3 larvae are 460–510 μm long and, in molluscan intermediate hosts, remain enclosed in the L_1 and L_2 sheaths.

Many terrestrial and aquatic snails and slugs can serve as intermediate hosts (Chen 1979, Otsuru 1979). Important snails for transmission are the giant African snail, *Achatina fulica* and *Pila* spp.. More recently, another edible snail, *Ampullarium canaliculatus*, was found to be naturally infected in Japan and Taiwan.

Animals that acquire L_3 larvae by eating infected molluscs may act as paratenic (transport) hosts and may transmit *A. cantonensis* to humans. Known paratenic hosts are toads, frogs, freshwater prawns, land planarians and land crabs. The yellow tree monitor has also been described as an epidemiologically important paratenic host in Thailand.

When ingested by rats, L_3 larvae exsheathe and penetrate into the intestinal wall, reaching the heart via the portal system and the inferior vena cava. Larvae then reach the left ventricle through the pulmonary circulation. Some migrate to the brain directly, whereas others migrate first through other organs or tissues. In either case, L_3 larvae reach the CNS within 2–3 days, after which they migrate within the brain and grow. The larvae moult twice, to become young adults that migrate through brain tissue to the subarachnoid space. Approximately 26–29 days after infection the worms, now 11.5–13.0 mm long, penetrate cerebral veins and return to the pulmonary arteries via the heart. The worms now grow rapidly and females lay eggs from around day 35. L_1 larvae appear in the faeces 40–42 days postinfection.

In non-permissive hosts, including man, L_3 larvae reach the CNS and moult twice, developing into young adults. They die in the brain without returning to the heart and lungs, causing serious eosinophilic meningoencephalitis.

Although *A. cantonensis* has been recovered from the lungs of 3 patients it seems unlikely that it can develop to sexual maturity in humans. Experimentally, young adult worms have been recovered from the heart and lungs of immunosuppressed mice (Yoshimura et al. 1982, Sugaya and Yoshimura 1988, Sasaki et al. 1993) but it is still unclear whether full maturity is reached.

4 TRANSMISSION AND EPIDEMIOLOGY

A. cantonensis infection can occur at any age, even in

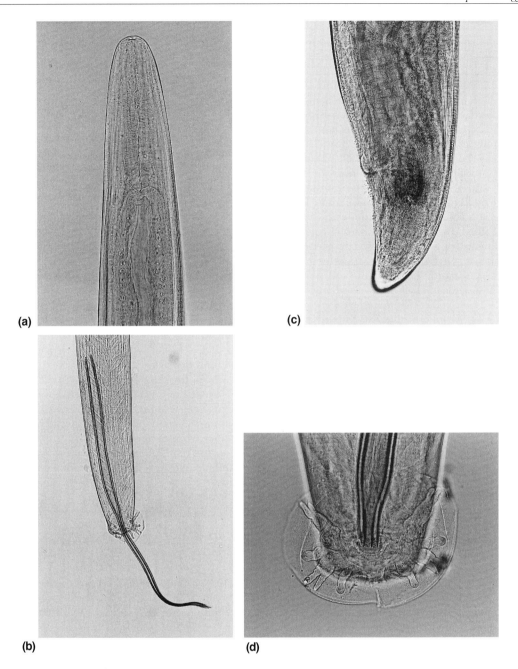

Fig. 34.1 *Angiostrongylus cantonensis.* (a) Anterior end of male (× 123). (b) Posterior end of male, showing copulatory bursa and spicules (× 61). (c) Posterior end of female, showing rectum and vulva (× 123). (d) Copulatory bursa of male, dorsal view (× 248).

young infants (Shih et al. 1992). Humans are infected by the following routes: (1) ingestion of L$_3$ larvae in raw or undercooked intermediate or paratenic hosts, (2) by drinking infected water and (3) oral contact with hands contaminated with larvae released from molluscs. Infections can be established in rodents by various routes including lacerated, abraded or intact skin. Theoretically, therefore, humans may also acquire infections through the skin.

In Taiwan most infections occur in aboriginal children, and are acquired by eating infected giant African snails; 80% of cases are in children under 14 years old (Chen 1979). The overall snail infection rate

is 28%, but snails of size >60 mm show 65% infection. In contrast, infections in Thailand are commonly seen in adult males, who often eat chopped raw *Pila* snails with vegetables as an accompaniment to alcoholic drinks. The overall snail infection rate has been calculated as 20%, but it was as high as 73% in some areas (Teekhasaenee, Ritch and Kanchanaranya 1986). Infection generally occurs during the rainy months.

Most of the cases reported in Japan have originated from the Ryukyu Islands, where patients have become infected by eating fresh toad liver or raw slugs as medicines (Otsuru 1979). Freshwater prawns, or sauces containing them, are responsible for infections acquired in the Pacific Islands, while in New Caledonia, infections are linked to accidental ingestion of infected small planarians (or fragments of these) on vegetables (Ash 1976). In Micronesia, land crabs and mangrove crabs act as paratenic hosts (Alicata 1965). L_3 larvae shed in slug mucus on lettuce may be a source of human infection in Malaysia (Heyneman and Lim 1967). Initial reports of *A. cantonensis* in rodents and molluscs were restricted to tropical and subtropical areas (Alicata and Jindak 1970), but it has since been found in many other countries.

Cerebral and ocular infections in humans have been confirmed in Hawaii, Japan, China, Taiwan, Thailand, Vietnam, Malaysia, Indonesia, Vanuatu, American Samoa and the Ivory Coast (Cross 1987). Suspected angiostrongyliasis has also been reported in Australia, Fiji and New Orleans. Cases are common in Taiwan, Ponape island, Tahiti island and New Caledonia and thousands of cases occur every year in Thailand.

It was previously thought that the spread of *A. cantonensis* was linked to dissemination of the giant African snail (Alicata and Jindrak 1970), but this snail does not occur in many of the new endemic areas. This suggests that if infected rats are present, the lifecycle of this parasite may easily become adapted to indigenous molluscs (Cross 1987).

5 CLINICAL MANIFESTATIONS

These are primarily associated with meningeal irritation and cerebral damage (Table 34.1). Symptoms develop 3–36 days postinfection.

Severe headache is the most common symptom (occurring in 86–99% of patients). It initially occurs intermittently but later becomes more frequent. Nausea or vomiting, fever (<38°C), constipation, malaise and anorexia are frequent (Yii 1976). Less common symptoms are cough, neck stiffness, paresthesia, weakness of extremities, muscle twitching, diplopia, strabismus and facial paralysis. Patients often present with abnormal (usually decreased) tendon reflexes, Kernig's sign, Brudzinski's sign, sometimes with absence of abdominal reflexes and eye muscle paralysis.

The disease is self-limiting and recovery usually occurs within 4 weeks. Serious cases sometimes result in coma, paralysis of the extremities, urinary incontinence or retention, profuse salivation, convulsions and the persistence of symptoms (Prociv and Tiernan 1987). Fatality ranges from 0.5% (Thailand) to 3% (Taiwan).

Eosinophilic radiculomyeloencephalitis has been reported, characterized by peripheral and spinal fluid eosinophilia, severe radicular pain, weakness and hyporeflexia of the legs and dysfunction of the bladder and bowels (Kliks, Kroenke and Hardman 1982). Patients may exhibit transient hypertension and lethargy and some become comatose. In eosinophilic myelomeningoencephalitis, patients develop a generalized maculopapular rash followed by myalgia, marked paresthesia, fever and headache, with progressive weakness, particularly of the legs rather than the arms. Some patients may progress to coma and die (Witoonpanich et al. 1991).

Infected mice usually develop paralysis of the extremities, ataxia, circling and torticollis at around day 20 postinfection. They develop degenerative or necrotic Purkinjé cells that subsequently disappear from the cerebellum, suggesting a Gordon-like phenomenon (Fig. 34.2) (Yoshimura et al. 1988, Yoshimura, Sugaya and Ishida 1994). Eosinophils in the spinal fluid and those around degenerating worms exhibit degranulative changes (Fig. 34.3). Eosinophil peroxidase has been detected in the spinal fluid of infected guinea pigs (Perez et al. 1989). Therefore, neurological disorders in eosinophilic meningoencephalitis are probably due not only to mechanical damage caused by migrating worms, but also to the neurotoxicity of eosinophil-derived basic proteins.

Ocular angiostrongyliasis has been reported from Thailand, Taiwan, Vietnam, Indonesia, Japan and Papua New Guinea, worms being found in the anterior chamber, retina and other sites. This form is rarely accompanied by meningoencephalitis (Nelson et al. 1988). L_3 larvae migrate to the base of the brain, move anteriorly into the orbit and finally penetrate the eye via the cribriform plate (Teekhasaenee, Ritch and Kanchanaranya 1986). Intracerebral migration may also cause optic nerve injury. Worms measuring 500 μm–18.6 mm have been found in the anterior chamber, vitreous humour and posterior pole of the eye, provoking a variety of symptoms (Scrimgeour, Chambers and Kaven 1982, Teekhasaenee, Ritch and Kanchanaranya 1986). Blindness may develop in rare cases.

6 PATHOGENESIS AND PATHOLOGY

Parasites, usually young adult worms, are found mostly in the medulla, pons and cerebellum and in the adjacent leptomeninges (Jindrak 1975) (Fig. 34.4). Some worms are alive at post mortem, whereas others are disintegrating. The number of worms varies but may reach several hundreds. Reactions are rarely seen around live worms, but dead worms are often surrounded by infiltrates of polymorphs and eosinophils, or by a zone of suppurative necrosis or granulomatous tissues. Migrating tracks (infiltrates of macrophages, foreign-body giant cells, plasma cells, eosinophils) are found near to worms and at some distance away. Nerve cells near tracks show central chromatolysis and cytoplasmic axonal swelling and blood vessels show perivascular cuffs of eosinophils, lymphocytes and plasma cells.

The leptomeninges are infiltrated with leucocytes, infiltration being marked over the cerebellum, pons and medulla. Worms are commonly seen within the underlying nerve tissue and the vessels, particularly veins, are dilated. The subarachnoid space is widened. Worms are found on the surface of the pia mater and foreign-body giant cells are found in the subarachnoid space near to parasites as well as more remotely. Cases

Table 34.1 Frequency of symptoms/signs among patients with eosinophilic meningitis or meningoencephalitis due to *A. cantonensis* infection

Symptom/sign	No. of cases (percentage)	
	Punyagupta et al. (1975) (484 Thailand cases)	Yii (1976) (114 Taiwanese cases)
Headache	477 (99)	98 (86)
Sensory impairment (lethargy, coma and confusion)	30 (6)	104 (91)
Vomiting or nausea	425 (88)	94 (83)
Fever	177 (37)	91 (80)
Constipation	–	87 (76)
Malaise	–	81 (71)
Anorexia	–	73 (64)
Neck stiffness	312 (64)	45 (40)
Cough	–	62 (54)
Paraesthesia	181 (37)	32 (28)
Abdominal pain	–	39 (34)
Weakness or paralysis of extremity	4 (1)	26 (23)
Diplopia	184 (38)	11 (10)
Strabismus	–	11 (10)
Muscle twitching	–	15 (13)
Irritability	–	9 (8)
Aching of body and extremities	30 (6)	–
Urinary incontinence or retention	2 (1)	7 (6)
Facial paralysis	20 (4)	–
Convulsion	17 (4)	3 (3)

of eosinophilic radiculomyeloencephalitis show a markedly swollen brain, intensely engorged meningeal vessels and diffuse subarachnoid haemorrhage. Numerous worms are found in sections of the spinal cord but not the brain (Kliks, Kroenke and Hardman 1982). The most striking findings are multiple haemorrhage tracks and cavities caused by worms migrating in the brain parenchyma and spinal cord (Witoonpanich et al. 1991).

7 DIAGNOSIS

Eosinophilic pleocytosis (Table 34.2) and a history of eating molluscs are indicative. Spinal fluid eosinophilia develops at around day 12 postinfection, peaking at days 25–30 (Punyagupta, Juttijudata and Bunnag 1975). Opening pressure is raised to >200 mm H_2O. Spinal fluid is usually clear or slightly cloudy but not xanthochromic (Table 34.2). The white blood cell count in the fluid range from 150 to 2000 μl^{-1}, of which eosinophils exceed 10% in 95% of patients and usually represent 20–70% of the total white cells (Weller 1993). Protein is slightly elevated but glucose is normal (Table 34.2).

Diagnosis should not depend on the identification of larvae in spinal fluid; among 257 cases in Taiwan, worms were found in only 25 patients (Chen 1979). Worm recovery is improved if patients sit upright for some time before sampling (Cross 1987).

According to Punyagupta, Juttijudata and Bunnag (1975), most patients had peripheral eosinophilia

>10% and 43% showed eosinophilia of 21–50%. Blood eosinophilia did not correlate with cerebrospinal fluid eosinophilia or with the clinical course. Over half of patients (56%) showed leucocytosis >10 000 mm^{-3}. Chest X ray findings are normal and a computed tomographic scan is usually free from abnormalities (Koo, Pien and Kliks 1988).

Many serological tests have been used to support the diagnosis (Koo, Pien and Kliks 1988). With partially purified antigens, enzyme-linked immunosorbent assay (ELISA) detects significantly higher IgM and IgE levels in serum than in the spinal fluid (Yen and Chen 1991). Immunoblot analyses for detecting serum antibodies to female worm antigens are also useful (Akao et al. 1992). Tests are complicated by possible cross-reactions between *A. cantonensis* and other nematodes; purified antigens with high specificity and sensitivity should improve this situation. Shih and Chen (1991) described 2 monoclonal antibodies that recognize a 91 kDa antigen in excretory-secretory (E-S) products of L_3 larvae, and they used an enzyme-linked fluorescent assay to detect circulating antigen in the serum and cerebrospinal fluid.

Cerebrospinal fluid eosinophilia often occurs in other helminth infections. In Thailand, it is especially important to distinguish between cerebral and ocular angiostrongyliasis, gnathostomiasis and cysticercosis, all of which are endemic (Teekhasaenee, Ritch and Kanchanaranya 1986).

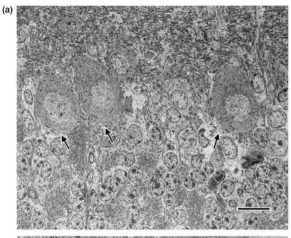

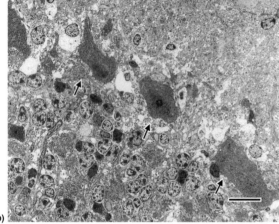

Fig. 34.2 Purkinjé cells (arrows) of the cerebellum from a normal ddY mouse (a) and from an infected ddY mouse at 25 days postinfection (b). Purkinjé cells in the infected mouse are small and irregular shaped, with pyknotic nuclei. Bar = 10 μm.

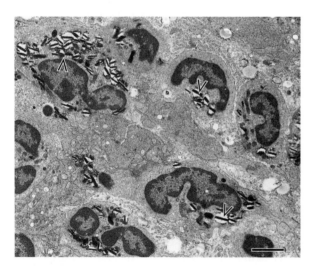

Fig. 34.3 Electron micrograph of eosinophils in a granulomatous reaction around degenerative *A. cantonensis* worms in a cerebellar fissure of a ddY mouse at 25 days postinfection. Eosinophils show marked degranulative changes, i.e., loss of matrix material from specific granules (arrowheads). Bar = 2 μm.

8 CONTROL

Thiabendazole and levamisole have been used to treat eosinophilic meningitis but their effectiveness is still doubtful. Symptoms may worsen during treatment (Bowden 1981) and anthelminthics should be used with caution, as most of the pathogenesis is ascribed to dead or dying worms (Cross 1987). Corticosteroids may alleviate some symptoms of increased intracranial pressure and relieve allergic reactions. Lumbar puncture may relieve severe headache. Treatment of ocular angiostrongyliasis depends on surgical removal of the parasite. A 2% isoptocarpin solution may prevent the worm from entering the deeper parts of the eye (Widagdo et al. 1977).

In order to prevent disease, ingestion of infected hosts and water or vegetables contaminated with L3 larvae must be avoided. Larvae are killed by freezing at −15°C for >12 h or by boiling for 2–3 min (Alicata 1967). The practice of eating toads or slugs for medical purposes (Otsuru 1979) should be prohibited. Controlling the spread of infected rats and molluscs to areas currently free of *A. cantonensis* will restrict further spread of the parasite. Trends towards increased travel, importation of food and movement of refugees from endemic areas are all factors which suggest that awareness of this infection must be raised.

ANGIOSTRONGYLUS COSTARICENSIS MORERA AND CÉSPEDES, 1971

9 INTRODUCTION

A. costaricensis was discovered in the mesenteric arteries of patients in Costa Rica by Morera and Céspedes (1971), who established it as the cause of abdominal angiostrongyliasis. It has subsequently been reported from Latin America, USA and, more recently, from Africa (Baird et al. 1987). In humans, adult worms lay eggs that can embryonate but not hatch. *A. costaricensis* therefore seems to be more adapted to humans than *A. cantonensis*, because it attains sexual maturity (Morera and Céspedes 1971).

10 MORPHOLOGY

A. costaricensis lacks a buccal capsule and the excretory pore is located slightly posterior to the oesophago-intestinal junction (Morera 1973). Adult males measure 17.4–22.2 mm × 0.28–0.31 mm. The club-shaped oesophagus is 0.182–0.225 mm long. Spicules are of equal length, measuring 0.318–0.330 mm. The gubernaculum has 2 branches, the bursa is symmetrical and well developed. Behind the cloaca are 3 papillae (Fig. 34.5). Adult females measure 28.2–42.0 mm × 0.322–0.35 mm and the oesophagus is 0.23–0.26 mm long.

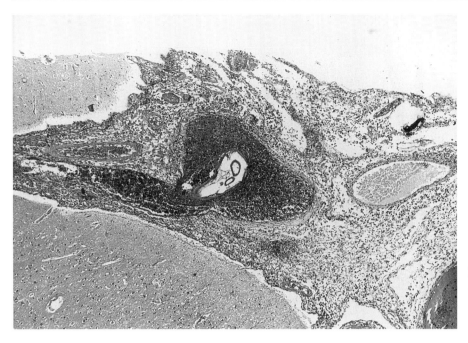

Fig. 34.4 Cross section of *Angiostrongylus cantonensis* in a blood vessel of the subarachnoid space of a human patient (× 47).

Table 34.2 Differential diagnosis of cerebrospinal fluid from patients with angiostrongyliasis cantonensis or gnathostomiasis spinigera

	Angiostrongyliasis (5 cases)	Gnathostomiasis (39 cases)
Colour	Clear or slightly cloudy	Slightly turbid, xanthochromic and bloody
Leucocytes mm^{-3}	Increased 840–3750 (2039)[a]	Increased 110–3000 (920)
Eosinophils (%)	Very high 35–85 (71)	High 15–90 (54)
Protein (g/l)	Slightly increased 0.45–1.25 (0.68)	Increased Not bloody, n = 29: 0.43–1.80 (0.80) Bloody, n = 6: 3.45–9.00 (4.96) Xanthochromic, n = 4: 1.15–3.60 (2.17)
Glucose (g/l)	Normal 0.32–0.62 (0.49)	Normal 0.018–1.00 (0.51)
Opening pressure (mm)	Increased 210–360 (280)	Increased 90–350 (200)

Data from Schmutzhard et al. (1988). [a]Range (mean).

The anus measures 0.060–0.065 mm and the vulva is situated 0.24–0.29 mm from the tip of the tail. The uterine tubules arise near the oesophago-intestinal junction and spiral around the intestine.

11 LIFE-CYCLE

Although the cotton rat, *Sigmodon hispidus*, is the most important natural final host in Costa Rica, 11 additional rodents can also carry infection. Coatimundi, marmosets and dogs can also serve as final hosts (Morera 1985, Brack and Schröpel 1995). In Brazil small rodents other than cotton rats are important final hosts (Graeff-Teixeira et al. 1990). L_1 larvae from the final hosts enter slugs, develop to the L_3 stage and are frequently shed into the mucus (Morera 1973). The most important intermediate host in Costa Rica, Ecuador and Nicaragua is the slug *Vaginulus plebeius*, infection rates reaching 85% (Morera 1985, Duarte et al. 1992). Other molluscs are also susceptible.

When cotton rats ingest infected slugs, the larvae penetrate the intestinal wall and migrate to the lymphatics. They complete their moults within 7 days. Young adult worms (measuring 3.8–4.4 mm long) migrate to the mesenteric arteries by day 10 and reach maturity and release eggs from day 18. Eggs deposited in the intestinal wall develop and hatch, the L_1 larvae appearing in faeces 24 days postinfection (Morera 1973).

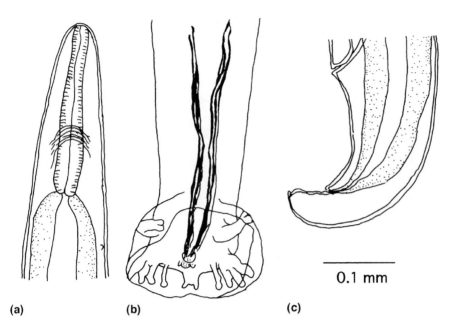

Fig. 34.5 *Angiostrongylus costaricensis.* (a) Anterior end of the body. (b) Posterior end of male, showing spicules and bursa. (c) Posterior end of female, showing rectum and vulva. (Adapted from Ohbayashi 1979).

(a) (b) (c)

0.1 mm

12 TRANSMISSION AND EPIDEMIOLOGY

Transmission to humans occurs by ingesting infected slugs, either intentionally or by the accidental ingestion of slugs hidden on vegetables. Larvae shed by slugs can also contaminate hands and food items. L_3 larvae can enter abraded (but not unabraded) skin of the cotton rat (Ubelaker, Caruso and Peña 1981).

A. costaricensis is widespread in the American continent, from the USA to northern Argentina. Human infections have been reported from California to Argentina (Hulbert, Larsen and Chandrasoma 1992). Incidence is particularly high in Costa Rica, numbering some 650 cases annually, or 18 cases/100 000 inhabitants (Morera 1994). Infection is twice as frequent in males as females and occurs predominantly in children under 13 years (99% of cases), especially in wet months (Loría-Cortés and Lobo-Sanahuja 1980). In Brazil, the incidence of infection is still increasing.

13 CLINICAL MANIFESTATIONS

Symptoms are localized in the abdominal regions, the parasite usually being present in the ileo-caecocolic branches of the anterior mesenteric artery (Morera 1985). Clinical manifestations appear c. 14 days post-infection. Most patients complain of abdominal pain in the right iliac fossa and right flank and palpation and rectal examinations are painful. Fever lasting for 2–4 weeks is common. Occasionally anorexia, vomiting, diarrhoea and constipation are seen. Patients usually show palpable tumour-like masses in the lower right quadrant and these are often confused with malignant tumours. Haematologically, there is significant leucocytosis and eosinophilia (Table 34.3).

Radiology usually reveals abnormalities in the terminal ileum, caecum and ascending colon. Contrast medium demonstrates spasticity, filling defects and irritability at the caecum and ascending colon. Fluoroscopy shows Sterling's sign. The intestinal lumen becomes narrow. When the liver is affected, pain is localized in the upper right quadrant and hepatomegaly is noticeable. Leucocytosis and eosinophilia are usually higher when there is liver involvement than in the intestinal form of the disease, and liver enzymes may be elevated.

14 PATHOGENESIS AND PATHOLOGY

Pathogenesis is attributed either to adult worms in the mesenteric arteries or eggs in the intestinal wall (Morera 1985). Worms damage arterial endothelia, causing thrombosis and distal necrosis. In humans, eggs fail to hatch but provoke local inflammatory reactions with numerous eosinophilic granulomas and ulceration, causing necrotic lesions and thickening of the intestinal wall. The intestinal lumen becomes narrow and restricts passage of faecal material.

Hepatic lesions are produced by larvae that invade the peritoneal cavity and migrate to reach branches of the hepatic artery. Larvae cause thromboses and the subsequent inflammation destroys the arterial walls (Vázquez, Sola and Boils 1994). Ectopic infection in the liver may also to occur (Morera 1985). Adult worms may block the testicular arteries and cause extensive necrosis (Ruiz and Morera 1983).

15 DIAGNOSIS

Diagnosis is difficult, because L_1 larvae are not discharged in stools. In endemic areas, physicians must pay special attention to appendicitis-like symptoms in children with prominent eosinophilia. Serological tests have been employed, including ELISA and latex

Table 34.3 Frequency of clinical symptoms and signs in patients with abdominal angiostrongyliasis

Symptom/sign	No. of cases (%)	
	Loría-Cortés and Lobo-Sanahuja (1980) (116 Costa-Rican cases)	Graeff-Teixeira et al. (1991) (13 Brazilian cases)
Abdominal pain	98 (85)	13 (100)
Fever	93 (80)	10 (77)
Abdominal tenderness	79 (68)	–
Anorexia	71 (61)	8 (61)
Malaise	–	7 (58)
Abdominal tumour	59 (51)	4 (31)
Vomiting	52 (45)	5 (38)
Abdominal rigidity	51 (44)	–
Painful rectal examination	50 (43)	–
Weight loss	–	5 (38)
Diarrhoea	40 (34)	1 (8)
Nausea	–	4 (31)
Constipation	16 (13)	5 (38)
Hepatomegaly	3 (3)	–
Testicular tumour	1 (1)	–
Jaundice	1 (1)	–

agglutination. Radiological findings of a mass in the right lower quadrant, thickening of the intestinal wall at the ileo-caecal region and a narrowed intestinal lumen are also suggestive (Loría-Cortés and Lobo-Sanahuja 1980). Definitive diagnosis depends on the examination of biopsy specimens or surgical resections.

16 CONTROL

Surgical treatments are generally required for definitive cure, but mild disease may resolve spontaneously (Graeff-Teixeira, Camillo-Coura and Lenzi 1987). The following chemotherapeutic regimens are recommended: (1) thiabendazole in combination with diethylcarbamazine, (2) thiabendazole alone, or (3) high dose mebendazole.

Prevention is the best management. Children in endemic areas must wash their hands before eating. Inspection and thorough washing of vegetables and related foods before consumption are recommended.

TERNIDENS DEMINUTUS RAILLIET AND HENRY, 1909

17 INTRODUCTION

Ternidens deminutus is found in Southern Africa, where it infects the large intestines of primates (baboon, vervet monkey, humans), and in parts of Asia where it has been reported only in monkeys.

18 CLASSIFICATION AND MORPHOLOGY

This genus belongs to the order Strongylida, and the superfamily Strongyloidea. Adult males measure 6–13 mm long, and adult females are 9–17 mm. There is a buccal capsule with 3 deep-set teeth and a mouth with a mouth-collar. The anterior end has 4 submedian papillae and 2 lateral amphids. Males have cup-shaped copulatory bursa, 2 spicules and a gubernaculum. Females have protuberant vulva slightly anterior to the anus. The eggs are frequently misdiagnosed as hookworm eggs (and hence are known as 'false hookworm'), but their measurements (81.5×51.8 μm) are slightly larger (Goldsmid 1968). The L_3 larva has paired sphincter cells at the oesophageal-intestinal junction.

19 LIFE-CYCLE

Eggs hatch into L_1 larvae in 2–3 days. Subsequently, they moult to L_2 larvae in 2–3 days and to L_3 filariform larvae in 8–10 days (Goldsmid 1971).

20 TRANSMISSION AND EPIDEMIOLOGY

Infection is by oral ingestion of L_3 larvae. Cases have been noted in Comoros, Mauritius and Southern Africa, from the Congo to the Republic of South Africa. A maximum prevalence of 87% was recorded in Rhodesia (Rogers and Goldsmid 1977).

21 CLINICAL MANIFESTATIONS AND PATHOLOGY

L₃ larvae penetrate the mucosa of the large intestine and moult, the L₄ larvae producing nodules or ulceration. L₄ larvae then moult to the adult stage. If worm loads are heavy, anaemia might result, although *T. deminutus* was not considered to be a blood-sucker by Boch (1956).

22 DIAGNOSIS

T. deminutus and hookworm L₃ can be differentiated morphologically, or by egg volume (Goldsmid 1968). An indirect fluorescent antibody test, using frozen sections of adult worms has been used to distinguish *T. deminutus* from hookworm infections (Rogers and Goldsmid 1977).

23 CONTROL

Thiabendazole and albendazole give cure rates of >90% (Goldsmid 1972, Bradley 1990). Accidental ingestion of the 3rd stage infective larvae should be avoided.

OESOPHAGOSTOMUM SPECIES

24 INTRODUCTION

Although principally parasitic in the large intestines of ruminants and swine, some species of *Oesophagostomum* parasitize monkeys and apes. Larvae produce nodules in the intestinal wall and cause diarrhoea, anaemia and intussusception. Human oesophagostomiasis occurs predominantly in Africa, with some cases reported in Indonesia, China and South America. Five species are known in humans (Polderman et al. 1991), *O. bifurcum* being the most common in Africa and Asia (Blotkamp et al. 1993). *O. aculeatum* occurs in South East Asia.

25 CLASSIFICATION AND MORPHOLOGY

This genus belongs to the order Strongylida and the superfamily Strongyloidea. *O. bifurcum* has a mouth surrounded by an oral collar. The cephalic end has a ventral groove and an excretory pore and the club-shaped oesophagus is 0.58–0.63 mm long. Adult males measure 8.6–15.1 mm long. The copulatory bursa is trilobate, the dorsal lobe small. Spicules are 1.02 mm long, and a gubernaculum is present. Adult females are 11.0–16.8 mm long. The vulva and anus are located 0.36–0.62 mm and 0.17–0.26 mm, respectively,

from the tip of the tail. Eggs measure 58–69 × 39–47 μm, and are indistinguishable from *Necator americanus*.

26 LIFE-CYCLE

Eggs develop to the L₁ stage in one or 2 days at 30°C. The larvae moult twice in 7 days to produce the L₃ stage (712–950 μm) which has triangular intestinal cells and a very long, finely tapered tail of the sheath.

Infection occurs by oral ingestion of L₃ larvae, which produce nodules in the large intestine wall. After further development, they return to the intestinal lumen, attach to the mucosa and develop into adult worms. Eggs are discharged in the faeces.

27 TRANSMISSION AND EPIDEMIOLOGY

Oral infection is the most likely route, but infection through the skin is also possible (Ross, Gibson and Harris 1989).

The prevalence of *O. bifurcum* in northern Togo and Ghana has been calculated as 14.2% in males and 20.1% in females (Polderman et al. 1991). Infection was epidemic in 38/43 villages and prevalence was high (up to 59%) in small isolated villages. Infection was rare in children <5 years old, but high levels were found in individuals >5 years old (Krepel, Baeta and Polderman 1992).

28 CLINICAL MANIFESTATIONS AND PATHOLOGY

L₃ larvae penetrate the intestinal wall and produce a solitary, tumour-like inflammatory mass or abscess (helminthoma), measuring one to 2 cm. This is usually located in the ileo-caecal region, but can be present in other organs and in the abdominal wall. The presence of a helminthoma and abdominal pain are major symptoms of the disease. Multiple abdominal masses or nodules containing greyish-green pus and a single immature worm may be present. Intense rectal bleeding and subsequent anaemia have been recognized but most cases are totally asymptomatic (Ross, Gibson and Harris 1989). Oesophagostomes occasionally produce subcutaneous nodules caused by direct skin penetration of L₃ larvae or by vascular dissemination of larvae from the bowel (Ross, Gibson and Harris 1989).

29 DIAGNOSIS

Clinical diagnosis is not necessarily easy and oesophagostomiasis has frequently been misdiagnosed as carcinoma, appendicitis, amoeboma and other aetiologies. Although principally a self-limiting disease, unnecessary radical surgery has frequently been performed. Leucocytosis and blood eosinophilia are not very useful and diagnosis can often be made only by laparotomy (Barrowclough and Crome 1979).

Barium enema examination is useful for detecting a filling defect on the mucosal surface of the large intestine. Harada-Mori test-tube culture technique is used to obtain L_3 larvae for morphological identification. ELISA for worm-specific IgG4 antibody has a specificity of >95% (Polderman et al. 1993). Body wall and internal structures help to identify worms in histological sections.

30 CONTROL

Albendazole and pyrantel pamoate give cure rates >80% (Krepel et al. 1993). Accidental oral ingestion of L_3 larvae should be avoided.

TRICHOSTRONGYLUS SPECIES

31 INTRODUCTION

At least 10 trichostrongylid species are capable of parasitizing humans. Most species are normally found in herbivores, human infections being accidental, but most *T. orientalis* infections have been recorded in humans. Human infections are prevalent in Iran.

32 CLASSIFICATION AND MORPHOLOGY

This genus belongs to the order Strongylida, superfamily Trichostrongyloidea. The worms are minute and delicate, measuring c. 4–8 mm long. The head is unarmed and lacks a distinct buccal capsule. The male bursa has long lateral dorsal rays that are poorly developed. Spicules are yellowish brown, stout and their chrysanthemum-flower-leaf shape is useful for species differentiation. A gubernaculum is present. The female vulva is situated midway along the body. Eggs resemble hookworm ova, but are longer and narrower (measuring $75–91 \times 39–47$ μm), with one end more pointed than the other. They are discharged at the 16–32 cell stage (Fig. 34.6).

33 LIFE-CYCLE

Eggs develop in 1–2 days and then hatch. L_1 larvae moult to L_2 larvae in 2–3 days and to the ensheathed filariform L_3 larvae in 7–8 days. L_3 larvae are resistant to desiccation. When ingested by humans with vegetables or drinking water the larvae develop in the intestinal mucosa, moulting twice and developing into adult worms in c. 4 weeks. Percutaneous infection may occur.

34 TRANSMISSION AND EPIDEMIOLOGY

Trichostrongylus infections have been reported from every continent. Infective larvae are relatively resistant to environmental pressures, and infections are thus prevalent even in relatively cold areas. In Iran, 9 species have been recorded from humans; in central Iran, the incidence of *T. orientalis* and *T. colubriformis* has been recorded as 67% (Ghadirian and Arfaa 1975). In this region of the world, it is common for women to mould animal dung into solid masses, to be dried and burnt as fuel. This practice may be important in the transmission of animal *Trichostrongylus* to humans. Human infections with *T. orientalis* are principally acquired by eating vegetables contaminated with nightsoil. In Japan, *T. orientalis* infection was previously common in cold areas, the prevalence in Aomori Prefecture in 1975 being c. 19%, but the current figure is estimated to be very low (unpublished data).

35 CLINICAL MANIFESTATIONS AND PATHOLOGY

Trichostrongylids penetrate into the intestinal mucosa, producing redness, erosion and local bleeding. Patients present with epigastric pain, diarrhoea, anorexia, nausea, dizziness and generalized fatigue or malaise (Otsuru and Ito 1972). If worm loads are light patients may be asymptomatic, but heavy worm loads are associated with the development of anaemia, and the entry of worms into the biliary tract, provoking cholecystitis.

36 DIAGNOSIS

Stool examinations are used to detect ova. Harada-Mori cultures are used to obtain L_3 larvae for morphological differentiation. Several methods for detecting ova or larvae should be used, because females discharge only a small number of eggs daily.

37 CONTROL

Pyrantel pamoate, bephenium hydroxynaphthoate and 1-bromo-naphthol are effective. Ingestion of fresh vegetables or pickles contaminated with L_3 larvae should be avoided. Caution must be used when handling animal dung to prevent infection with animal trichostrongylids.

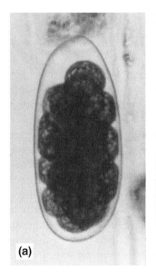
(a)

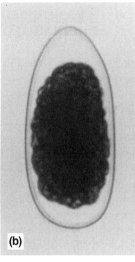
(b)

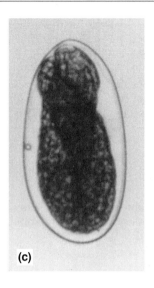
(c)

Fig. 34.6 *Trichostrongylus orientalis* eggs. (a) As seen in fresh faeces. (b) At the morula stage of embryonation. (c) With developed rhabdtiform larva. (× 600).

ANISAKIS AND RELATED SPECIES

38 INTRODUCTION

Anisakids live in the stomach of marine mammals. *Anisakis simplex* was first discovered as a cause of larva migrans by van Thiel, Kuipers and Roskam (1960) who noted a nematode larva in the intestinal wall of a patient suffering from acute abdomimal pain after eating raw herrings. The larva was identified as *Eustoma rotundatum* but the disease was later named 'anisakiasis' (van Thiel 1962). Prior to this discovery, cross-sections of a nematode-like parasite had frequently been recognized in Japanese patients suffering from acute terminal ileal enteritis, with prominent eosinophilic infiltration and severe allergic tissue reactions. These specimens were initially identified as *Ascaris* larvae. Later, *Anisakis* larvae were removed under gastric endoscopy (Namiki et al. 1970) and since then, many cases of gastric anisakiasis have been reported in Japan, linked to the habit of eating raw fish (sashimi or sushi). Anisakiasis has most frequently been found in Japan, followed by the Netherlands (where infections are acquired from ingesting raw herrings). The increasing popularity of 'sushi bars' has contributed to the spread of infections in the USA and Europe. Anisakid larvae parasitic to humans are *Anisakis simplex, A. physeteris, Pseudoterranova decipiens* and *Contracaecum osculatum, A. simplex* and *P. decipiens* being the most important.

39 CLASSIFICATION AND MORPHOLOGY

The genus *Anisakis* belongs to the order Ascaridida, family Heterocheilidae and subfamily Anisakinae. *P. decipiens* was initially called *Ascaris decipiens,* was subsequently transferred to the genus *Porrocaecum, Ter-* *ranova* or *Phocanema* and finally to the genus *Pseudoterranova* (Gibson 1983).

A. simplex L$_3$ were initially called *Anisakis* type-I larva. The larvae have a dorsal lip and 2 subventral lips orally, with a boring tooth on the dorsal lip. The excretory pore opens at the base of the subventral lips. The oesophagus is composed of 2 parts; the preventriculus and a relatively long ventriculus, with an oblique ventriculo-intestinal junction. The tail is short and rounded, with a mucron (Fig. 34.7). Larvae measure 28.40 × 0.45 mm on average. *A. physeteris* was initially called *Anisakis* type-II larva. These measure 27.80 × 0.61 mm on average, have a short ventriculus, a horizontal ventriculo-intestinal junction and a long tapering tail without a mucron (Fig. 34.7).

L$_3$ larvae of *P. decipiens* measure 32.6 × 0.8 mm on average and are yellowish brown. The ventriculus partly overlaps the intestinal caecum posterior and there is a mucron at the tail end (Fig. 34.7). In Japan, *P. decipiens* was previously called *Terranova* type A larva.

Anisakis species have a unique morphology in cross-sections; clear Y-shaped lateral cords (Fig. 34.11), cuticular lateral alae absent, 60–90 muscle cells/quadrant and 60–83 columnar intestinal cells. *P. decipiens* larvae have >100 intestinal cells and butterfly like lateral cords (Oshima 1972).

40 LIFE-CYCLE

Figure 34.9 summarizes the life-cycles of *A. simplex* and *P. decipiens.* Adult worms live in the stomachs of marine mammals. Eggs (40 × 50 μm) are discharged with the faeces, then the larvae moult once into the L$_2$ stage, which hatch when ingested by euphausiid krill and develop into the L$_3$ stage. When infected krill are eaten by squids or marine teleosts, e.g. salmon, cod, herring and mackerel, the larvae encyst in the viscera or muscles (Fig. 34.8) but do not develop further. When these paratenic hosts are eaten by marine mammals, the L$_3$ larvae moult twice in the stomach and develop into adult worms. In Japan, *A. simplex* larvae

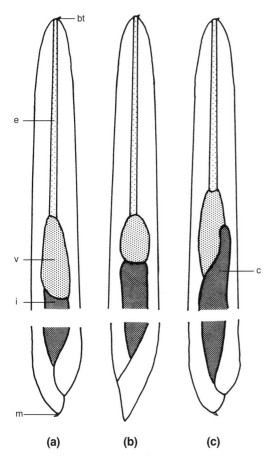

Fig. 34.7 Diagram of the anterior and posterior end of (a) *Anisakis simplex,* (b) *A. physeteris* and (c) *Pseudoterranova decipiens.* bt, boring tooth; e, oesophagus; v, ventriculus; c, caecum; i, intestine; m, mucron. (Adapted from Koyama et al. 1969).

have been found in 164 species of fish and one squid species and adult worms have been found in 26 cetacean species and 12 species of pinnipeds. Marine mammals may be infected by ingesting crustacean intermediate hosts. Humans are not suitable hosts; L_3 or L_4 larvae are found but never adult worms.

Isopods and mysids serve as intermediate hosts for *P. decipiens.* Cod, haddock, halibut, greenling, pollack and other fish serve as paratenic hosts (Fig. 34.9). L_3 larvae have been found in 9 species of fish in Japanese waters and 11 species in Californian waters (Ishikura et al. 1992). Seals, sea lions and walruses act as definitive hosts (Fig. 34.9). Adult worms have been recovered rarely from humans.

41 TRANSMISSION AND EPIDEMIOLOGY

Anisakiasis is linked to the ingestion of raw or undercooked marine fish or squids. Many fish are involved in *A. simplex* transmission in Japan (Fig. 34.8) (Oshima and Kliks 1987, Kino et al. 1993). Pacific cod and halibut are important for transmission of *P. decipiens* in Japan. Other important sources of infection include rockfish, salmon and red snapper in the USA

(Kliks 1983, Oshima 1987) and herring in Europe (van Thiel 1976).

Human anisakiasis has been reported from many countries in Asia, northern Europe and South America. In Japan a total of 20 582 cases were reported between 1980 and 1993 (Ishikura et al. 1993) but only 660 cases were reported from other countries by the end of 1992. In Japan, 93% of cases involved the stomach and only 4.4% were intestinal. In other countries intestinal anisakiasis accounts for a much larger percentage of cases. The annual incidence in Japan >1500 cases. Changes in dietary habits may account for the escalation of anisakiasis in the USA where >50 cases have been reported.

42 CLINICAL MANIFESTATIONS

Clinical manifestations can be severe if a secondary infection induces a strong immediate hypersensitivity reaction around the site of worm penetration. Mild clinical symptoms result from local foreign body formation during a primary infection. The disease is also classified into gastric, intestinal and extra-gastrointestinal (ectopic) anisakiasis. The last form is caused by larvae that penetrate into the abdominal cavity, entering abdominal organs or tissues and provoking inflammatory foci.

Acute gastric anisakiasis occurs c. 6 h after the ingestion of raw seafood (Deardorff, Kayes and Fukumura 1991). Larvae normally parasitize the fundus of the stomach, especially the greater curvature (Fig. 34.10). Symptoms are summarized in Table 34.4. Rarely, gastric anisakiasis may cause severe chest pain or angina-like pain (Sugano et al. 1993) that is often misdiagnosed as gastric ulcer, cancer or polyp.

Intestinal anisakiasis usually develops within 2 days after infection and occurs in any region between the duodenum to the rectum, most frequently in the ileal region (Matsui et al. 1985). Symptoms (Table 34.4) last for one to 5 days and then lead to ileus. Acute intestinal anisakiasis may cause ascites. The disease is frequently misdiagnosed. Patients usually have no pyrexia but develop moderate leucocytosis and, in some cases, eosinophilia (4–41%) (Ohtaki and Ohtaki 1989, Ishikura 1990, Deardorff, Kayes and Fukumura 1991).

P. decipiens larvae are less invasive than *A. simplex,* are frequently expelled by vomiting and rarely cause intestinal anisakiasis (Oshima 1987). Instead, they often provoke a tingling throat syndrome, associated with larval migration from the stomach to the mouth. In contrast, *A. simplex* larvae readily penetrate the gastrointestinal wall and invade the abdominal cavity, provoking peritonitis and intruding into various organs and tissues. Ectopic anisakiasis is usually mild and most cases are discovered accidentally during surgery (Ishikura et al. 1992).

Single worm infection is common but multiple infections occur, for example c. 50 *A. simplex* larvae were recovered from a Japanese patient (Takamuku, Iino and Fujino 1994).

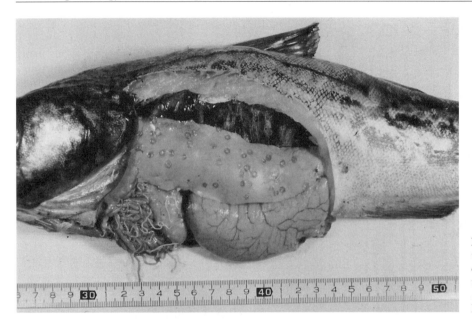

Fig. 34.8 *Anisakis simplex* third-stage larvae encapsulated in the liver of the pollack, *Theragra chalcogramma*. (Courtesy of Dr K. Ishida).

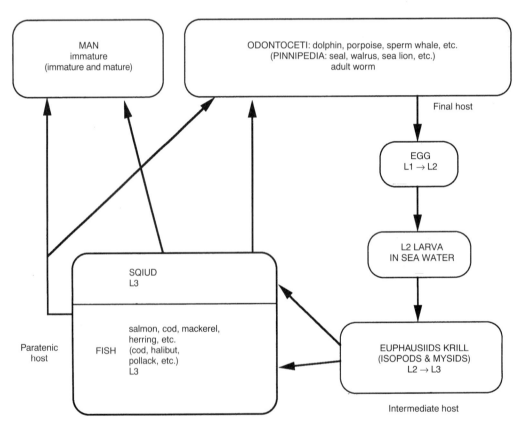

Fig. 34.9 Life-cycle of *Anisakis simplex* and *Pseudoterranova decipiens*. Names in brackets refer to host of *P. decipiens*. L_1, L_2, and L_3: the first-, second- and third-stage larvae. (Adapted from Oshima 1987).

43 PATHOLOGY

Initially, lesions are infiltrated mainly by neutrophils, with a few eosinophils and foreign body giant cells. There is little oedema, fibrinous exudation, haemorrhage or vascular damage. Within the first week there may be oedematous thickening of the submucosa and infiltration by numerous eosinophils and other cells

(Fig. 34.11). In chronic gastric and intestinal anisakiasis, necrotic and haemorrhagic abscesses with eosinophilic infiltration may be present. Eosinophilic infiltration becomes less extensive after 6 months and lymphocyte infiltration predominates. Degenerative worms may be surrounded by foreign body giant cells. In more advanced stages (6 months to one or more years) the abscess or granulomatous inflammation

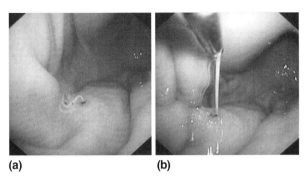

(a) **(b)**

Fig. 34.10 *Anisakis* larvae just penetrating into the stomach mucosa (a) The larva being removed with biopsy forceps of the endoscope (b) (Courtesy of Dr I. Sato).

may be replaced by granulation tissue with some eosinophil infiltration. Fragments of the degenerated worm are usually, but not always, present.

44 DIAGNOSIS

Clinical manifestations are not specific and therefore diagnosis is difficult, especially of intestinal or extra-gastrointestinal anisakiasis. When patients complain of abdominal pain, nausea and vomiting, their dietary history immediately prior to the onset of the symptoms should be determined. If raw seafood has been eaten, diagnostic measures must be performed.

44.1 Endoscopy

Endoscopy is useful for gastric anisakiasis and sometimes for duodenal anisakiasis (Kliks 1986). The site of larval penetration is oedematous, with various degrees of hyperaemia, erosion and bleeding. The penetrating *Anisakis* larva can be easily removed endoscopically with biopsy forceps (Fig. 34.10).

44.2 Radiology

Radiology is effective for diagnosing intestinal anisakiasis. Double-contrast, barium-filled roentgenographic images reveal coiled or thread-like filling defects. Oedematous, thickened, narrowed and obstructed areas in the gastrointestinal walls are present (Sugimachi et al. 1985, Matsui et al. 1985). *Anisakis* infection may also cause a vanishing tumour of the stomach.

44.3 Immunodiagnosis

Although several serological tests are used their application has limitations because of cross-reactions with other nematodes and because low levels of specific antibody may be present in acute anisakiasis. Nevertheless, immunodiagnosis is essential for chronic infections, intestinal and extra-gastrointestinal anisakiasis. Takahashi, Sato and Ishikura (1986) established 2 monoclonal antibodies, one of which (An2) recognized a specific epitope in the intestine, muscle cells and E-S products of the larvae. A micro-ELISA assay using this antibody has been developed (Yagihashi et al 1990). Antilarval *A. simplex*-specific IgG, IgA and IgM antibodies are detectable 4–5 weeks after the onset of disease; specific IgE antibody can be detected as early as one to 7 days. An immunoblot assay, using E-S antigens of *A. simplex* larvae and detecting IgA or IgE antibodies specific for E-S antigens of the larvae, is also useful (Akao, Ohyama and Kondo 1990).

Table 34.4 Clinical symptoms of patients with gastric or intestinal anisakiasis

	No. of cases (%)	
Symptom/sign	Gastric (363 cases)	Intestinal (124 cases)
Epigastric pain	228 (62.8)	16 (12.9)
Generalized abdominal pain	7 (1.9)	12 (9.7)
Lower abdominal pain	14 (3.9)	56 (45.2)
Epigastric distention	19 (5.2)	1 (0.8)
Abdominal bloating	3 (0.8)	13 (10.5)
Nausea	63 (17.4)	26 (21.0)
Vomiting	34 (9.4)	45 (36.3)
Heart burn	9 (2.5)	–
Anorexia	8 (2.2)	–
Tumour	8 (2.2)	8 (6.5)
General fatigue or malaise	7 (1.9)	1 (0.8)
Blood vomitus	7 (1.9)	–
Diarrhoea	5 (1.4)	14 (11.3)
Other peritoneal irritation symptoms	1 (0.3)	18 (14.5)
Urticaria	4 (1.1)	–
Asymptomatic	21 (5.8)	6 (4.8)

Data from Totsuka (1974).

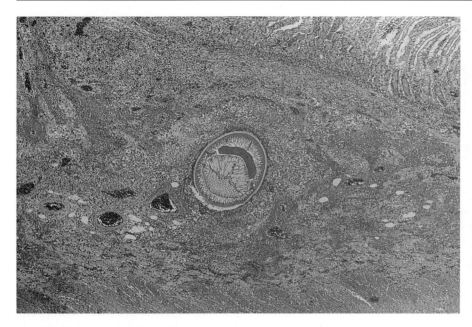

Fig. 34.11 Cross section of an *Anisakis* larva invading the submucosa of the ileum. Note the characteristic 'Y-shaped' lateral cords and the rennette cell, and intense cellular infiltration around the larva (× 47).

45   CONTROL

Gastric endoscopy is effective for locating and removing penetrating larvae. If diagnosis is confirmed and there is no ileus, surgical treatment is not necessary. Instead, supportive treatment is recommended until the larvae die and are absorbed. In experimental animals this occurrs within 3 weeks (Jones, Deardorff and Kayes 1990).

Thorough cooking and adequate freezing of seafood are easy and practical preventive measures. In the Netherlands, legislation (The Green Herring Law) requires fresh herring to be frozen to at least −20°C for 24 h before release to the public. Fish should be cooked so that the internal temperature reaches 60°C or higher for 10 min. Seafood should be frozen at −20°C for 3–5 days (Sakanari and McKerrow 1989, Deardorff, Kayes and Fukumura 1991). At room temperature, *Anisakis* larvae can survive for many days in vinegar, and for one day in soy sauce or Worcester sauce. The larvae may be harmed, but not killed, by gastric fluid.

GNATHOSTOMA SPECIES

Owen (1836) collected worms from a stomach wall tumour of a tiger in the London Zoological Gardens and named them *G. spinigerum*. The genus now contains 12 distinct species, 4 of which (*G. spinigerum, G. hispidum, G. doloresi* and *G. nipponicum*) are zoonotic in South East Asia and the Far East.

G. spinigerum is the most important species in Asia, causing cutaneous, cerebrospinal and ocular lesions. *G. hispidum* was first found to cause human cutaneous gnathostomiasis in Japan (Tsushima et al. 1980), and many cases have subsequently been reported. *G. doloresi* and *G. nipponicum* have also been shown to provoke creeping eruption in humans in Japan (Ogata,

Imai and Nawa 1988, Ando et al. 1988). *G. hispidum, G. doloresi* and *G. nipponicum* usually provoke creeping eruption and rarely affect deeper tissues. They differ from *G. spinigerum* in not causing long-term (>10 years) recurrent cutaneous lesions and they have not been recognized outside Japan.

GNATHOSTOMA SPINIGERUM OWEN, 1836

46   INTRODUCTION

Gnathostoma spinigerum was first discovered in 1889 in Thailand and named *Cheiracanthus siamensis* n. sp., later identified as *G. spinigerum*. Subsequently, many human cases have been reported from various South East Asian countries, Japan and China. In Thailand, eosinophilic-encephalitis, myelitis, radiculitis and subarachnoid haemorrhage caused by *G. spinigerum* are often confused with eosinophilic meningoencephalitis caused by *Angiostrongylus cantonensis*; differential diagnosis is therefore important in this country.

47   CLASSIFICATION AND MORPHOLOGY

This genus belongs to the order Spirurida, superfamily Gnathostomatoidea. The adult males and females are 12–30 mm long and 15–33 mm long, respectively. The head-bulb bears 8–11 rows of cuticular hooklets. The anterior body has toothed spines. The posterior body is naked apart from the presence of minute terminal spines. Males have 4 pairs of large papillae in the caudal alae and 4 pairs of small ventral papillae around the cloaca. Spicules are unequal in length, one being 3–4 times longer than the other.

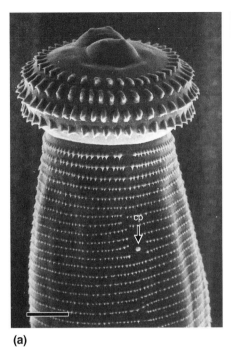

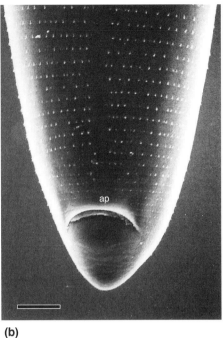

Fig. 34.12 Advanced third-stage larva of *Gnathostoma spinigerum*. (a) Anterior end. cp, cervical papilla. Bar = 30 μm. (b) Ventral surface of the terminal end. ap, Anal pore. Bar = 20 μm. (Courtesy of Dr M. Koga).

(a)

(b)

The vulva is situated just behind the middle of the body. Eggs (measuring 69.3 × 38.5 μm on average) are oval, brownish and unsegmented with a transparent knob-like thickening at one pole.

Advanced L_3 larvae are 3–4 mm long (Fig. 34.12 and Table 34.5). The body is entirely covered with cuticular spines. The morphology of the intestinal epithelial cells of the larvae is shown in Table 34.6.

48 LIFE-CYCLE

G. spinigerum adult worms occur naturally in the cat, dog and many other carnivores. In northern Thailand,

4.1% of 2940 dogs evaluated had adult worms in stomach nodules (Maleewong et al. 1992). Eggs laid in these nodules pass into the gastric lumen through a small aperture and are discharged into the faeces. L_1 larvae develop in the eggs and moult to the L_2 stage (Fig. 34.13) after which the eggs hatch. L_2 larvae are ingested by an aquatic crustacean (*Cyclops*), after which they develop in the haemocoel and moult into the early L_3 stage in 6–10 days.

When early L_3 larvae are ingested by freshwater fish they penetrate into the gut, reaching the muscle and developing into the advanced L_3 larvae, measuring 2.8–5.2 × 0.3–0.8 mm. These lie coiled and encysted by connective tissues (Daengsvang 1982). If hosts with

Table 34.5 Differential diagnosis of advanced third-stage larvae of 4 species of *Gnathostoma*

Species	No. of hooklets on head-bulb				Remarks	Reference
	1st row	2nd row	3rd row	4th row		
G. spinigerum	43.2	44.8	46.7	52.3	The number of hooklets in each row is more than 40, increasing posteriorly	Miyazaki (1960)
G. hispidum	38.3	40.5	41.8	46.0	The number of hooklets gradually increases posteriorly. The 1st row of hooklets are smaller than the others	Akahane et al. (1982)
G. doloresi	38.3	37.9	35.6	35.7	The number of hooklets in each row is fewer than 40, decreasing posteriorly. The hooklets in the 1st row are especially small	Mako and Akahane (1985)
G. nipponicum	37.0	37.1	41.0	–	Lack the 4th row of hooklets	Ando et al. (1988)

Table 34.6 Differential diagnosis in cross-section of the abdominal region of advanced third-stage larvae of 4 species of *Gnathostoma*

Species	No. of muscle cells/quadrant	Number	Intestinal cell shape	No. of nuclei
G. spinigerum	10–15	21–29	Columnar	0–7 (mostly 3–7)
G. hispidum	11–15	19–31	Spherical	0–2 (mostly 1)
G. doloresi	11–15	18–28	Spherical	0–3 (mostly 2)
G. nipponicum	10–14	10–14	Columnar	0–4 (1 in 50% of cells)

After Ando et al. (1991).

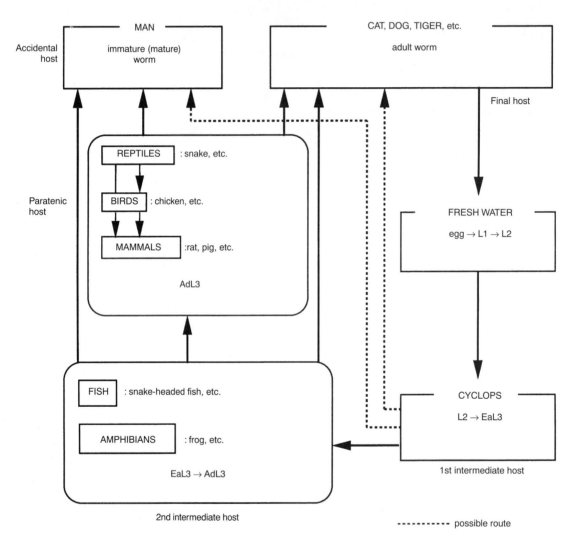

Fig. 34.13 Life-cycle of *Gnathostoma spinigerum*. L_1 and L_2, the first- and second-stage larvae; EaL_3, early third-stage larva; AdL_3, advanced third-stage larva.

L_3 larvae are eaten by paratenic hosts (reptiles, birds or mammals), the larvae encyst again. Advanced L_3 larvae have been found in 44 species of vertebrates in Thailand and in 36 species of animals in Japan. Rusnak and Lucey (1993) have listed the many species that can serve as natural and experimental hosts.

When advanced L_3 larvae are ingested by a final host they excyst in the stomach, then penetrate the gastric wall to the peritoneal cavity to reach the liver. Subsequently, they migrate through the host and, 4 weeks later, they return to the stomach, penetrating the gastric wall from the outside to form a tumour that connects with the stomach lumen through a small aperture. The adult worm develops within 4.5–6 months after infection. Although the adult stage can develop in humans, the worms cannot return to the stomach (Miyazaki 1991).

49 TRANSMISSION AND EPIDEMIOLOGY

Infections are normally acquired by ingestion of 2nd intermediate or paratenic hosts or, possibly, by drinking water containing infected *Cyclops* or free L$_3$ larvae. Although the most important source of infections is snake-headed fish in both Thailand and Japan, many other species of fish, amphibia, reptiles, birds and mammals are possible sources. People from Thailand often become infected by eating raw or fermented fish flesh, or raw or undercooked chicken flesh. Fresh water fish and chickens are major sources of human infections in Japan. The incidence of infection in snake-headed fish varies, but overall ranges from 44 to 99% (Daengsvang 1982). In Thailand, the incidence in freshwater eel has been reported to reach 80–100%, thus both the eel and snake-headed fish are epidemiologically important. Three possible human cases of prenatal infections have been documented (Rusnak and Lucey 1993).

Advanced L$_3$ larvae can penetrate the intact skin of mice, rats and cats, complete penetration occurring within 30 min. Human infections may also be acquired by this route (Rusnak and Lucey 1993).

Human gnathostomiasis has been recorded from 19 countries, predominantly in Asia, especially Thailand and Japan. In Thailand, infections mainly occur in the rainy seasons (Punyagupta, Bunnag and Juttijudata 1990) and are most prevalent in females, aged 20–25, whereas in Japan, they are most prevalent in males in their twenties (Daegnsvang 1982). The youngest recorded case in Japan was an infant less than 2 years old.

50 CLINICAL MANIFESTATIONS AND PATHOLOGY

Gnathostomiasis spinigera has cutaneous and visceral forms and the latter is divided into pulmonary, gastrointestinal, urogenital, ocular, otorhinolaryngeal and cerebral forms (Rusnak and Lucey 1993). Patients develop various prodromes, e.g. general malaise, anorexia, urticaria, vomiting, epigastric pain, diarrhoea and fever in about the first 5 days postinfection, i.e. when L$_3$ larvae excyst, penetrate into the peritoneal cavity and migrate through the liver. Right upper quadrant pain may be experienced. The larvae then migrate to various parts of the body, most frequently to muscle and subcutaneous tissues. A specific cutaneous symptom, i.e. migrating intermittent swelling, usually develops within one month after infection, but may sometimes occur one or 2 years later. During this process, tissues or organs are mechanically injured by the migrating worms and probably also by the toxins they release (Miyazaki 1960). The lesions thus become enlarged, with allergic inflammation around infected foci. Worms in human tissues are not encysted.

In cutaneous gnathostomiasis, migrating swelling frequently appears first in the abdominal area, after which the lesion migrates at random. Worms move at about one cm per hour in human skin. Swellings are rather hard, variable in size and mostly erythematous. Skin lesions are normally painless apart from light or moderate itch. Swellings last one to 2 weeks and then disappear, another swelling appearing elsewhere. Migrating swellings may recur intermittently for up to 10–12 years. Worms migrating near the body surface may cause creeping eruption, cutaneous abscesses or cutaneous nodules, from which the worms can often be resected. Inflammatory foci with profound eosinophilic infiltration are commonly seen in the skin lesions.

Migrating worms in deeper tissues produce visceral gnathostomiasis and serious symptoms may develop, depending on the organs or tissues affected (Rusnak and Lucey 1993). An acute or chronic inflammatory reaction occurs around invading worms and local haemorrhage, necrosis, oedema, fibrosis and tumour formation may occur. When the lungs are affected, respiratory symptoms occur. Involvement of the gastrointestinal tract is rare and usually asymptomatic, only being found incidentally at surgery. Urogenital involvement is also rare. Ocular involvement presents as pain and visual impairment, with a variety of signs (Teekhasaenee, Ritch and Kanchanaranya 1986). Involvement of the ear, nose and throat is always preceded by facial swellings; worms may extrude from tissues and there may be dyspnoea and difficulty in swallowing. The prognosis of gnathostomiasis with CNS involvement is poor and the infection is sometimes fatal (Punyagupta, Bunnag and Juttijudata 1990). A common clinical symptom in this form is radiculomyelitis, typically characterized by excruciating radicular pain associated with a burning sensation, which may last for one to 5 days as the worms migrate from the nerve root. When a cranial nerve or a cervical nerve is affected, the patient develops severe headache, convulsion, vomiting, paraesthesia and unconsciousness, followed by paralysis or weakness of the extremities. In Thailand, differential diagnosis between cerebral angiostrongyliasis and gnathostomiasis is required, because both involve marked eosinophilia in the spinal fluid (Table 34.2).

Initially patients show peripheral leucocytosis and 5–96% eosinophilia, but both these signs later gradually decrease. Patients with ocular gnathostomiasis show normal haematology. Cerebral gnathostomiasis usually shows xanthochromic cerebrospinal fluid with numerous leucocytes, especially lymphocytes and eosinophils (8–98%), and some erythrocytes. Protein in the spinal fluid is unchanged or slightly elevated, whereas glucose is normal (Table 34.2). Computed tomography of the head is useful for diagnosis of intracranial haemorrhage or obstructive hydrocephalus. Death is usually due to direct involvement of the brain stem and massive haemorrhage in this area; mortality ranges from 8 to 25% (Rusnak and Lucey 1993).

51 DIAGNOSIS

If biopsy specimens or sections containing worms are available, diagnosis can be made morphologically (Tables 34.5 and 34.6). Recovery of worms is not always possible and therefore serological tests have also been employed. An ELISA test using crude extract of advanced L_3 larvae or their E-S products is used for detecting antigen specific IgE (Soesatyo et al. 1987) or IgG antibody (Tuntipopipat et al. 1989) in sera or spinal fluid. A 24 kDa glycoprotein antigen from advanced L_3 larvae is specific to *G. spinigerum* and is thus useful for immunodiagnosis (Nopparatana et al. 1991, Tapchaisri et al. 1991). E-S antigens from advanced L_3 larvae give a better diagnostic result than crude somatic extracts. Detection of circulating antigens seems to be unreliable (Tuntipopipat et al. 1989).

52 CONTROL

There are currently no effective therapeutic measures other than surgical removal of worms, which is not always feasible. Effective anthelminthics are unavailable and supportive, symptomatic and anti-inflammatory treatments are recommended. Preventive measures include avoidance of raw or inadequately cooked hosts that may contain L_3 larvae and avoidance of drinking water that may contain infected *Cyclops*. L_3 larvae are killed by boiling for 5 min or freezing at −20°C for 3–5 days (Schantz 1989, Rusnak and Lucey 1993). Use of gloves or frequent washing of hands while handling food is recommended to prevent possible larval penetration of the skin. Relatively recent increases in world travel and importation of food mean that greater awareness of gnathostomiasis spinigera is required, even in the USA and European countries.

GNATHOSTOMA HISPIDUM FEDTSCHENKO, 1872

53 INTRODUCTION

Gnathostoma hispidum was discovered in 1872 in wild pigs in Turkestan and in domestic pigs in Hungary. Since then it has been found in pigs in Germany and many Asian countries (Daengsvang 1982). Two doubtful human cases were described in 1924 and 1949, and 4 cases of creeping disease were more recently found in Japan (Tsushima et al. 1980). Subsequently, a further 79 cases of cutaneous gnathostomiasis due to *G. hispidum* have been recognized in Japan (Ando 1992).

54 MORPHOLOGY

Adult worms live in the stomach wall, singly or in groups of a few worms, without producing a tumour. Males are 20 mm long and females are 25 mm long. Fresh specimens are red. The head-bulb bears 9–12 rows of cephalic hooklets and the entire body surface is covered with cuticular spines. Eight pairs of papillae are located caudally in the male worm, whereas the female has one pair of papillae. Eggs resemble those of *G. spinigerum* but are slightly larger, (72×40 μm). Advanced L_3 larvae from humans measure c. 900 μm (Tables 34.5 and 34.6).

55 LIFE-CYCLE

Eggs shed in swine faeces release L_2 larvae in c. 2 weeks. If ingested by *Cyclops* they moult into early L_3 larvae in c. 8 days. These develop into advanced L_3 larvae in 2nd intermediate or paratenic hosts (e.g., fish, amphibians and rodents) and become encysted in their muscles. Prevalence in loaches from the Beijing and Nanjing areas has been estimated at 12% and 6% respectively (Akahane, Iwata and Miyazaki 1982). In China, advanced L_3 larvae have been found in 14 species of freshwater fish, frogs, snakes, chickens and rats, the incidence in snakes being 100% (Chen and Lin 1991). The prepatent period in pigs varies from 3 to 6 months. Unlike *G. spinigerum*, *G. hispidum* cannot mature in humans. Experimentally, cats and rats can be infected by skin penetration of advanced L_3 larvae.

56 TRANSMISSION AND EPIDEMIOLOGY

Humans acquire infections by eating raw loaches containing early L_3 larvae or by consuming various vertebrates containing advanced L_3 larvae. All human infections in Japan have come from loaches imported from China, Korea and Taiwan.

57 CLINICAL MANIFESTATIONS AND PATHOLOGY

Clinical symptoms develop 3 weeks to 3 months after infection. Initially, patients complain of anorexia, diarrhoea and abdominal pain. All cases in Japan showed creeping eruption or mobile speckled erythema and a few showed also migratory intermittent swellings. Creeping eruption with erythema and itch normally occurs on the trunk or extremities. Morita et al. (1984) classified the disease into 5 types: (1) skin creeping eruption, on trunk and extremities, (2) migrating tracks on the liver, (3) migrating speckled erythema, (4) cerebrospinal form and (5) Löffler's syndrome revealed by transient pulmonary infiltration on X ray. Blood leucocytosis and eosinophilia (up to 84%) commonly occur, peaking 1–2 months after infection. Serum IgE levels are highly elevated. Clinical manifestations normally disappear within 3 months and never recur.

Monkeys experimentally infected with larvae from loaches yielded 64% encysted advanced L_3 larvae after 466 days (Koga, Ishibashi and Ishii 1988). This suggests that encysted larvae may survive in human musculature for long periods.

58 DIAGNOSIS

Morphological diagnosis (Table 34.6) is possible using resected whole worm specimens or sections. Patients with creeping eruption and peripheral eosinophilia, and a history of eating raw loaches from endemic areas, should be examined for antignathostome antibody. Crude *G. spinigerum* antigens are commonly used in Japan, because *G. hispidum* antigens are unavailable.

59 CONTROL

No effective drugs are available. Ingestion of raw loaches from endemic areas or flesh from chickens fed with loaches should be avoided.

GNATHOSTOMA DOLORESI TUBANGUI, 1925

60 INTRODUCTION

Gnathostoma doloresi was first discovered by Tubangui (1925) in the stomach wall of a pig in the Philippines. Later, it was also noted in pigs in India by Maplestone (1930) and it has subsequently been recovered from domestic pigs and wild boars in many Asian countries. The first human infections (with creeping eruption) were found by Ogata, Imai and Nawa (1988) in Japan. All 8 patients had a history of eating local freshwater fish. Larvae were found in the skin of 3/8 patients. A total of 25 human cases have been noted to date, all adults from Japan.

61 MORPHOLOGY

Adult worms occur singly or in groups of 2–3 worms in the gastric walls of domestic pigs or wild boars, inserting the anterior body into the thickened gastric wall. Males are 20 mm long and females are 34 mm long. The posterior half of the body is thicker than the rest. Worms are covered with cuticular spines, except for a small area at the tail end of the male. Males have 8 pairs of caudal papillae. Eggs are 61.3 × 30.9 μm on average, with transparent knob-like bulges at both ends.

Advanced L_3 larvae are c. 3 mm long. The head-bulb has 4 rows of cephalic hooklets, those in the 1st row being extremely small. The average number in

each row is <40 (Table 34.5). The morphological characteristics of cross-sections are presented in Table 34.6.

62 LIFE-CYCLE

The incidence of infection in wild boars in Japan was 70% with an average of 7 worms per boar (Nawa and Imai 1989); in Thailand the incidence in pigs was 2.1–8.7% (Daengsvang 1982).

Eggs shed into the faeces develop to the L_2 stage. These develop in cyclops to the early L_3 stage. If cyclops are eaten by amphibians, advanced L_3 larvae develop. Snakes that feed on these 2nd intermediate hosts can act as paratenic hosts. The prevalence in the poisonous snake *Agkistrodon halys* has been recorded as 100% (Imai et al. 1988). A pig infected with advanced L_3 larvae from *A. halys* shed eggs 58 days after infection (Imai et al. 1989).

63 TRANSMISSION AND EPIDEMIOLOGY

In Japan, freshwater fish are probably the major source of human infections.

64 CLINICAL MANIFESTATIONS AND PATHOLOGY

Before cutaneous symptoms develop, patients may experience prodromes (such as fever, 'cold-like' symptoms, vomiting, abdominal pain, weakness and malaise). Infections normally provoke creeping eruption with local pain and itch on the skin, particularly the trunk, and migratory swellings sometimes develop (Quincke's oedema). Creeping eruption leaves pigmentation in the skin. Histopathologically there is prominent eosinophil infiltration. Total serum IgE may be elevated and patients may show peripheral eosinophilia (6–67%).

Miyamoto et al. (1994) reported a case of pulmonary involvement in a patient with right chest pain and high fever. Clinical examination showed eosinophilia (18%), elevated IgE, a nodular lesion on r-S_4 as revealed by plain X ray and computed tomography and anti-*G. doloresi* antibody. No cutaneous lesions developed. The authors also described a case with an ileus due to an eosinophilic nodular lesion around migrating larvae in the colonic subserosa.

65 DIAGNOSIS

Various serological tests employ *G. doloresi* crude extracts as an antigen. If excised skin containing migrating worms is available, the species may be identified by the morphology of whole worms or cross-sections (Tables 34.5 and 34.6).

66 CONTROL

No effective drugs are available. The best treatment is to excise worms from the skin lesions, if this is possible. No fatal cases have been reported. It is advisable to avoid eating raw freshwater fish from local rivers in endemic areas.

GNATHOSTOMA NIPPONICUM YAMAGUTI, 1941

67 INTRODUCTION

This species was first found in the oesophagus of weasels in Japan, and was mistakenly identified as *G. spinigerum*. It was subsequently renamed *G. nipponicum* by Yamaguti (1941) and has since been found in weasels in various regions of Japan (incidence of 40%). The species may also exist in China.

Ando et al. (1988) reported patients in Japan with creeping eruption after eating raw loaches; a *G. nipponicum* larva was found in a skin biopsy specimen. Since then, at least 8 patients with similar gnathostomiasis have been reported.

68 MORPHOLOGY

Adult worms live singly or in groups in a hard tumour of the oesophageal wall of the weasel, located 2–3 cm from the stomach. The anterior body is embedded and the posterior lies free in the lumen. Adult males are 20–23 mm long and females are 29–34 mm long. The anterior body is covered with cuticular spines, as in *G. spinigerum*, but there are no spines caudally in the female. There are also differences in the shape of the spines of *G. nipponicum* and *G. spinigerum* (Miyazaki 1960, 1991). The caudal alae of the male have small cuticular spines and 8 pairs of papillae. Eggs measure 72.3×42.1 μm on average, with a transparent knob-like bulge at one end.

Advanced L_3 larvae are found encysted in the muscles of the 2nd intermediate or paratenic hosts. They have only 3 rows of hooklets on the head-bulb (Table 34.5). Morphological features of the cross-sections of the larvae are presented in Table 34.6.

69 LIFE-CYCLE

L_2 larvae released from fully developed eggs are eaten by cyclops and moult to early L_3 larvae. When cyclops are eaten by loaches the larvae develop to the advanced L_3 stage and encyst. Several species of freshwater fish, amphibians and mammals can act as 2nd intermediate hosts and several species of reptiles, birds and mammals act as paratenic hosts (Ando et al.

1992). Weasels experimentally infected with advanced L_3 larvae shed eggs 3 months after infection. Ferret and mink also serve as experimental hosts.

70 TRANSMISSION AND EPIDEMIOLOGY

Humans acquire infections by ingesting raw or inadequately cooked loaches or catfish.

71 CLINICAL MANIFESTATIONS AND PATHOLOGY

All 8 cases studied to date developed creeping eruption on the abdomen, waist and hip areas. The patients had all ingested loaches or various freshwater fish 3 to 4 weeks before the onset of symptoms. Some had peripheral eosinophilia (maximum 29%); leucocytosis was not always seen.

72 DIAGNOSIS

Excised worms or resected skin specimens can be used for morphological identification (Tables 34.5 and 34.6). Some patients show a positive serological reactions, but data are still scanty.

73 CONTROL

Excision of worms is the best therapeutic measure if feasible. Mebendazole was effective for stopping the creeping eruption (Taniguchi et al. 1991). Eating raw freshwater fish must be avoided in endemic areas.

SPIRUROID TYPE X LARVA

Since 1991, many human cases have been reported from Japan of a creeping disease caused by the type X larva of suborder Spirurina. This larva was first described by Hasegawa (1978) and has subsequently been recovered from human skin, intestinal wall (especially ileum) and the anterior chamber of the eye. The adult stage has not been identified. Kagei (1991) suggested that the larvae of Spiruroid nematodes other than the Spiruroid type X larva may cause cutaneous or visceral larva migrans.

Spiruroid type X larvae measure $6.7–8.0 \times 0.08–0.10$ mm, with 2 tubercles at the tail and 2 pseudolabia at the head. Larvae detected in sections of resected skin are 80–100 μm in diameter with characteristic cuticular annulations and intracuticular striae. The muscle layer is polymyarian-coelomyarian. Lateral cords are large and Y-shaped. The oesophagus has muscular and glandular parts, the latter filled with minute granules that resemble secretory granules or vacuoles. The intestine has 5–6 columnar intestinal cells.

These larvae have been found in marine fish which are therefore possible sources of human infections. Some species of squid also harbour type X larvae. Firefly squids are probably the most important source of human infections, because they are the type most frequently eaten raw in Japan. Spiruroid type X infections in humans occur predominantly during winter to spring seasons.

The disease is classified into ocular, cutaneous and intestinal (ileus) forms. Cutaneous symptoms develop as early as 2–9 days after eating raw squids (Shinozaki et al. 1993). There is usually only a transient, linear or meandering erythema, without significant leucocytosis or eosinophilia. Some cases showed a significant rise of serum total IgE levels.

Effective therapeutic measures are unavailable. Most patients with ileus undergo surgical resection of the intestinal lesions and confirmed diagnosis is then made. It is recommended that firefly squids are frozen at −32°C for 30 min or more to prevent infection.

REFERENCES

Akahane H, Iwata K, Miyazaki I, 1982, Studies on *Gnathostoma hispidum* Fedchenko, 1872 parasitic in loaches imported from China (in Japanese with English abstr), *Jpn J Parasitol*, **31**: 507–16.

Akao N, Ohyama TA, Kondo K, 1990, Immunoblot analysis of serum IgG, IgA and IgE responses against larval excretory-secretory antigens of *Anisakis simplex* in patients with gastric anisakiasis, *J Helminthol*, **64**: 310–18.

Akao N, Kondo K et al., 1992, Antigens of adult female worm of *Angiostrongylus cantonensis* recognized by infected humans, *Jpn J Parasitol*, **41**: 225–31.

Alicata JE, 1965, Biology and distribution of the rat lungworm, *Angiostrongylus cantonensis*, and its relationship to eosinophilic meningoencephalitis and other neurological disorders of man and animals, *Adv Parasitol*, **3**: 223–48.

Alicata JE, 1967, Effect of freezing and boiling on the infectivity of third-stage larvae of *Angiostrongylus cantonensis* present in land snails and freshwater prawns, *J Parasitol*, **53**: 1064–6.

Alicata JE, Jindrak K, 1970, *Angiostrongylosis in the Pacific and Southeast Asia*, Charles C Thomas, Springfield, 1 and 105.

Ando K, 1992, Gnathostomiasis in Japan (in Japanese), *Rinsho Derma (Tokyo)*, **34**: 517–26.

Ando K, Hatsushika R et al., 1991, *Gnathostoma nipponicum* infection in the past human cases in Japan, *Jpn J Parasitol*, **40**: 184–6.

Ando K, Tanaka H et al., 1988, Two human cases of gnathostomiasis and discovery of a second intermediate host of *Gnathostoma nipponicum* in Japan, *J Parasitol*, **74**: 623–7.

Ando K, Tokura H et al., 1992, Life cycle of *Gnathostoma nipponicum* Yamaguti, 1941, *J Helminthol*, **66**: 53–61.

Ash LR, 1976, Observations on the role of mollusks and planarians in the transmission of *Angiostrongylus cantonensis* infection to man in New Caledonia, *Rev Biol Trop*, **24**: 163–74.

Baird JK, Neafie RC et al., 1987, Abdominal angiostrongylosis in an African man: Case study, *Am J Trop Med Hyg*, **37**: 353–6.

Barrowclough H, Crome L, 1979, Oesophagostomiasis in man, *Trop Geogr Med*, **31**: 133–8.

Blotkamp J, Krepel HP et al., 1993, Observations on the morphology of adults and larval stages of *Oesophagostomum* sp. isolated from man in northern Togo and Ghana, *J Helminthol*, **67**: 49–61.

von Boch H, 1956, Knötchenwurmbefall (*Ternidens deminutus*) bei Rhesusaffen, *Z Angew Zool*, No. **2**: 207–14.

Bowden DK, 1981, Eosinophilic meningitis in the New Hebrides: Two outbreaks and two deaths, *Am J Trop Med Hyg*, **30**: 1141–3.

Brack M, Schröpel M, 1995, *Angiostrongylus costaricensis* in a black-eared marmoset, *Trop Geogr Med*, **47**: 136–8.

Bradley M, 1990, Rate of expulsion of *Necator americanus* and the false hookworm *Ternidens deminutus* Railliet and Henry, 1909 (Nematoda) from humans following albendazole treatment, *Trans R Soc Trop Med Hyg*, **84**: 720.

Chen ER, 1979, Angiostrongyliasis and eosinophilic meningitis on Taiwan: A review, *NAMRU-2-SP-44*, 57–73.

Chen HT, 1935, Un nouveau nematode pulmonaire, *Pulmonema cantonensis* n.g.n.sp., des rats de Canton, *Ann Parasitol*, **13**: 312–7.

Chen QQ, Lin XM, 1991, A survey of epidemiology of *Gnathostoma hispidum* and experimental studies of its larvae in animals, *Southeast Asian J Trop Med Public Health*, **22**: 611–7.

Cross JH, 1987, Public health importance of *Angiostrongylus cantonensis* and it relatives, *Parasitol Today*, **3**: 367–9.

Daengsvang S, 1982, Gnathostomiasis, *CRC Handbook Series in Zoonoses, Section C. Parasitic Zoonoses*, vol 2, ed Steele JH, CRC Press, Cleveland, 147 and 180.

Deardorff TL, Kayes SG, Fukumura T, 1991, Human anisakiasis transmitted by marine food products, *Hawaii Med J*, **50**: 9–16.

Duarte Z, Morera P et al., 1992, *Angiostrongylus costaricensis* natural infection in *Vaginulus plebeius* in Nicaragua, *Ann Parasitol Hum Comp*, **67**: 94–6.

Ghadirian E, Arfaa F, 1975, Present status of trichostrongyliasis in Iran, *Am J Trop Med Hyg*, **24**: 935–41.

Gibson DI, 1983, The systematics of ascaridoid nematodes: a current assessment, *Nematode Systematics Association Special Volume*, vol 22, eds Stone AF, Platt HM, Khalil LE, Academic Press, London, 321 and 338.

Goldsmid JM, 1968, The differentiation of *Ternidens deminutus* and hookworm ova in human infections, *Trans R Soc Trop Med Hyg*, **62**: 109–16.

Goldsmid JM, 1971, Studies on the life cycle and biology of *Ternidens deminutus* (Railliet & Henry, 1909), (Nematoda: Strongylidae), *J Helminthol*, **45**: 341–52.

Goldsmid JM, 1972, Thiabendazole in the treatment of human infections with *Ternidens deminutus* (Nematoda), *S Afr Med J*, **46**: 1046–7.

Graeff-Teixeira C, Camillo-Coura L, Lenzi HL, 1987, Abdominal angiostrongyliasis – an under-diagnosed disease, *Mem Inst Oswaldo Cruz*, **82**: 353–4.

Graeff-Teixeira C, Camillo-Coura L, Lenzi HL, 1991, Clinical and epidemiological aspects of abdominal angiostrongyliasis in southern Brazil, *Rev Inst Med Trop São Paulo*, **33**: 373–8.

Graeff-Teixeira C, de Avila-Pires FD et al., 1990, Identificação de roedores silvestres como hospedeiros de *Angiostrongylus costaricensis* no sul do Brasil, *Rev Inst Med Trop Sao Paulo*, **32**: 147–50.

Hasegawa H, 1978, Larval nematodes of the superfamily Spiruroidea. A description, identification and examination of their pathogenicity, *Acta Med Biol*, **26**: 79–116.

Heyneman D, Lim BL, 1967, *Angiostrongylus cantonensis*: Proof of direct transmission with its epidemiological implications, *Science*, **158**: 1057–8.

Hulbert TV, Larsen RA, Chandrasoma PT, 1992, Abdominal angiostrongyliasis mimicking acute appendicitis and Meckel's diverticulum: Report of a case in the United States and review, *Clin Infect Dis*, **14**: 836–40.

Imai JI, Akahane H et al., 1989, *Gnathostoma doloresi*: Development of the larvae obtained from snakes, *Agkistrodon halys*, to adult worms in a pig, *Jpn J Parasitol*, **38**: 221–5.

Imai JI, Asada Y et al., 1988, *Gnathostoma doloresi* larvae found in snakes, *Agkistrodon halys*, captured in the central part of Miyazaki Prefecture, *Jpn J Parasitol*, **37**: 444–50.

Ishikura H, 1990, Clinical features of intestinal anisakiasis, *Intestinal Anisakiasis in Japan. Infected Fish, Sero-immunological Diagnosis, and Prevention*, eds Ishikura H, Kikuchi K, Springer-Verlag, Tokyo, 89 and 100.

Ishikura H, Kikuchi K et al., 1992, Anisakidae and anisakidosis, *Progress in Clinical Parasitology*, vol 3, ed Sun T, Springer-Verlag, New York, 43 and 102.

Ishikura H, Sato S et al., 1993, Anisakiasis – its outbreak and present status (in Japanese), *Clin Parasitol*, **4**: 152–5.

Jindrak K, 1975, Angiostrongyliasis cantonensis (eosinophilic meningitis, Alicata's disease), *Topics on Tropical Neurology*, ed Hornabrook RW, FA Davis, Philadelphia, 133 and 164.

Jones RE, Deardorff TL, Kayes SG, 1990, *Anisakis simplex*: histopathological changes in experimentally infected CBA/J mice, *Exp Parasitol*, **70**: 305–13.

Kagei N, 1991, Morphological identification of parasites in biopsied specimens from creeping disease lesions, *Jpn J Parasitol*, **40**: 437–45.

Kino H, Watanabe K et al., 1993, Occurrence of anisakiasis in the western part of Shizuoka Prefecture, with special reference to the prevalence of anisakid infections in sardine, *Engraulis japonica*, *Jpn J Parasitol*, **42**: 308–12.

Kliks MM, 1983, Anisakiasis in the western United States: Four new case reports from California, *Am J Trop Med Hyg*, **32**: 526–32.

Kliks MM, 1986, Human anisakiasis: an update, *JAMA*, **255**: 2605.

Kliks MM, Kroenke K, Hardman JM, 1982, Eosinophilic radiculomyeloencephalitis: An angiostrongyliasis outbreak in American Samoa related to ingestion of *Achatina fulica* snails, *Am J Trop Med Hyg*, **31**: 1114–22.

Koga M, Ishibashi J, Ishii Y, 1988, Experimental infection in a monkey with *Gnathostoma hispidum* larvae obtained from loaches, *Ann Trop Med Parasitol*, **82**: 383–8.

Koo J, Pien F, Kliks MM, 1988, *Angiostrongylus (Parastrongylus)* eosinophilic meningitis, *Rev Infect Dis*, **10**: 1155–62.

Koyama T, Kobayashi A et al., 1969, Morphological and taxonomical studies on Anisakidae larvae found in marine fishes and squids (in Japanese with English abstr), *Jpn J Parasitol*, **18**: 466–87.

Krepel HP, Baeta S, Polderman AM, 1992, Human *Oesophagostomum* infection in northern Togo and Ghana: epidemiological aspects, *Ann Trop Med Parasitol*, **86**: 289–300.

Krepel HP, Haring T et al, 1993, Treatment of mixed *Oesophagostomum* and hookworm infection: effect of albendazole, pyrantel pamoate, levamisole and thiabendazole, *Trans R Soc Trop Med Hyg*, **87**: 87–9.

Loría-Cortés R, Lobo-Sanahuja JF, 1980, Clinical abdominal angiostrongylosis. A study of 116 children with intestinal eosinophilic granuloma caused by *Angiostrongylus costaricensis*, *Am J Trop Med Hyg*, **29**: 538–44.

Mackerras MJ, Sandars DF, 1955, The life history of the rat lungworm, *Angiostrongylus cantonensis* (Chen) (Nematoda: Metastrongylidae), *Aust J Zool*, **3**: 1–25.

Mako T, Akahane H, 1985, On the larval *Gnathostoma doloresi* found in a snake, Dinodon semicarinatus from Amami-Oshima Is., Japan [in Japanese with English abstract], *Jpn J Parasitol*, **34**: 493–9.

Maleewong W, Wongkham C et al., 1992, Detection of circulating parasite antigens in murine gnathostomiasis by a two-site enzyme-linked immunosorbent assay, *Am J Trop Med Hyg*, **46**: 80–4.

Maplestone PA, 1930, Nematode parasites of pigs in Bengal, *Records Ind Mus*, **32**: 77–105.

Matsui T, Iida M et al., 1985, Intestinal anisakiasis: Clinical and radiologic features, *Radiology*, **157**: 299–302.

Miyamoto N, Mishima K et al., 1994, A case report of serologically diagnosed pulmonary gnathostomiasis, *Jpn J Parasitol*, **43**: 397–400.

Miyazaki I, 1960, On the genus *Gnathostoma* and human gnathostomiasis, with special reference to Japan, *Exp Parasitol*, **9**: 338–70.

Miyazaki I, 1991, *An Illustrated Book of Helminthic Zoonoses*, International Medical Foundation of Japan, Tokyo, 368 and 402.

Morera P, 1973, Life history and redescription of *Angiostrongylus costaricensis* Morera and Céspedes, 1971, *Am J Trop Med Hyg*, **22**: 613–21.

Morera P, 1985, Abdominal angiostrongyliasis: A problem of public health, *Parasitol Today*, **1**: 173–5.

Morera P, 1994, Importance of abdominal angiostrongylosis in the Americas, *8th Int Congr Parasitol (Izmir, Turkey, Oct 1994) Abstr*, **1**: 34.

Morera P, Céspedes R, 1971, *Angiostrongylus costaricensis* n. sp. (Nematoda: Metastrongyloidea), a new lungworm occurring in man in Costa Rica, *Rev Biol Trop*, **18**: 173–85.

Morita H, Segawa T et al., 1984, Gnathostomiasis cases caused by imported loaches (in Japanese with English abstr), *J Nara Med Assoc*, **35**: 607–19.

Namiki M, Morooka T et al., 1970, Diagnosis of acute gastric anisakiasis (in Japanese), *Stomach and Intestine*, **5**: 1437–40.

Nawa Y, Imai JI, 1989, Current status of *Gnathostoma doloresi* infection in wild boars captured in Miyazaki Prefecture, Japan, *Jpn J Parasitol*, **38**: 385–7.

Nelson RG, Warren RC et al., 1988, Ocular angiostrongyliasis in Japan: A case report, *Am J Trop Med Hyg*, **38**: 130–2.

Nopparatana C, Setasuban P et al., 1991, Purification of *Gnathostoma spinigerum* specific antigen and immunodiagnosis of human gnathostomiasis, *Int J Parasitol*, **21**: 677–87.

Ogata K, Imai JI, Nawa Y, 1988, Three confirmed and five suspected human cases of *Gnathostoma doloresi* infection found in Miyazaki Prefecture, Kyushu, *Jpn J Parasitol*, **37**: 358–64.

Ohbayashi M, 1979, Hunting parasites in Thailand (in Japanese), *J Hokkaido Vet Med Assoc*, **23**: 3–15.

Ohtaki H, Ohtaki R, 1989, Clinical manifestation of gastric anisakiasis, *Gastric Anisakiasis in Japan. Epidemiology, Diagnosis, Treatment*, eds Ishikura H, Namiki M, Springer-Verlag, Tokyo, 37 and 46.

Oshima T, 1972, *Anisakis* and anisakiasis in Japan and adjacent area, *Progress of Medical Parasitology in Japan*, vol 4, eds Morishita K, Komiya Y, Matsubayashi H, Meguro Parasitol Museum, Tokyo, 301 and 393.

Oshima T, 1987, Anisakiasis – Is the sushi bar guilty?, *Parasitol Today*, **3**: 44–8.

Oshima T, Kliks M, 1987, Effects of marine mammal parasites on human health, *Int J Parasitol*, **17**: 415–21.

Otsuru M, 1979, *Angiostrongylus cantonensis* and angiostrongyliasis in Japan, *NAMRU-2-SP-44*, 74–117.

Otsuru M, Ito J, 1972, Genus *Trichostrongylus* in Japan, *Progress of Medical Parasitology in Japan*, eds Morishita K, Komiya Y, Matsubayashi H, Meguro Parasitol Museum, Tokyo, 421 and 463.

Owen R, 1836, Anatomical description of two species of *Entozoa* from the stomach of a tiger (*Felis tigris* Linn.) one of which forms a new genus of Nematoidea, *Gnathostoma*, *Proc Zool Soc London*, **47**: 123–6.

Perez O, Capron M et al., 1989, *Angiostrongylus cantonensis*: Role of eosinophils in the neurotoxic syndrome (Gordon-like phenomenon), *Exp Parasitol*, **68**: 403–13.

Polderman AM, Krepel HP et al., 1991, Oesophagostomiasis, a common infection of man in northern Togo and Ghana, *Am J Trop Med Hyg*, **44**: 336–44.

Polderman AM, Krepel HP et al., 1993, Serological diagnosis of *Oesophagostomum* infections, *Trans R Soc Trop Med Hyg*, **87**: 433–5.

Prociv P, Tiernan JR, 1987, Eosinophilic meningoencephalitis with permanent sequelae, *Med J Aust*, **147**: 294–5.

Punyagupta S, Bunnag T, Juttijudata P, 1990, Eosinophilic meningitis in Thailand. Clinical and epidemiological characteristics of 162 patients with myeloencephalitis probably caused by *Gnathostoma spinigerum*, *J Neurol Sci*, **96**: 241–56.

Punyagupta S, Juttijudata P, Bunnag T, 1975, Eosinophilic meningitis in Thailand. Clinical studies of 484 typical cases probably caused by *Angiostrongylus cantonensis*, *Am J Trop Med Hyg*, **24**: 921–31.

Rogers S, Goldsmid JM, 1977, Preliminary studies using the indirect fluorescent antibody test for the serological diagnosis of *Ternidens deminutus* infection in man, *Ann Trop Med Parasitol*, **71**: 503–4.

Rosen L, Chappell R et al., 1962, Eosinophilic meningoencephalitis caused by a metastrongylid lung-worm of rats, *JAMA*, **179**: 620–4.

Ross RA, Gibson DI, Harris EA, 1989, Cutaneous oesophagostomiasis in man, *J Helminthol*, **63**: 261–5.

Ruiz PJ, Morera P, 1983, Spermatic artery obstruction caused by *Angiostrongylus costaricensis* Morera and Céspedes, 1971, *Am J Trop Med Hyg*, **32**: 1458–9.

Rusnak JM, Lucey DR, 1993, Clinical gnathostomiasis: Case report and review of the English-language literature, *Clin Infect Dis*, **16**: 33–50.

Sakanari JA, McKerrow JH, 1989, Anisakiasis, *Clin Microbiol Rev*, **2**: 278–84.

Sasaki O, Sugaya H et al., 1993, Ablation of eosinophils with anti-IL-5 antibody enhances the survival of intracranial worms of *Angiostrongylus cantonensis* in the mouse, *Parasite Immunol*, **15**: 349–54.

Schantz PM, 1989, The dangers of eating raw fish, *N Engl J Med*, **320**: 1143–5.

Schmutzhard E, Boongird P, Vejjajiva A, 1988, Eosinophilic meningitis and radiculomyelitis in Thailand, caused by CNS invasion of *Gnathostoma spinigerum* and *Angiostrongylus cantonensis*, *J Neurol Neurosurg Psychiatry*, **51**: 80–7.

Scrimgeour EM, Chambers BR, Kaven J, 1982, A probable case of ocular angiostrongyliasis in New Britain, Papua New Guinea, *Trans R Soc Trop Med Hyg*, **76**: 538–40.

Shih HH, Chen SN, 1991, Immunodiagnosis of angiostrongyliasis with monoclonal antibodies recognizing a circulating antigen of mol. wt 91,000 from *Angiostrongylus cantonensis*, *Int J Parasitol*, **21**: 171–7.

Shih SL, Hsu CH et al., 1992, *Angiostrongylus cantonensis* infection in infants and young children, *Pediatr Infect Dis J*, **11**: 1064–6.

Shinozaki M, Akao N et al., 1993, Detection of type X larva of the suborder Spirurina from a patient with a creeping eruption, *Jpn J Parasitol*, **42**: 51–3.

Soesatyo MHNE, Rattanasiriwilai W et al., 1987, IgE responses in human gnathostomiasis, *Trans R Soc Trop Med Hyg*, **81**: 799–801.

Sugano S, Suzuki T et al., 1993, Noncardiac chest pain due to acute gastric anisakiasis, *Digest Dis Sci*, **38**: 1354–6.

Sugaya H, Yoshimura K, 1988, T-cell-dependent eosinophilia in the cerebrospinal fluid of the mouse infected with *Angiostrongylus cantonensis*, *Parasite Immunol*, **10**: 127–38.

Sugimachi K, Inokuchi K et al., 1985, Acute gastric anisakiasis. Analysis of 178 cases, *JAMA*, **253**: 1012–3.

Takahashi S, Sato N, Ishikura H, 1986, Establishment of monoclonal antibodies that discriminate the antigen distribution specifically found in *Anisakis* larvae (type I), *J Parasitol*, **72**: 960–2.

Takamuku M, Iino H, Fujino T, 1994, A case of gastric anisakiasis showing multiple infection of larvae in a large gastric ulcer (in Japanese), *Clin Parasitol*, **5**: 74–5.

Taniguchi Y, Hashimoto K et al., 1991, Human gnathostomiasis, *J Cutan Pathol*, **18**: 112–5.

Tapchaisri P, Nopparatana C et al., 1991, Specific antigen of *Gnathostoma spinigerum* for immunodiagnosis of human gnathostomiasis, *Int J Parasitol*, **21**: 315–9.

Teekhasaenee C, Ritch R, Kanchanaranya C, 1986, Ocular parasitic infection in Thailand, *Rev Infect Dis*, **8**: 350–6.

van Thiel PH, 1962, Anisakiasis, *Parasitology*, **52 (suppl.)**: 16–7.

van Thiel PH, 1976, The present state of anisakiasis and causative worms, *Trop Geogr Med*, **28**: 75–85.

van Thiel PH, Kuipers FC, Roskam RT, 1960, A nematode parasitic to herring, causing acute abdominal syndromes in man, *Trop Geogr Med*, **2**: 97–113.

Totsuka M, 1974, Human anisakiasis 3. Epidemiology (in Japanese), *Fish and* Anisakis, ed The Japanese Society of Scientific Fishery, Kohsei-sha-Kohsei-kaku, Tokyo, 44 and 57.

Tsushima H, Numata T et al., 1980, Gnathostomiasis cutis probably infected in Hiroshima city, *J Hiroshima Med Assoc*, **33**: 1183–7.

Tubangui MA, 1925, Metazoan parasites of Philippine domesticated animals, *Philippine J Sci*, **28**: 11–37.

Tuntipopipat S, Chawengkiattikul R et al., 1989, Antigens, antibodies and immune complexes in cerebrospinal fluid of patients with cerebral gnathostomiasis, *Southeast Asian J Trop Med Public Health*, **20**: 439–46.

Ubelaker JE, Caruso J, Peña A, 1981, Experimental infection of *Sigmodon hispidus* with third-stage larvae of *Angiostrongylus costaricensis*, *J Parasitol*, **67**: 219–21.

Vázquez JJ, Sola JJ, Boils PL, 1994, Hepatic lesions induced by *Angiostrongylus costaricensis*, *Histopathology*, **25**: 489–91.

Weller PF, 1993, Eosinophilic meningitis, *Am J Med*, **95**: 250–3.

Widagdo, Sunardi et al., 1977, Ocular angiostrongyliasis in Semarang, Central Java, *Am J Trop Med Hyg*, **26**: 72–4.

Witoonpanich R, Chuahirun S et al., 1991, Eosinophilic myelomeningoencephalitis caused by *Angiostrongylus cantonensis*: A report of three cases, *Southeast Asian J Trop Med Public Health*, **22**: 262–7.

Yagihashi A, Sato N et al., 1990, A serodiagnostic assay by microenzyme-linked immunosorbent assay for human anisakiasis using a monoclonal antibody specific for *Anisakis* larvae antigen, *J Infect Dis*, **161**: 995–8.

Yamaguti S, 1941, Studies on the helminth fauna of Japan. Part 35. Mammalian nematodes (2), *Jpn J Zool*, **9**: 409–38.

Yen CM, Chen ER, 1991, Detection of antibodies to *Angiostrongylus cantonensis* in serum and cerebrospinal fluid of patients with eosinophilic meningitis, *Int J Parasitol*, **21**: 17–21.

Yii CY, 1976, Clinical observations on eosinophilic meningitis and meningoencephalitis caused by *Angiostrongylus cantonensis* on Taiwan, *Am J Trop Med Hyg*, **25**: 233–49.

Yoshimura K, Sugaya H, Ishida K, 1994, The role of eosinophils in *Angiostrongylus cantonensis* infection, *Parasitol Today*, **10**: 231–3.

Yoshimura K, Sato K et al., 1982, The course of *Angiostrongylus cantonensis* infection in athymic nude and neonatally thymectomized mice, *Z Parasitenkd*, **67**: 217–26.

Yoshimura K, Sugaya H et al., 1988, Ultrastructural and morphometric analyses of eosinophils from the cerebrospinal fluid of the mouse and guinea pig infected with *Angiostrongylus cantonensis*, *Parasite Immunol*, **10**: 411–23.

DRACUNCULIASIS

R Muller

Dracunculiasis is an ancient disease quoted by many classical authors and possibly mentioned in the Old Testament. For the last few years there has been a world eradication campaign and this chapter has been written in the light of this campaign (Anon, Hopkins and Ruiz-Tiben 1991, Cairncross 1992, Muller 1992, Chippaux 1994). It is hoped that it will be superfluous in the next edition.

1 MORPHOLOGY

The mature female of the dracunculoid nematode, *Dracunculus medinensis*, (Linnaeus, 1758) Gallandant, 1773, measures 500–800 mm × 1.0–2.0 mm. The mouth has a triangular oval opening surrounded by a quadrangular cuticularized plate, and an internal circle of 4 double papillae. The vulva opens halfway down the body but is non-functional in the mature worm. The uterus has an anterior and a posterior branch; it is filled with 1–3 million embryos and occupies the entire body cavity (pseudocoel), the gut being completely flattened (Muller 1971).

Males recovered from experimental infections in animals measure 15–40 × 0.4 mm. The tail has 4(3–6) pairs of preanal and 4–6 pairs of postanal papillae; the subequal spicules are 490–750 μm long with a gubernaculum measuring about 117 μm. The males probably die in the tissues before the females mature but have only doubtfully been seen in human infections.

2 LIFE CYCLE

In the human body each female worm takes about one year to mature and moves to the surface of the skin. It provokes a blister at the anterior end which bursts and leaves an ulcer through which about 5 cm of the worm is extruded, particularly after immersion in water (Fig. 35.1a). Many thousands of larvae are released into the water where they can live for only a few days; for further development they have to be ingested by small freshwater crustacea (cyclops). The larvae moult twice in the body cavity and are infective in about 2 weeks. If cyclops are ingested in drinking water, released larvae penetrate the human intestinal wall and male and female worms mate in the connective tissues in about 3 months.

3 TRANSMISSION AND EPIDEMIOLOGY

Dracunculus infection is prevalent in 16 countries of West and Central Africa just south of the Sahara (Benin, Burkina Faso, Chad, Cote d'Ivoire, Ethiopia, Ghana, Mali, Mauritania, Niger, Nigeria, Sudan, Togo and Uganda; and with very small foci in Cameroon, Kenya and Senegal) (Muller 1991, Cairncross 1992, Chippaux 1994). It also occurs in India and Yemen, with a recent isolated outbreak in Libya. The disease has been eliminated or has died out in Central African Republic, Guinea Bissau, Iran, Pakistan and Saudi Arabia in recent years.

Dracunculiasis is typically a disease of rural communities which obtain their drinking water from ponds (or, in India, from large step wells), where cyclops can breed (Fig. 35.2). In all areas transmission is markedly seasonal and in most parts of Africa and India the maximum incidence coincides with the planting season, resulting in great economic hardship. In semi-desert (Sahel) areas of Africa (Burkina Faso, Chad, northern Cameroon, Mauritania, Niger, northern Nigeria, Senegal and Sudan), drinking water is

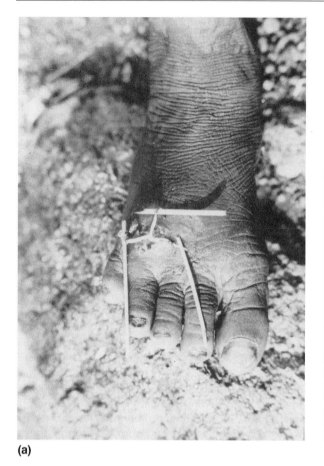

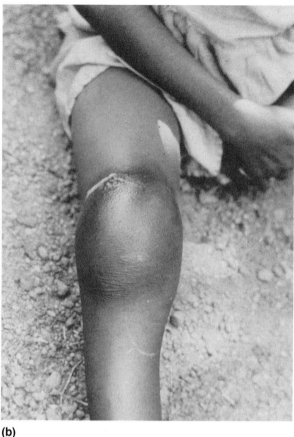

(a)

(b)

Fig. 35.1 (a) Foot of child with 3 worms emerging which are being wound out on sticks (by courtesy of Dr Ahmed Tayeh). (b) Knee of girl, with guinea worm emerging, which has become secondarily infected and swollen.

obtained from ponds during the rainy season but from deep (safe) wells for the rest of the year when the ponds are dry. However, in the humid (Guinea) savanna regions of West Africa where rainfall exceeds 150 cm per year (Benin, Cote d'Ivoire, Ghana, southern Nigeria and Togo) there is almost no transmission during the rainy season (July to September) when ponds turn into streams and cyclops densities are low because of the large volume and turbidity of the water. Similarly, infection is highest during the dry season in step wells in India. The life history of the parasite is well adapted to provide the maximum chances of transmission as the female takes almost exactly a year to mature and release its larvae.

4 LOCATION IN HOST

One to many adult female worms emerge from the subcutaneous tissues, usually of the foot or lower limbs, but sometimes from any part of the body.

5 CLINICAL MANIFESTATIONS AND PATHOLOGY

In most patients the first physical sign is the local lesion, accompanied by an intense burning pain usu-

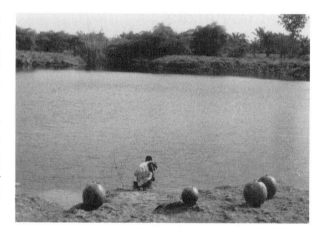

Fig. 35.2 One of many large artificial ponds constructed in Nigeria for drinking water and agriculture which is transmitting both dracunculiasis and schistosomiasis.

ally relieved by immersion of the affected limb in water. The blister fluid is bacteriologically sterile and contains numerous white cells and larvae. In uncomplicated cases, the worm emerges from the subsequent ulcer over a few weeks and then the lesion rapidly heals; thus, if there is only one worm present, patency will last for only 4–6 weeks. Unfortunately, secondary infection along the track of the worm in the tissues is very common, often with spreading cellulitis, and approximately 40% of patients will be totally incapacitated for an average of 6 weeks (Fig. 35.1b). More serious and permanent damage can follow the bursting of a worm in the tissues or as the result of bacterial infection, e.g. ankylosis of joints in about 1% of cases or occasionally tetanus.

Dracunculiasis is unusual among infectious diseases in that the parasite does not appear to stimulate a protective response, so that the same individual can be reinfected year after year.

6 DIAGNOSIS

6.1 Clinical and parasitological diagnosis

Patients in an endemic area usually have no doubt of the diagnosis, as soon as, or even before, the first signs appear. Local itching, urticaria, and a burning pain at the site of a small blister are usually the first signs of infection. The blister bursts in about 4 days and active larvae, obtained by placing cold water on the resulting small ulcer, can be recognized under a low-powered microscope.

6.2 Immunological diagnosis

Immunological methods are not useful in practice. ELISA and SDS PAGE/Western blotting worked well in one trial for patent infections (Bloch, Simonsen and Vennerwald 1983) and the fluorescent antibody test using deep frozen first stage larvae diagnosed pre-patent infections in monkeys (Muller 1971).

7 TREATMENT

7.1 Surgery

Guinea worms have been wound out on sticks since antiquity (e.g. in the Rig Veda of about 1350 bc). Provided that bacterial infection or other complications have not occurred, regular winding out of the worm on a small stick, combined with sterile dressing and acriflavine cream, usually results in complete expulsion in about 4 weeks with little loss of mobility. Treatment should be commenced as soon after emergence as possible (Magnussen, Yakuba and Bloch 1994). Sometimes worms can be seen and surgically removed before emergence while there is no tissue reaction against them.

7.2 Chemotherapy

There is no evidence that any chemotherapeutic agent has a direct action against guinea worms. However, many compounds, including thiabendazole, niridazole, metronidazole, mebendazole and albendazole, have been reported as hastening the expulsion of worms and may act as anti-inflammatory agents. Iver-mectin had no action against pre-emergent worms (Issaka-Tinorgah et al. 1994).

8 THE ERADICATION CAMPAIGN

The eradication of dracunculiasis from the world was adopted as a sub-goal of the Clean Drinking Water Supply and Sanitation Decade (1981–90) and was formally endorsed by the United Nations World Health Assembly in 1986 and 1989. If the original aim of complete eradication by the end of 1995 had been achieved, this chapter would have been superfluous. However, the task is likely to take quite a while longer, particularly in Ethiopia and Sudan. Nonetheless, the prevalence and distribution of infection have diminished markedly in the last few years: worldwide there were about 3.5 million cases in 1986, 1 million in 1989 but only 100 000 in 1994. Disease is likely to be eliminated from Asia in the near future with no cases in Pakistan and only a handful in India since 1994 (Hopkins et al. 1995). The situation in African countries is not so far advanced but active campaigns are being carried out in almost all endemic countries and some are at the stage of case containment (see Fig. 35.3). In Nigeria and Ghana for instance, new cases have reduced markedly since 1988, and in all African countries except Sudan on average 68% of cases were contained for the first 2 months of 1996 (i.e. all larvae were prevented from reaching ponds).

The first priority has been to have accurate figures on the distribution and prevalence in each endemic country. Because infected persons rarely report to health clinics, passive surveillance is almost useless (identifying less than 3% of cases) and trained teams of community workers are necessary to visit each village and obtain the necessary information. These teams have to be carefully monitored and when trained can also be associated with other primary health care initiatives, such as control of malaria and diarrhoeal diseases and immunization campaigns.

Once active surveillance measures have been initiated there are various possible interventions based on knowledge of the life cycle of the parasite.

The provision by governments and aid agencies of safe drinking water from tubewells is a priority in rural areas of Africa and Asia. UNICEF aims to provide one borehole for every 200 persons in suitable geological regions by the year 2000. In some areas traditional, usually hand built, draw wells can be equally effective and in all, cisterns can be constructed for storing rainwater (Fig. 35.4).

Health education interventions by local health workers form a very important component of any control or eradication campaign. Interventions being made include:

1 Filtering or boiling all drinking water. Boiling water is not usually feasible because fuel is a scarce commodity but filters are playing an important role in all countries now mounting campaigns. The donation by the manufacturer of monofilament nylon nets, which are long lasting, have a

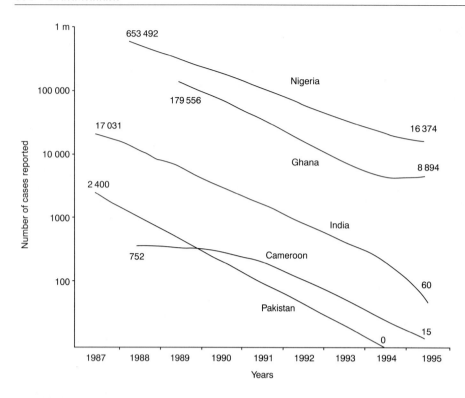

Fig. 35.3 Decrease in numbers of cases of guinea worm infection reported each year in 5 countries which have active campaigns (note log scale). The campaign in India started in 1980.

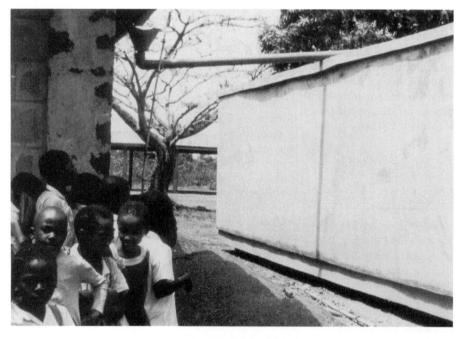

Fig. 35.4 Cistern built at a school in Nigeria to store rainwater for use during the dry season.

regular pore size, are easily washed and dry quickly, is proving of great help in sieving out cyclops.

2 Persuading or preventing infected persons with an emerging worm from entering the water source (containment). This is particularly important when prevalence has been greatly reduced (the current motto is 'detect every case, contain every worm'). Bandaging very early lesions can help to prevent subsequent immersion in the water.

3 Treating water sources. The chemical treatment of ponds can prove a useful adjunct to other meas-

ures, particularly when there is only a low level of transmission remaining. The insecticide temephos added to ponds at a concentration of 1 ppm will kill cyclops for 5–6 weeks and has low toxicity to mammals and fishes. In areas with a long transmission season, it has to be added a few times a year. The amount of temephos estimated to be needed for total eradication in Africa has been donated by the manufacturer.

9 ZOONOTIC ASPECTS

Female worms of the genus *Dracunculus* have been reported as emerging from a wide range of mammals and reptiles from many parts of the world, both endemic and non-endemic for the human disease. Those found in reptiles clearly belong to other species but the situation in regard to those in mammals is not clear. For instance guinea worm is common in wild carnivores in North America and the species was named *D. insignis* by Leidy in 1858 but there is very little morphological evidence for separating this from the human species.

There have been 2 documented cases of clearly zoo-notic infections, from Japan in 1986 and from Korea in 1926. In both cases the patients had eaten raw fresh-water fish which have been proved experimentally to be capable of acting as paratenic hosts.

In most highly endemic areas occasional infections in dogs and donkeys with what is presumably the human parasite have been reported but there is no evidence that they have any part in maintaining transmission. The parasite can still be found in dogs in the formerly endemic areas of Tamil Nadu in India and the central Asian republics of the former Soviet Union, but no new human cases have been reported, so it is not thought that this will be a problem once world eradication has been achieved.

REFERENCES

Anon, (monthly), Guinea Worm Wrap-Up, Centers for Disease Control, Atlanta, GA.

Bloch P, Simonsen PE, Vennerwald BJ, 1983, The antibody response to *Dracunculus medinensis* in an endemic human population in northern Ghana, *J Helminthol*, **67**: 37–48.

Cairncross S, 1992, Guinea Worm Eradication: A Selected Bibliography, Bureau of Hygiene and Tropical Diseases, London.

Chippaux J-P, 1994, Le Ver de Guinée en Afrique: Methodes de Lutte pour l'Eradication, ORSTOM, Paris.

Hopkins DR, Ruiz-Tiben E, 1991, Strategies for dracunculiasis eradication, *Bull WHO*, **69**: 533–40.

Hopkins DR, Azam, M et al., 1995, Eradication of dracunculiasis from Pakistan, *Lancet*, **346**: 621–4.

Issakah-Tinorgah A, Magnussen P et al., 1994, Lack of effect of ivermectin on prepatent guinea-worm: a single-blind, placebo-controlled trial, *Trans R Soc Trop Med Hyg*, **88**: 346–8.

Magnussen P, Yakubu A , Bloch P, 1994, The effect of antibiotic- and hydrocortisone-containing ointments in preventing secondary infections in Guinea worm disease, *Am J Trop Med Hyg*, **51**: 797–9.

Muller R, 1971, *Dracunculus* and dracunculiasis, *Adv Parasitol*, **9**: 73–151.

Muller, R, 1991, *Dracunculus* in Africa, *Parasitic Helminths and Zoonoses in Africa*, eds Macpherson CNL, Craig PS, Unwin Hyman, London, 204–23.

Muller R, 1992, Guinea worm eradication: four more years to go, *Parasitol Today*, **8**: 387–90.

INDEX

Note: Page numbers in *italics* refer to major discussions. *vs* denotes differential diagnosis or comparisons.

Readers referring to individual parasitic species are also advised to refer to the entries for both the genus and the respective infection.